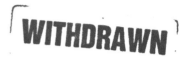

Avian Medicine and Surgery

Avian Medicine and Surgery

ROBERT B. ALTMAN, DVM
Co-Director, A & A Veterinary Hospital, Inc.
Franklin Square, New York
Adjunct Associate Professor, Zoological Medicine
University of Pennsylvania
College of Veterinary Medicine
Philadelphia, Pennsylvania

SUSAN L. CLUBB, DVM
Diplomate, American Board of Veterinary Practitioners (Avian Practice)
Staff Veterinarian, Parrot Jungle and Gardens
Miama, Florida
Consultant, Pretty Bird International,
Pet Joint Advisory Council, Loro
Parque, Tenerife, Spain

GERRY M. DORRESTEIN, DVM, PhD
Associate Professor in Avian, Exotic Animal, and Wildlife Pathology
Utrecht University
Faculty of Veterinary Medicine, Department of Pathology,
Section of Exotic and Laboratory Animals
Utrecht, The Netherlands

KATHERINE QUESENBERRY, DVM
Diplomate, American Board of Veterinary Practitioners (Avian Practice)
Service Head
Avian and Exotic Pet Medicine
The Animal Medical Center
New York, New York

Ronald S. Futral, CMI
Medical Illustrator

W.B. SAUNDERS COMPANY
A Division of Harcourt Brace & Company
Philadelphia   London   Toronto   Montreal   Sydney   Tokyo

W.B. SAUNDERS COMPANY
A Division of Harcourt Brace & Company

The Curtis Center
Independence Square West
Philadelphia, Pennsylvania 19106

Library of Congress Cataloging-in-Publication Data

Avian medicine and surgery / edited by Robert B. Altman.—1st ed.

    p.   cm.

ISBN 0–7216–5446–0

1. Avian medicine.   2. Birds—Diseases.   3. Birds—Surgery.
    I. Altman, Robert B.

SF994.A95 1997
636.6'8—dc20   95–4641

AVIAN MEDICINE AND SURGERY   ISBN 0–7216–5446–0

Last digit is the print number: 9   8   7   6   5   4   3   2   1

Preface

The knowledge generated about avian medicine over the past decade has stimulated tremendous interest in this field of veterinary medicine. The immense growth in the pet bird industry, including feeds, cages, and supplies, and the increased interest and advances in captive breeding and aviculture have placed immense pressure on the veterinary profession to keep up with the demand for services. Veterinarians who are involved with any or all aspects of this industry have been charged with the task and responsibility of meeting these needs. The demand for expertise in avian medicine currently exceeds the supply, and many more veterinarians are seeking comprehensive means of gaining knowledge of avian medicine.

Our goal for this book is to provide a means to gain knowledge in both basic and advanced clinical avian medicine and aviculture in a user-friendly manner. *Avian Medicine and Surgery* is written in a problem-oriented approach, which simplifies researching a clinical case or disease process and provides a practical means of finding information related to avian medicine. This approach is of particular value to the beginning avian practitioner because it offers easy and rapid access to information sought without requiring a great deal of background knowledge.

Avian medicine is still in its infancy, and it is difficult to keep pace with and incorporate changes and advances while adhering to a publication schedule. We have tried to incorporate as many of the more recent developments as possible during the production of this book, but we acknowledge that even with this effort, developments have occurred that we have been unable to include. We do feel, however, that the information in this book will provide comprehensive background information that will serve well as a basis for evaluating the most recent developments.

Avian Medicine and Surgery was very much a group effort of four editors, each with a very different background and area of expertise. We believe that these differences worked to our advantage in preparing *Avian Medicine and Surgery* by providing very different perspectives from which to evaluate information. These differences also emphasize that it is no longer possible for one person to have expertise in all areas of avian medicine—the field is now too vast.

ROBERT B. ALTMAN, D.V.M.
SUSAN L. CLUBB, D.V.M.
GERRY M. DORRESTEIN, D.V.M., PH.D.
KATHERINE E. QUESENBERRY, D.V.M.

Acknowledgments

We wish to thank the developmental editors, Sandra Valkhoff, Nellie McGrew, and Les Hoeltzel at W.B. Saunders Company for their support and patience during the production of this book, and Ray Kersey, senior editor, for his belief in this project. We thank Ron Futral for his expertise and patience in producing the illustrations. We thank Adina Rae Freedman for her unselfish dedication, expertise, and support in preparation of many of the manuscripts and for helping to coordinate time schedules for editors and authors. Above all, we thank all the authors who have contributed their time and knowledge, without which *Avian Medicine and Surgery* would not be possible.

Contributors

Robert B. Altman, DVM
Co-Director, A & A Veterinary Hospital Inc, Franklin Square, New York; Adjunct Associate Professor of Zoological Medicine, College of Veterinary Medicine, University of Pennsylvania, Philadelphia, Pennsylvania
General Surgical Considerations; Soft Tissue Surgical Procedures; Radiosurgery (Electrosurgery); Beak Repair, Acrylics

Louise Bauck, BSc, DVM, MVSc
Director of Veterinary Services, Hagen Avicultural Research Institution, Montreal, Quebec, Canada
Avian Dermatology; Toxic Diseases

R. Avery Bennett, DVM, MS
Diplomate, American College of Veterinary Surgeons; Assistant Professor of Zoo and Wildlife Medicine, University of Florida, College of Veterinary Medicine, Gainesville, Florida
Orthopedic Surgery

Mary B. Brown, MS, PhD
Associate Professor, Department of Pathobiology, College of Veterinary Medicine, University of Florida, Gainesville, Florida
Mycoplasmal Infections

James W. Carpenter, MS, DVM
Diplomate, American College of Zoological Medicine; Associate Professor, Exotic Animal, Wildlife, and Zoo Animal Medicine Service, Department of Clinical Sciences, College of Veterinary Medicine, Kansas State University, Manhattan, Kansas
Zoonotic Diseases of Avian Origin; Cranes

Robert Clipsham, DVM
Exotic Medicine Consultant/Clinician, Thousand Oaks, California
Beak Repair, Rhamphorthotics

Susan L. Clubb, DVM
Diplomate, American Board of Veterinary Practitioners (Avian Practice); Staff Veterinarian, Parrot Jungle and Gardens, Miami Florida; Consultant, Pretty Bird International, Pet Industry Joint Advisory Council, Loro Parque, Tenerife, Spain

Laws and Regulations Affecting Aviculture and the Pet Bird Industry; Embryology, Incubation, and Hatching; Psittacine Pediatric Husbandry and Medicine; Aviculture Medicine and Flock Health Management

Christine Davis, BS, BA
Avian Behavior Consultant, Writer, Lecturer; "The Bird Lady," Sierra Madre, California
Behavior; Behavioral Problems

Gerry M. Dorrestein, DVM, PhD
Associate Professor in Avian, Exotic Animal, and Wildlife Pathology, Utrecht University, Faculty of Veterinary Medicine, Department of Pathology, Section of Exotic and Laboratory Animals, Utrecht, The Netherlands
Diagnostic Necropsy and Pathology; Avian Cytology; Bacteriology; Respiratory System: Physiology of Avian Respiration; The Gastrointestinal Tract: Physiology of Digestion; Nervous System: Physiology of the Brain and Special Senses; The Endocrine System: Physiology of the Endocrine System; Cardiovascular System: Physiology of the Avian Cardiac System; Musculoskeletal System: Physiology of the Musculoskeletal System; Avian Dermatology: Physiology of Avian Dermatology; Urogenital Disorders: Physiology of the Urogenital System; Metabolism, Pharmacology, and Therapy; Passerines; Pigeons and Doves

Frank Enders, DVM
Staff Veterinarian, Loro Parque, Tenerife, Spain
Ultrasonography

Martha L. Ewing, MS, DVM
Company Veterinarian, Case Farm of North Carolina Inc., Morganton, North Carolina
Mycoplasmal Infections

Keven Flammer, DVM
Diplomate, American Board of Veterinary Practitioners (Avian Practice); Associate Professor, Non-Domestic Avian Medicine, Department of Companion Animal and Special Species Medicine, College of Veterinary Medicine, North Carolina State University, Raleigh, North Carolina
Chlamydia

Alan M. Fudge, DVM
Diplomate, American Board of Veterinary Practitioners (Avian Practice); Director, Avian Medical Center of Sacramento; Director, California Avian Laboratory, Citrus Heights, California
Avian Clinical Pathology—Hematology and Chemistry

Edward J. Gentz, MS, DVM
Instructor, Department of Clinical Sciences, College of Veterinary Medicine, Cornell University, Ithaca, New York
Zoonotic Diseases of Avian Origin

Helga Gerlach, Prof. Dr. Med. Vet. Dr. habil
Retired from Faculty of Veterinary Medicine, Ludwig Maximilians University, Munich, Germany
Galliformes; Anatiformes

Ellis C. Greiner, MS, PhD
Professor of Parasitology, Department of Pathobiology; Service Chief, Clinical Microbiology and Parasitology, Veterinary Medical Teaching Hospital, College of Veterinary Medicine, University of Florida, Gainesville, Florida
Parasitology

Joy Halverson, DVM, MPVM
Director of Product Development, Zoogen, Inc., Davis, California
Nonsurgical Methods of Avian Sex Identification

James M. Harris, DVM
Owner and Medical Director, Montclair Veterinary Clinic and Hospital, Oakland, California
The Human-Avian Bond; Grief and Bereavement

Darryl J. Heard, BVMS, PhD
Assistant Professor, Wildlife and Zoological Medicine Service, College of Veterinary Medicine, University of Florida, Gainesville, Florida
Anesthesia and Analgesia

Elizabeth V. Hillyer, DVM
Medical writer and editor
Physical Examination; Respiratory System: Clinical Manifestations of Respiratory Disorders

Manfred Hochleithner, DVM
Diplomate, European College of Avian Medicine and Surgery; Lector, Veterinary Medicine, University of Vienna; Head, Tierklinik Strebersdorf, Vienna, Austria
Endoscopy

Heidi L. Hoefer, DVM
Diplomate, American Board of Veterinary Practitioners (Avian Practice); Staff Veterinarian, Avian and Exotic Pet Service, The Animal Medical Center, New York, New York
The Gastrointestinal Tract: Diseases of the Gastrointestinal Tract

Jan Hooimeijer, DVM
Avian Veterinarian Practitioner, Bird Clinic Meppel, Meppel, The Netherlands
Pigeons and Doves

Jeffrey R. Jenkins, DVM
Diplomate, American Board of Veterinary Practitioners (Avian Practice); President, Avian and Exotic Animal Hospital, Inc., San Diego, California
Hospital Techniques and Supportive Care; Avian Critical Care and Emergency Medicine

Thomas J. Kern, DVM
Diplomate, American College of Veterinary Ophthalmologists; Associate Professor of Ophthalmology, College of Veterinary Medicine, Cornell University, Ithaca, New York
Disorders of the Special Senses

Maria E. Krautwald-Junghanns, DVM, PhD
University Lecturer; Head, Bird Clinic, Institute for Avian Diseases, University of Giessen, Giessen, Germany
Ultrasonography

Jerry LaBonde, MS, DVM
Owner, Avian and Exotic Animal Hospital, Englewood, Colorado
Toxic Diseases

Winston C. Lancaster, PhD
Postdoctoral Research Fellow, Department of Zoology, University of Aberdeen, Aberdeen, Scotland
Systematics

David M. McCluggage, DVM
Owner, Chaparral Animal Health Center, Longmont, Colorado
Bandaging

James R. Millam, PhD
Associate Professor, Department of Avian Sciences, University of California, Davis, California
Reproductive Physiology

Michael Miller, MS, VMD
Diplomate, American Board of Veterinary Practitioners (Canine and Feline Practice); Director, Cardiology-Ultrasound Referral Service, Thornton, Pennsylvania
Cardiovascular System: Cardiac Disease

Barbara L. Oglesbee, DVM
Diplomate, American Board of Veterinary Practitioners (Avian Practice); Assistant Professor, Department of Veterinary Clinical Sciences, The Ohio State University, College of Veterinary Medicine, Columbus, Ohio
Differential Diagnosis; Mycotic Diseases; The Endocrine System: Diseases of the Endocrine System

Glenn H. Olsen, DVM, MS, PhD
Veterinary Medical Officer, U.S. Department of Interior, Patuxent Environmental Science Center, Laurel, Maryland; Former Assistant Professor, Louisiana State University, School of Veterinary Medicine, Baton Rouge, Louisiana
Embryology, Incubation, and Hatching; Cranes

Susan Orosz, PhD, DVM
Diplomate, American Board of Veterinary Practitioners (Avian Practice); Associate Professor, Avian and Exotic Animal Medicine, Department of Comparative Medicine, College of Veterinary Medicine, The University of Tennessee, Knoxville, Tennessee
Respiratory System: Anatomy of the Respiratory System; The Gastrointestinal Tract: Anatomy of the Digestive System; Nervous System: Anatomy of the Central Nervous System; The Endocrine System: Anatomy of the Endocrine System; Cardiovascular System: Anatomy of the Cardiovascular System; Musculoskeletal System: Anatomy of the Musculoskeletal System; Avian Dermatology: Anatomy of the Integument; Urogenital Disorders: Anatomy of the Urogenital System

David N. Phalen, DVM, PhD
Assistant Clinical Professor, Zoological Medicine Service, Department of Large Animal Medicine and Surgery, Texas A&M University, College Station, Texas
Viruses

Katherine Quesenberry, DVM
Diplomate, American Board of Veterinary Practitioners (Avian Practice); Service Head, Avian and Exotic Pet Service, The Animal Medical Center, New York, New York
Musculoskeletal System: Disorders of the Musculoskeletal System; Neoplasia: Treatment of Neoplasia

Patrick T. Redig, DVM, PhD
Associate Professor, Department of Small Animal Clinical Sciences; Director, The Raptor Center, College of Veterinary Medicine, University of Minnesota, St. Paul, Minnesota
Raptors

Karen Rosenthal, DVM, MS
Diplomate, American Board of Veterinary Practitioners

(Avian Practice); Staff Veterinarian, Avian and Exotic Pet Service, The Animal Medical Center, New York, New York
Nervous System: Disorders of the Avian Nervous System; Cardiovascular System: Cardiac Disease

T. E. Roudybush, MS
President, Roudybush, Inc., Sacramento, California
Nutrition; Nutritional Disorders

Robert E. Schmidt, DVM, PhD
Zoo/Exotic Pathology Service, West Sacramento, California
Neoplasia: Neoplastic Diseases; Immune System

Bonnie J. Smith, DVM, PhD
Assistant Professor, Virginia-Maryland Regional College of Veterinary Medicine, Blacksburg, Virginia
Radiology

J. M. Smith, DVM
Owner, Avian Health Services, Placerville; Staff Veterinarian, Roudybush, Inc., Sacramento, California
Nutritional Disorders

Stephen A. Smith, DVM, PhD
Assistant Professor, Virginia-Maryland Regional College of Veterinary Medicine, Blacksburg, Virginia
Radiology

Brian L. Speer, DVM
Diplomate, American Board of Veterinary Practitioners (Avian Practice); Owner, Oakley Veterinary and Bird Hospital, Oakley, California
Urogenital Disorders: Diseases of the Urogenital System

Robert Stonebreaker, DVM
Owner, Mobile Veterinary Services; Associate Veterinarian, Del Mar Veterinary Hospital, Del Mar, California
Ratites

Thomas N. Tully, Jr., DVM, MS
Assistant Professor, Veterinary Clinical Sciences, Louisiana State University School of Veterinary Medicine, Baton Rouge, Louisiana
Formulary

Amy B. Worell, DVM
Diplomate, American Board of Veterinary Practitioners (Avian Practice); Director, All Pets Medical Centre, West Hills, California
Toucans and Mynahs

Contents

Color Section

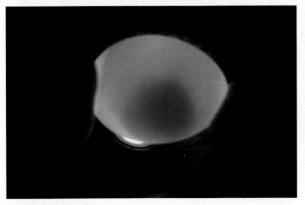

Figure 5-2

Infertile egg with no visible development. Airsac is on the right.

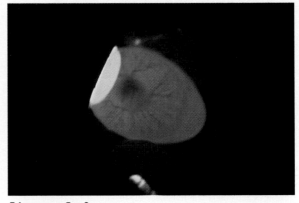

Figure 5-3

Normal parrot embryo in the first trimester of development. Developing embryo is in the center of the developing vascular system. At this stage the beating heart is clearly visible.

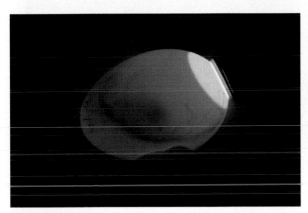

Figure 5-4

Blood ring indicates early embryonic death.

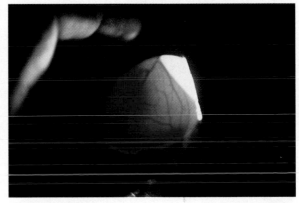

Figure 5-5

Eclectus parrot egg at 21 days' incubation. Dense area in the small end of the egg represents the embryo, and vasculature is well developed at this stage.

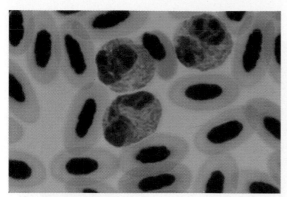

Figure 11–1

Heterophils. Rod-shaped granules are a hallmark of heterophils, but osmotic changes and staining differences may result in a cytoplasm ranging from orange to blue, with indistinct granules. Heterophils are variable in shape and show a nonhomogeneous cytoplasm. (Amazon 250×)

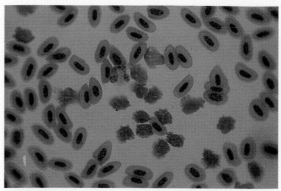

Figure 11–2

Smudge cells. These structures are usually ruptured leukocytes because of less-than-ideal smear technique. A coverslip-to-coverslip smear consistently produces fewer artifacts than a slide-to-slide smear. (cockatiel 100×)

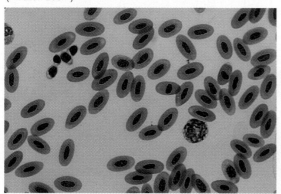

Figure 11–3

Toxic heterophils. Toxic changes can occur in birds that are fighting an infection. A variety of changes can include nuclear hypersegmentation and cytoplasmic vacuoles, but a more consistent finding is the presence of basophilic cytoplasmic inclusions. (blue and gold macaw 100×)

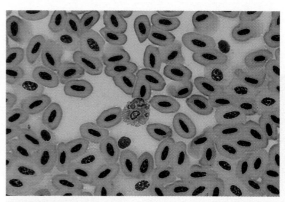

Figure 11–4

Eosinophil. The classic avian eosinophil seems to be the exception rather than the rule. Note the round, pink cytoplasmic granules and the round cell shape. (heron 100×)

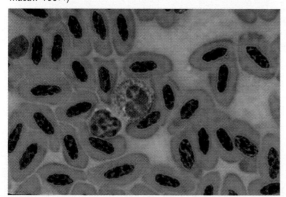

Figure 11–5

Eosinophil. Rules that can usually assist the technician in differentiating eosinophils from heterophils are: (1) homogeneous cytoplasmic color, (2) distinct nuclear/cytoplasmic contrast, and (3) round cell shape. This eosinophil shows the occurrence of bluish cytoplasm. Round granules may not be visualized. (cockatoo 100×)

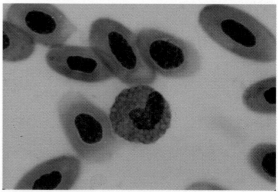

Figure 11–6

Eosinophil. This cell follows the rules listed in Figure 11–5. (eagle 250×)

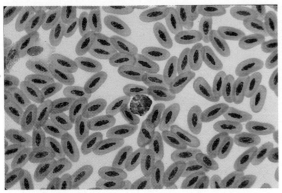

Figure 11-7

Basophil. The classical avian basophil is easy to recognize with the "concord grape" basophilic granules. Variations can include washed-out, degranulated, and artifact changes. Basophil morphology can vary greatly among common species of avian patients. (Amazon 100×)

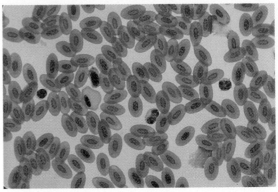

Figure 11-8

Lymphocytes. Avian lymphocytes resemble mammalian counterparts. (Amazon 100×)

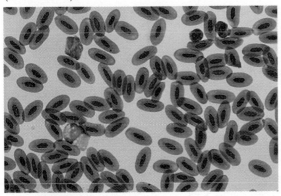

Figure 11-9

Monocytes. These cells can sometimes be difficult to differentiate from large lymphocytes. Abundant gun-metal cytoplasm, with variable shape, nonhomogeneous color, occasional vacuoles, and the absence of azurophilic cytoloplasmic granules are some characteristics of monocytes. Automated flow cytometry tabulation of avian blood typically demonstrates a higher number of monocytes, when compared with results of the manual method of counting. (Amazon 100×)

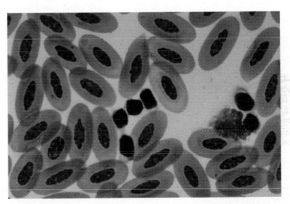

Figure 11-10

Thrombocytes and normal erythrocytes. Avian thrombocytes are nucleated and can be mistaken for small lymphocytes. Mature erythrocytes are elliptical in shape with uniform cytoplasmic color. Less mature erythrocytes appear rounder in shape, possess a bluer cytoplasm, and typically have a more prominent nucleus.

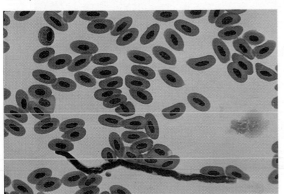

Figure 11-11

Microfilaria. Larval form of a typically nonpathogenic filarid, formerly common in imported cockatoos and selected psittacine species. (Moluccan cockatoo 100×)

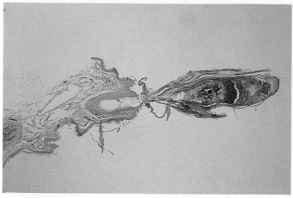

Figure 12–3

Sulphur-crested cockatoo *(Cacatua galerita galerita)*. New developing feathers with constrictions at the base—psittacine beak and feather disease (PBFD). Histologic examination shows bleeding and necrosis (4χ).

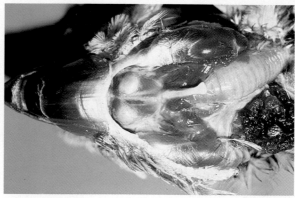

Figure 12–4

Blue-fronted Amazon *(Amazona aestiva)*. Submandibular salivary glands with metaplasia resulting from vitamin A deficiency.

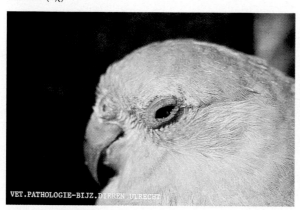

Figure 12–5

Red-rumped parrot *(Psephotus haematonotus)* (yellow strain) with pox lesion on the eyelids.

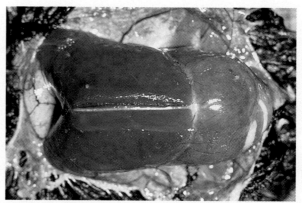

Figure 12–6

Red-fronted parakeet *(Cyanoramphus n. novaezelandiae)* with extremely enlarged liver, leukosis.

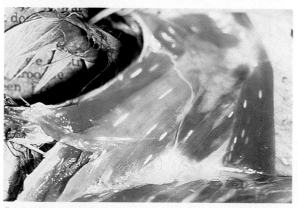

Figure 12–7

Blue-fronted Amazon *(Amazona aestiva)* with white striation in the leg muscles, *Sarcosporidia* species.

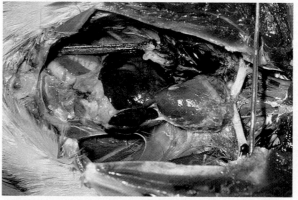

Figure 12–8

Blue and gold macaw *(Ara ararauna)* with organ displacement after perforation of the air sacs with a wooden stick. Postmortem.

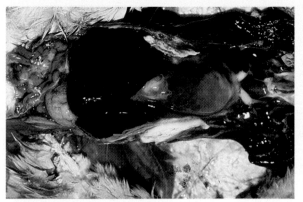

Figure 12-9

African grey parrot *(Psittacus erithacus)*. Both caudal thoracic air sacs are filled with mycotic material; aspergillosis.

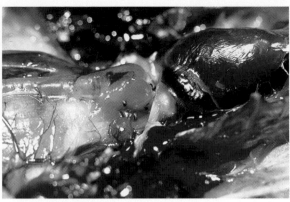

Figure 12-10

Gouldian *(Chloebia gouldiae)* finch with a cervical air sac with mites *(Sternostoma tracheacolum)*.

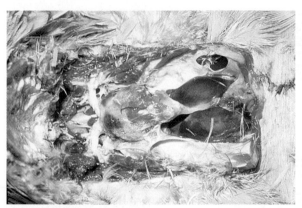

Figure 12-11

Yellow-fronted Amazon *(Amazona ochrocephala)*. Air sacs are filled with food after forced feeding.

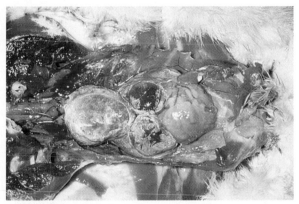

Figure 12-12

Galah *(Eolophus r. roseicapillus)*. Urate deposits are on the pericardium and liver; visceral gout.

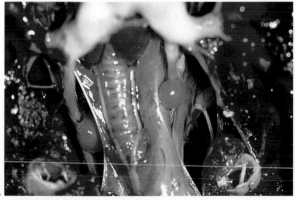

A   B

Figure 12-13

African grey parrot *(Psittacus erithacus)* with enlarged parathyroid glands, secondary hyperparathyroidism. *(A)* normal, *(B)* pathologic.

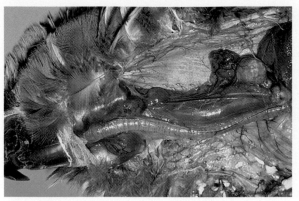

Figure 12–14

Yellow-collared macaw *(Ara auricollis)* with Salmonella "abscesses" along the neck.

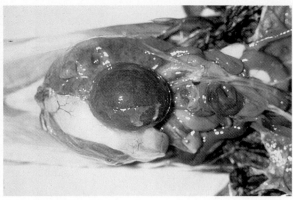

Figure 12–15

Red-fronted parakeet *(Cyanoramphus n. novaezelandiae)* with enlarged spleen, leukosis.

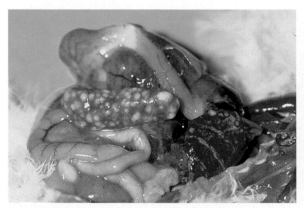

Figure 12–16

Canary *(Serinus canaria)* with enlarged spleen with yellow necrotic foci, yersiniosis.

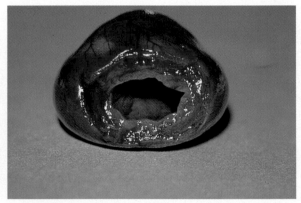

Figure 12-17

Cockatiel *(Nymphicus hollandicus)* with eccentric hypertrophy of the heart.

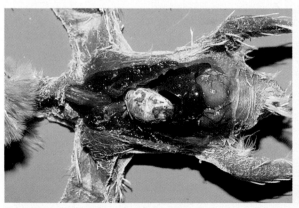

Figure 12–18

Canary *(Serinus canaria)* with pericarditis and uricemia.

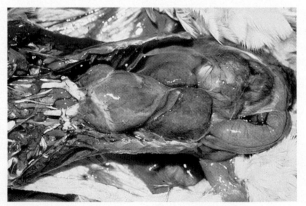

Figure 12–19

African grey parrot *(Psittacus erithacus)*, with heart decompensation in combination with liver fibrosis and hydrops ascites.

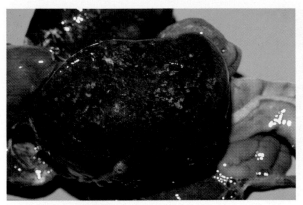

Figure 12-20

African grey parrot *(Psittacus erithacus)* with an enlarged liver with necrotic foci, herpesvirus infection (Pacheco's disease).

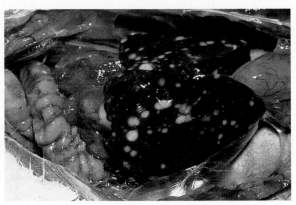

Figure 12-21

Imperial pigeon *(Ducula* species) with focal yellow proliferative foci, avian tuberculosis.

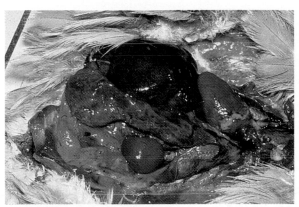

Figure 12-22

Scarlet macaw *(Ara macao).* Liver has small round necrotic foci, yersiniosis.

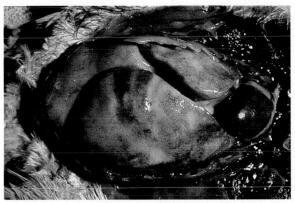

Figure 12-23

Mealy Amazon *(Amazona farinosa)* with enlarged yellow liver, fatty liver.

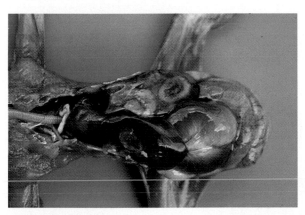

Figure 12-24

Peacock chicken *(Pavo cristatus)* with necrotic areas in the liver, histomoniasis (blackhead).

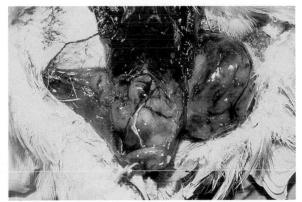

Figure 12-25

Budgerigar *(Melopsittacus undulatus)* with adenocarcinoma of the kidneys.

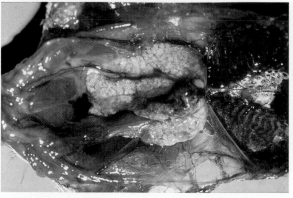

Figure 12–26

Canary *(Serinus canaria)*. An accumulation of urate crystals is in the collecting tubules of the kidney after deprivation of water.

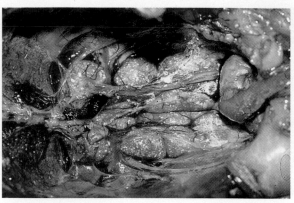

Figure 12–27

Blue and gold macaw *(Ara ararauna)*. Juvenile bird had renal gout after vitamin D$_3$ imbalance.

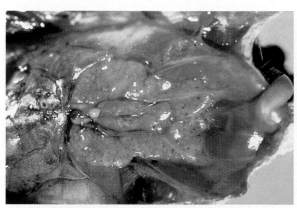

Figure 12–28

Canary *(Serinus canaria)*. Chronic nephritis after ingesting mycotoxins.

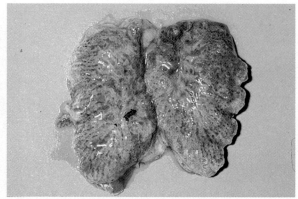

Figure 12–30

Blue-fronted Amazon *(Amazona aestiva)* with acute mycotic infection with *Mucor* species, lung edema.

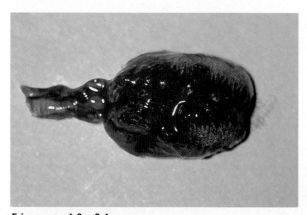

Figure 12–31

Lovebird *(Agapornis roseicollis)* with acute hemorrhagic pneumonia, polytertrafluoroethylene (Teflon) toxicosis.

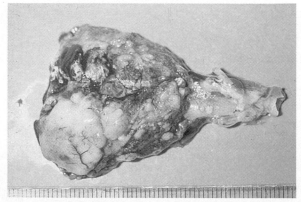

Figure 12–33

Yellow-fronted Amazon *(Amazona ochrocephala)* with proliferative granulomas in the lung, tuberculosis.

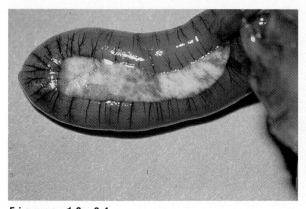

Figure 12–34

Ringneck dove *(Streptopelia semitorquata)*. Pancreatitis after a paramyxovirus infection.

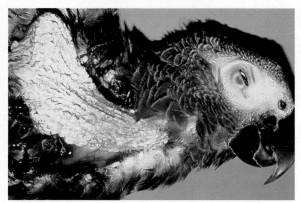

Figure 12–35

African grey parrot *(Psittacus erithacus)* with crop candidiasis.

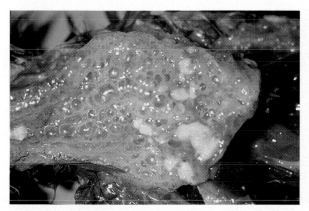

Figure 12–36

Hanging parrot *(Loriculus* species). There is thickening of the crop wall with necrotic foci, trichomoniasis.

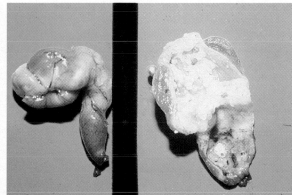

Figure 12–39

Budgerigar *(Melopsittacus undulatus)*. Changes of the stomach due to megabacterial infection.

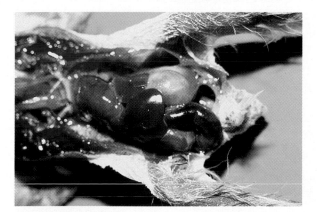

Figure 12–40

Chinese nightingale *(Leiothrix lutea)*. Hemorrhagic diatheses with the intestines filled with blood after 24 hours of fasting.

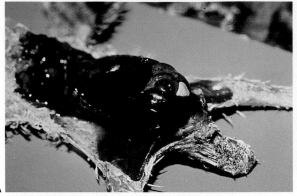
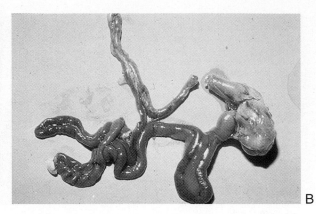

Figure 12–41

(A,B) Budgerigar *(Melopsittacus undulatus)*. Juvenile bird with hemorrhagic enteritis, *Giardia lamblia* infection.

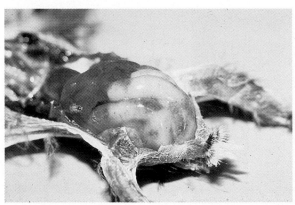

Figure 12–42

Black siskin *(Carduelis spinus)*. Duodenum with thickened and edematous wall with local hemorrhagic areas, coccidiosis.

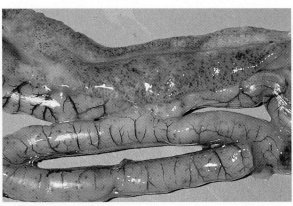

Figure 12–43

Backyard chicken *(Gallus domesticus)*. Enteritis with a thickened wall, coccidiosis, *Eimeria acervulina*.

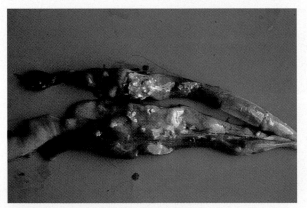

Figure 12–45

Peacock *(Pavo cristatus)*. Pseudomembraneous, necrotic typhlitis, histomoniasis (blackhead).

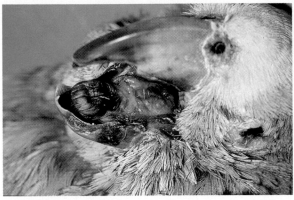

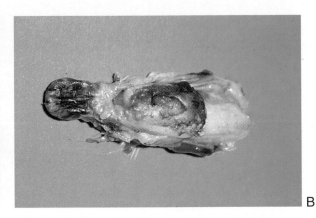

A **B**

Figure 12–46

(A,B) Yellow-fronted Amazon *(Amozona ochrocephala)*. Chronic proliferative lesion with necrosis, (bovine) tuberculous lesion. *(A)* tongue in situ, *(B)* tongue lesion.

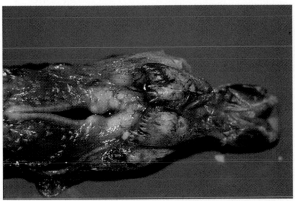

Figure 12–47

Sulphur-crested cockatoo *(Cacatua g. galerita)*. Metaplastic changes of the lingual salivary glands and tracheal orifice, vitamin A deficiency.

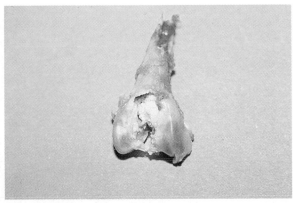

Figure 12–48

Military macaw *(Ara militaris)*. Proliferative granuloma with necrosis in the distal femur, tuberculosis.

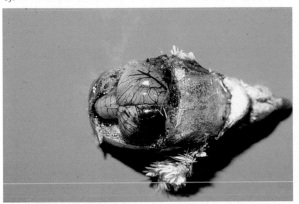

Figure 12–49

Pigeon *(Columba livia)* with hemorrhages on the brain surface, dimetridazole (emtryl) intoxication.

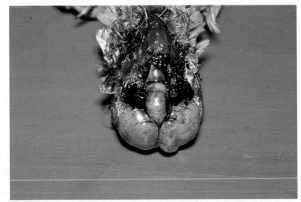

Figure 12–50

Malga parrot *(Psephotus varius)* with free blood inside the skull, trauma.

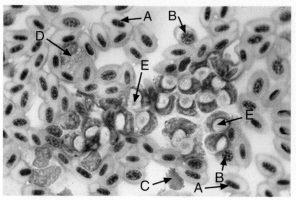

Figure 15-1

Atoxoplasmosis in a goldfinch *(Carduelis carduelis)* liver. A, mature erythrocyte; B, young erthrocyte; C, "smudge" cell; D, toxic heterophil; E, monocyte with one *Atoxoplasma* trophozoite.

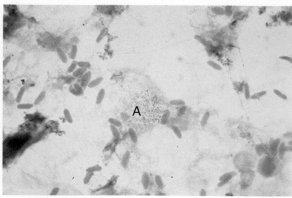

Figure 15-4

Chlamydiosis in a golden-manteled rosella *(Platycercus eximius cecilae)*, lung (Stamp stain). A, "Cloud" of red intracytoplasmic inclusions inside macrophages.

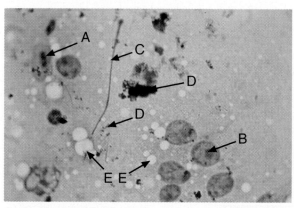

Figure 15-5

"Artifacts" in Jardine's parrot *(Poicephalus g. gulielmi)*, liver. A, Erythrocyte; B, liver cell nucleus; C, nuclear filament; D, stain precipitates; E, degeneration vacuoles. Notice the background staining of the liver cell cytoplasm with mitochondria.

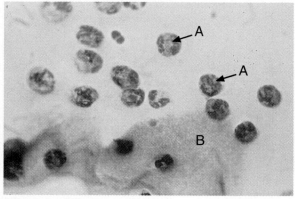

Figure 15-6

Toxic heterophils (joint salmonellosis) in a pigeon *(Columba livia)*, wing joint synovia; A, Toxic heterophils; B, protein-containing synovia.

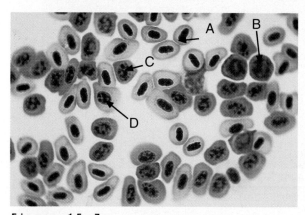

Figure 15-7

Erythroblastosis in a canary *(Serinus canaria)*, lung. A, Mature erythrocyte; B, erythroblast (=rubriblast); C, polychromatic erythrocyte (=rubricyte); D, reticulocyte.

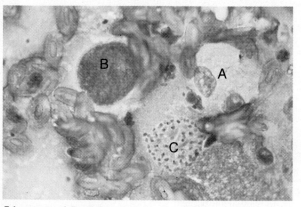

Figure 15-13

Coccidiosis in a black-headed siskin *(Spinus i. icteria)*, duodenum. A, Epithelial cell; B, macrogamont; C, microgamont.

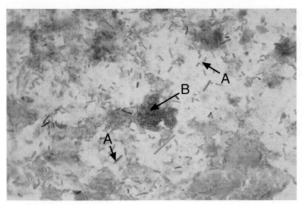

Figure 15-15

Chlamydiosis in a mealy Amazon parrot *(Amazona farinosa)*, rectum (Stamp stain). A, Rod-shaped bacteria; B, "cluster" of red intracytoplasmic inclusions. Notice in the background many "individual" red elementary bodies.

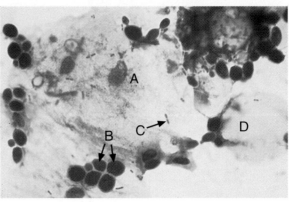

Figure 15-17

Regurgitation in a green-winged macaw *(Ara chloroptera)*, syrinx. A, Squamous epithelial cell; B, yeasts; C, rod-shaped bacteria; D, starch.

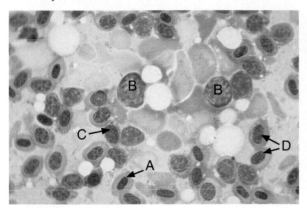

Figure 15-22

Anemia (blood-sucking mites) in a canary *(Serinus canaria)*, liver. A, Mature erythrocyte; B, erythroblast; C, polychromatic erythrocyte; D, reticulocyte.

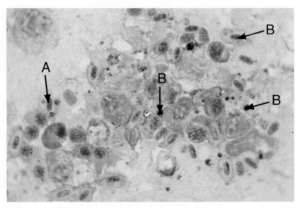

Figure 15-24

Plasmodium infection in a redpoll *(Acanthis flammea)*, spleen. A, infected erythrocyte; B, *Plasmodium* pigment.

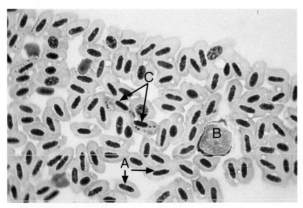

Figure 15-25

Leucocytozoon and *Plasmodium* in a sunbird *(Nectarinia* species), blood smear. A, Erythrocyte; B, *Leucocytozoon;* C, erythrocyte with *Plasmodium.*

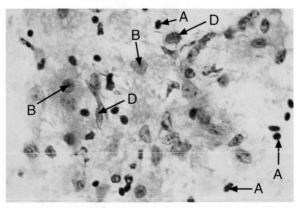

Figure 15-28

Tuberculosis in an Old World kestrel *(Falco tinnunculus)*, liver, (Ziehl-Neelson stain). A, erythrocyte; B, liver cell nucleus with postmortem changes; D, *Mycobacteria* (red, acid-fast stained rod-shaped bacteria).

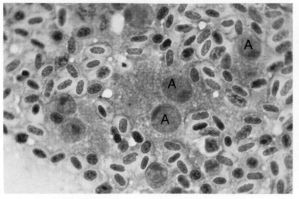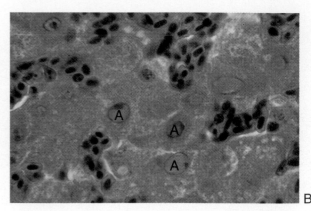

Figure 15–30

(A) Herpes virus inclusion bodies in a sulphur-crested cockatoo *(Cacatua galerita)*, liver; impression (Hemacolor). A, Liver cell nucleus with nucleolus pushed aside. *(B)* Herpesvirus inclusion bodies in a sulphur-crested cockatoo *(Cacatua galerita)*, liver. Hemalum-eosin stain (oil). Liver cell nucleus with nucleolus pushed aside.

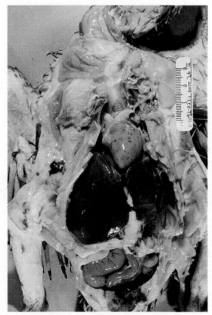

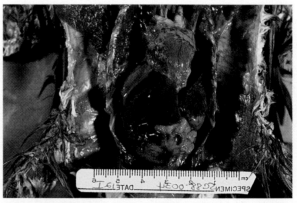

Figure 19–5

Amazon parrot with Pacheco's disease. Although an uncommon lesion, a diffusely yellow liver in a parrot dying with few premonitory signs should make the practitioner suspicious of Pacheco's disease. (Photograph kindly provided by Dr. David Graham.)

Figure 19–4

Nestling scarlet macaw with avian polyomavirus disease. There is a generalized pallor of the skin and muscles. The liver is moderately enlarged and there are numerous epicardial and subcutaneous hemorrhages.

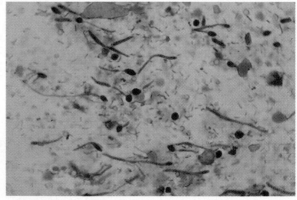

Figure 26–8

Hyphae formation in the crop of a young cockatiel with candidiasis (Gram's stain of a crop swab).

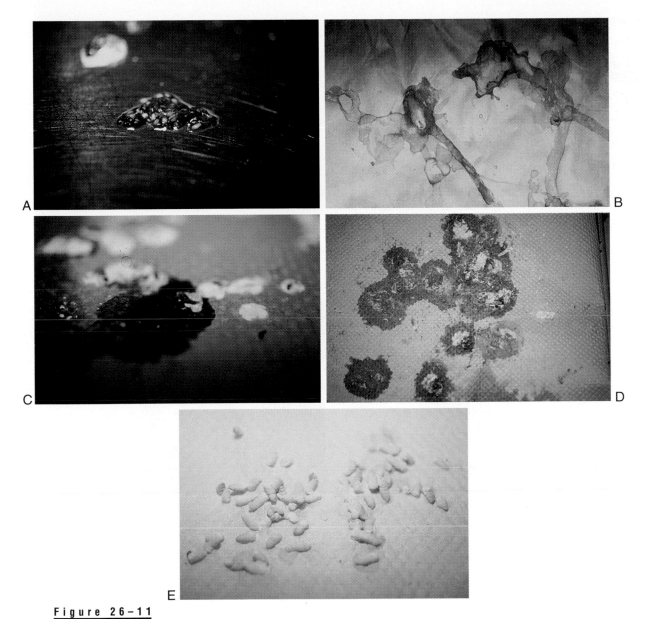

Figure 26-11

Abnormal psittacine droppings. *(A)* Whole millet seeds are visible in the feces of this cockatiel with neuropathic gastric dilation. *(B)* Hematuria in an Amazon parrot with acute lead poisoning. *(C)* Hematochezia in a parrot with a cloacal mass. *(D)* Biliverdinuria in a macaw with chlamydial hepatitis. *(E)* Maldigestion in a budgerigar.

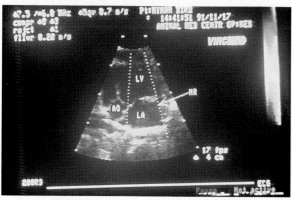

Figure 29-12

Two-chamber color flow Doppler echocardiographic image of a mynah bird with congestive heart failure. Enlarged ventricular chambers are present, as is the mitral regurgitation (MR) depicted here as a blue jet fluid. (LA = left atrium, LV = left ventriculus, AO = aorta.)

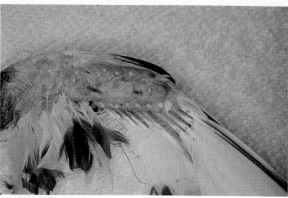

Figure 32-17

Xanthomatosis affecting the wingtip of a parakeet. This lesion was apparently pruritic (treated with amputation).

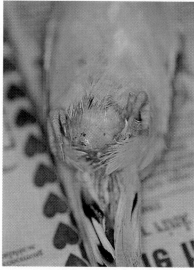

Figure 32-18

Fatty infiltration into the skin of a parakeet with a hernia. Note the quilted appearance. Xanthomatous changes may follow or accompany other symptoms.

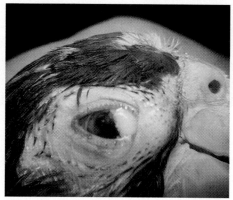

Figure 41-3

An exudative plug lies in the fornix of the medial canthus of a red-lored Amazon parrot *(Amazona autumnalis)*. The exudative mass can be expressed by applying pressure at the medial canthus.

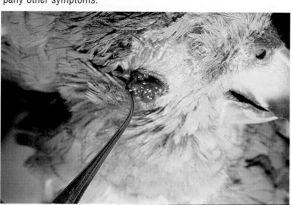

Figure 41-5

Grape-like conjunctival papillomas extruding from beneath the lower eyelid of an Amazon parrot responded well to radiosurgical excision.

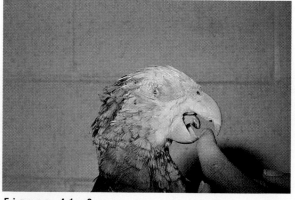

Figure 41-9

A draining fistula in the eyelid of a yellow-nape Amazon *(Amazona ochrocephala auropalliata)* 2 months after eye enucleation.

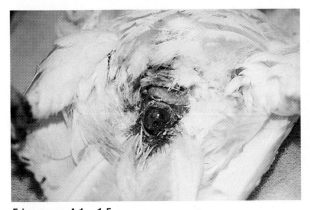

Figure 41–15

(A) Prolapsed cloaca in a cockatoo. Note the rectal opening.

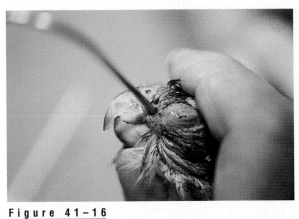

Figure 41–16

(C) The cannula passes into the infraorbital diverticulum beneath the eye.

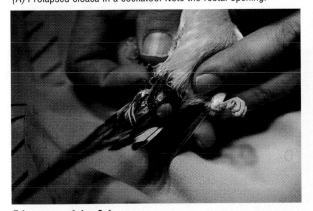

Figure 41–21

(B) Egg-bound budgerigar *(Melopsittacus undulatus)* as seen in position 1.

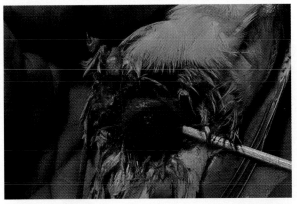

Figure 41–21

(C) The egg is in the pelvic canal and cloaca as seen in position 2.

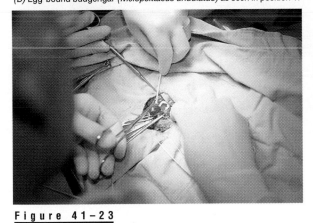

Figure 41–23

An egg-bound bird with an intraabdominal egg (position 3). The egg is removed by a transabdominal approach. The uterus was incised and the egg content aspirated, followed by removal of the shell and closure of the uterus.

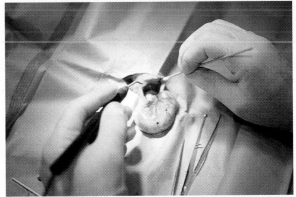

Figure 41–24

A cockatiel *(Nymphicus hollandicus)* with a uterus full of liquefied yolk material (pyometra).

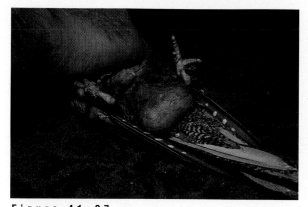

F i g u r e   4 1 – 2 7

(A) Abdominal hernia in a cockatiel *(Nymphicus hollandicus)*.

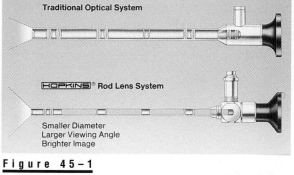

F i g u r e   4 5 – 1

Anatomy of a rigid endoscope showing the benefits of the Hopkins Rod Lens System patented by Karl Stroz GmbH. (Courtesy of Karl Storz Veterinary Endoscopy America, Inc.)

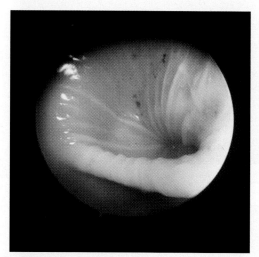

F i g u r e   4 5 – 2

Normal crop of a blue-fronted Amazon parrot. The crop mucosa is covered by clear mucus and some food particles. Observe the opening into the thoracic esophagus.

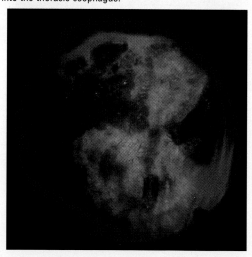

F i g u r e   4 5 – 3

Figures 45–3, 45–4 and 45–5 are endoscopic views of the lung from a lateral approach. The endoscope is within the caudal thoracic air sac. Figure 45–3 shows mild inflammation. In addition to normal lung tissue, an increase in number of small vessels because of inflammatory reaction can be observed.

F i g u r e   4 5 – 4

Severe inflammation. Only small areas of normal lung tissue can be seen. The red coloration indicates inflammation.

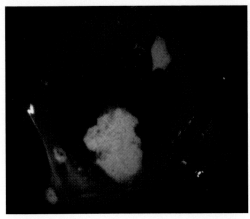

Figure 45–5

As differential diagnosis to the view in Figure 45–3, a sharp border between normal lung tissue and pathologic coloration can be seen. This can be observed after blood aspiration.

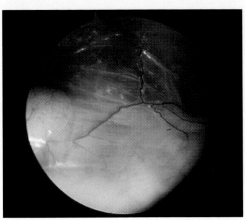

Figure 45–6

Diagnosis of air sac lesions can be performed easily using an endoscope. For an etiologic diagnosis, samples (biopsy, cultures) have to be taken to differentiate common diseases. In this figure, mild inflammation can be recognized because the air sac appears cloudy instead of clear, and vessels can be observed on the air sac surface. Among many bacterial diseases, this apperance can be observed also in chlamydiosis, *Salmonella* infection, or early states of aspergillosis.

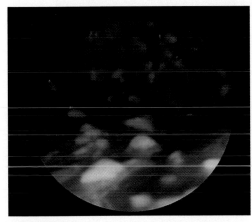

Figure 45–7

Caseous granulomas of an owl's air sac. Examination of a biopsy sample indicated mycobacteriosis.

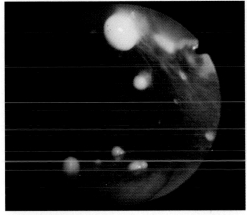

Figure 45–8

The granuloma-like masses in this buzzard contained only normal fat. This presentation should be considered in the differential diagnosis of a disease process.

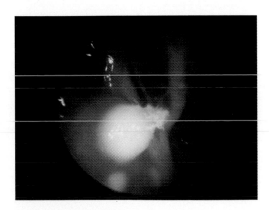

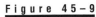

Figure 45–9

A clearly visible *Aspergillus* granuloma in a sulphur-crested cockatoo.

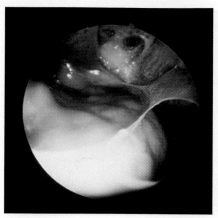

Figure 45-10

If an enlarged proventriculus is suspected, care must be taken when introducing the endoscope. After the endoscope passes the abdominal wall, the enlarged proventriculus containing seeds can be observed.

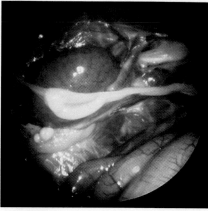

Figure 45-11

Organs in situ in an inactive female European buzzard. Note the dorsal ligament of the oviduct. This picture also demonstrates the importance of identifying all structures during routine sexing. The form and structure of the cranial part of the oviduct can easily be mistaken for a testicle. Therefore, the triangle including the adrenal gland, gonad, and kidney should always be identified.

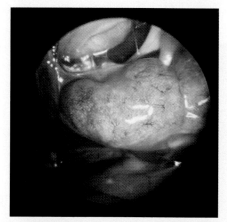

Figure 45-12

Disease of the kidneys can be observed in 8 to 10% of birds showing no clinical signs during routine surgical sexing. Urate stasis can be recognized by spots in the kidney. (Compare with the kidney shown in Fig. 45-11.)

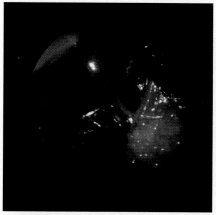

Figure 45-13

An enlarged spleen in a female African grey parrot. The speckled coloration can often be seen in psittacine birds but has no clinical significance.

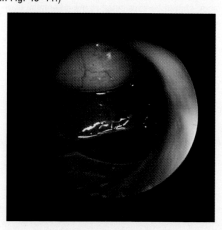
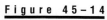

Figure 45-14

Visualization of the caudal edge of the left liver lobe using a ventral approach.

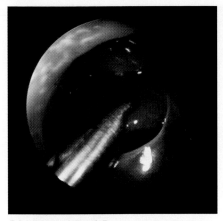

Figure 45-15
Liver biopsy can easily be performed.

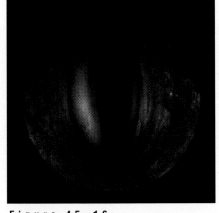

Figure 45-16
Inflammation of the trachea and the syrinx.

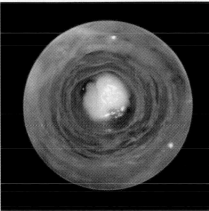

Figure 45-17
The trachea is nearly completely obstructed from an *Aspergillus* granuloma. Inflammation and swelling of the tracheal mucosa can be observed.

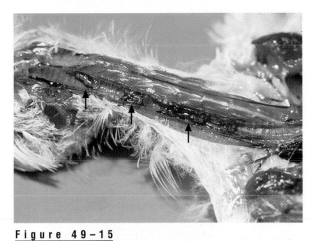

Figure 49-15
Canary *(Serinus canaria)*; trachea filled with *Syngamus* worms *(arrows)*.

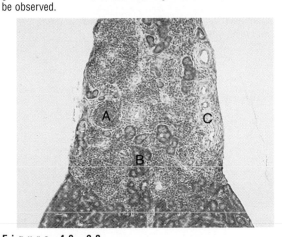

Figure 49-20
Sidney waxbill *(Estrilda temporalis)*; pancreatitis caused by paramyxovirus type 3. (a) lymph follicles; (b) exocrine pancreatic tissue; (c) area of fibrosis.

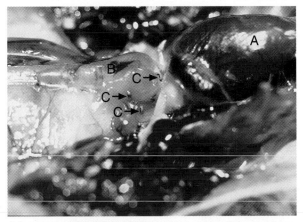

Figure 49-25
Lady Gouldian finch *(Chloebia gouldiae)* air sac mites *(Sternostoma tracheacolum)*. (a) heart; (b) syrinx; (c) mites.

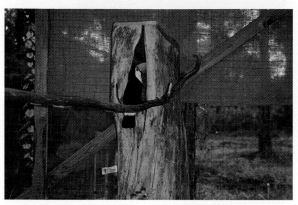

Figure 51–1

A breeding male toco toucan inspects his nest. Natural logs are ideal nest sites for breeding toucans.

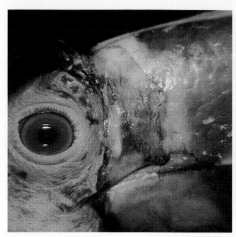

Figure 51–2

This toucan was severely injured when introduced to an unknown aggressive bird. Intraspecific aggression may also occur in the breeding season when the male attacks the female.

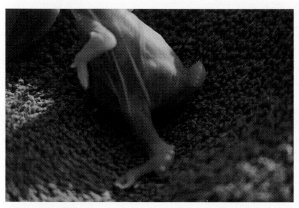

Figure 51–3

Spurred heel pad on the caudal tarsometatarsus of a toucan chick.

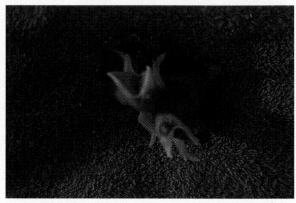

Figure 51–4

Hatchling toucans have smooth pink skin that is so thin that it is possible to visualize many internal organs.

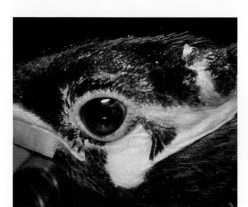

Figure 51–5

Avian poxvirus infection in a hill mynah.

The Normal Bird

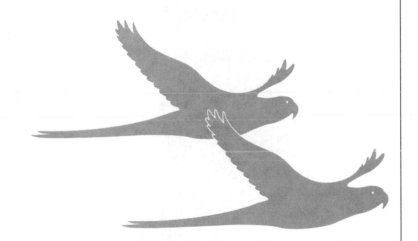

Winston C. Lancaster

1

Systematics

Birds represent the most abundant and diverse class of air-breathing vertebrates. With some 9700 species, birds inhabit every continent and occupy virtually every habitat with the exception of the deep seas. In an attempt to impose order upon this complexity, science categorizes birds on the basis of morphology, whether it be the structure of feathers and bones or that of DNA. Morphologic features also bear upon the lives that birds lead. Although most birds are united by having forelimbs adapted for flight, modes of flight vary radically and encompass hovering, soaring, dives at high speeds, sustained flights covering great distances, and the underwater flight of some sea birds. Diet also varies widely and is reflected in the morphology of the beak from the probing beak of nectar feeders, to the complex sieves of filter feeders, to the sharp hooked beaks of predators. Often overlooked by laymen, the feet and legs of birds also show exquisite adaptation to locomotion and feeding. These suites of characteristics form the foundation of our classification of birds, but also illustrate how birds function in their environment.

In times past, when avian medicine was limited to poultry, systematics had little practical application. However, the explosive popularity of birds as companion animals and interest in aviculture and exotic species created the need for a greater familiarity of bird diversity on the part of the clinician. In this chapter current concepts in the systematic classification of birds are outlined along with characteristics and relationships of the orders and families of birds most frequently encountered in veterinary practice.

CURRENT TRENDS IN AVIAN SYSTEMATICS

Schemes of taxonomic classification are intended to reflect evolutionary descent. Wetmore[1] presented the systematic arrangement of birds that is in common usage (Table 1–1), which is based primarily on gross morphologic characteristics. The members of most groups in this classification have sufficient anatomic similarities to represent plausible monophyletic taxa (i.e., all descended from a common lineage). It has, however, proven difficult to decipher phylogenetic relationships between high level taxa using classical morphologic criteria. In an attempt to clarify relationships, Sibley and his colleagues[2, 3, 4] presented a classification based on DNA-DNA hybridization. They developed a method to quantify differences between the DNA of species, and consider that these differences reflect the degree of genomic divergence. The more similar the DNA, the more closely related species were considered to be. Based on pair-wise comparisons of approximately 1700 species, clusters of species emerged that define taxonomic groups. The investigators established a level of difference that was considered sufficient to define separate families. Clusters with greater difference were designated as higher taxa (e.g., suborder, order). Assuming a constant rate of modification in DNA, quantified genomic divergence was used to estimate the period of time that elapsed since species shared a common ancestor. Houde[5] criticized the assumption of constant rates of DNA evolution, noting that variations in tempo of change in DNA may be sufficient to introduce ambiguity in the clustering of taxa.

The greatest differences between molecular and

Table 1–1

MAJOR ORDERS AND FAMILIES OF EXTANT BIRDS

Struthioniformes
  Struthionidae
    Ostrich, monotypic
Rheiformes
  Rheidae
    Rheas, two species
Casuariiformes
  Casuariidae
    Cassowaries, three species
  Dromaiidae
    Emu, one species
Apterygiformes
  Apterigidae
    Kiwis, three species
Tinamiformes
  Tinamidae
    Tinamous, 45 species
Sphenisciformes
  Spheniscidae
    Penguins, 16 species
Gaviiformes
  Gaviidae
    Loons, four species
Podicipediformes
  Podicipedidae
    Grebes, 20 species
Procellariiformes
  Diomedeidae
    Albatrosses, 14 species
  Procellariidae
    Shearwaters, Fulmars, 55
    species
  Hydrobatidae
    Storm petrels, 20 species
Pelecaniformes
  Pelecanidae
    Pelicans, seven species
  Sulidae
    Gannets and boobies, nine
    species
  Phaethontidae
    Tropicbirds, three species
  Phalacrocoracidae
    Cormorants, 29 species
  Fregatidae
    Frigatebirds, five species
  Anhingidae
    Darters, four species
Ciconiiformes
  Ardeidae
    Herons and bitterns, 60 species
  Ciconiidae
    Storks, 17 species
  Threskiornithidae
    Spoonbills and ibises, 31 species
  Phoenicopteridae
    Flamingos, 4 species
Anseriformes
  Anatidae
    Ducks, geese and swans, 147
    species
Falconiformes
  Cathartidae
    New World vultures, 7 species
  Pandionidae
    Osprey, 1 species
  Falconidae

Falcons and caracaras, 60 species
Accipitridae
  Kites, Old World vultures,
  harriers, hawks, eagles, and
  accipiters, 217 species
Galliformes
  Cracidae
    Guans and curassows, 42 species
  Tetraonidae
    Grouse, 16 species
  Phasianidae
    Pheasants and quail (domestic
    chickens), 180 species
  Numididae
    Guineafowl, seven species
  Meleagridae
    Turkeys, two species
Gruiformes
  Turnicidae
    Buttonquails, 16 species
  Gruidae
    Cranes, 15 species
  Rallidae
    Rails, 129 species
  Otidae
    Bustards, 22 species
Charadriiformes
  Jacanidae
    Jacanas, seven species
  Charadriidae
    Plovers, 62 species
  Scolopacidae
    Sandpipers, 81 species
  Laridae
    Gulls, 45 species
  Sternidae
    Terns, 42 species
  Alcidae
    Auks, 22 species
Columbiformes
  Columbidae
    Pigeons and doves, 300 species
Psittaciformes
  Loriidae
    Lories and lorikeets, 55 species
  Cacatuidae
    Cockatoos, cockatiels, 18 species
  Psittacidae
    Parrots, 257 species
Cuculiformes
  Musophagidae
    Turacos, 22 species
  Cuculidae
    Cuckoos and anis, 128 species
Strigiformes
  Strigidae
    Owls, 124 species
  Tytonidae
    Barn owls, 10 species
Caprimulgiformes
  Captimulgidae
    Nightjars, 70 species
Apodiformes
  Apodidae
    Swifts, 80 species
  Trochilidae
    Hummingbirds, 320 species

Trogoniformes
  Trogonidae
    Trogons, 35 species
Coraciiformes
  Alcedinidae
    Kingfishers, 87 species
  Meropidae
    Bee-eaters, 24 species
  Bucerotidae
    Hornbills, 45 species
Piciformes
  Capitonidae
    Barbets, 76 species
  Rhamphastidae
    Toucans, 40 species
  Picidae
    Woodpeckers, 200 species
Passeriformes
  Funariidae
    Ovenbirds, 220 species
  Formicariidae
    Antbirds, 230 species
  Tyrannidae
    Tyrant flycatchers, 375 species
  Pipridae
    Manakins, 53 species
  Hirundinidae
    Swallows, 74 species
  Alaudidae
    Larks, 75 species
  Laniidae
    Shrikes, 69 species
  Bombycillidae
    Waxwings, eight species
  Troglodytidae
    Wrens, 60 species
  Mimidae,
    Mockingbirds, 30 species
  Muscicapidae
    Thrushes, babblers, Old World warblers, etc.,
    approximately 1400 species
  Paridae
    Tits, 46 species
  Sittidae
    Nuthatches, 21 species
  Nectariniidae
    Sunbirds, 116 species
  Emberizidae
    New World sparrows, tanagers, etc., 552 species
  Parulidae
    Wood warblers, 119 species
  Vireonidae
    Vireos, 43 species
  Icteridae
    Blackbirds and orioles, 94 species
  Fringillidae
    Finches, canaries, etc., 148 species
  Estrilidae
    Waxbills, 124 species
  Ploceidae
    Weavers, weaver sparrows, etc., 145 species
  Sturnidae
    Starlings and mynahs, 106 species
  Paradisaeidae
    Birds-of-paradise, 43 species
  Corvidae
    Crows, ravens, magpies, and jays, 113 species

morphologically based classifications lie in the relationships between higher categories (e.g., orders); the placement of species within families changed little. Some differences between molecular and traditional interpretations of avian systematics remain controversial.[19] Although these questions are of an academic interest, they have little bearing on the practice of avian medicine.

SPECIES CONCEPTS

Of greater interest to the clinician is the controversy over species concepts. The species is the only taxonomic unit that exists in the physical world. Higher level taxonomic categories are mental constructs that facilitate discussion and, it is hoped, reflect historic and genetic relationships. Their utility lies in a hierarchic arrangement whereby the myriad species can be organized to render biologic diversity into manageable units. The composition of taxa[9] and polemics over contending theories have little relevance to the medical practitioner until they are applied to species. At this level, alternative concepts can yield startlingly different results. It is, therefore, of practical value to the clinician to understand the differences between the major species concepts.

The prevalent species definition of modern zoology is the biological species concept proposed by Mayr.[6] He defined species as groups of interbreeding, natural populations that are reproductively isolated from other such groups. Later, Mayr added that most species occupy distinct ecological niches.[7] Most simply stated, this means that different species do not interbreed and if they should happen to, they are unlikely to produce viable offspring. For most species that clinicians encounter, this is self-evident and of little practical value. Species concepts have their greatest utility when applied to relationships that are not obvious.

We identify species by physical characteristics that are a manifestation of the genotype. Where closely related but genetically distinct populations naturally encounter one another, physical, behavioral, and ultimately genetic differences segregate dissimilar gene pools. Differences may not be obvious, but studies can sometimes establish if interbreeding occurs and whether one or more species is involved. Thus, reproductive isolation can be applied as a definitive test. Ambiguities that arise in

the biologic species concept often center on disjunct ranges, either geographic or temporal. Tests of reproductive isolation in natural settings are seldom possible. Determinations, therefore, must be based on whether differences between the populations are of a similar magnitude as differences known to operate as reproductive isolating mechanisms between populations with overlapping ranges. Inevitably, this involves a degree of subjectivity.

Wide-ranging species can also be a source of ambiguity. Regional populations often show morphologic variation and are considered polytypic. Distinct populations can be named as subspecies, designated by a trinomen (e.g., *Amazona amazonica amazonica*, the mainland subspecies of the orange-winged Amazon parrot). Subspecies must, by definition, be capable of interbreeding. Therefore, morphologically distinct populations can produce viable offspring. Some species show a gradual clinal variation so that no line can be drawn to separate discrete subspecies, although distinct differences may be apparent in individuals from extremes of the range. To further complicate the matter, clear reproductive isolation can exist in the absence of discernible morphologic variation. Two or more species are considered sibling species if they are not readily distinguishable morphologically, yet reproductive isolation is maintained.[8] Eastern and western meadowlarks are virtually indistinguishable, except by call.[9] This is an important isolating mechanism in birds, however the two are considered separate species. These and other complications have led to the proposal of alternative species concepts.

A theory with adherents in many disciplines is the phylogenetic species concept. As defined by Cracraft,[10] a species is "the smallest diagnosable cluster of individual organisms within which there is a parental pattern of ancestry and descent." This approach differs significantly from the biological species concept, both in philosophy and methodology. Some consider its procedural basis to be more rigorous and consistently applicable. The criterion of reproductive isolation is eliminated. Species are based solely on sets of morphologic characteristics common to all individuals within a group that is considered to be monophyletic. Proponents of the phylogenetic species concept contend that it offers an objective analysis of speciation not dependent on predictions of reproductive isolation where evidence is unavailable. Species are the basal evolutionary units.[11]

There have been few comprehensive applications of this concept to birds, but one has produced interesting results. Cracraft[12] presented a phylogenetic review of the birds-of-paradise. Although clinicians seldom encounter these birds, the study provides an instructive example. Native to New Guinea, Australia, and adjacent islands, the family Paradisaeidae is well known for its numerous species, disjunct populations, and bewildering array of geographic variation. Previous interpretations have named 40 to 42 species and 88 to 90 subspecies. Basing his interpretation on the smallest groups of individuals with consistently diagnosable features, Cracraft arrived at 90 species. The Paradisaeidae, however, tend to be highly sexually dimorphic, with ornate males and plain females. In some of the new species females may not be clearly separable. Species are defined regardless of the possibility that gene flow may occur between them. If this concept were uniformly applied to birds, most subspecies could be elevated to species, thus increasing the number of species many-fold. Although this would present few therapeutic dilemmas to the veterinarian, it could introduce significant new complications to aviculturalists and agencies charged with the development and implementation of wildlife policy. Advocates of the phylogenetic species concept argue that this would be a more accurate reflection of the breadth of genetic diversity, focus attention on the results of evolution, and bring consistency to hierarchic ordering. Detractors contend that it ignores biologic criteria (reproduction), may rely on trivial characters as diagnostic keys to species, and is simply typological.

HYBRIDIZATION AND CONSERVATION MANAGEMENT

The biological species concept notwithstanding, interbreeding between unquestionably different species occurs. Approximately 10% of bird species have been known to breed with another species in nature and produce hybrid offspring, but the frequency is not uniformly distributed among orders. Ducks and geese show the greatest propensity to hybridize (over 40%); galliformes, woodpeckers, and hummingbirds also have a high incidence. Conversely, in over one-half the orders, hybridization rates range from 0 to 3%. Hybridization has important implications in aviculture, conservation, and evolutionary biology. Recent investigators of wild populations of Darwin's finches observed hybrids that were not only fertile, but actually exhibited superior fitness as compared with the parent species.[13] Hybridization has long been known as a means of speciation in plants, but its importance in animals bears further inquiry. Hybridization is used by aviculturalists as a tool for the creation of unusual colors and new varieties of birds. The inbreeding that sometimes occurs can result in unintended genetic aberrations, and clinicians should be alert to this possibility.

Perhaps the greatest area of controversy surrounding hybridization is in conservation biology. O'Brien and Mayr[14] discussed the implications of strict (and sometimes inaccurate) interpretation of the definitions and policies on hybrids, in relation to the management of endangered plants and animals. As amended, the Endangered Species Act of 1973 affords protection to species, subspecies, and populations. However, the US Fish and Wildlife Service has established the precedent that hybrids between endangered species, subspecies, and populations are not eligible for legal protection. The biological species concept specifies that subspecies and populations, because they are below the species level, are capable of interbreeding within their own species. Although inbreeding is not inconsistent with the status of these categories, it is considered as a basis for removal of legal protection. O'Brien and Mayr[14] contend that a policy that discourages protection of hybrids between species is appropriate. Genetic interchange below the species level, however, is part of the ongoing natural process, and policies affecting wild plants and animals should reflect biological realities. Conversely, Grant and Grant[13] suggest that depletion of a species increases the chance of hybridization owing to the scarcity of conspecific mates. Therefore, species in greatest need of protection are the ones most likely to hybridize. The question becomes even more complex as applied to programs of captive breeding and the reintroduction of species into formerly occupied ranges. The implications of hybridization in birds will continue to be a source of practical and theoretical controversy, and has importance far beyond the initial appearance of endless, pedantic bickering.

Uncertainties in the taxonomic status of populations can affect management policy. The scarlet macaw, in danger of extinction in Central America, is listed in CITES (Convention on International Trade in Endangered Species of Wild Fauna and Flora), Appendix 1, thus prohibiting international trade. This species is abundant in the Amazon Basin, but without recognition of separate subspecies (assuming that they exist), CITES protection is applied to the entire species.

Although often difficult to implement and defend, conservation policy should operate at the population level until details of taxonomic affinities can be thoroughly investigated. The importance of thorough systematic investigation in the development of conservation policy is demonstrated by the history of management of the tuatara, a unique New Zealand reptile.[15] Early studies of the tuatara recognized two species, one separated into two subspecies. However, legal designation of all populations as a single species hindered management of some island populations. In the absence of management based on true diversity, one species was reduced to a single, threatened population and one of its subspecies may be extinct. Situations such as this illustrate the critical role of taxonomy in the formulation and implementation of conservation policy.

A SURVEY OF SELECTED ORDERS

In recognition of the enormous diversity of birds, it is beyond the scope of this chapter to describe each of the orders listed in Table 1–1. For that, the reader is referred to the comprehensive systematic treatments that are available for most orders. Herein are described relationships and general characteristics of birds frequently encountered by clinicians.

Ratites

The term *ratites* refers collectively to four extant orders of flightless birds, the Struthioniformes, Rheiformes, Casuariiformes, and Apterygiformes. Until recently, ratites were seldom encountered by veterinarians outside zoos. However, the recent upsurge of interest in commercial production of ostriches

and other species has made them increasingly common. Although placed in separate orders, ostriches, rheas, cassowaries, emus, and kiwis are considered to be more closely related to each other than to any other birds. Ratites are restricted to the southern continents, and DNA-DNA hybridization studies indicate that South American tinamous are the closest flighted relative.[3] All are flightless, having reduced wings and sternal keels, and weakly developed pectoral musculature. In the absence of flight, muscular power is concentrated in the hind limbs for terrestrial locomotion. The distinctive feet of ostriches have only two toes. Others have three toes; the innermost toe of cassowaries is armed with a long, sharp, and potentially lethal claw. Ostriches, rheas, and emus inhabit open country and savannas, whereas cassowaries are residents of rain forests of New Guinea and northern Australia. Kiwis live in the forests of New Zealand. Ratites are mostly herbivorous, although the diet varies widely. A long digestive tract helps to process plant matter. In the rheas, two caecae function in the bacterial fermentation of cellulose. Unlike other ratites, kiwis are nocturnal and subsist on earthworms and soil invertebrates which they secure with their long, probing beaks.[16]

Anseriformes

The Anseriformes consist primarily of ducks, geese, and swans, which are members of the family Anatidae. These familiar waterfowl are characterized by flattened, blunt beaks and webbed feet with a hind toe, but show great diversity in plumage, range, diet, and natural history. Diet varies widely and is often reflected in the morphology of the beak and legs. Ducks are often divided into groups based on feeding habits. Dabblers feed by tipping the body up and extending the head below the water in search of aquatic vegetation, seeds, and small invertebrates on the bottom of shallow pools. The wings are large in relation to their bodies, and their legs are placed farther forward than other ducks. This allows dabblers to spring directly into flight, either from land or water. Diving ducks swim underwater to feed on aquatic vegetation, invertebrates, and fish. Legs are usually placed far to the back of the body. This facilitates underwater propulsion, but makes divers awkward on land. The relatively short wings are adapted to swift flight, but require divers to run across the surface to gain sufficient speed to become airborne.[17]

Many species have elaborate mating displays. Waterfowl typically copulate in the water and, unlike most birds, males have a penis. Nests are typically constructed of material immediately surrounding the site (e.g., sedges and grasses), but some species nest in cavities. Incubation does not begin until the last egg is laid, but once begun, the female is reluctant to leave the nest.[18] Ducks often practice brood parasitism, laying eggs in the nests of conspecifics or other species. Precocious young leave the nest soon after hatching and follow the parents, able to search for their own food.[19]

Waterfowl have a long history of association with humans, and ducks have been independently domesticated twice. Natives of South America domesticated the muscovy duck prior to the arrival of Europeans. The mallard is the ancestor of all other breeds of domestic ducks. Geese were also independently domesticated in Europe and China.[17]

Falconiformes

The diurnal birds of prey—eagles, hawks, and falcons—traditionally compose the order Falconiformes.[1] In molecular classifications, however, they are placed in the large Ciconiiformes, along with shore birds, gulls, waders, and penguins, among others. Raptors are equipped with hooked beaks and powerful talons used to dispatch prey. Female raptors are larger than males in most species, the difference being most pronounced in falcons and the least in vultures.[19] Raptors have long been used by humans in the sport of falconry, which began approximately 4000 years ago in the Middle East. Commonly encountered families are the Falconidae —the falcons and caracaras—and the Accipitridae —the kites, hawks, accipiters, and eagles. The osprey is the sole member of the family Pandionidae.

Falcons have a notched beak and long, pointed wings.[17] They are noted for swift flight and often take birds in flight, although smaller species such as the kestrel frequently feed on large insects. Falcons are known to dive or swoop on their prey at great speeds, striking with toes fully extended.[19] Prey is usually retrieved from the ground. Kites, hawks, eagles, and accipiters are diverse in size,

form, and natural history, ranging from small, agile, forest-dwelling sharp-shinned hawks to huge golden eagles. Prey include insects, birds, small mammals, reptiles, and fish. Ospreys are fish specialists and often hover briefly before plunging into the water after prey.

Galliformes

A diverse order of six families, the Galliformes include the familiar domestic chicken and turkey, prized game birds such as pheasants, grouse, and quail, and the unusual megapodes and curassows. Galliformes are typically ground-dwelling birds; few are accomplished fliers. Feet, with three forward-facing toes and an elevated hind toe, are adapted for terrestrial locomotion, and most species are poorly suited for perching.[20] They are, however, efficient at scratching the ground for food, which includes seeds, leaves, fruits, and a variety of invertebrates.

Perhaps the most unusual nesting behavior of any birds is seen in the Megapodiidae, who build large mounds of vegetation in which eggs are laid. Heat for incubation is generated by the fermentation of the plant matter.[16] Other families have more conventional nesting patterns, usually nesting on the ground. Hatchlings are precocious, most able to feed themselves shortly after hatching. In ptarmigans, young fledge in as little as 10 to 12 days, with flight sufficient to escape predators; they are independent in 8 to 10 weeks. The chicks of megapodes are independent from the time of hatching and can fly within 24 hours.[19]

The most important domestic fowl are members of the family Phasianidae, which includes pheasants, peafowl, and chickens. Descended from the red jungle fowl (*Gallus gallus*) of southern Asia, chickens may have been in domestication for 6000 years.[16] Hybridization is known to occur in the Phasianidae, both above and below the generic level; however, fertility of intrageneric hybrids is low. Hybridization in the wild is considered rare, and *Gallus* appears to exhibit no intrageneric hybrid fertility.[21]

Columbiformes

The order Columbiformes is primarily composed of pigeons and doves, which are usually placed in a single family, the Columbidae. There is no systematic difference between pigeons and doves; the words have different linguistic origins and are applied arbitrarily. The commonly known rock dove (*Columba livia*) is the ancestor of virtually all domestic and feral pigeons that range worldwide. Columbids vary in size from the diminutive diamond dove and dwarf fruit dove, near the size of sparrows, to the crowned pigeons, which approach the size of a hen turkey.

Some species feed primarily in trees or shrubs, subsisting on fruit, buds, flowers, and leaves. Others feed exclusively on the ground, searching for seeds and small invertebrates. In most species, feeding occurs both above ground level and on the ground. These species take a variety of food, including small invertebrates. Food items are usually swallowed whole, because beaks are not well adapted to bite food or husk seeds.[22]

Most species roost and nest in trees, but some have adapted to nest on cliffs and rock shelters or on the ground, and have established themselves in treeless environments. Domestic and feral pigeons descended from cliff nesters. Incubation requires 2 to 4 weeks. Pigeons nourish newly hatched young with pigeon milk or crop milk. Under stimulation by the hormone prolactin, the lining of the two-chambered crop thickens and is sloughed off and regurgitated to nestlings for about the first 3 or 4 days. The crops of adults can be infected by the flagellated protozoan *Trichomonas*, which can prove fatal if passed to the young. This infection can also be passed to predators of infected birds.[16]

Psittaciformes

In the words of Sibley, "Parrots are parrots. They seem to have no close living relatives and there is no doubt about what is and what is not a parrot."[23] Forshaw and Cooper[24] recognized three families with six subfamilies.

Overall, parrots are characterized by two morphologic features. First, all have a strong, hooked maxilla with a flexible attachment to the skull; the short mandible fits under the maxilla. Second, parrots have dexterous zygodactyl feet (two digits point forward and two are oriented backwards). These morphologic traits form the basis of some distinctive behaviors. Using the hooked beak as a

third appendage, most species are agile climbers. Strong feet are used to manipulate fruit and seeds, which are torn apart or husked by the beak. By these features, psitticines are well adapted as arboreal fruit- and seedeaters, although insects form part of the diet in some species. Worldwide, the distribution of psittacines is primarily tropical, extending into south temperate areas. Few species range into north temperate habitats.

The three families of psittacines are Loriidae (lories and lorikeets), Cacatuidae (cockatoos), and Psittacidae (parrots and parakeets). The Loriidae have an Australasian and Oceanic distribution. They feed mainly on nectar, pollen, and fruit. The tongue, tipped with papillae, is adapted for feeding on pollen, and the ventriculus is weakly muscled. Cockatoos have an Australasian and Oceanic distribution. They are characterized by an erectile crest, a heavy bill to feed on fruits, seeds, and insects, and a thick-walled, muscular ventriculus to accommodate this diet. Parrots and parakeets constitute the largest group, being divided into four subfamilies. This family is most diverse in South and Central America and Australasia, but also occurs in Africa and Asia.[24]

Most psittacines are cavity nesters, using holes in trees or termite mounds or in the ground, usually with little or no lining. An interesting exception are monk parrots, which build large communal nests of twigs and branches; each pair occupies a separate chamber. Clutch size ranges from two to four white eggs in larger species and up to eight in smaller species. Incubation ranges from 16 to 35 days. The young are altricial. Smaller species fledge in 3 to 4 weeks, whereas some macaws require 3 to 4 months.[24]

Strigiformes

Owls are immediately recognizable by their upright posture, hooked beak, and forward-facing eyes in a flat, facial disc. Feet are equipped with sharp talons and a reversible outer toe. Of the two families, the barn owls (Tytonidae) are characterized by a heart-shaped face, long legs, and small orbits.[25] Members of the family Strigidae have round facial discs, but otherwise are diverse in size and habitats. Along with large eyes sensitive to low light, owls have an acute sense of hearing. Facial discs serve as large sound receptors to funnel sound into the sensitive ears. These adaptations help owls locate prey in faint light.[26] Nocturnal birds of prey are often encountered by wildlife rehabilitators. While hunting along roadsides, these birds are often involved in collisions with automobiles. Head injuries may damage the delicate temporal bones and sclerotic rings of the eyes in the owl, which can result in complex neurologic deficits. Such impairments may render these birds incapable of obtaining food in the wild.

Owls prey on mammals, birds, fish, other small vertebrates, and insects. Small prey are swallowed whole and the bones, hair, and other indigestible parts are regurgitated as pellets. Cast pellets are often used by biologists to analyze the diets of owls and occasionally as a tool to sample small mammal populations.

Most species nest in cavities, some in burrows. Abandoned nests of eagles are occasionally used. As many as twelve eggs may be laid in some species, but clutch size can vary based on food availability. Incubation lasts an average of 30 days and fledging about 8 weeks.[16]

Piciformes

The Piciformes are a diverse order of six families. Of these, the toucans (family Rhamphastidae) have become popular cage birds. Distributed from Southern Mexico to Argentina, toucans are best known for their oversized, unmistakable bills. Like all members of the order, toucans have zygodactyl feet. The large, lightweight bill is used to pick fruit, but they also feed upon insects, lizards, and the nestlings of other birds. Toucans nest in cavities. Altricial young hatch in about 15 days and take up to 7 weeks to fledge.[16]

Passeriformes

The Passeriformes include some 5200 species in 74 families, over one-half of the world's birds. Feet are well adapted for perching, with three forward-facing toes and a strong hind toe. The size range is great, from some flycatchers and finches less than 10 cm in length and weighing only a few grams, to ravens, which can exceed a length of 60 cm and a

weight of 1.5 kg. Some forms that are popular cage birds are noted here.

Mynahs are members of the starling family (Sturnidae) and are native to Southern Asia. The most popular captive species is the hill mynah (*Gracula religiosa*), which is well known for its ability to mimic human speech. In the wild, hill mynahs feed on insects, fruit, and small vertebrates, and nest in tree cavities.[27] Domestic canaries are descended from the Island Canary, *Serinus canaria* (family Fringillidae) which is native to the Azores, and the Madiera and Canary Islands west of Portugal and North Africa. Still common on their native islands, canaries have adapted to altered habitats as well as native woodlands.[27] Numerous species of small finches are popular pets. Species such as the Gouldian and zebra finches of Australia and waxbills of Africa are members of the family Estrilidae.

Increased interest in aviculture and birds as companion animals together have fueled the growth of avian medicine as a discipline. Conservation of avian diversity bridges the gap between medicine and pure science, and systematics lies at the heart of the current renaissance of biological diversity. Far from being an archaic vestige of Victorian science, systematic biology works at the cutting edge of biotechnology, evolutionary theory, and conservation policy.

References

1. Wetmore A: A classification for the birds of the world. Smith Misc Coll 139:1–37, 1960.
2. Sibley CG, Ahlquist JE: Phylogeny and classification of birds based on the data of DNA-DNA hybridization. Curr Ornithol 1:245–292, 1983.
3. Sibley CG, Ahlquist JE, Monroe BL Jr: A classification of living birds of the world based on DNA-DNA hybridization studies. Auk 105:409–423, 1988.
4. Sibley CG, Ahlquist JE: Phylogeny and Classification of Birds: A Study in Molecular Evolution. New Haven, Yale University Press, 1990.
5. Houde P: Critical evaluation of DNA hybridization studies in avian systematics. Auk 104:17–32, 1987.
6. Mayr E: Speciation phenomena in birds. Am Nat 74:249–278, 1940.
7. Mayr E: Populations, Species, and Evolution. Cambridge, MA, Belknap Press, 1970.
8. Mayr E: Animal Species and Evolution. Cambridge, MA, Harvard University Press, 1963.
9. Farrand A (ed): The Audubon Society Master Guide to Birding, vol. 3. New York, Alfred A. Knopf, 1983.
10. Cracraft J: Species concepts and speciation analysis. Curr Ornithol 1:159–187, 1983.

11. McKitrick MC, Zink RM: Species concepts in ornithology. Condor 90:1–14, 1988.
12. Cracraft J: The species of the birds-of-paradise (Paradisaeidae): Applying the phylogenetic species concept to a complex pattern of diversification. Cladistics 8:1–43, 1992.
13. Grant PR, Grant BR: Hybridization of bird species. Science 256:193–197, 1992.
14. O'Brien SJ, Mayr E: Bureaucratic mischief: Recognizing endangered species and subspecies. Science 251:1187–1188, 1991.
15. Daugherty CH, Cree A, Hay JM, Thompson MB: Neglected taxonomy and continuing extinctions of tuatara (*Sphenodon*). Nature 347:177–179, 1990.
16. Brooke M, Birkhead T (eds): The Cambridge Encyclopedia of Ornithology. Cambridge, UK, Cambridge University Press, 1991.
17. Teres JK: The Audubon Society Encyclopedia of North American Birds. New York, Wings Books, 1991.
18. Johnsgard PA: Waterfowl of North America. Bloomington, Indiana University Press, 1975.
19. Ehrlich PR, Dobkin DS, Wheye D: The Birders Handbook. New York, Simon & Schuster, 1988.
20. Johnsgard PA: The Grouse of the World. Lincoln, University of Nebraska Press, 1983.
21. Johnsgard PA: The Pheasants of the World. Oxford, Oxford University Press, 1986.
22. Goodwin D: Pigeons and Doves of the World. Ithaca, Cornell University Press, 1983.
23. Sibley CG: Phylogeny and classification of birds from DNA comparisons. Acta XX Cong. Int. Ornithol 20:111–126, 1991.
24. Forshaw JM, Cooper WT: Parrots of the World. Melbourne, Lansdowne Press, 1973.
25. Burton JA (ed): Owls of the World. Dover, NH, Tanager Books, 1984.
26. Konishi M: Listening with two ears. Sci Am 268:66–73, 1993.
27. Perrins CM (ed): The Illustrated Encyclopedia of Birds. New York, Prentice-Hall, 1990.

James R. Millam

2

Reproductive Physiology

Of the approximately 8700 avian species, the most typical can be described as neotropical, diurnal, monogamous, altricial, aerial, and seasonally breeding. Most companion psittacine species resemble a "typical" bird in these respects. But much of our understanding of reproductive physiology comes from a small number of domesticated gallinaceous species, which tend to be precocial, polygynous, ground-nesting, incapable of sustained flight, and with greatly expanded fecund periods. Nonetheless, physiologic processes underlying reproductive management of poultry species often appear to be the same as those underlying management of companion birds. Since the Wild Bird Conservation Act of 1992 prohibited importation of companion birds into the US, captive propagation is the sole means of meeting the demand for the companion bird trade in the US. But reproductive efficiency with current management techniques is low, particularly for larger species.[1]

The goal of this chapter is to facilitate improved reproductive efficiency and well-being of companion birds in captivity by relating how neuroendocrine regulation of reproduction is influenced by management procedures. The chapter focuses on the limited experimental evidence on psittacines and otherwise on relevant gallinaceous and passerine species. The chapter is meant to be complementary to the recent review by Joyner[2] on normal and abnormal reproductive anatomy and physiology of companion birds. References emphasize other significant reviews.

PERCEPTION OF DAYLENGTH

Most temperate-clime species use the increasing daylengths of winter and spring as a proximal or initial predictive cue for stimulating gonadal growth,[3] although, remarkably, neither the eyes nor the pineal gland is required for birds to detect changes in daylength[4] (see Follett[5] for general discussion of avian reproductive physiology). The encephalic photoreceptors by which daylength is perceived occur deep in the brain, near the lateral ventricles in the telencephalon and in the tuberal hypothalamus in the diencephalon. Immunohistochemical evidence in pigeons (*Columba livia*) and chickens indicates that some neurons in these areas contain an opsin-like protein similar to that contained in retinal photoreceptors.[6] Some of the opsin-like protein–containing neurons also co-stain for the avian prolactin-releasing factor, vasoactive intestinal polypeptide (VIP), suggesting a potential role for VIP-containing neurons in mediating daylength information (see later). Some of these neurons may also be immunopositive for either gonadotropin-releasing hormone (GnRH) or contact neurons containing GnRH,[7] thus suggesting the possibility that the same neurons that can detect photostimulation may also participate in the GnRH stimulation of pituitary gonadotropins.

SPECTRAL RESPONSE OF ENCEPHALIC PHOTORECEPTORS

The encephalic or "deep brain" photoreceptors have a spectral response similar to that of retinal photoreceptors, as judged by the serum luteinizing hormone (LH) response of Japanese quail (*Coturnix japonica*) to photosexual stimulation with monochromatic light.[8] When equal fluxes of different wavelengths of light reaching deep brain photoreceptive areas were compared in their ability to stimulate LH release, blue-green light was more effective than red-orange light. These findings at first appear to conflict with reports in poultry indicating that red-orange light is most effective in stimulating gonadal growth.[9] However, this apparent contradiction is the result of the relatively greater transmission efficiency of red light in tissue. Although encephalic photoreceptors are approximately 20 times more sensitive to blue-green than red-orange light, the latter colors traverse tissue approximately 30 times more efficiently.[8] The fortunate implication of greater blue-green receptor sensitivity and greater red-orange transmission efficiency is that most readily available fluorescent, incandescent, and sodium vapor lamps provide ample spectral coverage for photosexual stimulation in enclosed facilities.

LIGHTING INTENSITY

Even brightly artificially lit rooms (200–300 lux) do not approach outdoor light intensities (10,000–300,000+ lux). Indeed, the difficulty of providing high intensity lighting indoors has tended to constrain research to lower intensity ranges. In poultry, although egg production is generally greater for hens housed under natural lighting, little influence of light intensity on egg production is observed if intensities are above that required for comfortable reading by humans (approximately 20 lux).

Japanese quail assess light intensities during different portions of a daily photoschedule (e.g., 12 hours of 300 lux: 12 hours of 5 lux) and interpret the more and less intense portions as subjective day and night, respectively. Thus, quail can interpret a 12-hour period of low intensity light (dim light, approximately 5–10 lux) as daytime, if it is paired with a 12-hour period of darkness, or as nighttime, if it is paired with a 12-hour period of much brighter light. Similarly, dim light can be either sexually stimulatory (15 hours dim: 9 hours dark), or inhibitory (9 hours bright: 15 hours dim), depending upon the light intensity in other parts of the photoschedule.[10]

Furthermore, quail can interpret ambiguous intermediate light intensities as day or night, depending upon the relative intensity of other parts of the photoschedule. For example, a lighting schedule of 8 hours dark: 4 hours dim: 8 hours bright: 4 hours dim, is interpreted as a short daylength (8 hours

day: 16 hours night). But reducing the light intensity of the 8-hour bright portion converts the interpretation to that of long daylength[11] (16 hours day: 8 hours night). These considerations may be important for companion birds subjected to the often highly variable light intensities and durations experienced in homes.

CRITICAL DAYLENGTH

Compared with temperate-clime species, daylength may be predicted to exert little influence on breeding of tropical species in the wild. But in captivity and in the absence of other predictive cues, daylength manipulation can often stimulate reproductive activity in tropical and even equatorial species. Some equatorial species such as the African stonechat (*Saxicola torquata*) respond readily to daylength changes in captivity.[12] Gwinner and Dittami point out that because of the ellipsoid shape of the earth, time of sunrise at the equator can vary annually by as much as 20 minutes, thereby providing potentially significant seasonally varying photoperiodic cues.[12]

The sexual stimulatory effects of long daylengths are exerted when photosensitive birds (see later) are exposed to light during a restricted time of day, termed the "photosensitive phase." The photosensitive phase, which is circadian in nature, typically occurs from approximately 13 to 17 hours after subjective light onset or dawn (i.e., it is entrained by dawn). The length and phase (in relation to dawn) of the photosensitive phase are highly species-specific and can only be determined experimentally. Although precise photosensitive periods have not been determined for psittacines, long daylengths stimulate reproductive activity in cockatiels[13] (*Nymphicus hollandicus*) and blossom-headed parakeets[14] (*Psittacula cyanocephala*), and both species develop photorefractoriness. Numerous anecdotal and field accounts support these observations.

Research on several species demonstrates that "long" daylengths need not consist of continuous periods of light (see Murton and Westwood[15] for review). It is sufficient that a portion of the day be interpreted as "dawn" (usually light onset or the period of increasing light intensity just prior to sunrise) and that light then occurs during the photosensitive phase. For example, a photoschedule of 4 hours light: 9 hours dark: 1 hour light: 10 hours dark would likely be perceived as having a 14-hour daylength, even though only 5 hours of the 24-hour period would be lit because the 1 hour of light would occur during the photosensitive phase.[5]

Figure 2–1 illustrates the testicular response of Japanese quail to such "skeleton" light schedules.[16] One practical implication of this is that care should be taken that birds maintained on short daylengths, either to establish photosensitivity or to prevent photosexual stimulation, should not be exposed to even brief periods of light during their photosensitive phase.

PHOTOSENSITIVITY

Before they can respond to long daylength stimulation, birds must be in a physiologically photosensitive state. In the wild, photoperiodic species typically gain photosensitivity by exposure for several weeks or months to the short and declining daylengths of late summer and fall. In captivity, this is often achieved by exposure to short daylengths (e.g., 10 hours light: 14 hours dark) for several weeks. During exposure of starlings (*Sturnus vulgaris*) to short daylengths, hypothalamic neurons containing GnRH increase in both number and size.[17] In this sense, exposure to short daylengths can be thought of as "pro" gonadal in that the neuroendocrine potential for responding to long daylength stimulation is achieved by exposure to short daylengths (for review see Nicholls and co-workers[18]). The dissipation of photorefractoriness in rose-ringed parakeets (*Psittacula krameri*) by exposure to the declining daylengths of autumn may also be a factor in the occurrence of pair formation and increased serum LH levels that occur at that time of year.[19, 20]

PHOTOSTIMULATION AND PHOTOREFRACTORINESS

Exposure of photosensitive Japanese quail to long daylengths stimulates secretion of GnRH from hypothalamic neurons. Excised hypothalamic fragments cultured in vitro from quail photostimulated a few hours earlier showed increased release of

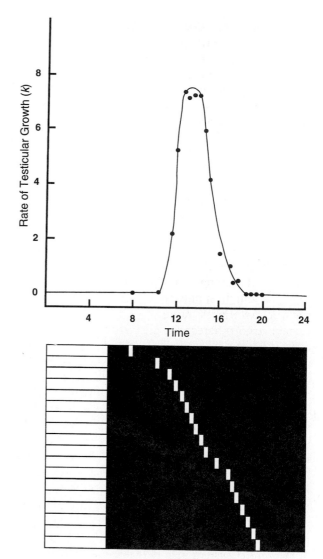

Figure 2 – 1

Testicular growth rate, k, of groups of Japanese quail exposed to various photoschedules. Each photoschedule consists of a 6-hour portion of light plus 15 minutes of light interspersed at different times of the "night." The photosensitive phase for Japanese quail extends from approximately 12 to 16 hours after onset on the 6-hour light period. (Redrawn from Follett BK, Sharp PJ: Circadian rhythmicity in photoperiodically induced gonadotropin release and gonadal growth in the quail. Nature 223:968–971, 1969.)

GnRH.[21] Increased GnRH release, most likely the avian variant of GnRH occurring in the preoptic/septal region ([Gln^8]GnRH; chicken GnRH I [cGnRH I]), leads to increased gonadotropin secretion and gonadal growth. For many species, however, exposure to long daylengths also initiates processes that lead to the regression of gonadal tissue, even in the face of long daylength stimulation. The condition when long daylengths fail to stimulate gonadotropin secretion is termed "photorefractoriness." Whether and when photorefractoriness develops is highly species-specific. Not all photoperiodic species develop photorefractoriness (e.g., pigeons), and some species (e.g., Japanese quail) may maintain gonads in a mature state until daylengths begin to shorten, although daylength may remain of a duration that was clearly gonadostimulatory earlier in the season. The latter is termed "relative photorefractoriness."[22]

The development of photorefractoriness is likely mediated by the secretion of thyroid hormones. Changes in serum levels of thyroid hormones correlate with the development of photorefractoriness in starlings. If starlings are thyroidectomized prior to long daylength stimulation, they do not develop photorefractoriness; rather, their gonads grow and remain large, whereas the gonads of sham-operated control birds held under the same long daylengths grow large but then spontaneously regress. Treatment of such thyroidectomized birds with thyroid hormones will initiate photorefractoriness and induce gonadal regression. Likewise, photorefractory starlings held on long days (with regressed gonads) show spontaneous gonadal regrowth if they are thyroidectomized. These observations led Nicholls and coworkers[18] to suggest that thyroid hormones may be essential for proper assessment of daylength.

How thyroid is functionally involved in the development of photorefractoriness is not known, but photorefractoriness is also associated with changes in the GnRH system in some species. For example, in starlings, photorefractoriness is associated with a decline in the number and size of cGnRH I–containing neurons.[17]

Numerous studies in passerine and poultry species show that photorefractoriness develops sooner if daylengths are longer.[18] For example, gonadal involution occurs sooner in turkey hens (*Meleagris gallopavo*) exposed to 20-hour daylengths than in sibling hens exposed to 14-hour daylengths, although hens exposed to 20-hour-long days show a greater rate of lay prior to becoming photorefractory.

Cockatiel pairs typically become photorefractory after laying two clutches.[23] However, whether exposure to short daylengths is necessary to restore photosensitivity is not clear. Simply removing nest boxes for several weeks may be sufficient to restore the capacity to lay eggs—exposure to short daylengths is not required. This suggests that cockatiels may become refractory not to light, per se, but to the nest box, which is an important sexual stimulus for cavity nesters.

Some species (for example, many songbirds and gamebirds) reach somatic maturity within several weeks or months of hatching. If such birds were hatched in early spring in the wild, they would be exposed to photostimulatory daylengths later in the summer that would be expected to stimulate gonadal development. However, these birds are photorefractory from hatch, and, just like adult birds that show postnuptial photorefractoriness, they require exposure to a period of short daylengths before gaining the ability to respond to long daylengths. The phenomenon is termed "juvenile photorefractoriness."

RATE OF CHANGE OF DAYLENGTH

Gradually changing daylengths are natural, and some evidence suggests that rate and direction of change may exert effects that are independent of absolute daylength. For example, a photostimulatory but gradually decreasing daylength may provide less gonadotropic drive than a photostimulatory but gradually increasing daylength. So-called step-down lighting programs are used to retard sexual development of poultry housed in semienclosed (not "light controlled") housing. These programs turn lights on before dawn and/or after dusk during a time of the year when natural daylengths are increasing. Declining daylengths are then presented by turning lights on progressively later in the morning and/or earlier in the evening.[9] Lighting schedule changes are typically made at weekly intervals. Step-down lighting programs have not yet been tested in psittacines.

RELATION OF LIGHTING SCHEDULES TO MELATONIN

The pineal gland (aka, epiphysis cerebri) is a biologic clock in birds that transmits its timekeeping information by the phasic secretion of melatonin. The neuroanatomic distribution of melatonin receptors varies considerably among species, but includes the suprachiasmatic nucleus, another important biologic clock,[24, 25] as well as visual processing areas. In birds, as in most vertebrates, circulating melatonin levels are elevated at night and low during the day. Excised chicken (*Gallus domesticus*) pineal glands cultured in vitro and exposed to light-dark cycles show changes in melatonin output that mimic in vivo pineals exposed to the same stimuli. The rhythmic output of melatonin in such preparations remains entrained to phase-shifts in environmental lighting and is self-sustained under constant darkness.[26] Thus, pineal glands are capable of both independent photoreceptive and timekeeping functions.

The pineal gland is believed responsible for the circadian rhythm of locomotion, as pinealectomized house sparrows (*Passer domesticus*), but not sham-operated controls, become arrhythmic when held in constant darkness; that is, subjective day/night differences in locomotor activity are no longer discernible. If pineals from light-dark–entrained donor birds are surgically implanted in pinealectomized recipients, rhythmicity is restored and the phase of the donor is established in the recipient.[27] Melatonin may also be important for the ability of some species to become torporific when they are food-deprived and/or exposed to low nighttime temperatures.[28]

Despite the central role of the pineal gland and melatonin in these circadian rhythms (besides, undoubtedly, a host of other rhythms), a clearly defined role for melatonin in reproductive physiology has yet to be established. Several studies have found associations between changes in pineal gland histology and reproductive activity, but pinealectomy has generally failed to alter photosexual responses appreciably. However, administration of a melatonin antiserum prior to light offset or dusk in Japanese quail held under short days induced some degree of gonadal growth.[29]

Many seemingly contradictory data regarding pineal function and reproduction may have arisen in the past because, at least in some galliforms, not all circulating melatonin arises from the pineal gland. Underwood and coworkers[30] showed that in Japanese quail a substantial amount of circulating melatonin is produced by the retina. Thus, previous work reporting negative effects of pinealectomy must be reevaluated.

Pineal morphologic types vary considerably among psittacines, and, as with other birds, associations between pineal activity and reproduction have been reported. Fairly large doses of melatonin administered to captive-breeding blossom-headed parakeets induced gonadal involution.[31] Prasadan and Kotak[32] found ultrastructural changes in rose-ringed parakeet pineal glands, which were associated with periods of increased metabolic or secretory activity over the breeding cycle, although periods of heightened activity were neither entirely in or out of phase with gonadal activity or annual changes in daylength.

CIRCANNUAL RHYTHMS

Daylength manipulation is almost universally used to control reproduction in commercial poultry operations, but the degree of control exerted by light-dark cycles is far from complete. Controlled lighting can retard or advance the onset of egg-laying in laying strains of chickens by only a couple of weeks.[9] Lighting can exert greater control on sexual maturity in other poultry species (e.g., turkeys, chukar (*Alectoris chukar*), Japanese quail). For most species, the tendency for cyclic gonadal growth and regression can only be modulated by daylength, not strictly controlled.

Few investigators have studied circannual rhythms of reproductive activity under constant lighting conditions (e.g., constant 12 hours light: 12 hours dark). Gwinner and Dittami[12] demonstrated circannual rhythms of gonadal growth and regression in several passerine species held under unchanging photoperiods of 12 hours light: 12 hours dark. Their research also demonstrated that as length of the light phase departs from 12 hours, the circannual cycle of growth and regression is greatly altered. For example, starlings held on daylengths of less than 12 hours showed quite slow rates of testicular growth, and testicular regression was often incomplete. In contrast, exposure to daylengths greater than 12 hours resulted in more rapid rates of testicular growth and prolonged periods of testicular regression.

NUTRITION

The role of nutrition in reproduction has been extensively studied in opportunistic breeders such as the African red-billed quelea (*Quelea quelea*).[15] There is no doubt that nutrition, in a general sense, influences gonadotropic drive (e.g., refeeding of fasted chickens increases serum LH levels).[33] Whether nutritional factors can act as breeding cues for companion birds that are already feeding on a nutritionally complete diet is not known. However, changing from a diet consisting of only millet to a nutritionally complete diet at the time of nest box presentation did not appreciably enhance reproductive performance of cockatiels over that of controls.[13]

The specific appetite for calcium (Ca), best studied in poultry species, is the most dramatic example of a specific nutritional requirement for reproduction. In chickens, a specific Ca appetite occurs in association with ovulation and in relation to light offset. Hens show a specific appetite for Ca within approximately 2 hours of light offset only on days when ovulations occur.[34] It is not clear what factor is responsible for this appetite. The increased need for Ca for shell calcification is associated with the estrogen induction of calcium-binding protein. But poultry, which tend to lay daily over a laying period of several months, likely have a much higher dietary requirement for Ca than do companion birds, which lay thinner shelled eggs (associated with cavity nesting), lay less frequently (typically every other day rather than daily), and in most husbandry situations lay only one or two clutches per breeding season (rather than hundreds of eggs). Thus, the dietary requirement for Ca for egg-laying in cockatiels is judged to be less than 1% (see Roudybush, Chapter 3).

HUMIDITY AND RAINFALL

Serventy[35] reviewed reports noting positive relationships between rainfall or correlates of rain and sexual activity of wild Australian desert species including budgerigars (*Melopsittacus undulatus*) and Bourke's parrots (*Neophema bourkei*). Many anecdotal reports likewise suggest that birds appear to enjoy being sprayed with water or lay eggs after exposure to misting, the sound of rain, or high humidity. Whether birds perceive rain by physical cues (sight, tactile stimulation), by an increase in rain-stimulated food availability, by the possibility of increased relative humidity, and/or by other

means is not clear. Few experimental studies have been done.

SOCIAL CUES

Social cues can contribute to sexual stimulation, particularly in monogamous and colonial companion birds. Conspecific calls induce gonadal growth in budgerigars,[36, 37] and male "soft warble" calls particularly stimulate ovarian development in budgerigars.[38] Cockatiel reproductive activity is stimulated roughly in proportion to the extent of social contact with mates (i.e., pairs permitted full contact are more likely to inspect nest boxes and lay eggs than are pairs physically separated yet permitted visual and auditory contact, pairs with auditory contact only, or pair members without any mate access).[39] Ovarian development in ring doves (*Streptopelia risoria*) is stimulated by perception of the female's own calls. An auditory pathway in doves links the midbrain auditory nucleus (nucleus intercollicularis) with a cGnRH I-rich area of the anterior hypothalamus[40]; thus, sexually relevant calls may have direct input to cGnRH I neurons in female ring doves.

Auditory stimulation of sexual development may not necessarily be from species-specific calls. Sound cues,[41] as well as cyclic feeding schedules,[42] can entrain locomotor rhythms of house sparrows. European quail (*Coturnix coturnix coturnix*) male "crows" can stimulate sexual development in females held on 6 hours light: 18 hours dark,[43] but gonadal growth in quail is also stimulated by playing recorded commercial radio sounds prior to light onset.[44, 45] We noted that radio sound played during the dark phase elicited a degree of locomotor activity in many birds similar to that observed during a pulse of light or light onset, although the gonadal response, as judged by the size of the quail's cloacal gland area, was not as robust as in response to long daylength stimulation. These observations may account for potential cross-species sexual stimulation of birds held in mixed species aviaries.

VOLITION

Because force-pairing is akin to rape in violating female choice, it is not surprising that females are often aggressive toward males when force-paired.

For example, canvasback females (*Aythya valisineria*) allowed to self-select mates in captivity breed readily, but females kill potential mates with whom they are force-paired.[46]

For monogamous birds, forming a pair bond is often a prerequisite for sexual development. Cockatiels force-paired (confined in 0.33 m × 0.33 m × 0.67 m cages) at the time of photostimulation and nest box presentation showed less reproductive activity than cockatiels force-paired 6 weeks earlier, permitting a pair bond to form. Reproductive performance was evaluated in previously paired cockatiels (pairs that had produced fertile eggs together in a previous breeding trial) which had been force-paired with new mates and separated from each other for 6 weeks. When reunited with their previous mates at the time of photostimulation and nest box presentation, reproductive performance was not impaired.[47] This was interpreted to mean that formation of a new pair bond (during the 6 weeks of being force-paired with a novel mate) did not disrupt the sexually facilitating effects of a previously established pair bond.

EARLY LEARNING

Early learning can be critical for conferring sexual efficacy on otherwise neutral stimuli. Hand-reared cockatiel chicks that were deprived of exposure to either nest boxes or adult conspecifics during the brooding and fledging periods showed impaired reproductive performance as adults.[48] In their first breeding trial, such cockatiels tended not to inspect nest boxes, and eggs from pairs containing hand-reared males were usually infertile. However, hand-reared females were more likely to lay eggs than parent-reared females, perhaps because of a reduced stress reaction to animal caretakers. The negative effects of hand-rearing on fertility and nest box use were partially reduced in the subsequent breeding trial, supporting the view that early learning is not necessarily irreversible. However, if chicks imprint on their habitat, nest boxes provided to adults may have greater sexual efficacy if they match those from which chicks fledge. Zebra finches (*Taeniopygia guttata*) were shown to alter adult preference for nesting substrate based on early experience.[49]

Whereas sexual efficacy can be conferred on neutral stimuli by early learning, early learning may also be involved in inhibition of reproduction. The trauma experienced by birds captured in the wild and shipped under adverse conditions may well produce the equivalent of an avian post-traumatic stress disorder in which there is prolonged hyperreactivity to stressors.[50] This may explain why some species of wild-caught parrots are often reported to require several years in captivity before they breed, whereas birds reared in captivity often mature at a relatively young age.

Intrusion of humans on captive wild birds not yet habituated to captive conditions is obviously stressful. In mammals, neuropeptides that mediate stress, such as corticotropin-releasing factor (CRF), impinge on GnRH neurons, thereby providing a neuroanatomic basis by which psychological activation of the CRF-ACTH-corticosterone axis could inhibit GnRH activity. CRF nerve terminals are also collocalized with cGnRH I cell bodies in some areas of turkey hen brain, although whether they have synaptic contact is not known.

It may be possible to improve captive reproductive success by habituating chicks to humans at an early age. We found that relatively little human handling of parent-reared orange-winged Amazon (*Amazona amazonica*) chicks during the brooding phase (approximately 20 minutes daily handling for a 3-week period beginning about day 35) is sufficient to render them quite tame at fledging.[51] Whether these birds will breed as adults, or, if so, if they will remain tame to humans, is not known.

INTERACTION OF ENVIRONMENTAL FACTORS

Sexually stimulatory input to the cGnRH I system provided by auditory or visual access to mates is probably additive with input provided by other environmental cues. For example, cockatiels are maximally stimulated, as judged by serum LH levels and a variety of reproductive performance measures, only when given access to a nest box, photostimulated, and provided full access to a mate. Individual birds without full mate access and without nest boxes are less likely to lay eggs, and they have lower LH levels.[39] Similarly, starlings provided with nest boxes in an outdoor aviary have higher LH levels and greater testicular size than those without nest boxes.[52] Birds integrate diverse cues in determining the timing and intensity of their reproductive effort, and breeding is probably maximally stimulated when a constellation of environmental factors are all propitious. This suggests that if essential or minimal environmental requirements for breeding of a species are not known, it may still be possible to maximize sexual stimulation by an assemblage of environmental manipulations judged likely to be propitious.

Cockatiels are more likely to lay eggs when presented with an assemblage of environmental manipulations consisting of increases in temperature, humidity, plane of nutrition, and photostimulation.[13] This approach identified a set of environmental conditions that were then used as positive control conditions for testing whether individual manipulations were essential. Photostimulation was found to be a sufficient cue for stimulating reproduction in cockatiels. A similar approach was used to stimulate egg-laying in wild-caught orange-winged Amazon parrots that had not previously laid eggs in captivity.[53] Amazon pairs exposed to numerous manipulations (separation into same-sex flocks prior to photostimulation, then pair reunification at the time of nest box presentation; addition of fruit to diet; restricted nest box entrance; daily misting; and slightly deeper nest boxes) were more likely to lay eggs than controls provided with nest boxes only. Once pairs had produced eggs, however, nest box presentation alone was sufficient to elicit egg-laying in the subsequent breeding trial.

GnRH NEURONAL SYSTEMS

Birds are typical of most vertebrates in having multiple forms of GnRH. In birds there are at least two forms, cGnRH I[54] and cGnRH II[55] ([His[5], Trp[7], Tyr[8]]GnRH). The former is well established as being involved in gonadotropin release. The cGnRH I cell bodies extend from the preoptic area of the brain dorsally and caudally to the septal region. Based on evidence from rats, perhaps most of these neurons project to the median eminence (ME). Axons of these cells also extend to other parts of the brain where they may be involved in coordinating reproductive behavior with gonadal function.[56]

There are several subgroups of cGnRH I cell bodies. Whether some subgroups are preferentially innervated to respond to particular environmental inputs or to support particular gonadotropic functions is a current research question. Subgroups of GnRH cells in some female mammals appear to be selectively activated during ovulation; others are involved in chronic pulsatile secretion of GnRH.

The cGnRH II cells occur near the midbrain central gray area and in the caudal lateral hypothalamus.[56] Although cGnRH II fibers innervate several brain areas associated with reproduction (e.g., preoptic area, septum), cGnRH II fibers do not extend to the ME. A function for this neuropeptide in birds has not been established, although cGnRH II is equal to or more active than cGnRH I in stimulating gonadotropin release in in vitro pituitary preparations[57] and after injection in chickens.[58]

GnRH DOWN-REGULATION

Chicken pituitary cells in vitro require pulsatile GnRH stimulation for gonadotropin release; constant exposure leads to receptor down-regulation.[57] Thus, treatment of laying chickens with a long-acting depot formulation of the superactive GnRH agonist leuprolide acetate (Lupron, TAP Pharmaceuticals) reduces gonadotropin output, which stops egg production, causes gonadal involution, and leads to molting.[59] Leuprolide treatment also reversibly prevents egg-laying in cockatiels[60] and may be useful in applications in which a temporary reduction in gonad size is required.

Although both pulsatile and nonpulsatile GnRH treatments have been used to stimulate gonadotropin release and gonadal development in several nonavian vertebrates, this approach has not been successful in birds. However, ovarian development and egg-laying were achieved in nonphotostimulated Japanese quail by administration of crude preparations of gonadotropins.[61]

PITUITARY HORMONES

The avian pituitary is comprised of six or seven histologically distinct cell types, each of which is associated with the production and secretion of particular pituitary hormones.[62] The composition of cell types within the pituitary can change with reproductive condition. In principle, the same level of hypothalamic output can elicit quite different amounts of pituitary hormone output because of changes in type and sensitivity of pituitary cells in different reproductive conditions. For example, the pituitary of an incubating turkey is larger and has more prolactin-producing cells than that of an egg-laying turkey. As a result, the ability of releasing hormones such as GnRH and VIP to stimulate, respectively, LH and prolactin release in in vitro pituitary preparations depends both on the reproductive condition of pituitary donors and the steroid hormones to which the preparations are exposed.[63, 64]

Furthermore, the avian pituitary may produce not just one molecular form of a hormone but rather an array of related hormones, isoforms, each with different target organ potencies. Some isoforms of chicken LH show substantial potency by radioimmunoassay but have little potency in a granulosa cell bioassay.[65] Different isoforms may partially account for the range of potencies of various purified gonadotropin preparations in stimulating steroidogenesis in chicken ovarian tissue.[66] Distinct forms of turkey prolactin have likewise been isolated,[67] each with different potencies in radioimmunoassays, radioreceptor assays, and bioassays. These observations point out the interpretational hazards of experimental results based on poorly validated assays.

TESTICULAR STIMULATION BY GONADOTROPINS

The pulsatility of GnRH release has been inferred from the pulsatile release of LH seen in castrated cockerels[68] and intact turkey males.[69] Circulating testosterone levels in turkey toms also may reflect pulsatile testicular stimulation by LH, although LH peaks and testosterone peaks are often not synchronous.[70] These findings point out the hazards in interpreting single-point measurements of testosterone level in individual animals. Nonetheless, average testosterone values for groups show characteristic changes that often, but not invariably, reflect gonadal size.

As in mammals, testicular size may be determined by the amount of follicle-stimulating hormone (FSH) stimulation. Evidence in chicken hens[71] and roosters[72] shows that FSH secretion from the pituitary may be under the influence of negative feedback control of an avian inhibin. The discovery of

inhibin and its FSH-specific effects on the pituitary offers an explanation of how stimulation by a single GnRH could provide hormonal drive for two gonadotropins that may circulate at quite different levels.

Wingfield and coworkers[73] emphasized the importance of ecologic niche and behavior in controlling circulating testosterone levels in male birds. He suggested in the "challenge hypothesis" that, whereas a critical minimal amount of testosterone is required for competence of spermatogenesis, in the mature testes levels of testosterone above that minimum may be regulated by the extent and success of aggressive encounters with other males. These observations suggest that reducing male-male interactions in an aviary could reduce testosterone levels of a male parent, which could improve male parenting performance.

Examination of field data from species representing a range of male investment in parental care suggested further refinement of the challenge hypothesis. Behavioral interactions may be especially important in controlling the highly variable levels of testosterone seen in males of monomorphic species showing biparental care of eggs and young. In these species, high testosterone levels, which may aid in increased aggressiveness for territorial defense and mate guarding, may be incompatible with parental care. In contrast, in polygynous species with minimal male parental investment, it may be disadvantageous to have testosterone under as much behavioral control and, in fact, less plasticity is seen. Our data on testosterone levels of orange-winged Amazon males in various reproductive stages support the view that testosterone levels may be suppressed during incubation and brooding, although they were quite high and variable, as evidenced by high standard errors, during nest inspection and egg-laying (Fig. 2–2).

OVULATION

In the chicken, ovulation occurs in association with high levels of serum LH and progesterone, which begin to rise some 4 to 7 hours prior to ovulation. During this time a positive feedback relationship exists between LH and progesterone such that the serum increases in these hormones are nearly coincident. Although premature ovulatory surges can be elicited with either LH or progesterone injections,

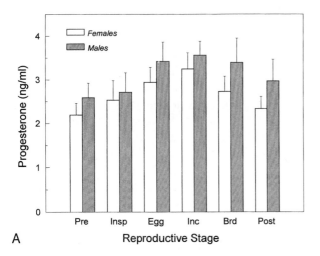

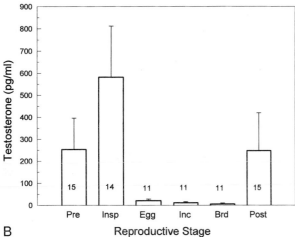

Figure 2–2

Serum progesterone (*A*, males and females) and testosterone (*B*, males only) levels of captive orange-winged Amazons at different stages of the reproductive cycle. (Pre = before nest box presentation; Insp = one day after nest box inspection; Egg = on the day the second egg was laid; Inc = 3 weeks after the first egg was laid; Brd = 7 weeks after the first egg was laid; Post = after chicks had fledged and nest boxes were removed.) (From Kenton B, Millam JR: Photostimulation and serum steroids of orange-winged Amazon parrots. Proceedings of the Annual Conference of the Avian Veterinary Association, Reno, NV, 1994:435 (Abstract).

natural initiations in many species are typically restricted in time to a so-called open period. During the open period, an ovulatory surge is initiated if the largest follicle is sufficiently mature to secrete a postulated "maturation factor."[74, 75] That serum progesterone derives primarily from the granulosa cells of the largest follicle[76, 77] may support the view that progesterone is the postulated follicular maturation factor.

Factors determining when the open period occurs are not well understood, although light offset time, the transition from light to dark, correlates well with oviposition time over a wide range of photoschedules.[78] In the absence of photoperiodic cues, several other cues such as feeding schedules, temperature cycles, or sound cues can exert entraining influences on oviposition rhythms.

Oviposition interval is largely species-typical and shows considerable variation both within and among species. Cockatiels are typical of many psittacines in laying at intervals of 2 days, although under propitious conditions in captivity it is not unusual for individual cockatiels to lay at daily intervals for several days.[13]

HYPOTHALAMIC CONTROL OF OVULATION

Cyclicity of gonadotropin release for ovulation is characteristic of female vertebrate reproduction. In female birds, cyclicity results from exposure of the brain to organizing steroid hormones during embryonic development. The locus of cyclic gonadotropin control in mammals is the preoptic area of the brain. Lesion and deafferentation studies indicate that the preoptic area is also involved in ovulation in chickens (for review, see Van Tienhoven[79]). The preoptic area is also an effective site for brain injections of progesterone to induce ovulation in chickens.[80] Davies[81] found that lesions of the supraoptic region, just caudal to the preoptic area, specifically disrupted ovulations in Japanese quail, whereas preoptic area lesions blocked gonadal growth generally (see Sharp[82] for review). As noted above, turkey preoptic and supraoptic areas contain cGnRH I cell bodies, cGnRH II nerve fibers,[56] and estrogen,[83] and progesterone[84] receptors have also been found in these areas in chickens.

CLUTCH TERMINATION

In poultry species, and probably in other indeterminate egg-layers, egg-laying continues until rising serum prolactin levels signal a transition from egg production to egg incubation. The increase in serum prolactin is strongly associated with parental behavior in both females and males in several avian species, although in ring doves prolactin is not associated as much with the initiation as the maintenance of incubation and brooding. The neurochemical regulation of incubation and prolactin secretion has been most thoroughly studied in turkeys by El Halawani and Rozenboim.[85] The transition from egg-laying to incubation in turkeys is most likely initiated by tactile stimulation of the defeathered and edematous brood patch, which forms in response to ovarian steroid exposure.

Tactile stimulation, most naturally by eggs, via a multisynaptic pathway, probably stimulates activity of serotonergic neurons that participate in a neuroendocrine reflex arc leading to increased prolactin secretion. Serotonin, in turn, is believed to stimulate hypothalamic VIP-containing neurons that project to the median eminence.[86] As mentioned earlier, VIP is a prolactin-releasing hormone in birds.

In galliforms, high prolactin levels are associated with gonadal regression. Prolactin may act centrally to inhibit cGnRH I secretion, because intraventricular infusion of even microgram quantities of prolactin induces incubation behavior in turkeys.[87] Prolactin may also exert peripheral effects by antagonizing the steroidogenic actions of luteinizing hormone.[88] High prolactin levels are also associated with incubation behavior, characterized by prolonged nesting bouts in turkeys, a species in which only the female incubates. High prolactin levels are also associated with profound anorexia in chickens and turkeys. During the course of incubation, chicken hens may lose 20% of their body mass.[89] At the end of incubation, exposure of nesting hens to turkey poults causes prolactin levels to fall.[90] Exposure to brooded chicks also appeared to inhibit serum LH in Gifujidori chickens, because both LH and estradiol levels increased following removal of chicks at either 1 or 3 weeks of age.[91]

Particular prolactin levels characterize each phase of reproduction in the turkey and appear to be controlled by distinct proximal factors at each stage of the reproductive cycle.[92] Initially, prolactin levels are slightly elevated by photoperiodic stimulation. They are further increased by exposure to ovarian steroids and increased further in response to tactile brood patch stimulation. Finally, they decline in response to exposure to poults. To what extent prolactin may fulfill similar functions in psittacine species is not known. Serum levels of prolactin in cockatiels, however, show a pattern typical of other monogamous species in which both parents incu-

bate (Fig. 2–3); levels are elevated during egg-laying, further elevated during incubation, lower but still relatively high during brooding, and fall to pre-laying levels after brooding.[93]

MANIPULATION OF CLUTCH LENGTH

Egg production in turkeys can be increased beyond the natural clutch length of perhaps 12 to 18 eggs by interventions that disrupt the sequelae of events outlined earlier. The most common method of intervention is egg removal. By this means hens in commercial turkey flocks often lay more than 100 eggs during a 6-month period of lay. Likewise, egg removal from cockatiels can increase production from a natural clutch length of four to seven eggs to 30 or more eggs in a 2-month period.[13] Surgical

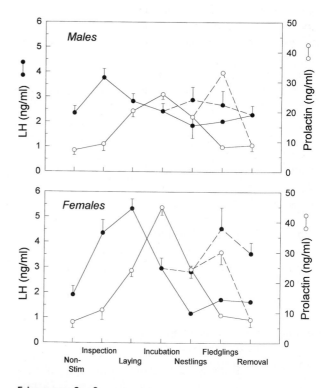

F i g u r e 2 – 3

Plasma luteinizing hormone and prolactin levels of cockatiels during the reproductive cycle of pairs laying one or two clutches. Dashed lines represent birds laying a second clutch. Sample sizes range from three to 11 when standard error bars are present and one to two when they are absent. (From Myers SA, Millam JR, El Halawani ME: Plasma LH and prolactin levels during the reproductive cycle of the cockatiel [*Nymphus hollandicus*]. Am Comp Endocrinol 73:85–91, 1989.)

denervation of the turkey hen brood patch also prevents incubation behavior and thereby increases egg production over sham-operated controls.[94] Antagonizing increases in serotonergic activity with drugs such as para-chlorophenylalanine can also prevent incubation and increase egg production in turkey hens.[95] In addition, immunizing turkey hens against VIP reduces prolactin levels and thereby maintains egg production in hens that would otherwise incubate.[96]

Cockatiels, however, are unlike turkeys and are typical of many psittacines in that incubation begins while clutches are still being formed. For example, a cockatiel that lays a clutch of seven eggs over a 12-day period and begins incubating after the second egg is laid has an active ovary during approximately one-half of the total incubation time of the first two eggs. If prolactin is acting to inhibit cGnRH I release, either prolactin must remain low during incubation or prolactin levels must rise slowly during the course of incubation, reaching inhibitory levels as the number of eggs in the clutch increases. These possibilities were tested in cockatiels by artificially manipulating rate of clutch accrual by removing or adding eggs to nest boxes as clutches were being formed. Indeed, serum prolactin levels rose slowly over the course of incubation; addition or removal of eggs, respectively, decreased or increased egg production of hens, suggesting that clutch length may indeed be limited by high prolactin levels in cockatiels as it is in turkeys.[97] In cockatiels, as in several species showing biparental care, prolactin levels are elevated in males in a manner comparable to that in females.[93]

Some evidence suggests that high levels of testosterone are incompatible with parental care; thus, incubating or brooding Bengalese finch (*Lonchura striata*) males with high prolactin levels may be expected to have low testosterone levels.[98] As mentioned earlier, testosterone levels in orange-winged Amazon males are strikingly reduced during incubation and brooding.[99]

CONCLUSION

Reproductive efficiency of captive psittacines using prevailing management strategies is abysmally low compared with efficiency in poultry species. A typical flock of 100 domestic turkeys, consisting of 90 females and 10 males, may be expected to produce 9000 poults or more in a 6-month production period, but a flock of 100 Amazon parrots, 50 females and 50 males, may be expected to produce from 50 to 100 chicks in the same period, even assuming that the Amazon flock is sexually mature, sexually competent, and effectively pair-bonded. This very rough and somewhat farcical comparison illustrates that management for captive propagation of parrots is probably far from being optimized, at least as judged by current standards of poultry production. However, there is considerable ecologic and economic incentive to improve reproductive efficiency of captive propagation. Improvement will be most effectively pursued by a better understanding of how environmental, social, and hormonal factors influence neuroendocrine control of reproductive events.

References

1. Clubb S, Clubb KJ, Phillips S: Aviculture: an alternative to trade in wild-caught birds. In Schubot RM, Clubb KJ, Clubb S (eds): Psittacine Aviculture. Loxahatchee, FL, Avicultural Breed Research Center, 1992.
2. Joyner KL: Theriogenology. In Ritchie BW, Harrison GJ, Harrison LR (eds): Avian Medicine: Principles and Application. Lake Worth, FL, Wingers Publishing, 1994.
3. Wingfield JC: Environmental and endocrine control of avian reproduction: An ecological approach. In Mikami S, Homma K, Wada M (eds): Avian Endocrinology. New York, Springer-Verlag, 1983.
4. Siopes TD, Wilson WO: Extraocular modification of photoreception in intact and pinealectomized Coturnix. Poult Sci 53:2035–2041, 1974.
5. Follett BK: Birds. In Lamming G (ed): Marshall's Physiology of Reproduction, ed 3. Edinburgh, Churchill Livingstone, 1984.
6. Silver R, Witkovsky P, Horvath P, et al: Coexpression of opsin and VIP-like-immunoreactivity in CSF-contacting neurons of the avian brain. Cell Tissue Res 253:189–198, 1988.
7. Saldanha CJ, Leak RK, Silver R: Detection and transduction of daylength in birds. Psychoneuroendocrinology 19:641–656, 1994.
8. Foster RG, Follett BK: The involvement of a rhodopsin-like photopigment in the photoperiodic response of the Japanese quail. J Comp Physiol A 157:519–528, 1989.
9. Ernst RA, Millam JR, Mather FB: Review of life-history lighting programs for commercial laying fowl. World Poult Sci 43:45–55, 1987.
10. Meyer WE, Millam JR, Bradley FA: Photostimulation of Japanese quail by dim light depends upon photophase contrast, not light intensity. Biol Reprod 38:536–543, 1988.
11. Meyer WE, Millam JR: Plasma melatonin levels in Japanese quail exposed to dim light are determined by subjective interpretation of day and night, not light intensity. Gen Comp Endocrinol 82:377–385, 1991.
12. Gwinner E, Dittami J: Photoperiodic responses in temperate

zone and equatorial Stonechats: a contribution to the problem of photoperiodism in tropical organisms. In Follet BK, Ishii S, Chandola A (eds): Endocrine System and the Environment. New York, Springer-Verlag, 1985.

13. Millam JR, Roudybush TE, Grau CR: Influence of environmental manipulation and nest-box access on reproductive activity in captive cockatiels (*Nymphicus hollandicus*). Zoo Biol 7:25–34, 1988.

14. Maitra SK: Influences of length of photoperiod on testicular activity of the blossomheaded parakeet *Psittacula cyanocephala*. J Yamashina Inst Ornithol 19:28–44, 1987.

15. Murton RK, Westwood NJ: Avian Breeding Cycles. New York, Oxford University Press, 1977.

16. Follett BK, Sharp PJ: Circadian rhythmicity in photoperiodically induced gonadotrophin release and gonadal growth in the quail. Nature 223:968–971, 1969.

17. Foster RG, Plowman G, Goldsmith AR, et al: The LH-RH system of male European starling: Photoperiod induces changes to a possible multifunctional peptide system. Basic Appl Histochem 32:95–102, 1988.

18. Nicholls TJ, Goldsmith AR, Dawson A: Photorefractoriness in birds and comparison with mammals. Physiol Rev 68:133–176, 1988.

19. Krishna Prasadan TN, Kotak VC, Sharp, PJ, et al: Environmental and hormonal factors in seasonal breeding in free-living male Indian rose-ringed parakeets (*Psittacula krameri*). Horm Behav 22:488–496, 1988.

20. Sailaja R, Kotak VC, Sharp PJ, et al: Environmental, dietary, and hormonal factors in the regulation of seasonal breeding in free-living female Indian rose-ringed parakeets (*Psittacula krameri*). Horm Behav 22:518–527, 1988.

21. Perera AD, Follett BK: Photoperiodic induction in vitro: The dynamics of gonadotropin-releasing hormone release from hypothalamic explants of the Japanese quail. Endocrinology 131:2898–2908, 1992.

22. Follett BK, Nicholls TJ: Influences of thyroidectomy and thyroxine replacement on photoperiodically controlled reproduction in quail. J Endocrinol 107:211–221, 1985.

23. Martin SG, Millam JR: Nest box selection by floor laying and reproductively naive captive Cockatiels (*Nymphicus hollandicus*). Appl Anim Behav Sci 43:95–109, 1995.

24. Brooks DS, Cassone VM: Daily and circadian regulation of 2-[I-^{125}]iodomelatonin binding in the chicken brain. Endocrinology 131:1297–1304, 1992.

25. Lu J, Cassone VM: Pineal regulation of circadian rhythms of 2-deoxy[C-^{14}]glucose uptake and 2[I-^{125}]iodomelatonin binding in the visual system of the house sparrow, *Passer domesticus*. J Comp Physiol A-Sen Neural Behav Physiol 173:765–774, 1993.

26. Binkley S, Riebman J, Reilly K: The pineal gland: A biological clock *in vitro*. Science 202:1198–1201, 1978.

27. Zimmerman N, Menaker M: The pineal gland: A pacemaker within the circadian system of the house sparrow. Proc Natl Acad Sci 76:999–1003, 1979.

28. Saarela S, Reiter RJ: Function of melatonin in thermoregulatory processes. Life Sci 54:295–311, 1994.

29. Ohta M, Kadota C, Konishi H: A role of melatonin in the initial stage of photoperiodism in the Japanese quail. Biol Reprod 40:935–941, 1989.

30. Underwood H, Binkley S, Siopes T, Mosher K: Melatonin rhythms in the eyes, pineal bodies, and blood of Japanese quail (*Coturnix coturnix japonica*). Gen Comp Endocrinol 56:70–81, 1984.

31. Chakraborty S: A comparative study of annual changes in the pineal gland morphology with reference to the influence of melatonin on testicular activity in tropical birds, *Psittacula*

cyanocephala and *Ploceus phillippinus*. Gen Comp Endocrinol 92:71–79, 1993.

32. Prasadan RNK, Kotak VC: Fine structure of the free-living parakeet pineal in relation to the breeding cycle. J Pineal Res 15:122–131, 1993.

33. Millam JR, El Halawani ME: Serum prolactin and luteinizing hormone levels during an induced pause in domestic fowl. Poult Sci 65:1004–1010, 1986.

34. Hughes BO: A circadian rhythm of calcium intake in the domestic fowl. Br Poult Sci 13:485–493, 1972.

35. Serventy DL: Biology of desert birds. In Farner D, King J (eds): Avian Biology, vol I. New York, Academic Press, 1971.

36. Ficken RW, van Tienhoven A, Ficken MS, Sibley F: Effect of visual and vocal stimuli on breeding in the budgerigar (*Melopsittacus undulatus*). Anim Behav 8:104–106, 1960.

37. Brockway BF: The effects of nest-entrance positions and male vocalizations on reproduction in budgerigars. Living Bird, First Ann Cornell Lab Ornithol, Ithaca, NY, 1962, pp 93–101.

38. Brockway BF: Stimulation of ovarian development and egg laying by male courtship vocalization in budgerigars (*Melopsittacus undulatus*). Anim Behav 13:574–578, 1965.

39. Shields KM, Yamamoto JT, Millam JR: Reproductive behavior and LH levels of cockatiels (*Nymphicus hollandicus*) associated with photostimulation, nest-box presentation and degree of mate access. Horm Behav 23:68–82, 1989.

40. Cheng MF, Zuo M: Proposed pathways for vocal self-stimulation: Met-enkephalinergic projections linking the midbrain vocal nucleus, auditory-responsive thalamic regions and neurosecretory hypothalamus. J Neurobiol 25:361–379, 1994.

41. Menaker M, Eskin A: Entrainment of circadian rhythms by sound in *Passer domesticus*. Science 154:1579–1581, 1966.

42. Hau M, Gwinner E: Circadian entrainment by feeding cycles in house sparrows. J Comp Physiol 170:403–409, 1992.

43. Guyomarc'h C, Richard J-P: Role of social signals in photoperiodic control of reproduction in European Quail (*Coturnix coturnix coturnix*). In Morgan E (ed): Chronobiology and Chronomedicine. New York, Peter Lang, 1988.

44. Millam JR, El Halawani ME, Burke WH: Effect of cyclic sound cues on sexual development in nonphotostimulated Japanese quail. Poult Sci 64:169–175, 1985.

45. Li ZZ, Burke WH: Influence of 12 hours of sound stimuli on gonad development and plasma luteinizing hormone in Japanese quail (*Coturnix coturnix japonica*) exposed to 6 hours of daily light. Poult Sci 66:1045–1052, 1987.

46. Bluhm CK: Mate preferences and mating patterns in Canvasback Ducks (*Aythya valisneria*). In Gowaty A, Mock DW (eds): Avian Monogamy. Ornithol Monogr 37:45–56, 1985.

47. Yamamoto JT, Shields KM, Millam JR, et al: Reproductive success of force-paired cockatiels (*Nymphicus hollandicus*). Auk 106:86–93, 1989.

48. Myers SA, Millam JR, Roudybush TE, Grau CR: Reproductive success of parent-reared vs hand-reared cockatiels (*Nymphicus hollandicus*). Auk 105:536–542, 1988.

49. Sargent TD: The role of experience in the nest building of the Zebra Finch. Auk 82:48–61, 1965.

50. Yehuda R, Antelman SM: Criteria for rationally evaluating animal models of posttraumatic stress disorder. Biol Psychol 33:479–486, 1993.

51. Davis WL, Millam JR: Handling of parent-reared chicks (abstract). Proc Ann Conf Assoc Avian Vet, Reno, NV, 1994, p 422.

52. Gwinner H, Gwinner E, Dittami J: Effects of nestboxes on LH, testosterone, testicular size, and the reproductive behavior of male European starlings in spring. Behaviour 103:68–82, 1987.

53. Millam JR, Kenton B, Jochim L, et al: Breeding Orange-winged Amazon parrots in captivity. Zoo Biol 14:275–284, 1995.

54. Miyamoto K, Hasegawa Y, Mingegishi T, et al: Isolation and characterization of chicken hypothalamic luteinizing hormone-releasing hormone. Biochem Biophys Res Commun 107:820–827, 1982.

55. Miyamoto K, Hasegawa Y, Nomura M, et al: Identification of the second gonadotropin-releasing hormone in chicken hypothalamus: Evidence that gonadotropin secretion is probably controlled by two distinct gonadotropin-releasing hormones in avian species. Proc Natl Acad Sci USA 81:3874–3878, 1984.

56. Millam JR, Faris PL, Youngren OM, et al: Immunohistochemical localization of chicken gonadotropin-releasing hormones I and II (cGnRH I and II) in turkey hen brain. J Comp Neurol 333:68–82, 1993.

57. Millar RP, Milton RC, Follett BK, King JA: Receptor binding and gonadotropin-releasing activity of a novel chicken gonadotropin-releasing hormone ([His^5, Trp^7, Tyr^8]GnRH) and a D-Arg^6 analog. Endocrinology 119:224–231, 1986.

58. Sharp PJ, Dunn IC, Talbot RT: Sex differences in the LH responses to chicken LHRH-I and -II in the domestic fowl. J Endocrinol 115:323–331, 1987.

59. Dickerman RW, Bahr JM: Molt induced by gonadotropin-releasing hormone agonist as a model for studying endocrine mechanisms of molting in laying hens. Poult Sci 68:1402–1408, 1989.

60. Millam JR, Finney HL: Leuprolide acetate reversibly prevents egg laying in Cockatiels. Zoo Biol 13:149–154, 1994.

61. Wakabayashi S, Kikuchi M, Wada M, et al: Induction of ovarian growth and ovulation by administration of a chicken gonadotrophin preparation to Japanese quail kept under a short-day regimen. Br Poult Sci 33:847–858, 1992.

62. Mikami S: Avian adenohypophysis: Recent progress in immunocytochemical studies. In Mikami S, Homma K, Wada M (eds): Avian Endocrinology. New York, Springer-Verlag, 1983.

63. Knapp TR, Fehrer SC, Silsby JL, et al: Gonadal steroid-mediated alteration of luteinizing hormone secretion by anterior pituitary cells of young turkeys. Gen Comp Endocrinol 68:449–455, 1987.

64. Knapp TR, Fehrer SC, Silsby JL, et al: Gonadal steroid modulation of basal and vasoactive intestinal polypeptide-stimulated prolactin release by turkey anterior pituitary cells. Gen Comp Endocrinol 72:226–236, 1988.

65. Krishnan KA, Proudman JA, Bahr JM: Purification and partial characterization of isoforms of luteinizing hormone from the chicken pituitary gland. Comp Biochem Physiol Biochem Mol Biol 108:253–264, 1994.

66. Robinson FE, Etches RJ, Anderson-Langmuir CE, et al: Steroidogenic relationships of gonadotrophin hormones in the ovary of the hen (*Gallus domesticus*). Gen Comp Endocrinol 69:455–466, 1988.

67. Corcoran DH, Proudman JA: Isoforms of turkey prolactin: Evidence for differences in glycosylation and in tryptic peptide mapping. Comp Biochem Physiol B Comp Biochem 99:563–570, 1991.

68. Wilson SC, Sharp PJ: Episodic release of luteinizing hormone in the domestic fowl. J Endocrinol 64:77–86, 1975.

69. Bacon WL, Long DW, Kurima DP, et al: Coordinate pattern of secretion of luteinizing hormone and testosterone in mature male turkeys under continuous and intermittent photoschedules. Poult Sci 73:947–952, 1994.

70. Bacon WL, Proudman JA, Foster DN, Renner PA: Pattern of secretion of luteinizing hormone and testosterone in the sexually mature male turkey. Gen Comp Endocrinol 84:447–460, 1991.

71. Johnson PA: Inhibin in the hen. Poult Sci 72:955–958, 1993.

72. Lewis WM, Muster KM, Marin TL, et al: Evidence for inhibin in roosters (abstract). Biol Reprod 40[Suppl 1]:109, 1989.

73. Wingfield JC, Ball GF, Dufty A, et al: Testosterone and aggression in birds: Tests of the "challenge" hypothesis. Am Sci 75:602–608, 1987.

74. Fraps RM: Egg production and fertility in poultry. In Hammond J (ed): Progress in the Physiology of Farm Animals, vol 2. London, Butterworths, 1950.

75. Fraps RM: Photoregulation in the ovulation cycle of the domestic fowl. In Benoit J, Assenmacher I (eds): La Photoregulation de la Reproduction chez les Oiseaux et les Mamiferes. Colloques Int Centre Nat Recherche Sci 172:281–295, 1970.

76. Shahabi NA, Bahr JM, Nalbandov AV: Effect of LH injection on plasma and follicular steroids in the chicken. Endocrinology 96:969–975, 1975a.

77. Shahabi NA, Norton WH, Nalbandov AV: Steroid levels in follicles and the plasma of hens during the ovulatory cycle. Endocrinology 96:962–968, 1975b.

78. Etches RJ: The ovulatory cycle of the hen. CRC Rev Poult Biol 2:293–318, 1990.

79. Van Tienhoven A: Neuroendocrinology of avian reproduction, with special emphasis on the reproductive cycle of the fowl (*Gallus domesticus*). World Poult Sci 37:156–176, 1981.

80. Ralph CL, Fraps RM: Induction of ovulation in the hen by injection of progesterone into the brain. Endocrinology 66:269–276, 1960.

81. Davies DT: The neuroendocrine control of gonadotrophin release in the Japanese quail. III: The role of the tuberal and anterior hypothalamus in the control of ovarian development and ovulation. Proc R Soc Lond [Biol] 206:401–423, 1980.

82. Sharp PJ: Hypothalamic control of gonadotrophin secretion in birds. In Nistico G, Bolis L (eds): Progress in Nonmammalian Brain Research, vol III. Boca Raton, FL, CRC Press, 1983.

83. Kawashima M, Kamiyoshi M, Tanaka K: Estrogen receptor binding in the hen hypothalamus and pituitary during the ovulatory cycle. Poult Sci 72:839–847, 1993.

84. Kawashima M, Kamiyoshi M, Tanaka K: Changes in progesterone receptor binding of preoptic hypothalamus during an ovulatory cycle of the hen. Poult Sci 73:855–863, 1994.

85. El Halawani ME, Rozenboim I: The ontogeny and control of incubation behavior in turkeys. Poult Sci 72:906–911, 1993.

86. Mauro LJ, Elde RP, Youngren OM, et al: Alterations in hypothalamic vasoactive intestinal peptide-like immunoreactivity are associated with reproduction and prolactin release in the female turkey. Endocrinology 125:1795–1804, 1989.

87. Youngren OM, El Halawani ME, Silsby JL, Phillips RE: Intracranial prolactin perfusion induces incubation behavior in turkey hens. Biol Reprod 44:425–431, 1991.

88. Camper PM, Burke WH: The effects of prolactin on gonadotropin induced rise in serum estradiol and progesterone of the laying turkey. Gen Comp Endocrinol 32:72–77, 1977.

89. Sherry DF, Mrosovsky N, Hogan JA: Weight loss and anorexia during incubation in birds. J Comp Physiol Psychol 94:89–98, 1980.

90. Wentworth BC, Proudman JA, Opel H, et al: Endocrine changes in the incubating and brooding turkey hen. Biol Reprod 29:87–92, 1983.

91. Kuwayama T, Shimada K, Saito N, et al: Effects of removal of chicks from hens on concentrations of prolactin, luteinizing hormone and oestradiol in plasma of brooding Gifujidori hens. J Reprod Fertil 95:617–622, 1992.

92. El Halawani ME, Burke WH, Millam JR, et al: Regulation of prolactin and its role in gallinaceous bird reproduction. J Exp Zool 232:521–530, 1984.

93. Myers SA, Millam JR, El Halawani ME: Plasma LH and prolac-

tin levels during the reproductive cycle of the cockatiel *(Nymphus hollandicus)*. Gen Comp Endocrinol 73:85–91, 1989.

94. Book CM, Millam JR, Guinan MJ, Kitchell RL: Broodpatch innervation and its role in the onset of incubation in the turkey hen. Physiol Behav 50:281–285, 1991.

95. El Halawani ME, Silsby JL, Fehrer SC, Behnke EJ: Reinitiation of ovulatory cycles in incubating female turkeys by an inhibitor of serotonin synthesis, p-chlorophenylalanine. Biol Reprod 28:221–228, 1983.

96. El Halawani ME, Silsby JL, Rozenboim I, Pitts GR: Increased egg production by active immunization against vasoactive intestinal peptide in the turkey *(Meleagris gallopavo)*. Biol Reprod 52:179–185, 1995.

97. Millam JR, Zhang B, El Halawani ME: Number of eggs in nest influences subsequent egg production and correlates inversely with plasma prolactin concentration in cockatiels (Abstract). Annual Meeting of American Society of Zoology, San Antonio, TX, 1990.

98. Seiler HW, Gahr M, Goldsmith AR, Guttinger H-R: Prolactin and gonadal steroids during the reproductive cycle of the Bengalese finch *(Longchura striata* var. *domestica,* Estrildidae), a nonseasonal breeder with biparental care. Gen Comp Endocrinol 88:83–90, 1992.

99. Kenton B, Millam JR: Photostimulation and serum steroids of orange-winged Amazon parrots (Abstract). Proc Ann Conf Assoc Avian Vet 1994:435, 1994.

T. E. Roudybush

3

Nutrition

Nutrition is the science that interprets the relationship of food to the functioning of the living organism. The living organisms considered here are cage and aviary birds, which simplifies our task in discussing this relationship. Although the available information in this field has expanded rapidly in the last decade, it is still filled with conjecture, guesswork, and, at best, educated estimates of actual nutrient requirements.

NUTRIENTS AND REQUIREMENTS

Nutrients are simply materials that nourish the body. Essential nutrients are those that must be supplied in the diet for the normal functioning of the body. The requirement for a nutrient is based on a set of interactions between many variables such as species, physiologic state, gender, other nutrients in the diet, and environmental factors. To find the requirements of a species under all possible conditions is clearly beyond the scope of the most ambitious research efforts. For simplicity the nutrient requirements in a context of species and physiologic state are reviewed, assuming that other nutrients are available in reasonable amounts and that the environment is benign. Severe environments and disease states can push the nutrient requirements of a bird beyond that which would be considered normal.

TOXICITY AND DEFICIENCY

Toxicity and deficiency are the high and low limits on the levels of nutrients in the diet. Toxic levels of most nutrients are possible to achieve if the diet is not carefully formulated. For some nutrients that are required as a significant portion of the diet, as little as a 50% overage can result in toxicity. As a general rule, there is little room to add large excesses of the nutrients that comprise significant proportions, 0.1% or more, of the diet. Trace minerals are often toxic at 50 to 100 times the requirement. The next most potentially toxic nutrients are the fat-soluble vitamins, particularly vitamins A and D, followed by the water-soluble vitamins.

A nutrient is usually considered to be deficient in the diet when the addition, or increase in amount, of the nutrient improves performance or relieves some pathologic condition.

Nutritional imbalances occur when an excess of one nutrient interferes with the normal metabolism of another nutrient. This can be overcome by either adding the limiting nutrient or reducing the interfering nutrient. For example, when any one of the branched chain amino acids—valine, leucine, or isoleucine—is present in large excess, it interferes with the transport of the others that share the same transport mechanism. The transport mechanism is flooded by the amino acid present in excess, keeping the others from being transported. This shows up metabolically as a deficiency of the other two branched chain amino acids, because they do not reach the sites where they are needed in amounts adequate for normal metabolic processes. This competition for the common transport mechanism can be balanced either by a reduction in the amount of the amino acid present in excess or by addition of the other two.

POULTRY MODEL

The most useful and valuable information on the nutrient requirements of any bird comes from poul-

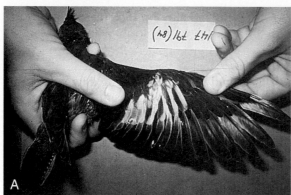
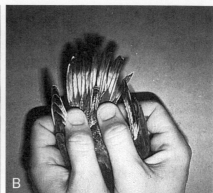

Figure 3 – 1

(A) The more distal feathers on the wing of this cockatiel show achromatosis due to a choline deficiency. Riboflavin deficiency may also produce achromatosis in growing cockatiels. *(B)* The tail feathers of the cockatiel show achromatosis due to a choline deficiency. Contour feathers do not show achromatosis.

try research. Poultry requirements have been determined over decades of research in a large number of laboratories and have been field-tested in billions of commercial and backyard birds.

The application of information from poultry to other species requires caution. The nutrients required by poultry and other birds are likely to be the same, with some minor exceptions.

Qualitatively, poultry are good models for other birds. Quantitatively, however, the requirements of other birds for a nutrient may differ markedly from the needs of poultry. For example, growing poultry require choline in relatively large amounts, but only minor amounts are required for growth in cockatiels. The signs of choline deficiency in poultry are growth retardation and perosis,[6] whereas cockatiels show only achromatosis of wing and tail feathers (Fig. 3–1).[7] Lysine deficiency in poultry results in achromatosis of the wing feathers,[6] whereas no achromatosis of any type is observed in cockatiels[8] or pigeons[9] fed lysine-deficient diets (Figs. 3–2, 3–3).

Poultry are clearly poor models for estimating the requirements of other birds for some nutrients. Water is the most critical nutrient for an animal under almost any condition. In poultry, water intake is regulated by the bird, even at hatch. In altricial birds, water and food are supplied to the chick in amounts regulated by the parent or hand-feeder. Water requirements and tolerances change with age in cockatiels, and thus water requirements must be known and followed throughout hand-feeding.[10]

Poultry are also poor models for calcium require-

ments in other birds. Even in breeding poultry, which require less calcium than birds producing table eggs, the level of calcium recommended in the diet is 2.25% or higher.[6] Cockatiels have been shown to lay large numbers of normal eggs when fed diets containing as little as 0.35% calcium.[11]

Ascorbic acid, which can be synthesized from glucose in most animals, is not required in the diets of poultry. Red-vented bulbuls, however, develop scurvy when fed diets low in ascorbic acid and recover when supplemented.[2] The willow ptarmigan requires large amounts of ascorbic acid for growth.[5]

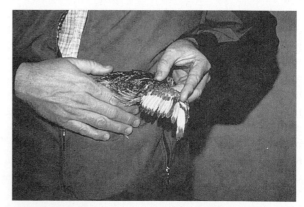

Figure 3 – 2

Achromatosis in Japanese quail fed a lysine-deficient diet. Note the one dark feather that grew after the feather it replaced was removed. Achromatosis of this type occurs in growing birds of some species, but does not occur in cockatiels or rock doves.

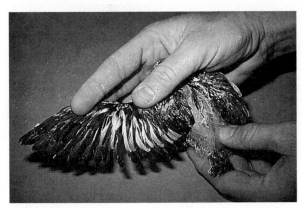

Figure 3-3

This cockatiel chick was fed deficient levels of lysine from hatch. This deficiency would have produced achromatosis in dark breeds of chickens, turkeys, and quail (see Fig. 3–2), but does not do so in cockatiels or rock doves. The white feathers that are seen are the normal white wing patch. More distal feathers show normal pigmentation.

PHYSIOLOGIC STATES

Physiologic state is a major determinant of the nutrient requirements of a bird. Normal functions of birds, such as growth and reproduction, increase nutrient needs above maintenance levels. This increased need for nutrients may not be uniform for all nutrients. For example, the increased requirement for calcium for egg-laying exceeds the increased need for other minerals. When increasing the nutrient levels of the diet, specific effects of the physiologic state must be considered.

Reproduction

The degree of nutritional stress faced by a bird when it produces eggs is directly related to the number of eggs produced. In many species the number of eggs laid at any one time is small, and nutrients can likely be taken from body stores. With sustained egg production the stress is greater. In cockatiels fed seed diets, supplementation was necessary to continue high levels of production for more than 2 weeks and to maintain hatchability.[13] If cockatiels are stimulated to lay for more than 2 weeks, body stores of vitamins are depleted. When cockatiels were fed diets low in calcium, hens laid two to four eggs of normal shell thickness and shell

conductance before both parameters deteriorated.[11] Again, body stores were depleted. This shows that the nutrients needed for more than four eggs are not stored by cockatiels and that nutrition is important when even this small number of eggs is laid. Eggs that are laid by hens experiencing a deficiency of vitamins due to an unsupplemented seed diet would be expected to experience mortality in the middle one-third of incubation.

Nutritional requirements for the chick are higher than for the adult that feeds it. Diets fed to adults while they are rearing chicks must be formulated to meet the requirements of the chick.

Growth

With the exception of certain disease states, the greatest nutritional stress that most birds will experience is that of growth. Growth, unlike sustained egg production, cannot be stopped before completion without the potential for permanent damage to the bird.

Stunting can occur when growth is limited, and stunting has been produced in cockatiels fed low-protein diets.[10] The shape of the growth curve is important even if birds appear to be normal. Cockatiels that grow slowly to their 5-week body weights experience difficulty weaning, may fail to wean, or may fail to balance food and water intakes. Cockatiels younger than 1 week of age appear unable to mobilize body tissue in the face of inadequate food intake.[13] When fed a diet devoid of protein, these chicks did not lose weight but maintained their weights until death. In precocial chicks, a loss of one-third to one-half of their initial weight would be expected before death. These observations point out the usefulness of growth data.

In fast-growing species, daily weight records are needed. Altricial chicks that fail to grow are often in as much physiologic stress as are precocial chicks during weight loss.

Body weight data can demonstrate a problem long before other clinical signs are apparent. Physical and developmental parameters can also be observed to determine whether birds are growing at a reasonable rate. Psittacine chicks that are roughly halfway between hatch and peak body weight should have plump wings and feet. Chicks fed deficient diets do not. The shape of the growth curve is also an indicator of proper growth. Altricial chicks grow rapidly, exhibiting almost linear growth until they reach peak body weight. They then experience a small decline in weight before weaning. If the overshoot is not present or the growth phase is not linear, there are problems during growth. Standard growth curves for a variety of species of birds would be useful for evaluating the growth of chicks under a variety of conditions. Data need to be maintained so that an increasing number of such growth curves can become available.

Feed efficiency can be used to evaluate the adequacy of the diet. Chicks that are offered balanced diets in adequate amounts efficiently use the food they ingest to gain weight; the amount of feed needed for each unit of gain is small. Chicks fed deficient diets use food inefficiently; their rate of gain is low, and the amount of food needed to produce a unit of gain is high. To evaluate the diet, it is necessary to measure feed efficiency, supplement the diet, and remeasure feed efficiency. If feed efficiency improves, the diet was deficient.

Columbiformes are unique among birds because parents produce crop milk. Crop milk is rich in fat and protein and low in carbohydrate, unlike the seeds and grains that form the basis of most dove and pigeon diets. When squab are taken to hand-rear, the chicks frequently die with impacted guts as a result of the accumulation of undigested complex carbohydrates. When squab are fed a diet containing no complex carbohydrates, this does not occur.[25]

Maintenance

Maintenance of adult birds is the least demanding physiologic state a bird experiences. For each calorie of intake, the adult has the lowest requirement for essential nutrients. In some cases, the absence of a nutrient may result in no clinical signs for years. The absence of vitamin B_{12} in humans has been shown to take as long as 13 years to result in clinical signs.

At the other end of the nutritional spectrum is the problem of nutritional excess. There is little evidence to demonstrate the long-term effects of moderate levels of most nutrients during maintenance, but it is reasonable to reduce those nutrients that may result in stress if they are above adequate

levels. Protein can be reduced to 6 to 8% of the diet in birds if the amino acid profile is balanced.[13] A level of 10 to 12% is commonly used for birds fed a seed diet. This is substantially lower than the 20% protein used in growing birds and may be helpful in limiting kidney stress in adults. Calcium and other minerals may also need to be limited, but exact levels have not been determined. There is some evidence that calcium levels as low as 0.1% are safe.

THE NUTRIENTS

Energy

Energy is not a specific nutrient, because it is not present in the diet as a specific chemical compound. But energy is essential and is present as substrates that are metabolized to yield compounds needed to drive cellular reactions. The ratios of dietary components determine energy concentration in the diet, allowing regulation of dietary energy density. Birds regulate food intake to obtain required energy. Dietary composition will regulate energy intake only when the energy density of the diet is so low that the bird is unable to ingest and digest enough food to maintain its normal energy intake.

There are three major sources of energy in the diet—fat, carbohydrate, and protein. They yield respectively 9.0, 4.0, and 4.0 kilocalories of metabolizable energy per gram. Metabolizable energy is the gross energy of food minus the energy lost in feces, urine, and expelled gases. It represents the amount of energy that can be extracted from food minus the amount of energy excreted in byproducts produced in the metabolism of the food. The major byproduct in birds is uric acid or urate, which is formed from the excretion of nitrogen from protein.

Because the bird regulates food intake with energy density, intake of any nutrient is regulated by that energy density and the concentration of the nutrient in the diet. Therefore, a diet that is high in energy (i.e., high in fat) must also be high in all other essential nutrients to be adequate. For example, a diet containing 20% protein and 3.75% fat was found to be adequate for growth in cockatiels.[10] To maintain the amount of protein per calorie in the diet at a constant level, more protein needs to be added to the diet as fat is increased and carbohydrate is decreased. When the amount of carbohydrate nears zero and the amount of fat reaches 60%, protein needs to be increased to 30% of the diet to maintain adequacy. Protein is then increased 1.5 times. All other essential nutrients would need to be increased by the same factor to maintain their original calorie-to-nutrient ratios.

Carbohydrate

Carbohydrate has been shown to be essential in the diets of chickens.[15, 16] The requirement is low, and a deficiency in birds fed a practical diet is unlikely. The glycerol moiety of triglycerides in the fat of the diet is used to form glucose by gluconeogenesis and is adequate to supply most of the carbohydrate needed if no other source of carbohydrate is present.

Protein

The requirement for protein is actually the requirement for the amino acids contained in the protein. This requirement can be broken down into two components: (1) the essential amino acids that the bird either cannot make or cannot make fast enough to meet its needs, and (2) the nonessential amino acids or enough amino nitrogen to synthesize them. A diet must supply all of the essential amino acids needed for that stage of the bird's life. The rest can be supplied by almost any combination of amino acids or amino nitrogen.

To simplify the concept of protein and amino acid requirement, the term "protein requirement" is often used, assuming that the amino acid profile of the protein contains enough essential amino acids to meet the requirements of the bird. This is often not the case. Meeting the protein requirements of a bird requires careful formulation. In most feedstuffs there is a limiting essential amino acid, resulting in a deficiency even when the total protein requirement is met. In some proteins there is more than one limiting amino acid, and each one must be considered. In the feedstuffs usually used for birds, the common limiting amino acids are lysine, methionine, and tryptophan (Fig. 3–4). They must be supplemented either by mixing complementary proteins or by adding the pure amino acid. Lysine

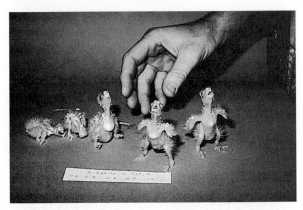

F i g u r e 3 – 4

Cockatiel chicks respond to increasing levels of dietary lysine until a level of 0.8% is reached. Further increases do not enhance growth. These chicks were fed a diet containing crystalline amino acids instead of protein and are not robust as would be expected of birds fed adequate protein. Even though the chicks suffered from acid-base balance problems and high osmotic pressures across the gut, they did respond to lysine in the diet.

and methionine are both available in the pure form for use in feeds. Tryptophan has recently become available, and its use in feed formulation is beginning.

Fat

Fat is essential in the diets of birds that have been tested. The requirement is small, and deficiency is unlikely in a practical diet (Fig. 3–5). The addition of fat to the diet to supply energy is common and affects the palatability, texture, and the bird's intake of the diet.

Vitamins

Vitamins are organic trace nutrients that have either cofactor or hormone functions in the body. The possible exception to this is vitamin E, which acts primarily as an antioxidant, although it is thought to have other functions. Vitamins have traditionally been divided into fat- and water-soluble groups, because this difference in solubility results in greater storage times in the fat-soluble vitamins. The vitamins that act as hormones in some of their functions are fat-soluble.

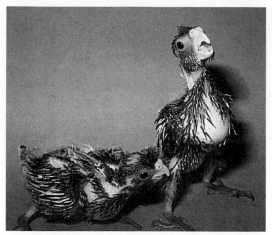

F i g u r e 3 – 5

Chicks fed differing levels of fat in the diet did not differ in growth rate if the ratio of calories to essential nutrients was not varied. The chick on the left was fed over 63% fat, whereas the chick on the right was fed 3.75% fat.

Fat-soluble Vitamins

The fat-soluble vitamins are so named because of their solubility in lipid. By attaching these vitamins to dextran, they can be made dispersible in water. Sometimes these are erroneously called the "water-soluble form." The resulting mix can be clear or cloudy and often colors the drinking water.

Unlike water-soluble vitamins, some fat-soluble vitamins have essential functions besides cofactor functions.

Vitamin A. Vitamin A is a fat-soluble vitamin found in many fruits and vegetables but missing in most seeds. Vitamin A functions as a cofactor in vision, but it also acts as a hormone, interacting directly with the genome to promote the expression of certain genes important in the normal differentiation of cells. Vitamin A deficiency often results in sinus infections. The epithelial lining of the sinus is subject to exposure to a variety of airborne pathogens. Vitamin A deficiency causes squamous metaplasia of the epithelial lining, resulting in reduced ability to resist pathogen colonization.

Fat-soluble vitamins are stored in the liver. These vitamins must be mobilized from their stores to be useful to the bird. In one preliminary experiment, cockatiels that were abruptly changed from a high vitamin A diet to a low vitamin A diet died with levels of liver vitamin A comparable to those of control birds that had been maintained on a high vitamin A diet. The problem of mobilization of vitamin A from stores and the required frequency of supplementation deserves further study.

Vitamin D$_3$. Vitamin D$_3$ (cholecalciferol) is the form of vitamin D that is used by birds. Vitamin D$_2$ (ergocalciferol) is used by mammals but birds use it only $\frac{1}{30}$ to $\frac{1}{40}$ as well as vitamin D$_3$. Cholecalciferol is synthesized when 7-dehydrocholesterol in the skin is struck by ultraviolet light. This cholecalciferol is absorbed through the skin or ingested during preening. Under most conditions of adequate light, birds do not require vitamin D in the diet, except during growth and egg-laying. Like the steroid hormones and vitamin A in some of its functions, vitamin D acts like a hormone rather than a cofactor. It acts directly on the genome to cause the expression of specific genes that produce the proteins causing the effects of vitamin D. The net effect of vitamin D is the mineralization of bone, through a complex mechanism that involves interactions with a number of other hormones. Vitamin D deficiency during growth causes rickets, in which both the bones and the beak fail to calcify and become soft and rubbery. Adult birds produce shell-less or thin-shelled eggs. Eventually the bones of vitamin D–deficient laying hens demineralize and the birds become unable to stand as a result of osteomalacia.

Vitamin E. Vitamin E functions mainly as an antioxidant, interacting with selenium, which functions in the repair of oxidized tissues. Vitamin E and selenium spare each other in the diet and therefore need to be considered together in stating the requirement; neither can be absent from the diet. Vitamin E also functions in unknown ways unrelated to its antioxidant activity. Efforts to use antioxidants to replace the activity of vitamin E in these functions have failed. This further complicates the determination of the requirement of vitamin E.

Large amounts of polyunsaturated fat in the diet increase the vitamin E requirement. Fortunately, oilseeds, the main source of polyunsaturated fats in the diets of many birds, are also rich in vitamin E. In adult birds fed mostly seed or fruit and vegetable diets, vitamin E deficiency is unlikely. In prepared diets such as pellets and extruded diets, the level of vitamin E must be carefully maintained. Significant reductions in the cost per ton of feed can be achieved by reducing vitamin E to marginal levels.

Levels between 10 and 25 IU/kg of diet are recommended for poultry.

Signs of vitamin E deficiency in poultry include encephalomalacia, exudative diathesis, and muscular dystrophy. Because of the sparing effect of selenium on vitamin E, the level of selenium as well as the level of vitamin E should be considered in diagnosis and treatment of disorders related to vitamin E deficiency.

Vitamin K. The role of vitamin K in the clotting of blood has long been recognized. As the mechanism by which vitamin K contributes to blood clotting has become understood, other functions of vitamin K have been observed or speculated. Vitamin K is a cofactor in the post-translational carboxylation of specific glutamyl residues. The carboxylated glutamyl residues are calcium-binding, which explains the role of calcium in blood clotting. The question of whether vitamin K acts on other proteins in the same way was raised by the elucidation of this reaction. In bone matrix, at least one other reaction of this type is found. Deficiency of vitamin K has been shown to result in skeletal abnormalities in humans. The calcium-binding protein in question was first found in chicken bone; therefore, the possibility that similar skeletal abnormalities may occur in other birds is apparent.

Water-soluble Vitamins

The water-soluble vitamins, unlike the fat-soluble vitamins, are generally required in the diet because they are cofactors for enzymatic reactions essential to the normal functioning of metabolism, and because they cannot be made by the animal. Most of them have relatively short storage times, and so must be provided to the animal at regular, frequent intervals. Few of them have been studied in non-poultry bird species.

Thiamin. Vitamin B_1 was discovered using chickens as experimental animals. Thiamin is found in large amounts in grain and so is unlikely to be deficient in most practical diets. Diets containing large proportions of a polished grain such as rice may be low in thiamin and may be improved by using brown instead of white rice. In birds fed large amounts of raw fish or fish that has had an opportunity to sit without inactivation of the enzyme thiaminase, thiamin deficiency may occur.

The probability of a reduction in thiamin as a result of thiaminase activity is dependent upon a number of factors, including the species of fish fed.

Thiamin deficiency in poultry results in polyneuritis. In a single case of feeding polished rice to adult cockatiels, head tremors occurred before the experiment was discontinued. These signs were consistent with the early polyneuritic signs observed in poultry.

Riboflavin. Vitamin B_2 is often limiting in practical diets, although its relatively low price makes it unlikely to be limiting in prepared diets. Riboflavin deficiency in growing poultry is characterized by retardation of growth, diarrhea, and leg paralysis. It is often suggested that curled toe paralysis, as found in riboflavin-deficient chickens, is seen in riboflavin deficiency in other species. In preliminary work with cockatiels, chicks fed diets low in riboflavin did not show curled toe paralysis, but did show achromatosis of wing feathers. In chickens, turkeys, and quail, achromatosis has been considered pathognomonic for lysine deficiency. Achromatosis in cockatiels has not been related to lysine deficiency.

The requirement for riboflavin for normal production of eggs is higher than for maintenance. Chickens fed marginal levels of riboflavin lay reduced numbers of eggs, and the eggs experience increased mortality during the second week of incubation. In experiments with cockatiels in which pairs were fed seed mixes either unsupplemented or supplemented with multiple vitamins, eggs were removed for artificial incubation to encourage laying. Unsupplemented pairs laid fewer eggs beginning the second week of production, and hatchability was significantly lower. In seed diets fed to laying birds, riboflavin is likely to be limiting.

Niacin. Niacin deficiency—pellagra or "black tongue disease" in chickens—is historically associated with corn diets. The niacin in corn is bound, making it unavailable for absorption from the gut, and corn is relatively low in tryptophan, which can act as a precursor of niacin. Pellagra has also been associated with diets high in millet, owing to high levels of the amino acid leucine. Leucine at high levels interferes with the conversion of tryptophan to niacin. Diets high in corn or millet need to be supplemented with niacin.

Biotin. Biotin deficiency, like niacin deficiency, is associated with particular cereals, wheat and barley. Biotin deficiency is implicated in fatty liver and kidney syndrome, which has caused mortality as high as 30% in chickens fed diets based on wheat or barley. This problem is easily overcome by supplementation. Mold in the diet may increase the requirement for biotin, possibly by the production of antimetabolites. In addition, rancid dietary fat may increase the need for dietary biotin by destruction of the vitamin.

The signs of biotin deficiency are complex and variable. In chicks dermatitis of the feet, necrosis of the toes, mandibular lesions, and swollen eyelids are seen. Both poults and chicks may show hock problems with bending of the metatarsus. Embryos from biotin-deficient eggs show micromelia, syndactyly, and parrot beak.

Folic Acid. Folic acid functions in single carbon metabolism, but is of great interest in birds as a cofactor in the synthesis of purines. Uric acid, the main purine synthesized by birds, is the avian vehicle for the excretion of nitrogen. Folic acid is found in many foods, but diets for cage and aviary birds may fail to include these foods. Deficient growing chickens show slow growth, poor feathering, failure of feathers to pigment normally, and anemia. Folic acid deficiency reduces egg production and hatchability. Embryos show bending of the tibiotarsus, defects of the mandible, syndactyly, and hemorrhages.

Vitamin B$_{12}$. Vitamin B$_{12}$ is not found in significant quantities in plants and so was called the "animal protein factor." It is stored for long periods of time (years in some cases) in the liver.

Vitamin B$_{12}$ is required for maximal growth in chickens and turkeys. Deficiency results in anemia and gizzard erosion. Perosis and fatty heart, liver, and kidney may also occur. Vitamin B$_{12}$–deficient eggs hatch poorly. Embryos show hemorrhages and edema. Some birds may obtain part of their vitamin B$_{12}$ from bacterial synthesis in the gut, but this source is neither consistent nor reliable. Birds should have supplemental vitamin B$_{12}$, particularly when fed diets containing only plant materials.

Pantothenic Acid. Pantothenic acid is a component of coenzyme A, which acts as an acyl carrier in metabolism. When coenzyme A is ingested, it is digested and the free pantothenic acid is absorbed and incorporated into new coenzyme A. Pantothenic acid that is not incorporated into coenzyme A is quickly eliminated in the urine. Pantothenic acid is found in adequate amounts in seeds and is unlikely to be deficient in most practical diets.

Pantothenic acid deficiency in poultry results in growth retardation and ragged feathering. At 12 to 14 days dermatitis is apparent. The dermatitis is seldom as severe as in a biotin deficiency. In cockatiels fed a diet low in pantothenic acid, mortality frequently occurred abruptly near the age of maximal growth, about 3 to $3\frac{1}{2}$ weeks of age. Chicks that survived had a complete absence of feathers on the body but normal feathering on the wings and tail (Fig. 3–6). Cockatiel chicks fed diets essentially devoid of pantothenic acid died within 7 to 10 days of hatch.[13] Pantothenic acid–deficient chicken eggs exhibit significant embryo mortality during the last few days of incubation. Chicks that do hatch are frequently too weak to survive.

Pyridoxine. Vitamin B$_6$ is essential in a number of reactions related to nitrogen or amino acid metabolism. A deficiency of pyridoxine is unlikely when birds are fed a practical diet.

Growing chickens deficient in pyridoxine show reduced appetite, neurologic signs, and slow growth. Chicks become excitable, showing random running accompanied by constant cheeping and convulsions. These violent convulsions lead to exhaustion and death.

Ascorbic Acid. Ascorbic acid or vitamin C is among the most interesting of the vitamins in avian nutrition. Ascorbic acid is essential as a cofactor in a large number of enzymatic reactions. Hemorrhage, the classic sign of scurvy, is the result of the inability to maintain collagen and elastin in blood vessel walls because of the lack of ascorbic acid as a cofactor. Most animals do not require dietary ascorbic acid. It appears that most birds and mammals can make ascorbic acid from glucose and that those species that require dietary ascorbic acid have lost this ability.

In mammals, there is a clear taxonomic relationship between the requirement for ascorbic acid and the degree of evolution of the animal.[3] In birds a similar relationship exists. Those birds that are thought to require ascorbic acid in the diet are all passerines[1–4] except one—the willow ptarmigan, a galliform.[5] This illustrates that any particular species must be tested to see if it requires ascorbic acid.

Ascorbic acid is safe to use, so in doubtful situations it should be administered. Species that have been shown to require ascorbic acid include the

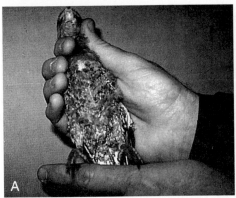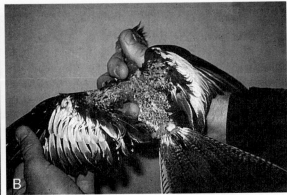

Figure 3-6

(A) This newly weaned cockatiel was exposed to a mild pantothenic acid deficiency during growth. At weaning it was fed a diet adequate in pantothenic acid. All the feather growth on the body was the result of that week of feeding adequate pantothenic acid. *(B)* The back of the cockatiel.

willow ptarmigan[5] and the red-vented bulbul.[2] Suspect species are the other bulbuls, and the more evolved passerines.[1, 3, 4] Species that do not appear to require ascorbic acid include chickens, turkeys, quail, cockatiels, Alexandrine parakeets, hummingbirds, ducks, geese, partridge, and pheasants. Individual species may require ascorbic acid in the diet, although they are represented in the groups listed above.

Minerals

Minerals in feed formulation must be carefully regulated and evaluated for possible interactions with other nutrients and to avoid toxic levels. Although vitamins and many of the minerals are trace nutrients, they must be considered in quite different ways in the diet. Vitamins are susceptible to destruction primarily by oxidation. Minerals are difficult to destroy and suffer either from binding to some matrix such as a chelate or another mineral (which makes them unavailable) or from dietary imbalances that interfere with their absorption or transport within the body. Mineral levels must be carefully controlled because of their relative toxicity. Minerals fed at 50 to 100 times the requirement may cause clinical signs in birds. Vitamins are usually at least 100 times less toxic and so can be added in large excess and still have a good margin of safety.

Calcium

The requirement for calcium in the diets of birds under maintenance conditions is controversial. Although levels as high as 1.0% of the diet have been recommended, no published experiments support this recommendation. In *Nutrient Requirements of Poultry,* even growing birds are fed as little as 0.55% calcium and birds under holding conditions between bouts of laying are fed as little as 0.5% calcium.[6] Nonlaying hens maintained calcium balance on as little as 0.02% calcium,[17] and male chickens maintained balance on less, although the authors concluded that 0.02% calcium was adequate. Until more data are available, a level of 0.1% calcium appears to be adequate.[18]

There is no evidence for a requirement of more than 1.0% calcium for laying in most cage and aviary birds. In experiments with cockatiels, 0.35% calcium was found to be adequate to maintain shell thickness, conductance, and egg production compared with these factors in birds fed higher or lower levels of calcium.[11] In chronic layers, a level of 0.35% calcium is recommended to maintain bone integrity if laying cannot be stopped.

A level of 0.9% calcium appears to be adequate for growth if balanced with 0.6% available phosphorus. There are no controlled studies verifying this, but many birds have been raised on 1.0% calcium without bone abnormalities. Toxic levels of calcium occur at levels only slightly above the requirement in birds that have been tested. In various experiments levels of 1.2%,[19] 1.35%,[20] and 2.5% all were shown to result in poorer performance than lower levels of calcium in growing chickens. A level of 2.5%[19] calcium resulted in high morbidity and mortality in pullets between 8 and 20 weeks of age.[19] The calcium intake of growing cage and aviary birds should probably be limited to no more than 1.2% of the diet unless specifically indicated by unique conditions.

Phosphorus

The requirement for phosphorus in the avian diet is closely coupled with that of calcium. With the exception of egg-laying birds, the ratio of calcium to available phosphorus should be 2:1 within relatively narrow bounds. In the case of laying poultry, the level of available phosphorus in the diet should not exceed 0.8%.

Levels higher than this are toxic, independent of the level of calcium. Phosphorus availability in plant sources is variable depending upon the major form of the organically bound phosphorus. Generally, phosphorus from plant sources is 30 to 40% available.

Sodium

Sodium in the diet is frequently reduced to minimal levels to reduce moisture in the feces. Because the level of sodium in most feedstuffs is low compared to the requirements of poultry, there is the possibility of a deficiency. In poultry a sodium deficiency results in decreased egg production, poor growth, and cannibalism.

Potassium

Potassium is not likely to be deficient in most practical diets because of its high level in most feedstuffs. Deficiency of potassium in poultry diets results in high mortality and retarded growth of chicks. It causes reduced egg production and decreased shell thickness in laying hens.

Copper

Copper is a cofactor in the crosslinking of lysine residues in elastin. Dissecting aneurysm of the aorta, microcytic hypochromic anemia, and cardiac hypertrophy can occur in copper deficiency. Bone deformities have been observed, and New Hampshire and Rhode Island red chickens have been shown to have reduced feather pigmentation.

Iodine

Iodine is essential for synthesis of thyroid hormones. An iodine deficiency can result in goiter and reduction in the production of thyroid hormones, which leads to poor growth and egg production and smaller egg size. Laying hens fed low iodine diets produce low iodine eggs, which have low hatchability, and possibly embryos with goiter.

Selenium

Selenium is required in the diet even in the presence of large amounts of vitamin E. Low selenium diets can result in poor growth and increased mortality of chicks. The level of selenium in grains varies with the selenium content of the soils in which the grains are grown. Selenium supplementation of feeds is regulated by federal laws limiting the amount of selenium that can be added and the concentration of the supplement to be used.

Iron

Most grains are adequate in iron for growth in poultry. The level of 350 ppm iron in corn is several times the requirement of 40 to 80 ppm iron for growing poultry. The problem of excess iron in the diets of some birds still requires research to determine the actual maximal tolerance level of iron. A maximum of 100 ppm has been suggested, but experimental feeding of various levels of iron has not yet confirmed that dietary iron level is closely associated with iron storage disease. Iron deficiency results in microcytic, hypochromic anemia. In red-feathered chickens, a deficiency of iron results in a failure to deposit normal red pigments.[21]

Manganese

Manganese deficiency in poults and chicks results in perosis. Deficiencies of choline or biotin may play a role in perosis, and thus the signs of manganese deficiency may be complicated by nutrient interactions. Excess dietary calcium or phosphorus may also complicate a manganese deficiency by reducing the absorption of manganese. In laying birds, a manganese deficiency results in reduced egg production and shell strength. Eggs hatch poorly and embryos exhibit shortening of the long bones, parrot beak, and wiry down. Many feedstuffs are low in manganese compared with the requirement for growth in poultry. Unsupplemented diets may result in a deficiency of manganese.

Magnesium

Magnesium is found in more than adequate amounts in most feedstuffs, rendering a deficiency unlikely. High levels of calcium and phosphorus can reduce absorption of magnesium and produce or exacerbate deficiencies. Chicks deficient in magnesium show lethargy and poor growth. At some levels of magnesium, chicks show neuromuscular signs, leading to convulsions and a comatose state. In laying hens, magnesium deficiency results in poor egg production, poor hatchability, and eventually a comatose state.

Zinc

Zinc has a large number of cofactor functions that are essential to normal metabolism. A zinc deficiency results in retarded growth and frayed feathers in growing birds. The long bones of the legs and wings are shorter and thicker than normal with a thickening of the hock joint. Laying hens fed zinc-deficient diets have reduced egg production and hatchability. Embryos from zinc-deficient eggs have a wide variety of skeletal abnormalities.

Chlorine

Chlorine is unlikely to be deficient because of its relatively high concentration in feedstuffs used in practical diets. The main function of chlorine is in acid-base balance, in which it is balanced against bicarbonate to maintain the proper pH. Chlorine deficiency results in mortality, hemoconcentration, and poor growth. Chlorine-deficient chicks show a nervous condition resembling tetany, and they fall forward when stimulated by a sharp noise.

PROPERTIES OF SPECIFIC FEEDSTUFFS

A large variety of feedstuffs are used in the feeding of cage and aviary birds. These feedstuffs cannot be examined exhaustively in the space offered here, but some of the properties of concern can be reviewed in a general way.

Simple Sugars

Simple sugars fed to carnivorous birds that subsist mainly on fat and protein for their energy may lead to elevated blood sugar levels. Whether this is acceptable or not depends on the situation and on the biology of the bird, but clearly it is a nutritional consideration.

Simple sugars offer a ready substrate for *Candida* growth. In general, the use of simple sugars should be minimized to reduce *Candida* infection; however, birds such as hummingbirds, lories, and sunbirds tolerate and even seem to require large amounts of sugar in their normal metabolism. In each case the biology of the bird must be considered before choosing a specific diet.

Some sources of simple sugars commonly used in diets are sugar (sucrose), corn syrup, honey, molasses, jellies and jams, punch and juices, and a variety of foods prepared for human consumption.

Milk Products

Milk products can be either a concentrated source of essential nutrients or a source of dietary problems.

Lactose is a specific product of mammals and as such had not been ingested by birds until humans made milk available to them in large amounts during this century. Birds that have been tested cannot digest lactose and suffer from diarrhea when the diet reaches a level of 10 to 30% on a dry weight basis. Thus, lactose in milk products should be avoided when possible. When a milk product is used, the total amount of lactose in the diet should be limited.

Some of the milk products that contain significant amounts of lactose include dried skim milk, which is 50% lactose and dried whey, which can reach 70% lactose. These and other milk products provide protein and trace nutrients that can enhance marginal diets. In these cases they can be useful supplements, but in most cases other sources of the missing nutrients can be found and offer safer methods of supplementation.

Some milk products contain little or no lactose. Cheese manufacturing extracts the fat, protein, and some of the trace nutrients from milk, leaving most of the lactose in the whey. Yogurt is fermented milk in which the lactose has been converted to lactate. In experiments with dried skim milk and dried yogurt, the performance of chickens was improved when yogurt was used instead of milk.[22]

Animal Byproducts

Animal byproducts include processed whole animals or animal parts. Some of the common products are meat meal, fish meal, meat and bone scraps, fish solubles, blood meal, feather meal, and bone meal. Animal byproducts are frequently used in the commercial feed industry as inexpensive sources of well-balanced protein, phosphorus, and other trace nutrients. They are generally produced by a cooking process that renders the product sterile at the end of manufacture. But these products are frequently sources of pathogen contamination resulting from recontamination after cooking. The raw materials from which they are made are usually high in pathogens.[23] Rendering plants are not usually run in such a way as to prohibit human and machine traffic between the finished product and the raw material brought in for rendering. In surveys of such products, as much as 80% has been found to contain significant numbers of pathogens. This industry is largely unregulated, and finished products are not tested for contamination. Until verifiably clean supplies of the products can be obtained, animal byproducts should be considered sources of contamination in feeds.

Seeds

Seeds have historically been used as the major food of a variety of birds and were considered adequate for maintenance and, in some cases, for breeding birds. Seeds can be part of a balanced diet for most cage and aviary birds, but they require supplementation to avoid nutritional disease.

Oil Seeds

Oil seeds are so named because most contain 50% fat or more. They are a rich source of energy, which can be beneficial if the bird is active or kept in cold conditions (Fig. 3–7). In sedentary birds this high fat level can result in obesity. The high fat dilutes the rest of the nutrients and the bird, eating for energy, may reduce consumption, resulting in nutritional deficiencies. High levels of polyunsaturated fat in the diet also increase the need for vitamin E, but oil seeds are rich sources of vitamin E.

Safflower seeds have a seed rich in fat and protein like the other oil seeds. Safflower is more bitter than the other oil seeds. It has frequently been considered to be a better seed than sunflower, because it was thought that sunflower seeds contain papaverine. In fact, neither safflower nor sunflower seeds contain papaverine.

Sunflower seeds have long been used to feed a variety of birds. In some cases they are the main source or sole source of food. Sunflower seeds are high in fat and can lead to obesity. Sunflower seeds of various cultivars have different levels of fat. As a

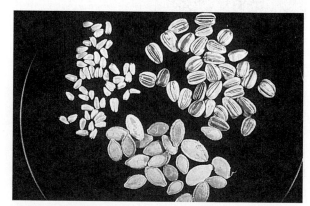

F i g u r e 3 – 7

Oil seeds. Left, safflower; right, sunflower; bottom, pumpkin.

general rule, the darker the sunflower seed the more fat it contains. Although the protein in sunflower seeds is relatively well balanced, a diet composed predominantly of sunflower seeds does not provide adequate, balanced nutrition.

Peanuts are another oil seed commonly fed to birds. Like other oil seeds, peanuts are a rich source of energy, which can lead to dietary imbalances. Peanuts are highly susceptible to mycotoxin contamination due to growth conditions in the field. Peanuts sold for human consumption must meet Food and Drug Administration (FDA) requirements of less than 20 parts per billion of aflatoxin. Peanuts sold for pet consumption are less subject to regulation and are thus more likely to be contaminated.

Non-oil Seeds

The other seeds commonly fed to birds might be called the non-oil seeds. These seeds store most of their energy as starch and are thus lower in energy and protein. This may result in a similar calorie-to-protein ratio as in oil seeds.

Various types of millet are used in seed mixes. Millet is inexpensive and readily available (Fig. 3–8). It is too low in total protein and several other essential nutrients for growing birds.

Canary seed is commonly used to increase the amount of protein in the mix. Canary seed appears to be high in protein, but some of the analyses of

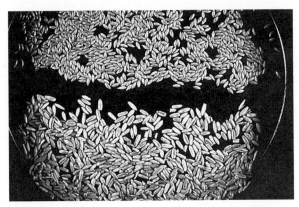

F i g u r e   3 – 9

(Bottom) Oat groats (hulled oats). *(Top)* Canary seed. The occasional rough smaller seed in the canary seed is a canary seed missing the hull.

canary seed differ in their results. For such a common seed it is poorly characterized.

Hulled oats or oat groats, ranging from 15 to 17.5% protein, are also used to increase protein in a seed mix (Fig. 3–9). Being a common feedstuff for domestic animals, they are readily available.

Limiting Nutrients

Most seeds are deficient in some essential nutrients. Vitamin B_{12} is low or absent in almost all plant materials. In the seeds used in most seed mixes, the following vitamins are usually limiting: riboflavin, niacin (except in sunflower seeds), folic acid, vitamin A, and, in cases where it is needed, ascorbic acid. The most limiting amino acids in most seeds are lysine, methionine, and tryptophan. The minerals likely to be limiting in seeds are calcium, manganese, sodium, and, in some cases, copper, zinc, iodine, and selenium.

Annual Harvest

Most seeds are harvested annually, leading to a cycle of progressively older seeds until the next harvest. At some time during the year at least a portion of the seeds in a seed mix are 1 year old or older. The nutrients that are most affected by aging are the vitamins, which lose activity owing to oxidation, and fat, which becomes rancid. This aging

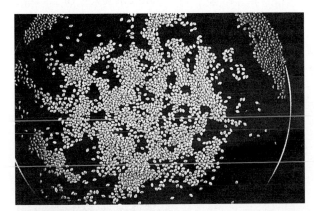

F i g u r e   3 – 8

Red millet and other millets are common seeds in seed mixes. They are non-oil seeds rich in carbohydrates and relatively low in protein. They require supplementation to assure adequacy even in adult diets.

process can lead to reduced nutrient concentration, usually depleting the most easily oxidized nutrients first. Oxidation can be limited by reducing temperature and oxygen in the storage environment. This is seldom done in bulk storage. Packaging seeds for freshness is effective only after the seeds enter the package. Seed that is 1 year old will not improve by being maintained in a nitrogen atmosphere or held at low temperatures. The practice of packaging old seed in freshness packaging to reduce oxidation is questionable. This type of packaging can, however, reduce the possibility of insect infestation.

Insects that infest feed are of little importance to the health of the bird, but are pests in the home or aviary. Two of the most common insect problems are *Tribolium,* a flour beetle, and moths—the Indian meal moth and the Mediterranean flour moth. *Tribolium* can be controlled by freezing, which kills it, or by fumigating feed with commercial safe fumigants or with carbon dioxide in the form of dry ice. *Tribolium* often survives refrigerator temperatures or carbon dioxide atmospheres maintained in polyethylene bags. Polyethylene allows exchange of gases with the atmosphere, causing carbon dioxide to be lost and oxygen to replace it in the bag.

The Indian meal moth and the Mediterranean flour moth both infest feed by laying eggs near the surface. The eggs hatch into caterpillars. The caterpillars move about in the feed, leaving a silk thread trailing behind them. This thread then binds the feed into lumps, often referred to as webby feed. The webs can clog small bulk-style feeders and deprive the bird of food. These moth larvae can be controlled by the same measures as for *Tribolium* and by the use of *Bacillus thuriengiensis* (BT) spores. BT spores germinate in the guts of caterpillars and eventually kill them. Birds fed BT or fed caterpillars infected with BT are unaffected.

BT is applied as a wettable suspension, Dipel, most commonly available as a product used in gardens. To treat 50 pounds of feed, 1 heaping tablespoon of Dipel is mixed with about one-half cup of water. This mixture is misted onto the feed and mixed by hand. This does not cause molding of the feed unless the feed is already near the level of moisture required to grow mold.

Sprouted Seeds

Many aviculturists like to feed sprouted seeds to their birds, mainly because most birds seem to rel-

ish them. Germination does affect the nutrition of the seed, and research shows that the effects vary with different species of seed. The most consistent changes are a decrease in phytate phosphorus, an increase in available phosphorus, and increased protein digestibility. Increases and decreases in vitamin and mineral levels appear to be highly dependent on species studied.[26–30] The decrease in phytate phosphorus may be significant to mineral and protein utilization. High levels of phytate phosphorus interfere with availability of calcium, magnesium, zinc, iron, and protein because of the formation of insoluble complexes that are not readily absorbed. Sprouted seeds can be an important source of microbial contamination unless antimicrobial agents are used in the sprouting medium. Chlorine at 50 ppm has been shown to reduce contamination.[31]

Fruits and Vegetables

Fruits and vegetables vary in composition, but they are generally high in water and trace nutrients and low in energy. They supply the nutrients that are likely to be low in seed diets while not diluting the diet with excess calories. Feeding fruits and vegetables can create a sanitation problem because fruits spoil easily and offer a substrate for *Candida* growth under some conditions.

Manufactured Foods

Feeding manufactured foods to birds has recently become an increasingly popular practice. The benefits and problems of these feeds must be understood.

The most important issue of a manufactured food is whether it is eaten. In the section on feeding behaviors, the conversion of a bird from one food to another is discussed. Birds familiar with seeds may not initially recognize pellets as food.

Assuming that the food is eaten, the next most important consideration is the composition of the food. Manufactured foods offer the ability to control the composition of the diet, and the bird no longer has the option to choose among many foods offered. The manufactured food should be formulated based on what is known about cage and aviary bird nutrition and other avian (usually poultry) nutrition. Treats that may upset the balance of the manufactured food should be limited; only small amounts of a high-energy treat may be offered, whereas a much larger amount of a low-energy treat may be offered.

Pellets

Pellets are one type of manufactured food, produced by steam cooking a mash and forcing it through a die to produce the pellet. High temperatures and pressures kill most of the bacteria present, but the feed is not sterilized and thus care must be taken to start with uncontaminated ingredients. Vitamin and mineral premixes are used to provide nutrients that are low in the major feedstuffs included in the formulation. Pellets can be crumbled between rollers to break them down to sizes that can be consumed by small birds. The crumbles can be screened to select a range of sizes for birds of various sizes. The feed can then be packaged and shipped without the long storage that can occur with seeds.

Extruded Products

Extruded products are similar to pellets except that they are subjected to higher temperatures and pressures and must be ground much finer for extrusion. The greater energy required for manufacture results in higher costs. The energy content of extruded diets can be slightly higher than that of pelleted diets using the same mash composition.

BEHAVIOR AND FOOD

Behavior is a basic aspect of nutrition. The only nutrients that are available to a bird are those that it chooses to consume. Diets that allow the bird to selectively consume food items with different nutrient values are possibly the most common source of malnutrition seen today. The interaction of diet and food consumption needs to be understood before a balanced feeding program can be instituted or a current feeding program can be evaluated.

Chick Feeding

Budgerigars have been shown to feed their chicks in order from youngest to oldest during a single feeding.[24] The reason for this behavioral adaptation was at first obscure, but when the need for higher proportions of water in the diets of younger chicks was shown,[10] it became apparent. Many altricial birds such as the budgerigar consume food and water that they store in their crops and later regurgitate for their chicks. This food is the sole source of nutrition for the chicks and must include the proper proportions of each nutrient, if the chicks are to grow to their potential. How parents achieve this balance is not understood in detail for any nutrient, but the method by which parents deliver the proper proportions of water is partially understood. The crop is a dilation of the esophagus that holds food and water until they either are passed into the gut or are regurgitated for feeding. The food in the crop settles as it sits and stratifies into layers that contain more water at the top and less water near the bottom. By feeding the youngest chick first, the parent takes the water-rich layers off the top of the crop first and ensures that the youngest chicks receive the highest proportions of water from the material in the crop. It is not known whether parents regulate the ratio of food to water as the chicks grow or whether the increased capacity of the chicks to receive food causes the stratification of the contents of the crop to become insignificant in older chicks.

Chicks seek food by begging. This behavior stimulates the parent to seek and deliver food to the chick. Observations made during experiments to determine protein requirements in cockatiels[10] indicate that begging behavior is one of the possible signs of the adequacy of a diet for chicks.[13] Chicks that were fed diets containing 10% or 15% protein begged more frequently and more vigorously than chicks that received an adequate diet containing 20% protein. Chicks that received a diet containing 35% protein rejected feeding and regurgitated food at many feedings, particularly when chicks had reached peak body weight. Caution must be used, however, in assuming that feed rejection or regurgitation indicates that a diet is toxic. There are other causes of diet rejection, such as shrinkage of the crop at peak body weight, disease, environmental changes, improper food temperature, and weaning.

As a chick grows, it goes through stages in which the incidence and vigor of begging change. When a chick reaches peak body weight, the capacity of the crop is reduced and meal size must be reduced to compensate.[13] Many hand-feeders do not observe this change because chicks that are fed deficient diets or those that are fed less food than is needed to meet their requirements do not reach peak body weights. These birds reach weaning weights only by continuing to gain after they should have begun weight loss. Such chicks usually experience late weaning even though they reach the same weights as chicks fed adequate diets.[12] When a chick weans, it may continue to beg and to be fed by the parent or hand-feeder. These meals are not necessary but appear not to cause harm and not to inhibit weaning.

Food Acceptance

Food acceptance is of prime importance in the treatment of nutritional disease and in the management of a variety of infections treatable with antibiotics in the food or water. The ability to change the diet of a bird is an advantage under many conditions. Food recognition is the first factor in food acceptance. Food that is novel is often not recognized as food and so is not consumed. In cockatiels when their familiar food was replaced with a novel food, 90% of the birds accepted the novel food in 48 hours. The other 10% did not accept the food and further exposure did not increase acceptance. After returning the old food for 2 weeks, the birds that did not accept the food the first time were again exposed to the novel food. Of these birds, 90% accepted the new food.[13] As long as the new diet is palatable, repeated exposure is one method to cause birds to accept a new diet.

Particle size is an important consideration in the acceptance of food by a bird. If particles are too large, small birds will not be able to ingest the food and will starve to death. Larger particles may be fed to larger birds, but are not needed. In cockatiels, the particle size that resulted in the least amount of waste was the smallest size that the cockatiels would consume.

Birds are often classified according to their feeding habits as being carnivorous, omnivorous, or granivorous. Some omnivorous and granivorous birds change their feeding habits when feeding chicks. Cockatiels that did not eat bread when not raising chicks readily ate bread when they were feeding chicks.[13] This plasticity of food intake can be used to advantage when changing the food of birds. Novel foods that are more readily accepted during chick feeding can be maintained in feeders, and old foods can be allowed to become diminishing portions of the diet.

Palatability of food for birds is poorly understood. It does not appear that there is any general food type or flavor that is universally accepted. In general, birds do tend to selectively eat higher fat food items. Medications in feed tend to reduce palatability.

Weaning

The weaning process is poorly understood, but a few of its characteristics have been studied in cockatiels. Weaning is a response to physiologic processes related to growth. Chicks experiencing poor growth during the weeks preceding peak body weight usually wean late, even though they have compensated for this poor growth and have reached the same preweaning weight as chicks experiencing early rapid growth.[12] The single most important aspect of weaning is that birds be allowed to grow at their potential so that the processes of maturation can occur in their normal time sequence (Figs. 3–10, 3–11).

The process of actively consuming food instead of begging is not learned. Chicks having no experience with food that is available for consumption wean as early as chicks that have had long experience with food. Of chicks that were hand-fed to the age of weaning without access to other food, one-third weaned immediately upon presentation of food that they could consume on their own.[13]

Some defects of food intake and weaning are related to poor growth during the phase of rapid growth preceding peak weight. Groups of cockatiel chicks that grew poorly had a high incidence of individuals that drank to the exclusion of eating when both food and water were available. Many chicks failed to wean and eventually died when hand-feeding was discontinued. In control chicks that were allowed to grow rapidly to their peak weights, no such problems were found.[13]

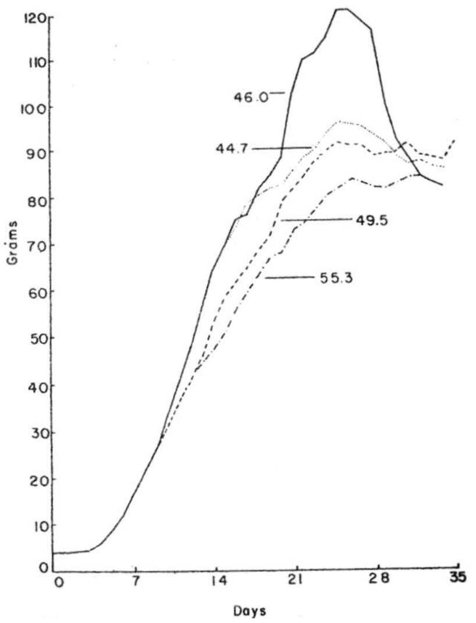

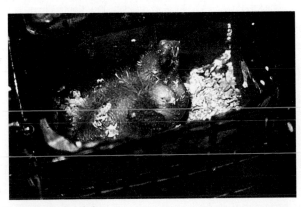

Figure 3-10

Weaning ages in days of cockatiels that grew at different rates. The differences in growth were produced by varying the rate of feed intake. Some chicks in the lower two groups failed to wean and are not included in the data.

Water Availability

Water availability is essential for feed consumption to occur. Cockatiels were observed to be weaning late on one occasion. It was found that they had not learned to use the waterer. When water was offered in a bowl instead of a waterer, the chicks ate and drank on their own.[13]

FEED STORAGE

The principle of feed storage is relatively simple: keep feed cool and dry. Mold growth can occur when feed moisture reaches 15%. Feed absorbs moisture from the air and reaches 15% moisture at an ambient humidity of 85% or higher. Moisture can also stratify in feed if air movement is low or if the feed is stored against a cool or impervious surface. In these cases, although the total moisture content of the feed is not enough to allow mold growth, local high concentrations can occur and may allow mold growth. This mold then produces more moisture as a result of the oxidation of the food.

Feed should be stored in a low humidity atmosphere, up off floors, and in areas with good air circulation. Mold inhibitors are used in some feeds to reduce the possibility of mold growth. Mold inhibitors are of variable effectiveness, depending on both their composition and environmental conditions. At best, they can be expected to reduce or delay mold growth. Proper storage is still essential.

Another method to reduce mold growth and other types of feed spoilage is keeping feed cool. Feed will keep twice as long at 20°C as it will at 30°C, four times as long as at 40°C, eight times as long as at 50°C, and so on. Nutrients such as polyunsaturated fats and vitamins will be preserved longer if kept cool.

Antioxidants are another tool in the preservation of feed. They interrupt the oxidation of nutrients and are oxidized themselves in the process. They are effective in preventing oxidation until they are significantly reduced in concentration themselves.

Exotic Gases

Some products are now packaged in containers in exotic atmospheres such as nitrogen or carbon dioxide. If sufficient oxygen is removed, this serves to reduce oxidation of fats and vitamins. A carbon dioxide atmosphere kills insects and their eggs.

Vermin

Vermin control in feed is a management problem. Almost any feed storage area is subject to the occa-

Figure 3-11

A normal cockatiel at about 12 days of age. Note the plump wings, which are usually a sign of good growth. Weighing birds is a better indicator, however.

sional visit from rodents or insects. An occasional visit differs from an infestation, however. Ongoing control programs are necessary to maintain premises free from vermin infestation. The methods of control vary, but sanitation is an effective method of limiting the need for other measures.

Verifying Claims

Claims are often made that a feed is complete or balanced for birds. These claims are impossible to substantiate for nonpoultry species with the information now available to us. Efforts to represent feeds as proven, complete, balanced, or the exact nutrition a bird requires are misleading.

References

1. Roy RN, Guha BC: Species differences in regard to the biosynthesis of ascorbic acid. Nature 182:319, 1958.
2. Roy RN, Guha BC: Production of scurvy in a bird species. Nature 182:1689, 1958.
3. Chaudhuri CR, Chatterjee IB: L-ascorbic acid synthesis in birds: Phylogenetic trend. Science 164:435, 1969.
4. Chatterjee IB: Evolution and the biosynthesis of ascorbic acid. Science 182:1271, 1973.
5. Hanssen I, Grav HJ, Steen JB, Lysnes H: Vitamin C deficiency in growing Willow Ptarmigan (*Lagopus lagopus lagopus*). J Nutr 109:2260, 1979.
6. National Research Council: Nutrient Requirements of Poultry, 8th rev ed. Washington, DC, National Academy Press, 1984.
7. Roudybush T: Growth, signs of deficiency, and weaning in cockatiels fed deficient diets. Proc Assoc Avian Vet 333, 1986.
8. Roudybush TE, Grau CR: Lysine requirement of cockatiel chicks. Proc. 34th Western Poultry Dis Conf, Davis, CA, 113, 1985.
9. Grau CR, Roudybush TE, et al: Obscure relations of feather melanization and avian nutrition. World Poult Sci 45:241, 1989.
10. Roudybush TE, Grau CR: Food and water interrelations and the protein requirement for growth of an altricial bird, the cockatiel (*Nymphicus hollandicus*). J Nutr 116:552, 1986.
11. Roudybush TE, Grau CR, Limberg LA: Unpublished observations.
12. Roudybush T: Weaning of cockatiels. Proc. 35th Western Poultry Dis Conf, 162, 1986.
13. Roudybush T, Grau CR: Unpublished observations.
14. Roudybush T: Unpublished observations.
15. Renner R, Elcombe AM: Metabolic effects of feeding "carbohydrate free" diets. J Nutr 93:31, 1967.
16. Brambila A, Hill FW: Effects of glucose supplementation of high lipid diets based on free fatty acids for the growing chicken. J Nutr 91:261, 1967.
17. Rowland LO Jr, Sloan DR, Fry JL, Harms RH: Calcium requirement for bone maintenance of aged non-laying hens. Poult Sci 52:1415, 1973.
18. Norris LC, Kratzer FH, Lin AB: Effect of quantity of dietary calcium of maintenance of bone integrity in mature white Leghorn chickens. J Nutr 102:1085, 1972.
19. Scott ML, Nesheim MC, Young RJ: Nutrition of the Chicken. Ithaca, NY, ML Scott and Associates, 1969, p 276.
20. Smith H, Taylor JH: Effect of feeding two levels of calcium on the growth of broiler chickens. Nature 190:1200, 1961.
21. Davis PN, Norris LCF, Kratzer FH: Iron deficiency studies in chicks using treated isolated soybean protein diets. J Nutr 78:445, 1962.
22. Simhaee E, Keshavarz K: Comparison of gross protein value and metabolizable energy of dried skim milk and dried yoghurt. Poult Sci 53:184, 1974.
23. Riemann H, Bryan FL: Food-Borne Infections and Intoxications, ed 2. New York, Academic Press, 1979.
24. Stamps J, Clark A, Kus B, Arrowood P: The effects of parent and offspring gender on food allocation in budgerigars. Behavior 101:177, 1987.
25. Yang M, Vohra P: Protein and metabolizable energy requirements of hand-fed squabs from hatching to 28 days of age. Poult Sci 66:2017, 1987.
26. Reddy N, Balackrishnan C, Salunkhe D: Phytate phosphorus and mineral changes during germination and cooking of black gram (Phaseoluss mungo) seeds. J Food Sci 43:540–543, 1978.
27. Harmuth-Hoene A, Bognar A, Kornemann U, Diehl J: Der einfluss der keimung auf den nahrwert von weizen, mungbohnen, und kichererbsen. Z Lebensm Unters Forsch 185(5):386–393, 1987.
28. El-Mahdy A, Moharram YY, Abou-Samaha O: [Influence of germination on the nutritional value of lentil seed.] Z Lebensm Unters Forsch 181(4):318–320, 1985.
29. Yun-Yun D, Fields M: Germination of corn and sorghum in the home to improve nutritive value. J Food Sci 43:1113–1115, 1978.
30. Chen L, Wells C, Fordham J: Germinated seeds for human consumption. J Food Sci 40:1290–1294, 1975.
31. Hsu D, Leungt H, Finney P, Morad M: Effect of germination on nutritive value and baking properties of dry peas, lentils, and faba beans. J Food Sci 45:87–92, 1980.

Susan L. Clubb

4

Laws and Regulations Affecting Aviculture and the Pet Bird Industry

Regulations, laws, treaties, customs, and rules of ethics and etiquette allow us to coexist in relative harmony. Myriad regulations—international, federal, state, and local—affect aviculturists and pet bird dealers or suppliers, thereby influencing the supply of birds for aviculture and pets. These regulations will therefore have an effect on the practice of avian medicine. An in depth knowledge of regulations and the legislative basis behind them is not essential to the practitioner, but familiarity with them as a point of reference is important so the practitioner and client can avoid unintentional noncompliance.

International trade in avian species is regulated under the Convention on International Trade in Endangered Species of Wild Fauna and Flora (CITES). Various aspects of the importation of birds into the US come under the auspices of five government departments, the Department of Agriculture (USDA), the Department of Interior (USDI) Fish and Wildlife Service (USFWS), the Department of Treasury (Customs), the Department of Justice (enforcement of the regulations of other departments), and the Department of Health and Human Services (US Public Health Service). Additional regulatory forces affect the trade and possession of some species of exotic birds in the US. Possession of native birds is also regulated.

Each item mentioned here contains volumes of information that cannot possibly be detailed in this text. Practitioners need to be aware of the complexity of dealing with myriad regulatory pressures.

HISTORY OF THE US BIRD TRADE

Estimates by the Pet Industry Joint Advisory Council (PIJAC) place US bird populations at 40 to 50 million, with pet birds in 15% of American homes. The majority of these birds are small, highly domesticated species (budgerigars, canaries, cockatiels) that are bred in the US.

Records dating back to 1901 indicate a steady stream of imports rarely dropping below the 300,000 birds-per-year mark, except for a period of years from 1943 to 1967 during which no records were available. Psittacine imports were banned during this time; however, other species were allegedly being imported.[1] According to records from the US Bureau of Biology Survey and reported by Richard Banks, 14,409,140 birds were imported into the US between 1901 and 1942, an average of 350,000 per year, of which 71% or 10,186,248 were canaries. No data are available on mortality rates during this period.[1]

Import of wild or delicate species was facilitated by the advent of air transport following World War II. Prior to this, passage by ship was difficult for delicate species but was still used for many birds well into the 1960s.

In the years between the creation of the USDA quarantine system for imported birds in 1974 and passage of the Wild Bird Conservation Act in 1992, 300 to 900 thousand wild-caught birds were imported into the US each year, approximately 75% of which were exotic, wild-caught birds. Many dis-

45

eases and health problems were delineated during that time, some of which continue to have an impact on aviculture in the 1990s. Since passage and implementation of the Wild Bird Conservation Act, aviculture must supply the pet industry's demand for exotic as well as common domesticated birds. Future regulatory changes may allow limited importation of wild-caught birds under programs of sustainable utilization.[1, 5]

The Effects of Disease on the Importation of Birds

The history of the pet bird industry is often interwoven with that of major diseases such as psittacosis and Newcastle disease. Psittacosis was named by a French physician, Morange, who described it as a disease of humans and parrots and associated it with parrots imported from Argentina. Later it became known as parrot fever. A decade of worldwide investigation in the 1930s revealed information on the etiology and epidemiology of psittacosis in humans and birds. In 1929, pandemic psittacosis occurred in the US with a concurrent worldwide outbreak, which was traced back to infected parrots from Brazil and Argentina sent by ship to Europe and North America. A ban on the importation of psittacines was implemented in 1942 in response to reports of a high incidence of psittacosis; however, other species were still being imported. Ornithosis was described in 1938 in poultry, and many human cases were subsequently traced to domestic poultry sources, especially from turkey processing plants.[1, 2]

Researchers at the Hooper Foundation (Paul Arnstein, Karl Meyer, and B. Eddie) in the 1960s developed protocols in conjunction with the US Public Health Service for the treatment of psittacosis in birds. In 1968, treatment centers were established overseas where birds were held and treated for 45 days prior to importation.[2]

The second disease to affect the pet bird industry was viscerotropic velogenic Newcastle disease (VVND). Newcastle disease was first recognized by Doyle, in 1926, in Newcastle, England. It was almost simultaneously reported in Java and Korea. The disease disappeared shortly afterward in England but remained endemic in Southeast Asia. It is theorized that Newcastle disease began to spread from Asia around the world. As the various forms of the disease were recognized, the virulent Asiatic form, Doyle's form, became known as VVND. Psittacine birds traveling aboard sailing ships were thought responsible for the spread of the disease to Europe and South America between 1926 and 1942. An epornitic of a very virulent strain of VVND reached every continent between 1968 and 1972.

VVND was reportedly introduced by imported mynahs and psittacines into an exotic bird aviary in California, and spread to neighboring chicken farms, resulting in a widespread VVND outbreak. The 1972 outbreak in California resulted in the first test of disease control by eradication on a national basis. The fear of reentry of VVND resulted in the establishment of the USDA quarantine system for all imported birds in 1974. At that time the Public Health Service program of foreign treatment centers was abandoned. VVND has been reported from virtually every country exporting birds; however, it is most prevalent in birds from Southeast Asia and Central America, with softbilled birds having an especially high incidence.[3, 4]

REGULATION OF INTERNATIONAL TRADE IN BIRDS

International treaties, most notably CITES, regulate the movement of birds in international trade. There are other factors, however, that determine the availability of species for the pet trade. The majority of countries in which psittacine birds are found prohibit their exportation. Many export only pest species. Some operate under quota systems wherein pest species predominate. Most levy taxes on all birds exported.[7]

The Lacey Act, a US law enacted in 1908 "to support the state laws for the protection of game and birds" has evolved over the years into a complex set of laws that prohibit the trade in any wildlife, or wildlife product that is taken or possessed in contradiction to another law. This includes any species protected by foreign laws, international treaty, US laws, state or local ordinances, or Indian tribal law. Species that are removed from their native country where they are protected and imported from a second country could be seized by USFWS, and the importer can be prosecuted under the Lacey Act. The Lacey Act has been amended on several occasions. The Tariff Act of 1930 added the enforcement of foreign wildlife laws. A second major Lacey Act amendment in 1949 prohibited the importation of wild animals or birds under conditions known to be inhumane or unhealthful.

The first truly comprehensive amendment of the Lacey Act came in 1981. The 1981 amendments expanded and refined all aspects of the law including a strengthening of enforcement procedures.[8–11] Simply stated, under the Lacey Act, it is unlawful to import, export, transport, sell, receive, acquire, or purchase, in interstate or foreign commerce, any fish or wildlife or plant taken or possessed in violation of any state law, foreign law, treaty, or regulation of the US or in violation of any Indian tribal law. These laws are enforced primarily by the USFWS, a branch of the Department of Interior. The transport of animals into the US is also governed under the Lacey Act (50 CFR, part 13).[11]

The Injurious Wildlife provisions of the Lacey Act prohibit importation, transportation, or acquisition, without a permit, of certain animals (or their eggs) that have been determined to be injurious wildlife.[11]

CITES (Convention on International Trade in Endangered Species of Wild Fauna and Flora)

CITES is an international treaty that in 1994 comprised 115 signing countries, including the US, which began implementing the treaty in 1975. CITES relates only to international trade in plants and animals and has no jurisdiction in internal affairs of the parties to the treaty.[7, 8]

International trade was recognized years ago as a major threat to many wildlife species. In 1963 the International Union for the Conservation of Nature called for an international treaty regulating trade and developed the first draft. Eighty countries concluded the draft in March 1983 in Washington, DC. In 1975 the treaty was ratified by 10 of the original signatories in Berne, Switzerland (the depository nation for the convention).[7]

The structures created by the CITES treaty include the Conference of the Parties (COP), the Secretariat, and the Management Authorities and Scientific Authorities of each party. The COP meets every 2 years and has the power to adopt rules or procedures, approve the budget of the Secretariat, adopt changes to the appendices, and adopt recommen-

dations to improve the effectiveness of the Convention. Within the COP exists a complex system of procedures and committees including the Standing Committee, which assists the Secretariat in carrying out its functions and establishing the agenda and procedures for the meeting of the COP.[7]

The Secretariat was established by the treaty as a function of the United Nations Environment Program (UNEP). UNEP is a UN body established by the Stockholm Conference on the Human Environment in 1972. It has a governing council of over 40 nations and serves essentially as a stimulator and instigator of environmental research, planning, and management. For several years UNEP contracted out the Secretariat function to the International Union for Conservation of Nature (IUCN). The Secretary General and his staff are UN employees. The Secretariat is relatively independent and answers primarily to the Standing Committee and the Parties (COP). Each party country has a scientific and management authority.[7]

Plant and animal species are listed by CITES in Appendices I, II, and III. Those species that are considered to be endangered are listed in Appendix I, and no international commercial trade is permitted except under exceptional circumstances. Those species that are judged to be currently capable of tolerating commercial exploitation, but that may be threatened by trade, are listed in Appendix II. All psittacine birds with the exception of the budgerigar, cockatiel, and Indian ringneck parakeet are listed in Appendix II, except for those listed in Appendix I. (The African ringneck is listed in Appendix III.) Appendix III includes species that any party identifies as being subject to regulation within its jurisdiction for the purpose of preventing or restricting exploitation. Trade in any listed species, or products of a listed species, between signing countries requires a permit.[7, 8, 11]

Procedures for amending the treaty or appendices are complex. Any party to the treaty may propose an amendment, which must be submitted to the Secretariat at least 150 days prior to the meeting. The Secretariat then circulates the proposals with recommendations. Amendments are adopted by two-thirds majority of those parties present and voting and enter into force 90 days later. The Berne Criteria—adopted at the first meeting in 1976—established standards for the addition of species to Appendix I, II, or III.[7]

Specimens of animal species in Appendix I bred in captivity for commercial purposes can be treated as if they were Appendix II species (COP, Costa Rica, 1979). However, for such trade to take place, the breeding facility must be certified by the COP for each species involved (COP, Ottawa, Canada, 1987).[7]

As CITES membership has increased, so have the number and complexity of issues the convention has attempted to resolve. Parties must make informed decisions as to the level of trade that populations of wildlife species can support with insight into the biology and ecology of these species. Often producer countries lack the scientific expertise to make these decisions and they are made on purely political grounds.[7]

International Air Transport Association (IATA)

IATA is an international organization of airlines established to standardize air transport policies. The IATA Live Animal Board is responsible for formulation and update of guidelines. The board meets every 2 years to revise the IATA Live Animal Regulations, an approximately 150-page document that details packing and shipping requirements for many types of animals. These guidelines are developed in conjunction with CITES, the pet industry, veterinarians, and other interested parties and are sensitive to the needs of animals as well as airlines.

The regulations cover virtually every order of animals from elephants to insects, with detailed illustrations and descriptions of shipping containers. Other general information includes sections on animal behavior, lists of prohibited species, labeling requirements, disinfection of aircraft, feeding and watering requirements, sedation and euthanasia, segregation, and persons accompanying shipments. The regulation book also has an extensive section on CITES, including a list of countries party to CITES and the management authority for each country.

IATA has some 119 active member airlines worldwide with 24 additional associate members and 83 additional participating carriers. Sixteen countries have accepted these regulations either by legislation or by issuance of a permit authorizing air carriers to carry live animals in accordance with these regulations. In 1991, the US adopted portions of the Live Animal Regulations as the US Humane and Healthful Transport Regulations as enforced under the Lacey Act.[8, 11]

NATIONAL LEGISLATION AND REGULATIONS

Endangered Species Act

The provisions of the Lacey Act are augmented by the US Endangered Species Act (ESA), enacted in 1973 to halt the serious decline in numbers of many species of wild animals and plants. The ESA provides two levels of protection for listed species. Species considered to be in danger of extinction are listed as "endangered" and are provided the most stringent protection. Species likely to become endangered are listed as "threatened" and are protected by less restrictive regulations. Administration of the ESA is shared by the USFWS and the National Marine Fisheries Service (NMFS).[8, 11]

Possession of and commercial activities involving legally acquired endangered or threatened wildlife that take place entirely within one's state of residence are not prohibited by the act. For interstate sales, however, both the buyer and the seller must obtain permits from USFWS. Advertisements for sale of endangered species in publications that have interstate circulation must include a warning that an endangered/threatened species permit is required to purchase the listed animal.

The Captive Bred Wildlife (CBW) Regulation became effective in 1979, making it easier to conduct activities that enhance the propagation or survival of eligible captive-bred wildlife listed under the ESA. To transport, deliver, receive, sell, or offer captive-bred wildlife for sale in interstate commerce, both the buyer and the seller must be registered for the families or species of wildlife involved. Each transaction must document that the animal was born in captivity in the US and must reveal the buyers' and sellers' CBW permit numbers. At the time of writing, the CBW regulations were under revision by USFWS.[8, 11]

Twenty-six species of psittacines are included in the list of Endangered and Threatened Wildlife and Plants and covered by the Act (50 CFR, part 17.17). (For a copy of the current list, write to USFWS, 4401 Fairfax Dr., Arlington VA 22203.)

Importation of Birds

The importation of birds falls under the auspices of three government departments. All birds imported into the US are subject to quarantine regulations under the Department of Agriculture's Animal and Plant Health Inspection Service—Veterinary Services (USDA-APHIS-VS) regulations (50 CFR, part 9).[8, 11]

USDA Regulation of Imports

Eight privately owned and USDA-supervised quarantine stations were established in 1974, and the number subsequently grew to a high of 96 in 1979. The number of privately owned stations has decreased since that time, and in recent years many have been converted to use for the importation of ratite hatching eggs and quarantine chicks. The USDA also owns and operates commercial and pet bird quarantine stations.[8, 11]

Privately owned quarantine stations are operated under the supervision of USDA-APHIS. All birds entering the US are required to undergo a 30-day quarantine, during which they are tested for poultry lethal disease. The only disease of serious consideration is VVND; however, USDA is on the alert for any new threat to the US poultry industry. The quarantine station must be approved prior to issuance of the permit to import birds.

Current regulations dictate that all psittacines are fed a medicated ration containing 1% chlorotetracycline during the 30-day quarantine. Tissues are collected from all birds that die during the first 16 days (up to 150 a day) and are submitted to the national Veterinary Services Laboratory in Ames, Iowa for virus isolation. A representative sample of birds are also swabbed for virus isolation. Virus isolation is accomplished in embryonated chicken eggs. Isolates are tested by hemagglutination and hemagglutination-inhibition tests for the presence of Newcastle disease virus. Isolates are pathotyped in chickens. If VVND is isolated, all birds in the station must be euthanized or reexported.[11]

Procedures for the importation of ratite and hatching eggs vary significantly from those for other exotic birds. Only eggs can by imported through privately owned stations. These eggs must be unincubated and must undergo 45 days of incubation in the quarantine station. The 30-day quarantine period begins when the last chick hatches. Live birds can only be imported through government stations in New York, Miami, or Honolulu, and ostriches entering these stations cannot exceed 3 feet in height. These regulations were promulgated in 1992 in response to requests to allow imports. All imports of ratites were stopped in 1990 when ticks capable of carrying heart water fever were found on imported ostriches.[11]

The demand for APHIS services for the supervision of quarantine stations is declining rapidly as a result of passage of the Wild Bird Conservation Act of 1992. At the time of writing, USDA quarantine regulations are under revision.

US Fish and Wildlife Service Inspection and Regulation of Imports

Avian imports also come under the scrutiny of the Department of Interior under the auspices of the USFWS enforcement of the Wild Bird Conservation Act, the Lacey Act, the ESA, and the CITES treaty. CITES export permits must be presented along with the Declaration of Importation form (filed by importers or their brokers shortly after arrival) and the USDA Permit to Import Birds. The numbers and species of birds are then fed into the USFWS "LEMIS" data system for correlation. If they do not agree or if there is suspicion of noncompliance with any regulation, the country of origin is contacted through the US State Department. If there is reason to suspect misidentification, USFWS agents enter a station to inspect. In addition, import documents must pass inspection by US Customs and the Department of the Treasury.

The Wild Bird Conservation Act of 1992

The Wild Bird Conservation Act was signed into law on October 23, 1992. The stated purpose of the Wild Bird Conservation Act (WBCA) is to promote the conservation of exotic birds by encouraging wild bird conservation and management programs in the country of origin; by ensuring that all trade in such species is biologically sustainable and to the benefit of the species; and by limiting imports of exotic birds when necessary to ensure that exotic wild bird populations are not harmed by removal for the trade. Under the WBCA importations of all CITES-listed birds are prohibited except under specific exemptions. The WBCA applies to the importation of all bird species not indigenous to the 50 United States while exempting game bird families and orders (Phasianidae, Anatidae, Struthionidae, Rheidae, and Gruidae).[13]

The WBCA placed an immediate moratorium on 10 heavily traded psittacine species. The act provided for a 1-year phaseout of imports of all CITES-listed avian species, after which all imports of wild-caught CITES-listed species would be prohibited unless the species was on a list of species approved for import.[13]

For wild-caught birds to be listed on the approved list, USFWS must determine that (1) CITES is being effectively implemented for the species in every country of origin; (2) measures recommended by CITES committees are implemented; (3) there is a scientifically based management plan that provides for the conservation of the species and its habitat; and (4) the methods of capture, transport, and maintenance minimize the risks to the bird's health and welfare. A list of species of wild-caught birds that are managed under a strict program of controls in the country of origin, and for which it has been determined that trade can be sustainable, will also be developed. Birds included on the list can be imported only from the approved country.[13]

For captive-bred birds, the USFWS is required to determine that either (1) only captive-bred birds are in trade for that species, or (2) the birds were bred in an USFWS-approved facility. The USFWS will maintain a list of captive-bred, CITES-listed species that can be imported without a permit. These species must be commonly bred in captivity, and cannot be in legal or illegal trade. Captive-bred birds that are not included on the "clean list" can only be imported from breeding facilities that are approved by USFWS.[13]

The USFWS may issue import permits for any exotic bird for scientific research, as personally owned pet birds, for zoologic display, or for cooperative breeding programs designed to promote the conservation of the species in the wild by enhancing the propagation and survival of the affected species.[13]

The Exotic Bird Conservation Fund was established under the WBCA to be used for conservation of birds in their country of origin. Money for the fund will come from fines, forfeitures, donations, and appropriations. The fund is designed to support wild bird research and management programs.

The WBCA established significant penalties for violators, including civil penalties up to $12,000 for some infractions and up to $25,000 for others, as well as misdemeanor and felony criminal penalties.[13]

At the time of writing regulations to enforce the WBCA were being promulgated.[13]

Animal Welfare Act

The Animal Welfare Act as administered today by the US Department of Agriculture evolved over the years from the original Laboratory Animal Welfare Act of 1966. The Regulatory Enforcement and Animal Care (REAC) division of USDA is assigned responsibility for the performance of functions under the act. Covered under the act is any live dog, cat, nonhuman primate, guinea pig, hamster, rabbit, or any other warm-blooded animal that is domesticated or wild, and being used for research, testing, experimentation, exhibition, or as a pet. Excluded in the promulgation of regulations enforcing the act are birds, rats, mice, horses, and other farm animals such as poultry and livestock. Animals are covered in research facilities, in commerce, pet stores, exhibits of all types, and breeding facilities.

In 1992 a coalition of animal welfare and humane groups brought a successful suit against USDA to require that enforcement of the Animal Welfare Act include birds. On appeal by USDA-APHIS-VS, the judgment was overturned in 1994.

Bald Eagle Protection Act

The Bald Eagle Protection Act prohibits taking, possession, sale, importation, exportation, and transportation of bald and golden eagles. It is administered by the USFWS. Possession of eagles requires a permit. Moulted feathers must be retained and returned to the USFWS.

Feather Import Quota

Part of the Tariff Acts of 1930 and 1962, the Feather Import Quota limits the commercial importation of feathers from seven species of birds under a quota system, which is administered by the Department of the Interior. These regulations are being revised and incorporated into regulations promulgated to enforce the WBCA of 1992.

Migratory Bird Treaty Act

The act regulates banding and marking and taking, possession, transportation, and sale of migratory birds and their nests, eggs, parts, or products. The list of birds protected by the Migratory Bird Treaty Act is extensive, and includes most of the species found in North America. It is administered by the Department of the Interior. Any protected birds held in captivity must be reported annually to the USFWS. Member facilities accredited by the American Zoological Association (formerly the American Association of Zoological Parks and Aquariums, AAZPA) are exempt from the annual reporting requirement.

Miscellaneous Factors Affecting the Bird Trade

State Bird Ban Laws

These laws include bans on the sale of imported or wild-caught birds. After the surprise enactment of a ban against the sale of wild-caught birds in New York State in 1985 (which became effective in 1986), similar legislation was introduced around the country. Critics of the New York bill predicted the emergence of smuggled birds and concurrent introduction of disease into the state if the bill was passed. In 1987, New York was one of six states in which VVND was diagnosed in association with smuggled yellow-naped Amazons. A similar bill was adopted in New Jersey in 1991. Similar legislation was introduced in eight states between 1985 and 1989 (Pennsylvania, Michigan, California, Connecticut, Massachusetts, New Jersey, Illinois, and Maryland) but failed to be enacted.

Local—City and County—Ordinances

Local zoning ordinances pose the most immediate threat to the possession of birds. City and county

ordinances may also prohibit ownership of a variety of animal and bird species. These ordinances, as well as state laws restricting ownership of certain species, are detailed in the Controlled Wildlife Series.[11]

Improvement Plans

In 1983, a small group of workers, inspired by the highly successful, voluntary National Poultry Improvement Plan (NPIP), attempted to develop a similar program for pet birds. Despite intensive efforts, the plan was greeted with suspicion by aviculturists as government intrusion into their aviaries. Widely accepted now, NPIP was likewise poorly accepted initially.

The Maryland Cage Bird Improvement Plan (MBIP) was approved by the Maryland State Legislature in 1986. It was a voluntary, self-governing program developed by breeders, pet shops, and veterinarians in association with the University of Maryland Cooperative Extension Service, Maryland Department of Agriculture, Maryland Department of Health and Hygiene, the poultry industry, and the State Legislature. The MBIP became inactive in 1992.

The Model Aviculture Program

The Model Aviculture Program (MAP) is a voluntary program for the certification of aviculturists through inspection by avian veterinarians. MAP is designed to improve the care and breeding of exotic birds. The program is not run by state or federal agencies; it is governed by a board of directors consisting of aviculturists and avian veterinarians. This program is designed to provide a high or low profile to bird breeders. Confidentiality is an integral part of each aspect of the program. Inspection involves facilities, management practices, and record-keeping.

Nongovernment Organizations Affecting Aviculture and the Pet Industry

Many large and powerful humane and conservation groups influence elected officials in all levels of the government and serve as watchdogs over the industry.

IUCN (International Union for the Conservation of Nature and Natural Resources—the name was recently changed to the World Conservation Union), founded in 1948, is a network of governments, nongovernment organizations, scientists, and other conservation experts, who have joined together to promote the protection and sustainable use of living resources. IUCN monitors the status of ecosystems and species around the world, plans conservation action, promotes such action by governments, and provides assistance and advice necessary for achievement of such action.

IUCN Species Survival Commission and Trade Specialist Groups work through the Center for Environmental Education in Cambridge, England. They review proposals to CITES for adequate trade and scientific data and make recommendations to the COP. IUCN also publishes the *Red Data Book* (lists of endangered species) and the *Significant Trade in Wildlife Reports* (see the suggested reading list).

Bird Life International, formerly the ICBP (International Council for Bird Protection), also based in Cambridge, predates the IUCN but now primarily handles bird-related issues for the IUCN.

UNEP (United Nations Environment Programme) was established in 1972. Its mandate is to keep the world environmental situation under review to ensure that emerging environmental problems of international significance receive appropriate consideration by governments, and to safeguard the environment for the benefit of future generations. The ultimate aim of UNEP's activities is to promote development that is environmentally sound and sustainable.[7]

WWF (World Wide Fund for Nature, previously World Wildlife Fund) is an international conservation foundation based in Switzerland. The scope of WWF is the conservation of the natural environment and the ecologic processes essential to life on earth. WWF aims to create awareness of threats to the environment and to generate and attract on a worldwide basis the strongest possible moral and financial support for safeguarding the living world. WWF, with its international and national trustees, also provides a bridge for the conservation movement to the business community. WWF through its subgroup TRAFFIC (Trade Records Analysis of Flora and Fauna in Commerce) monitors trade and has played a major role in the development of CITES.

The World Conservation Strategy (1980) is a plan prepared by IUCN, with the advice, cooperation, and financial assistance of UNEP and WWF. It provides an intellectual framework and practical guidance for conservation actions needed to conserve living resources for sustainable development. It details major threats to the environment, the obstacles to achieving conservation, the strategy to solve conservation problems, and an international plan to coordinate use of the global commons and the requirements for sustainable development. The 1990 revision of the World Conservation Strategy was entitled Caring For Earth.

PIJAC (Pet Industry Joint Advisory Council), through its counsel, Marshall Meyers, is the only unified voice of the pet industry. A nonprofit organization based in Washington, DC, PIJAC monitors legislation adverse to the pet industry, provides information to industry members, represents the pet industry to government agencies and conservation groups, and serves as a lobby for pet industry interests. PIJAC has been a nongovernmental observer to CITES since 1979 and has played an active role in the CITES transport working group and the CITES significant trade study. PIJAC strongly encourages cooperation between the pet industry and the veterinary community.

Cooperative Working Group on Bird Trade

In the summer of 1988, amid growing international concern about depleted wild bird populations and high mortality rates associated with the international trade in wild-caught birds, the WWF convened the Cooperative Working Group on Bird Trade. This diverse committee represented a broad spectrum of organizations with interests in the bird trade —organizations with strong differing views and objectives. For 1½ years, the Working Group analyzed imports of exotic avian species into the US and reviewed federal procedures and controls that are related to such imports. The Group concluded that the procedures and performance of the responsible federal agencies failed to adequately meet the requirements and intent of the Endangered Species Act, the Lacey Act, the Animal Welfare Act, and CITES, nor do they meet the real needs of aviculture and the pet industry.

The Group recognized that habitat loss and local use as well as international trade threatened the survival of both individual avian populations and entire species. It concluded that the US, as one of the principal consumers of wild-caught birds for the pet trade, should reduce its reliance on wild avian populations and, within an agreed-upon time frame, replace wild-caught birds with captive-bred birds for the pet trade. The members of the Working Group were not opposed to limited imports of wild-caught birds for captive breeding of exotic avian species within the US or abroad, because imports will be critical to the survival of the species in the wild and to the long-term health of the pet bird industry.

On the basis of its findings, the Working Group drafted comprehensive recommendations that address all aspects of the wild-bird trade. These recommendations were ultimately used to draft legislation, which culminated in passage of the WBCA of 1992, although humane and animal rights group pressures resulted in the stricter provisions adopted in the WBCA.[12]

References

1. Nilsson G: The Bird Business, A Study of the Commercial Cage Bird Trade. Washington, DC, Animal Welfare Institute, 1981.
2. Code of Federal Regulations (CFR) part 11, 1-1-85 ed. Animal and Plant Health Inspection Service, USDA Subchapter A, Animal Welfare, 1985.
3. Francis DW: Newcastles and psittacines. Proc 8th Calif Poult Health Symp, Davis, CA, 1974.
4. Hanson RP: Newcastle disease. In Diseases of Poultry, ed 7. Ames, Iowa, Iowa State University Press, 1978.
5. TRAFFIC USA Report, Washington, DC, World Wildlife Fund, 10(3) October 1990.
6. Page L: Avian chlamydiosis (ornithosis). In Hofstad MS, Barales HJ, Calnek BW, et al, eds: Diseases of Poultry, ed 7. Ames, Iowa, Iowa State University Press, 1978.
7. IUCN Species Survival Commission: CITES—A Conservation Tool, ed 4. Prepared for the 9th meeting of the Conference of the Parties, 7–18 November, 1994.
8. Bean M: The Evolution of National Wildlife Law. New York, Praeger Publishers, 1983.
9. 50 CFR, part 13. Lacey Act, Humane and Healthful Transport of Animals.
10. Fitzgerald S: International Wildlife Trade, Whose Business Is it? Washington, DC, World Wildlife Fund, 1989.
11. Controlled Wildlife. University of Kansas, Lawrence, KS, Association of Systematics Collections, Museum of Natural History, 1984. Estes C, Sessions K: Volume I, Federal Permit Procedures. Estes C, Sessions K: Volume II, Federally Controlled Species. King S, Schrock JR: Volume III, State Wildlife Regulations.
12. Findings and Recommendations of the Cooperative Working Group on Bird Trade. Washington, DC, World Wildlife Fund, 1990.
13. Wild Bird Conservation Act of 1992. Public Law 102-440 (HR 5013), October 23, 1992.

Suggested Reading

Endangered Birds of the World, The ICBP Bird Red Data Book. Compiled by Warren B. King, Smithsonian Institution Press, Washington, DC, 1981.

Significant Trade in Wildlife: A Review of Selected Species. In CITES, Appendix II, Volume 3, Birds, Tim Inskipp, Steven Broad, and Richard Luxmore. Compiled by IUCN Conservation Monitoring Center, 219c Huntington Road, Cambridge, UK, 1988.

The Endangered Species Handbook, 2nd ed. Greta Nilsson, Animal Welfare Institute, P.O. Box 3650, Washington, DC 20007, 1985.

The Bird Business—A Study of the Commercial Cage Bird Trade. Greta Nilsson, Animal Welfare Institute, P.O. 3650, Washington, DC 20007, 1981.

Endangered Parrots. Rosemary Low, Blindfold Press, Link House, West Street, Pole, Torsi BH15, 1LL UK, 1984.

CITES, Identification Manual (5 volumes), Volume III. Aves Editor Peter Dollinger, Secretariat of CITES, Lausanne, Switzerland, 1985.

Proceedings of the Conference of the Parties (CITES)
    1st meeting—Berne, Switzerland, 1977
    2nd meeting—San Jose, Costa Rica, 1979
    3rd meeting—New Dehli, India, 1981
    4th meeting—Gaborone, Botswana, 1983
    5th meeting—Buenos Aires, Argentina, 1985
    6th meeting—Ottawa, Canada, 1987
    7th meeting—Lausanne, Switzerland, 1989
    8th meeting—Kyoto, Japan, 1992
    9th meeting—Ft. Lauderdale, Florida, 1994

For Further Information

American Federation of Aviculture, P.O. Box 56218, Phoenix, AZ, 85079–6218 Tel 602–484–0931

Animal and Plant Health Inspection Service (APHIS)—US Department of Agriculture, Federal Building, Hyattsville, MD 20782 Tel 301–436–8097 Fax 301–436–8818

Convention on International Trade in Endangered Species of Wild Fauna and Flora (CITES)—Secretariat—15 Chemin des Anemones, Case Postale 456, 1219 Chatelaine, Geneva, Switzerland. Tel (41) 22 979 9139 Fax (41) 22 797 3417

International Air Transport Association, IATA Building, 2000 Peel Street, Montreal, Quebec, Canada H3A 2R4

Model Aviculture Program, P.O. Box 1657, Martinez, CA 94553

Pet Industry Joint Advisory Council (PIJAC), 1220 19th St., N.W., Washington, DC 20036 Tel 1–800–553–PETS Fax 202–293–4377

TRAFFIC USA—World Wildlife Fund, 1250 24th St., N.W., Washington, DC 20037 Tel 202–293–4800 Fax 202–775–8287

US Fish and Wildlife Service, 4401 Fairfax Dr., Room 420, Arlington, VA 22203 Tel 800–358–2104 Fax 202–358–2281

World Conservation Monitoring Center, TRAFFIC International and IUCN Species Survival Commission, 219c Huntington Road, Cambridge CB3 0DL, United Kingdom, Tel (44) 1233 277 966 Fax (44) 1233 277 845

World Conservation Union—International Union for the Conservation of Nature and Natural Resources, 1196 Gland, Switzerland.

Glenn H. Olsen
Susan L. Clubb

5

Embryology, Incubation, and Hatching

Proper incubation and hatching is vital for aviculture success. Veterinarians must have an understanding of embryology and incubation procedures to assist the aviculturist with minimizing embryonic mortality and providing neonatal care. We work with a broad range of species but most of what is known about incubation is derived from poultry. For other groups, such as waterfowl and psittacines, more information is becoming available. For rare and endangered species, or species not commonly found in captivity, little is known, and information must be gleaned from successes and problems with other species.[1]

EMBRYOLOGY

The ovum of an avian egg includes the yolk, which is produced by the ovary. The protoplasm containing the nucleus floats above the yolk and under the plasma membrane. Upon ovulation the ovum moves through the fimbria and, shortly after ovulation, into the oviduct. Fertilization takes place in the upper infundibulum and the first cleavage occurs 4 to 5 hours after ovulation. Rapid cell division follows as the yolk passes down the oviduct. Albumin, the inner and outer shell membranes, and finally the shell are applied.[2, 3]

Embryonic development begins prior to laying. When the egg is laid, an embryo already consists of 2000 to 60,000 cells in the form of a circular disc

called a "blastula," which is in the process of gastrulation. Gastrulation is the stage in embryonic development in which the blastula folds into itself to form the embryonic gut. The resultant embryo is visible on the surface of the yolk shortly after laying.[4] A fertile unincubated egg can be distinguished from an infertile egg by selective staining of the blastula (embryo) at the time of laying. The trained eye may also be able to recognize an embryo, especially if death occurs after a few days of incubation.[2–4]

The egg membranes, the amnion, chorion, and allantois, are sheets of living tissue that develop from the embryo itself. A pouch-like outgrowth of the digestive system encircles the yolk to form the yolk sac. In the last one-third of the incubation period the embryo produces enzymes to digest the yolk and transport nutrients through its blood vessels. The amnion and chorion develop as folds of the body wall and surround the embryo.[2] The amnion develops into a fluid-filled sac in which the embryo grows, allowing movement. The allantois, an extention of the digestive tract, fuses with the chorion to form a compound membrane, the chorioallantoic membrane (CAM). The CAM is filled with many blood vessels, necessary for exchange of oxygen and carbon dioxide through the shell. All of these critical developmental stages occur within the first one-half of the incubation period. The embryo is most susceptible to adverse conditions or trauma during this time.[2]

54

INCUBATION TECHNIQUES

The success of incubation and hatching techniques is indicated by fertility and hatchability rates. Fertility is the percentage of eggs found to be fertile, as indicated by evidence of embryonic development. Hatchability is the percentage of fertile eggs that hatch.

Candling is the oldest and most frequently used method to monitor embryonic development. The term "candling" dates this technique to the days when a candle was the light source used in the procedure. A candling lamp may consist of an electric light source within a box or a small bright flashlight. Light passes through a raised circular opening within a rim of rubber or flexible plastic. The egg is held tightly against the rim. With the large end (air cell) against the rim, the egg is rotated to identify different structures inside. The light source must be adequate for viewing but not so strong or hot that it will damage the egg. It must be used in a dark room. A 40-watt bulb at 4 cm (1.5 inches) from the egg will work well with chicken-sized eggs. Abnormal shell development may affect visibility as well as hatchability (Fig. 5–1). For smaller eggs, a lower wattage bulb is recommended. Colored or spotted eggs are difficult to candle. In a newly laid egg the air cell is very small,

the albumin clear, and the yolk appears yellow (see Color Fig. 5–2). Embryonic development appears as a darker area. In early development, the vascular ring is often visible as a red circle, and the embryo as a small dark or red spot within the blood ring (see Color Fig. 5–3). The beating heart is usually visible by the end of the first third of incubation.

The air cell is the lightest colored part of the egg, usually found in the blunt end of the egg. With practice, infertile, dead, or damaged eggs can be identified (see Color Figs. 5–4 and 5–5). Cracks are more visible during candling. Seal cracks with a small amount of paraffin, beeswax, or white glue. (Avoid products containing acetone because it is toxic to the embryo.) Eggs should be candled once or twice weekly and damaged or dead eggs removed from the nest or incubator.[4, 6]

Egg Hygiene

Improper egg handling contributes to decreased hatchability and can foster certain types of disease. An incubation temperature of 99.5°F (37°C) is ideal for bacterial growth.[6, 7] Eggs should always be handled with clean or gloved hands.

The egg is laid at the body temperature of the hen and begins cooling immediately. As the egg cools, its contents contract and a negative partial pressure forms, drawing air into the egg, forming the air cell. During the cooling process, contaminants on the shell (such as bacteria, fungi, and viruses) can be drawn into the egg.[2, 4, 6]

Egg contamination can be reduced in the nest and during egg collection. Offer only fresh, suitable nesting material to the parent birds. Keep the nest clean and dry because wet, rotting bedding can be a source of *Aspergillus* spores. Keep the cage clean; parent birds can track fecal contamination back into the nest on their feet and feathers. Eggs to be artificially incubated should be collected as soon as possible after laying to help reduce the chances of contamination. In some species, and in aviaries using some incubation equipment, artificial incubation from day 1 may not be recommended.[8] Both the collection basket and the aviculturist's hands should be clean. Take care to ensure that eggs are not chilled when they are moved from the nest to

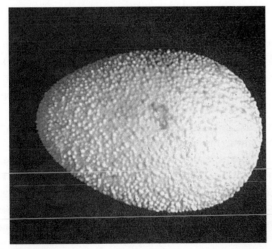

Figure 5–1

Egg with abnormal calcium deposition laid by a scarlet macaw with salpingitis.

the incubator, especially if the hen has already started to set.

Washing Eggs

Washing eggs, if done properly, can reduce contamination; however, improper washing may result in contamination. For species such as ostriches and psittacines, routine washing is not recommended.[5, 7] Washing may remove the protective cuticle layer on the outer shell. Bacteria enter the pores of a wet egg more readily than those of a dry egg. Washing can be beneficial if the egg has visible contamination, such as adherent fecal material.[4]

To avoid causing further contraction of the egg contents and movement of contaminated water into the egg, always use water that is warmer than the egg (110°F, 43°C). Higher temperatures (43–60°C) have been used successfully on eggs for short periods (3–5 minutes) but can be dangerous for small eggs. Detergents or disinfectants are added to the wash water (e.g., 10% povidone-iodine added to warm water to make a 1% solution, or chlorhexidine, sodium hypochlorite, quaternary ammonia, and phenolic disinfectants have all been used).[1] The use of detergents and some disinfectants can be harmful to passerines and other species with small porous shells. Cleaning by gently scraping with a bristle brush or sanding is also effective in removing gross organic debris clinging to the shell.[4]

Fumigation

Fumigating both eggs and incubator is an effective method for disinfecting both. Egg fumigation is most effective shortly after laying. Fumigation of eggs after incubation has begun can result in toxicity unless levels of fumigants are reduced. Place eggs in an incubator and allow them to warm. Then, inside the incubator, mix 0.33 ml of 40% formalin and 0.175 g of potassium permanganate (per cubic foot of incubator space) in a clean glass jar. Allow the gaseous fumigant cloud to remain in contact with the eggs and inner incubator surfaces for 20 to 30 minutes before exhausting the fumigant to the outside.

Use caution! Do not inhale the fumigant mixture. It is carcinogenic and may cause severe irritation to the skin, eyes, and respiratory tract. Perform fumigation only in a well-ventilated room and leave the room while fumigation is in progress. Safety badges should be worn to detect dangerous levels of formalin that may be present in the air. The U.S. Department of Occupational Safety and Health Assessment (OSHA) may prohibit the use of fumigants in the workplace.

Egg Storage

Storage of eggs before incubation may be used to synchronize incubation and hatching, and to produce even-age chicks. Hatch synchronization is important for neonatal care of precocial species but may not be of importance for altricial species. Store eggs at 12.8 to 18.3°C (55–65°F)[2, 3] and 75% relative humidity. Chicken egg hatchability is reduced by about 2% per day when stored. Storage may result in unacceptable losses in nondomestic species.[1, 4, 5]

Egg storage for more than one week is not recommended. Warming the eggs to 27°C (80°F) for 5 minutes and turning each egg 90 degrees may improve hatchability, because this reportedly mimics the behavior of some wild birds that lay large clutches that hatch simultaneously.[4] Other authors argue that egg turning when eggs are stored for less than a week is not required.[5]

ARTIFICIAL INCUBATION

As desirable as parental incubation may be, in some cases this is not possible and the aviculturist must rely on artificial incubation (Table 5–1). Artificial incubation may be used to increase production by encouraging multiple clutching. It may be necessary when incubating birds are lost, when removing eggs from wild nests or nests in large flight cages, and when inappropriate incubation behavior is observed in parent birds. Artificial incubation may be needed until suitable parents are available.

A variety of commercial incubators are available. Small, tabletop units are practical and cost-effective for the small aviculture collection. Incubators range

T a b l e 5 – 1

INCUBATION AND HATCHING TIMES FOR COMMON PSITTACINES (Forced Air Incubation)

Species	Length of Incubation (days)	Pip to Hatch (hours)
Macaws		
(*Ara* spp.)	26	24–48
Hyacinth macaw		
(*Anodorhynchus hyacinthinus*)	26–28	24–72
Conures		
(*Pyrrhura* spp. and *Aratinga* spp.)	23–24	24–48
Grey parrots		
(*Psitticus* spp.)	26–28	24–72
Senegal parrots		
(*Poicephalus senegalus*)	24–25	24–48
Eclectus parrots		
(*Eclectus roratus*)	28	24–72
Monk parakeets		
(*Myiopsitta monachus*)	23	24–48
Budgerigars		
(*Melopsittacus undulatus*)	18	12–36
Cockatiels		
(*Nymphicus hollandicus*)	21	24–48
Yellow Amazons		
(*Amazona ochrocephalia*)	28–29	24–48
Other Amazons		
(*Amazona* spp.)	24–26	24–48
Cockatoos		
(*Cacatua* spp.)		
Large cockatoos	26–29	24–48
Small cockatoos	23–25	24–48
Palm cockatoos	28–30	48–96
(*Probosciger aterrimus*)		
Lories		
(*Eos* spp., *Lorius* spp., *Chalcopsitta* spp.)	26–27	24–36
Lovebirds		
(*Agapornis* spp.)	22	24–48
Caiques		
(*Pionites* spp.)	25	24–48
Pionus parrots		
(*Pionus* spp.)	25–26	24–48

Data from Jordan,[6] Joyner,[7] and Clubb and Phillips.[8]

in size from these tabletop units to large walk-in units that hold thousands of eggs (Fig. 5–6).

Incubation Temperature

Temperature and humidity requirements differ with the species of bird and may vary with the microenvironment within the incubator and the room environment in which the incubator is housed. If the species is commonly hatched in captivity, incubation requirements may be published. If incubation information is unavailable, the following guidelines may be useful: small eggs are incubated at 37°C (99.5°F), whereas larger eggs require lower temperatures, usually 0.25 to 0.50°C less.[1] Ostriches are incubated at 36.0 to 36.4°C (96.8–97.5°F).[5] One author feels that cockatoos and macaws do well at slightly below 37°C, while galahs (rosebreasted cockatoos) and Australian parakeets do best at (98.7°F).[6]

Temperature requirements are critical, especially during the first one-third of the incubation period. A temperature elevation of as little as 1.0°C can kill an embryo in the first one-third of incubation. A marginally higher temperature during incubation increases the incidence of late-dead embryos. Embryos that survive to hatch are small and weak, and many have unhealed navels or exposed yolk sacs. Elevated incubation temperature also increases the incidence of crossed or scissor bills, curled toes, and wry necks. Temperature is less critical in the last one-third, as the embryo gains some ability for thermoregulation. During this period a slight elevation of incubation temperature may produce only a hatch earlier than expected.[2, 4]

Temperatures lower than recommended during incubation will result in developmental problems as well that vary in severity based on the margin of error. A slight lowering of temperature each day has little effect on the embryo other than a possible

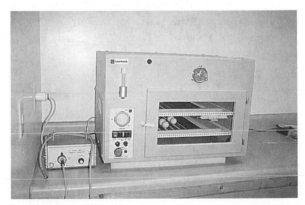

F i g u r e 5 – 6

Table-top incubator with automatic turning device. A halogen light source with fiberoptic light cable is ideal for candling eggs in the incubator without handling them.

slight delay in hatching. However, a low temperature throughout incubation increases the incidence of late-dead embryos. Chicks surviving to hatch are weak, with large, soft bodies resulting from a large yolk sac, and have weak legs and a poor sense of balance. Hatching is delayed and may take several days.[2, 4]

Humidity

Relative humidity requirements for proper incubation vary with species but, generally, they are not as critical as proper incubation temperature. An embryo has some ability to compensate for differences in humidity, particularly during the last one-third of the incubation period. During this period the embryo actually swallows amniotic fluid and remaining albumin to compensate for water loss resulting from low incubation humidity. Low relative humidity, especially in the first one-third of the incubation period, interferes with proper mobilization of eggshell calcium required for bone development and may result in a stunted embryo. In late incubation, low relative humidity results in dehydration of the embryo. Albumin appears glue-like in consistency, and the kidneys fail because of insufficient water. This often results in the death of the embryo just before entering the air cell. Increased humidity levels during incubation result in eggs with small air cells and soft, edematous chicks with increased incidence of poor umbilical seal and exposed yolk sacs. Embryonic mortality can result from inadequate space in the air cell for pipping.

Egg Weights

Eggs naturally lose weight during incubation because of metabolism and evaporation of water. The rate of weight loss is dependent upon environmental humidity but also varies as a result of shell porosity, air flow, and temperature, so that even in a single species individual variability in weight loss occurs. A useful technique to monitor the health of eggs is to weigh them periodically and chart the weight loss. A mathematical relationship exists between shell porosity, incubation time, and relative humidity. During the entire incubation period, acceptable total weight loss averages 13% (11–16% range). Weight loss varies with the incubation stage, generally being greater during both early and late incubation. However, even during these periods, weight loss should not vary by more than 3% from expected. Air cell size, determined through candling, is also proportional to weight loss and can be used by experienced persons to monitor water loss. If humidity is too low, the air cell is larger than normal; conversely, high humidity results in a smaller than expected air cell.

Turning

Eggs require turning for proper incubation and hatching. Parent birds on average turn an egg every 35 minutes. Turning eggs is required to prevent adhesions of the embryo to the shell membranes. Inadequate turning results in early-dead or malpositioned, late-dead embryos. During artificial incubation, eggs should be rotated at least five times daily. The better quality commercial incubators, including some of the smaller tabletop models, have mechanical turners and timers to automatically rotate eggs.

EMBRYONIC MORTALITY

The egg and developing embryo are very susceptible to unfavorable environmental conditions. Considering the complexity of the developmental process it is surprising that so few defects occur during incubation. Research using fruit flies, frogs, and mice has shown that radiation (x-rays), ultraviolet rays, temperature changes, and a variety of chemical substances induce alterations in development of the embryo. The type of defect that occurs depends more upon the stage of development of the embryo at the time of exposure to the teratogenic agent than on the agent used. Such observations have led to the concept of critical periods in development, when particular organs or systems are developing rapidly and are most susceptible to interference.[2, 4]

In poultry, 33% of embryonic mortality occurs during the first critical period (first week of incubation), and approximately 60% occurs during the hatching period, with little mortality during other periods. In one study of psittacine embryonic mortality, similar patterns of mortality were observed in psittacine eggs.[2, 4, 9]

Many factors are responsible for mortality during the first week of incubation, including rough egg handling, improper incubation parameters when artificial incubation is used, failure of the parents to properly incubate eggs, high or low temperatures in the nest, inbreeding or genetic abnormalities, eggborne infection, and contamination. Artificial incubation parameters that may result in early embryonic mortality include improper temperature or humidity levels, excessive vibration, improper egg turning, and poor ventilation, leading to buildup of carbon dioxide.

A blood ring, which is extravasation of blood into a ring surrounding the remnants of the embryo and embryonic circle of blood vessels, indicates early embryonic death.

The period of least mortality and risk to the embryo is midincubation. Improper incubation parameters, especially overheating, are the most common risks. Nutritional deficiencies in breeding stock, eggborne infections, and toxins such as chemical fumes around the incubation area may also result in mortality.

HATCHING

Hatching is a complex process. Problems during incubation may be reflected in mortality at hatching. As an egg nears hatching, the head of the embryo shifts within the egg. From its position in the narrow end of the egg the head moves up under the right wing, with the tip of the beak pointed toward the air cell. Carbon dioxide levels in the embryo begin to rise because the allantoic circulation no longer has the capacity to meet embryonic needs. The rising carbon dioxide levels produce spasms or twitching in the embryo's neck muscles, which forces the egg tooth on the tip of the beak to puncture the air cell membrane. Internal pip occurs when the chick breaks through the chorioallantoic membrane and its head enters the air cell. At that time, the embryo has direct access to air and begins gulping it. As this happens, the lungs begin to

function in air exchange, and a right-to-left ventricular shunt closes. In species that vocalize, a gentle peeping sound may be emitted by the embryo. The elevated carbon dioxide levels that produce contractions of the neck muscles, and the struggle associated with hatching, also cause abdominal contractions that slowly pull the yolk sac into the abdominal cavity.

Pipping

As an embryo breathes from the air cell, the gaseous exchange through the shell is unable to meet the demand. Gradually, the carbon dioxide levels rise as high as 10%, inducing even stronger muscle contractions. These contractions eventually force the beak through the shell, creating the pip hole and increasing the air circulation to the embryo. Elapsed time between entering the air cell and pipping ranges from as little as 3 hours to as long as 3 days, depending on the species.[4] For most psittacine species this interval is 24 to 48 hours (see Table 5–1). Knowledge of hatching sequence and time intervals for a species is important to diagnose hatching problems and to determine if intervention is appropriate to help produce a viable chick.[11] Opening an air cell too soon interferes with other aspects of the hatching process that require elevated carbon dioxide levels (Fig. 5–7).

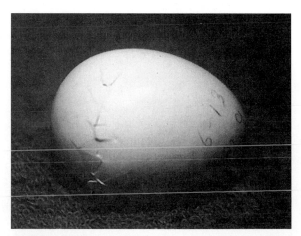

F i g u r e   5 – 7
Embryo is cutting out of the shell, moving in a typical counterclockwise fashion.

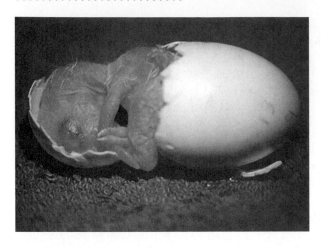

Figure 5–8

Blue and gold macaw chick emerging from the egg.

The Hatch

When the chick's head is in the air cell, activity alternates between jerking head movements and prolonged contractions of the head and back. The head movement further chips the shell, while the contractions of the neck and back help draw remaining exteriorized yolk sac into the body. Contractions force the body to rotate slightly in a counterclockwise direction. This rotation positions the head over a new section of the shell. As the chick rotates and further pips at the shell, it makes a circular pattern of connected holes in the cap or wide end of the egg. This chipping away the shell is referred to as "cutting out." Finally, during one of the contractions, the head is pushed against the weakened shell and forces open the top of the egg (Figs. 5–8 and 5–9). The chick then proceeds to kick free. The time between pipping and kicking free is species-dependent and ranges from 0.5 hours to 3 days. The normal interval for most psittacines is less than 24 hours. After hatching, the exhausted chick will rest and dry. As the chick dries, the sheaths around the down feathers are shed, and this is sometimes referred to as "incubator fluff."

Critical Stages of Development

In the absence of disease that is transmitted through the ovary or oviduct infection, the egg is essentially

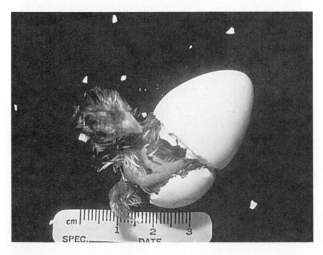

Figure 5–9

Masked bobwhite quail chick kicking free in normal hatch.

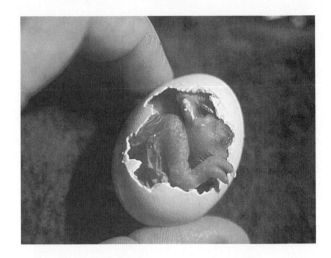

F i g u r e   5 – 1 0

Malposition with head in the small end of the egg. (malposition 2.)

a sterile package. After laying, however, the egg is exposed to environmental and handling factors that can result in mortality from contamination or trauma.[4]

Hatching is another critical developmental stage and is the time of highest mortality. Mortality at this time may be related to improper hatchery environment, such as low humidity or temperature fluctuations (possibly caused by a concerned aviculturist who opens the incubator or hatcher door too frequently). Chicks that pip a blood vessel, rupturing it during pipping, can die from the resulting hemorrhage. They are usually malpositioned and typically are found in poultry embryo malposition 4 (see Table 5–2), with the head rotated away from the air cell. In this position the chick is unable to pip into the air cell.[9]

Some embryos fail to hatch when malpositioned (Table 5–2). There are several causes for malpositioned embryos, some of which are correctable. If the head is in the small end of the egg (malposition 2) the egg may have been set small end up, or it may have been incubated horizontally (Figs. 5–10 and 5–11). With a small embryo or round egg, the embryo may be located crosswise in the egg and may try to hatch on the side of the egg. Other causes of malpositioned embryos include failure to turn the egg sufficiently, excess carbon dioxide levels, low oxygen levels, and delays in development.[7] Described malpositions of psittacine birds are similar to those of poultry (Figs. 5–12 and 5–13).

FACTORS REDUCING HATCHABILITY

Embryonic mortality can occur during any stage of development, from the time of egg formation in the

T a b l e   5 – 2

CLASSIFICATIONS OF MALPOSITIONED POULTRY EMBRYOS

Number	Posture of Embryo	Outcome
1	Head between the thighs	Early normal position for embryo Will result in death if development is delayed
2	Head in small end of egg	Only lethal about 50% of time; good success if hatching is assisted
3	Head to left (under left wing)	Lethal
4	Body rotated along long axis of egg with head away from the side of the egg, not in the air cell	Because the beak is pointed away from the air cell, position is often fatal
5	Feet over the head	Embryo cannot kick to rotate the body when cutting out; therefore often fatal unless assisted
6	Head over right wing instead of under	Usually has live hatch without serious complications
7	Embryo lying crosswise in egg	Seen with small embryos or spherical eggs; often have other defects, fatal

Data from Brown,[4] Joyner,[7] Clubb and Phillips,[8] and Olsen and Duvall.[11]

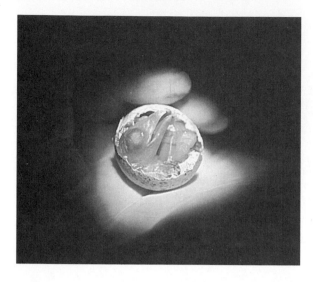

Figure 5-11

Head over right wing (malposition 6) in a Hawaiian crow embryo.

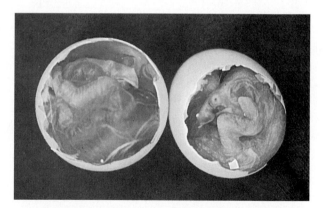

Figure 5-12

Embryo on right (yellow-crowned Amazon) shows normal position. Embryo on left (umbrella cockatoo) is malpositioned with the head under the left wing. (malposition 3.)

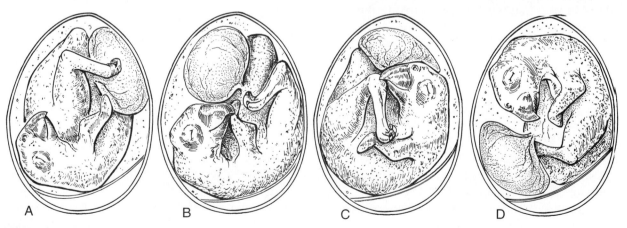

A   B   C   D

Figure 5-13

Malpositions of psittacine birds. (*A*) Normal position. (*B*) Beak rotated away from air cell. (*C*) Back of chick is toward air cell with head near large end of egg. (*D*) Head at small end of egg. (From Schubot RM, Clubb KJ, Clubb SL: Psittacine Aviculture Perspectives, Techniques, and Research. Loxahatchee, FL: Aviculture Breeding and Research Center.)

oviduct until hatching. Detailed records of incubation parameters, parental health, previous production by the pair, and egg handling techniques complement the necropsy determination. Reduced hatchability may be due to parental age, nutrition, or genetics.

Parental Age

Both fertility and hatchability are known to change with the age of the parent birds. Young and old parent birds often have reduced hatchability. For young parents, this may be the result of an immature reproductive tract, inexperience, or behavioral problems. In older birds, underlying health problems, nutrient exhaustion, poor shell quality, or deficiencies related to chronic conditions may contribute to reduced hatchability.

However, age is a species-relative factor. In commercial chicken, duck, pheasant, and quail flocks, reproductively active birds are not maintained beyond two breeding seasons. Certainly this is not true in longer-lived birds such as cranes, psittacines, and raptors. At the Patuxent Environmental Science Center, an Andean condor pair were still reproductively active when the male was 44 and the female 31 years old. A whooping crane pair is still reproductively active and producing viable eggs at 31 years for the male and 24 years for the female. Macaws have been reported to breed successfully at 35 years of age.[10] Generally, the longer the species takes to reach sexual maturity, the longer its active breeding life.

Inherited Factors

The genetic material an embryo receives from its parents' egg or sperm is sometimes defective. Genetic defects may be expressed at some point in the embryo's development. The most obvious defects are malformations seen at hatching. An especially high rate of embryonic malformation is seen in ostrich chicks, which may be related to genetics or incorrect incubation. But in other cases, embryonic development may proceed to a certain point and then cease. Determining the cause of death in some of these cases can be difficult and is based on eliminating other causes of mortality. Using genetic epidemiology to correlate the ratio of similarly dead embryos with hereditary factors is also helpful.

Genetically lethal traits are usually recessive genes. The incidence of genetic defects can increase when inbreeding birds for desirable traits or when breeding endangered species in which low founder flock numbers and genetic bottlenecks are frequent problems.

Embryonic mortality or deformity may also be the result of teratogenic factors such as pesticide exposure. An apparently normal-looking embryo may have died from lethal traits that prevented it from metabolizing certain nutrients or synthesizing compounds required for normal development.

Dietary Factors

A number of dietary deficiencies can contribute to poor hatchability. Minor deficiencies in the female bird can be magnified over the course of a breeding season, especially if multiple clutching techniques are used to maximize the pair's reproductive potential. The most obvious deficiency is a general lack of nutrients or a debilitated state in a laying bird (or, to a lesser extent, a male bird). However, such cases are not common because ovulation is usually inhibited to conserve nutrients for the adult bird.[11]

Some vitamins are extremely important for proper embryonic development. Dietary levels of vitamins sufficient for maintenance of an adult bird for a period of time without clinical signs of disease may be insufficient for the laying female and may result in deficiencies in her eggs.[11, 12]

Marginal deficiencies in vitamin A can lead to poor hatchability. However, deficiencies of vitamin A in a laying bird on a balanced diet or one in which synthetic vitamin A is added are rare.

Of the B vitamin group, deficiencies in thiamine (B_1), niacin, biotin, and pantothenic acid are rare. Riboflavin (B_2) is extremely important for incubation, and large quantities are found in egg white. Deficiencies reduce hatchability, causing curly toe paralysis and clubbed down feathers in the embryos that survive to hatch. The quality of the diet may be adequate to prevent clinical signs in the laying bird but insufficient for the embryo.[11, 12]

Pyridoxine (B_6) is also important for hatchability and early chick growth. Pyridoxine is needed for the breakdown and synthesis of proteins. Laying birds on high protein diets have increased demand for B$_6$, which may result in egg deficiencies. Simple deficiencies of B$_6$ may result in embryonic death with no definitive signs. However, a more common appearance of B$_6$ and manganese deficiency in poultry is perosis, with soft developing bones and slipped gastrocnemius tendons. Vitamin B$_6$ is commonly found in nature, and marginal deficiencies are more common than absolute deficiencies.[12]

Folic acid is required for proper synthesis of red blood cells. Deficiencies result in early embryonic death because of failure of blood to form properly. Folic acid is synthesized by bacteria in the intestines; therefore, natural deficiencies are uncommon. However, laying birds on antibiotic therapy can rapidly develop deficiencies in eggs being laid at the time of therapy. Cyanocobalamine (B$_{12}$) is also required for proper blood formation in embryos, with reduced hatchability even with minor deficiencies. This vitamin is produced by both bacteria and molds, and synthetic B$_{12}$ is added to bird rations.

Vitamin D is required for proper calcium and phosphorus metabolism. Marginal deficiencies in an egg interfere with the embryonic mobilization of eggshell calcium and lead to embryonic deaths. In the laying female bird, insufficiencies in vitamin D can lead to abnormal calcium metabolism for normal eggshell formation. Most birds exposed to natural sunlight or ultraviolet light can manufacture their own vitamin D (as D$_3$).[11, 12]

Deficiencies in vitamins C, E, and K are rare in pet birds.

Infectious Agents

Investigating possible microbiologic agents as causative factors in episodes of reduced hatchability is important. A number of bacterial agents in addition to *Chlamydia* and some viruses are pathogenic to avian embryos. When signs seen in association with embryonic mortality are consistent with one of these agents, every effort should be made to isolate and identify the pathogen. Direct ovarian (transovarian) transmission as well as transmission through shell penetration by pathogens can result in disease. Transovarian transmission of many poultry pathogens is well documented, including that of

Salmonella (S. pullorum, S. enteritidis, S. gallisepticum), Mycoplasma, viruses of the leukosis/sarcoma group, adenoviruses (group I and egg drop syndrome), and avian encephalomyelitis virus.[13] Notably, investigators of transmission of some diseases important to nondomestic birds have failed to demonstrate transovarian transmission of chlamydiosis, *Mycobacteria* infection, pox, and Newcastle disease.

Salmonellosis is a common cause of embryonic mortality and loss of chicks shortly after hatching. Postmortem lesions include an enlarged congested liver with the normal yellow-orange colored liver streaked with areas of hemorrhage, coagulated yolk material, a congested and enlarged spleen, and congested kidneys. Pinpoint necrotic foci may be found in the liver. Pericarditis is also seen. Bacterial culture is necessary for a positive identification.[1, 12]

Staphylococcus species are common bacterial pathogens. The avian embryo can be highly susceptible to some strains of staphylococci but resistant to other strains. Infected wounds on parent birds or on the hands of the aviculturist can lead to infected eggs. The organism proliferates readily in the environment of a mechanical incubator. Infection can result in death within 48 hours or less, especially with some strains of *S. aureus.* Embryonic mortality is known to decrease with increasing age of the embryo at first exposure.[12, 13]

Staphylococcus bacteria have been isolated from the brain, kidney, liver, and heart of dead embryos. Postmortem lesions include hemorrhagic encephalosis plus hemorrhage, and necrosis of nervous tissues throughout the body. Frequently, hemorrhage is seen in the kidney and liver. In addition, some structural distortion occurs in liver tissue. Hemorrhage and pericarditis characterize cardiac lesions, especially with *S. epidermis* infections.[12, 13]

Prevention of *Staphylococcus* infections in parent birds requires that people handling eggs minimize embryonic exposure to this pathogenic agent. Feeding low levels of antibiotics, especially such products as penicillin or chlortetracycline, increases the possibility of developing resistant *Staphylococcus* strains. Therefore, this practice should be avoided unless indicated by a more pressing disease problem (such as chlamydiosis requiring a treatment regimen of tetracyclines).

Streptococcus faecalis, commonly found as normal flora in the intestinal tract of many bird species, can be a cause of embryonic mortality. A laying bird's ovary can become infected, resulting in the *S. faecalis* organism entering the forming egg. Contamination of the egg in this manner may lead to a 20 to 50% mortality rate. Culturing eggs is important to identify the causative agent and carrier hens.

Escherichia coli can enter the egg through the shell, if there is contamination of the shell with feces containing the bacteria. Dirty nests and contaminated pens or cages are sources of contamination. Parent birds in dirty pens can track feces onto eggs from feet or feathers.

E. coli may also enter the egg from infections in the reproductive tract of the female bird. Aviary dust can be a source of contamination. Dust from poultry houses has been found to have 10^5 to 10^6 bacteria per gram. Low brooding temperature also contributes to higher incidence of *E. coli*–infected eggs (Fig. 5–14).[12]

The most common site of *E. coli* infection is the yolk sac. Yolk sac contents may appear yellow-green or yellow-brown and watery in consistency. There may be an associated omphalitis, with the yolk sac wall appearing edematous. Histologically, the outer connective tissue layer is followed by a layer of inflammatory cells characterized by heterophils and macrophages, then a layer of giant cells, and finally a layer of necrotic heterophils and bacteria next to the yolk materials.[14]

Many infected embryos die late in incubation or shortly after hatching. The incidence of infection causing death is greatly reduced by 6 days after hatching in both cranes and chickens. Post-hatching yolk sac infections (omphalitis) and poor weight gain in young nestlings are associated with *E. coli* infections acquired during incubation. Mushy duck disease, in which the duckling appears edematous, can be the result of several bacterial agents, but *E. coli* is most common and is isolated in 70% of such cases.

Reducing fecal contamination and dust in the aviary and incubator rooms is important for control. There is no recommended treatment for infected eggs. However, fumigating or disinfecting eggs shortly after laying is commonly used for poultry and reduces the incidence of *E. coli* infections.[14] Cracked eggs are more likely to become infected and serve as a source of infection for other eggs in the nest or incubator. Discarding cracked eggs or sealing the crack as soon as possible helps prevent contamination and the spread of disease.

Mycoplasma infections are transmitted with the egg and reduce hatchability. The role of *Mycoplasma* infections in cage birds is not as well documented as it is for poultry. *Mycoplasma* can spread to the egg from an infected oviduct or from the semen of infected male birds. Transmission from contaminated facilities or equipment is not well documented.[15]

The infection is commonly seen in upper respiratory passages and clavicular and thoracic air sacs. Catarrhal or caseous exudates are characteristic gross lesions. By day 13 post infection, 37 to 100% of turkey eggs will show air sac involvement. Other gross lesions include dwarfing, generalized edema, liver necrosis, enlarged spleens, and joint abscesses. Joint involvement occurs as subcutaneous periarticular granulomas with necrotic centers, bordered by epithelioid cells and some giant cells.

Treatment of eggs for *Mycoplasma* infections is possible. Tylosin (0.5–1.0 mg/dose) is injected into the air cell at the start of incubation. A small hole is drilled into the egg using a fine surgical burr. This is often best done by rotating the drill bit or burr by hand to avoid breaking delicate eggs. The hole is sealed afterward with a drop of beeswax. A combination of lincomycin and spectinomycin is also effective for egg injection.[16] Dipping eggs in antibiotic solutions is effective in reducing the incidence of disease. Eggs are first warmed to 35 to

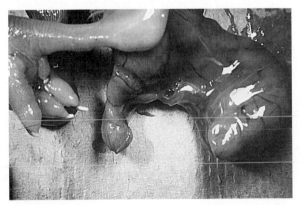

Figure 5 – 1 4

Consolidation of yolk material due to *E. coli* infection in a full-term dead-in-shell crane embryo.

37°C then dipped into an antibiotic solution maintained at 2 to 8°C for 5 to 20 minutes. Antibiotics of choice include tylosin (1000–3000 ppm or 1–3 mg/ml) or gentamicin (400–1000 ppm or 0.4–1.0 mg/ml), plus a disinfectant (such as quaternary ammonium at 250 ppm). Dilute in sterile water.

A third treatment technique that has proved effective to break the transmission cycle of *M. gallisepticum* and *M. synoviae* is to take eggs from a room temperature environment (26.5°C) and place them in a forced-air incubator. Then the temperature is elevated to 46°C for 12 to 14 hours before returning to room temperature or normal incubation temperature. This technique inactivates the *Mycoplasma* organisms but has the disadvantage of reducing hatchability by 8 to 12%.

In 1934 *Chlamydia psittaci* was found to be an egg-borne pathogen in parakeets. The organism can be isolated from the ovary of the female bird and from eggs. Chlamydiosis results in embryo death in 5 to 12 days. Characteristic pathologic findings include congested or grossly hemorrhagic yolk sac membranes.[1, 4]

Several viral diseases have been documented as adversely affecting avian embryos. Budgerigar herpes is transmitted within the egg and causes reduced hatchability. Avian paramyxovirus (Newcastle disease) will enter eggs contaminated with infected fecal material. Transmission from an infected female bird is possible, but usually viremic female birds cease laying. Embryos infected with paramyxovirus are retarded in growth and show defects in the neural tube, eye lenses, auditory vesicles, visceral arches, limb buds, and olfactory pits.[4] Embryo mortality approaches 100% with all Newcastle disease strains.

Aspergillus species is the most important fungal pathogen of eggs. Spores originate from an outside source or another infected egg. The disease is especially a problem in forced-air incubators. Embryos either die before hatching or are weak, gasping, and dyspneic at hatching. Nervous system symptoms and diarrhea are less common occurrences in embryos that survive to hatching. Typical lesions found at necropsy include small yellow foci in the lungs,[17] bronchial plugs,[18] and air cell plaques.[19] The fungus grows readily on the air cell membrane. Cultures should be taken from lesions in the lung or air sac and from the air cell membrane (Fig. 5–15).

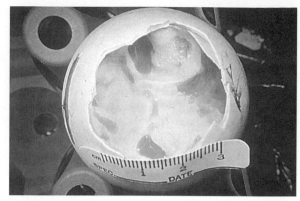

Figure 5–15

Aspergillus infection in the membranes between the embryo and the air cell resulted in death of this Canada goose embryo.

Treatment of eggs infected with *Aspergillus* is not currently feasible. However, prevention of infection is possible. Incubators should be cleaned and fumigated between groups of eggs. Individual eggs should be candled frequently to monitor viability and dead eggs removed quickly to minimize potential for the spread of aspergillosis as well as other diseases.

Parasitism

The primary effect of parasites on egg development is indirect. Parasitic infestations, if severe, reduce the nutritional status of the adult bird and lead to deficiencies in eggs laid by these birds.

Several species of parasites have been documented to occur within eggs. Adult ascarids are occasionally found within eggs. These worms enter the forming egg by reverse peristalsis, moving from the cloaca up the oviduct.[20] The fluke *Prosthogonimus ovatus* is found in the oviduct of Galliformes and Anseriformes. The fluke may be found within the egg but, more often, fluke infestation leads to abnormal shell formation (failure to form a shell or soft-shelled eggs).[21]

Other parasitic infections have been documented only experimentally. Eggs inoculated with *Coccidia* show 100% mortality at day 3, 80% mortality at day 12. Lesions seen in coccidial infections include microcephalus (64% of eggs examined), anomalies of the central nervous system (60%), microphthalmia (53%), atrophy of the lower body (47%), abnormal limb development (46%), and lordosis (34%).[13] Certainly, cracked eggs present the potential for *Coccidia* to enter the egg. Therefore, as with bacterial infections, care must be taken to avoid fecal contamination, clean eggs that are contaminated with feces, and seal cracked eggs.

Plasmodium has been experimentally inoculated into eggs, resulting in death within 9 days. Necropsy findings included green-colored liver, spleen, and embryonic membranes.[13] *Plasmodium* theoretically could be inoculated into an egg in the oviduct as a result of hemorrhage from the female bird in the formation of a blood spot. The fact that this apparently does not occur may be the result of some natural immune mechanism.

Toxic Substances

With the plethora of oil spills around the world, veterinarians are frequently called upon to save oiled birds and advise others on the impact of oil on wildlife. In addition, occasionally caged birds, especially those in outside aviaries, are exposed to petroleum products. The initial reports of reduced hatchability associated with petroleum products on feathers was with terns and gulls.[22, 23] Originally, oil toxicity in eggs was believed to result from oil coating the eggshell and preventing proper gaseous exchange between the embryo and the environment. Work in the last 15 years has shown that even small amounts of oil (1–10 μl), when deposited on the eggshell, can penetrate the egg and be embryotoxic or teratogenic.[24–29] In one study, as little as 0.3 μl of a commercial grade oil used on roadways killed 50% of developing mallard embryos (Fig. 5–16).[30] Typical lesions seen in eggs exposed to crude oil include extensive edema, enlarged heart and spleen, and hepatic necrosis.[31–33] Polychlorinated biphenyls (PCBs) and dioxins can also be toxic to embryos.[42]

Mineral oil, often used in the preparation of medicinal ointments, can be transferred from an incubating female bird to her eggs, reducing hatchability.[34] The primary mechanism appears to be blockage of shell pores by the oily preparations. Therefore, caution should be exercised when prescribing oil-based preparations to actively laying or nesting birds or in egg-bound birds.

Some insecticides have long been known to be toxic to birds and their eggs. Organophosphate insecticides cause malformed embryos with defects including scoliosis, lordosis, and possible reduction in total length of the entire vertebral column (Fig. 5–17, *A* and *B*).[35] With exposure to parathion, these defects are most pronounced in the cervical region. Diazinon exposure results in incomplete caudal ossification and stunting of embryonic growth. Of the common insecticides, carbaryl, malathion, permethrin, and phosmat are relatively nonembryotoxic if used properly in small amounts.[35]

Herbicides, once thought to be nontoxic to vertebrates, have proved to be equally or more toxic than insecticides when applied to eggs (Fig. 5–18). Paraquat and trifluralin are two highly embryotoxic herbicides in studies using mallard eggs.[35] Trifluralin exposure causes beak defects, whereas paraquat produces extensive edema, exencephaly, or anencephaly.[35]

Components of automotive exhaust are harmful to avian embryos. Carbon monoxide at 100 ppm is known to decrease hatchability by 21%, and at 200 ppm a reduction in hatchability of 83% was seen.[36] Carbon monoxide decreases embryonic growth while producing hypertrophy of the liver, spleen, and heart. Serum albumen is increased, globulin decreased, hematocrit increased, serum alanine transfer increased, and lactic dehydrogenase increased.[37, 38] Other components of automotive exhaust are considered hepatotoxic. Exposure of avian embryos to exhaust gases causes increased heart and liver-to-body weight ratios. Catalytic converter–treated exhaust has smaller effects on these organs and on embryo hatchability as compared with untreated exhaust.[37]

Dietary selenium in excess of 4 ppm reduces hatchability and is teratogenic. The naturally occurring organic form of selenium, selenomethionine, when present in excess in the diet of a laying female, accumulates in eggs but does not always produce clinical disease in the female bird. Malformations seen in embryos include ectodactylia, hydrocephaly, microphthalmia or anophthalmia, and beak defects (Figs. 5–19 and 5–20).[39, 40]

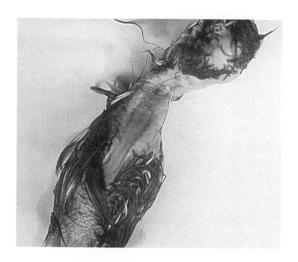

Figure 5–16

Rachischisis and encephalitis in a mallard duck embryo experimentally exposed to crude oil. (Courtesy of David Hoffman.)

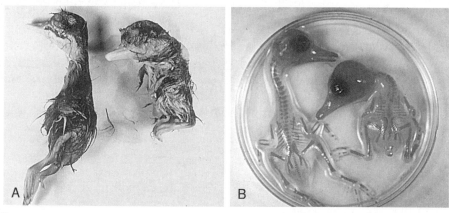

Figure 5–17

A. Normal (*left*) and abnormal (*right*) 18-day-old mallard embryos. Abnormal chick shows shortened axial skeleton, cervical lordosis, and subcutaneous edema associated with experimental application of low-level organophosphate insecticide to the shell. (*B*) The same embryos cleared to illustrate skeletal deformities. (Courtesy of David Hoffman.)

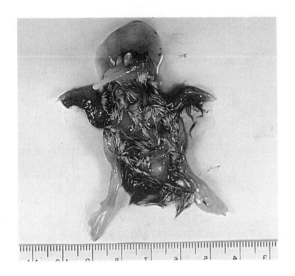

Figure 5–18

Extensive edema and an encephaly in a mallard duck embryo associated with herbicide application to the shell. (Courtesy of David Hoffman.)

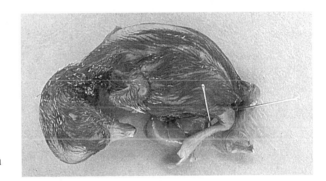

Figure 5–19

Selenium toxicity is evident by deformed toes and microphthalmia in a coot embryo. (Courtesy of David Hoffman.)

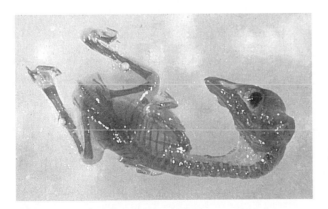

Figure 5–20

Mallard duck embryo with soft tissue cleared and bones stained, showing malformation of the feet caused by selenium toxicity. (Courtesy of David Hoffman.)

Some antibiotics are known to affect avian embryonic development. Penicillin causes hemorrhage and edema of the limbs and head.[41] Exposure to tetracycline-type antibiotics produces stunted embryos through the inhibition of skeletal mineralization and erosion of long-bone cartilage. Chloramphenicol also inhibits embryonic growth, but does not produce malformed embryos. Sulfa drugs lead to multiple embryo problems including granular degeneration of urinary tubules, enlarged head, micro- or macrophthalmia, beak hypoplasia, knee and toe joint amylosis, and regressive changes in liver cells.[13] Most of the research has been performed with the older antibiotics. Any embryotoxic or teratogenic effects of the newer antibiotics have not been discovered. The best advice is to use caution when giving any antibiotic to a laying female bird or one about to lay and to advise the client of a possible risk in such therapy.

References

1. Olsen GH: Problems associated with incubation and hatching. Proc Assoc Avian Vet, 1989, pp 262–267.
2. Romanoff AL: The Avian Embryo. New York, Macmillan, 1960.
3. Kosin IL: Macro and microscopic methods of detecting fertility in unincubated hen's eggs. Poult Sci 23:266–269, 1944.
4. Brown AFA: The Incubation Book. Hindhead, Surry, England, 1979.
5. Stewart J: Ratites. In Branson WR, Harrison GJ, Harrison LR (eds): Avian Medicine: Principles and Applications. Lake Worth, FL, Wingers Publishing, 1994, pp. 1284–1326.
6. Jordan R: Parrot Incubation Procedures. Pickering, Ontario, Silvio Mattacchione, 1989.
7. Joyner KL: Theriogenology. In Branson WR, Harrison GJ, Harrison LR (eds): Avian Medicine: Principles and Application. Lake Worth, FL, Wingers Publishing, 1994, pp 748–804.
8. Clubb S, Phillips A: Psittacine embryonic mortality. In Psittacine Aviculture, Perspectives, Techniques and Research. Loxahatchee, FL, Publication of the Avicultural Breeding and Research Center, 1992.
9. Clubb KJ, Swigert T: Common sense incubation. In Psittacine Aviculture, Perspectives, Techniques and Research. Loxahatchee, FL, A Publication of the Avicultural Breeding and Research Center, 1992.
10. Clubb S, Clubb K: Reproductive life span of macaws. In Psittacine Aviculture, Perspectives, Techniques and Research. Loxahatchee, FL, A Publication of the Avicultural Breeding and Research Center, 1992.
11. Olsen GH, Duvall F: Commonly encountered hatching problems. Proc Assoc Avian Vet, 1994, pp 379–385.
12. Olsen GH, Nicolich JM, Hoffman DJ: A review of some causes of death of avian embryos. Proc Assoc Avian Vet, 1990, pp 106–111.
13. Romanoff AL, Romanoff AJ: Pathogenesis of the Avian Embryo. New York, Wiley-Interscience, 1972.
14. Gross WB: Miscellaneous bacterial diseases. In Hofstad

MS, Barnes HJ, Calnek BW, et al (eds): Diseases of Poultry. Ames, IO, Iowa State University Press, 1984, pp. 257–282.
15. Yoder HW Jr: *Mycoplasma gallisepticum* infection. In Hofstad MS, Barnes HJ, Calnek BW, et al (eds): Diseases of Poultry. Ames, IO, Iowa State University Press, 1984.
16. Truscott RB, Ferguson AE: Can J Compar Med 39:235–239, 1975.
17. Eggert MJ, Barnhart JV: A case of egg-borne aspergillosis. J Am Vet Med Assoc 122:225, 1953.
18. Clark DS, et al: Aspergillosis in newly hatched chicks. J Am Vet Med Assoc 124:116–117, 1954.
19. O'Meara DC, Chute HL: Aspergillosis experimentally produced in hatching chicks. Avian Dis 3:404–406, 1959.
20. Hungerford TG: Diseases of Poultry, Including Cage Birds and Pigeons, 4th ed. Sidney, Australia, Angus and Robertson, 1969.
21. Kingston N: Trematodes. In Hofstad MS, Barnes HJ, Calnek BW, et al (eds): Diseases of Poultry. Ames, IO, Iowa State University Press, 1984, pp 668–690.
22. Rittinghaus H: On the direct spread of oil in a seabird sanctuary. Ornithol Mitt 8:43–46, 1956.
23. Birkhead TR, Lloyd C, Corkhill P: Oiled seabirds successfully cleaning their plumage. Br Birds 66:535–537, 1973.
24. Albers PH: Effects of external applications of fuel oil on hatchability of mallard eggs. In Wolfe DA (ed): Fate and Effects of Petroleum Hydrocarbons in Marine Ecosystems and Organisms. New York, 1977, pp 158–163.
25. Szaro RC, Albers PH: Effects of external application of No. 2 fuel oil on common eider eggs. In Wolfe DA (ed): Fate and Effects of Petroleum Hydrocarbons in Marine Ecosystems and Organisms. New York, 1977, pp 164–167.
26. Dieter MP: Acute and chronic studies with waterfowl exposed to petroleum hydrocarbons. In Hall C, Preston W (eds): Program Review Proceedings of Environmental Effects of Energy/Related Activities on Marine/Estuarine Ecosystems. Washington, D.C., EPA-60017-77-111:35–42, 1977.
27. Hoffman DJ: Embryotoxic effects of crude oil in mallard ducks and chicks. Toxicol Appl Pharmacol 46:182–190, 1978.
28. Coon NC, Albers PH, Szaro RC: No. 2 fuel oil decreases embryonic survival of great black-backed gulls. Bull Envir Contam Toxicol 21:152–156, 1979.
29. Szaro RC: Bunker C fuel oil reduced mallard egg hatchability. Bull Envir Contam Toxicol 22:731–732, 1979.
30. Hoffman DJ, Albers PH: Evaluation of potential embryotoxicity and teratogenicity of 42 herbicides, insecticides, and petroleum contaminants to mallard eggs. Arch Envir Contam Toxicol 13:15–27, 1984.
31. Couillard CM, Leighton FA: Comparative pathology of Prudhoe Bay crude oil and inert shell sealants in chicken embryos. Fund Appl Toxicol 13:165–173, 1989.
32. Couillard CM, Leighton FA: Sequential study of the pathology of Prudhoe Bay crude oil in chicken embryos. Ecotoxic Envir Safety 19:17–23, 1990.
33. Couillard CM, Leighton FA: The toxicopathology of Prudhoe Bay crude oil in chicken embryos. Fund Appl Toxicol 14:30–39, 1990.
34. Hartung R: Some effects of oiling on reproduction of ducks. J Wildl Manag 29:872–874, 1965.
35. Hoffman DJ: Embryotoxicity and teratogenicity of environmental contaminants to bird eggs. Rev Envir Contam Toxicol 115:39–89, 1990.
36. McGrath JJ, Moffa JV: System to evaluate the influence of chronic exposure to CO on the hatching eggs of the white leghorn chicken. J Air Pollut Cont Assoc 22(2):123, 1972.
37. Hoffman DJ, Campbell KI: Embryotoxicity of irradiated and

nonirradiated automotive exhaust and carbon monoxide. Envir Res 15:100–107, 1978.

38. Baker FD, Tumasonio CF: Carbon monoxide and avian embryogenesis. Arch Envir Health 24:53–61, 1972.

39. Hoffman DJ, Heinz GH: Embryotoxic and teratogenic effects of selenium in the diet of mallards. J Toxicol Envir Health 24:477–490, 1988.

40. Heinz GH, Hoffman DJ, Gold LG: Impaired reproduction of mallards fed an organic form of selenium. J Wildl Manag 53:418–428, 1989.

41. Gentry RF: The toxicity of certain antibiotics and furazolidone for chicken embryos. Avian Dis 2:76–82, 1958.

42. Rice CP, O'Keefe P: Sources, pathways and effects of PCBs, dioxins and dibenzofurans. In Hoffman DJ, et al (eds): Handbook of Ecotoxicology. Boca Raton, FL, Lewis Publishers, 1995, p 424.

Susan L. Clubb

6

Psittacine Pediatric Husbandry and Medicine

In any field of animal management, proper husbandry dramatically reduces or eliminates medical or disease problems. Nursery management and hand-feeding techniques for neonatal psittacine birds have improved dramatically in recent years. With improved husbandry and nutrition, catastrophic infectious disease and overt malnutrition occur less frequently. Developmental, congenital, and specific nutritional abnormalities are being delineated and differentiated from infectious or management-related problems.

Psittacine birds are altricial—born naked, with eyes closed, helpless, and totally dependent on the parent or foster for food and warmth. Neonates lack a fully competent immune system and are more susceptible to disease than older birds. Genetics, incubation techniques, and nutrition all affect the early survivability and growth of the chick.

Chicks may be raised by their parents, by foster parents of the same or other species, or by humans. Each rearing technique has advantages and disadvantages.

PARENT-REARED CHICKS

It is often assumed that parent-raised chicks are preferred as breeding birds because behavior learned from the parents may increase reproductive success. Further study is needed to confirm this theory. Myers and coworkers[2] found that parent-raised male cockatiels were more likely to inseminate females than hand-raised cockatiels, and that hand-raised cockatiels laid more eggs than parent-raised birds but often failed to lay them in the nest. Birds bred for reintroduction into the wild may also benefit from behaviors learned in parent-rearing. Parent-raising relieves the aviculturist of considerable time-consuming work and expense. Recent research with Amazon parrots indicates that removing and handling chicks while in the nest (12 days and older) for 15 to 30 minutes daily can produce tame chicks.[1–3]

Many breeding pairs exhibit poor parenting habits, including eating eggs, traumatizing chicks, and failing to feed chicks. Some pairs abandon eggs or chicks following a disturbance in the aviary. Chicks may be exposed to disease in the aviary or nest box. Chicks left in the nest after the emergence of pin feathers are often difficult to tame and adapt to use as pets. Chicks in the nest are potentially exposed to hazards such as extremes of weather, predators, pest species, and parasites. Chicks that fledge from the nest may be injured in initial flight attempts or abandoned on the floor of a flight.[1]

FOSTERING

Fostering refers to moving eggs or chicks from the parents' nest to that of a foster parent. Fosters may be of the same or other species. Some highly domesticated species adopt virtually any egg or chick. In most cases fostering of eggs is preferable to fostering hatchlings or larger chicks. Fostering may be used to increase production of some pairs by using pairs that are otherwise nonproductive. Diseases such as bordetellosis may be spread from nest to nest by fostering or by foster parents that are asymptomatic carriers of disease.[1, 40]

PROBLEMS OF PARENT-REARED CHICKS

Parenting is both an instinctual and learned process. Psittacine birds often fail in initial attempts to raise their young. Most inexperienced pairs improve performance with subsequent clutches. Eggs from pairs that are habitually bad parents should be removed for fostering or artificial incubation.[1]

Parent-reared chicks should be monitored frequently for problems that may be associated with parental neglect, aggression, and adverse environmental conditions. Pairs that are accustomed to frequent nest box inspection usually allow examination of chicks. Large psittacines, especially macaws, however, become very protective and even injure chicks in response to nest examination. Parent-fed chicks will have food in the crop most of the time. Chicks that have no food in the crop or are cool to the touch may have been abandoned. Examine chicks for bite wounds, especially around the beak, extremities, and the back, which may indicate parental abuse.[1]

Prolific, highly domesticated species such as cockatiels and lovebirds frequently lay another clutch of eggs prior to the fledging of their chicks. The chicks are often abused by plucking and pecking. Psittacines typically lay every second or third day and begin sitting with the first or second egg. In large clutches, older chicks may be much larger than younger chicks, sometimes twice the size or larger. Smaller chicks may be crushed or may not be able to compete adequately for food. Removal of older chicks for hand-rearing helps younger chicks receive adequate parental care.[1, 4]

Neonatal mortality may indicate management-related problems or disease. A nest box that is too hot, too cold, wet, has inadequate bedding, or is infested with vermin may cause abandonment. Rats or snakes may kill or consume chicks. Nest boxes should be cleaned after fledging of each clutch. Pine shavings make excellent nesting material and should be deep enough to keep eggs and chicks off the floor of the box. Cedar shavings should be avoided because aromatic oils may irritate the eyes and respiratory mucosa. Corn cob bedding should be avoided because it molds with minimal moisture. Soil, peat, and leaves should also be avoided.[1, 4]

Inadequate nutrition, such as calcium-deficient diets for breeders, may lead to fractures or splayleg deformities in chicks. The incidence of these injuries may be potentiated by rapid growth and inadequate nest material. Chicks may also traumatize each other, most frequently biting the face, beak, and wing tips.[1]

Infectious and parasitic disease often result in nestling mortality. Bacterial and yeast infections are especially prevalent in the hot summer months when heat stress and rapid growth of bacteria lead to secondary infections. Closure of boxes may be indicated until cooler weather arrives. Sick chicks should be removed from the nest for hand-feeding. Management should be examined to detect possible sources of contamination such as dirty water bowls or spoiled soft foods. In some instances chicks may be treated in the nest. If parents are tolerant of disturbance, chicks can be dosed individually, or chicks can be treated by supplying medicated soft foods to the parents. Chlamydiosis, polyoma virus, and psittacine beak and feather disease can also result in nestling mortality.[1]

Parasites may plague chicks in the nest. Protozoal endoparasites, including *Giardia* and *Trichomonas*, may cause morbidity and mortality, especially in cockatiel and budgerigar nestlings. *Hexamita* infestation also occurs frequently in cockatiel chicks. Whether *Hexamita* is a pathogen in nestlings or proliferates in the face of other disease or management problems is unknown.[1]

Red mites (*Dermanyssus gallinae*) and Northern fowl mites (*Ornithonyssus sylviarum*) may infest nest boxes. They feed on chicks at night, resulting in anemia and sometimes mortality. Ants and bees may build nests within a nest box, driving out its avian inhabitants. These problems can usually be controlled by adding a small amount of 5% carbamate dust to nest material. In areas where cockroaches live and possibly carry *Sarcocystis falcatula,* a potential hazard in adding insecticides to nest material is that cockroaches may die and be eaten by the adults or nestlings, resulting in infection with *Sarcocystis.* Mosquitoes may torment chicks in the nest and can transmit parrot pox. The use of repellents has not been satisfactory. Fogging in the aviary with water-base pyrethrum insecticides is helpful in reducing mosquito populations. When used according to directions, the insecticides pose no known toxicity problem for the birds.[1]

PRINCIPLES OF HAND-REARING AND NURSERY MANAGEMENT

Neonatal psittacines are totally dependent upon their foster parents for a suitable, sanitary environment. Given appropriate housing and good nutrition, they will thrive. For a clinician to evaluate disease outbreaks or failure to thrive, an understanding of basic management principles is necessary.

Large commercial aviaries find it essential to establish nursery facilities that can be managed to control disease. In such facilities, some personnel can be assigned to care for chicks other than those caring for adults. Ideally, the nursery facility has separate rooms for artificially incubated chicks and those pulled from the nest. Small common species such as conures, budgerigars, cockatiels, and lovebirds are typically pulled from the nest at 1 to 2 weeks of age. These species have often been implicated as carriers of infectious diseases and should be kept separated from, and fed after, larger species that were artificially incubated. A separate room ideally supplied with separate air flow should be available for isolation of sick chicks.[4]

For the small aviary, an elaborate nursery facility and separate nursery personnel are not cost-effective, and the aviculturist typically cares for the adults as well as the chicks. A practical nursery room can be provided in the home. Chicks are often kept in the kitchen, which may be a problem because of temperature fluctuations, high level of human activity, and the potential for production of toxic fumes. A spare bedroom is preferable, especially if water is available. A visit to the aviary and inspection of the nursery will help the clinician to assess pediatric problems.[4]

ASSESSING THE NEONATE AND ITS ENVIRONMENT

The neonate is a product of its environment. The history of the nursery is as important if not more important than the history of the chick. Examine growth and or weight records, if available. Assess the incubation history. Did the chick hatch in a nest or an incubator? Breeding and production history of parents should be considered. Are other chicks affected?[4, 5]

Assess the nursery environment and husbandry. Are brooder or room temperature and humidity appropriate? What type of bedding and primary containers are used? What is the diet and is it appropriate for the species? What feeding utensils are used and how are they cared for? Review hand-feeding techniques and the sanitation program.[4, 5]

Ideally, each aviculturist develops records of growth rates that are "normal" for chicks in their nursery (Fig. 6–1). Growth rates vary depending on diet, food volumes, and feeding frequency. Chick size and growth rate also vary according to the size of the parents and sex of the chick and according to whether it was fed by the parents, and thus no single published chart will be appropriate for each individual chick.[4–8]

Evaluate the sanitation program for the nursery. The feeders should be observed to detect potential contamination of formula and utensils or for practices that may result in spread of disease from chick to chick. Incubation and hatcher and brooder sanitation should be reviewed. Review pest-control practices and procedures for moving chicks into the nursery.[4, 6]

To detect sources for food-borne contamination,

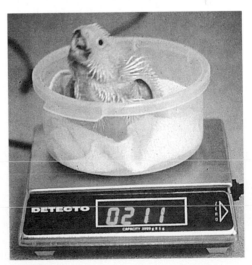

Figure 6–1

Frequent weighing of chicks helps the aviculturalist and veterinarian assess the health and growth of psittacine chicks.

review methods of storing formula, disinfecting and rinsing feeding utensils, handwashing, and cleaning surfaces. Water-related contamination is especially prevalent in farms utilizing well water; however, water filtration systems and pipelines can also present problems, especially if water filters are not changed with appropriate frequency. Ensure that food is not contaminated by inappropriate use of feeding utensils. Feeding all chicks with a single syringe or spoon is a common means of spreading disease.[6]

Assessing the Neonate

An understanding of normal growth and development is essential in assessing the health of a neonate. Assessing the neonate without consideration of the environment can lead to erroneous conclusions. Improper or malfunctioning incubation or brooder equipment, improper use of hand-feeding formulas, and poor sanitation must be considered. Upon physical examination, the veterinarian should determine if the general size and condition of the chick is appropriate for the species and age.

Physical proportions, posture, and plumage development of the chick may reveal nutritional, husbandry, or developmental problems. Pectoral musculature is poorly developed and weight is better assessed by evaluating the back, toes, and wings. The posture and stance of chicks varies by species. In general, Asian parakeets and cockatiels stand tall and are active. Macaws tend to remain recumbent unless feeding. Cockatoos generally sit up often with the head bowed in front. Conures and African parrots often lie on their backs kicking in the air if startled. In evolution, such behavior was necessary as a defensive posture; it is the only way a chick can defend itself when the parents are away from the nest.[4, 6]

Disproportion such as an excessively large head, thin extremities, and a small body indicate stunting (Fig. 6–2). Skin color and texture must be assessed. For most species the normal skin is pinkish yellow (Fig. 6–3) with adequate subcutaneous fat deposits; however, skin pigmentation varies with species and age. Pale skin may indicate hypothermia, shock, or anemia. Reddish coloration may indicate thin skin without adequate subcutaneous fat, or a sick, dehydrated, or stunted chick. Flaky dry skin is common

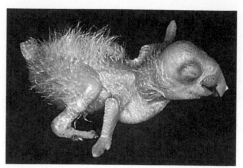

F i g u r e 6 – 2

This chick is underweight and thin and has dark red skin and dehydration resulting from bacterial infection and stunting.

in some species, especially eclectus parrots and macaws, but it may indicate low environmental humidity or excessive brooder ventilation.[4, 6]

Examine the beak for symmetry, brachygnathism or prognathism, lateral deviations, bite wounds, or excoriations. Examine the eyes for discharge, swelling, scabbing, or blepharospasm. Clear discharge may be present when eyes are opening. The age for eye opening will vary with the species. For macaws it is 14 to 28 days; for cockatoos it is 10 to 21 days; for Amazons it is 14 to 21 days.

Ears are generally open at hatching in Old World psittacines. Ears are closed at hatching in neotropical psittacines, opening at 10 to 30 days. Abnor-

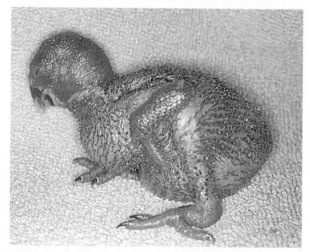

F i g u r e 6 – 3

A normal chick is well filled out and has adequate subcutaneous fat deposits to give the skin an opaque pink-yellow color. Skin pigmentation may be present, as in this eclectus parrot chick.

mally small ear openings are often found in macaws and may lead to infection. Delayed ear and eye opening may occur in stunted chicks. Examine nares for wetness, blood, or exudate.[8]

Examination of the oral region may be difficult because of the pumping behavior of chicks associated with the feeding response. The oral cavity should be examined for abnormal color (hyperemia, pallor), excess fluid or mucus, plaques, or signs of trauma. Some chicks, especially if malnourished or hungry, pump excessively on objects in their environment, often ingesting bedding or injuring the soft tissue at the commissures of the beak, or the mouths of chicks nearby.[6, 9]

Examine the crop for tone, foreign bodies, and thickness and volume of contents. Swelling or discoloration of the crop and surrounding tissues may indicate a burn or puncture. Thick mucosa or white discoloration may indicate candidiasis. Normal feeding response should be elicited by digital stimulation at the lateral commissures of the beak. The smooth muscle wall of the crop periodically contracts, causing visible waves of motility. Hypermotility or hypomotility may be evident with some diseases.[6, 9]

Examine the spine, body, and neck for abnormal curvature. Examine wings and legs for skeletal defects, swelling, wasting, skin lesions, fractures, entwining fibers, asymmetry, and deviations. Visualization through the skin of some internal organs, including liver, supraduodenal loop of the intestine, yolk sac, and lungs is possible. Transillumination of the abdomen may be useful in evaluating the size of the liver and presence of ascites or hemorrhage. The abdomen is typically large and the ventriculus is prominent and protruding, especially in the eclectus parrot. The yolk sac is not fully absorbed until 5 to 7 days after hatching but is usually not visible after 3 to 4 days. Examine the umbilicus for infection, poor seal, protrusion or hernia, or accumulation of fecal material. The umbilicus should be healed by 5 to 17 days of age. Rectal atresia is evident when a hatchling fails to defecate and resolves after dilation with a small swab. Pasting of the vent may result in constipation.[6, 9, 10]

Auscultation of the heart and airways is performed over the pectoral muscles, lateral aspect of the caudal thoracic air sac, trachea, and back. Heart rates are rapid, 180 to 400 beats per minute, and respiratory rates are generally 20 to 60 breaths per minute. Arrhythmias, dull or overly loud heart sounds, or murmurs may indicate congenital defects or heart disease. Harsh wet sounds may indicate aspiration or respiratory infection. Rapid panting may be present in chicks that are overheated, obese, or in pain, especially with abdominal pain.[6, 9, 10]

The condition of the feathers is indicative of the suitability of the diet and hand-feeding techniques, as well as the health of the chick. Feathers that are not emerging properly or the presence of feathers with stress marks or color abnormalities may indicate problems (Fig. 6–4). Stunted macaws often lack down and have delayed emergence of covert feathers on head and body. Hemorrhage in feather shafts or deformity of emerging feathers may indicate disease such as polyomavirus infection or psittacine beak and feather disease (PBFD) or may result from malnutrition or trauma. For example, drying with a hot hair drier held too close to the chick can result in coagulation of blood in the blood feathers and retention of necrotic tissue along the shaft of the feather as it matured (Fig. 6–5), which may be mistaken for clinical signs of PBFD. Systemic disease or drug therapy may also result in feather development abnormalities. Rapid growth and metabolic changes occurring at the time the wing coverts emerge make the wing covert feathers around the elbow the most common site for stress marks.[6]

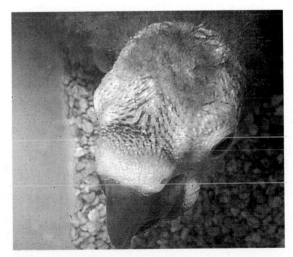

F i g u r e 6 – 4

Abnormal feather emergence can be seen in stunted chicks.

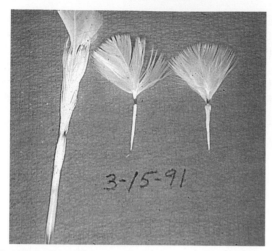

Figure 6–5

Hemorrhage in feather pulp associated with drying a cockatoo chick with a hot hair dryer.

Laboratory Diagnostics

Laboratory diagnostics are essential tools in psittacine pediatrics; however, a presumptive diagnosis and remedial measures must often precede confirmation of the diagnosis. Bacteriology testing is especially useful because neonates frequently succumb to bacterial and fungal infections.

Bacteriology of Intestinal Microflora

Aerobic bacteria, anaerobic bacteria, and fungi make up the intestinal microflora of most animals. The "normal" microflora of psittacine chicks has historically been thought to consist of primarily gram-positive bacteria including *Lactobacillus, Bacillus, Corynebacterium, Streptococcus,* and *Micrococcus* species, and *Staphylococcus epidermidis.* Gram-negative bacteria, including *Escherichia coli,* and *Klebsiella, Enterobacter, Pseudomonas,* and *Salmonella* species, are generally considered potential pathogens. Yeast are often present in low numbers but overgrowth in response to disease, mismanagement, or antibiotic therapy is common.[11-13]

Theoretically, at the time of hatching a chick should be sterile. The chick develops a bacterial flora as it is exposed to bacteria in food or the nursery environment. Some gram-negative bacteria, such as *E. coli, Klebsiella,* and *Enterobacter,* can be found as part of the microflora of clinically healthy chicks and adults, and their isolation does not necessarily require therapy. Judgement as to the necessity of treatment of these chicks must balance clinical evaluation, other diagnostic tests, environmental parameters, and a liberal dose of clinical experience.[11-13]

Cultures of the crop and cloaca may be used to assess the microflora of the chicks as well as to evaluate the level of environmental contamination in the nursery. Treatment of chicks without correction of the contamination problems typically results in reinfection or exacerbation of problems in neonates. High levels of gram-negative bacteria in asymptomatic chicks may result in disease at times of stress such as shipping and weaning. Gram's staining may be useful if a quick presumptive diagnosis is necessary or if economics limit diagnostic testing. Poor correlation of diagnosis with culture results may occur because of nonviable yeast in formulas, the presence of anaerobes, or variable staining qualities of organisms. Cytologic examination may also be valuable.[11-13]

As in adults, blood collection in volumes approximately equal to 1% of body weight (1 ml = 1 g) is safe. For example, in a 200-g chick, up to 2 ml can be collected. Typically only 1 ml of blood is necessary for hematology and blood chemistry tests, especially in chicks that have a low hematocrit and excellent plasma yield. Jugular venipuncture is practical for most chicks weighing 50 g or more. Nail clips may also be used but may result in urate contamination or clotting as well as pain.[12]

Hematology and blood chemistry test results must be assessed using normal values that are appropriate for the age of the chick. As with mammals, values in juvenile birds can vary significantly from those of adults. In a study of hematologic and biochemical parameters of juvenile eclectus parrots, cockatoos, and macaws, a number of parameters were found to vary significantly from published values for adult birds. In all three groups an initial relative anemia, leukocytosis, and heterophilia was observed. Red blood cell parameters including red blood cell count, hemoglobin, hematocrit, and mean corpuscular hemoglobin concentration (MCHC) were initially low, increasing with age. White blood cell values were initially higher than in adults and were higher in macaws than in cockatoos and eclectus parrots. A transition from heterophilia to lymphocytosis was found in juvenile eclectus parrots and cockatoos as they matured. In general, sodium, chlorine, calcium, urea, uric acid, cholesterol, aspartate transaminase, total protein, albumin, and globulin all varied from adult values and increased with age. Potassium, phosphorus, and alkaline phosphatase decreased with age.[14–16]

For radiographic interpretation, the clinician must also understand development. Chicks normally have relatively large livers, little air sac space, a large proventriculus, large fluid-filled intestines, and large hearts in comparison with adults. Growth plates typically close around the time of fledging.[17]

DIETS AND FEEDING

A plethora of commercial hand-feeding formulas is now available, making hand-rearing psittacines much easier. Poultry nutrition has been extensively researched and is typically used as a point of reference in formulation of diets for psittacines. Limited research in psittacine nutrition has delineated numerous differences that exist between psittacines and poultry.[18–22]

Although the minimum nutrient requirements for most psittacines are unknown, if a diet has been used successfully to raise a significant number of chicks to weaning in good health, it must be considered to be complete and adequate for growth of that species. Numerous handmade formulas have also been used extensively with varying degrees of success. It is theorized that secretions from the upper gastrointestinal (GI) tract present in regurgitated parental food enhance the growth of parent-fed psittacine chicks over that of incubator-hatched chicks hand-fed the same diet.[4, 19, 23]

Proper preparation of formula is vital to success. Bacterial infections associated with contamination of water systems are common. If in doubt, boil water for 10 minutes before formula preparation. Poor utensil sanitation, improper formula storage, or inappropriate feeding techniques may result in morbidity. Formula should be stored dry, and only the quantity needed for a meal should be prepared. Remaining formula should be discarded.[4]

Growth rate will be greatly affected by caloric intake. Caloric intake varies with type of formula fed, especially fat content, percent solids, feeding frequency, and volume fed.

The consistency of the diet varies because of the method of manufacture, type of grains used, and presence or absence of digestive enzymes that liquefy formulas or thickeners such as corn starch. When first feeding a formula and periodically thereafter, the feeder should calculate percent solids to ensure proper dietary concentration.

$$\frac{\text{Weight of dry formula}}{\text{Weight of mixed formula} \times 100} = \text{Percent solids}$$

The concentration or percent solids content of the formula affects intestinal transit time as well as the availability of all nutrients. Too high percent solids slows intestinal transit time, whereas too low percent solids results in inadequate caloric intake or too rapid intestinal transit time. Hatchlings have traditionally been fed more dilute formulas (as low as 5% solids) or only fluids in initial feedings. This author recommends feeding regular formula of 10% solids initially. Older babies should be fed 20 to 30% (ideally 23–27%) solids. The experienced hand-feeder may elect to feed smaller chicks first, feeding the more watery food off the top. Others may prefer a more precise increase of percent solids on a schedule such as follows:

1st day—10% solids
2nd day—12% solids
3rd day—15% solids
4th day—18% solids
5th day—20% solids

By the 6th or 7th day most chicks should be eating 23 to 25% solids.

Feeding Schedule

Hatchlings grow more rapidly if initially fed around the clock. Such a feeding schedule, however, is very demanding on the human foster parent. Significant numbers of most psittacine species commonly kept in captivity have been raised successfully with an 18-hour feeding schedule. Some difficult or delicate species may require feeding through the night (Table 6–1).[4]

A practical feeding schedule for hatchlings can be based on 7 feedings a day at approximately 6 AM, 9 AM, 12 noon, 3 PM, 6 PM, 9 PM, and 12 MN. Smaller species or weak or dehydrated chicks should be fed between these feedings so that they are fed each 1½ hours initially. As the chick grows

T a b l e   6 – 1

TROUBLE-SHOOTING IN HAND-FEEDING

Crop Does Not Empty

Infection—Bacterial, viral, mycotic
Crop and gut stasis—systemic disease
Food or chick too cold
Chick dehydrated
Too high or low percent solids
Excessive dietary fat/protein
Crop atony—stretched crop from overfeeding
Foreign body consumption, impaction
(Some chicks' crops never completely empty)

Crop Emptying Too Fast

Hypermotile intestine—diarrhea
Low percent solids
Inadequate food volume
(Older chicks' crops may empty rapidly, leaving
   the chick normal and well nourished)

Chick Not Growing

Infection
Environmental or dietary contamination
Malnutrition (diet inappropriate for species)
Inadequate food intake (inadequate volume and/or
   feeding frequency)
Chick too cold
Too high temperature—dehydration
Congenital or incubation-related problems

Chick Vomiting

Normal crop shrinkage—weaning
Food too hot or cold
Overfeeding—obese
Infection—bacterial/viral/yeast
Gout—kidney disease
Vitamin D toxicity
Polyomavirus infection
Foreign body ingestion
Food allergy

Chick Will Not Eat

Food too hot or too cold
Chick stressed—frightened
Chick thinks it's ready to wean
Lockjaw
Chick does not like taste of food
Chick is overweight

Chick Begs Excessively

Malnutrition
Inadequate feeding volume or frequency
Low percent solids
Chick too cold
Kidney disease
Continuous light—too long photoperiod
Too high protein
Chick spoiled
Infection—viral/bacterial/yeast

Chick Too Thin

Malnutrition—diet inappropriate for species
Inadequate food volume
Inadequate feeding frequency
Infection or other illness
Low percent solids
Stunting

Chick Too Fat

Food too high in calories for species
Excessive volume or frequency of feeding

Chick Pale

Too cold
Anemic
Sudden blood loss or internal or intestinal
   hemorrhage
Hepatic hematoma
Chick in shock
Umbrella cockatoo chicks are often pale at 2–3
   weeks of age

Chick's Skin Too Red

Too hot
Infection
Dehydration
Inadequate subcutaneous fat—stunting

Dry Skin

Dehydration
Low environmental humidity
Excessive ventilation in brooder
Low dietary fat
Malnutrition—low fat diets
Often seen in normal chicks of some species (e.g.,
   eclectus)

Beak Malformed

Congenital abnormality
Improper handling/hand-feeding
Improper calcium:phosphorus ratio
Injury
Vitamin D deficiency
Idiopathic developmental

Splay Leg

Congenital abnormality
Inadequate bedding/slippery surface
Parents sitting too tight on chicks
Injury
Improper calcium:phosphorus ratio
Vitamin D deficiency
Premature or incomplete growth plate closure
Femoral rotational deformity

Crooked Toes

Congenital abnormality
Possible dietary deficiency in parents
Standing on hard flat surfaces—cockatoos
Inadequate dietary calcium

Crooked Neck/Back

Congenital abnormality—possibly hereditary
Inadequate dietary calcium
Injury

Chick Will Not Sit Up

Normal in some species
Injury—fracture
Inappropriate bedding—slippery
Fear
Spinal deformity—scoliosis

Chick Lies on Back

Normal in some species
Neurologic problem
Fear or fright response in some older chicks

Chick Throws Head Over Back

Crooked neck—congenital or developmental
Neurologic problem

Bloody Bedding

Abrasion of skin of feet and wingtips
Low environmental humidity
Abrasive bedding—rough toweling
Hyperexcitable chick
Blood in stool—intussusception
Injury
Polyomavirus infection

Dark (Wine-colored) Stains on Bedding

Normal metabolite in urine of some species
   (Greys, Amazons, Pionus)

Chick Eats Bedding

May be associated with malnutrition
Inappropriate bedding
Inadequate feeding—hunger
Ready to wean

Chick Swallows Tube

Tube too short
Tube slips easily off syringe

Food Pasted to Chick's Face

Sloppy feeding
Inadequate cleaning
Chick regurgitating on itself or cage mate

Abdominal Distention

Normal in parent-raised chicks
Chick too fat
Liver enlarged
Infection
Fatty liver
Ascites
Congenital heart defect
Congenital liver defect
Low blood protein
Viral serositis
Proventricular dilatation
Cloacal atresia in hatchling
Constipation—pasted vent

Jaw Will Not Open

Bordetella infection
Fear—possibly associated with rough handling or
   trauma

Lesions in Mouth

Candidiasis
Bacterial stomatitis
Vitamin A deficiency
Pox virus infection
Bite wounds from siblings
Trichomonas

Table 6–1

TROUBLE-SHOOTING IN HAND-FEEDING *(Continued)*

Crop Feels Thick and Doughy

Candidiasis
Dehydration
Crop stasis
Too high percent solids
Ingested bedding

Dark Lines Visible on Abdomen

Dark intestinal contents (often hemorrhagic)
Infection
Starvation—gut stasis

Swelling/Scab at Umbilicus

Poor umbilical seal
Infection
Normal umbilical scab—drops off when 3–10
    days old

Red Mass, Intestine Protruding From Rectum

Intussusception
Cloacal prolapse

Toes Swollen or Constricted

Twine-threads wrapped around digits
Constricted toe syndrome

Eyes Swollen

Infection
Foreign body
Stunted—eyes appear prominent
Congenital deformity with prominent eyes or
    enlarged anterior chamber—lutino Indian
    ringnecks
Lacrimal sac infection—abscessation

Eyes Fail to Open at Proper Time

Stunted growth
Lids sealed—low humidity
Congenital abnormality

Ear Full of White Material

Stunted growth
Infection

Delayed Feather Emergence

Stunted growth
Malnutrition
PBFD
Polyomavirus infection
Temperature too high?

Indented Lesions on Beak

Bites from cage mates
Beak tip caught in cage wire
Beak too soft—low calcium diet

Bloody Lesions Inside Mouth

Bite wounds from siblings
Pharyngeal puncture

Swelling and Discoloration of Head, Neck, and Crop

Bite wounds from siblings
Pharyngeal or esophageal puncture
Crop burns
Subcutaneous emphysema

Ballooning of Skin

Subcutaneous emphysema—rupture of air sac
Distention of cervicocephalic airsac
Air-gulping

Air in Crop

Air-gulping
Slow feeding, swallowing air with food
Forcing air into crop with syringe
Fermentation of food in crop

Diarrhea

Infection—viral/bacterial/yeast
Parasitism—protozoa, worms

Contamination of food/water
Malnutrition
Intussusception
Intestinal hemorrhage—starvation
Excessive milk products
Excessive vegetables or fruits in diet
Abrupt change in diet
Food allergy

Polyuria

Low percent solids
Vitamin D toxicity
Congenital kidney disease
Chronic kidney disease
Polyomaviral infection
Too high mineral content in food

Nasal Discharge

Too cold
Sinusitis
Foreign body in nostrils
Vitamin A deficiency
Choanal atresia
Infection—*Bordetella, Mycoplasma, Chlamydia,*
    other bacterial
Aspiration of food
Dusty environment
Low environmental humidity
Allergies?

Labored Breathing, Panting

Aspiration of food
Chick too hot
Infection—pneumonia
Ascites
Obesity
Adbominal pain

Hemorrhage When Feather Pulled

Polyoma—sometimes other systemic infections
Possible vitamin K deficiency

and the crop expands in capacity, the 9 AM, 3 PM, and 9 PM feedings can be dropped. If the crop empties between feedings, the chick can be "topped off" with supplemental feeding. Continue at four feedings until pin feathers are mostly in and opening. At this time the chick's schedule can usually be reduced to three or two feedings. Start to offer solid food. When chicks are in a cage, have food present. When chicks are interested in the food, the schedule should be reduced to one or two feedings daily.

Feeding Volumes

Most chicks can be fed 10 to 12% of their body weight per feeding. Cockatoos have smaller crops

and are more efficient in food conversion, and thus they should be fed 10% or less if too heavy (Fig. 6–6). Macaws can usually hold more food and may be fed 12 to 14% of their body weight per feeding.

Commercial diets are formulated to optimize nutrient levels for a broad range of species. Some species, however, may require significantly different nutrient levels for optimal growth. For example, cockatoo and Amazon parrot chicks exhibit good growth on a diet much lower in nutrient density (percent fat) than macaw chicks. Cockatoos and Amazon parrots fed large quantities of high-fat diets often develop hepatic lipidosis. Macaws require a diet higher in fat and/or large volumes of food to meet their caloric requirements for growth. Hyacinth macaws (*Anodorhynchus hyacinthinus*),

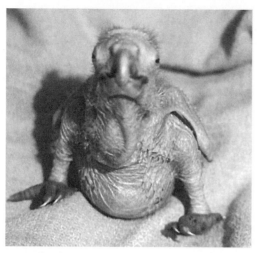

Figure 6–6

Cockatoo chicks in general are more efficient in using calories than neotropical species. Overfeeding may result in obesity and fatty liver disease. This chick has excellent weight without obesity.

green-winged macaws *(Ara chloroptera)* and Queen of Bavaria conures *(Aratinga guarouba)* have better growth on a 15% fat formula.

Hypervitaminosis D and/or hypervitaminosis A may occur if commercial diets are supplemented with vitamins.[37]

DISEASES AND DISORDERS

Developmental and Husbandry Problems

Stunting is poor growth rate or failure to thrive. It may be clinically obvious or may be subclinical in a chick that grows slowly and may experience weaning crisis because of subnormal weight at the onset of weaning. Stunting is often related to poor husbandry, malnutrition, or inexperienced feeders and is usually reversible if diagnosed and corrected early. Stunting associated with inadequate caloric intake may result from inadequate feeding volume or frequency, malnutrition or dietary imbalance, inadequate caloric density of the diet, or excess water in the diet.[10]

Stunted birds appear thin and the head is often disproportionately large. Toes and wings are thin, eye and ear opening may be delayed, and eye slits may open high on the orbit or above the orbit. The skin may be dry, thin, wrinkled, and without

adequate subcutaneous fat. Abnormal patterns of feather emergence, slow emergence, scant down, and stress bars of feathers frequently occur.[10]

Other causes for stunting are enteric bacterial and fungal infections, viral infections such as polyomavirus infection, suboptimal environmental temperature, and excessively long light cycles.[10]

Beak and leg deformities may be multifactoral in etiology. Dietary imbalance, such as improper calcium-to-phosphorus ratio or vitamin D deficiency, too rapid growth rate, or stunting may increase the incidence of these deformities. Trauma may cause or contribute to leg deformity.

Lateral leg deformities, "splay leg," may occur if chicks are placed on slippery surfaces, or if hens sit on chicks, especially if nesting material is inadequate. Green-stick or folding fractures can cause leg deformities. Premature or unilateral closure of the lateral diaphysis may result in lateral deformity of the stifle. Lateral deformity of the stifle may result in rotational deformity of the femur (Fig. 6–7).[24, 25]

If detected at a young age most leg deformities can be corrected by packing the chick tightly with towels or paper towels (Figs. 6–8, 6–9). This is

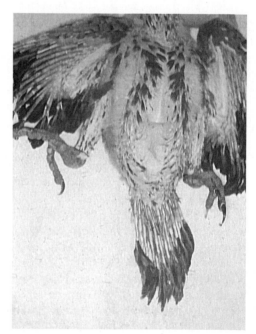

Figure 6–7

This blue and gold macaw chick had unilateral splay leg deformity caused by premature lateral closure of the growth plate of the cranial tibiotarsus and rotational deformity of the femur, both of which were corrected surgically.

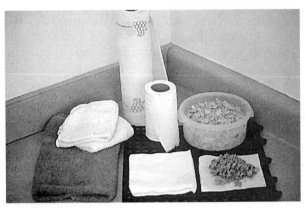

Figure 6 – 8

Suitable substrates for neonates include paper towels, cloth towels, and manufactured paper ball bedding. Older chicks may be placed on rubber mats (Dri-Dek), plastic coated welded wire, or pine shavings (for those birds that are unlikely to ingest the pine shavings).

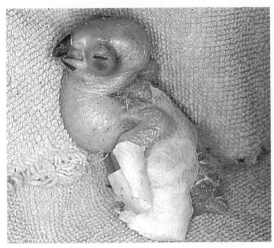

Figure 6 – 10

Many deformities of the legs can be corrected at an early age by taping, hobbling, or packing chicks in toweling.

accomplished by forming a deep cup of toweling and placing the chick inside in a vertical position. Toweling must be changed frequently. Taping the legs together as with a hobble, taping legs around a pad such as a sponge or sanitary napkin, or placing legs through holes cut in a piece of foam rubber or in traction devices may be used for deformities that do not respond to packing alone (Fig. 6–10). Care should be taken to avoid applying tape directly to the leg and to avoid vascular compromise in a rapidly growing chick with bandages that quickly become too tight. Packing reduces struggling and provides a normal upright stance.[24, 25]

More severe leg defects may require a fixed brace. Braces may be formed from pliable splint material (Figs. 6–11 to 6–13) (Sam splint, Jorgenson Laboratorics, Loveland CO) or can be made from the bottom of a plastic bottle that is cut with the bottom and two side bars intact. The brace has a flat bottom and a vertical extension on each side to which the legs are taped. The chick is placed inside

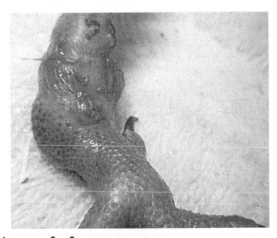

Figure 6 – 9

Toes and legs may become wrapped in strings from frayed towels. Removal of the strings and topical application of dimethyl sulfoxide (DMSO) is usually sufficient to resolve the problem. If scab formation results in constriction, surgical intervention is necessary.

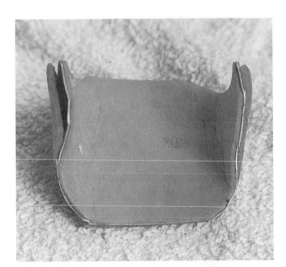

Figure 6 – 11

U-shaped splint made from Sam splint, a malleable metal with foam padding on each side. (Courtesy of Everett Butler.)

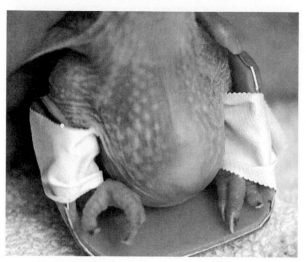

Figure 6-12

This splint can be used for correction of several types of leg deformities, including luxation of the stifle and hyperextension of the stifle. (Courtesy of Everett Butler.)

(the brace must be slightly wider than the chick) and the legs taped to the side bars to provide a normal position. Care must be taken to avoid pressure points. Pack the chick for comfort and to prevent struggling. In general, the younger the age at which correction is initiated, the more successful it

will be. Tiny neonates are typically allowed a week or two of growth before splinting but respond well to packing or hobbling.[24, 25]

Luxation of the stifle (Fig. 6–14) can be a particularly difficult problem. The tibiotarsus is typically luxated and rotated medially with medial luxation of the patellar ligament. In a recent case, a moluccan cockatoo chick with a luxated stifle at the time of hatching had the deformity corrected using a Sam splint.[24]

Surgical correction may be indicated for some leg deformities, especially rotational deformities, but surgery should not be pursued until bones are adequately calcified. In a report of two cases of splay leg, both rotational deformity of the femur and premature closure of the lateral aspect of the growth plate of the proximal tibiotarsus were diagnosed. The growth plate was cauterized medially to stop further uneven growth. Femoral rotation was corrected by midshaft osteotomy and retrograde placement of an intermedullary pin. To prevent rotation, the entire leg was immobilized in a bandage, and the chicks were suspended in a sling postoperatively. Medial stifle luxation can also be repaired surgically by open reduction and tacking of the patellar ligament laterally.[10] (See Chapter 42, Orthopedic Surgery.)

Lateral deviations of the maxilla, often referred to as "scissors beak," are often observed in macaws (Fig. 6–15) and less frequently in other species. The

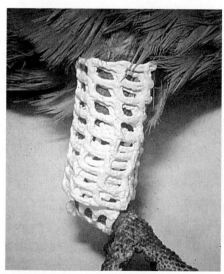

Figure 6-13

Fractures of the tibiotarsus, or correction of folding tibiotarsus fractures, can be immobilized by external splints; however, splints may be changed each week to allow for growth.

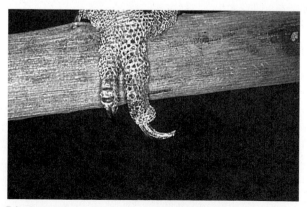

Figure 6-14

Lateral luxation of the distal phalanx of the third toe is frequently observed in heavy-bodied cockatoo chicks that stand on hard, flat surfaces, especially those given calcium-deficient diets. If detected early, luxation can be corrected by splinting, supplemental calcium, and trimming the nails. In older chicks, surgical correction may be required.

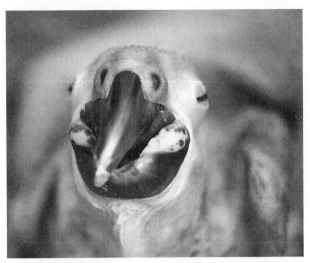

Figure 6–15

Lateral deviation of the maxilla in a hyacinth macaw chick. Note the thickened and raised point on the left side of the mandibular occlusal surface that is forcing the maxilla to the right. (Courtesy of Everett Butler.)

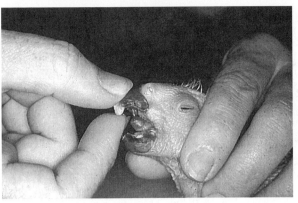

Figure 6–17

The majority of cases of mandibular prognathism can be corrected by physical therapy applied as shown, one to three times daily. Prior to physical therapy, the occlusal surfaces of the maxilla and mandible should be trimmed with cuticle clippers or ground with a Dremel drill.

beak may deviate either to the left or right, may deviate from the frontal bones or cere, or may simply deviate at the tip. Lateral deviations of the maxilla are often blamed on feeding technique (i.e., feeders approaching the same side of the mouth at each feeding). In several studies, however, it has been shown that whereas feeders typically pass food only on one side, the beak may deviate to either side. Many cases are actually initiated by an irregular occlusal surface of the mandible that, upon occlusion, forces the maxilla to one side. In some cases this uneven occlusal surface has resulted from

a frenulum-like ridge of thicker beak tissue lying slightly to the left or right of the midline. The initial deviation results in uneven wear. Trimming of the occlusal surface of the mandible and the application of digital pressure to the beak once or twice daily will correct the defect in most cases if initiated early enough. Once the beak is calcified, application of acrylic corrective devices must be used (see Chapter 44A).[24, 26]

Mandibular prognathism or maxillary brachygnathism occurs primarily in cockatoos (Figs. 6–16, 6–17). Causes may be developmental and/or traumatic, possibly potentiated by dietary calcium deficiency. Most can be corrected by digital manipulation before the beak is calcified (Fig. 6–18). In small cockatoo chicks, the inside occlusal surface of the

Figure 6–16

Mandibular prognathism in a 2-week-old umbrella cockatoo chick.

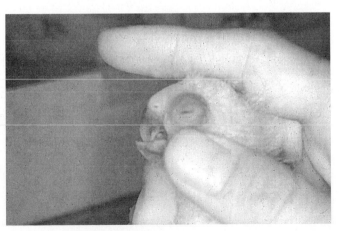
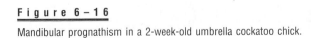

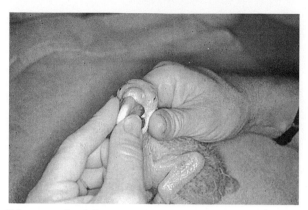

Figure 6–18

Physical therapy used to correct lateral deviation of the maxilla. Pressure is applied to the beak two to three times daily as needed. The occlusal surface of the mandible should be trimmed if necessary to correct irregularities in the surface.

beak has soft cartilage flanges that can be trimmed with cuticle clippers to help in physical therapy for correction. In older chicks with some calcification of the beak, the inside occlusal surface of the maxilla and the external occlusal surface of the mandible can be ground with a Dremel drill. Correction of deformity after calcification of the beak may be achieved by application of an acrylic prosthesis (see Chapter 44A) (Figs. 6–19, 6–20).[10, 24, 26]

Deformities of toes causing a lateral deviation of

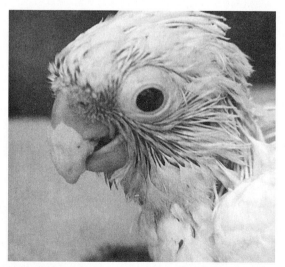

Figure 6–19

Acrylic device used to correct cases of mandibular prognathism that do not respond to trimming and physical therapy. (Courtesy of Everett Butler.)

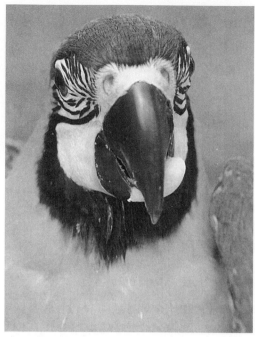

Figure 6–20

Acrylic device used to correct lateral deviations of the maxilla. (Courtesy of Everett Butler.)

the last phalanx of the third and sometimes the second toes may be associated with inadequate dietary calcium and may be potentiated by the chick standing on a hard flat surface. Forward deviation of the first or fourth toes can be corrected, if detected at an early age, by taping the toes in a normal position.[10, 21]

Neck deformities such as torticollis and twisting or lateral deviations may be corrected by use of a padded neck brace (Fig. 6–21) held in place with Velcro or by taping the neck into the corner of a square bowl. The neck brace can be removed for feeding and for massage therapy, which may also be beneficial.[10, 24]

A poor umbilical seal may be associated with incubation at an excessively high incubation temperature. External yolk should be tied off and removed. The open umbilicus should be sutured and swabbed with a tamed iodine preparation.[10]

A retained yolk sac may be associated with improper incubation parameters, weak hatch, or other factors that result in poor neonatal development in the first week of life (Fig. 6–22). Fasting in the first 24 hours is not necessary in psittacines and may in

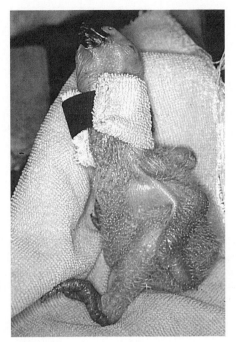

Figure 6-21
Neck brace made of a wash cloth and Velcro fastening strip to straighten the crooked neck of an African grey parrot chick.

the sinuses. If fluid that is flushed through the nostrils does not exit the choana, suspect atresia. Surgical repair has not been described.[38]

Digestive disorders are the most common problems observed in neonatal psittacines. Digestive disorders and reduced intestinal motility are the most common or most obvious clinical signs observed in a variety of systemic disorders. Gram-negative bacterial infections often accompanied by candidiasis are the most common, but the signs may also be seen with viral infections, malnutrition, or inappropriate environmental conditions. Reduced intestinal motility results in slow crop emptying, crop impaction, and "sour crop." Fluids may be absorbed in a dehydrated chick, leaving a hard ball of food in the crop.[6, 9, 10]

Gut transit time may be affected by diet and environment. Percent solids is known to affect gut transit time; higher percent solids prolongs gut transit time. Some types of fiber may also affect gut transit time; more research is needed in this area. Crop washes and transfer of normal flora from the adult to the chick are often advocated but can result in transmission of disease. Dietary supplementation

fact be detrimental. Most yolk should be absorbed within the first 5 to 7 days of life. After approximately a week, retention of yolk should be considered abnormal. The chick may develop toxicity due to degradation of yolk material, even if no infection is present. Yolk sac retention is typically not a specific disorder but rather a sign of other problems. Bacterial infection of the yolk may remain from infection within the egg. Because of the chicks' tiny size, yolk sac removal is not practical in psittacines. In some cases thought to have a fatal prognosis, aspiration of yolk with a syringe has been accomplished and some chicks have survived.[6, 9, 10, 25, 27]

Congenital heart diseases such as ventricular septal defect have been diagnosed on postmortem examination of chicks. Cardiomyopathy has also been observed.

Congenital atresia of the choana has been reported in an African grey and an umbrella cockatoo. The author has observed several cases in African grey parrots and a hybrid macaw. In this disorder the sinuses fill with exudate as drainage through the choana is obstructed. Diagnosis is by flushing

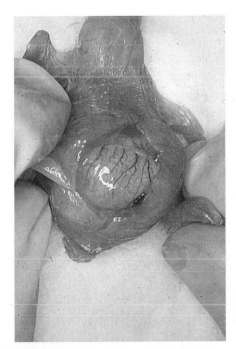

Figure 6-22
Normal sized yolk sac in a 1-day-old chick. A retained yolk sac is usually the result of other developmental, husbandry, or disease problems.

with *Lactobacillus* and other probiotics has been reported with mixed results. Hand-feeding formulas that are heavy with particulate matter may remain in the crop after fluids are absorbed.[9, 28]

Air-gulping may occur during feeding or before or after feeding. Birds that swallow air may not be fed adequate volumes of food because the crop appears to be full when it is not. Birds may be burped by extending the neck and applying gentle pressure to the upper crop, or air may be released by passing a tube. Training birds to feed rapidly or feeding by tube may help reduce the effects of air-gulping.[6, 10]

Regurgitation of small amounts of formula after feeding is normal in birds that are weaning and in which the crop is shrinking. The most common cause of regurgitation in preweaning birds is overfeeding. If a chick regurgitates a portion of formula (for example, 5 ml of a 30-ml feeding) the volume should be reduced. Overweight chicks frequently regurgitate. Some birds, such as African grey parrots, may regurgitate if fed cold food.[4, 6]

Primary crop disorders include impaction, mycotic or bacterial ingluvitis, and consumption of foreign bodies. Crop atony or flaccid crop may occur as a result of stretching of the crop wall by overfeeding. Providing physical support with a bandage "crop bra" is beneficial.[6, 10]

Enteritis is often associated with bacterial infection, osmotic imbalance, bacterial endotoxin production, mucosal disease, or hypermotility. Severe intestinal hypermotility may result in intussusception. Affected chicks often exhibit melena or frank blood in the stool. Mild intussusception is evident on contrast radiography films. Oral antibiotic therapy and oral administration of barium may be helpful. In severe intussusception, protrusion of the ileum from the cloaca appears as a dark tube up to an inch in length and is typically fatal. Surgical intervention is usually unrewarding because of vascular compromise; however, a successful technique for jejunostomy and jejunocloacal anastomosis has been reported.[6, 10, 36]

Pasted vents resulting from fecal accumulation may be caused by dirty bedding or diarrhea.

Foreign body pneumonia may result from aspiration of formula. Training birds to feed rapidly reduces the chances of aspiration. Coughing after feeding may be associated with aspiration of minute particles of food during feeding and is often associated with vocalization during feeding. Chicks nearing weaning are more prone to aspiration because they often resist feeding prematurely.[6, 10]

TREATMENT OF THE CRITICALLY ILL NEONATE

Samples for diagnostic evaluation should be collected before initiation of therapy. Delay of therapy until results are available may be fatal.[9, 10]

Parenteral therapy is necessary in birds exhibiting intestinal stasis; however, the potential for tissue trauma in very small birds should not be discounted. Antifungal therapy should always accompany antibiotic use to prevent overgrowth of *Candida albicans*.[9, 10]

Chicks with intestinal stasis often become dehydrated. Oral rehydration therapy may be provided using commercially available products, lactated Ringer's solution, or dilute cereal preparations.[6, 9, 10]

Fluids may be administered subcutaneously, intramuscularly, or interosseously. An interosseous catheter may be placed in the femur even in small chicks. Fluid deficit may be estimated by clinical signs.

5% dehydration—subtle tenting of skin and loss of elasticity

10–12% dehydration—skin tents and has a muddy appearance

12–15% dehydration—bird is in shock, with generalized systemic depression and near-moribund condition

Calculate fluid requirement for replacement

Normal body weight × percent deficit (in decimal value) + maintenance requirement

(Maintenance is estimated at 50 ml/kg/day.)

Fluids may be administered through an interosseous catheter using a microdrip intravenous infusion set that administers 60 drops/ml.[6, 10]

Nutrients can be supplied by the enteral or parenteral route. In cases of intestinal stasis, bypassing the crop by passage of a tube directly into the proventriculus is often advocated. This can be dangerous because of potential for puncture of the proventriculus, and if the bird has intestinal stasis the food may remain in the proventriculus. Surgical placement of a feeding tube directly into the duodenum has been reported. The effects of hyperalimentation using interosseous catheters has been assessed in adult birds.[43] The use of metoclopramide (Reglan, AH Robbins), 0.2 to 0.4 mg/kg twice or three times daily for 2 to 3 days, preferably by subcutaneous administration, has been helpful.[6, 10]

Crop lavage may be necessary in chicks exhibiting intestinal stasis. Milking the crop contents out with the chick held upside down is rapid but may result in aspiration. Crop lavage can be accomplished by flushing the crop with warm water, massaging to break up contents, and removing contents with a tube. Antibiotics and antifungal drugs should be added to the empty crop before administration of oral fluids. If the crop is not empty in 12 to 24 hours, the crop should again be flushed and parenteral antibiotics and fluids administered. A sling-type bandage "crop bra" is a useful adjunct to therapy.[6, 10]

The addition of enzymatic preparations for predigestion of formula has been reported with mixed results. In a study using healthy eclectus parrot chicks, no difference was observed in growth be-

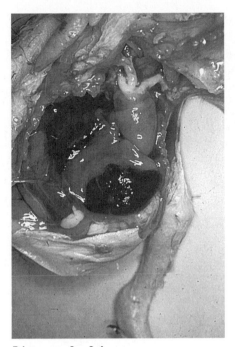

Figure 6–24

Hepatoma in chick shown in Figure 6–23.

tween treated birds and controls. Enzymatic supplements may be helpful in sick chicks. One danger is that formula with enzymatic additives appears more liquid than without. An aviculturist may inadvertently feed formula that is too high in percent solids when adding enzymes.[29, 30]

TRAUMATIC PROBLEMS

Hepatic hematoma (Figs. 6–23, 6–24) may result from blunt trauma such as from the chick being dropped, or by trauma incurred by the chick being picked up with digital pressure placed on the liver. Therapy consists of blood transfusion, vitamin K administration, and fluid administration.[10]

Chicks housed together often damage each other's beaks in attempted feeding behavior (Fig. 6–25). Puncture of laminae of the beak, especially the maxilla, may occur from chicks trying to feed each other. Depression defects should be corrected by lifting the depressed flap until it is flush with the surface of the laminae and providing a protective patch of acrylic that will fall off as the beak heals. Bite wounds inside the mouth, usually in perilingual

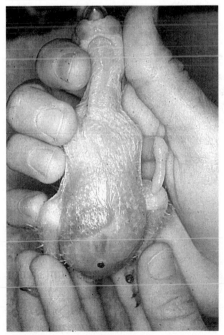

Figure 6–23

Hepatoma (hematoma of right lobe of liver) in a 2-week-old macaw chick visible through the skin.

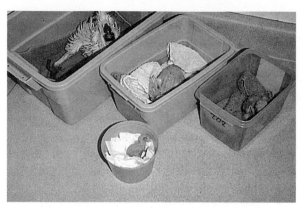

F i g u r e 6 – 2 5

Housing chicks separately in suitable containers aids in identifying very small chicks, monitoring weight and feces, and avoiding beak damage that occurs when chicks try to feed from each other. Although there are no known behavioral problems associated with housing chicks separately, some aviculturalists prefer to keep siblings together for the psychological benefits of companionship.

tissue, also result from chicks attempting to feed each other.[10]

Fracture of the tip of the maxilla (Fig. 6–26) occurs when a chick has hooked its beak over wire and is pulled away. Some can be repaired by pinning and acrylic fixation.[10]

Circumferential constriction defects of the toes resemble fiber constriction but typically consist of scar tissue. Constriction occurs most frequently on the last phalanx of the fourth digit (lateral back toe). It occurs most frequently in macaws, eclectus, and African grey parrots. A similar condition in human infants, termed amniotic band syndrome, is theorized as being associated with a remnant of the amnion. Swelling occurs distal to the constriction and progresses to formation of fluid-filled vesicles. Auto-amputation results as the constrictive band extends deeper and avascular necrosis occurs. Low environmental humidity is suspected as being contributory and may occur with the use of very hydroscopic bedding material. If detected early, constriction can be alleviated by massage, warm water soaks and application of dimethyl sulfoxide (DMSO). Surgical repair consists of making longitudinal, full-thickness incisions through the band and elevating tissue laterally and medially out of the constricted area. Close with everting suture patterns to stabilize the toe and prevent recurrence. Bandage for a few days, then use massage and DMSO.[9, 10, 24]

Crop burns (Fig. 6–27) are caused by feeding formula that is too hot (in excess of 110° F) or by contact with a heat lamp or heating pad. Skin cov-

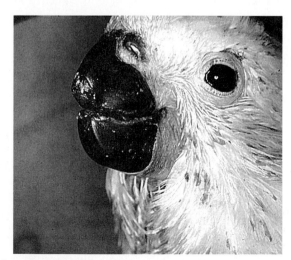

F i g u r e 6 – 2 6

Fracture of the tip of the maxilla in a Moluccan cockatoo chick. This occurred when the chick was pulled out of a cage while it was holding the wire with the beak. If avulsion is not complete, the tip may be immobilized by pinning and sealing with acrylic.

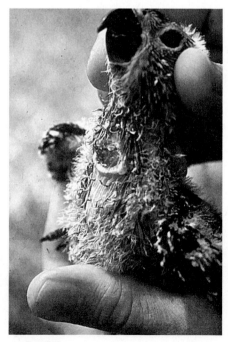

F i g u r e 6 – 2 7

Necrosis following a third-degree burn of the crop. Surgical repair should be delayed until the wound begins to leak.

ering the crop initially blisters then scabs in a few days. Lesions usually appear on the most ventral, central aspect of the crop. Mild cases (first-degree burns) result in edema and erythema. Second-degree burns result in blistering that may not be apparent until a day or more after the burn. Necrosis and sloughing follow third-degree burns. Scabs should be left intact and the wound allowed to contract until the crop leaks. In premature intervention, viable tissue cannot be discriminated from nonviable tissue and debridement may cause more loss of tissue or a tiny nonfunctional crop. Debride the wound and close using a two-layer closure. In very large defects the crop tissue alone may be closed, then bandaged allowing the skin to granulate over the crop, or after a short period of healing the surrounding skin may be undermined and pulled over the crop. This allows maximal crop capacity. Therapy should include prophylactic antibiotic and antifungal therapy, anti-inflammatory drugs, and/or topical vitamin E or aloe ointments.[6, 9, 10, 24]

Esophageal and pharyngeal punctures result from hand-feeding accidents often with injection of food into subcutaneous tissues (Fig. 6–28). Esophageal punctures occur in birds being fed with a metal or rubber feeding tube and occur at the midpoint of the neck where the esophagus is narrow and has the greatest curvature. Pharyngeal punctures result from feeding with a syringe and occur in buccal tissue usually to the right of the tongue. Subcutane-

ous deposition of food results in cellulitis, toxemia, and usually death without surgical intervention.

Locate the most ventral point of the food deposit by transillumination. Drain and flush the wound. Large wounds in the mouth may require closure by suture or tissue glue. Postoperative antibiotics, antifungal drugs, anti-inflammatory drugs, and flushing is required. Small amounts of food may be walled off, forming abscesses, which should be removed after healing is complete.[6, 9, 10, 24]

Idiopathic stifle luxation may be present at hatching or may be noticed later. The tibiotarsus and patellar ligament luxate medially, the foot rotates medially, and contraction of tendons occurs. The dislocation can usually be reduced manually but will not stay in place. Repair in very small chicks can be accomplished by splinting with a platform-type splint taking care to tape the tarsometatarsus so that it is pointed cranially. In older birds, open reduction is required, tacking the patellar ligament laterally and stabilizing the joint with lateral sutures from the tibiotarsus to the lateral condyles of the femur. Splint postoperatively with a spica splint rigid enough to stabilize against medial rotation. Such a splint may be constructed of Vetwrap, tape, and Sam splint.[24]

Fractures

Folding fractures are common in chicks that have metabolic bone disease or protein deficiency. Internal fixation is not recommended in poorly calcified bones. Improper splints may cause deformation of other bones. Limbs splinted in abnormal positions may cause malformation of adjacent bones or joints or contraction of tendons. The most common sites are the distal third of the tibiotarsus, with the bone bowing cranially, and the distal femur, with the bone bowing craniodorsally. Under anesthesia the fracture should be manually refractured, straightened, and splinted. If the bones have calcified, a wedge osteotomy may be necessary to straighten the bone. The bone is often shortened, but not significantly.[24]

The most common fracture site is the midshaft tibiotarsus from legs or bands being caught in wire floors. Splinting is usually sufficient, with care to loosen the splint after 1 week in rapidly growing

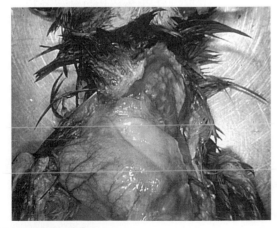

Figure 6 – 2 8

Subcutaneous deposition of food and cellulitis following rupture of the esophagus with a feeding tube.

chicks. Fractures usually heal in 2 weeks in well nourished chicks.[10, 24]

Concussions may occur during a chick's clumsy initial flight attempts. Keep chicks in a cool dark place and treat with corticosteroids.

Trauma to blood feathers from heat or sharp or blunt trauma may result in hemorrhage in the shaft. Traumatized feathers may resemble feathers from birds clinically affected with PBFD.[10]

MISCELLANEOUS CONDITIONS

Kidney disease (Fig. 6–29) is common in some species, especially in red-bellied macaw chicks *(Ara manilata)* (Fig. 6–30), which exhibit a high incidence of uremia and visceral gout. Other chicks, especially cockatoos, are often presented as poor-doers that continually cry. Uric acid levels often range from 5 to 12. (Normal uric acid values increase with age from 0.2–3.2 for 30-day-old cockatoos to 2.0–8.5 for 6-month-old cockatoos.) Many of these chicks have gram-negative bacterial infections. Chicks often respond to treatment with allopurinol.[14–16]

Idiopathic wine-colored discoloration of the urates (Fig. 6–31) is a frequent occurrence in juvenile (2–5-week-old) Amazon, African grey, and Pionus parrots and does not appear to be clinically

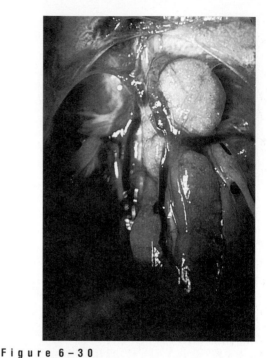

F i g u r e 6 – 3 0

Congenital absence of the right kidney and nephrosis of the left kidney in a red-bellied macaw *(Ara manilata)*. Visceral gout is common in chicks of this species. (Courtesy of Frank Enders.)

significant. These pigments darken after being passed in the urine as if they are photosensitive or react with oxygen or with some bedding, such as paper toweling. They may be associated with carotenoid pigments in corn.[10]

Dietary imbalances such as excessive protein or vitamin D_3 have been associated with gout. Clinical evidence indicates other factors must be involve and further investigation is necessary. Macaws are particularly susceptible to vitamin D_3 toxicity, which causes nephrocalcinosis and calcification of other soft tissues. Polyomavirus infection in the chronic form can cause nephritis and cystic kidneys. Polyuria is normal in hand-fed psittacines given very watery diets.[6, 10, 24]

Eye Problems

Corneal scratches from clutch mates or foreign bodies under the lids are the most common ophthalmic problems. *Mycoplasma* has been implicated in conjunctivitis of cockatiel chicks but is poorly docu-

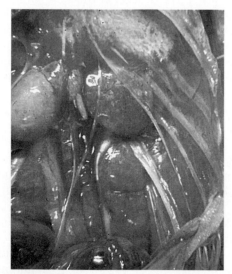

F i g u r e 6 – 2 9

Cystic kidney in a chick with chronic polyomavirus infection.

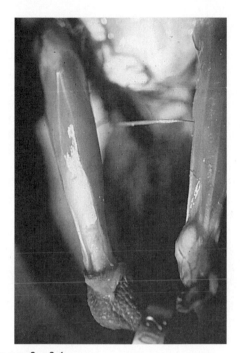

Figure 6-31

Urate deposits in fascia of legs in a rainbow lorie chick *(Trichoglossus hematodus)* with visceral gout. (Courtesy of Frank Enders.)

mented. Congenital abnormalities include micro-ophthalmia, atresia of the lids, and congenital cataracts. A moluccan chick had bilateral, mature congenital cataract. Sight was restored by bilateral cataract surgery at 5 months of age. Congenital lens opacity in cockatoo chicks may be associated with excessive incubation humidity causing edema of the lens. Most cases resolve spontaneously.[6, 10]

ANESTHETIC CONSIDERATIONS

Gas anesthesia is rapid and safe. Chicks should be fasted long enough to empty the crop to avoid reflux of food into the mouth. Anesthetic concentrations are equal to or higher than those used for adults. Chicks are especially susceptible to chilling during anesthesia.[31]

PHARMACOLOGY

Drug therapy in the neonate may be accompanied by adverse effects resulting from differences in drug disposition and organ function. Absorption of drugs from the gastrointestinal tract may be affected by pH-dependent passive diffusion and by gastric emptying time. Percutaneous absorption may be substantially increased in newly hatched chicks, as in human infants, because of an underdeveloped epidermal barrier and increased skin hydration. The total body water as a percentage of the total body weight in a hatchling is estimated to be 30 to 40% higher than in adult birds. Extracellular water, interstitial water, blood volume, and plasma volume are all higher in the neonate, which may affect drug distribution. Drug metabolism is substantially slower in infants compared with older chicks and adults. Renal excretion of antibiotics such as aminoglycosides is not as efficient in neonatal animals, which may prolong the drug half-life. With the higher percentage of body fluids and reduced elimination, aminoglycosides should be used in slightly higher doses and less frequently than in adults. The blood-brain barrier is also more permeable in neonates than adults.[32, 33]

There is evidence that some adverse effects of drugs are more common in neonates. The combination of ticarcillin and tobramycin was reported to be hepatotoxic in cockatoo chicks. Articular cartilage erosions associated with quinolones in some species have not been reported in psittacines despite widespread use. Stonebreaker reported diarrhea, regurgitation, GI bleeding, ingluvial ulcers, myalgia, myopathies, respiratory distress, and overgrowth of beta hemolytic gram-positive bacteria. In an 8-month study of water-administered enrofloxacin in pigeons, dosages up to 800 ppm produced dose-dependent embryonic mortality and joint alterations. This dosage and duration, however, do not constitute a normal clinical application.[32–34]

Oral doxycycline or trimethoprim sulphate in lovebirds and macaws is reported to cause vomiting, facial flushing, and depression. Large amounts of calcium in young birds are reported to cause nephrocalcinosis, visceral gout, parathyroid dysfunction, and retarded growth. Vitamin D_3 overdosage may result in visceral gout and soft tissue calcification, especially in macaws and to a lesser degree in conures and Amazon parrots. Chronic vitamin A overdosing may result in osteodystrophy and parathyroid hypertrophy. In debilitated young birds, cephalosporins may cause hepatotoxicity and renal toxicity.[32]

In dehydrated patients, in which peripheral circulation is compromised severely, the uptake and elimination of drugs may be slowed. Neonatal birds are frequently medicated orally in conjunction with feedings. Severely ill chicks should receive parenteral therapy because of the prevalence of intestinal stasis. Subcutaneous administration may reduce myositis.[32]

Some drugs administered to breeding birds may be detrimental to eggs or chicks. Chloramphenicol in doses as low as 0.5 mg per egg causes marked inhibition of embryonic growth. Penicillin can cause edema and hemorrhage in the wings, legs, and head of chicken embryos. Tetracyclines can cause decreased embryo size and embryonic limb size as well as inhibition of mineralization of long bones and cartilage. Certain sulpha drugs may induce embryonic deformities. Several antiparasitic drugs and insecticides are reportedly toxic to young birds.[32] Excess vitamin D_3 supplementation in breeding macaws may result in embryonic and renal calcinosis and mortality.[41]

INFECTIOUS DISEASES

Chicks that hatch in the nest are more likely to become exposed to infectious agents than chicks hatched in an incubator and raised in a nursery containing only incubator-hatched chicks.

Direct transovarian transmission of some poultry pathogens have been documented, such as *Salmonella (S. pullorum, S. enteritidis, S. gallisepticum)*, *Mycoplasma,* viruses of the leukosis/sarcoma group, adenoviruses and encephalomyelitis virus. Transmission of PBFD in artificially incubated eggs has been reported. Transovarian transmission of polyoma virus has been reported in budgerigars.[42] Improper egg handling techniques can result in transmission of some pathogens by penetration of the shell.[35]

Bordetella avium infection has been associated with a "lockjaw" syndrome in hand-fed psittacines, especially cockatiels. The bacterium invades from the sinuses into skeletal muscle of the mandible, resulting in lockjaw. The disease is transmitted from asymptomatic carrier parents to chicks. Horizontal transmission can occur in the hand-feeding nursery. Antibiotic therapy is unrewarding.[36]

Infectious diseases of most importance in the nursery and nest include polyomavirus infection, PBFD, psittacine proventricular dilatation syndrome/avian viral serositis, psittacine pox, and chlamydiosis. These diseases are covered in Chapters 18 and 19.

Aspergillosis or brooder pneumonia caused by *Aspergillus fumigatus* is occasionally reported in psittacines. It occurs most frequently in macaws as a disseminated infection or miliary granulomatous pneumonitis. Gross contamination of air sources should be suspected, especially air conditioner ducts and filters and brooder fans. Particulate bedding, especially corn cob bedding and, to a lesser extent, pine shavings, may become contaminated when soiled with feces. Emptying pans inside the nursery building may grossly contaminate the air and result in outbreaks.[39]

References

1. Clubb K, Clubb S: Management of psittacine chicks and eggs in the nest. In Schubot RM, Clubb K, Clubb S (eds): Psittacine Aviculture, Perspectives, Techniques and Research. Loxahatchee, FL, Avicultural Breeding and Research Center, 1992, pp 15/1–15/6.
2. Myers SA, Millam JR, Roudybush TE, Grau CR: Reproductive success of hand-reared vs. parent-reared cockatiels (*Nymphicus hollandicus*). Auk 105:536–542, 1988.
3. Millam JR. U.C. Davis Amazon breeding project. Proc Assoc Avian Vet, Reno, 1995, pp 403–415.
4. Clubb K, Clubb S: Psittacine neonatal care and handfeeding. In Schubot RM, Clubb K, Clubb S (eds): Psittacine Aviculture, Perspectives, Techniques and Research. Loxahatchee, FL, Avicultural Breeding and Research Center, 1992, pp 11/1–11/12.
5. Clipsham R: Introduction to psittacine pediatrics. Vet Clin North Am Small Anim Pract 21:1361–1392, 1991.
6. Flammer K, Clubb SL: Neonatology. In Ritchie BW, Harrison G, Harrison, L (eds): Avian Medicine: Principles and Application. Lake Worth, FL, Wingers Publishing, 1994, pp 804–841.
7. Hanson JT: Handraising large parrots, methodology and expected weight gains. Zoo Biol 6:139–160, 1987.
8. Phillips A, Clubb SL: Psittacine neonatal development. In Schubot RM, Clubb K, Clubb S (eds): Psittacine Aviculture, Perspectives, Techniques and Research, Loxahatchee, FL, Avicultural Breeding and Research Center, 1992, pp 12/1–12/26.
9. Joyner KL: Theriogenology. In Ritchie BW, Harrison G, Harrison L (eds): Avian Medicine: Principles and Application. Lake Worth, FL, Wingers Publishing, 1994, pp 748–804.
10. Clubb SL, Wolf S, Phillips A: Psittacine pediatric medicine. In Schubot RM, Clubb K, Clubb S (eds): Psittacine Aviculture, Perspectives, Techniques and Research. Loxahatchee, FL, Avicultural Breeding and Research Center, 1992, pp 16/1–16/26.
11. Drewes LA, Flammer K: Preliminary data on aerobic microflora of baby psittacine birds. Proc Jean Delacour/Int Foundation for Conservation of Birds, Int Symp on Breed Birds in Captivity, Los Angeles, 1983, pp 73–81.

12. Flammer K, Drewes LA: Environmental sources of Gram-negative bacteria in an exotic bird farm. Proc Jean Delacour/Int Foundation for the Conservation of Birds, Int Sympos Breeding Birds in Captivity, Los Angeles, 1983, pp 83–93.

13. Worell AB: Pediatric bacterial diseases. Semin Avian Exotic Pet Med 2(3):116–124, 1993.

14. Clubb SL, Schubot RM, Joyner K: Hematological and serum biochemistry reference intervals in juvenile eclectus parrots *(Eclectus roratus)*. J Assoc Avian Vet 4:218–225, 1991.

15. Clubb SL, Schubot RM, Joyner K: Hematological and serum biochemistry reference intervals in juvenile cockatoos. J Assoc Avian Vet 5:5–16, 1991.

16. Clubb SL, Schubot RM, Joyner K: Hematological and serum biochemistry reference intervals in juvenile macaws. J Assoc Avian Vet 5:154–162, 1991.

17. Joyner KL: Psittacine pediatric diagnostics. Semin Avian Exotic Pet Med 1:11–21, 1992.

18. Roudybush TE, Grau CR: Solid food requirements for hand-rearing cockatiels. American Federation of Aviculture Watchbird 11(3):40–45, 1984.

19. Nearenberg DS, Roudybush TE, Grau CR: Hand-fed vs parent-fed cockatiels, a comparison of chick growth. Proc 34th Western Poultry Dis Conf, 1985, pp 109–112.

20. Roudybush TE, Grau CR: Food and water interrelations and the protein requirement for growth of an altricial bird, the cockatiel *(Nymphicus hollandicus)*. J Nutr 116:552–559, 1987.

21. Roudybush TE: Growth, signs of deficiency, and weaning in cockatiels fed deficient diets. Proc Assoc Avian Vet, 1986, pp 333–340.

22. Grau CR, Roudybush TE: Protein requirement of growing cockatiels. Proc 34th Western Poultry Dis Conf, 1985, pp 107–108.

23. Hagen M: Nutritional observation, hand feeding formulas, and digestion in exotic birds. Semin Avian Exotic Pet Med 1(1)3–10, 1992.

24. Clipsham R: Noninfectious diseases of pediatric psittacines. Semin Avian Exotic Pet Med 1(1):22–23, 1992.

25. Clipsham R: Correction of pediatric leg disorders. Proc Assoc Avian Vet, 1991, pp 200–204.

26. Wolf S, Clubb S: Clinical management of beak malformations in handfed psittacine chicks. In Schubot RM, Clubb K, Clubb S (eds): Psittacine Aviculture, Perspectives, Techniques and Research. Loxahatchee, FL, Avicultural Breeding and Research Center, 1992, pp 17/1–17/11.

27. Cambre RC: Indications and techniques for surgical removal of the avian yolk sac. J Zoo Wildl Med 23:55–61, 1992.

28. Clubb SL: The effects of selected parameters on intestinal transit time in handfed cockatiels and Quaker parakeets. Proc Assoc Avian Vet, Reno, 1995, pp 165–173.

29. Skidmore D, Clubb S: Effects of dietary supplementation of digestive enzymes in handfed eclectus parrots *(Eclectus roratus)*. In Schubot RM, Clubb K, Clubb S (eds): Psittacine Aviculture, Perspectives, Techniques and Research. Loxahatchee, FL, Avicultural Breeding and Research Center, 1992, pp 13/1–13/3.

30. Joyner K: The use of a Lactobacillus product in a psittacine handfeeding diet, its effect on normal aerobic microflora, early weight gain and health. Proc Assoc Avian Vet, 1988, pp 127–138.

31. Altman RB: Neonatal and pediatric surgery. Semin Avian Exotic Pet Med 1(1):34–39, 1992.

32. Dorrestein GM: Avian pediatric pharmacology. Semin Avian Exotic Pet Med 2(3):110–115, 1993.

33. Sturkie PD: Avian Physiology, ed 3. New York, Springer-Verlag, 1976.

34. Stonebreaker R: Husbandry and medical management of the nursery. Proc Assoc Avian Vet, 1991, pp 161–166.

35. Calnek BW, Barnes CW, Beard WM, et al (eds): Diseases of Poultry, ed 9. Ames, Iowa State University Press, 1991.

36. VanDer Heyden N: Jejunostomy and jejunocloacal anastomosis in macaws. Proc Assoc Avian Vet, 1993, pp 72–77.

37. Takeshita K: Hypervitaminosis D in baby macaws. Proc Assoc Avian Vet, 1986, pp 341–346.

38. Greenacre CB, Watson E, Ritchie BW: Congenital atresia of the choana in an African Grey parrot and an umbrella cockatoo. J Assoc Avian Vet 7:19–22, 1993.

39. VanDerHayden N: Aspergillosis in psittacine chicks. Proc Assoc Avian Vet, 1993, pp 207–212.

40. Clubb SL, Homer BL, Pisani J, Head C: Outbreaks of bordetellosis in psittacines and ostriches. Proc Assoc Avian Vet, 1994, pp 63–68.

41. Speer BL: Pediatric medical management. In Abramson J, Speer BL, Thomsen JB (eds): The Large Macaws, Their Care, Breeding and Conservation. Fort Brigg, CA, Raintree Publications, 1995, pp 361–372.

42. Ritchie BW: Avian viruses, function and control. Lake Worth, FL, Usingers Publishing, 1995.

43. Degernes LA, Davidson GF, Barnes J, White D. A preliminary report on intraosseous total parenteral nutrition in birds. Proc Assoc Avian Vet, 1995, pp 25–26.

Christine Davis

7

Behavior

PET PSITTACINE BEHAVIOR

Understanding Pet Bird Behavior

Understanding natural behavior is important. Yearly, many thousands of birds are abused, abandoned, or neglected because of unrealistic expectations of their owners. Client education can greatly decrease such incidents.

Birds are among the oldest living species on the planet; their earliest known relatives were dinosaurs. Genetically, even a hand-fed, domestically bred bird has not been altered or domesticated to be a companion to man, and its reactions to various environmental stimuli will reflect that.

Domestically *bred* pertains solely to the *environment* in which the bird was hatched, and does not relate to behavioral alteration (i.e., domestication through selective long-term breeding). It is therefore unrealistic to expect *domesticated behavior* from a bird as a part of its natural reaction to various stimuli within a domestic environment.

Common Behavioral Characteristics of the Psittacine

Birds are emotionally and intellectually as diverse as human beings; however, the average large hookbill exhibits *emotional* behaviors corresponding to those of a 2- to 3-year-old human child and never progresses beyond that point. Expected "negative" emotional responses and behaviors are inclusive of, but not limited to, short attention spans; hyperactivity; possessiveness of people and property; extreme self-centeredness; a need to control others in their environment; and an appreciation of dramatic emotional displays, regardless of whether they are positive or negative in nature. Expected "positive" emotional responses and behaviors are inclusive of, but not limited to, extreme intelligence, need for social (flock) interaction, playfulness, and childlike affection for primary individuals within their environment.

Common behavioral characteristics must be considered when interacting with the pet psittacine. For example, expecting a particularly hyperactive bird to sit and entertain itself for long periods of time, without occasional diversions, can lead to undesirable behaviors, such as screaming and feather picking. Interactive playtimes and brief, intermittent displays of affection can be used to easily accentuate the positive aspects of the bird's behavior, and avoid reinforcing those of a negative nature.

Intellectually, the larger hookbills possess sophisticated visual and auditory comprehension concepts (e.g., of categories: color; shape; material [same and different; bigger and smaller]; and of number) comparable to those of a 5- or 6-year-old human child. Because of its emotional and intellectual capabilities, a bird is not the desired choice for individuals who need a low-maintenance companion. As with children, the bird's development is directly contingent upon environmental stimuli provided by the people in the household. The larger birds are a lifelong commitment and should be considered as such.

Clients should understand that expecting the veterinarian to also be a qualified behaviorist is similar to expecting a family physician to also be a psychologist. The veterinarian is professionally trained for the heavy responsibility of saving the animals' lives. Even if knowledgeable in the area of behavior, most veterinarians simply do not have the time to work with behavior problems in addition to all of their other duties.

The Bird's Natural Environment

In the wild, the flock is primarily a *protective* unit, and affiliation with others is essential to the survival of each individual. The need for social interaction, although extremely important, is secondary to the instinct for survival. Psittacine behavior will reflect this. Consequently, birds do not fare well as "ornamental objects" and need social interaction, human or animal, to prevent the development of undesirable behaviors, such as screaming (often the result of separation anxiety) and nervous feather picking.

Many psittacine species are prey animals in the wild and react accordingly to situations *perceived* to be threatening, even in a domestic environment. Any startling occurrence, such as unfamiliar or sudden movements or sounds, may elicit panic or aggression—the classic "flight or fight" response. Many biting episodes are a direct result of the bird's reaction to a situation that it *perceives* to be dangerous.

Destroying foliage and fruit is a natural part of food gathering and social behavior in the wild. The forest's vegetation is continually replenished in this manner. Destructive behavior also occurs in the domestic environment. Drapes and furniture offer an accessible substitute for jungle vegetation, as do the practices of flinging food and tearing apart cage substrate.

Screaming, especially at daybreak and dusk, is a normal activity in the wild, essential in keeping track of companions at those particular times and at various intervals throughout the day. In a domestic environment, screaming behavior can often be instinctive, and behavior modification may be needed to alleviate it. Some birds, such as many of the conure species, are frequently predisposed to loud vocal displays. The prospective owners should be informed of this possibility and urged to choose a quieter type of bird if they live in an apartment building or housing units within proximity to others.

Basic characteristics of the more commonly seen genera and species should be learned to better educate clients who may be choosing a first or second bird. Some birds *are* predisposed to certain behaviors, both positive and negative.

Wild-Caught Versus Domestically Bred Birds

Genetically, birds are wild animals, and this is reflected in their behavior, whether they are wild-caught or domestically bred.

Wild-caught birds are *wild* animals, adapted to a wild environment, and captured for exportation. They often have difficulty being tamed into good companions and are not advisable as pets, especially for the novice. They are seldom the "bargain" they seem to be. Domestically bred birds are *wild* animals that have been hatched in captivity, usually hand-fed by human beings, and socialized to a domestic environment. Few species have been domesticated. Most are wild animals who are *socialized* to interact within a domestic environment. In contrast, dogs and cats have been genetically "programmed," or domesticated, for many thousands of years, specifically to be companions to human beings. Expecting consistently "domesticated" behavior patterns in a psittacine, whether wild-caught or domestically bred, is unrealistic, as well as unfair to the bird.

Avian "Politics" in the Wild

Being fundamentally wild animals, birds have no concept of the owner/pet relationship. *They can only interact with their human companions on the same level in which they would interact with other flock members.* This can be a source of problems for the unwary new bird owner. Most flocks function according to a hierarchic arrangement, which can often be visually discerned (in the wild) by the grouping of more dominant birds in the higher branches with less dominant individuals occupying correspondingly lower branches. Many birds naturally seek the most dominant position in their environment and are very comfortable there. This is merely a reasonable element of survival within the flock and has little to do with the bird's like or dislike of the people in a household. Unfortunately, people inadvertently create problems with regard to this natural predisposition.

To ensure desirable behaviors, it is essential that the people implement clear parameters and guidelines for the bird. Most problems are the result of the fact that people do not do this. In a domestic environment, many owners place the bird in relatively high locations, unwittingly bestowing upon them the role dominant to all others within their "flock," including human beings. Biting and screaming are two behaviors that can result if a dominant bird becomes frustrated with its human "subordinates" and their lack of "proper" social deference. In the wild, subordinant companions would understand the superior bird's position and would never step beyond the bounds of social propriety. Punitive measures, such as biting, on the part of the dominant individuals are then seldom necessary. Relatively mundane human activities, such as eating or visiting with others without the dominant bird's direct participation or physical proximity, can result in screaming if the bird has not been taught to behave otherwise. The dominant bird *expects* to be included in all flock activities. Vocal or physical displays are often misconstrued by the owners as aggressive or "spoiled" behavior, instead of being recognized as a natural consequence of environmental conditioning implemented by the human members of the household and exacerbated by a genetic predisposition to those particular reactions.

Most psittacines are primarily monogamous in nature, and they resent anyone (human or animal) encroaching upon their relationship with their mate. In such situations, physical displays of aggression, often directed at the very person they love, are commonplace, especially in the more assertive species, such as conures, Amazons, and macaws. It is commonly felt that this is an order to motivate, or warn, the beloved individual to take flight and leave the situation. In the wild, this would be understood by an avian companion; mates would avoid being in a position to be bitten in the first place.

Basic Guidelines for Motivating Desirable Behaviors

Traditional exercises in "behavior modification" have consisted of dominating the bird into submis-

sion. Unfortunately, even if humanely conveyed, most people become too aggressive when in a dominant role. Finesse can easily replace dominance, provided that the bird's behavior is clearly understood.

Birds as wild animals have absolutely no concept of the master/pet relationship familiar to common domesticated species. Taking into consideration the emotional and intellectual capabilities of the psittacine, it becomes easy to understand that behavior control or modification can be implemented from a gentle, loving, parental/child perspective, without resorting to punitive or confrontational methods. Most behavior problems, in humans *and* animals, are the result of lack of clear parameters. Inconsistent boundaries reap inconsistent results in controlling or molding behavior. A system of loving, "parental" control can be implemented in which the bird's behavior is gently molded toward the desired results with absolutely no confrontation. When the bird understands that the human is the "parent" and the bird is the "child," aggressive displays are no longer considered appropriate *by the bird* and will disappear.

When the bird's head level is above midbreast level to the person, *it gains dominance in direct relationship to its height.* If the head is lower, the bird will feel threatened by close, even normal, movement within the environment. When the top of the bird's head is kept at midbreast level to the human, it feels comfortable and familiar, such as when the mother bird places her breast over her young to keep them warm and protected. Many aggressive birds quickly accept this loving interaction and become extremely tractable with relatively little additional manipulation.

The bird should be trained to stay on a play gym or perch when outside of the cage, and not be allowed to wander around the home. This is similar to keeping small children in their own yard. The perch inside the cage, as well as separate play gyms or T stands, should be placed so that the top of the bird's head is at the same midbreast level to a human standing in front of the bird.

Simple Corrective Techniques

Corrective techniques are usually of little or no value if the reason for the bird's behavior is not understood and managed. As with children, what is perceived as a correction to one bird has little or no effect on another. Corrective measures should always be inevitable and instantaneous. Inconsistent practices yield inconsistent and sloppy results.

In a well-socialized bird, banishment from the flock, by placing it in its cage (covered or uncovered) or in a room away from its human "flock" for 5 to 10 minutes can be sufficient to motivate the bird to interact in a more positive manner.

It is important to understand what constitutes a correction. Ignoring the bird is considered a negative situation by the sociable bird; however, *people often unknowingly "punish" their well-behaved birds by ignoring them when they are quietly behaving themselves!*

Positive Reinforcement

Without the balance of offering positive reinforcement for positive behaviors, such as quietly playing, corrective behaviors will not be effective and can actually be considered somewhat abusive to the bird. Positive reinforcement for a sociable individual can be as simple as a look or a verbal interaction ("good bird" or "pretty bird"), or as obvious as a food treat, the tickling of a favorite spot, or short periods of interactive playtime.

Pet owners must take care that the bird is not inadvertently rewarded for negative behaviors. This is a common problem. Birds are extremely visual, and looking at them, even in a negative manner, is usually construed as a reward, even if it is meant as a correction for an undesirable behavior. Scolding the bird and stalking angrily into the room, offers the bird much-loved theatric displays. Many people actually *reward* negative behaviors on a regular basis and then wonder why the bird persists in "misbehaving," not realizing that they have "trained" it to do so.

Positive reinforcement should be frequently lavished upon the bird, even for extremely simple behaviors, such as sitting quietly and playing on the play gym. *Rewards should always greatly outweigh corrections.* In this manner, the bird will naturally be led in the positive direction.

HISTORY-TAKING FOR BEHAVIOR MODIFICATION PURPOSES

Why Take a History?

Behavior modification is an intricate and sophisticated process. Unfortunately, many individuals knowledgeable in other aspects of companion birds often refuse to recognize the intricacies of behavior and resort to simplistic solutions that do not work. Unfortunately, this practice has led to many birds being sold or abandoned because the simple techniques were ineffective.

Most undesirable behaviors can be resolved; however, there is no simple "dosage" of modification. Like a mathematic equation, *all* components of the problem must be discovered and incorporated into the process, or there will be only partial resolution (or no resolution at all) of the offending behavior.

Assessing Behavior

Often, perceived problems are actually normal avian behaviors, which some clients expect to be more like those of dogs and cats. Using "shotgun" corrective techniques without a clear understanding of contributing factors is irresponsible and usually confusing to the bird. If the behavior is deemed to be a problem, a detailed history of both the physical *and* emotional environment (changes, stimuli, dissension, etc.) must be taken.

The historian must not overlook the obvious. Is the bird bored or hungry? Have there been any changes, even seemingly minor ones, in the environment? Is it molting or breeding season? Is the bird in pain? Is the client inadvertently reinforcing the bird's behavior, at least part of the time?

In many of the cases, there are sensitive issues in the client's life that are directly contributing to the problem. Birds are flock creatures who react profoundly to environmental stimuli of all kinds, including human emotions.

History-taking must be done in strictest confidence and in a nonjudgmental, compassionate manner. Berating clients, even if it seems that they "deserve" it, will only make them turn a deaf ear to suggestions and certainly will not help the bird in any way.

The Practitioner's Role in Educating the Client

Frustrated from being confronted with conflicting advice regarding behavior, the bird owner often approaches the veterinarian for an expert's opinion. If the practitioner exhibits a clear understanding of the unique, sometimes bewildering behavior of birds and conveys to the owner much-needed insight, a feeling of trust in the veterinarian's skills develops in the client. Once behaviors are clearly understood, it becomes evident that psittacine behavior is extremely logical and that everything birds do makes sense when considered in context with their origins.

As a result of understanding the complexity of avian behavior, clients become receptive to seeking the assistance of an avian behaviorist in working with their birds, instead of abusing, neglecting, or discarding them. An animal companion whose behavior is understood is deeply loved and valued and receives proper veterinary care and husbandry.

Behavior modification in any creature, especially one as intelligent as the psittacine, is a profession requiring an extensive knowledge of wild animal behavior, as well as human behavior. In most situations, the major component in modifying avian behavior actually consists of retraining the human beings in the environment. A program is devised in which all of the factors contributing to the behavior are determined, and then assessed according to their importance. By using a combination of many different techniques specific to the individual situation, problem elements in the environment are decreased or, when possible, eliminated. Regardless of the program devised by the behaviorist, it will fail if the client is not clear and consistent with the execution of its various elements. Only after *that* process is completed and only if there are absolutely no other alternatives can humane and appropriate corrective techniques be considered and, possibly, employed. In most cases, modification of undesirable behaviors is not instantaneous. Often the longer the behavior has been in existence, the longer it may take to eliminate it.

Behavior modification is *work* and needs to be taken seriously if success is desired. Clients may want the bird to change its behavior, but the bird itself usually does not *want* to change. This does not mean that they *cannot* change, only that they

will, like humans, initially resist the process. The age of the bird is irrelevant. Most behave appropriately when their parameters are made clear and consistent and there are no other avenues available to them.

Eventually, as with humans, dogs, cats, and other domesticated creatures, the proper raising of the bird during its socially and intellectually formative stages will eventually eliminate much of the need for behavior modification.

Birds are not "objects," nor are they genetically "programmed" to be companions to humans. They are intelligent, sentient individuals who need to be respected and treated with love, understanding, and compassion. It is unfair to expect behaviors of them that they cannot comfortably perform; however, when loved *for what they are*, and when given clear, consistent guidelines and respected as integral family members, they can be the source of a lifetime of pleasure, companionship, and enjoyment.

Suggested Reading

Athan, Mattie-Sue, "Guide to a Well Behaved Parrot," Barron's Educational Series, 250 Wireless Blvd., P.O. Box 8040, Hauppauge, N.Y. 11788.

Barber, Theodore Xenophon, Ph.D, "The Human Nature of Birds," St Martin's Press, New York. 1993.

Blanchard, Sally (ed), "The Pet Bird Report," avian behavior newsletter, 2236 Mariner Square Dr., #35, Alameda, CA 94501.

Davis, Christine, "Avian Behavior," "Companion Bird Medicine," Burr, Elisha W., (ed). Iowa State University Press, Ames, Iowa. 1987. pp 28–32.

Davis, Christine, "Parrot Psychology and Behavior Problems," "Veterinary Clinics of North America," Rosskopf, Walter J., Woerpel, Richard W., (eds). November, 1991. pp 1281–1288.

Davis, Christine, "The Well-Mannered Parrot," "The Complete Bird Owner's Handbook," Gary A. Gallerstein, DVM. Howell Book House, New York. 1994. pp 81–92.

Doane, Bonnie Munro and Qualkinbush, Thomas, "My Parrot, My Friend," Howell Book House, New York. 1995.

Kaufman, Kenn, "The Subject is Alex," Audubon, September–October, 1991. pp 52–58.

Munn, Charles A., "Macaws," National Geographic, Vol. 185, No. 1, January, 1994. pp 118–140.

"Parrot Trick Training—The Course," 647 W. Harvard St., Glendale, CA 91204. (818) 246-1617.

Warshaw, Jennifer, "The Parrot Training Handbook," Parrot Press, 357 Sunnyslope Dr., Fremont, CA 94536. 1-800-729-7734.

Video

"Alex The Grey," Wasatch Avian Education Society. Can be ordered from: "Alex The Grey," C/O WAES, P.O. Box 540753, North Salt Lake, UT 84054. (800) 525-2177. All profits from sale of video are donated to avian research and education.

Susan L. Clubb

8

Aviculture Medicine and Flock Health Management

Passage of the Wild Bird Conservation Act of 1992 has transformed American aviculture, shifting the supply of birds for pet and avicultural consumers from reliance on wild-caught imported birds to aviculture. Economics of the pet bird industry are also changing with the changing political and social climate. Predictions of price increases after passage of the act have not materialized. As aviculture matures as a cottage industry, maintaining the health and increasing the productivity of avicultural flocks will be vital to success. Veterinarians can play a major role in enhancing avicultural profitability and production.

Aviculture medicine differs from companion avian practice in several very important ways. Flock health and management is the primary concern. Establishing an etiologic diagnosis or preventing the introduction of infectious disease is of primary importance. The aviculturist usually is knowledgeable in providing home care; hospitalization is not cost-effective. Attention to the maintenance of appropriate biosecurity must also be considered to avoid the veterinarian's becoming the vector for disease between clients' facilities.

Confidentiality is of utmost importance, because rumors concerning disease problems in an aviculture facility can permanently and irreparably damage a facility's reputation. Staff must be counseled on strict professional behavior and in maintaining client-doctor confidentiality.

Economics must always be considered, especially when dealing with a commercial flock. Increased production usually coincides with decreasing sale prices for individual birds. The commercial aviculturist, like any livestock producer, often operates on a relatively slim margin of profit, which can be profoundly affected by disease or management problems. Understanding the economics of the pet bird industry is vital for a successful aviculture practice.

THE VETERINARIAN'S ROLE IN AVICULTURE MANAGEMENT

An understanding of the principles of aviculture management as well as avian medicine and disease is needed for a veterinarian to work with an aviculturist as a management team. A veterinarian who provides routine preventive care and has an understanding of the facilities and collection of the aviculturist can be invaluable in making quick management decisions in the face of a disease outbreak. In this section the veterinary services that can most benefit aviculture are outlined.

New Bird Examination

The addition of new birds to an established aviary always carries with it the risk of introduction of disease. New birds that are misrepresented (not accurately sexed or sold as a result of previous reproductive failure) constitute a potential loss to the aviculturist by occupying space that could be used for productive pairs. A new bird examination should include confirmation of sex and diagnostic testing as indicated by the client's needs, the bird's species, source of the birds, and physical examination results.

Aviary Visits

Annual flock examination can assist in detection of flock problems, establishing identification systems, confirmation of identification and sex, clarification of records, assessment of physical condition as an indicator of suitability of diet and husbandry, correction of health and management problems, and elimination of nonproductive individuals. A review of the health problems of previous years and selective testing of suspect animals can assist in epidemiologic tracing of problems. An assessment of age may be helpful in understanding reproductive failure.

Biosecurity must be paramount to avoid being a mechanical vector of disease. The veterinarian should visit only one facility a day, preferably in the morning prior to hospital cases, or plan for cleanup or wearing of protective clothing between aviaries.

Providing Emergency Care

An experienced aviculturist is the first person involved in providing emergency care. The client should be well schooled in provision of first aid and recognizing signs of illness that require veterinary intervention. The veterinarian assists the aviculturist in preparing a first aid kit, in preparation for nursing and transporting an ill bird, and in providing the proper environment for nursing care after an ill or injured bird is stable. The experienced aviculturist should also know how to collect appropriate samples and provide supportive care in the event that the veterinarian cannot immediately attend to an ill bird. Helping aviculturists deal with those problems within their capabilities encourages them to involve a veterinarian in management of the collection.

Advisor on Husbandry

Husbandry advice should be directed to the level of experience of the aviculturist. Successful aviculturists have vast experience in animal husbandry and have studied the behavior of their birds. They often understand intuitively that problems exist but require veterinary assistance in identification of problems and implementing control programs. To gain compliance with therapeutic programs, the veterinarian must be aware of the daily problems faced by the breeder, and the demands that some procedures (such as treatment protocols that may be very time-consuming or disruptive) may place on available time, labor, and resources.

Assist with Incubation and Pediatric Problems

Veterinarians can play a role in evaluation of incubation failures and nursery management. The art of successful incubation entails extensive experience. Subtle problems in egg handling, especially prior to incubation or in early incubation, can result in developmental abnormalities that may not be expressed until the time of hatching. A definitive cause of embryonic mortality is often elusive. Ideally, all fertile eggs that fail to hatch should be examined in an attempt to detect patterns of mortality, which may be helpful in detecting problems associated with incubation. A veterinarian who is experienced in nursery management can provide valuable consultation to prevent the development of clinical disease related to husbandry or nutritional problems.

Establish a Preventive Medicine Program

Quarantine procedures, infectious disease (viral, bacterial, and fungal) testing or prophylaxis plans, parasite control techniques, pest control, identification systems, and first aid procedures should be discussed (Table 8–1). The aviculturist should establish a relationship with the veterinarian in advance of problems so that fast action can be taken in case of disease outbreaks. An isolation area for new and sick birds should be available and protocols established for management of these areas. Storage for medical supplies and equipment should be discussed.

Table 8–1

FIRST AID SUPPLIES TO BE KEPT ON HAND BY AN AVICULTURIST

Isolated area with cage and provision for supplemental heat and humidity
Balanced electrolyte solutions
Feeding tubes and syringes
Selection of emergency medications and dosage recommendations, as prescribed by attending veterinarian
For wound care, bandage materials including nonsticking elastic bandage material, adhesive tape, nonstick wound pads, antibiotic ointments, hydrogen peroxide, or iodine solutions
Scissors and forceps
Coagulants for bleeding nails
Clean container for transporting sick or injured bird

Evaluate Reproductive Failure

Veterinarians can help aviculturists introduce or adopt a reproduction record system. Reproductive failure may be multifactoral and the causes elusive. The veterinarian working in unison with the aviculturist may be able to determine physical, hormonal, nutritional, behavioral, and psychological causes of reproductive failure and institute remedial measures (Table 8–2).

Table 8–2

EVALUATION OF REPRODUCTION FAILURE IN PSITTACINES

1. Review health and production records and take detailed history
2. Perform physical examination and appropriate diagnostic tests as indicated by results
3. Re-evaluate sex determination techniques for monomorphic birds. If in doubt, laparoscopy should be used to verify sex and visually evaluate the reproductive system and other organ systems
4. Evaluate suitability of husbandry practices
    a. Is diet appropriate, balanced, and accepted?
    b. Is caging appropriate?
    c. Is nest box secure, dry, clean, free of pests, and placed appropriately in the cage?
    d. Are secure perches available for copulation?
    e. Is shelter or protection from elements appropriate for the climate and location?
    f. Is the cage or aviary protected from disturbance by visitors, pests, pets, etc?
5. Evaluate behavior
    a. Is one bird of a pair, or in a colony, exhibiting excessive aggression?
    b. Does the pair exhibit a strong pair bond?
    c. Has the pair been observed in copulation?
    d. Does the pair show an interest in or inspection of the next box?
    e. Do the birds exhibit signs of stress, fear, or unrest in the present location?
    f. Do birds quarrel with or display to birds in adjacent cages?

AN INTRODUCTION TO AVICULTURE

To serve as part of the aviary management team, a veterinarian must understand some of the principles of aviculture. The needs of aviculturists vary widely depending on their level of experience, the species being bred, and the aviculturists' status as hobbyists or commercial producers.

The primary goal of a commercial breeder is profitable production of companion birds. The breeder must select species that are productive in captivity, adapt well to the environment in which they are kept, are popular in the trade, and are suitable companion animals. Rare or endangered species, species that inherently make poor pets, species that are difficult avicultural subjects, or species that have extraordinary housing requirements are not suitable for the commercial breeder. Increases in housing density that may contribute to economy also contribute to the incidence and potential severity of disease outbreaks; therefore, there is the necessity of closer monitoring of a facility for potential health hazards.

Hobbyists usually specialize in a species or group of species, producing birds for exhibition, for the pure pleasure of aviculture, or for the more altruistic goals of establishing or preserving a species in captivity. Hobbyists typically sell offspring to offset the costs of maintenance of their collection. Profit is not typically the primary motive. Many aviculturists may start as hobbyists and turn that hobby into a profitable business as they gain expertise with the proper species and individual birds for their aviaries.

BIRD ACQUISITION

Selection of appropriate species increases breeding success and provides better satisfaction and economic rewards for the aviculturist. Inexperienced aviculturists have little concept of which species they will ultimately be breeding and often acquire and sell many birds, prior to settling upon species that are right for their aviaries.

Choosing species that are adaptive to the region and climatic conditions increases success. For example, species that inhabit dry, high altitude environments may be unduly stressed and more susceptible to disease when housed in outdoor aviaries in a warm humid climate, such as when attempting to breed the plum-headed pionus in South Florida.

Sources of birds for captive breeding include imported wild-caught birds; captive-bred juvenile birds; surplus birds, either wild-caught or captive-bred, that are being eliminated from another aviculturist's aviaries; or unwanted pets. Until recently, aviculturists have depended upon wild-caught birds for the majority of their breeding stock. Future imports (into the US) of species listed by the Convention on International Trade in Endangered Species of Wild Fauna and Flora (CITES) are restricted. Wild-caught birds for captive breeding are limited to those aviculturists who are willing to participate in cooperative breeding programs.

Because recent imports are no longer available in large quantities, the aviculturist must rely on long-term captives or captive-bred birds for breeding stock. These birds cannot be considered disease-free and may introduce diseases such as polyoma, proventricular dilatation, or psittacine beak and feather disease (PBFD). Wild-caught birds that have been nonproductive are often offered. Often, re-pairing or changing the environment for these birds results in breeding success. Some individuals or pairs, however, are refractory to adaptation to captivity.

The purchase of captive-bred birds for breeding stock is a logical alternative for many species. It is common for gallinaceous and columbiform birds. Some psittacine and passerine species have adapted well to captivity, and the success of breeding captive-bred birds has been demonstrated. For the larger psittacine species, however, the productivity of many species, especially of hand-raised individuals, has not been well demonstrated. For captive-bred birds, inbreeding is often a problem.

As in the purchase of birds for resale or as pets, care must be taken to avoid the purchase of smuggled birds, which pose an unacceptable disease risk as well as a legal risk. Bargain-priced birds should be looked upon with suspicion. The buyer should attempt to gain as much information as possible prior to buying a bird for breeding. The first question to ask the potential seller would be "why is this bird/pair being sold?". Other questions include the source of the bird. If it is wild-caught, does the seller know the country of origin and who the importer was? Has the bird been sold numerous times, and if so why? If captive-bred, who bred the

bird, was it parent-raised or hand-raised, and when was it hatched? If the bird is represented as captive-bred but is not closed-banded, why? Can the parents be identified for genealogic purposes? What is the health history of this bird, its parents, and the flock of origin? Has the bird exhibited aggressive behavior to people or other birds? (For example, male cockatoos are often sold after they have killed their mate.) How and when was sex determined? If a proven pair is being sold are the birds identified and can breeders' records be produced? This type of information often is withheld because of fear that disclosure will lose the sale.

CULLING

Culling is a vital tool for management of breeding stock. The subject of culling has emotional repercussions, especially when dealing with birds considered pets, and with birds that represent endangered species. In reality, maintaining birds for breeding stock that are not vigorous, that fail to adapt to captivity, or that are not of the best genetic stock is a detriment to the future of aviculture and to the species. Birds should not be considered disposable, but we must also consider the importance of selective breeding in aviculture success.

Purchasing culled breeding stock, especially birds represented as proven breeders, carries with it a degree of risk. Birds are often culled because they failed to breed. Laparoscopic examination of these birds is important. Birds sold as part of an entire collection that is being sold are less likely to be misrepresented.

Dealing with culled birds can strain veterinary ethics. Euthanasia of valuable birds because of a poor reproductive record or a poorly understood medical problem (such as cloacal papillomatosis) is not acceptable to many people. Resale of these birds without disclosure is equally unacceptable and can strain the client/veterinarian relationship. It is inadvisable for the veterinarian to represent both the buyer and seller in a bird transaction unless both parties are present at the time of examination. Although the purchase of culled breeding stock should be looked upon with suspicion, movement of healthy pairs to a new environment often results in breeding.

Culled breeding birds can often be placed or

sold as pets. Older birds that have exceeded their reproductive potential can make excellent companions. They are content to be more sedate and quiet than young or sexually active birds, therefore adapting to life in the home.

QUARANTINE AND ACCLIMATION

Quarantine facilities vary tremendously. In many aviaries, there is no space for strict segregation of new arrivals. Birds in quarantine should be housed separately in an enclosed or, if outdoor, screened facility for a minimum of 30 days, and often longer. Birds in quarantine should be cared for by a person who either has no contact with the established collection, or who takes care of established birds prior to servicing the quarantine facility, or who showers and changes clothes after servicing the birds in quarantine. Off-premises quarantine, such as holding new birds in the home of a neighbor, is a practical means of quarantine.

Household options for quarantine should be in a room that does not contain existing birds and that can be serviced after other birds are attended, without traffic flow directly into existing housing. Absolute minimal segregation is a separate cage, physically separated as much as possible, with separate handling of bowls. A bird in the same airspace with established birds is not in quarantine. The aviculturist must understand that quarantine does not ensure that new birds are not asymptomatic carriers of parasitic, bacterial, or viral pathogens.

Veterinarians should standardize the new bird examination and quarantine testing program to the needs and resources of the aviculturist and the species. Minimal screening includes a thorough physical examination, cloacal culture, and evaluation of a blood smear. Complete blood count, *Chlamydia* testing, and blood chemistry profile are useful to detect birds that require more extensive evaluation. Specific diagnostic screens may be employed, including enzyme-linked immunosorbent assay (ELISA) tests or deoxyribonucleic acid (DNA) probes for *Chlamydia*, polyomavirus, and PBFD virus. Direct or flotation examination for internal parasites is essential if birds will be placed in flights or colonies where establishment of parasitism will be difficult to control. In species other than psitta-

cines, a direct and flotation fecal examination and crop swab for trichomoniasis is recommended. Routine worming of new birds, (for nematodes and cestodes, depending upon the species) should be considered. Thin birds, especially those species susceptible to proventricular dilatation syndrome, should be examined radiographically. Some diseases that are characterized by an asymptomatic carrier state are easily missed, even with routine testing, including Pacheco's parrot disease, giardiasis, fluke infestation, and proventricular dilatation syndrome.

Acclimation

Acclimation begins when the bird arrives in the facility. Small birds often refuse food for several days, and large birds may refuse to eat for up to 1 week, especially those that previously were pets. New birds should be weighed upon arrival and watched for weight loss. Initiating gavage feeding hastily should be avoided if weight loss is not dramatic to avoid unnecessary stress, especially in frightened birds. The bird should initially be given the previous diet and slowly changed to the diet offered by the aviculturist. Change in water may also cause temporary intestinal upset. Note that small birds such as canaries die within 48 hours if they do not eat.

If the bird is to be housed outdoors, it should be acclimated to environmental temperatures. Tropical birds should be placed in outdoor facilities in northern temperate climates during the summer to allow acclimation before being exposed to winter temperatures. Bare skin areas may be sunburned when birds are placed in outdoor facilities and exposed to direct sunlight. Birds on chlortetracycline therapy may suffer photosensitization. Exposed areas such as eye rings, facial patches in macaws and exposed skin in feather-plucked birds eventually "tan" and show color changes indicative of melaninization or deposition of other protective pigmentation. Biting insects may also cause dermatologic reactions that can become quite severe in the new arrival. Housing of affected birds indoors until the severity of such reactions subsides may be helpful. Antigens for desensitization are not available. Sensitization to pollens or resins of plants may also occur.

Identification

Records should be established at the time the bird enters the aviary. As much medical history as possible should be obtained from the seller. Many aviculturists are becoming involved in establishment of stud books and cooperative breeding programs. Identification of individuals while recording all existing information when it is most available could be invaluable in the future.

Each new bird should be permanently identified at the time of entrance into the aviary. Electronic identification using implantable transponders is ideal, allowing permanent unalterable identification with minimal risk to the bird.* Incorporation of the transponder number into medical, genealogic, and breeding records allows accurate records to follow a bird throughout its lifetime. Closed bands should be used as an adjunct to, or replacement for, transponders. Properly fitting closed bands are an indication (not proof) that a bird was bred in captivity, and bands allow immediate visual identification as well as an indication of the source of the birds.

Permanent identification using closed bands or implantable transponders is required for export of captive-bred birds (from the US) of CITES-listed species. Unfortunately, the numbers often wear off closed bands; large birds may collapse them, resulting in foot injury; or bands may become caught on loose cages wires. These disadvantages should not preclude the serious aviculturist from closed banding, nor should they encourage the veterinarian to remove those bands.

Open bands are the least desirable means of identification but are preferable to no identification. Rolled steel bands used for imported birds have sufficient tensile strength to preclude complete closure. These bands always have a slight gap between the ends, making the risk of entanglement higher than for closed bands. An alternative to removal of open bands is to close them as tightly as possible, thereby reducing the risk of the gap slipping over cage wire. The numbers are more durable on steel

open bands than on breeders' closed bands, which are usually made of aluminum.

The importance of individual identification was graphically presented in the aftermath of Hurricane Andrew's assault on South Florida in August, 1992. Many birds escaped from damaged aviaries and could not be identified for recovery by their owners.

FACILITY DESIGN AND HOUSING

The aviary must be designed for safety, security, sanitation, ease of maintenance, and meeting the psychological needs of the bird. No single formula exists for successful aviculture other than housing healthy pairs in a way that they feel secure and remain healthy. Happy, healthy birds are more likely to breed.

Outdoor aviaries are commonly used in southern regions, whereas breeders in northern climates and city dwellers usually house their birds indoors.

Indoor Aviaries

Indoor aviaries have the advantages of easier pest control; ability to manipulate lighting, temperature, and humidity factors; and protection from the elements and theft. Routine care is not affected by seasonal changes, rainfall, and weather conditions. Disturbance by nocturnal predators or other wildlife and introduction of disease by wild birds is eliminated.

Indoor facilities are usually less spacious than outdoor aviaries. High population density increases the potential for the spread of disease. The lack of seasonal cycling of light and other climatic factors may affect breeding success. Cost per unit of housing as well as maintenance costs are typically higher for indoor facilities. Indoor areas require more cleaning to prevent accumulation of feces, food wastes, and dust as well as preventing stagnation of the air. The potential hazard that dust poses for human health should also be considered.

When planning an indoor avicultural facility, ease of cleaning must be paramount. Drainage to allow hosing or pressure washing must be considered. If floor drains are installed, they must be of adequate size to prevent blockage by feed (especially seed, which sprouts in drains) or debris. Floor drains may

---

*Companies marketing electronic identification systems in the US are Infopet Identification Systems, Inc., distributing Trovan equipment, 517 West Travelers Trail, Burnsville, MN 55337 Telephone 612–890–2080; and American Veterinary Identification Systems (AVID), 3179 Hamner, Suite 5, Norco, CA 91760 Telephone 714–371–7505; and Destron IDI, 2545 Central Avenue, Boulder, CO 80301 Telephone 303–444–5306.

be used by pests, especially rats, to enter a facility. Design to reduce excessive movement around or under birds during cleaning may be important to reduce disturbance.

Good air quality reduces stress and the spread of disease. The use of ventilation fans, air filters, and ozone generators should be considered for improvement of air quality. Provision of full spectrum light should be used to enhance activation of vitamin D_3 and to enhance well-being. In dry climates or during northern winters, supplemental humidity, by air humidifiers or misters, may be required for the comfort of tropical species.

Outdoor Aviaries

Outdoor aviaries are more common in southern states and provide a more natural setting for birds. Outdoor aviaries are usually more spacious because of decreased per unit construction and maintenance costs. Natural seasonal weather variations may stimulate reproduction. The beneficial effects of fresh air and sunshine to health and productivity may play a role in aviculture success.

Disadvantages include the inability to control climatic factors when the weather is inclement, difficulty in pest control, the potential for bird noise to irritate neighbors, and increased risk of theft. Some birds may exhibit sensitivity to biting insects or other allergens. Predation and the potential for introduction of disease by wild animals pose some risk. Protection of food bowls and nest boxes from heavy rains poses some problems.

Some of the disadvantages of both approaches can be corrected by using combination indoor/outdoor facilities, in which birds can be allowed outside in good weather.

Aviary Design and Planning

Site selection and preparation is the first step in outdoor aviary planning and construction. Location of aviaries and support buildings; flow of traffic through the aviaries; source of water and electric power; the effects of noise on neighbors; and the potential for disturbance of the birds by people, animals, and traffic must be considered. Aviculturists must evaluate drainage, weather protection, and

windbreaks for protection from the elements. Roofs should maximize protection of nest boxes and food bowls from rain.

Privacy is provided by the use of vegetation or fences, or by placement of birds as far as possible from roads or houses. Shade should be used appropriately. Desert species may prefer a more sunny, open aviary whereas forest species may feel more secure in wooded or secluded aviaries.

Security from predators that prey upon the birds or spread disease must be provided. Raccoons, opossum, foxes, cats, dogs, and rats may injure birds, frighten them into self-inflicted injuries, or introduce disease. Electric fences help to exclude wild predators from aviaries. Dogs are often used to exclude predators. Poorly trained, noisy, or excitable dogs may reduce production by killing, disturbing, or frightening birds. A fenced kill zone, where dogs are housed surrounding bird holding areas, may reduce some pest control and predator problems.

When outdoor housing is chosen, the effects of climatic factors are more critical. Species that evolved in a vastly different climate may be unsuitable for inclusion in the breeding collection. Birds that are housed outdoors and exposed to natural sunlight should not require supplemental vitamin D_3. Macaws are especially susceptible to vitamin D toxicity, which can be potentiated by supplementation of the vitamin to birds that receive natural sunlight.

Caging

Breeding birds can be housed in either suspended cages or flights. A suspended cage is elevated on poles or suspended from the ceiling and is not entered by the caretaker. Suspended cages have the advantages of being simple to construct, easy to clean, inexpensive, and easy to modify or move if necessary. Birds have less exposure to their feces and accumulated food, and thus disease and parasite control is simplified. Larger cages and perches placed above eye level of the caretaker contribute to security and contentment of the birds housed within (Table 8–3).

Flight cages extend to the floor or ground. They are aesthetically pleasing to people. They provide more space for large, shy or aggressive species,

T a b l e 8 – 3

SUGGESTED SIZES* FOR SUSPENDED CAGES AND NEST BOXES FOR BREEDING PSITTACINE BIRDS

	Cage (feet)	Nest Box (inches)
Large macaws	6 × 6 × 12 5 × 5 × 10	16 × 48 × 16
Large cockatoos, medium macaws, obese Amazons	4 × 4 × 8 6 × 6 × 8	36 × 12 × 12
Amazons, African grey parrots	2 × 2 × 6 4 × 4 × 4	24 × 12 × 12
Pionus, mini-macaws	2 × 3 × 8	18 × 12 × 12
Conures, caciques	2 × 2 × 6 2 × 2 × 4	18 × 12 × 12
Small conures, cockatiels	2 × 2 × 3 2 × 2 × 4	16 × 10 × 10
Lovebirds, parrotlets, budgies	2 × 2 × 3 2 × 2 × 2	8 × 6 × 6

*Cage and box dimensions are height × width × depth.

and provide more space for exercise. Disadvantages include difficulty in sanitation and pest and parasite control. Caretakers walking from flight to flight can track disease organisms or parasites.

Furnishing Cages and Flights

Furnishings should be placed so enclosures can be serviced with minimal disturbance and labor. Efficiently designed feeders reduce contamination, reduce dumping by the birds, prevent or reduce perching on bowls, and protect food from rain. Alcove feeders or basket feeders can be used.

Adequate cage doors allow capture of birds with minimal chasing. Enclosures can be made escape-proof with safety aisles or suspended safety netting. A portable catching cage or drape can be suspended over the door surrounding the catcher to reduce the chance of escape in cases of outside suspended cages that lack safety doors or aisles. Adequate space or double wiring between cages or flights prevents fighting between neighboring pairs.

Nest boxes should be mounted in or on the cage in such a way to facilitate easy and frequent examination. Placement on the same end as the feeding/watering station allows simultaneous feeding and nest box examination. Very shy birds may be more comfortable if the nest box is away from high traffic areas.

Some aviculturists believe that species such as

Amazons require visual isolation around the nest box, whereas other species, such as cockatoos, are less affected by visual contact with conspecifics. These differences may arise from flocking behavior and the existence or lack of communal nesting in the species.

Nest boxes must be constructed so that water does not soak through. They must be shielded from rain or direct sunlight, which may cause overheating. Nest boxes may be constructed of many materials, plywood being the most common. Pressure-treated plywood should not be used because of the potential of ingestion of toxins. Wire lining reduces nest box chewing; however, chewed wires can produce dangerous projections that could damage eggs or injure chicks or adults. Plastic or metal barrels have the advantages of being more permanent and they can be disinfected; however, they are more susceptible to environmental temperature variations. Nesting materials can contribute to disease problems. The use of potting soil, corn cob bedding, or hay may contribute to fungal growth. Pine shavings are recommended for nesting material.

Perches must be secure for successful copulation. Natural wood perches with variable diameter and surface textures provide optimal exercise for feet. However, unless very hard woods such as manzanita or Australian pine are used, wood perches are rapidly destroyed by many psittacines. Very large or flat perches, used to avoid frequent replacement, may cause pressure lesions on the ventral surfaces of the hocks. More permanent perches may be made from polyvinylchloride (PVC) or steel pipe, concrete, rolled wire, and some synthetic materials. Some foot and leg problems may be associated with long-term perching on hard perches, especially in cold climates where chilling of the feet may occur. Alternative perching must be provided. A concrete perch helps keep nails trimmed.

AVICULTURE MANAGEMENT

Managing Intraspecific Aggression

Unpredictable aggression of a bird toward its mate is a common cause of mortality for species such as cockatoos. It most frequently involves a male cockatoo, which with or without previous signs of aggression attacks or kills its mate. Aggression may

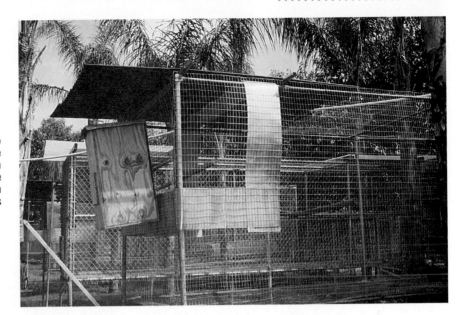

F i g u r e 8 – 1

Sheetmetal barriers can be used to provide a safe haven surrounding the nest box for a hen that is paired with an aggressive male. When his wings are clipped he cannot climb up to the perch and nest box. The hen can fly to his perch to be bred.

occur at any time of year but is more common early in the breeding season. In species or pairs that exhibit this behavior, preventive management may reduce the chance of losing a bird.

Many breeders routinely clip the wings of male cockatoos prior to the breeding season so that they are less able to catch the female. Special boxes with two entrances and baffled interiors may help reduce the chance of the male trapping the hen in the box. A promising cage alteration has been designed in which a sheetmetal strip is placed as a barrier around the box and a perch in front of the box. This keeps the wing-clipped male from climbing up to the box (Figs. 8–1, 8–2). The hen can fly down to the male for breeding.

In males that have a history of biting the hen, an acrylic or rubber bumper can be attached to the tip of the maxilla to reduce the chance that he can inflict a fatal injury. These tips are only temporarily effective, because they loosen and fall off with beak

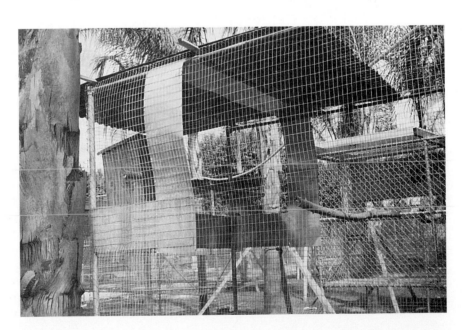

F i g u r e 8 – 2

Sheetmetal barriers.

growth. Bumpers typically last 2 to 8 weeks, but this time period may be adequate to prevent aggression in the early breeding season.

Diets and Nutrition

Proper nutrition is vital to aviculture success. Diets should be complete and balanced for optimal health and reproduction. Establishing a species in captivity often requires an understanding of the feeding habits of the species in the wild and preferences of captive birds to meet nutritional requirements and provide psychological stimulation to enhance breeding success. Several goals should be met when formulating diets for captive breeding birds, including meeting the known or perceived nutritional requirements; maintaining good food hygiene; providing psychological enrichment by offering variety; affording ease of preparation; and minimizing labor, waste, and expense.

A wild parrot must forage for its food. In its quest for food a bird may ingest a varied diet, which may include fruits, flowers, buds, pollen, seeds, grains, roots, and some live foods. Many of these foods are seasonally available. In tropical or subtropical zones, seasonality of food and breeding seasons may be associated with wet and dry seasons. The seasonal provision of extra soft foods prior to the onset of the breeding season may stimulate reproduction. This practice is often referred to as "flushing."

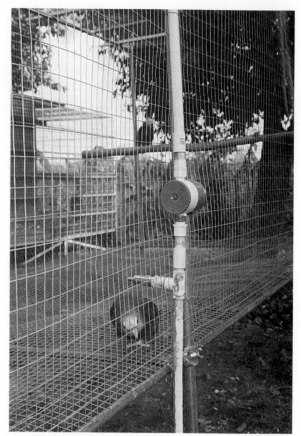

Figure 8-3

A nipple drinker (Lixit) can be used to provide fresh water at all times without using bowls. The gray sprinkler timer above the drinker provides periodic showers from overhead sprinklers.

Planning a Health Maintenance Program

A health maintenance program is necessary for each aviary, while considering problems that are common in the aviary and endemic problems in the locality. For example, birds housed in outdoor aviaries in southern coastal states must be provided with protection against the introduction of opossum (if Old World psittacine species are housed in the aviary) to prevent the inevitable introduction of sarcocystosis. Controlling biting insects is important to prevent or limit introduction of pox viruses as well as reduce insect bite hypersensitivity.

Annual examinations should be done in the nonbreeding season, typically in the fall. The veterinarian should limit the numbers of assistants and visitors when visiting an aviary so that disturbance is minimized.

Sanitation is vital to good health; however, the level of hygiene must be balanced against the disturbance associated with it. Designing cages so that cleaning and maintenance are minimized saves labor and limits disturbances that can reduce the chances of successful reproduction in shy birds. Frequent disinfection of cages is not necessary if healthy birds are permanently housed within and organic debris is not allowed to build up in the cage.

Good food hygiene practices prevent the spread of food-borne pathogens. Storage of feed in closed garbage cans prevents infestation by insects or rodents. Hygiene is especially important when dealing with soft or fresh foods with high water content in which spoilage is rapid. Sprouts are considered highly beneficial and stimulating by many aviculturists, but routine cultures usually reveal gram-negative bacteria and fungi. Rinsing sprouts in dilute hypochlorite or chlorhexidine solutions prior to feeding can reduce bacterial and fungal contamination. Likewise, fruits and vegetables support microbial growth if left too long in a cage, especially in a warm, humid climate. Feeding programs should be designed so that removal of food from a cage is easy. For example, use of a commercial coleslaw machine to grind and blend vegetables allows for easy removal of uneaten food by simply hosing the remains out of the cage.

Water offered to birds must be potable and provided fresh daily. Water bowls should be washed as necessary and as indicated by algae growth and food or fecal deposition in the bowl. Vitamins should not be added to drinking water because they oxidize rapidly and promote bacterial growth.

Automatic waterers reduce labor and ensure that birds have a clean, fresh supply of water at all times (Figs. 8–3, 8–4). Contamination from food or fecal deposition in water is eliminated. Contamination of water lines can occur, and frequent flushing of water lines is important to maintain good water quality (Fig. 8–5). Water should be flushed through lines daily as part of the maintenance routine. Periodic flushing of water lines with hypochlorite or iodophors may be necessary. Reliance on automatic waterers without a visual check to assure they are working every day can result in mortality from system failures. Water bottles are less susceptible to contamination than bowls; however, bottles can be a reservoir for bacteria if not cleaned frequently or appropriately.

The use of foot baths is often considered an important aspect of a disease control program. They are probably of minimal value as long as people are not entering flight cages; more attention should be focused on the cleanliness of objects that directly contact birds, such as clothing, nets, and hands. Nonetheless, the veterinarian must take precautions when going from one premises to another to avoid transmission of pathogens on contaminated footwear. Washing shoes or boots after leaving an aviary, or the use of disposable plastic shoe covers, is a good preventive measure. The proper disinfection of equipment is especially important because items such as nets, restraint devices, and instruments come into direct contact with birds and can serve as fomites.

Air conditioners and ventilation systems may be foci for bacterial and fungal growth in an indoor facility. In a California finch breeding facility, the source of recurrent bacterial infections was traced to an air conditioner filter that supported the growth

Figure 8–4

The water system pictured here consists of a polyvinyl chloride (PVC) pipe running over the cage. The pipe is drilled with holes so water drips into the cage. A sprinkler timer system allows the water to flow for 3- to 20-minute periods each day. This system allows birds to drink without bowls and without contacting the water line, which could result in contamination.

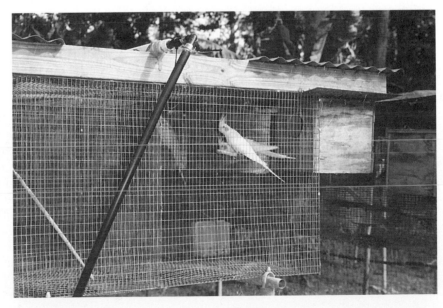

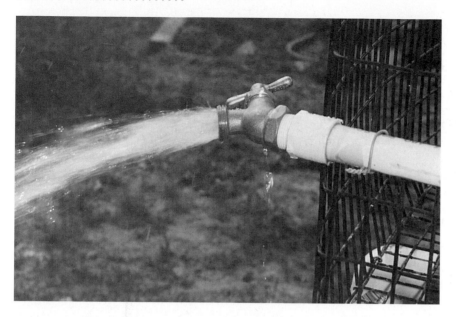

Figure 8–5

It is vital that water lines for automatic watering system can be easily flushed to dislodge bacterial plaques. The flushing system is best fitted on a timer for frequent flushing.

of *Pseudomonas.* In another facility, *Aspergillus* was disseminated through an air conditioner filter that was not changed with necessary frequency.

Daily washing of food bowls is not practical in many avicultural facilities. Soiled bowls, however, are a source of contamination, and a system must be established to wash bowls as frequently as necessary to maintain a reasonable level of sanitation (Fig. 8–6). Bowls should either be washed with

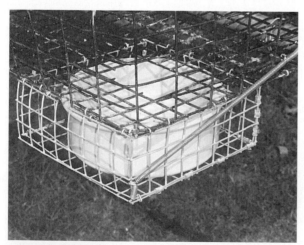

Figure 8–6

Basket feeders allow changing bowls without opening cage doors. The basket is mounted under a hole in the cage floor. If it is mounted above the floor, it has a hole in the top. The opening is large enough for the bird to insert its head but is too small to allow escape.

soap and water and returned to the same cage, or, if washed in a group, they should be washed then disinfected. For ease of washing, a series of tubs can be set up, the first with detergent and hot water, followed by a rinse, followed by immersion for the recommended period of time in a properly diluted disinfectant solution, followed by a second rinse and air drying on a rack. A commercial dishwasher is a viable alternative if organic debris can be adequately removed.

Nest boxes, at a minimum, should be thoroughly cleaned annually, and nest material should be changed after each clutch if chicks were allowed to hatch in the nest (Fig. 8–7). The dark, damp interior of a nest box can provide an ideal environment for the proliferation or dissemination of pathogens. Wood nest boxes should be destroyed if the inhabitants develop viral or serious bacterial diseases, such as psittacine pox, polyoma, or salmonellosis. Problems such as dead-in-shell embryos, contaminated eggs, and chicks hatching with infections may be directly traced to a moist nest box and transport of bacterial agents through eggshell pores.

Wire floor cages allow feces and food debris to fall through or to be hosed out of the cage, limiting unnecessary disturbance associated with overzealous cleaning. Excessive organic debris should not be allowed to build up in a cage.

Facilities should be maintained in a clean, sanitary condition. All surfaces should be cleaned of

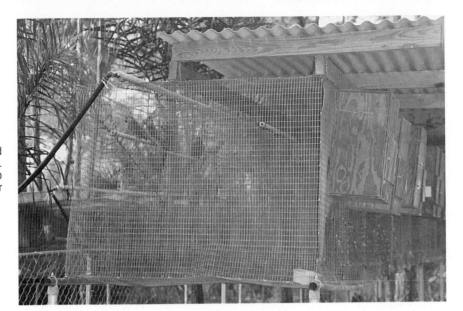

Figure 8–7

Roofs suspended above nest boxes and food bowls protect them from rain. Corrugated PVC roofing does not absorb heat in the summer. Note the drip/timer water system as in Figure 8–4.

organic debris prior to disinfection. Disinfectants should be used according to label instruction; stronger solutions are not more effective. The constant use of powerful disinfectants in the absence of a disease threat may not be beneficial and can be potentially harmful. Chlorine bleach should only be used in well-ventilated areas, and a 5% solution is effective for most uses.

PEST CONTROL

Insect and rodent pests are vectors for disease and parasites and are a source of irritation and disturbance for breeding birds. Cockroaches transmit *Sarcocystis falcatula* from opossum feces and can contaminate a bird's food and nest or can be eaten by a bird, resulting in fatal illness. Control of roaches, especially in outdoor facilities in southern coastal climates, is challenging if not impossible. The use of insecticides alone is not likely to be effective; the potential exists that they may cause toxicity in birds. Biologic control methods are preferable, such as attempting to limit or eliminate breeding sites, or keeping insectivorous animals, such as chickens or geckos, in a bird compound to consume insects (Fig. 8–8). The use of flightless chicken breeds, such as silky chickens, is recommended so that the chickens are not able to roost on the cages of parrots.

Ants can transmit some parasites such as the proventricular worm *Dispharynx*. Ants can also reduce food consumption by swarming food bowls or build nests in nest boxes. Control procedures should include baiting of nests and trails, keeping facilities clean, and avoiding foods that attract ants into cages. The incidence of mites and lice is low in captive psittacines, but they may be introduced into an aviary by wild birds. The red mite (*Dermanysis gallinae*), however, can be troublesome in aviculture. The mite is nocturnal and hides during the day in crevices in aviaries and nest boxes, and thus control cannot be achieved without treating the environment. Red mites can kill chicks by weakening from exsanguination. Carbaryl powder 5% has been used successfully for the control of mites inhabiting nest boxes without apparent harm to chicks or adults. Mosquitos can also be a problem for chicks in nest boxes.

Rodents and Predators

Rats entering an aviary at night can not only spread disease, but also can disturb nesting birds and on occasion kill birds. In a survey on one breeding farm in South Florida, 50% of resident rats were found to be carrying *Salmonella* species.

In Southern US coastal areas, rats are particularly a problem in the fall when populations seem to

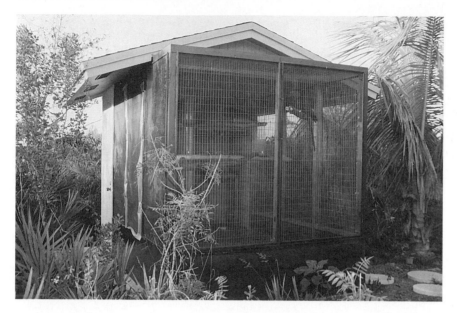

Figure 8–8

This isolated aviary, constructed for a pair of hyacinth macaws, is screened to prevent entry of biting insects and is equipped with a burglar alarm. Feeding and nesting areas are sheltered, but the open end of the flight allows exposure to sun and rain.

rise. Biologic control methods appear to be most effective. Attempts should be made to build in such a way as to discourage nesting in or around the aviary. For example, the use of concrete slabs under aviaries appears to provide additional cleanliness under suspended cages, but rats almost invariably tunnel and nest under these slabs. Cages suspended on poles can be fitted with rat guards, or the poles can be greased to prevent climbing. Sheetmetal guards can be wrapped around trees to prevent nesting in trees by rats or use of trees by predators to cross fences. Bait boxes should be used as needed and with caution.

Snakes occasionally enter cages and eat small birds, but they rarely attack larger species. If an aviculturist is breeding small birds outdoors, such as finches, the cage should be constructed with small wire or screened to prevent entry of snakes.

Large predators such as opossum, raccoons, cats, and dogs should be carefully excluded from the aviary (Fig. 8–9). Electric wires running along the top or bottom of a perimeter fence that is buried at the bottom is a very effective means of control. Aviculturists must observe the perimeter of the enclosure to ensure that overhanging trees do not provide access to aviary roofs from points outside the perimeter.

Wild birds may also be problematic in an outdoor aviary, especially pigeons and doves, which may transmit *Chlamydia* to psittacines.

Preventive Medicine

Routine preventive medicine programs can be designed around a detailed health history of the collection. Many parasites can be excluded from an aviary by screening of new birds, and annual deworming of all birds may yield some benefit, especially if food- or water-borne medications can be used, which do not result in stress. Testing of all or a portion of the birds may help to reveal the need for deworming and the choice of medication. If birds are handled for annual examinations, the opportunity exists for deworming.

Annual prophylactic treatment for chlamydiosis is often advocated, even in the absence of a diagnosis of chlamydiosis. If the birds are housed outdoors and exposed to wild birds, especially pigeons, this may be necessary and quite beneficial. Treatment should be delayed until the nonbreeding season, usually the fall for most species. Egg production typically is reduced or stopped, and chicks that hatch from eggs laid during treatment may exhibit abnormalities.

Commercially available oil emulsion adjuvant vaccines for Pacheco's parrot disease and *Salmonella* infection can be very beneficial in populations at risk. These vaccines were developed for use in wild-caught imported birds to prevent catastrophic disease outbreaks. In an aviculture collection, the benefits of vaccination must be weighed against the

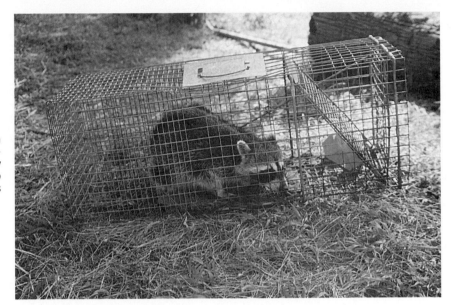

Figure 8–9

Live trapping of predators can be useful in controlling raccoons and opossum. Raccoons must be relocated many miles away (at least 10 miles) and may still return to the farm. Sardines, cat food, and eggs make good baits.

potential for granulomatous reactions to oil emulsion adjuvants.

Disinfectants should be used judiciously in aviaries. All disinfectants are potentially toxic. All are ineffective if organic debris is present, and thus cleaning with detergents and water prior to disinfection is necessary. The least toxic disinfectant for the need should be chosen. Bleach diluted at the rate of one part bleach to 20 parts water is very effective; however, bleach should never be mixed with other chemicals because toxic chlorine gas may be liberated. Increasing the water temperature increases the efficacy of chlorine. Chemical burns result if birds come into contact with bleach, and some birds attempt to ingest bleach if allowed to.

An appropriate response taken in the face of a disease outbreak can dramatically alter the outcome. When dealing with an individual bird, isolation and the provision of specific therapy is indicated. In an aviculture setting, the flock must take priority. Containment of spread, or demonstrating the source and implementing control procedures, is the primary consideration. Ideally, management changes or biologic control measures can be instituted in preference to drug therapy.

Selling Birds

Offering a liberal warranty may be used as a sales tool. However, as a perishable product, long-term guarantees given on the health or life of birds, especially unweaned birds, can be difficult to provide. Presale testing for selected infectious diseases such as polyoma virus, PBFD, or chlamydiosis may help assure the buyer of good health. However, for birds entering commercial trade, the cost of such testing is often declined because an initial negative test does not rule out exposure after testing, testing during incubation periods, or false negative test results. The best guarantee of good health logically stems from a stable flock of known health history and good husbandry practices.

Pet shops and breeders often require veterinary examination within a certain period of time to activate a guarantee. A suggested guarantee may be 14 to 30 days with a postpurchase examination within the first 7 days to activate the guarantee. A no-question return policy should be in place for birds found unsuitable for purchase by the buyers' veterinarian. The veterinarian must practice good judgment in recommending return and not reject birds for frivolous or unsubstantiated reasons.

Suggested Reading

Alderton DA: The Atlas of Parrots. Neptune City, NJ, TFH Publications, 1991.
Jordan R: Parrot Incubation Procedures. Pickering, Ontario, Canada, Silvio Mattacchione and Co, 1989.
Low R: Parrots, Their Care and Breeding. Poole, England, Blandford Press, 1980.

Schubot RM, Clubb KJ, Clubb SL: Psittacine Aviculture. Loxahatchee, FL, Avicultural Breeding and Research Center, 1992.

Silva T: Psittaculture, The Breeding, Rearing and Management of Parrots. Pickering, Ontario, Canada, Silvio Mattacchione & Co, 1991.

Snyder NFR, Wiley JW, Kepler CB: The Parrots of Luquillo; Natural History and Conservation of the Puerto Rican Parrot. Los Angeles, Western Foundation of Vertebrate Zoology, 1987.

Voren H, Jordan R: Parrots, Handfeeding and Nursery Management. Pickering, Ontario, Canada, Silvio Mattacchione and Co, 1992.

Woolham F: The Handbook of Aviculture. Poole, England, Blandford Press, 1987.

Joy Halverson

9

Nonsurgical Methods of Avian Sex Identification

THE IMPORTANCE OF AVIAN SEX IDENTIFICATION

Many species of birds exhibit little or no external evidence of gender. Many more are sexually dimorphic (male and female appear different) as adults but are monomorphic as juveniles. The majority of psittacine birds, the most common birds seen by avian veterinarians, are monomorphic throughout their lives. The lack of external sexually dimorphic features presents a challenge to veterinarians and aviculturists wishing to breed birds in captivity.

Sex identification is important in birds for a variety of reasons. From a clinical standpoint, knowledge of a bird's sex can play an important role in the differential diagnosis of disease. Common problems of the female reproductive tract can be eliminated in a known male bird. Sick birds are often presented in an advanced state of illness, and none of the available methods of sex identification is appropriate by that time. Prior knowledge of the bird's sex can reduce the number of differential diagnoses that must be rapidly considered.

Birds undergo behavioral changes as they mature; these changes can be better understood if the sex of the bird is known. Behavior plays a major role in a client's relationship with the pet and can alter dramatically as the bird matures. For example, an affectionate, hand-raised, male parrot may attempt, as he matures, to assume a dominant relationship over the owner by biting. A veterinarian may therefore advise the client to take steps to prevent this predictable behavior by firmly maintaining a dominant role (see Chapter 7).

The gender of a bird is important when introducing it or new birds into a household or aviary. In the wild, birds can escape from territorial disputes; escape is not possible in a cage or even a large aviary. Certain species of psittacines (such as Mollucan cockatoos) are prone to injuring their mates and should be carefully watched not only on introduction but when courting behaviors are displayed. Knowledge of a bird's gender can provide important insight into such behaviors.

Knowledge of a bird's sex enhances the bond between a client and the bird. Awareness of an animal's sex is part of "knowing" it. It is normal and healthy to anthropomorphize pets to a certain extent and to assign particular personality traits to gender. Longstanding pet bird owners usually think their bird is a given sex and may be reluctant to hear otherwise; others are thrilled to hear their suspicions confirmed. New bird owners want their birds to become an important part of their lives, and knowledge of the sex enhances that potential bond.

The knowledge of a bird's gender is an absolute prerequisite for breeding any bird species in captivity. Most psittacine birds exhibit territoriality in their nesting behavior and must have a clearly defined territory to breed successfully in captivity. Therefore, most aviculturists establish breeding pairs in single cages and do not give birds the opportunity to choose their mates, as would happen in the wild. In addition, many aviculturists buy and sell birds among each other and must know the sex before they decide which birds to keep and which to sell.

Scientific studies of sexually monomorphic wild bird populations can be greatly enhanced by identi-

117

fication of gender. Population demographics such as colony nesting behaviors or family dynamics can be much more informative when observers know the gender of the birds under study.

MORPHOLOGIC METHODS OF SEX IDENTIFICATION

External secondary sexual characteristics, although subtle, can be useful in sex identification of birds. Although many species of birds exhibit obvious sexual dimorphism such as plumage color (e.g., sexually mature *Psittacula* species) or the size and color of wattles, combs, or spurs, many others exhibit more subtle evidence. Birds of prey, such as owls, are a good example. Females are generally larger than males, but sex can be determined more precisely with careful measurements of the skull, foot pads, and other anatomic features.

Caution should be exercised in relying absolutely on subtle secondary sexual characteristics for sex identification in birds. Many of these characteristics are variable and can be influenced by nongenetic factors (e.g., nutrition). Moreover, evidence suggests that some of these characteristics may be determined hormonally, whereas others may be genetically determined and are independent of the bird's hormonal status.[1] A classic example is the "black hen" ostrich, which has black plumage typical of a male but the cloacal morphology and sex chromosome constitution of a female. In birds, the male is the "neutral sex" and "femaleness" is imposed on the plumage by the presence of ovarian hormones. A genetically female ostrich with inactive ovaries has black plumage rather than the drab brown of the normal female.

Sex Identification by Cloacal Morphology

Cloacal morphology (vent-sexing) is the most widely used indicator of avian gender. The morphology of the cloaca can be markedly different in some birds, such as adult ostriches, or very subtle and almost indistinguishable, as in psittacines. Rapid, accurate vent-sexing of poultry is a skilled profession that has been passed down to successive generations. However, the age at which chicks are sexed is fundamentally important; in poultry, vent-sexing is performed within the first day of hatch.

Later in the chick's life the distinguishing features are drawn farther up into the vent and cannot be seen.

Vent-sexing is currently the most common means of sexing ostriches and emus. Ostrich and emu breeding is a growing industry internationally, and there is a large demand for accurate sex identification. Published reports describe the distinguishing features of cloacal morphology in ratites and other species.[2, 3] However, the accuracy of vent-sexing in ratites is highly variable. Certainly, hard-won experience plays a large role in accuracy. Anecdotal reports are common that emu sexing is most accurate before the bird is 3 months of age, but it is still quite problematic for many emu breeders.

Sex Identification by Gonad Morphology

The most direct means of assessing the sex of birds is direct visualization of the primary gonads. The methodology is discussed in Chapter 45.

LABORATORY METHODS OF SEX IDENTIFICATION

The inaccuracy, inconvenience, and risk of morphologic methods of sex identification in birds has led to the development of several laboratory methods. All methods currently available are based on examining either the hormone status or the sex chromosome status of the bird to determine gender.

Sex Identification by Hormone Analysis

In the late 1970s, a radioimmunoassay measuring steroid hormones in the droppings was developed and offered commercially.[4] The testing procedure measured estrogen conjugate and testosterone levels and reported their ratio (E:T ratio). The test's accuracy varied with the age and species of the bird, and commercial introduction was not successful. More recent literature reports refinement of this method; a fluoroimmunoassay is used and only estrogen conjugates are measured.[5] This method was reported 87% accurate (13/15) in adult cockatiels. The test is not commercially available at this time.

Sex Identification by Genetic Analysis

Commercially available laboratory tests for sex identification are based on examination of avian sex chromosomes by several techniques. A bird's sex is determined by the sex chromosomes it inherits from its parents. Male birds have two identical sex chromosomes (ZZ), whereas females have one Z chromosome and one W chromosome (ZW). Birds are different from mammals in that the female carries the heteromorphic sex chromosome; thus, it is the female's genetic contribution that determines the sex of the offspring. The genetic mechanism of sex determination in birds is controversial; scientists have not yet established whether one or more genes on the W chromosome is the "master switch" (as is the case in mammals with the Y chromosome) or whether the balance of Z chromosomes to autosomes (non–sex chromosomes) determines gender.[1] These details are only relevant, however, in the rare cases of abnormal chromosome numbers or translocations. In birds with normal chromosome constitution, the morphologic or deoxyribonucleic acid (DNA) sequence differences between the Z and W chromosome can be exploited to determine the sex of an individual.

Sex Identification by Chromosome Analysis

During metaphase in cell division, the chromosomes can be examined by light microscopy (karyotyping). In many birds, the W chromosome can be distinguished from the Z chromosome and other chromosomes by size and staining characteristics. To perform chromosome analysis for sex identification, cells capable of division (commonly, feather pulp epithelial cells or blood leukocytes) are collected and cultured. Cultured cells are arrested in metaphase and treated so that they can be examined individually.

The accuracy of chromosome analysis is highly dependent on the skill of the investigator and varies in published reports from 68 to 100%.[6, 7] Advantages of sex identification by chromosome analysis are the absence of risk to the bird, accuracy at any age, and the possibility of detecting large chromosome defects. Disadvantages are the cost and inconvenience of sample shipping, lack of availability of a blood feather, sample loss due to bacterial contamination, and laboratory processing time (12 to 14 days minimum). In addition, the sex of ratite birds cannot be determined by chromosome analysis at this time. The sex chromosomes of ratites cannot be easily distinguished from one another by light microscopy.

Sex Identification by DNA Analysis

The course of gonad development in the embryo is guided by genetic messages. These messages are encoded by the molecule DNA, which forms a bivalent, helical chain and combines with other molecules to make up the chromosomes. All the proteins that build and regulate the developing embryo are encoded by DNA, which is made up of four nucleotides (bases); the genetic messages that cause a male and a female to develop differently reflect differences in the sequence of bases that encode these messages. In the last two decades a number of techniques have been developed to examine the variations in DNA sequences, and hence to examine the genetic differences between animals.

DNA is a powerful tool for analysis because of its unique biologic properties. When the bivalent chain is pulled apart, the separate DNA strands are chemically unstable and will find similar DNA strands with which to bind. A labeled DNA sequence cloned from a conserved gene of the sex chromosome(s) will find similar sequences in sample DNA and bind to them, allowing them to be identified. The ability of DNA to recognize similar target DNA sequences in a sample has yielded several different methods of sex identification.

The most widely used DNA method is restriction fragment length polymorphism (RFLP).[8, 9] A labeled gene sequence found on the sex chromosomes of most avian species tags DNA fragments produced by digestion with restriction enzymes (bacterial enzymes that cut DNA sequences at specific sites). Genetic differences between the Z and W chromosome result in DNA fragments of different size; the characteristic length of tagged sequences reveals the sex chromosome constitution of the sample bird (Fig. 9–1). The examination of both sex chromosomes and the internal controls (species-specific patterns, examination of both Z and W chromosomes) implicit in the technique make RFLP extremely accurate (100% in a double-blind study) for avian sex identification.

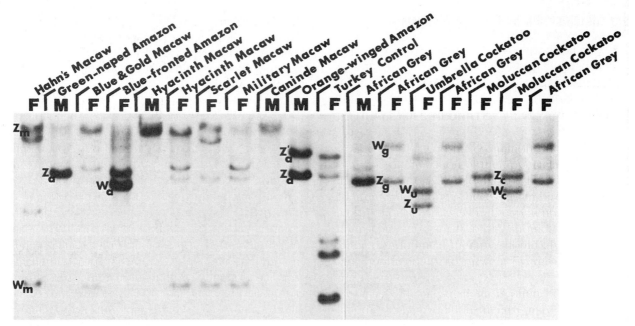

Figure 9–1

Sex identification by RFLP DNA analysis. Sample DNA is cut by restriction enzymes into fragments that are separated by size via electrophoresis. DNA fragments from the sex chromosomes are highlighted with a DNA probe. The variation in the size of the fragments reflects genetic differences between the sex chromosomes and gives a characteristic pattern for each species. The subscripts denote fragments from the Z and W chromosomes of macaws (m), amazons (a), African greys (g), umbrella cockatoos (u), and Moluccan cockatoos (c). Minor bands that are sex- and species-related have not been labeled.

Other methods of sex identification by DNA analysis include the use of repeated DNA sequences[10] (noncoding DNA sequences present in many copies) or families of such sequences.[11] Both methods are targeted exclusively at the W chromosome and identify sex by the presence or absence of a signal from the W chromosome. These methods can be performed at a lower cost than RFLP but they require strict external controls to prevent false-negative results.

Another method is based on the polymerase chain reaction (PCR), in which DNA sequences act as primers to amplify sex chromosome–specific DNA fragments. This method is very rapid (1 to 2 days) and also very accurate. The disadvantage of PCR is that primers are generally species-specific; thus, the method is less useful for sexing a wide cross-section of species. However, PCR-based sexing is available for certain individual species and is widely used for ostriches and emus.

The advantages of sex identification by DNA analysis are absence of risk to the bird, accuracy at any age, easy sample collection and shipment, and more rapid laboratory processing time (3 to 5 days) than chromosome analysis. Sex identification of ratites by DNA analysis is available because, despite the morphologic similarity of ratite sex chromosomes, DNA sequence differences have been identified. The major disadvantages of DNA analysis, like any laboratory technique, are the laboratory processing time required and problems such as poor sample collection and labeling.

CHOOSING THE BEST METHOD OF SEX IDENTIFICATION

The veterinarian should consider several factors when choosing a method of sex identification. Is the owner's interest casual or is there a plan to breed the bird? Is the bird too young to be surgically sexed accurately or safely?

As more birds are domestically bred and sold soon after weaning, veterinarians will see a larger proportion of young birds on initial presentation. Is the bird a good anesthetic risk? Are there potential conditions (tumors, chronic aspergillosis) that justify or contraindicate an invasive procedure? Many aviculturists believe that "breeding readiness" or sexual maturity can be estimated by visualizing the gonads; others believe that the gonads can rapidly change and that age and behavior are more reliable indicators.

Does the owner need the result by a given time (such as before a pending sale)? Vent-sexing, surgical sexing, chromosome analysis, and DNA analysis are available and have advantages and disadvantages. The choice of techniques depends on the species of bird, the veterinarian's skills and facilities, and the client's needs.

References

1. Halverson JL, and Dvorak J: Genetic control of sex determination in birds and the potential for its manipulation. Poult Sci 72:890–896, 1993.
2. Samour JH, Markham J, Nieva O: Sexing ratite birds by cloacal examination. Vet Rec 115:167–169, 1984.
3. Samour JH, Stevenson M, Knight JA, Lawrie AJ: Sexing penguins by cloacal examination. Vet Rec 113:84–85, 1983.
4. Bercovitz AB, Czekala NM, Lasley BL: A new method of sex determination in monomorphic birds. J Zoo Animal Med 9(4):114–124, 1978.
5. Tell LA, Lasley BL: An automated assay for fecal estrogen conjugates in the determination of sex in avian species. Zoo Biol 10:361–367, 1991.
6. Prus SE, Schmutz SE: Comparative efficiency and accuracy of surgical and cytogenetic sexing in psittacines. Avian Dis 31(2):420–424, 1987.
7. Valentine M: Chromosome analysis. In Stoodly J (ed): Genus *Amazona*. Portsmouth, UK, Bezels Publications, 1990.
8. Dvorak J, Halverson JL, Gulick P, et al: cDNA cloning of a Z- and W-linked gene in Gallinaceous birds. J Hered 83:22–25, 1992.
9. Halverson JL: Avian sex identification by recombinant DNA technology. Proc Assoc Avian Vet, Phoenix, Arizona, September 10–15, 1990.
10. Uryu N, Yoshiho N, Ito K: Determination of the sex of chickens by a biotin-labeled deoxyribonucleic acid probe. Poult Sci 68:850–853, 1989.
11. de Kloet DH, de Kloet SR: Molecular determination of the sex of parrots. Focus 14(3):106–108, 1991.

Diagnostics, Hospital Techniques, and Supportive Care

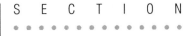

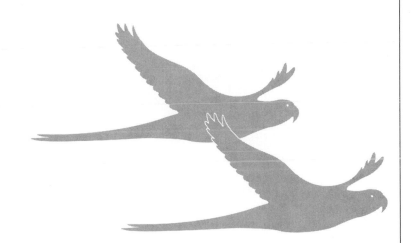

Elizabeth V. Hillyer

10

Physical Examination

A thorough patient history and physical examination provide important information with which to evaluate the husbandry for well birds and with which to make diagnostic and therapeutic plans for sick birds. Give yourself time to obtain a good history and to perform a thorough examination. Laboratory testing is ancillary. Indeed, laboratory test results are interpretable only within the context of the history and physical findings.

You must be familiar with the normal bird. This knowledge comes from carefully observing and examining your avian patients. Perform a complete examination of all birds, even well birds, scheduled for office visits. In this manner, the features of the normal bird become familiar, and, equally importantly, you will detect subclinical physical abnormalities. A systematic approach is important; establish a list of questions to ask each avian owner and develop a routine physical examination sequence. In this way, you are less likely to overlook abnormalities.

PRACTICAL CONSIDERATIONS

Recommend that all birds be examined at least once a year. Office visits for first-time and sick avian patients should be scheduled for at least ½ hour; allow enough time to obtain a complete history, make management recommendations, and perform the physical examination and preliminary diagnostic testing. Recheck and grooming visits can be shorter.

All birds should be transported to your office in a secure carrier or cage and should be confined while in the waiting room. Request that, if possible,

the owner transport the pet in its own cage so that you can directly evaluate the bird's environment, the droppings, and the cage sanitation. (Obviously this is not possible for larger birds.) Ask the client not to clean the cage for 12 to 24 hours before the visit so you can examine the droppings.

The examination room should be fully enclosed to contain any escapees. The room should be large enough to accommodate the veterinarian, an assistant, and the patient and its owner. Keep all equipment and supplies within closed cabinets or in covered containers so that escaped birds do not damage breakables or, conversely, damage themselves by landing in disinfectant solution, for example. You should be able to darken the room to aid in capture; a dimmer switch is ideal.

Basic equipment needed in avian practice is listed in Table 10–1. Store all potentially useful equipment safely within the avian examination room so it is rapidly accessible when needed. This precludes having to leave the room or having to lengthen the restraint period while searching for supplies. A good light source, such as a surgical light, is invaluable during the examination.

PATIENT HISTORY

The patient history is helpful in prioritizing the list of differential diagnoses for a sick patient. The history is equally important for healthy birds because details of management, particularly caging and diet, often reveal problems. Improper husbandry and poor sanitation are common underlying factors causing or promoting illness in captive avian species.

Table 10-1

EQUIPMENT FOR AVIAN PRACTICE*

Capture nets of varying sizes
Clean towels for restraint
Paper towels to restrain small birds
Ear protection equipment†
Magnifying loupe (4×)
Gram scales—a tub scale and a perch scale
Mouth specula
Grooming equipment (according to preferences; see text)—files, sharp nail
    clippers
Dremel drill
Ophthalmic cautery unit‡
Blood drawing equipment
Specimen containers for common diagnostic tests
Slides for Gram's stains
Culturettes and Mini-tip Culturettes
Chromosomal sexing equipment
Crop gavage tubes for sample collection
Injectable vitamins A and D
Medications commonly used in outpatients
Band removal equipment

*Equipment listed is in addition to the equipment standard to most practices, such as penlight, stethoscope, otoscope, gauze strips, cotton-tipped swabs, K-Y jelly, etc.
†Noisegard Hearing Protectors, Shoplyne, Cleveland, OH.
‡MDS, Inc., St. Petersburg, FL.

Establish a standard list of questions to ask of each owner. An avian history is typically more lengthy and more involved than that for dogs and cats because of management considerations. A written history form to be filled out before the office visit saves time and ensures that important questions will not be forgotten.[1] A sample history form is presented in Table 10–2. The written form gives clients something to occupy their time while waiting for the office visit and starts them thinking about the issues you consider important to their bird's health. The written answers will guide you in the direction to take for further questioning.

Birds tend to hide signs of illness until the disease process is advanced. In nature, this serves as an adaptive mechanism to avoid attracting predators. Owners may not notice the less obvious signs of illness, such as decreased vocalization or decreased activity, until they progress to more obvious signs, such as inactivity, persistent fluffing, or anorexia. It is often helpful to ask clients about *change*—whether there have been recent changes in the bird's environment and husbandry or in the bird's behavior. Changes in the bird's droppings may be more obvious to clients than changes in food and water intake.

Breeding behavior may be the clue to a medical problem, such as egg binding. Breeding behavior can include hiding in dark places; paper shredding; spending more time on the cage bottom; masturbating; increased territoriality; and regurgitating to mirrors, other birds, or the owner. The large droppings produced by female birds in breeding condition are often reported by owners as "diarrhea."

Signalment and Pet Status

Infectious disease is most common in aviary birds, newly acquired birds, or those that have been recently exposed to other birds—at a bird show or while being boarded, for example. Nutritional diseases are most common in older, long-term pets that are chronically malnourished or birds that are under heavy metabolic demands, such as growth, reproduction, and parenting. Toxicities and trauma are most common in birds allowed free access to the home; cage-mate trauma is most common in breeding situations.

Nutrition and Feather Care

Malnutrition is very common in pet avian species (see Chapter 30). It is important to question an owner about what the bird actually *eats*, rather than what foods are offered.

The health and appearance of the feathers reflect the bird's overall systemic health, environment, and diet. The appearance of the feathers is maintained by preening. Some birds, particularly young birds, may not preen themselves sufficiently. Access to a bath often stimulates preening and can have a dramatic effect upon the appearance of the feathers. Birds should be encouraged to bathe daily or at least two or three times a week, even during winter months. Some birds climb into a shallow pan of warm water or their water bowl; others enjoy being misted with a spray bottle. Many large psittacines enjoy showering with their owners. Baths should be given in the morning so that the feathers will dry over the course of the day.

Discourage owners from applying anything but warm water to the feathers. Commercial grooming or antiparasite sprays are ineffective and coat the feathers with foreign substances. Exposure to ciga-

SAMPLE AVIAN HISTORY FORM

Name: _____   Date: _____

Pet's Name: _____   Species: _____

How long have you owned your bird?
Age of bird (if known)?
Do you know the sex of your bird?
   Has your bird been sexed using chromosomal analysis (blood ☐ or feather ☐ test)?
   If female, has your bird ever laid eggs?   If so, how many and how often?
Where did you obtain the bird?
If there was a previous owner, how long was the bird with that owner?
Describe the bird's cage:
Where is the cage located?
   Any windows near the cage?
   Any air conditioner or heating vent near cage?
   What type of heating system is in your home?
   Do you have any humidifiers?
How much time does the bird spend out of the cage?
   Supervised?
Grooming: Do you clip the bird's wings?
   Do the nails require trimming?   If so, how often?
   Does the beak require trimming or filing?   If so, how often?
Do you give the bird baths or showers?
Do you ever apply anything other than water to the feathers or skin?
Diet: which of the following do you feed?
   Seed ☐ % of diet? ____ Type:
   Pellets? ☐ % of diet? ____ Type:
   Fresh foods? ☐ How often? _____
      Vegetables? ☐ How often? _____ Types:
      Fruits? ☐ How often? _____ Types:
      Meats? ☐ How often? _____ Types:
      Bread, rice, pasta, potatoes? ☐ How often? _____ Please specify:
      Dairy products? ☐ How often? _____ Please specify:
      Other? ☐ Please specify:
      Source of drinking water: tap water ☐ bottled water ☐
What are your bird's preferred food items?
Do you use a vitamin or mineral supplement?
   Type?
   In water ☐ or on seed ☐? How often? _____ Amount? _____
When did the bird last molt? _____ How often does it molt? _____
Is your bird around other birds?   If yes, how frequently and for how long?
Are any of these birds ill?
Has your bird been exposed recently to any new birds?
   Has it been boarded recently?
   Do you have any other pets?
   Are any of them ill?
Is your bird exposed to cigarette smoke?
If your bird is ill, please answer the following questions:
How long has the bird been ill?
Did the bird suddenly become ill, or has the illness come on gradually?
What signs have you noticed?
Is the bird eating any food?
Is the bird drinking water?
Are the droppings different from normal?
    If so, please describe them:
Is your bird making its normal sounds?
    If not, please describe the change(s):
If the bird spends time out of the cage, does it chew on furniture, any objects, or paint?
   Please specify:
   Does it have access to any plants?
Are any other pets or any humans in your household ill?
Have you given the bird any medications?
    If yes, please list type and for how many days:
Have you seen another veterinarian for this problem?
    If so, whom did you see?
Please describe treatment recommendations and list all medications:

rette smoke and cooking fumes also adversely affects the appearance of the feathers.

Caging

As a general rule, all pet birds should be caged when unsupervised. Birds left loose in the home have access to many potential foreign bodies and toxins, including jewelry, metallic objects, plants, leaded stained glass, curtain weights, and leaded paint in older homes. Free-flighted birds may land in hot foods or hot water, fly out of windows or doors, or get caught in ceiling fans or rodent glue traps. Psittacines can be quite destructive to furniture.

Birds of all sizes require proper caging and a clean environment. Small birds are often confined in a cage; therefore, that cage should be clean and adequately equipped to meet the bird's behavioral needs with appropriate perches, space for exercise, toys, and visual barriers.

Size and Type of Cage

Birds that spend most or all of their time in the cage should be in a relatively larger cage than birds that are frequently uncaged. The cage should be at least large enough for the bird to spread its wings. It should be appropriate for the size and type of bird, with perches placed so that the bird can get exercise. Most smaller psittacine and passerine birds enjoy horizontal space and the ability to hop from perch to perch. Some species, such as cockatiels, enjoy climbing and, therefore, do well in cages with horizontal bars.

Cages should be constructed such that the bars do not intersect in a **V**, where extremities can get trapped. In small cages with vertical bars and malpositioned perches, tail and primary feathers can become frayed from rubbing on cage bars. Older, ornate cages may be constructed of metals such as lead or copper that are toxic if ingested. Galvanized wire cages may contain zinc.

Perches

The best perches are of variable diameter because they promote exercise for the feet and toes. Natural, nontoxic tree branches are ideal. Manzanita and other hardwood perches can be purchased from pet stores. Alternatively, branches can be collected from local hardwood trees (nonsappy trees) and baked in an oven at 300°F for 30 to 45 minutes before use. To prevent fecal contamination, avoid placing perches over food and water bowls.

An abrasive perch (there are many brands, one of which is the Nail and Beak Conditioning Perch, RJR Pet Supplies, Jacksonville, FL) in the cage may help to keep the nails rounded and prevent overgrowth of nails and beak. The perch should be placed where the bird will use it frequently and should be of a circumference that is spanned a maximum of 270° by the bird's toes. Sandpaper perch covers are contraindicated because they can cause plantar abrasions and predispose to foot problems, such as pododermatitis. Moreover, they do not fulfill their intended purpose, which is to keep nails worn down.

Toys

Birds are active, inquisitive animals and do best in a varied environment with toys. All toys should be designed specifically for birds and made of nontoxic substances without small openings or chains in which a bird could trap a foot or wing.

Location of Cage

The cage should be located in a well-ventilated area but not exposed to temperature extremes or direct airflow from an air conditioner. Exposure to natural light (unfiltered through glass) is beneficial, with time in direct sun (with access to shade) on warm days. Use of a Vitalite or other artificial ultraviolet light is a less ideal alternative. Birds should not be housed in the kitchen because of potential exposure to greasy cooking fumes, which can coat the feathers, and to toxic aerosols emitted from overheated polytetrafluoroethylene nonstick cooking pan coatings, such as Teflon.

Cage Sanitation

Poorly cleaned cages, perches, mirrors, food dishes, and water bowls may harbor pathogenic microorganisms. If food is left on the cage bottom, the bird may feed on contaminated or spoiled food and be exposed to opportunistic organisms.

The best cage substrates are nontoxic, easy to clean, and flat so that the bird's droppings can be easily monitored. Examples include butcher paper, newsprint, and paper towels. Substrates to avoid include wood chips and corn cob particles, which can harbor microorganisms and cause gastrointestinal obstruction if consumed.

VISUAL EXAMINATION

The Cage

If the owner brings the bird's cage, evaluate it for size and shape, perch placement, and sanitation. Are the perches and food and water cups clean? What substrate is on the cage bottom? Observe the bird's droppings for color, consistency, and volume of urine, urates, and feces.

The Bird

While speaking with the owner and reviewing the history, carefully observe the bird in its cage or carrier. Small birds may arrive in a shoe box; shine a light into the box while opening the box lid slightly. Observe the bird's general attitude and posture. Most birds are stressed in the examination room and appear alert as an adaptive mechanism. If the bird appears depressed in this setting, chances are good that it is quite ill.

Is it fluffed or do its wings droop? Is it hanging by its beak from the side of the cage? These are abnormal postures. The bird should be standing straight on a perch, bearing weight symmetrically on its legs, alert and watching you. If the bird is not symmetrically weight-bearing, note the way in which it holds its feet. With an injury or fracture of a pelvic limb, the bird will usually hold the foot in a relatively normal but non-weight-bearing posture. With conditions causing paresis or paralysis, such as renal or gonadal tumors in budgerigars (*Melopsittacus undulatus*), the bird will often rest the plantar aspect of the tarsometatarsus, rather than the foot, on the perch or cage bottom (Fig. 10–1).[2]

Birds usually develop a wing droop after bony or

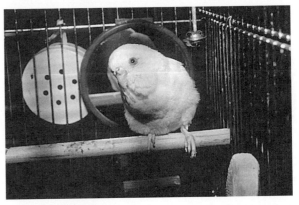

Figure 10–1

Budgerigar with left leg paresis as a result of a renal tumor impinging on the sciatic nerve. Note the way in which the bird is weight-bearing on the plantar tarsometatarsal region. This is unlike the clinical presentation in birds with fractures of the leg, which typically hold the foot in a normal position on the perch but without bearing weight on it.

soft tissue injuries to the wing. Note the way in which the bird holds the drooping wing. If a fracture is present, the position of the wing droop is often indicative of the bone involved. With a fracture at or distal to the middle of the radius and ulna, the primary wing feathers usually rest on the perch or ground. With a fracture between the midhumeral and midradius and ulnar regions, the wing droops but the primaries are typically off the perch or ground. With a fracture of the coracoid or shoulder joint, the wing usually droops and rotates so that the primaries are high over the dorsum.[3]

Are there any obvious physical abnormalities, such as a swelling in the region of the crop (Fig. 10–2) or pasted feathers around the head or vent? A swelling in the crop area could be a mass or, more likely, a full crop from delayed emptying. Clumping of head feathers, seen most commonly in budgerigars, usually represents regurgitated food or fluid that lands in the feathers when the bird shakes its head to clear its mouth, and then dries there. (The owner often does not realize that the bird has been regurgitating or vomiting.)

Is the bird's respiratory rate normal? Respirations should be barely perceptible. A tail bob with each respiration usually indicates lower airway disease; open-mouth breathing indicates severe dyspnea.

The appearance of the feathers reflects the bird's overall condition (Fig. 10–3). The feathers should be shiny and smooth and without frayed edges.

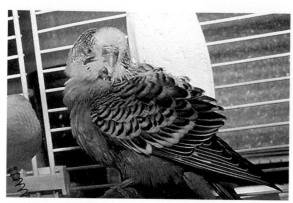

Figure 10–2

Four-year-old male budgerigar that was presented for inactivity and decreased appetite. Note half-closed eyes, fluffing of feathers, and large swelling in the crop region. This bird had severe crop stasis and regurgitation as a result of goiter. The bird responded well to in-hospital supportive care and parenteral iodine therapy.

The Droppings

Normal birds produce many droppings over the course of the day. Budgerigars (budgies) produce 25 to 50 droppings per day, whereas larger birds, such as Amazon parrots, produce 10 to 15 droppings per day. The avian gastrointestinal transit time is rapid, and some food items, particularly fruit, may pass through rapidly with minimal change in appearance. More than one owner has been alarmed by bright red or blue droppings, only to realize that the bird had just eaten beets or blueberries, for example.

The appearance of droppings varies between species and according to the diet. Birds, such as budgies, from arid climates tend to have small, dry droppings; fruit-eating birds, such as lories, tend to have wet, voluminous droppings. Any persistent change in the quantity, volume, or appearance of droppings is abnormal.

Normal avian droppings comprise three components—feces, urates, and urine—which are deposited into a common area in the cloaca and excreted simultaneously. The color of the feces depends on the diet; the urates are normally white; and the urine, if present or visible, is normally a clear liquid. In birds with diarrhea, the consistency of the feces is loose and the liquid portion of the droppings may increase. Anorexic birds have a reduced number of droppings with a small fecal por-

tion. Dehydrated birds have dry urates and scant to no urine. Always check the color of the urates. A pink to red or rust color of the urates usually indicates hemoglobinuria, seen most commonly with acute lead poisoning. With hepatic disease, the urates may be yellow or green. In Amazon parrots, lime green *urates* are seen most commonly with chlamydiosis, although this type of urates may be seen with other diseases that affect the liver or cause hepatic necrosis, such as salmonellosis, reovirus infection, Newcastle disease, Pacheco's disease, and bacterial septicemia. (Lime green *feces* with normal urates are not specific for any disease. A common mistake of avian clients and inexperienced clinicians is to link lime green feces with chlamydiosis.) Egg-laying female birds have less frequent but much larger droppings because of cloacal relaxation.

RESTRAINT

Approach to the Critically Ill Bird

Do not attempt to restrain birds that appear very weak or dyspneic; these birds can die from the

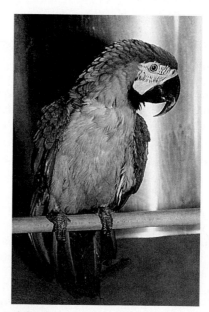

Figure 10–3

Blue and gold macaw with scruffy, ragged feathers. This bird's appearance improved dramatically with institution of daily baths (in this case by misting with warm water from a spray bottle), which stimulated the bird to preen. Other management changes included a larger cage and an improved diet.

stress of restraint. Inform the owner of the bird's fragile state and the available options for care. The ideal option is to admit the bird to the hospital and place it in a warm, humidified, oxygen-rich environment. Remove all perches and allow the bird to rest on a flat surface. Food and water should be made readily available except to birds with crop stasis or those that you anticipate anesthetizing soon. Preferred foods can be placed near the bird in a shallow cup or directly on the flat surface. Even anorexic birds may begin to eat and gain strength in such an environment.

With the bird in the hospital, you can do diagnostic testing and institute therapy in stages, allowing the bird to rest between periods of brief handling. Supportive care, such as vitamin and fluid therapy, is often indicated for these birds before diagnostic samples can be collected. A slow diagnostic approach is preferable to thorough sample collection that can result in the death of the bird.

Preparing for Restraint

The period of restraint should be as brief as possible to accomplish the necessary tasks. A trained assistant is invaluable and, for working with large birds, indispensable. The assistant should know not only how to hold the bird but also how to monitor it during restraint so that you can concentrate on the physical examination and collection of diagnostic samples. Monitoring should be continual throughout the period of handling, and the assistant should be allowed to concentrate on this task without distraction. Monitoring includes watching the bird's general demeanor, feeling its strength or lack thereof, and evaluating its respiratory rate. If it weakens or the respirations become slow or irregular, the bird should immediately be allowed to rest by placing it back in the carrier.

Before capturing the bird, develop a preliminary diagnostic and therapeutic plan and prepare your equipment accordingly. Lay out a mouth speculum and a lubricated cotton swab for examining the cloaca, for example. If the bird needs grooming, lay out the necessary equipment. If you plan to collect blood, prepare the syringe, alcohol cotton, and containers. If you plan to administer a medication, measure it out and place the syringe within reach.

Ear protection is suggested for all persons in the room when handling loud species, such as macaws. Headsets (Noisegard Hearing Protectors, Shoplyne, Cleveland, OH) are relatively inexpensive (about $15) and can be obtained at good hardware stores.

Capturing the Bird

Before capturing the bird, ascertain that the room is secure and that capture nets are available. Capture the bird out of its carrier or cage or, if necessary, from the table or floor. *Never* attempt to grab a bird from the owner's shoulder; this could result in a bad bite or injury as the bird grabs at its owner for safety. Dimming the lights often facilitates a quick capture.

The best equipment for capturing a psittacine or passerine bird is a clean towel. The towel hides your hand from the bird, giving you some protection and avoiding the bird's fright in seeing the hand advancing toward it. A paper towel is adequate for small birds, such as finches, budgerigars, cockatiels, and small conures. Larger birds are best captured with a clean cloth towel the size of a standard hand towel or bigger. Keep the hospital stocked with an abundant supply of inexpensive towels so they can be laundered after each use and replaced when torn. A towel can be ruined in a single session of restraining a large parrot.

Leather gloves can be used for handling raptors but are not appropriate for handling psittacine and passerine species. Gloves interfere with the mobility and agility of the handler, possibly resulting in an injury to the patient. Moreover, gloves cannot be properly disinfected between patients.

Certain birds, particularly Amazon parrots and macaws, will rapidly learn the meaning of a towel and will lie on their backs, making it difficult to catch their heads. Using a net to capture these birds and maneuver them so you can get them in a towel is often more rapid, safe, and humane than attempting to catch them with a towel. Tell the owner you are going to use a net and explain your reasoning. Skeptical owners can be convinced of the net's value when they see how it facilitates capture.

To take a small bird out of a shoebox, weighing tub, or other closed container, slide a paper towel under the lid so it covers the entire container as a second layer. In this way you can slip your hand between the paper towel and the lid and then catch the bird using the paper towel. If you try to slip your hand in without taking this precaution, the bird can escape through the opening next to your hand.

Psittacines

The first goal in capturing a psittacine bird is to restrain the head. Try to pin the head against a flat surface and work your hand around it dorsally so as to restrain it in your preferred way. Then restrain the wings against the body and lift the bird.

The most common mistake made by the inexperienced handler is to be too gentle and tentative. Birds tend to struggle more if lightly restrained than if firmly restrained and stretched. Hold the head with one hand, cupping the wings with that same hand, and hold the tarsometatarsal region with the opposite hand, placing the forefinger between the tarsometatarsi and applying enough stretch to fully extend the bird's neck and legs (Figs. 10–4 and 10–5). The key to good restraint is in stretching the bird. Do not apply any circumferential pressure to the bird's trunk; allow the sternum to lift with respirations. You can let the bird chew on the towel; this has a calming and distracting effect.

There are three common ways to hold the head—with the thumb and forefinger on either mandible; with a three-point hold using the thumb and third finger around the mandibles and the forefinger over the top of the head; and with the thumb and forefinger (medium-size to large birds) or fore-

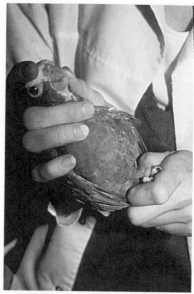

Figure 10–5

Psittacine restraint without a towel. Note the three-point hold on the head; this prevents the bird from turning its head. The bird's sternum is left unrestrained to facilitate respiration. If necessary, the feet can be pulled farther caudally to stretch the bird out.

finger and third finger (small birds) around the neck just under the mandibles. The last technique works well only if the bird's neck is extended. The three-point hold is useful for preventing side-to-side motion of the head, such as for an ophthalmic examination, but is difficult in large macaws.

Do not apply pressure on the bird's cheek. Macaws and African grey parrots (*Psittacus erithacus*), which have featherless skin on the cheeks, readily develop obvious bruising as a result of pressure.

Passerines

Dimming the lights is particularly helpful when trying to catch passerine birds, which often move more quickly than psittacines. The smallest passerines, especially finches and canaries, are held most securely with a bare hand after capture; you can transfer them out of the towel or catch them without a towel.

Restrain the bird's head by holding the neck between the forefinger and third finger rather than between the thumb and forefinger, which would leave a larger space from which escape is likely.

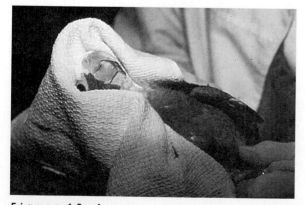

Figure 10–4

Psittacine restraint using a towel.

Cup the bird's body in the palm of your hand and stretch its neck gently by extending your fingers slightly. If necessary, stretch and restrain the legs as described above for psittacine birds.

Tame Birds

Most tame birds, unlike dogs and cats, do not allow a thorough physical examination as they stand unrestrained on the table. However, examination without capture and restraint is possible for some birds, such as pediatric patients and tame cockatoos. For these birds, touch and palpate them as though your examination were a petting session. Save potentially stressful portions, such as the oral and cloacal examinations, for last.

Sedation and Anesthesia

The physical examination can be performed in most birds without sedation or anesthesia. However, sedation may facilitate certain procedures while minimizing stress on the patient. Isoflurane administered by facemask is ideal for short procedures because it is relatively safe and provides rapid induction and recovery. If you anticipate using sedation or anesthesia soon, such as for obtaining radiographs, you can perform a more complete physical examination while the bird is anesthetized. This is a good time to do a complete oral examination. In larger birds, you can use a canine vaginal speculum to examine the cloaca.

Precautions

The process of examining avian patients carries a greater potential to cause physical harm than with dogs and cats. The most obvious danger is in overly stressing a bird with marginal reserves. Occasionally, apparently healthy birds suffer cardiac arrest and die during restraint; necropsy examination of these birds usually reveals previously asymptomatic pathology, such as cardiomyopathy. Other potential problems to avoid include injury to an extremity caught in a hole in the restraint towel and bruising of featherless facial skin (in macaws and African grey parrots).

WEIGHING THE BIRD

Weigh all birds at each examination. Having a record of weights is invaluable in assessing the avian patient's response to disease and to therapy. A current weight can be compared with previous weights. However, establishing whether an individual bird is at its appropriate weight is done by physical examination and palpation, not by comparison with published weight charts for the species. Birds, similar to humans, show great intraspecies variations in weight.

The use of metric weight scales is standard in avian practice. Hospital scales should be sensitive to 1- to 2-gram weight increments; less ideal but still useful are scales measuring in 5-gram increments. If possible, include two types of scales in the examination room—a perch scale for tame birds with clipped wings and a scale with a weighing tub for small, flighted, or untamed birds. Scales should tare to the weight of the weighing tub.

Tame birds can be weighed at any time during the examination on a perch scale or sitting in an open tub. Less tame birds can be weighed in a closed tub at the end of the physical examination. This allows you to prepare treatment or diagnostic equipment, if necessary, while the bird rests quietly in the tub.

PHYSICAL EXAMINATION

As described above, assess the bird's attitude, strength, respiratory rate and character, feather quality, and overall demeanor before beginning the hands-on physical examination. When the bird is physically restrained, rapidly assess its weight and hydration status. This gives a rough indication of its health and ability to withstand restraint. If the bird is dehydrated, thin, or obese, the period of restraint should be as short as possible.

Start a routine examination at the head and work back to the vent, examining the body in the following sequence: head and mouth, crop, pectoral muscles, lungs and heart (auscultation), abdomen, wings, dorsum and uropygial gland, legs, feet, and vent. As for other species, look at or touch every part of the body. Develop your own systematic routine.

Muscle Mass and Hydration Status

A bird in good body condition has rounded (convex), firm pectoral muscles with minimal subcutaneous adipose tissue. The appearance and feel of the pectoral muscle mass (breast muscles) can vary by species, age, and fitness level. Some of the cockatoos, such as lesser sulfur-crested cockatoos (*Cacatua sulphurea*), are normally quite slender and might be considered thin by the inexperienced clinician, especially if compared with a more muscular species, such as a double yellow-headed Amazon parrot (*Amazona ochrocephala oratrix*). Birds that fly are more muscular than those with clipped wings. Pediatric and geriatric patients may have relatively flabby, soft pectoral muscles.

If a bird is malnourished or loses weight, the pectoral muscles become smaller and the keel bone is prominent. The feet and legs may appear bony. Weight loss can be rapid, particularly in smaller birds, which can become cachexic in a matter of days.

Obesity is a common health problem in cage birds, particularly budgerigars and Amazon parrots. Obese birds develop large subcutaneous fat deposits that are most evident in the flanks and abdominal area. Budgerigars develop lipomas typically over the cranial sternum and crop region.

During the physical examination, be aware of the bird's demeanor and listen to its voice. Most birds resist restraint but become calmer with firm restraint. Most psittacines vocalize throughout the examination; however, excessive inappropriate vocalizing can indicate a neurologic problem. A high-pitched squeaky voice in a budgerigar may indicate goiter or another mass pressing on the syrinx.

Dehydration is assessed by examining the oral mucosa and tenting the skin over the feet or lifting the upper eyelid. The oral mucosa should be moist and pink, and the eyes should be moist. In severely dehydrated birds, the mucosa and eyes appear dry, the foot skin remains elevated when tented, the eyes appear sunken, and the upper eyelid does not fall back into place when lifted (Fig. 10–6).

Assess vascular perfusion by compressing the medial ulnar vein and then releasing it and watching the return of blood; slow refill and decreased turgor of the vein indicate dehydration or shock. To screen for anemia, check the color of the conjunctiva or the oral or cloacal mucosa; the color

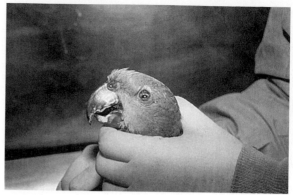

F i g u r e 1 0 – 6

Severely dehydrated Amazon parrot. Note the sunken eye and the lifted upper eyelid, which does not fall back into place as it would normally.

should be pink (although some psittacine species have black-pigmented oral mucosa).

Head and Neck

The structures of the head, including the eyes, ears, nares, cere, and beak, should be bilaterally symmetric. There should be no discharge from the eyes, nares, or choana. The ear canals should be open and clean; examine them with a small otoscope cone. The beak should be the proper length, firm, and not excessively flaky.

To examine the oral cavity of psittacines, hold a penlight near the beak; most birds try to bite the penlight, thereby giving you a good view of the mouth (Fig. 10–7). For uncooperative patients or to closely examine oral structures, use an oral speculum or loop strips of gauze on the upper and lower beaks and pull the mouth open gently. For passerine birds, hook a penlight on the tip of the upper beak and gently pry the beak open by pushing up with the penlight. The oral mucous membranes should be pink and moist; the tongue mucosa appears dry. Many species of bird have pigmented oral mucous membranes; however, these birds may have small unpigmented patches of oral mucosa where you can assess membrane color. The choanal slit in the dorsal soft palate should be bilaterally symmetric and bordered with straight, slender papillae.

Asymmetry in the structures of the head is usually

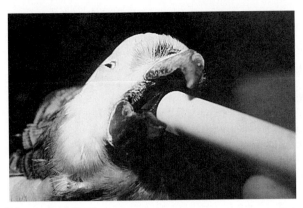

Figure 10-7

A preliminary oral examination is performed by allowing the bird to bite at a penlight.

An appreciation for the normal, species-specific appearance of the beak comes from experience. The beak should wear properly without need for trimming in a healthy bird on a good diet and offered toys and hardwoods to chew. A slightly overgrown or flaking beak is usually indicative of poor management or malnutrition, whereas gross overgrowth is usually indicative of underlying disease. An asymmetric beak is often the result of an injury or infection that damaged the germinative tissue. Sometimes the cause for beak overgrowth in pet birds is not identifiable, and periodic grooming may be necessary.

The beak of a normal, mature cockatoo has a dull, grayish appearance from the powder produced by the powder down and deposited on the beak during preening (Fig. 10–9). Psittacine beak and feather disease (PBFD) often affects the powder down feathers; therefore, the first obvious clinical sign in an infected cockatoo may be a black, shiny beak resulting from lack of powder. Longitudinal grooves in the beak originating at the nares may be the result of damage to germinative tissue from a past episode of severe rhinitis or sinusitis.

indicative of a problem. Birds with sinusitis may show periocular swelling in addition to hyperemia of the ear canals. Discharge from the nares or from the choanal slit is seen with rhinitis or sinusitis. A bad odor from the mouth is abnormal and could be associated with oral, pharyngeal, or nasal infection. Blunting and shortening of the choanal papillae are seen most commonly with hypovitaminosis A but can occur also with bacterial stomatitis. White oral plaques are seen with several different infectious and nutritional diseases (see Chapter 26). Keratin-filled oral swellings may result from hypovitaminosis A (Fig. 10–8). Oral papillomas are seen occasionally, particularly in macaws.

In budgies, an overgrown, asymmetric beak with exuberant, honeycomb-like tissue around the cere, eyes, and face is pathognomonic for *Knemidokoptes* mite infection. Brown hypertrophy of the cere is common in older, female budgies; the cause is unknown.

After examining the head, palpate the neck and crop region (Fig. 10–10). Any ingesta in the crop should be soft and fluctuant; individual seeds may

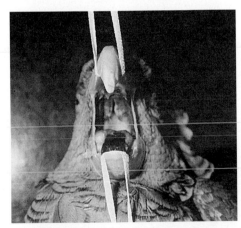

Figure 10-8

Amazon parrot with severe hypovitaminosis A. Note large keratinaceous swellings at the base of the tongue.

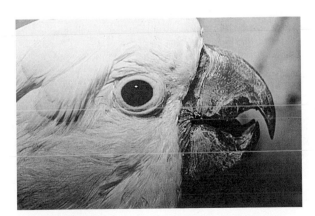

Figure 10-9

Normal powder on the beak of this cockatoo. Powder originates from the powder down and settles on the beak during preening.

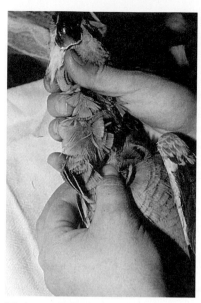

Figure 10–10

Palpation of the crop region.

be palpable. Distension of the crop by fluid or ingesta is usually abnormal and indicative of a crop-emptying problem, which is most common in pediatric patients and budgies with goiter. In a crop containing food, waves of peristalsis should be visible at the rate of one to two per minute.[4] A firm mass in the crop region could be a crop foreign body, ingluviolith, inspissated food within the crop, or, alternatively, an extraluminal mass in the subcutis. Transillumination of the crop and esophageal region may help in identifying abnormalities and determining the thickness of the crop wall, which should be very thin and translucent.

Trunk

Palpate the pectoral muscles to evaluate them for symmetry, firmness, and size. The keel bone (sternum) should be straight. Nutritional deficiencies can result in an S-shaped sternum; this is seen most commonly in pigeons and doves.

A loud, sharp clicking noise may be evident in conjunction with sternal movement, particularly in large psittacines. Although alarming, this noise is not abnormal and has been attributed to subluxation of a joint.[5]

Perform auscultation of the heart for rate and rhythm. The lower respiratory system is best assessed by close observation of the rate and character of respirations before, during, and after the restraint period. A pumping appearance to the respirations at rest before restraint is abnormal, as is an accompanying tail bob. Respiratory auscultation is less informative than in mammals because of differences in avian respiratory anatomy. Fluid noises and wheezing generally indicate severe respiratory disease.

Palpate the abdomen by placing a thumb and a forefinger on either side (Fig. 10–11). Abdominal palpation in birds is not as rewarding as for other species, but eggs and other masses may be palpable. Gently try to feel for the caudal border of the liver, which should be just under the sternum and, therefore, not normally palpable. In small passerine birds, wet down the feathers below the sternum with an alcohol swab to check for an enlarged liver visible through the skin.

The abdominal space in psittacines is normally very narrow (narrower than a finger width in budgerigars). Therefore, a widening of the distance between the caudal tip of the sternum and the pubis (sternopubic width) is often indicative of a space-occupying abdominal mass. In budgerigars with re-

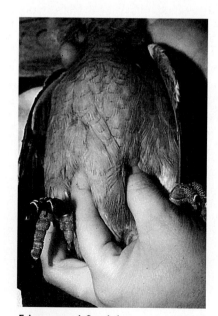

Figure 10–11

Abdominal palpation.

nal or gonadal tumors, the sternopubic width is frequently enlarged, and the gizzard may be pushed ventrally and caudally so that it is readily palpable and easily mistaken for a mass. You may be able to palpate the tumor with deep, dorsal palpation.

To examine the wings, pull each one out of the towel individually and palpate and examine it thoroughly. Particularly in canaries and cockatiels, check for feather cysts, which occur commonly on the wings. Palpate the dorsum of the bird under the towel. Examine the uropygial gland in species that have one. It should be bilaterally symmetric and is usually a yellow color. Infections, duct obstruction, and benign and malignant tumors of the uropygial gland are not uncommon, particularly in budgies.

Feathers and Skin

Throughout the course of the examination, inspect the feathers and the skin over the body and on the extremities. The feathers should be smooth and shiny; the skin should be soft, well hydrated, and translucent. Feathers grow in tracts called pterylae and normally cover the areas of unfeathered skin, which are called apteria. Occasionally, a client glimpses a (normal) featherless area and brings the bird to you for evaluation.

Unpreened, scruffy feathering can result from many different diseases; however, the most common causes in otherwise "healthy" birds are poor nutrition and insufficient bathing. Certain physical conditions, such as obesity and neurologic problems, may prevent birds from preening specific areas. Other birds may preen poorly and, at the same time, chew on their covert or flight feathers. (This is seen most commonly in some cockatoos, which shred the ends of their flight feathers.)

Legs and Feet

Palpate the muscle mass of the legs and examine the feet for symmetry. A neurologic problem can result in muscle wasting. If you suspect a fracture but have difficulty with palpation, part the feathers with an alcohol swab; bruising often marks the site of an underlying fracture. The bruises turn from burgundy-purple color to green after 2 or 3 days. Swelling of the legs or toes is abnormal and may

indicate infection or neoplasia. The grasping ability of the toes should be strong and bilaterally symmetrical.

Examine the skin of the feet. The scales should be smooth and not dry or flaky. Excessive flakiness can indicate a nutritional problem. *Knemidokoptes* infection in budgies causes honeycomb-like scaliness of the feet, as on the face, and abnormal growth of the nails. In canaries, *Knemidokoptes* infestation causes a common syndrome known as tassel foot, characterized by long, scale-like lesions on the feet and corkscrew nail growth. Erythema on the plantar aspect of the foot or toes is abnormal and is seen in birds with hypovitaminosis A or in obese birds, particularly those on inappropriate perches.

Nail overgrowth is not uncommon in the captive setting, particularly in birds restricted to their cages. This condition is often seen in conjunction with beak overgrowth.

Cloaca

The feathers around the cloaca should be clean and well preened. Pasting of the droppings around the cloaca is abnormal and is usually the result of diarrhea in conjunction with weakness or obesity preventing the bird from preening the area. Occasionally a bird has such severe matting of the feathers around the vent that the droppings can no longer pass. When the area is cleaned, the bird often excretes a large, malodorous dropping that had accumulated within the cloaca.

A cloacal papilloma check is a routine part of the physical examination for susceptible species, particularly for birds in breeding programs and those in multibird households. Susceptible species include most of the South American psittacines, particularly hawk-headed parrots (*Deroptyus accipitrinus*), Amazon parrots (*Amazona* species), and macaws of the *Ara* genus. Cloacal papillomatosis is uncommon in conures and hyacinth macaws (*Anodorbynchus hyacinthinus*). To check for cloacal papillomas, use a cotton-tipped swab that has been well lubricated with a sterile water-soluble jelly, such as K-Y lubricating jelly (Johnson & Johnson Consumer Products, New Brunswick, NJ). Gently insert the swab into the cloaca and then withdraw it partially to evert the mucosa, section by section,

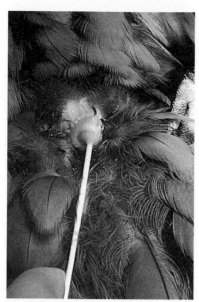

Figure 10-12

Examination of the cloacal mucosa using a cotton-tipped swab (see text for technique). Note the normal, glistening appearance of the mucosa and the straight smooth edge of the mucosal fold that is seen at the farthest distance from the cloaca.

for the full 360° (Fig. 10–12). The cloacal mucosa should be smooth and glistening; some species have linear mucosal ridges running parallel to the cloacal wall. An irregular mucosal surface or an obvious mass could represent papillomatous tissue. This abnormal tissue temporarily turns white when 5% acetic acid (white vinegar) is applied. Warn the owner that there may be a small amount of fresh blood on the first one or two droppings after the cloacal examination.

Pediatric and Geriatric Patients

The basic principles of avian physical examination apply to very young and very old birds also. Handle pediatric patients carefully to avoid regurgitation because they often have food in the crop. Babies should have a strong feeding response (pumping motion of the head) when you touch them around the beak. They should be well hydrated with pink, soft skin. They tend to be very bottom-heavy with a large, rounded abdomen.

Geriatric patients may show muscle wasting, joint stiffness, poor feather condition, and loss of skin tone and elasticity. Macaws over 40 years of age may develop cataracts and laterally rotated deformities of the carpi that resemble "helicopter wing" of poultry.[6]

Stamina and Length of Recovery

Most birds become stressed and tachypneic during the course of the physical examination. Amazon parrots often struggle, trying to flap their wings, the entire time. Macaws may also struggle continuously or may be still and then suddenly flap their wings at an unpredictable and inopportune moment.

Assess the bird's stamina during the restraint period and the length of the recovery period from handling. Malnourished and ill birds tire rapidly and recover slowly. Obese birds also tire rapidly because intra-abdominal adipose tissue interferes with respiration. Healthy birds, even those that become frenzied with handling, recover rapidly when allowed to rest. However, in hot, humid weather, even normal birds tire rapidly and recover more slowly. Normal canaries may lie on their sides for 30 to 60 seconds after being handled (warn the owner of this). With these considerations kept in mind, reduced stamina and prolonged rate of recovery can be early indicators of a health problem.

Determination of Age

Once birds reach adulthood, there is no reliable means of determining age. Some of the physical changes seen in geriatric macaws are similar to those seen in malnourished birds. Therefore, to establish at least the minimal age of an avian patient, record the bird's origins and ownership history. For example, birds imported as adults are at least 1 or 2 years older than the length of time they have been in the country.

Immature birds have a distinctive appearance and behavior that are recognized easily with experience. Their behavior patterns tend to be subordinate. The beaks of young birds are smooth and devoid of flaking. Budgerigars have horizontal black barring of the forehead and head feathers until a few months of age. Young macaws have dark gray to black irises that gradually lighten to white and then turn into the adult yellow color. Young African grey parrots have dark gray irises that gradually lighten to the adult white color.

GROOMING

Grooming of avian patients is frequently necessary and includes wing, beak, and nail trims. Many avian clinics offer grooming services separate from a regular office visit. Although these visits may be more expensive than a similar visit to a pet store, grooming at a clinic offers the advantage of experienced handlers and attention to good sanitation and the bird's health. All grooming equipment should be disinfected between birds.

After a nail or a wing trim, particularly if both are done simultaneously, birds often have an adjustment period during which they may slip off the perch or appear clumsy. Always warn the client of this.

Wing Trims

Many avian veterinarians recommend that all pet birds have their wings clipped to decrease the potential for accidents and escapes. Clipping the wings may also enhance a bird's pet quality by making it easier to tame and handle. Wing clipping is a temporary measure and must be repeated as the bird molts, dropping the cut feathers, and new flight feathers emerge. Always educate clients about this fact and never guarantee a wing clip; a clipped bird could theoretically ride an updraft of wind and escape. No bird, even with wings clipped, should be left loose out of doors for this reason.

There are several techniques of wing-trimming; however, some general principles apply to all techniques. The goal of a wing trim is to render the bird unable to fly but still able to glide slowly to the ground without falling. Clip both wings symmetrically so that the bird can keep its balance. Avoid clipping the wings too short! If a wing clip is too severe, the bird will fall and may sustain an injury. Young African grey parrots, in particular, seem prone to these injuries and, as a result, present with chronic, nonhealing sternal wounds with accompanying osteomyelitis.

The ideal wing clip varies according to species, age group, and individual physical build. Young birds and obese birds tend to be poor fliers and should have minimal wing clips. Amazons usually do best with intermediate wing clips. Macaws, cockatoos, and cockatiels tend to be light-bodied and often require the shortest wing clips.

The author clips the primaries in an arc such that the outermost primaries are cut the shortest and the inner primaries are left progressively longer until reaching the length of the secondary flight feathers (Fig. 10–13). This gives a cosmetic result when the bird stretches its wings. The severity of the clip is adjusted by the degree of arc and the length of the outermost primaries. Another cosmetically effective technique is to cut the primaries just shorter than the covert feathers so that the cut end is hidden from view. With this technique, the severity of the cut is adjusted by how many primaries are trimmed. Cut each feather individually and avoid blood feathers, which, when cut, usually continue to bleed until removed completely at the follicle.

Some cockatoos chew persistently on the cut ends of clipped flight feathers. This habit may stop when new feathers come in if the bird is allowed to remain full-flighted.

Beak Trims

For some birds, one or two beak trims may be necessary to correct a growth abnormality caused by *Knemidokoptes* or trauma, after which the beak may wear normally. For other birds, long-term, regular beak trimming or periodic filing to remove excessive flaking is necessary. (Perform complete health and nutritional evaluation of these birds.) A slightly abrasive perch in the cage for beak rubbing and hardwoods to chew may help the beak to wear normally (see the section on caging in this chapter).

Restraint for beak trimming is routine, with the bird wrapped in a towel. The clinician can steady the bird's head with one hand while trimming the beak with the other (Fig. 10–14). Beak trimming should be done carefully by slowly sculpting the beak back to its regular shape. Leaving the beak tip slightly long is preferable to shortening it excessively and causing it to bleed. The blood supply tends to be more distal than normal in beaks that have been chronically overgrown. If the beak bleeds, use an ophthalmic cautery unit to stop the bleeding and inform the owner that the beak will

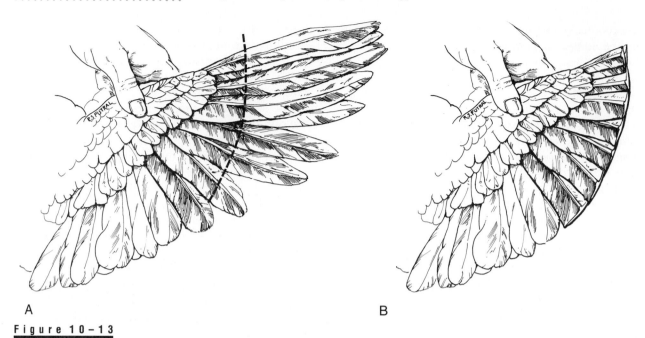

A   B

Figure 10–13

(*A* and *B*) One technique for trimming the wings whereby the primary wing feathers are cut in gradually increasing lengths so as to merge with the secondaries.

be painful for the next day or two. If using silver nitrate cautery, hold the beak firmly closed to prevent the bird from biting the nitrate stick or touching it with its tongue. If necessary, keep the bird in the hospital for a short time to observe it for recurrence of bleeding.

This author uses all manual tools for beak trims—folding fingernail and toenail manicure clippers, side-cutting wire cutters, and nail files of vari-

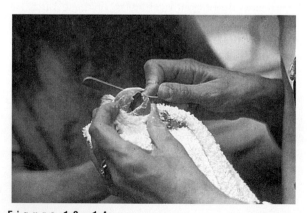

Figure 10–14

Filing the beak of an Amazon parrot using a nail file. Note restraint of the bird's head by the groomer.

ous textures ranging from rough to fine. In small birds, the human nail clippers work well and give good control for shaping the beak. A fine nail file can be used to finish the job if necessary. In large birds, the appropriately sized wire cutter or toenail clipper is used to clip the beak tip before first using a coarse grade and then progressively finer grades of nail files to smooth the beak. A Dremel drill with grinding stone can also be used to shape the beak, but it requires precise control to prevent overgrinding. The noise of the drill may be stressful to some birds.

Nail Trims

Nail overgrowth is very common in the captive setting, and periodic nail trims are necessary in many birds. It may be possible to keep the nails worn down by encouraging the bird to walk on a rough surface or by placing one slightly abrasive perch in the cage (see the section on caging). As previously discussed, sandpaper perch covers are contraindicated.

The mechanics of nail trimming in psittacines and passerines are relatively straightforward once you know the normal nail length. In smaller birds, the blood supply is often visible in the nail and helps in assessing proper nail length. Clip the nail just beyond where the blood supply stops. Most medium-size to larger birds have pigmented nails; for these birds, an appreciation of normal nail length comes with experience. Always have some type of cautery, such as silver nitrate sticks or ferric subsulfate powder, available within reach before you start to trim nails.

There are several methods of nail clipping. The author uses the folding human nail clippers for small birds through the size of a small conure. For large birds, a wire-loop type of ophthalmic cautery is useful because it cauterizes while cutting. Both disposable (Storz Sure-Temp Surgical Cautery, Storz Instrument Co., St. Louis, MO) and electric ophthalmic cauteries (MDS Inc., St. Petersburg, FL) are available (Table 10–1). Loop the wire around the place where you want to cut the nail, press the button to heat the cautery wire, and slowly pull the hot wire through the nail. Other nail trimming tools include sharp cat nail clippers, Resco nail clippers, and a Dremel drill to grind the nails.

References

1. Harris JM: Avian client compliance. Semin Avian Exotic Pet Med 2:2–6, 1993.
2. Murray MJ: The art of observation in caged bird medicine. In Proc 99th Annual Cal Vet Med Assoc, San Francisco, CA, pp 317–337, 1987.
3. Coles BH: Clinical examination. In Avian Medicine and Surgery. Boston, Blackwell Scientific Publications, 1985, pp 1–18.
4. Joyner KL: Psittacine pediatric diagnostics. Semin Avian Exotic Pet Med 1:11–21, 1992.
5. Harrison GJ, Ritchie BW: Making distinctions in the physical examination. In Ritchie BW, Harrison GJ, Harrison LR (eds): Avian Medicine: Principles and Application. Lake Worth, FL, Wingers Publishing, 1994, pp 144–175.
6. Clubb SL, Karpinski L: Aging in macaws. J Assoc Avian Vet 7:31–33, 1993.

Alan M. Fudge

11

Avian Clinical Pathology— Hematology and Chemistry

Laboratory diagnostics are invaluable tools for the clinician. Blood testing provides important information during a post-purchase or routine health examination, assessment of a sick bird, or reassessment of a patient after treatment.

AVIAN HEMATOLOGY

Leukocytes

Leukocyte Counts

Until recently, tabulation of avian leukocytes by automated methods was not possible because of the presence of nucleated erythrocytes and thrombocytes. Variability in leukocyte counts can occur as a result of assay method, sample collection and preparation, and shipping parameters such as time and temperature. Manual methods of counting avian leukocytes are commonly used. The direct manual hematocytometer method involves dilution of the blood sample with Natt and Herrick's solution. This solution differentially stains cell types so that they can be counted. The indirect manual hematocytometer method involves diluting the blood sample with phloxine (Unopette 5877, Becton-Dickinson), which stains only heterophils and eosinophils. Total leukocyte count is calculated from the differential count by a mathematical formula (see Appendix I). The indirect estimate of total leukocyte count from a blood film involves counting all leukocytes in several high-power microscopic fields and then multiplying the total by a specific factor (see Appendix I). This method relies on a high-quality, uniform blood smear. Calculations assume a constant erythrocyte-to-leukocyte ratio, requiring a proportional adjustment with out-of-range pack cell volume measurements.[1-3]

The hematocytometer methods, when done under controlled conditions (good technique, whole blood tested <12 hours after collection) probably provide the most reproducible results. Estimate of the leukocyte count from a blood film provides the best results when the smear is uniform, made with a 22- × 22–mm coverslip resulting in a monolayer of cells, and exhibits minimal presence of ruptured or "smudge" cells. In a commercial laboratory setting, the practitioner can optimize results by paying particular attention to sampling, handling, and shipping requirements.

Until recently, automated analysis of avian blood was limited to total erythrocyte counts by impedance measurement. Impedance measurement instrumentation precluded total and differential avian leukocyte tabulation because of interference of nucleated erythrocytes.

Laser flow cytometric commercial instrumentation is now available (Cell-Dyn 3500, Abbott Laboratories, Abbott Park, IL). A laser beam is focused at a 90° angle by a laminar flow stream of cells. Photodetectors measure laser light scatter at four angular intervals, which vary in cell size, complexity (nuclear to cytoplasm ratio), granularity, and nuclear lobularity.

Cell-Dyn software tabulates a total optical leukocyte count and a five-part leukocyte differential count by algorithm. Separate subsystems also tabulate erythrocyte, thrombocyte, and leukocyte counts by a cell-lysing impedance measurement of cell nuclei, and hemoglobin measurement by the cyanomethemoglobin assay.

By mid-1995, this author implemented laser flow cytometric technology for hematologic analysis of psittacines, passerines, waterfowl, and ratites. The presence of prominent thrombocytes in some species necessitates modifications in the veterinary software to differentiate these cells from lymphocytes. Early observations include slightly higher mean monocyte counts in normal patients. The phenomenon is commonly observed in automated human hemograms because of the tendency to undercount monocytes on a blood film. Sodium citrate appears to be the anticoagulant of choice when analyzing avian samples.

Leukocytosis

Leukocytosis occurs in birds as a result of disease or "stress." Stress leukocytosis occurs in a variety of avian species, including macaws, cockatoos,[4] African grey parrots, and ratites. The avian spleen does not appear to be the source of blood pooling.[5] Clinical observations indicate that leukocyte counts can increase markedly in excited birds compared with samples taken when the patient is "at rest."[4] "Stress hemograms" can also be observed in birds that have been recently treated with corticosteroids.[4, 6, 7]

Juvenile birds demonstrate a great variability in total leukocyte counts until 4 to 6 months of age. Elevated counts are common and must be interpreted with caution, because the bird may be normal.[8–12] The clinician should always carefully review the differential count and cell morphology to determine if illness seems likely. In the author's experience, young birds residing in pet stores before sale to the public tend to have higher-than-normal leukocyte counts in the absence of documentable disease. This may be the "stress hemogram" effect.[4, 6]

Disease-induced leukocytosis in birds occurs mostly as a result of infection. Degenerative and neoplastic disorders can inconsistently produce moderate elevations in the total leukocyte counts.

The clinician cannot easily differentiate diseases based solely on leukocytosis, but certain trends emerge. Mild leukocytosis correlates with bacterial, fungal, and chlamydial infections. Moderate elevations

can be caused by yolk peritonitis, granulomatous disease, and some phases of septicemia.[1, 2, 4, 13, 14]

Very high leukocyte counts (over 60,000 cells/μl) can occur with active chlamydiosis (especially in macaws), aspergillosis, or tuberculosis. The largest range of the total leukocyte count varies with the species. Leukocyte counts rarely exceed 20,000 cells/μl in budgerigars, 30,000 cells/μl in cockatiels, and 80,000 cells/μl in Amazon parrots. Leukocyte counts can exceed 150,000 cells/μl in macaws.[4, 7, 13] Leukemia must be included in the differential diagnosis of very high leukocyte counts. Although the actual occurrence is rare, this cannot be ruled out without repeated morphologic examination of peripheral and bone marrow elements.[1]

Leukopenia

Leukopenia must be interpreted in conjunction with knowledge of typical reference ranges for the species examined. Smaller birds tend to have lower normal leukocyte counts. In any species, a total leukocyte count less than 3000 cells/μl is considered abnormally low.

The primary diagnostic differential of avian leukopenia is sample artifact. Whole blood that clots before placement in anticoagulant yields reduced counts. Lysis of leukocytes before analysis because of excessive shipping and storage times can result in pseudoleukopenia. Poor quality blood films often display a high percentage of ruptured leukocytes or "smudge cells," which artifactually indicate a leukopenia when slide assessment is used to quantitate leukocytes.[6, 7]

True leukopenia usually stems from overwhelming bacterial infection, severe viral disease, or occasionally, toxic substances.[2, 4, 7, 15] In bacterial sepsis, a degenerative left shift becomes a heteropenia; the few cells that are seen are usually lymphocytes. Depending on the chronicity of the sepsis, this leukopenia may be accompanied by nonregenerative anemia. A feature of bacterial leukopenia is the presence of intracellular bacteria, which can be seen in the cytoplasm of heterophils or monocytes.[1] Classic presentations include cat-bite septicemia (*Pasteurella* species),[1, 15] sepsis from an abscess focus (*Staphylococcus* species, *Pseudomonas* species, *Salmonella* species, coliforms), and sepsis secondary to apparent viral immunosuppression. The prognosis for recovery is poor, even with aggressive intravenous antimicrobial therapy.

Viral leukopenia may appear similar, except that intracellular bacteria are absent. Very low leukocyte counts can be seen in neonatal and pediatric psittacine circovirus (psittacine beak and feather disease [PBFD]) infection. This is characterized by the presence of only a few lymphocytes seen in a blood film and accompanied by severe nonregenerative anemia.* Leukopenia may be present with psittacine herpesvirus (Pacheco's disease), although acute death is most typical of this disease, and ante mortem blood samples are rarely submitted. Birds with psittacine polyomavirus variably show leukopenia or leukocytosis. Psittacine viral serositis, a syndrome of unproven etiology, is not typically associated with leukopenia. Proventricular dilation syndrome (PDS, macaw wasting disease) is believed to be viral in origin, but a causative agent has not been confirmed. PDS does not usually produce leukopenia.

Normal Counts

A normal leukocyte count can occur in the disease-compromised bird. Chronic, low-grade infection can result in a normalizing of the leukocyte count.[4] Birds with degenerative disease or a neoplastic disorder may have a normal leukocyte count. The clinician should assess changes in the leukocyte morphology and the differential count when interpreting a normal leukocyte count in a sick bird.[1, 7]

Leukocyte Differential and Morphology

Granulocytes

The heterophil (see Color Fig. 11–1) is the most frequently observed leukocyte in an avian hemogram. Some cytochemical differences exist, but the heterophil most closely resembles the mammalian neutrophil in function.

Absolute heterophilia often is the primary contributor to leukocytosis. "Stress" heterophilia occurs for the same reasons as "stress" leukocytosis. The

*Fudge AM, unpublished data.

veterinarian can expect to see heterophilia in acute inflammatory and infectious processes, including chlamydial, bacterial, and fungal infections.[1, 2, 4, 13]

Relative heteropenia may be a normal finding in species with lower heterophil/lymphocyte ratios, such as Amazon parrots and canaries. Artifactual heteropenia can follow poor blood smear techniques, resulting in smudge cells. Differential diagnosis for absolute heteropenia includes bacterial sepsis and severe viral disease. In bacterial sepsis, immature heterophils with toxic and degenerative changes may be seen. The presence of intracellular bacteria indicates bacterial sepsis. Extracellular bacteria may be artifactual. In viral disease, the typical hemogram shows the virtual absence of heterophils, with lymphocytes predominating in number.[1, 2, 4, 13]

Heterophil morphology is important when evaluating the hemogram. A moderate amount of variability occurs in color tones, depending on the staining protocol used. Thus, morphologic changes are not universally agreed upon. Artifactual cytologic damage occurs commonly, mainly the result of poor technique, and is characterized by free nuclei, ruptured cells, and "smudges" (see Color Fig. 11–2). Toxic changes, however, are common in deteriorating infectious disease, particularly bacterial, fungal, or chlamydial infections. These cellular differences can include basophilic cytoplasmic inclusions, nuclear hypersegmentation, and cytoplasmic vacuolization (see Color Fig. 11–3). Toxic heterophils can be the only abnormal hematologic finding, but they are very significant clinically.[7] Granulocytic leukemia occurs in birds, although recognition can be difficult and may require bone marrow cytology and special stains for definitive diagnosis.

Immature heterophils occasionally occur in peripheral blood.[4, 7, 13] Bands and mesomyelocytes usually imply a worsening bacterial infection and indicate guarded prognosis.

Eosinophils

Eosinophils (see Color Fig. 11–4) are uncommon in the hemogram of many avian species and common in others. This cell can be difficult to differentiate from other granulocytes. Eosinophils are distinguished by their round shape, distinct nuclear/cytoplasmic contrast, and uniform cytoplasmic color (see Color Figs. 11–5 and 11–6). Granule shape and color vary greatly. The clinician should question an avian hemogram showing a high eosinophil count, because an inexperienced technician can easily mistake the pinkish heterophil for the avian eosinophil. The function of the avian eosinophil is poorly understood, but clinical observations can provide guidelines.[13, 16–18]

Eosinophilia is typically a relative change that reflects an increase in the percentage but not necessarily the absolute number of circulating eosinophils. Eosinophilia can be observed in a variety of alimentary tract parasitisms including giardiasis, ascaridiasis, and cestodiasis, but is not a consistent finding.[4] Suspected allergic, nonparasitic conditions such as allergic dermatitis or respiratory hypersensitivity may be accompanied by highly suggestive histopathologic changes, but are not associated with peripheral eosinophilia. Tissue sporozoa (Apicocomplexa including *Atoxoplasma, Toxoplasma, Sarcocystis*) and malarial forms (*Plasmodium, Hemoproteus*) are not associated with eosinophilia. Birds with resolving tissue damage (trauma, organ damage) can sometimes show increases in peripheral eosinophils.[4] The mechanism for this is unknown. Passerine birds with air sac mites (*Sternostoma*) variably present with eosinophilia. It is not known whether this is an allergic or "tissue damage" response.

Eosinopenia is not well documented in birds. In normal birds, peripheral eosinophils are rare. This is particularly true in New World psittacines. Abnormal eosinophil morphology is not generally recognized.

Basophils

Basophils (see Color Fig. 11–7) are uncommon in avian peripheral blood. Commonly, avian basophils resemble their mammalian counterparts,[1, 16, 17] but variability in appearance does occur among avian species. Basophils must be differentiated from toxic heterophils, which often have large amounts of variably sized basophilic cytoplasmic inclusions.

Basophilia is observed in birds with respiratory infections or resolving tissue damage.[4, 7, 13] Baso-

philia is common with active chlamydial infections, particularly in budgerigars and Amazon parrots.

Basopenia is not well documented, but many normal avian hemograms show no basophils. Abnormal morphology is limited to degranulation; the clinical significance is unknown. It is not clear how to determine degranulation from preparation and staining artifacts.

Mononuclear Cells

Lymphocytes. These occur at a higher frequency than all other leukocytes, except heterophils (see Color Fig. 11–8).[13] Some avian species are "lymphocytic," including Amazon parrots and passerine birds.[1, 4] Although there are two to three unique populations of lymphocytes based on size differences, these groups are not differentiated by the clinical laboratory.[1, 16]

Lymphocytosis is not common. An apparent relative lymphocytosis is normal for some avian species with a low heterophil/lymphocyte ratio, such as Amazon parrots and canaries. Absolute lymphocytosis may indicate lymphocytic leukemia, particularly if the total count is very high and the morphologic changes are also suggestive. In some stages of viral and chlamydial infections, absolute lymphocytosis may occur.

A relative lymphopenia appears to occur with marked heterophilia.[13] In fact, the heterophils are present in such large numbers that the relative lymphocyte count appears low. Absolute lymphopenia can occur in association with the pancytopenia observed in terminal viral infections, such as in a juvenile African grey parrot infected with circovirus.

Lymphocytes can appear reactive. Although not standardized, reactive changes include cytoplasmic blobbing and vacuolization, nuclear changes, and deep blue cytoplasm.[7] Marked reactive changes are usually associated with severe viral infections. Reactivity may also be associated with chlamydial infections and blood parasites.

Monocytes. These are rarely seen in avian peripheral blood smears (see Color Fig. 11–9). The actual incidence of monocytes in avian blood remains undetermined and will require standardized cytochemical methods to resolve.

Relative or absolute monocytosis is a hallmark of

chronic infection. In birds, this can indicate chlamydial, mycobacterial, fungal, granulomatous, or organ-reactive bacterial infections.[1, 4, 7, 16] In budgerigars, a relative monocytosis and basophilia may be the only abnormal hematologic result, and it is suggestive of chlamydiosis. In birds with aspergillosis or tuberculosis, the hemogram may be similar and includes leukocytosis and monocytosis.[4, 7] The stage of infection and host response in birds infected with *Aspergillus* species or *Mycobacterium* species may result in little or no hematologic changes.

Monocytopenia is not documented, but a low or zero monocyte count is normal for most species. Morphologic changes can include the presence of intracellular bacteria in septicemic birds. Monocytes can appear macrophagic in some severe chronic infections.

Leukocyte Parasites

Leucocytozoon species (see Fig. 6, Chapter 21) has been reported in a wide variety of birds including wild turkeys, waterfowl, and birds of prey.[19] Although these parasites can be quite numerous in the blood and destructive to the host cell, many investigators are undecided whether this organism causes disease.[1]

Atoxoplasma species is occasionally seen in the cytoplasm peripheral to mononuclear leukocytes, but is best diagnosed by organ (lung, liver, spleen) impression smears or zinc sulfate fecal flotation.[1, 20] High morbidity and mortality can occur in passerines, particularly canaries and mynahs.[21]

Thrombocytes

Thrombocyte counts are not routinely done in avian hematology because of problems with clumping. Campbell describes the use of Natt and Herrick's method for manual thrombocyte counts. He considers one to two thrombocytes per $100\times$ power field to be normal.[3] Clinical laboratories often report that thrombocytes are present and adequate, or that numbers appear decreased. The thrombocyte derives from a stem cell precursor, not a megakaryocytic cell type as seen in mammals. The avian thrombocyte can also participate in cellular defense functions.

Thrombocytopenia occurs in pancytopenic forms of some viral diseases, such as psittacine circovirus,* psittacine reovirus, and psittacine polyomavirus infections. Idiopathic thrombocytopenia, although not well documented, has been observed by clinicians. This may be viral in origin also or result from an as yet unknown cause. Increased clotting times may be observed in the avian patient. Thrombocytosis has not been documented.[13]

Erythrocytes

The avian erythrocyte is nucleated and larger in size than its mammalian counterpart. The increased size allows increased oxygen-carrying capacity to interact with the highly efficient avian respiratory exchange system.[22] The avian erythrocyte half-life ranges from 28 to 45 days, much shorter than that of the dog and cat.[13] This short half-life has important clinical implications, such as the rapid onset of nonregenerative anemia.[23]

Erythrocyte Counts

Automated erythrocyte counting has been possible using standard impedance counting equipment. Manual counts can be complicated by the presence of other nucleated cells and the tendency of samples to contain clots. Avian blood is very labile, particularly in ethylenediamine tetraacetic acid (EDTA), necessitating whole cell counts within a few hours of collection. Erythrocyte indices can be calculated if red blood cells (RBC), hemoglobin, and hematocrit are measured.[23]

In clinical practice, the most common methodology involves measuring the packed cell volume (PCV) or hematocrit. Using the PCV and erythrocytic morphologic changes, the clinician can assess erythrocyte status for the most commonly recognized disease problems.

The Abbott Cell-Dyn analyzes avian erythrocytes by impedance measurement, creating a histogram based on distribution of cells by volume. The mean corpuscular volume (MCV) is derived from this measurement. The hematocrit is calculated from the

---

*Fudge AM, unpublished data.

total RBC count and the MCV. In the author's experience, chilled citrate samples remain viable for erythrocytic analysis for up to 3 days with this technology.

Erythrocyte Morphology

Erythrocytic Polychromasia

Polychromasia refers to variation in erythrocyte coloration. This variation largely is related to cell maturation. The cytoplasm of a younger cell appears blue in Romanowsky stains; the mature form stains uniformly orange-pink (see Color Fig. 11–10). No standardized index of avian polychromasia is being used clinically. A slight degree of polychromasia is normal.[23] Increased polychromasia suggests an increased bone marrow response. Absence of polychromasia correlates with nonregenerative anemia and is characterized by all cells exhibiting the same coloration. This condition presents a guarded prognosis, pending resolution of the cause of the nonregeneration.[7, 15]

Erythrocytic Anisocytosis

Mature avian erythrocytes are oval-shaped and nucleated. Less mature cells are rounded in shape and more basophilic in color. Reticulocytes are normally present in peripheral blood at approximately 1 to 2% of the total erythrocyte count.[1, 23]

Anisocytosis describes the degrees of variability of cell size. Laboratories employ a variety of schemes to describe and quantitate the degree of anisocytosis. Automated erythrocytic analysis can result in a calculated measure of anisocytosis, the red cell distribution width (RDW%). The RDW% is a numeric expression of the coefficient of variability of the MCV. A typical normal psittacine RDW% is 10 to 11%. An increase in RDW% denotes an increase in anisocytosis.

Anemia

Anemia is evidenced by a decrease in the total erythrocyte count and PCV.[24] Deficiency anemias have been reported experimentally in poultry[25] but

are not recognized in exotic birds.[23] Because of the presence of iron in many dietary products fed to pet birds, it is unlikely that iron deficiency anemia would occur except with blood loss. Anemias can be classified as nonregenerative or regenerative, hemolytic, or blood-loss–related. Juvenile psittacines often have somewhat lower RBC counts and hematocrits than adults. Generally, these values should be within normal adult ranges at weaning.[8–12, 26]

Nonregenerative Anemia

Nonregenerative anemia is the most common type of anemia observed in birds. Disease conditions that reduce erythropoiesis cause nonregenerative anemia. These include infectious disease, cachexia, neoplasia, and certain toxicities.[4, 7, 23] The most common cause of nonregenerative anemia in pet birds is infectious disease.[7]

Nonregenerative anemia is common in both chronic and acute chlamydial infection.[4, 7] This condition can also be found in bacterial infections, sepsis, chronic granulomas (*Mycobacterium* species, *Escherichia coli,* and *Salmonella* species), *Aspergillus* granulomas, viral infections, and toxicosis.[7, 23, 24] An increase in RBC count, PCV, immature erythrocytes, anisocytosis, and polychromasia signifies cessation of nonregenerative anemia and indicates an improving prognosis.[23] Wasting diseases and neoplasia often result in anemia, because of catabolic influences.[4] Anemia as a result of chronic renal disease is uncommon.

Hemolytic Anemia

It is likely that autoimmune hemolytic anemia occurs in birds, but this is not well documented. Lead toxicosis damages the hemoglobin and results in premature lysis and removal of the damaged cells.[23, 24] Affected cells are seen in the peripheral blood with hypochromatic cytoplasm and erythrocytic ballooning. One hallmark of lead toxicosis is the vigorous regenerative response that occurs within hours of the toxic insult.[7] Basophilic stippling is not a typical finding with avian lead toxicosis.

Oil ingestion is a well-documented cause of hemolytic anemia and is one of the adverse effects suffered by birds residing in oil spill disaster zones.[23]

Blood Loss Anemia

Acute blood loss greatly concerns many pet bird owners. In reality, the highly effective avian clotting system, coupled with adequate exogenous vitamin K, prevents many bleeding episodes from becoming fatal. Severe trauma, organ rupture, aneurysms, and iatrogenic causes can result in severe blood loss. In an otherwise healthy bird, post-shock recovery from blood loss is rapid and effective. No significant storage pool exists in birds, but erythropoiesis increases dramatically within hours.[1, 23] As with cessation of nonregenerative anemia, recovery from blood loss anemia is characterized by increases in the RBC count, PCV, number of immature erythrocytes, as well as increased amounts of anisocytosis and polychromasia. Mitotic figures occur in the peripheral blood of birds experiencing a dramatic response to blood loss anemia.[13]

Conure bleeding syndrome is characterized by a rapid onset of weakness and somnolence. The conure may bleed from the mouth or cloaca. In some birds, the hemogram may suggest a responsive anemia with no visible bleeding, consistent with internal hemorrhage.[4] Cytologic changes seen with conure bleeding syndrome appear similar to those seen with lead toxicosis.[7] This syndrome may be associated with a calcium deficiency, which is supported by a finding of hypocalcemia in a historically calcium/vitamin D_3–deficient bird. Clinical response to parenteral calcium therapy strengthens this hypothesis.[4]

Polycythemia

Polycythemia is characterized by an elevated hematocrit and erythrocyte count. Relative polycythemia is caused by hemoconcentration as a result of dehydration.[24] The clinician must assess a sick bird clinically for hydration, in addition to reviewing and comparing analytes such as protein to the hematocrit. Species such as cockatiels normally can have high erythrocyte counts in the absence of disease. This perhaps is related to their natural desert habitat

and possible physiologic adaptation to low water intake.

Absolute polycythemia is signaled by an increase in erythrocyte numbers in the absence of clinical signs of dehydration or laboratory evidence of hemoconcentration.[24] Clinical causes of avian polycythemia center on hypoxia. Macaws can develop a respiratory hypersensitivity syndrome, which eventually reduces air exchange as a result of inflammatory and fibrotic changes.[27, 28]

Erythrocyte Artifacts

Errors in collecting, handling, and preparing avian blood samples can result in artifacts that affect erythrocyte appearance. The blood film should be made immediately during or soon after the blood collection from mixed anticoagulated blood. Failure to make an adequate blood film may result in ruptured and distorted cells. EDTA can cause distortion of erythrocyte shape if left in contact with whole blood for several hours.[1] Blood films that are shipped in packages containing formalin can be damaged by the fumes, resulting in staining artifacts.[1, 6] Stains containing excess sediment can create the appearance of erythrocytic inclusion bodies or parasites.

Erythrocytic Parasites

Infestation with *Plasmodium* species has been reported in many avian species. Clinical disease is important in a much narrower range of species. Mortality can occur in canaries, falcons, and pigeons. Diagnosis is aided by identifying gametocytes within erythrocytes. Organisms may not be present in peripheral blood, necessitating Wright's or Giemsa-stained preparations of the lungs, liver, and spleen.[1, 16–18] (See Figs. 21–3, 21–4, Chapter 21.)

Haemoproteus species (see Fig. 21–5, Chapter 21) is also widely distributed in a variety of avian species.[1, 19] At the height of pet bird importation, this parasite was most frequently seen in white cockatoos, green-winged macaws, and half-moon conures. In pet birds, documented disease from this parasite is rare.

The rickettsial organism *Aegyptianella* species appears as a black dot in the erythrocytic cytoplasm.

Aegyptianella has been most frequently seen in African grey parrots. Horizontal transmission in captivity has been suggested.[29] Clinical disease as a result of *Aegyptianella* is poorly documented.

Microfilaria are sometimes seen in peripheral blood smears (see Color Fig. 11–11). These parasites are usually *Chandelerella* species, *Splendidofilaria* species, or *Cardiofilaria* species (see Chapter 21). The microfilaria are actually the motile embryo and are the infective stage acquired by the vector.

CLINICAL BIOCHEMISTRY

Hematology often provides the clinician with insight about possible problems with an avian patient. Biochemical parameters, with a few exceptions, are not diagnostic but may indicate the degree of organ involvement. A critically ill bird may have biochemical parameters all within normal range. Conversely, a normal bird may show physiologic or artifactual changes in biochemical parameters that are not caused by medical conditions.

Iatrogenic artifacts are frequent causes of abnormally elevated biochemical values. Causes of avian biochemical artifacts include intramuscular injections, bacterial sample contamination, unseparated blood, clots, hemolysis, and some anticoagulants. The practitioner should avoid introduction of these artifacts and be able to interpret their effect on the biochemical profile (Table 11–1).[6, 30]

Enzymes

Lactic Dehydrogenase

Lactic dehydrogenase (LDH) activity occurs in cardiac and skeletal muscle, liver, kidney, and erythrocytes.[31] Somatic cellular damage and leakage results in increased LDH concentration in the blood. Of the most commonly measured avian enzymes, LDH tends to rise and fall most rapidly after an acute insult. As in mammals, LDH is not liver-specific.[31, 32] Physiologic and medical increases in enzyme concentration in nonhemolyzed samples originate in skeletal muscle and the liver, with occasional contributions from cardiac muscle. LDH released from the kidneys is largely excreted in the urine.[32]

Active or acute hepatocellular damage and leakage can elevate LDH blood concentration. Chronic liver disease or reduced hepatic function may or may not contribute to LDH elevation.[31] Skeletal muscle damage resulting from trauma, surgery, feather picking, or injection of irritant drugs can markedly elevate LDH concentration.[6] Injections of corticosteroids given several hours before withdrawal of a blood sample can dramatically increase blood concentration of LDH. Concentration decreases within hours of cessation of the insult, because of the short half-life of circulating avian LDH.

Sampling artifact probably represents the single most common cause of LDH elevation. Erythrocyte hemolysis releases intracellular LDH isoenzyme.[6] Blood collection techniques must be used that avoid or minimize hemolysis or clotting. Blood samples must be promptly centrifuged and the serum or plasma immediately decanted from the cell fraction.[7]

Decreases in LDH concentration are uncommon. Macaws normally have lower values than most other pet birds.[31, 33] Birds with end-stage liver disease, characterized by hepatocyte displacement through fibrotic or fatty changes, may have lower-than-average LDH values.

Aspartate Transaminase

Aspartate transaminase (AST, SGOT) is nonspecific for avian liver disease[31, 32] but is often used by clinicians as an indicator of liver status. Similar to LDH, tissue sources that cause elevations in blood concentration of AST are primarily liver, skeletal muscle, and cardiac muscle. AST has a longer half-life than LDH, and thus it remains elevated for a few days longer after the cellular insult has ceased.[31, 32] A common misconception is that AST elevation results from hepatocellular damage, when the elevation is often the result of other organ damage. Another incorrect belief is that when AST concentration returns to normal, the liver is healthy. The correct conclusion is that the hepatocellular (or other) insult may have ceased, but no information can be derived about remaining liver function (see Bile Acids). Some birds with advanced hepatocellular damage, usually characterized by replacement of much of the parenchyma with fibrous tissue, may

T a b l e   1 1 – 1

AVIAN BIOCHEMISTRY HELPERS

| Chemistry | High Value | | Low Value | |
	Artifactual	Medical	Artifactual	Medical
Bile acids	Lipemia, hemolysis—such samples should not be submitted	Loss of liver function even with normal enzymes	Lipemic samples that are chemically treated	Response to therapy
AST (SGOT)	Rare—seen in severe lipemia, 300–1000 U/L	Liver, muscle, or heart damage, 300–15,000 U/L		<50 U/L, end-stage liver disease
Uric acid	Severe lipemia, 15–150 mg/dl; dirty nail clip	Renal disease, gout, 15–150 mg/dl	Overhydration of sample or patient	End-stage liver disease
LDH	Sample hemolysis: 300–1200 U/L	Liver, heart, or muscle damage, 300–15,000 U/L	<50 U/L usually artifact (rare)	End-stage liver disease
Glucose	Improper dilution	Stress, 400–600 mg/dl; diabetes, 800–1500 mg/dl	<100 mg/dl, unseparated blood; bacterial contamination	<100 mg/dl, hypoglycemia
Calcium	>12.0 mg/dl, lipemia (cloudy because of other reasons), protein elevation, bacterial contamination	Hormonal disorders, egg production, metabolic disease, cancer	Use of EDTA (lavender top tube) for collection, bacterial contamination	<8 mg/dl, metabolic and nutritional disorders, lead poisoning
CPK	Stress, handling, minor trauma may cause elevations, 300–1000 U/L	600–25,000 U/L; muscle or heart damage, seizures, injections	<10 U/L, bacterial contamination	Rare
Phosphorus		Kidney failure	EDTA	
Cholesterol		Liver, metabolic disease		Liver disease, metabolic disease
Creatinine	Nonspecific chromogens	Kidney failure (rare)		
BUN	Hemolysis	Dehydration		
Potassium	Hemolysis	Adrenal disease; metabolic disease, severe illness	Overhydration	Adrenal disease; metabolic disease, severe illness
Plasma protein	Lipemia; non-temperature compensated refractometer	Inflammatory disease, dehydration	Nontemperature compensated refractometer	Wasting disease

Note: Avian biochemistry analysis is most useful when performed with the hemogram and other clinical information. Out of range values can be the result of medical reasons or artifacts. Artifacts are generally caused by the quality of the sample and can be affected by collection, processing, shipping, and patient status. Please take care to properly submit the sample for best results. This chart should be helpful as a guide to the practitioner to differentiate artifact from medical causes of out of range biochemical values.

From Fudge AH: Blood testing artifacts: Interpretation and prevention. Semin Avian Exotic Pet Med 3:2–4, 1994.

show an abnormally low concentration of plasma AST.[31]

Alanine Transaminase

Alanine transaminase (ALT, SGPT) is a liver-specific enzyme in mammals. Activity of this enzyme in avian livers is low. Elevation of ALT in association with liver disease in birds is rare, making this test inappropriate in avian patients.[31, 34]

Creatine Kinase

Creatine kinase (CK, CPK) is found in skeletal and cardiac muscle and nervous tissue. Clinical or physiologic elevations of CK are primarily attributed to changes in skeletal or cardiac muscle.[31, 32] Myocarditis can result in cellular damage and leakage of CK, resulting in very high values. Muscle wasting, vigorous physical activity, rough handling, irritating injections, surgery, and traumatic bite wounds can all cause marked elevations in this enzyme. The half-life of avian CK falls between that of LDH and AST.[32] Measurement of CK activity is most valuable in differentiating between liver or muscle origin of AST elevation. Artifactual decreases in CK activity can be caused by bacterial contamination of the sample during collection and processing, with multiplication of the bacteria during shipment in warm weather. Typically, cocci are the contaminants.

Glutamate Dehydrogenase

Glutamate dehydrogenase (GLDH) is an enzyme that has been largely studied only in cellular biology. This enzyme is closely bound to hepatocyte mitochondria and is specific for liver disease.[32] Elevations in GLDH activity are only seen with severe hepatocellular disease. Until recently, a test kit was unavailable in North America, but this test is now offered by a limited number of clinical laboratories.

Alkaline Phosphatase

Alkaline phosphatase (AP) is not useful in the diagnosis of avian liver disease.[31] Elevations in AP can be noted in bone maladies including fractures, cancer, and infection.

Gamma Glutamyl Transferase

Gamma glutamyl transferase (GGT) is not considered a sensitive indicator of hepatocellular damage in birds.[31, 34] Lumeij noted elevations of GGT in pigeons with experimentally induced liver disease, but GGT activity could not be measured in supernate of liver homogenates.[31] This study did not support GGT as a clinically useful test for detection of avian liver disease.

Amylase and Lipase

A variety of pathologic changes have been reported in the avian pancreas,[35] but a model equivalent to canine pancreatitis is not recognized in the avian species most frequently treated by veterinarians. Other than in domestic fowl, very little research has been done to assess amylase and lipase activities in

birds. Histopathology currently provides the best information about the pancreas. Endoscope-guided biopsy techniques offer great promise for sampling of pancreatic tissue.[36]

Renal Analytes

Uric Acid

The primary method for excretion of nitrogenous waste in birds is through the formation of uric acid in the liver. Uric acid is eliminated by tubular secretion only and is independent of glomerular filtration.[37]

Elevation in uric acid concentration is typically considered a sign of renal disease. In fact, clinicians do not have sensitive and effective analytes for avian renal function. When true moderate-to-severe elevation in plasma uric acid concentration is seen, significant tubular damage has already occurred.[32] Most diagnoses of renal disease are made on postmortem examination. Renal disease may be suspected in polyuric birds[38] with urinary casts on microscopic examination of urine sediment.[39]

Avian gout occurs as two different and possibly physiologically distinct mechanisms—an articular form and a visceral form. Articular gout is frequently accompanied by marked elevations in plasma uric acid concentration, whereas the concentration may be normal in visceral gout.

Slight elevations in uric acid concentration are commonly observed in dehydrated birds because of a prerenal increase in solute concentration. Values in the range of 10 to 20 mg/dl should always be rechecked after the patient has been clinically stabilized.

Artifactual elevation in uric acid concentration can be caused by lipemia, which falsely raises values determined by the photometric uricase method.[6] Blood samples taken from trims of soiled nails can also result in falsely elevated values. Hemolysis, however, does not appear to significantly affect uric acid assays.

Decreases in uric acid concentration occasionally may occur in birds with hepatic dysfunction. Birds with marked polydipsia and polyuria can have very low values. The exact mechanism for this is not known.

Creatinine

Creatinine is a normal constituent of avian urine but is formed in very small quantities compared with creatine. Creatinine can be removed by tubular secretion in birds, but clearance is variable. At normal plasma concentration this analyte is reabsorbed. Certain chemicals can inhibit reabsorption, whereas diuresis increases elimination.[37]

Clinically, elevation of creatinine concentration in pet birds has been associated with the feeding of high-protein diets, such as dog chow. Spurious elevations in creatinine concentration can be artifactually caused by nonspecific chromogens in avian plasma that interfere with the typical Jaffé reaction performed by clinical laboratories.[40] Creatinine, therefore, is not a particularly reliable indicator of avian renal function.

Urea

Urea is manufactured in very small quantities in birds. This analyte is completely filtered by the kidney and can be reabsorbed.[37] Urea is not particularly useful in assessing kidney function in birds, but Lumeij noted that elevations in this analyte are a useful indicator of prerenal dehydration.[32]

Metabolic Analytes

Calcium

Nutritional and metabolic problems involving calcium imbalances occur commonly in pet avian species. Assays of plasma calcium are limited in the assessment of clinical disorders. Therefore, the nutritional history is always important when considering differential diagnoses of possible calcium metabolic problems.

Birds uniquely develop new medullary bone under the influence of estrogen. They have a tremendous ability to absorb dietary calcium, which relies on the presence of exogenous vitamin D_3. Large quantities of circulating calcium can be taken up by the shell gland during egg formation. Elevation in blood calcium concentration occurs during egg production in the hen, partly because of increased quantities of circulating carrier proteins.[41]

Calcium assays rely primarily on the albumin dye-binding method and are sensitive to physiologic and sampling artifacts. Measured plasma calcium concentration is within normal range in most birds, even when the history and, physical, radiographic, or pathologic evidence suggest a calcium disorder.

Clinical signs associated with hypocalcemia include neurologic weakness and seizures, particularly in African grey parrots. Low blood protein concentration, particularly albumin, is often associated with hypocalcemia.[42] An important predisposing cause is an unsupplemented all-seed diet, which is high in phosphorus and low in calcium and vitamin D_3. African grey parrots are particularly susceptible to this condition because of their apparently reduced ability to mobilize bone calcium. Other species of pet birds that are fed similar diets are more prone to traumatic and pathologic bone fractures. Hypocalcemia is not normally associated with these cases.

Artifactual causes of low blood calcium are most common. Blood for avian chemical assays should never be collected into tubes containing EDTA. When this is done, calcium concentration is extremely low as a result of in vitro binding by the EDTA. Serum quality problems, including hemolysis and bacterial contamination, can lower the calcium value. Most blood calcium is protein-bound. The clinician should be careful to assess the total protein concentration in relation to the calcium assay.[6]

Physiologic hypercalcemia can occur during normal ovulation in the hen. Increased concentrations of carrier proteins are present in the circulating blood. Increased absorption of calcium and mobilization from the bones also are occurring during this time. Lipemia, which is a normal physiologic event during ovulation, can further artifactually elevate the photometric assay of plasma calcium.[41] Lipemia, which occurs with some hepatopathies, results in artifactual calcium elevation. Hemolysis and bacterial contamination[6] can also result in falsely elevated calcium values.

Phosphorus

Phosphorus metabolism in birds is similar to that in mammals. However, elevation in phosphorus concentration is not commonly noted in birds.[41] Renal disease is often subclinical until the bird is near death. Hyperphosphatemia, associated with apparent renal disease, is not commonly recognized clinically. Hypophosphatemia is also uncommon. Artifactual alterations in plasma phosphorus concentration are similar to those seen with calcium. EDTA and hemolysis can falsely depress values, whereas hemolysis and lipemia can falsely elevate values.

Iron

Disorders of iron metabolism are important problems in mynahs, toucans, and occasionally other species. Hemochromatosis is characterized by excess iron pigment in the liver and other organs and is associated with cellular pathology. One current theory suggests that this disorder results from excess absorption and uptake of dietary iron, rather than actual dietary iron content.[43] Plasma iron assays have been used to screen for this disease. However, clinical observations support the conclusion that the circulating iron concentration is neither diagnostic nor predictive of hemochromatosis. Furthermore, nonvisible sample hemolysis can contribute significantly to the total iron concentration. Measurement of plasma ferritin would be an ideal assay, but a commercial radioimmunoassay reagent is not currently available for clinical use. Assessment and diagnosis of hemochromatosis currently requires liver biopsy.[44–46]

Glucose

Birds maintain a much higher plasma glucose concentration (around 300 mg/dl) than mammals. Maintenance of avian glucose metabolism is predicated on pancreatic glucagon as the most important regulator.[47] The high metabolic demands of flight dictate readily available carbohydrates and rapid mobilization of free fatty acids.

Moderate transient hyperglycemia (up to 800 mg/dl) can occur with stress.[41] Diabetes mellitus, possibly as a result of glucagon excess, is characterized by persistent elevations of plasma glucose in excess of 900 mg/dl.[48, 49] Renal disease, including renal adenocarcinoma, may result in hyperglycemia.[49] True hypoglycemia in birds is typically the result of starvation. Values of glucose less than 150 mg/dl are usually life threatening.

Artifactual decreases in plasma glucose are common. Avian erythrocytes do not rapidly consume glucose,[50] but shipping unseparated blood can result in significant decreases in glucose values within 12 to 72 hours. Bacterial contamination of samples during collection and processing can also markedly reduce glucose values.

Electrolytes

The cellular functions of sodium and potassium in birds are very similar to those in mammals. Regulation of avian electrolytes occurs by the kidneys and is modulated by a variety of hormones.[41] Corticosterone, rather than cortisol, appears to be the primary avian glucocorticoid. Hypoadrenalcorticism, characterized by hypokalemia and decreased adrenocorticotropic hormone (ACTH) response, has been documented in pet birds.*

Electrolytes are not routinely measured, but electrolyte imbalances that result from organ dysfunction, alimentary tract disorders, and iatrogenic causes can occur. These changes parallel those seen in mammals.

Protein

Blood proteins are very important in maintaining metabolic homeostasis in birds. Proteins promote correct osmotic pressure to prevent extravasation of blood and maintain proper pH through a buffering effect. Protein fractions include albumin and the globulins. Albumin serves as a reserve protein and as a carrier for other molecules. Globulins include inflammatory proteins, clotting proteins, and immunoglobulins.[41]

Biochemical measurement of total protein concentration indicates that normal values in birds are approximately one-half of mammalian values. Measurement of total solids by refractometer has been reported as unreliable compared with chemical measurement by the biuret method.[40] Refractometric or chemical measurement can be complicated by chromogens and lipids in the sample. A high-quality temperature compensated refractometer,

---

*Fudge AM, unpublished data.

though, can provide a reasonable approximation of avian total protein.

No reliable biochemical method exists to measure avian albumin. Dye-binding methods fail to measure avian albumin adequately, resulting in abnormally low values in normal birds reported by clinical laboratories. Hence, globulin and albumin values are usually inaccurate as reported.[27, 32, 51]

Protein electrophoresis (EPH) remains the only reliable method to properly quantitate the main protein fractions. Inflammatory conditions such as egg yolk peritonitis, chlamydiosis, and tuberculosis show a reduced albumin-globulin (A-G) ratio. The gamma globulin fraction is typically two to three times normal in birds with active chlamydial infections.* Psittacine circovirus infections (PBFD) have been reported to show reduced prealbumin and γ globulin.[52] Although poorly documented in birds, increased A-G ratios are expected in many hepatic disorders and in wasting diseases, including starvation.[53]

Cholesterol

Reference ranges for cholesterol in pet birds are not well documented. Values in normal birds range from 180 to 250 mg/dl. Increased concentrations are seen in carnivorous birds. Sedentary pet birds on high-fat diets may have elevated values. Lipoprotein fractions are not commonly assessed clinically in pet birds. Elevations in triglyceride concentration have been documented in birds with lipemic blood samples.* Elevations in cholesterol occur in hypothyroidism. Atherosclerosis associated with hypercholesterolemia has been noted in pet birds.[54]

Bile Acids

Birds lack bilirubin reductase; instead, they excrete biliverdin into the bile. Small quantities of bilirubin are detectable in avian plasma, possibly because of nonspecific reduction. The biliverdin is unconjugated and does not accumulate in tissue. There are no commercial test kits available to measure avian biliverdin. Carotenoid pigments can contribute to yellow color in avian plasma, but controlled studies

have not ruled out pathologic contributions to plasma color.[55]

Bile acids are synthesized in the liver from cholesterol and assist in the digestion and absorption of fats. In seed-eating birds, chenodeoxycholic acid is the primary bile acid produced. Bile acids are stored in the gall bladder and released after a meal. Postprandial increases in bile acid concentrations have also been documented in birds without gallbladders. A majority of the excreted bile acids are reabsorbed by the small intestine, transported to the liver by portal veins, and recycled by the liver.

Elevations in bile acid concentrations are associated with reduced hepatic function. Clinical experience with bile acid assays indicate that this assay is a much more sensitive indicator of hepatic disease than measurement of liver-related enzymes.[56] Enzymes that measure hepatocellular damage often return to normal after an acute insult. Persistent loss of hepatic function is better indicated by measurement of bile acids. When single-point assays are done, the bird should be fasted for up to 12 hours[57] (raptors up to 24 hours).[58] The clinician may want to avoid fasting the seriously ill bird. Postprandial bile acid assays show moderate elevations in normal birds.[57, 59]

Elevations in bile acids do not indicate the type of hepatic pathology or dysfunction present. Persistent elevation of bile acids provides a strong indication for a liver biopsy.[43] A biopsy usually reveals the pathology, enabling the clinician to tailor specific therapy for the patient. Early recognition, diagnosis, and treatment of hepatic disease is the goal. Bile acid assays have allowed the clinician to recognize liver problems in birds that are otherwise clinically and biochemically normal.

Reference ranges have not been established for many species, but most birds appear to have fasting bile acid concentrations below 100 μmol/L. Amazon parrots have somewhat higher values.[59, 60] This author recommends liver biopsies in patients with values that repeatedly exceed 200 μmol/L. Patients with values exceeding 500 to 700 μmol/L are likely to already have advanced hepatic pathology.

Most laboratories use the photometric enzymatic assay rather than the radioimmunoassay (RIA) method.[43] Artifactual elevations can be caused by lipemia or hemolysis with the photometric method. Lipemia can be removed by ultracentrifugation.

---

*K. Quesenberry, personal communication.

Chemical treatment (Liposol) for lipemia results in artifactual depression of bile acid values.

PROFILING WITH AVIAN BLOOD PANELS

When evaluating blood test results, the clinician should first assess the hematologic data. Leukocyte parameters to consider include total leukocyte count, leukocyte differential, and leukocyte morphology.[61] A very low leukocyte count may suggest viral infection. Moderate leukocytosis could result from nonmedical stress, but should be considered in light of other hematologic parameters. Clinicians should note any relative or absolute increase in basophils, monocytes, or eosinophils. Heterophilia is common in avian hemograms. Band forms are relatively uncommon. Toxic heterophilic changes usually indicate chlamydial, bacterial, or fungal infection.

The erythrogram is assessed first by looking at total erythrocyte count, or the hematocrit in the absence of total count data. Anemia is most commonly characterized by nonregenerative changes, as indicated by erythrocyte indices or morphology (minimal anisocytosis and minimal polychromasia). An elevated total erythrocyte count could suggest hemoconcentration from dehydration or polycythemia from chronic obstructive respiratory disease. *Plasmodium* species is the only parasite of erythrocytes associated with clinical signs of disease, most commonly in passerine birds.

It is a misunderstanding that any enzyme elevation suggests liver dysfunction. However, many enzyme elevations are nonhepatic in origin. Assuming there are no plasma quality problems (hemolysis, lipemia, bacterial contamination), the clinician can use the following guidelines:

Moderate Elevations in AST, LDH, CK. LDH elevates and declines most rapidly, followed by CK and AST. This profile points to nonhepatic cellular damage and leakage, such as skeletal muscle or cardiac muscle. This profile does not rule out liver damage as a partial cause of AST and LDH elevation.

Moderate Elevation in AST, Normal LDH, Normal CPK. This pattern suggests two possibilities: (1) acute skeletal or cardiac muscle damage that occurred and ceased 2 to 4 days previously, or (2) the more likely conclusion that AST elevation stems from hepatic damage.

Normal AST, High LDH, Moderate Elevation in CK. This profile suggests skeletal or cardiac muscular insult commencing less than 24 hours before sampling. Subsequent resampling in 24 to 48 hours may show normal LDH, slight elevation in CK, and slight-to-moderate elevation in AST.

Normal AST, High LDH, Normal CK. It is not possible to determine whether LDH elevation is of hepatic or cardiac/skeletal muscle origin. Review the plasma or serum quality, because the most common cause of this profile is hemolysis resulting from sampling or processing errors.

Elevated AST, Elevated LDH, Normal CK. This profile most likely suggests hepatocellular damage.

Normal AST, Normal LDH, Normal CK. There is no evidence of current cellular damage of the heart, muscle, or liver. The clinician is unable to make any conclusion about the patient's liver function, only that no apparent damage is currently occurring.

Renal Assessment

Normal uric acid values do not prove that kidney function is normal, because uric acid is not a sensitive renal function test. Polyuria, endoscopic abnormalities, or radiographic changes should point the clinician toward further assessment, such as urinalysis or renal biopsy.

Glucose

In most profiles, the glucose concentration is normal. An elevation over 900 to 1000 mg/dl should direct the clinician to a possible diagnosis of diabetes mellitus. A very low value can result if a sample is left in contact with cells for 1 or more days, or from bacterial contamination that can occur during sampling and processing.

Calcium

In most profiles, the blood calcium level is normal. True increases can be seen during ovulation. A true decrease may correlate with neurologic signs or malnutrition. A normal value does not rule out metabolic bone disease or other disorders in calcium metabolism.

Protein

A true increase in plasma protein is seen in inflammatory disorders and with hemoconcentration resulting from dehydration. A true decrease is seen in acute blood loss, starvation, and protein-losing enteropathies.

The clinician should use hematology and biochemical profiles as tools. Pet bird owners often demand and expect a high level of care that correlates with the emotional bond rather than the purchase price of the bird. Breeding and production birds are often financially valuable as individuals or as a group. The information gained from these tests is invaluable in the diagnosis and medical management of many disease problems in all types of birds.

References

1. Campbell TW: Avian Hematology and Cytology. Ames, IA, Iowa State University Press, 1988.
2. VanderHeyden N: Evaluation and interpretation of the avian hemogram. Semin Avian Exotic Pet Med 3:5–13, 1994.
3. Campbell TW: Hematology. In Ritchie BW, Harrison GJ, Harrison LR (eds): Avian Medicine, Principles and Application. Lake Worth, FL, Wingers Publishing, 1994, pp 176–198.
4. Rosskopf WJ, Woerpel RW: Pet avian hematology trends. Proc Assoc Avian Vet, Chicago, IL, 1991, pp 98–111.
5. King AS, McLelland J: Birds: Their structure and function. London, Bailliere Tindall, 1984, p 234.
6. Fudge, AM: Blood testing artifacts: Interpretation and prevention, Semin Avian Exotic Pet Med 3:2–4, 1994.
7. Fudge AM: Avian hematology—identification and interpretation. Proc 1989 Annual Meeting Assoc Avian Vet, Seattle, WA, 1989, pp 284–292.
8. VanderHeyden N: The Hematology of Nestling Raptors and Psittacines. Proc 1986 Annual Meeting Assoc Avian Vet, Miami, FL, 1986, pp 347–354.
9. Clubb SL, Schubot RM, Joyner K, et al: Hematologic and serum biochemical reference intervals in juvenile cockatoos. J Assoc Avian Vet 5:16–26, 1991.
10. Clubb SL, Schubot RM, Joyner K, et al: Hematologic and serum biochemistry reference intervals in juvenile eclectus parrots. J Assoc Avian Vet 4:218–225, 1990.
11. Clubb SL, Schubot RM, Joyner K, et al: Hematologic and serum biochemical reference intervals in juvenile macaws (Ara sp.). J Assoc Avian Vet 5:154–162, 1991.
12. Clubb SL, Schubot RM, Wolf S: Hematologic and serum biochemical reference values for juvenile macaws, cockatoos, and eclectus parrots. In Schubot RM, Clubb SL, Clubb
K (eds): Psittacine Aviculture: Perspectives, Techniques and Research. Loxahatchee, FL, Avicultural Breeding and Research Center, 1992, pp 18–1 to 18–20.
13. VanderHeyden N: Hematology and plasma chemistry values in selected diseases of Amazon parrots. Proc Second Eur Symp Avian Med Surg, Utrecht, The Netherlands, Dutch Assoc Avian Vet, 1989, pp 357–364.
14. Dein FJ: Hematology. In Harrison GJ, Harrison LR (eds): Clinical Avian Medicine and Surgery. Philadelphia, WB Saunders, 1986, pp 174–191.
15. Zinkle JG: Avian hematology. In Jain NC (ed): Schalm's Veterinary Hematology. Philadelphia, Lea & Febiger, 1986, pp 256–273.
16. Dein FJ: Laboratory Manual of Avian Hematology. East Northport, NY, Assoc of Avian Vet, 1984.
17. Hawkey CM, Dennett TB: Comparative Veterinary Hematology. Ames, IA, Iowa State University Press, 1989.
18. Lind PJ, Wolf PL, Petrini KR, et al: Morphology of the avian eosinophils in raptors. J Assoc Avian Vet 4:33–38, 1990.
19. VanderHeyden N: Identification, pathogenicity and treatment of avian hematozoa. Proc 1985 Annual Meeting Assoc Avian Vet, Boulder, CO, 1985, pp 163–174.
20. Flammer K: Clinical aspects of Atoxoplasmosis in canaries. Proc Joint Meeting Assoc Zoo Vet, Assoc Veter, Turtle Bay, HI, 1987, pp 33–36.
21. Panigraphy B, Senne DA: Diseases of mynahs. JAVMA 199(3):378–381, 1991.
22. Fedde MR: Respiration. In Sturkie PD (ed): Avian Physiology. New York, Springer-Verlag, 1986, pp 202–208.
23. Dein FJ: Avian clinical hematology: Erythrocytes and anemia. Proc 1983 Annual Meeting Assoc Avian Vet, San Diego, CA, 1983, pp 10–23.
24. Jain NC: Clinical and laboratory evaluation of anemias and polycythemias. In Jain NC (ed): Schalm's Veterinary Hematology, ed 4. Philadelphia, Lea & Febiger, 1986, pp 563–576.
25. Austic RE, Scott ML: Nutritional diseases. In Calnek BW (ed): Diseases of Poultry. Ames, IA, Iowa State University Press, 1991, pp 45–71.
26. Joyner KL: Psittacine pediatric diagnostics. Semin Avian Exotic Pet Med 1:11–21, 1992.
27. Taylor M: Polycythemia in the blue and gold macaw—a report of three cases. Proc First Int Conf Zool Avian Med, Oahu, HI, 1987, pp 95–104.
28. Fudge AM, Reavill DR: Pulmonary artery aneurysm and polycythemia with respiratory hypersensitivity on a Blue and Gold macaw (Ara araruana). Proc Eur Conf Avian Med Surg, Utrecht, The Netherlands, 1993, pp 382–386.
29. Rosskopf WJ, Woerpel RW, Fudge AM: Aegyptienella-like parasites in an eclectus parrot in Southern California. Proc Assoc Avian Vet, New Orleans, 1992, pp 129–133.
30. Fudge AM: Avian practice tips. Vet Clin North Am, Nov, 1991, pp 1121–1134.
31. Lumeij JT: Avian clinical enzymology. Semin Avian Exotic Pet Med 3:14–24, 1994.
32. Lumeij JT, Wolfswinkel J: Tissue enzyme profiles of the budgerigar (Melopsittacus undulatus) (PhD thesis). In Lumeij JT (ed): A contribution to Clinical Investigative Methods for Birds with Special Reference to the Racing Pigeon (Columba livia domestica). Utrecht, University of Utrecht, 1987, pp 71–77.
33. Harris D: Laboratory testing in pet avian medicine. Vet Clin North Am, Nov, 1991, pp 1147–1156.
34. Campbell TW: Selected biochemical tests used to detect the presence of hepatic disease in birds. Proc Assoc Avian Vet, Miami, FL, 1986, pp 43–51.
35. Graham DL, Heyer GW: Diseases of the exocrine pancreas

in pet, exotic, and wild birds. Proc Assoc Avian Vet, New Orleans, 1992, pp 190–193.

36. Taylor M: Avian endoscopy. In Assoc Avian Vet Conf Guide Pract Labs, Nashville, 1993, pp 51–62.

37. Sturkie PD: Kidneys, extrarenal salt excretion and urine. In Sturkie PD (ed): Avian Physiology. New York, Springer-Verlag, 1986, pp 359–382.

38. Ekstrom D, Degernes L: Avian gout. Proc Annual Conf Assoc Avian Vet, Seattle, 1989, pp 130–138.

39. Rosskopf WJ, Woerpel RW, Lane RA, et al: The practical uses and limitations of the urinalysis in diagnostic pet avian medicine: With emphasis on the differential diagnosis of polyuria, the importance of cast formation in the avian urinalysis. Proc Assoc Avian Vet, Miami, 1986, pp 61–73.

40. Lumeij JT: The diagnostic value of plasma protein and non-protein nitrogen substances in birds (PhD thesis). In Lumeij JT (ed): A Contribution to Clinical Investigative Methods for Birds with Special Reference to the Racing Pigeon (Columba livia domestica). Utrecht, University of Utrecht, 1987, pp 80–87.

41. Jenkins JR: Avian metabolic chemistries. Semin Avian Exotic Pet Med 3:25–32, 1994.

42. Lumeij JT: Relation of calcium to total protein and albumin in the African grey parrot. Avian Pathol 19:661–663, 1990.

43. Dorrestein GM, Grinwis GM, Dominguez L, et al: An induced iron storage disease in doves and pigeons: A model for hemochromatosis in mynah birds. Proc Assoc Avian Vet, New Orleans, 1992, pp 108–112.

44. Worell AB: Diagnosis and management of iron storage disease in Toucans. Semin Avian Exotic Pet Med 3:38–40, 1994.

45. Worell AB: Serum iron levels in Rhampastids. Proc Assoc Avian Vet, Chicago, 1991, pp 120–130.

46. Ward RJ, Iancu TC, Henderson GM, et al: Hepatic iron overload in birds: Analytical and morphological studies. Avian Pathol 17:451–464, 1988.

47. Hazelwood RL: Carbohydrate metabolism. In Sturkie PD (ed): Avian Physiology. New York, Springer-Verlag, 1986, pp 303–325.

48. Murphy J: Diabetes in toucans. Proc Assoc Avian Vet, New Orleans, 1992, pp 165–170.

49. Lothrop C, Harrison GJ, Schultz D, et al: Miscellaneous diseases. In Harrison GJ, Harrison LR (eds): Clinical Avian Medicine and Surgery. Philadelphia, WB Saunders, 1986, pp 525–536.

50. Lumeij JT: A Contribution to Clinical Investigative Methods for Birds with Special Reference to the Racing Pigeon (Columba livia domestica) (PhD thesis). Utrecht, University of Utrecht, 1987, pp 26–30.

51. Anderson CB: Determination of chicken and turkey plasma and serum protein concentrations using refractometry and the biuret method. Avian Dis 33:93–96, 1989.

52. Jacobson ER, Clubb S, Simpson C, et al: Feather and beak necrosis in cockatoos: Clinicopathologic evaluations. JAVMA 189:999–1005, 1986.

53. Quesenberry K, Moroff S: Plasma electrophoresis in psittacine birds. Proc Assoc Avian Vet, Chicago, 1991, pp 112–117.

54. Johnson JH, Phalen DN, Kondik VH, et al: Atherosclerosis in psittacine birds. Proc Assoc Avian Vet, New Orleans, 1992, pp 87–93.

55. Hoefer HL: Bile acid testing in psittacine birds. Semin Avian Exotic Pet Med 3:33–37, 1994.

56. Lumeij JT, Meidam M, Wolfswinkel J: Changes in plasma chemistry after drug induced liver disease or muscle necrosis in racing pigeons (Columba livia domestica). Avian Pathol 17:865–874, 1988.

57. Lumeij JT: Fasting and postprandial bile acid concentrations in racing pigeons (Columba livia domestica) and mallards (Anas platyrhynchos). J Assoc Avian Vet 5:197–200, 1991.

58. Lumeij JT, Remple JD: Plasma bile acid concentrations in response to feeding in peregrine falcons (F. peregrinus). Avian Dis 36:1060–1062, 1992.

59. Hoefer HL, Moroff S: The use of bile acids in the diagnosis of hepatobiliary disease in the parrot. Proc Assoc Avian Vet, Chicago, 1991, pp 118–119.

60. Lumeij JT, Overduin LM: Plasma chemistry reference values in psittaciformes. Avian Pathol 19:235–244, 1990.

61. Fudge AM: Avian clinical biochemistry. In Rosskopf WJ, Woerpel RW (eds): Diseases of Caged and Aviary Birds. Baltimore, Williams & Wilkins, in press.

Gerry M. Dorrestein

12

Diagnostic Necropsy and Pathology

Athorough postmortem examination of birds that die or are euthanized is a necessary adjunct to good clinical practice.[2, 3]

There are several reasons for performing a necropsy. These can be finding the cause of death, confirming a diagnosis, investigating unsuccessful therapy, increasing knowledge, or satisfying curiosity. Diagnostic pathology is not limited to a necropsy. The pathologist uses the clinical history (including hematology, blood chemistry, therapeutic measurements), the gross description of the lesions, culture results, and other data as well as the cytologic and histologic appearance of the lesions to make a diagnosis. Absence of any of these or incorrect submission of tissues will hamper this process.

SUBMISSION OF CARCASSES OR SPECIMENS

If a practitioner has access to the services of an avian pathologist who will perform the gross necropsy, procedures should be established for the submission of the intact carcass. These specialists have the experience and training, and their work will yield the best results. Often the avian practitioner or technician performs the postmortem examination and submits appropriate tissue to a diagnostic laboratory. Based on the findings, material is collected and sampled for followup investigation. The quality of information received from such an examination is directly proportional to the quality and choice of the specimens submitted and the information that accompanies them.

To promote rapid cooling of the carcass, thoroughly soak the plumage in cold water to which a small amount of soap or detergent has been added to aid complete wetting of the plumage and skin. Any feathers that remain dry will provide insulation, retarding cooling of the carcass. Place the carcass in a plastic bag, squeeze out all excess air, seal or tie the bag, refrigerate, and contact the laboratory for further instructions.

If the carcass has been cooled immediately upon death and can be submitted to the laboratory within 72 to 96 hours of the time of death, it should be refrigerated (*not frozen*) and packed with sufficient ice or cool packs to keep it cold until arrival at the laboratory. If delivery to the laboratory is expected to be delayed beyond 96 hours, the carcass should be frozen immediately, rather than simply refrigerated. Frozen tissue specimens or carcasses must be packed with sufficient *dry ice* to keep them frozen until arrival at the laboratory.

Refrigerated or frozen specimens should be packed in a sturdy, insulated (Styrofoam) box and shipped to the laboratory by a private courier service that guarantees same-day or next-day delivery to the laboratory.

Most laboratories cannot receive specimens over the weekend; it is thus advisable not to ship refrigerated or frozen specimens on Fridays or weekends. Remember, it is crucial that sufficient refrigerant be packed with the specimen and that it be adequately insulated to ensure that it will remain cold (or frozen) until it is received by the laboratory.

In instances when the carcass is extremely small, such as embryos, nestlings, or very small adult birds, the entire carcass may be submitted for histologic examination. This is best accomplished by opening the body cavity, gently separating the viscera and fixing the entire carcass in formalin solution.[3]

Whether the practitioner is performing the necropsy or simply collecting diagnostic material, preparation must be done systematically. In cases of mortality in small aviary birds, the necropsy has to be considered as a part of the diagnostic workup. The correct selection of material for further examination and correct method of sampling, storage, and shipping of material increases the quality of results tremendously.

A written report of the necropsy findings helps the clinician to keep track of the disease status of the bird collection.

Even a negative finding is significant, because it means that all the things you have been looking for are not present.

EQUIPMENT

It is helpful to have a set of instruments designated for postmortem examinations; these should be thoroughly cleaned and sterilized after use. A separate room is advisable to perform the necropsy. One should not use instruments that are used around living birds. It is pertinent to use adequate protective clothes.

The *instrument pack* should include forceps, two scalpel handles (one for cutting, one for burning organ surfaces before taking a microbiology sample), necropsy knife, stout scissors and/or poultry shears (for cutting bones), and fine scissors for dissection. Tiny birds such as finches require fine instruments such as iris scissors. For large birds (e.g., ratites or waterfowl), instruments appropriate for large or small mammal necropsy including a vibrating (cast-cutting) saw may be used.

Other useful equipment is a gram scale, a hand lens or dissecting microscope, and tissues. In addition to instruments, one should have on hand

- 10% neutral buffered formalin (= 4% formaldehyde)
- 70% alcohol for wetting and disinfecting the feathers and skin
- 100% ethyl alcohol (for fixing specimens suspected of having gout)

- A bottle with saline (0.9% NaCl) with a pipette (for parasitologic examination)
- Appropriate containers

Other materials for ancillary diagnostic procedures include:
- Syringes and needles to obtain samples for serology, hematology, or cytology tests
- Clean glass slides for impression smears
- A stain set for cytology (e.g., DiffQuick, Hemacolor, Stamp, or Macchiavello's)
- Clean glass slides and coverslips for wet mounts (parasitology)
- Burner for heating and sterilizing one scalpel blade before taking a sample for microbiology testing
- Sterile swabs or culture tubes with appropriate transport media for bacterial, fungal, or chlamydial culture
- Transport media for chlamydial antigen demonstration (enzyme-linked immunoassay [ELISA])
- Petri dishes or freezer-proof tubes for submission of tissues for viral isolation

Clinicians may choose to have a camera available for documentation of gross lesions. A standard checklist and necropsy report form assist in recording observations (Table 12–1).

EUTHANASIA

The method of euthanasia may affect specimens submitted to the pathologist. High doses of barbiturates are caustic to tissues and cause crystallization in and on organs. This may be mistaken for early gout, but it also changes and masks macroscopic and microscopic alterations. In adequate dosage (e.g., pentobarbital 200 mg/kg body weight (bw) intraperitoneally) few alterations are seen.

The euthanasia agent can also be administered intravenously, intramuscularly, or into the spinal cord area at the base of the skull with the head flexed (in larger birds especially). Giving such agents slowly to effect is helpful to prevent undesired artificial changes. Collect hematologic samples prior to euthanasia. Larger samples may be obtained from the jugular vein or, under anesthesia, from direct heart puncture through the thoracic inlet. The blood may be centrifuged and serum submitted or saved and frozen pending necropsy re-

Table 12–1

NECROPSY REPORT FORM AND CHECKLIST

1. Bird species, weight, age/leg band number, sex, summarized history.
2. Date of necropsy, your name.
3. Macroscopy
   External Examination
      General body condition: muscle mass: robust, well muscled, moderately muscled, thin, emaciated, depot fat
      Feathers/integument/ectoparasites
      Palpation of skeleton
      Body openings/oral cavity
   Internal Examination
      Fat/subcutis/body wall
      Body cavities (air sacs/pleura/peritoneum)
      (Para)thyroids, thymus
      Spleen (size)
      Heart, aorta, other vessels
      Liver, gall bladder, bile ducts
      Reproductive system (gonads, reproductive tract)
      Respiratory tract (nasal/sinus, choanal, larynx, trachea, syrinx, air sacs, lungs)
      Urinary tract (kidneys, ureters) and adrenal glands
      Digestive tract (beak, tongue, oropharynx, esophagus, crop, proventriculus, gizzard, duodenum and pancreas, small intestine, yolk sac, ceca, rectum [colorectum], cloaca, bursa of Fabricius, vent)
      Special senses (eyes, ears, nares)
      Musculoskeletal system—muscles, skeleton (sternum, ribs, vertebrae, long bones), bone marrow, joints
      Brain, pituitary, spinal cord, meninges, peripheral nerves
4. Wet mounts (crop, rectum, etc.)
5. Cytology (liver, spleen, lung, rectum)
6. Chlamydiosis examination
7. Tentative (differential) diagnosis
8. Ancillary diagnostics: bacteriology, mycology, virology, parasitology, toxicology, others
9. Tissue saved:
10. Tissues submitted for histopathology:

sults. This may be helpful in diagnosis of endocrine disorders or viral infections. Routine hematologic tests may also be performed on these samples.

IMPRESSION SMEARS

Impression smears are a useful adjunct to a complete postmortem examination (see also Cytology). In our protocol, two sets of impression smears are made from liver, spleen, lung, and rectum. Organs with pathological changes are automatically added. In our routine for all Columbiformes and Psittaciformes an immunofluorescent staining (IFT) of impression smears for *Chlamydia* species of the same organs is done. In cases suspected of chlamydiosis (psittacosis or ornithosis), an IFT for *Chlamydia* is

far more reliable than routine histochemistry on fixed paraffin-embedded histologic sections. Tissue phases of parasites such as *Atoxoplasma* species, *Toxoplasma* species, *Plasmodium* species, *Haemoproteus* species, and *Leucocytozoon* species are more readily identified in impression smears of liver and spleen. In addition, the cytology of lymphoreticular and hematopoietic neoplasms is more diagnostic on impressions of liver, spleen, and bone marrow compared with histology.[2]

To make a good impression smear (actually a touch preparation), it may be easier to bring the slide to the tissue. Grasp a small piece of the tissue with forceps so that a fresh-cut, well-blotted surface faces upward. Lower the clean slide to the tissue, touching it lightly. Retract quickly without drawing the slide across the tissue. Make several "touch preps" on each slide. Impressions are generally more useful when air-dried. If other fixation is necessary (e.g., heat fixation for acid-fast stains), it can be done later. Exudate may be prepared for cytologic evaluation.

FIXATION FOR HISTOPATHOLOGY

The choice of tissues for histopathologic examination can be determined by several philosophies:

1. Economic reasons; this is a poor rationale. It is better to collect the tissues and, after consulting the pathologist, send in the selected tissues and keep the others "just in case."
2. Completeness; this is especially valid for scientific research. Collect all tissues listed in Table 12–2.[3]

Table 12–2

TISSUE ROUTINELY COLLECTED FOR HISTOPATHOLOGY

Skin (including feathers, follicles)	Crop	Pancreas*
	Proventriculus*	Ovary and oviduct (female)
Trachea	Ventriculus*	
Lung*	Duodenum*	Testes (male)
Air sac	Small intestine	Pectoral muscle
Heart*	Rectum	Bone marrow
Kidneys*	Ceca and cloaca	Cloacal bursa
Thyroid glands	Spleen*	Thymus
Parathyroid glands	Liver*	Brain
Adrenal glands	Gall bladder	Ischiatic
Esophagus	(if present)	(Sciatic) nerve

*Standard selection of tissues for routine histopathologic examination. Selection of additional tissues depends upon gross lesions observed at necropsy.

3. A standard selection completed with a choice based on the necropsy findings. This list is practical and will in most cases lead to sufficient diagnostic support. In Table 12–2, the standard selection is marked with asterisks (*).

Normally selected tissues are fixed in neutral-buffered formalin for histopathologic examination. Buffered 10% formalin penetrates only about 2 mm in 24 hours and thus the specimen must be less then 5 mm thick. Penetration is slower in very bloody, dense tissues (e.g., congested spleen or liver) and more rapid in relatively porous tissue (e.g., lung). Formalin does not penetrate well into the brain through the unopened calvarium or into the marrow of bone unless the bone has been cracked. The greatest problem with submission of fixed tissues is inadequate fixation because of prior severe autolysis or inadequate volume of fixative, allowing continuing decomposition. Initial fixation is achieved with 10 times the volume of formalin to volume of tissue. The amount of formalin may be reduced after 12 to 24 hours of fixation in preparation for mailing. Wet formalin-fixed tissue may be conveniently stored and shipped in plastic heat-sealed bags.

Other fixatives, such as those required for electron microscopy (EM) are unnecessary, since formalin-fixed tissue is easily refixed with glutaraldehyde and the main structures (including viruses) are preserved. Essential for this fixation for EM is very fresh tissue in tiny parts (cubic millimeters).

The number of tissues submitted to the histopathology laboratory may depend on the cost per tissue. If you do not send the complete set of tissues it is wise to save the rest in formalin while awaiting a diagnosis. If only grossly visible lesions or limited tissues are submitted, a diagnosis may not be possible. When specific lesions are observed at necropsy, the tissue specimen collected should include a small margin of normal tissue adjacent to the lesion. Too often, the limited tissues suggest a diagnosis that cannot be confirmed because other tissues have already been discarded.

Tissues for histopathology examination should not be frozen. Freezing creates crystals and ruptures cells, making histopathology virtually useless.

Tissues for toxicologic analysis should be frozen. They may be frozen at −20°C after being wrapped in aluminum foil. Freezing for virus isolation is best done at −70°C. If this cannot be accomplished, the tissues for viral isolation should be sent (by rapid mail) in sterile containers on wet ice.

AUTOPSY PROTOCOL

There are probably as many ways to dissect a bird as there are pathologists. Several procedures have been published.[1, 2, 3] Choose a procedure that is familiar and that feels comfortable; use it consistently. It is the standard admonition that each necropsy be performed in as regular and thorough a manner as can be summoned by the prosector and that a "complete" set of tissues and specimens be collected for subsequent histopathologic, parasitologic, toxicologic, serologic, and biochemical examination.[1] The veterinarian should review the appended detailed checklist of organs to be examined, observations to be made, of ancillary tests to be performed and specimens to be collected prior to disposal of the remains.

The following procedure and checklist is used at the Department of Pathology, Division of Avian and Exotic Animals in Utrecht, The Netherlands.

Before starting the necropsy procedure the packing material is to be inspected for the presence of mites or lice (Fig. 12–1).

History

Read the history (including identification, physical findings, medical history, and pertinent laboratory

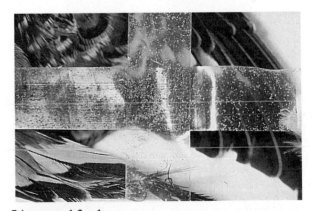

F i g u r e   1 2 – 1

Budgerigar *(Melopsittacus undulatus)*. Mites were on the glue side of the tape of the package.

data[3]) and summarize the most relevant data on your worksheet. Make a note of leg band numbers, transponders, or other identifying marks.

External Examination of the Carcass

First make a carcass identification based upon patient data (species, age, and color pattern) as well as leg band, tattoo, or microchip implant data.[3] Record information about general body condition, weight, muscle mass, joints, integument (including beak and nails), plumage (for defects, ectoparasites, feces), body orifices (eyes, ears, nostrils, and vent), uropygial gland, traumata, and abnormalities. Palpate the skeleton. The feeding status can be judged based upon the condition of the muscles on the keel and the filling of the crop and intestines. When presence of heavy metals is suspected (e.g., rifle bullets or ingested lead), survey radiographs may be taken (Fig. 12–2).

Examples of Alterations Found at External Examination

- Broken feathers because of feather picking; diagnosis—normal feathers on the head

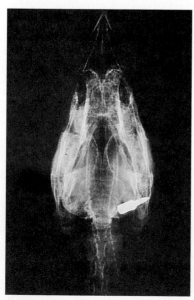

Blue and gold macaw *(Ara ararauna).* Radiograph of the skull shows a rifle bullet in the skull.

- Altered feathers with constrictions at the base caused by psittacine beak and feather disease (PBFD); diagnosis—histology of skin with feather follicles (Fig. 12–3; see also Color Fig. 12–3B); DNA test
- Feather and skin parasites
- Swelling above the eye or dilated nostrils with a plug due to vitamin A deficiency; diagnosis—histologic examination with metaplastic changes in salivary glands (see Color Fig. 12–4).
- Conjunctivitis and sinusitis related to ornithosis or psittacosis
- Conjunctivitis with pox lesions (see Color Fig. 12–5); diagnosis—cytology, histology, and culture
- Abdominal or other swellings (see Color Fig. 12–6), tumors, egg-related peritonitis
- Cloacal mucosal prolapse, papilloma; diagnosis—histology.

Preparation of the Bird

Small birds are wetted and plucked, all other birds should be wetted with alcohol 70% before the necropsy. This is done to allow for better visualization of the skin, to part the feathers to permit incision of the skin, to prevent loose feathers from irritating or harming the prosector (from zoonosis) and contaminating the viscera.

The bird is positioned on its back. In small birds the wings and legs are pinned to a dissecting board with nails or needles; large birds are fixed on a metal tray with pieces of rope.

Postmortem Examination

General procedures for conducting a thorough necropsy include the following:

- Use the gram scale for measuring the size of organs
- Open all tube-like structures
- Cut all parenchymatous organs in slices of 1.5 to 2 mm to find small focal lesions
- Keep tissue for formalin fixation at less than 3 to 4 mm in thickness (5 mm maximum)
- Keep the ratio of tissue to formalin to 1:10
- Collect tissue samples during the necropsy to prevent desiccation. Do not wait until the gross examination is finished

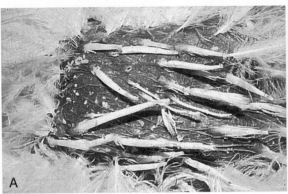 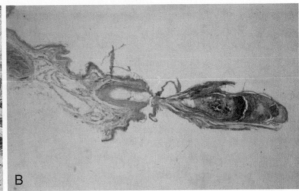

Figure 12-3

(A, B) Sulphur-crested cockatoo *(Cacatua galerita galerita)*. New developing feathers with constrictions at the base—psittacine beak and feather disease (PBFD). Histology examination shows bleeding and necrosis. *(A)* macroscopy, *(B)* histology (4×).

- Remember to collect and submit specimens from a broad spectrum of organs and systems
- Collect heart, lung, liver, spleen, kidney, gonad, and adrenal, and a piece of intestine (duodenum and pancreas) for histopathology
- When suspecting a viral problem, freeze the tissue as soon as possible to −70°C, or collect tissue on wet ice until shipment.

Step 1. An incision is made in the skin along the ventral midline from the mandible over the sternum to the cloaca. The skin is reflected to expose the subcutis, crop, pectoral muscles, keel, abdominal wall, leg muscles, and fat.

Watch for color of the muscles, parasites, subcutaneous hemorrhages, and edema. Judge the amount of food in the crop. In pigeons a vascular plexus in the deep layers of the cutis of the cervical region can be seen, *plexus venosus intracutaneus collaris*. This plexus can be mistaken for an extensive hemorrhage.

Examples

- Stripes in leg or breast muscle: sarcosporidiosis (see Color Fig. 12–7); diagnosis—cytology of such a stripe reveals the bradyzoites
- A large dark spot distal of the keel; swollen liver: diagnosis—see later.
- Changes of the skin: *Knemidocoptes*, yeast infection; diagnosis—wet mount and cytology smear

Step 2. Make an incision through the pectoral muscle along the sides and around the posterior border of the sternum through the abdominal muscles; cut with heavy rongeurs, scissors, or poultry shears through the ribs, coracoid bones, and clavicle to remove the sternum.

Examine the air sacs (Fig. 12–8; see also Color Fig. 12–8B) and pericardial sac, and make impression smears (if necessary). During dissection of the keel the air sacs are easily seen. Normal air sacs appear as glistening transparent membranes.

Examples

- Opaque air sacs: chlamydiosis; diagnosis—cytology with special staining
- Opaque air sacs: bacterial infection; diagnosis—rods or cocci in cytology smear; culture and sensitivity test
- Air sacs covered with white or yellow plaques: fungal infection; diagnosis—wet mount showing hyphae, culture
- Air sacs solid with white/yellow material (see Color Fig. 12–9): chronic fungal infection, mostly aspergillosis; diagnosis—wet mount showing hyphae, culture
- Air sacs, especially cervical and prescapular, with small black dots (see Color Fig. 12–10): *Sternostoma tracheocolum* infestation; diagnosis—magnifying glass and wet mount
- Air sacs, filled with food (see Color Fig. 12–11): forced feeding; diagnosis—wet mount and histology

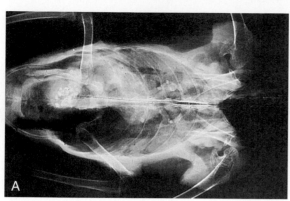
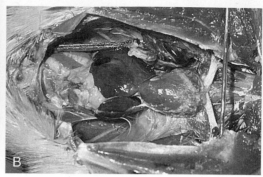

Figure 12-8

(A, B) Blue and gold macaw *(Ara ararauna)* with organ displacement after perforation of the air sacs with a wooden stick. *(A)* radiograph, *(B)* postmortem.

- Pericardial sac filled with fluid: inanition, cachexia; diagnosis—muscle wasting, edema and gelatinous fat tissue
- Pericardium covered with white chalky deposits (see Color Fig. 12–12); visceral gout; diagnosis—wet mount with crystals; often in combination with nephritis

Step 3. Identify the parathyroids and thyroid glands above and lateral to the syrinx along the carotid arteries. The liver is examined in situ (examples, see Step 7 later, on the liver).

Examples

- In budgerigars enlarged thyroid glands; diagnosis—histology
- Parrots (especially African greys): hyperparathyroidism (see Color Fig. 12–13); diagnosis—histology
- "Abscesses" (see Color Fig. 12–14): *Salmonella* or *E. coli* infections; diagnosis—rod-shaped bacteria in cytology, culture

Step 4. The spleen can be found by grasping the gizzard with forceps and rotating it toward the right side. This exposes the spleen in the angle between the proventriculus, gizzard, and liver. Examine, remove, and measure the spleen; make impression smears from a fresh-cut surface after blotting to remove excess of blood.

Examples

- Spleen swelling together with air sac opacity: chlamydiosis; diagnosis—see earlier
- Very large swollen and cherry red spleen in parrots, watch for herpes virus infection (Pacheco's disease) or *Sarcocystis* infection; diagnosis—liver necrosis with intranuclear inclusion bodies or protozoa, cytology, histology, IFT, virus isolation
- Swelling and pale: (bacterial) septicemia; diagnosis—cytology with bacteria, culture
- Multiple irregular yellow foci in the spleen: tuberculosis; diagnosis—the same foci in other organs, in imprint nonstaining rods, acid-fast. Differentiation avian/bovine strains by culture
- Large firm spleen (see Color Fig. 12–15): tumor; diagnosis—histology
- Enlarged friable spleen with multiple, miliary necrotic foci (see Color Fig. 12–16): salmonellosis, yersiniosis; diagnosis—the same foci in liver and ceca; imprint with rod-shaped bacteria; culture
- Homogeneous red enlarged spleen in canaries and finches: atoxoplasmosis; diagnosis—cytology
- Small, gray spleen: lymphoid depletion; stress, viral infection; diagnosis—cytology, histology, virus isolation

Step 5. Remove the heart with the carotids and thyroids attached and cut across the apex to check for an "open" lumen and to assess the thickness of the ventricular walls (see Color Fig. 12–17). Open the heart and large vessels and examine the valves and endocardial surface. Keep in mind that the right atrioventricular valve in birds is a muscular structure.

Examples

- Yellow plaques on the wall inside the large vessels; the vessels are stiff: arteriosclerosis; diagnosis—macroscopy, histology
- Epi- or endocardial hemorrhages: septicemia or agonal event; diagnosis—continue postmortem
- Gelatinous, serous pericardial fat: starvation, chronic illness; diagnosis—continue postmortem
- Pericardium covered with white chalky material (see Color Fig. 12–18): pericarditis uricemia; diagnosis—macroscopy, polaroid microscopy
- Changes (inflammation, necrosis) in the myocardium: myocarditis; diagnosis—cytology, histology, microbiologic isolation, continue postmortem
- Cardiomyopathy with muscle cysts: *Sarcocystis* infection; diagnosis—cytology, histology
- A enlarged lumen of the left ventricle and only little difference in thickness of the ventricle walls: heart failure (see Color Fig. 12–19); diagnosis—congestion of the lungs and/or liver

Step 6. To remove the viscera, cut the esophagus in the bifurcation of the trachea and with combined blunt and sharp dissection remove the viscera including the liver, leaving the lungs and kidneys. Do not cut the cloaca, but bend the viscera caudally.

Step 7. Separate liver from the viscera by holding the ligaments in the forceps and cutting them with scissors. Examine the gall bladder (if present). Make impression smears and a culture from the liver. For a thorough examination, slice the liver at regular intervals.

Examples

- Enlarged red variegated liver with pale areas: hepatitis; diagnosis—cytology with many inflammatory cells; histology
- Enlarged liver with necrotic foci: hepatitis by chlamydiosis, herpes virus infection (see Color Fig. 12–20); diagnosis—imprints, ELISA, culture, histology
- Very extensive acute liver necrosis: suspect periacute or acute hepatitis by bacterial septicemia, polyoma-, herpes, or reovirus; diagnosis—macroscopy, cytology, histology, virology, culture
- Focal yellow proliferation often with central necrosis (see Color Fig. 12–21): tuberculosis; diagnosis—see earlier
- Small round necrotic foci (see Color Fig. 12–22): salmonellosis or yersiniosis; diagnosis—imprints with rod-shaped bacteria; culture
- Evenly enlarged, often variegated, pale liver: leukosis; diagnosis—macroscopy (see Fig. 12–6); other organs are often included; cytology and histology
- Evenly enlarged, often variegated, pale soft liver: degeneration; diagnosis—cytology hepatocytes with vacuoles; histology
- Enlarged orange, yellow liver (see Color Fig. 12–23): fatty liver; diagnosis—macroscopy, cytology, histology with Sudan III stain
- Liver with necrotic ulcer (see Color Fig. 12–24): histomoniasis (black head); diagnosis—histology

Step 8. Examine the adrenals, gonads (determine sex) and genital tract, and the kidney with ureters in situ. Look for the thymus.

Examples

- A swelling inside the oviduct: egg binding, egg concrements; diagnosis—open the oviduct
- Irregular swellings related to kidney or gonads (see Color Fig. 12–25): tumor; diagnosis—macroscopy and histology
- Pale swollen kidneys with white striation (see Color Fig. 12–26): urate congestion; diagnosis—dehydration; histology (fixation 100% alcohol!)
- Irregular pale swollen kidney with white foci (see Color Fig. 12–27): "renal gout"; diagnosis—histology (fixation 100% alcohol)
- Irregular swollen kidney with multifocal abscesses: bacterial infection; diagnosis—histology, cytology, culture
- Enlarged red kidneys; acute nephritis; diagnosis—histology
- Pale, swollen, friable kidneys: kidney degeneration; diagnosis—histology

- White, firm, small kidneys (see Color Fig. 12–28): chronic kidney fibrosis; diagnosis—macroscopy; histology

Step 9. Free the lungs by applying gentle traction to the trachea and esophagus and cut the attachment to the ventral ribs and backbone at the thoracic inlet. This may be difficult because there is no pleural space in birds. Using blunt and sharp dissection frees the lungs and the kidneys, but look for the sciatic nerve in the middle division. Inspect the lungs and the kidneys. Watch for the thymus. Open the esophagus. To open the syrinx, trachea, and main bronchi a strip has to be cut out (Fig. 12–29); cut through the lungs at intervals; make an impression smear from the lungs. In our laboratory the kidneys are not routinely screened in cytology examinations.

Examples

- Dark-colored gray lungs (see Color Fig. 12–30): lung edema; diagnosis—on cut surface clear seral fluid
- Dark-colored wet red lungs: lung congestion; diagnosis—from a cut surface only blood; the lungs are supple and evenly bright red—watch

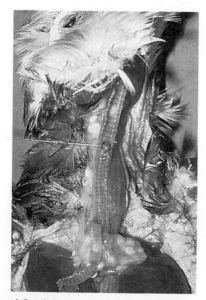

Figure 12–29

Cockatiel *(Nymphicus hollandicus)* after inhalation of millet seed.

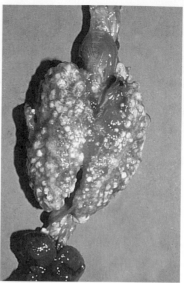

Figure 12–32

Yellow-fronted Amazon *(A. ochrocephala)* with subacute massive inhalation of *Aspergillus* spores, mycotic pneumonia.

for congestion in other organs and alterations of the heart. Think also of polytetrafluoroethylene (Teflon) toxicosis (see Color Fig. 12–31), acute mycotic infection, and *Sarcocystis* infection
- Dark, firm lungs often variegated with focal changes: pneumonic foci; diagnosis—cut surface, cytology (inflammation cells), histology
- Dark, supple, dry lungs: atelectasis; diagnosis—on cut surface only a dark color of the surface of the lung and dried up
- White or yellow foci scattered through the lungs (Fig. 12–32; see Color Fig. 12–33): aspergillosis, tuberculosis; diagnosis—wet mount with hyphae, acid-fast rods (in routine quick staining, non-stained rods); culture and histology
- Irregular scattered pneumonic foci: bacterial pneumonia; e.g., *Salmonella* species or *Yersinia* species; diagnosis—cytology and culture
- In the syrinx of parrots white material: syringal mycosis; based on metaplasia due to vitamin A deficiency; diagnosis—see aspergillosis
- In the trachea, red worms: *Syngamus* species, black dots; *Sternostoma* mites; mucous and fibrin; avipox

Step 10. Examine the "abdominal" viscera. Open and inspect the proventriculus and gizzard (with koilin layer). Examine the contents for foreign

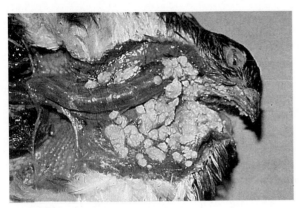

Figure 12–37

Pigeon *(Columba livia)* with diphtheric lesions in the crop, avipox.

bodies and heavy metals. The bowel should be opened by making longitudinal cuts at intervals to examine the contents and the wall for changes and parasites. Open and inspect the ceca when present. Look for the pancreas (see Color Fig. 12–34), bursa, and umbilical sac. Take the following samples:

> From the duodenum and rectum for parasitology (as well as direct examination on very fresh specimens for flagellates)
> From the rectum a smear for staining (DiffQuick)
> From the rectum for microbiology

Examples

Crop

- Thickened wall with white material (see Color Fig. 12–35): yeast infection; diagnosis—smear of the material, culture

- Thickened wall with gray-yellow material, sometimes with trapped air bubbles (see Color Fig. 12–36): trichomoniasis; diagnosis—wet mount, cytology, histology
- Local yellow necrotic ulcera (Fig. 12–37): pox lesions; diagnosis—macroscopy, histology, virus culture
- Local red mucosal thickening: papillomas; diagnosis—histology

Stomach (Proventriculus and Ventriculus)

- Dilated proventriculus and gizzard, often stuffed with seeds (sunflower) (Fig. 12–38): gastric dilatation syndrome; diagnosis—histology, (ganglio) neuritis
- An empty proventriculus with excess of mucus (see Color Fig. 12–39): "megabacteria"; diagnosis—wet mount and cytology
- Swollen red glands in proventriculus: *Tetrameres* species; diagnosis—parasitologic examination

Intestines

- Hemorrhagic contents duodenum: coccidiosis; diagnosis—wet mount, cytology
- Hemorrhagic, black contents in the entire small intestine (see Color Fig. 12–40): hemorrhagic diathesis; diagnosis—history (fasting for over 24 hours), macroscopy
- Hemorrhagic contents: lead intoxication, clostridial infection, *Pseudomonas* infection, *Giardia* species (see Color Fig. 12–41); diagnosis—lead in

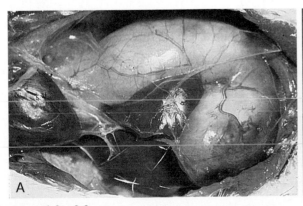
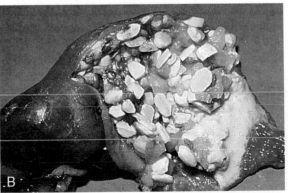

Figure 12–38

(A, B) Sulphur-crested cockatoo *(Cacatua g. galerita)* showing the dilated proventriculus and gizzard, stuffed with seeds, gastric dilatation syndrome. *(A)* dilated stomachs, *(B)* after opening of the stomachs.

gizzard, lead analysis of liver and kidneys, cytology, culture
- Pseudomembranous covering of the duodenal wall: hexamitiasis; in cranes; diagnosis—wet mounts, cytology, and histology
- Thickened wall with or without blood in the lumen: enteritis; diagnosis—wet mount and cytology, parasitology, microbiology. Beware: in small passerines rarely worms, often Coccidia species (see Color Figs. 12–42, 12–43); in psittacines very rarely Coccidia, often *Ascaridia* (Fig. 12–44)
- Clear watery contents in small intestine with flabby wall: hexamitiasis; diagnosis—fresh wet mount, cytology, histology
- Yellow nondigested starch and broken seeds in small passerines: *Cochlosoma* or *Campylobacter* species; diagnosis—fresh wet mount, cytology, selective culture
- Enlarged ceca with pseudomembranous to necropurulent content (see Color Fig. 12–45): typhlitis; diagnosis—Galliformes: histomoniasis, "black head"; diagnosis—cytology, histology (often with liver lesions)
- Ceca with nodular lesions: parasitic typhlitis; pheasants: *Heterakis isolonga*; diagnosis—worms and ova; histology

Cloaca

- Congested, swollen red mucosa: papilloma; diagnosis—histology

BEWARE: TRY TO ESTABLISH A RELATIONSHIP BETWEEN THE CLINICAL HISTORY AND THE POST-MORTEM FINDINGS

Step 11. Open the anterior part of the esophagus from the beak, make a wet mount. Remove the tongue and cut the salivary glands. Inspect the beak, choanae, and esophagus.

Examples

- See also crop/intestines (e.g., trichomoniasis, pox, candidiasis)
- Chronic, necrotic lesions especially in commissures (see Color Fig. 12–46): tuberculosis: diagnosis—cytology (acid-fast stain), histology, culture

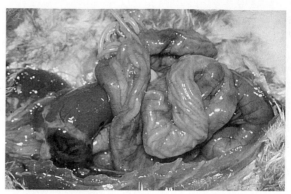

Figure 12–44

Red-rumped parakeet *(Psephotus haematonotus)*. The intestines are filled with nematodes, Ascaridia species.

- Tongue with yellow "abscesses" at the location of the salivary glands (see Color Fig. 12–47): metaplasia due to vitamin A deficiency; diagnosis—wet mount, diet history, histology

Step 12. Cut across the beak through the nostrils and sinuses.

Examples

- The presence of turbid mucus: sinusitis; diagnosis—wet mount, cytology, culture

Step 13. Inspect the joints, bones, bone marrow, brains. Joints of the wings, legs, and feet should be opened and examined. If exudate is present, both cytologic as well as microbiologic examination should be done. White, chalky deposits may represent urate deposition.

Bone marrow is most easily collected from the tibiotarsus for both cytology and histology examination. In bone marrow, tuberculosis lesions can be found (see Color Fig. 12–48); they are often visible on radiographs.

Examination of the nervous system and associated tissues is governed by the presence or absence of neurological or ocular disease.[3]

The brain may be removed by skinning the head, making a sagittal incision through the calvarium and removing the bony calvarium to expose the brain (see Color Fig. 12–49). When sampling for histology, it is often better to leave the brain inside the skull after opening it and to immerse the whole head in formalin.

Ecchymoses within the calvarium are a common agonal change and do not imply head trauma (see Color Fig. 12–50).

Step 14. The muscles of the legs and sciatic nerve running on the posterior surface of the femur should be examined.

Final Activities

1. Bacterial cultures are taken from the liver and the rectum and all abnormal organs, especially when bacteria are seen in the imprints! The following media are selected: blood agar, selective Enterobacteriaceae agar (brilliant green agar), or McConkey agar and serum broth.

The intestinal contents are collected in tetrathionate broth as an enrichment medium for *Salmonella* species. When special microorganisms are expected (e.g., anaerobes, *Campylobacter* species) contact the laboratory.

2. When a mycotic problem is suspected, a malt-agar or other selective culture medium is selected as well.

3. The impression smears are allowed to dry, stained with Hemacolor or DiffQuick and Stamp or Macchiavello's (for *Chlamydia*) stains, and examined by microscope with objective ×100 in immersion oil.

The slide for an immunofluorescence test (IFT) for *Chlamydia* is fixed in cold acetone (freezer −20°C) and sent to the laboratory.

4. *Positive* cytology results require sampling for *Chlamydia* ELISA.

5. Examine the wet preparations of gut contents.

6. Samples collected for ancillary diagnostics should be packed, labeled, and stored properly until shipment. See that each sample is provided with the essential documentation.[2]

7. Make a detailed report and use this to document the samples.

References

1. Graham DL: Check list for necropsy of the pet bird and preparation and submission of necropsy specimens—A mnemonic aid for the busy avian practitioner. Assoc Avian Vet: Introduction to Avian Medicine and Surgery, New Orleans, 1992, Dx7, pp 1–4.
2. Lowenstine LJ: Necropsy procedures. In Harrison GJ, Harrison LR (eds): Clinical Avian Medicine and Surgery. Philadelphia, WB Saunders, 1986, pp 298–309.
3. Latimer SL, Rakich PM: Necropsy examination. In Ritchie BW, Harrison GJ, Harrison LR (eds): Avian Medicine: Principles and Application. Lake Worth, FL, Wingers Publishing, 1994, pp 355–379.

Bonnie J. Smith
Stephen A. Smith

13

Radiology

Radiography is one of the most important diagnostic tools available to the avian veterinarian. Radiography is useful as a primary diagnostic technique, and also as an adjunct to other procedures in differentiation among possible diagnoses, monitoring the progression of clinical conditions, and evaluating effectiveness of treatments. Radiographing birds is simple, noninvasive, cost-effective, and generally well received by clients. With the exception of severely ill birds or those in respiratory difficulty, properly performed radiographic examination is minimally stressful to the patient. Excellent descriptions of the normal radiographic anatomy of psittacine species have been available for some time,[1] and more recent descriptions of numerous other species[2] have broadened the applicability of radiography in avian medicine.

This chapter provides a basic introduction to the use and application of radiography in avian medicine. An exhaustive treatment of avian radiographic diagnosis is beyond the scope of this chapter. However, familiarity with avian radiographic anatomic features as presented here, together with application of basic radiographic principles in the interpretation of avian radiographs, yield significant diagnostic and prognostic information to the practicing avian clinician. In all descriptions, radiographic terminology follows that approved by the American College of Veterinary Radiology.[3]

TECHNIQUES IN RADIOGRAPHY

Techniques for Optimal Detail

Partially related to the small body size of many patients, radiographic equipment must be fully rec-

tified to ensure consistent exposures. Following routine detail-enhancing principles, such as the use of a small focal spot, collimated beam, and high- or ultra-detail film, together with the shortest exposure times possible (1/30 to 1/60 second) is necessary to produce the most useful films. High-detail film is particularly recommended for use with small species. Intensifying screens may also be used. A methodology using human mammography techniques has been employed that provides excellent detail in radiographing avian patients.* Kodak Min-R single emulsion mammography film is used in single intensifying screen cassettes. Milliamperage settings of 1000 to 1200 together with short exposure times of 1/60 to 1/120 second and kilovolts peak settings of 40 to 50 kVp generally yield the best diagnostic-quality films.

Regardless of the system used, the cassette is placed directly on the tabletop, using neither a grid nor a bucky. The bird is positioned either directly on the cassette or on a thin plexiglass positioning board placed on the cassette. Certain commercially available positioning boards are equipped with various restraint aids, facilitating the optimal situation of requiring no handlers in the room during exposure.

Citation of specific values for radiographic technique is difficult because details vary with individual machines, films, and cassettes. Beyond variation in equipment, size differences among avian species prevent any single technique from applying in all instances. In general, use of either a feline technique or extremities charts is often adequate for birds the size of medium parrots. For smaller and larger species, adjustments are necessary in milliam-

---

*J. Stefanacci, personal communication.

peres and kilovolts peak (typically by 5–10 U), using as little kilovolts peak as possible to obtain the best contrast. Initially, trial and error must be used to tailor technique to individual machines. Once successful techniques have been achieved with individual equipment, a permanent record should be made and kept with the x-ray machine. Several detailed descriptions of useful techniques have been published,[4–9] and practitioners may use them as initial guidelines subject to their own modification.

Restraint

Opinions vary as to the need or advisability of chemical restraint during avian radiography. Both chemical and physical restraint have attendant advantages and disadvantages, and each may be preferable to the other based on individual circumstance. Despite the risks of anesthesia, some species as well as individuals of any species may be poor candidates for solely physical restraint. Physical restraint alone is unacceptable in birds that are highly stressed or struggling, or in those that have an injury that can be exacerbated by handling. Particularly, chemical restraint is often necessary with the larger, more fractious psittacine species. The nature of an individual of any species may also dictate the prudent use of chemical restraint. Each bird must be evaluated and appropriate restraint decided upon on an individual basis, giving simple physical restraint fair consideration first.

Judicious use of anesthesia can permit production of diagnostic quality radiographs without multiple exposures or risk of injury to an uncooperative patient. Because of the importance of positioning with completely extended limbs, anesthesia may be required if an inability to achieve extension becomes apparent during positioning. Inhalation anesthesia using isoflurane is by far the method of choice. Birds can be directly "masked down" and radiographed, and most recover quickly with minimal side effects from anesthesia. Injectable compounds may also be used, but for reasons related to their prolonged effect, slow reversibility, and minimal safety margin, injectable anesthetics are not the method of choice. (For a discussion of the use of anesthetics and tranquilizers in birds, see Chapter 46.)

Although required at times, chemical restraint or anesthesia during radiography has distinct disadvantages. Anesthesia in healthy birds can be unpredictable. In stressed or clinically ill birds or in birds with respiratory distress anesthesia can be an unacceptable risk. Furthermore, many sedatives and tranquilizers are respiratory depressants, and can thereby interfere with interpretation of the lungs and air sacs.

Although the use of physical restraint alone is fundamentally simple, appropriate care must nonetheless be taken in its use. Most difficulties or injuries associated with physical restraint are the result of stress on seriously ill patients or fractured bones due to improper restraint. The latter typically occurs in small birds and birds with metabolic bone disease, or in cases when an inexperienced handler is too forceful.

Many avian species can be successfully radiographed using only physical restraint, if handled with slow and gentle motions in a darkened, quiet room. Species that are not apt to struggle and/or become overly stressed while handled include smaller species up to the size of a cockatiel, as well as most raptorial species. Placing a mask or lightweight glove over the bird's head is often helpful. The use of positioning boards can allow handlers to leave the room during exposure. However, when the use of a board is not practical or possible, proper collimation of the beam, use of lead-lined protective gear by handlers, and avoidance of lead-gloved hands contacting the primary beam should confer safety to the handlers. Generally, two people are necessary to restrain the bird in the proper ventrodorsal (VD) position, although one person may suffice for restraining the bird in the lateral position. The manipulations and actual restraint must be brief to minimize chances of the bird beginning to move or struggle. Thus, no more than 2 to 3 minutes should ideally be required to complete both views.

Lightly applied masking tape can be an excellent restraint or positioning aid in species of all sizes, whether used alone or with chemical restraint. This is particularly true in the smallest species, where handling with lead-lined gloves is difficult and dangerous to the bird. Birds may be taped either directly to the film cassette or to a positioning board. Masking tape is preferred to other tapes, being easily applied, largely radiolucent, nonirritating to the bird's skin, and, most importantly, easily removed without damage to feathers. To restrain the bird in the VD or lateral position, tape is generally applied across the carpometacarpus, tarsometatarsus, and cranial cervical region. The advantage offered by placing tape over the body must be weighed against the detail desired in the imaging of soft tissues in the body cavity. If a body tape is applied, care must be taken not to place it so tightly as to restrict sternal movement and, thereby, breathing. Great care must also be taken in removal of tape. When removing tape from the wings, tape should be pulled from cranial to caudal direction so that the rachis of the feather is not bent. Furthermore, when feathers of any body region stick tightly to the tape, the feather should be gently pressed off the tape rather than the tape pulled off the feather, thus avoiding bending the rachis or pulling the calamus from the follicle. Such care is necessary because feather damage is permanent, and a damaged feather will not be replaced until the next moult.

Older literature describes other techniques of physical restraint such as placing the bird in stockinette, radiographing the bird as it sits on a perch, or placing the bird in a tube or wrap formed from old x-ray film, clear plastic, or other material. However, any method of radiographing a bird in a position with its limbs folded and/or superimposed over the body produces a largely unusable radiograph. This position produces superimposition of the long bones of all limbs on each other and on the body cavities, resulting in a jumbled mass of body parts that cannot be clearly distinguished. Neither bone nor soft tissue of any body region can be adequately evaluated with a bird in such a position.

Positioning

Correct positioning is absolutely critical in obtaining useful avian radiographs. Even slight rotation of the body produces artifactual changes in the radiographic image that may obscure or mimic important clinical signs. Failure to completely extend the limbs can produce difficulties in evaluation of the soft tissues of the body, as well as of the long bones and joints. Thus, meticulous positioning prevents the need for repeated exposures. Two views, the VD and lateral, are mandatory in avian radiography,

as with any species. Films should be exposed on inspiration when possible.

For the VD view of the body, the bird is placed in dorsal recumbency, and the bird's right side is identified with an appropriate marker. The keel of the sternum is placed directly over the vertebral column. On a properly positioned radiograph, the keel and the vertebral column are directly superimposed. The wings are symmetrically and almost fully extended with the carpometacarpus at the level of the shoulder; the pelvic limbs are symmetrically and fully extended without rotation. Extension of the limbs is necessary to permit proper interpretation of the body cavities. Correct limb positioning also permits evaluation of both shoulder regions and the proximal humerus, as well as both hip regions and proximal femurs on the VD body view. Optimal positioning includes extension of the neck.

Importance of proper positioning in the VD view of the body cannot be overemphasized; minor rotation of the body can convincingly mimic soft tissue disease (see the section on the gastrointestinal system). In small species, the entire body and extremities can often be imaged on a single film, with useful full-length VD views of the wings and craniocaudal (CC) views of the pelvic limbs obtained on the same film as the VD view of the body.

For the lateral view of the body, the bird is usually placed in right lateral recumbency and an appropriate film marker is used. The wings are extended over the back of the bird, with the dependent wing placed slightly cranial to the upper wing to permit differentiation of right from left. The pelvic limbs are fully extended and drawn as far caudally as possible to facilitate unobstructed evaluation of the abdominal soft tissue. Similar to the wings, the dependent limb is placed slightly cranial to the upper limb. Optimal positioning again includes extension of the neck. In the correctly positioned lateral radiograph, the scapulohumeral joints and the acetabula are superimposed. Unlike the VD view, the lateral views of the limbs produced on lateral body views are suitable for only cursory survey, even in small birds.

When the head or neck is the primary concern, separate radiographs of these regions should be prepared. Anesthesia is required when performing radiography of the head. If gas anesthesia is used, the handler can work quickly to prepare one view at a time by removing the cone from the bird's head, positioning the bird, and replacing the cone for a few moments prior to proceeding with the next view. Lateral, VD, and rostrocaudal ("face-on") views of the head are routinely prepared. In addition, an oblique view of the head, which permits separate visualization of each eye and orbital region, can be very useful in evaluating conditions such as head trauma and sinusitis.

To evaluate the wings, the VD view is prepared either as a part of the whole-body view of smaller birds, or as a separate exposure in larger birds. The CC view of the wing should be prepared as the second view. In the CC view, the wing may be aligned to superimpose the bones of the antebrachium and of the carpal and digital regions on the film, or rotated slightly to permit separate imaging of these bony elements. The CC view can be prepared by moving the x-ray tube to a horizontal position, placing the cassette in a vertical holder at table level, and then placing the bird in ventral recumbency while extending the wing in front of the cassette. If the x-ray tube cannot be rotated, this view can be obtained by placing the cassette at the edge of the table, and then holding the bird upside down with the body off the edge of the table with the head pointing toward the floor, and the cranial edge of the extended wing in contact with the cassette. Although this procedure is admittedly cumbersome, the advantages offered by having the second view of the wing far exceed the technical difficulties involved.

To evaluate the pelvic limbs in small birds, the CC view can be prepared as part of the whole-body VD view. Larger birds will require preparation of a separate film, obtained with the bird positioned essentially as for a VD view of the body. The mediolateral view of the pelvic limb is prepared separately, even in small birds. For the mediolateral view, the bird is placed in lateral recumbency with the desired limb in direct contact with the cassette. The limb is extended as far as possible in a directly ventral position, rather than extended caudally as in the lateral body view. The opposite limb is then drawn caudally, and the bird's body rotated slightly dorsally to completely remove the undesired limb from the final view.

The feet should be separately imaged when these extremities are the primary region of interest. Achieving proper positioning of each toe while concurrently concerned with positioning of the remain-

der of the limb for a VD or lateral view is time-consuming, difficult, and often counterproductive. Small pieces of tape may be applied to each claw to hold the toes separate from each other in both the dorsoplantar and lateral views of the feet.

NORMAL RADIOGRAPHIC ANATOMY

Thorough understanding of unique avian anatomic features is necessary for complete and correct interpretation of avian radiographs. Brief mention will be made here only of those features directly relevant to radiographic interpretation.

Axial Skeleton

The scleral ring of the eye (Figs. 13–1 to 13–6) is visible in most avian species, being smallest in pet species and largest in owls and diurnal raptors. Portions of the infraorbital sinus are often evident

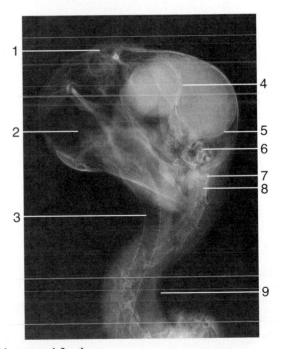

F i g u r e   1 3 – 1

Lateral (Le-Rt) view of the head of the Goffin cockatoo. Note the large, muscular tongue, typical of psittacine species. 1 = cere, 2 = entoglossum within tongue, 3 = trachea, 4 = caudal edge of orbit, 5 = caudal edge of cranial cavity, 6 = semicircular canals, 7 = atlas, 8 = axis, 9 = cervicocephalic air sac.

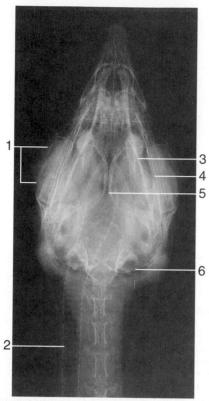

Figure 13–2

Ventrodorsal view of the head of the Goffin cockatoo. Note the large size of the eyes and their close approximation on the midline. Note also the relatively small size and flat orientation of the scleral ring (compare with Figs. 13–5 and 13–6). 1 = scleral ring, 2 = trachea, 3 = mandible, 4 = jugal (zygomatic) arch, 5 = medial orbital border, 6 = caudal edge of cranial cavity.

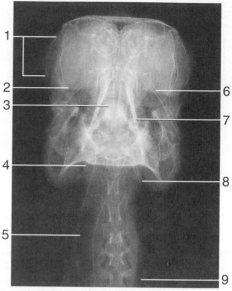

Figure 13–3

Rostrocaudal view of the head of the Goffin cockatoo. Care must be taken not to mistake the joint between the epi- and ceratobranchial bones for a fracture. 1 = scleral ring, 2 = edge of cranial cavity, 3 = tongue, 4 = ceratobranchial bone of hyoid apparatus, 5 = trachea, 6 = jugal (zygomatic) arch, 7 = mandible, 8 = epibranchial bone of the hyoid apparatus, 9 = cervicocephalic air sac.

radiographically. Cervical ribs are normally not imaged in conventional films. The fused vertebrae of the notarium, synsacrum, and pygostyle are visible in the VD view as specific regions of the spinal column (Figs. 13–7 and 13–9 to 13–11). Vertebral ribs are best visualized in the lateral view (Figs. 13–8, 13–12). The ossified sternal ribs are not always evident in the VD view, but in the lateral view (see Figs. 13–8, 13–12) are clearly visualized. The uncinate processes of the vertebral ribs are normally not seen. The keel of the sternum is visible on the lateral view (see Figs. 13–8, 13–12) as a ventral expansion of the sternum, and on the VD view (see Figs. 13–7, and 13–9 to 13–11) as a thin line superimposed over the vertebral column. The free caudal vertebrae are clearly distinguishable from the pygostyle (see Figs. 13–7 to 13–12).

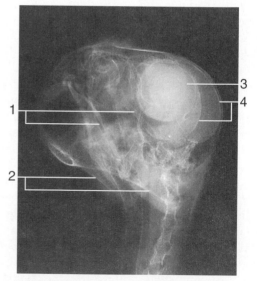

Figure 13–4

Oblique (LeD-RtVO) view of the head of the Goffin cockatoo. Note how the left ("upper") eye is imaged in its entirety, and how the entire anterior edge of the scleral ring can be viewed. 1 = jugal (zygomatic) arch, 2 = mandible, 3 = scleral ring, 4 = edge of cranial cavity.

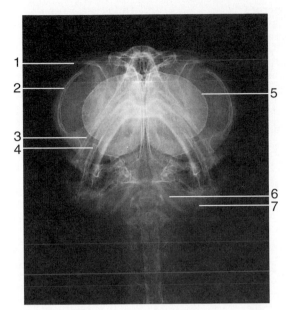

Figure 13–5

Rostrocaudal view of the head of the red-tailed hawk. Note the prominence of the lacrimal bone and the scleral ring (compare with Fig. 13–3). 1 = lacrimal bone, 2 = scleral ring, 3 = jugal (zygomatic) arch, 4 = mandible, 5 = lateral margin of cranial cavity, 6 = ceratobranchial bone of the hyoid apparatus, 7 = epibranchial bone of the hyoid apparatus.

Appendicular Skeleton

The most striking feature of the long bones is the normally thin nature of their cortices (Figs. 13–13 to 13–16). This appearance in a mammal of comparable size would indicate osteoporosis. The thin cortex is normal in birds, in part as a result of the invasion of the medullary cavity by air sacs. In reproductively active females, the endosteal and intramedullary density normally increase prior to the egg-laying part of the cycle.

The bones of the pectoral girdle are often best visualized in the views of the body. The coracoid bone is clearly visualized in both views (see Figs. 13–7 to 13–12). Owing to its function as a strut bracing the wing against the sternum, the coracoid bone must be carefully evaluated in cases of wing or thoracic trauma. The proximal region of the elongate scapula is evident in both views, but the distalmost region can be somewhat difficult to visualize in either view (see Figs. 13–7 to 13–12). The furcula (i.e., the two fused clavicles) are best imaged on the lateral view (see Figs. 13–8, 13–12), but can also be visualized on the VD view (see Figs. 13–7 and

13–9 to 13–11). The marked species-specific variations in its form are best appreciated on the lateral view. The ulna is larger and more robust than the radius, and the attachment sites of the secondary flight feathers to the ulna may be visible (see Fig. 13–13). The radial and ulnar carpal bones are imaged separately in the VD view, as are the alular, major, and minor metacarpal bones and digits (see Fig. 13–13).

In the pelvic limb, the termination of the fibula against the shaft of the tibiotarsus is often visible in the CC view, with the proximal interosseous space bridged to a varying degree by tissue of moderate radiodensity (see Fig. 13–16). The first metatarsal bone, being small, free, and located distally on the tarsometatarsus, must not be mistaken for a phalanx. Nearly all avian species have four toes, but the arrangement of the toes varies; in most species, one digit (I) is directed caudally and three digits (II

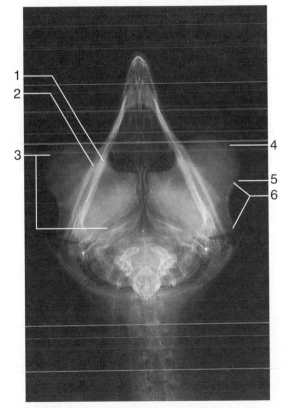

Figure 13–6

Ventrodorsal view of the head of the great horned owl. Note the immense size of the eyes, and the scleral ring. 1 = mandible, 2 = jugal (zygomatic) arch, 3 = antero-posterior dimension of the eye, 4 = cornea, 5 = limbus, 6 = scleral ring.

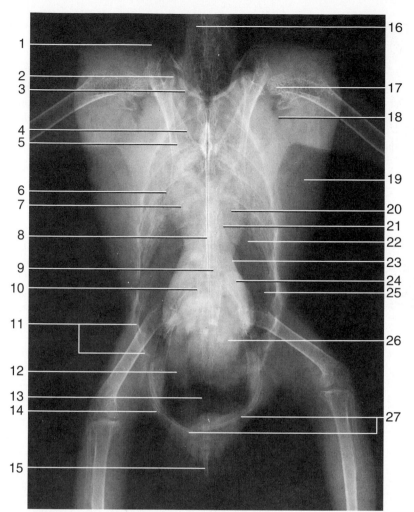

Figure 13–7

Ventrodorsal view of the body of the orange-winged Amazon parrot. 1 = shoulder extremity of coracoid bone, 2 = head of scapula, 3 = clavicle, 4 = medial margin of coracoid bone, 5 = dorsal (medial) margin of scapula, 6 = caudal extremity of scapula, 7 = vertebral rib, 8 = keel of sternum, 9 = region of cardiac apex, 10 = synsacrum, 11 = sternal ribs, 12 = intestinal loops, 13 = free caudal vertebrae, 14 = terminal process of ischium, 15 = pygostyle, 16 = trachea, 17 = humeral head, 18 = clavicular air sacs, 19 = pectoral muscles, 20 = heart, 21 = cranial margin of liver, 22 = lung, 23 = cardiohepatic angle. (Note that the lateral proventricular margin is not typically included in the cardiohepatic angle.) 24 = liver, 25 = overlap of caudal thoracic and abdominal air sacs, 26 = ventriculus containing grit, 27 = pubis (right and left).

to IV) cranially. However, psittaciform birds and some others have two digits (I and IV) directed caudally, and two directed cranially. Owls can voluntarily place their toes in either of these described positions. However, digits of species of common veterinary importance are characterized by an anatomic feature that permits positive identification of any toe independent of its placement; each digit possesses one more phalanx than the number of the digit itself. Thus, digit I has two phalanges, digit II has three, and so on. This feature provides a convenient way to specifically identify individual toes on the film.

Respiratory System

In the VD view, the trachea is visible coursing on the *right* side of the neck (see Figs. 13–2, 13–3, 13–5 to 13–7, 13–9 to 13–11). Toucans and mynah birds are characterized by a normal ventral deviation of the trachea just cranial to the thoracic inlet, which is visible in the lateral view. The syrinx of male ducks is modified into the syringeal bulla. This bony and cartilaginous structure is readily visible near the thoracic inlet on the VD view (see Fig. 13–10), and permits radiographic differentiation of the sexes in ducks. The syrinx of other species is not routinely visualized. The lungs are best visualized on the lateral view (see Figs. 13–8, 13–12). Cartilage in tertiary bronchioles produces a prominent stippled or honeycombed appearance that would be alarming in mammals. In the VD view (see Figs. 13–7 and 13–9 to 13–11), the peripheral lung fields are normally slightly more dense than the medial fields because of the concave shape of

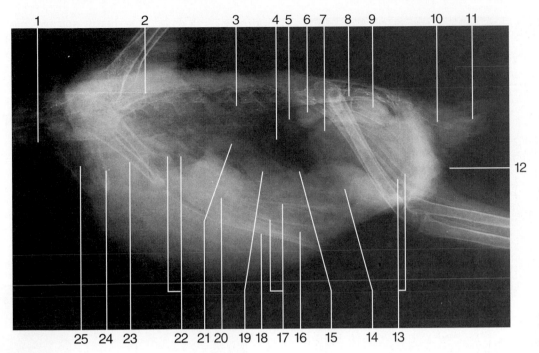

Figure 13-8

Lateral (Le-Rt) view of the body of the orange-winged Amazon parrot. Note the absence of a uropygial gland, typical of Amazon parrots. 1 = trachea, 2 = scapula, 3 = lung, 4 = overlap of caudal thoracic and abdominal air sacs, 5 = gonadal region, 6 = cranial division of kidney, 7 = intestinal loops, 8 = synsacrum, 9 = caudal division of kidney, 10 = free caudal vertebrae, 11 = pygostyle, 12 = vent, 13 = pubis (left and right), 14 = ventriculus, 15 = spleen, 16 = liver, 17 = sternal ribs, 18 = dorsal margin of keel, 19 = proventriculus, 20 = heart, 21 = thoracic esophagus joining proventriculus, 22 = great vessels of heart, 23 = coracoid bone, 24 = clavicle, 25 = crop containing ingesta.

the lungs. The nonexpansile lungs do not change in size on inspiration and expiration.

Portions of the cavities of several air sacs are visible, but their thin walls are not normally observed. The cervicocephalic air sac system is present in psittaciform (see Fig. 13–1), columbiform, and galliform birds and can cover much of the head and neck, sometimes imparting a false impression of subcutaneous emphysema. Diverticula of the clavicular air sac are visible interspersed among the shoulder muscles in the VD view (see Figs. 13–7 and 13–9 to 13–11). The caudal thoracic and the abdominal air sacs appear on the VD view (see Figs. 13–7 and 13–9 to 13–11) as prominent symmetric lucencies on either side of the thoracoabdominal viscera, and they change size noticeably with ventilatory movements. The right and left abdominal air sacs extend as far caudally as the lateral margins of the cloaca, with the right abdominal air sac often extending slightly more caudally than the left. On the lateral view (see Figs. 13–8, 13–12), the air sacs

are not as widely visualized, being restricted to a relatively small, roughly triangular lucent area bordered by the lungs dorsally, kidneys caudally, and proventriculus-ventriculus ventrally.

Cardiovascular System

In part because of the high avian metabolic rate and cardiac output, the heart is proportionately larger in birds than in comparably sized mammals. The base of the heart is normally visible radiographically on both the VD and lateral views (see Figs. 13–7 to 13–12), and the great vessels can also be visualized. End-on views of the great vessels must be distinguished from granulomas in the lung. The heart normally lies in contact with the sternum and extends from the second to the fifth or sixth ribs. Because the liver envelops the caudal half of the heart, the cardiac apex is not visible, but rather is superimposed with the liver. Normally, the superim-

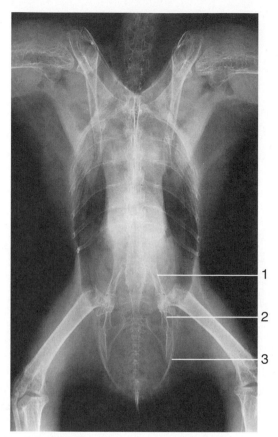

Figure 13-9

Ventrodorsal view of the body of the great horned owl. Note the absence of the cardiohepatic angle and the sculpturing of the ischium. 1 = ilium, 2 = ischium, 3 = pubis.

posed shadows of the heart and liver create an hourglass-shaped shadow in the VD view of most species of veterinary importance (see Fig. 13–7). This central constriction of the cardiac-liver shadow is referred to as the cardiohepatic angle or "waist." In species normally characterized by a cardiohepatic angle, widening or loss of the angle implies hepatomegaly. It is important that slight rotation of the bird's body during positioning for the VD view can convincingly mimic hepatomegaly by changing the appearance of the cardiohepatic angle in birds with entirely normal livers.

Certain species departing from this general description deserve mention. In owls (see Fig. 13–9), large psittacine species, and galliform species, the angle is typically absent; in ducks (see Fig. 13–10), the entire body form including the cardiohepatic

angle is elongate; and many macaws have a relatively small liver, resulting in VD radiographs giving a false impression of splenomegaly and cardiomegaly.

Gastrointestinal System and Related Organs

The crop is variably developed among species, being best developed in graminivorous and omnivorous species. The crop is sometimes visible as an air- or soft-tissue density (depending on content) just cranial to the thoracic inlet in both the lateral view and VD views. In the VD view, its exact position to the right or left of midline varies with its

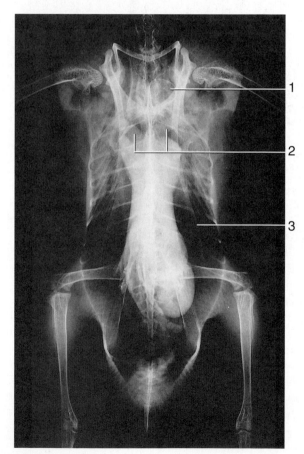

Figure 13-10

Ventrodorsal view of the body of a male mallard duck. Note the syringeal bulla in the region of the thoracic inlet. This structure is absent in females. Note also the elongated nature of the entire body silhouette including the cardiohepatic angle, and the prominence of the lateral sternal margin and of the vertebral and sternal ribs. 1 = syringeal bulla, 2 = great vessels, 3 = lateral margin of sternum.

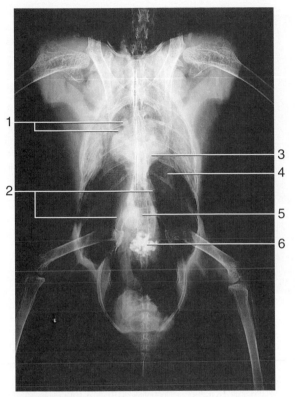

F i g u r e 1 3 – 1 1

Ventrodorsal view of the body of a blue and gold macaw. Note the relatively small size of the liver (typical of many macaws). The smaller liver together with the barrel-chested body form gives a false impression of splenomegaly and cardiomegaly, and enlarges the radiolucent areas of the air sacs. 1 = great vessels, 2 = right and left lateral margins of the liver, 3 = heart, 4 = lung, 5 = spleen, 6 = grit in ventriculus.

state of fullness. The thoracic esophagus is normally visualized only as it widens to join the proventriculus at the level of the cardiac base. The proventriculus is best visualized in the lateral view (see Figs. 13–8, 13–12) as an elliptical or funnel-shaped density dorsal to the liver and cranial to the ventriculus. The ventriculus is a large oval organ occupying most of the left caudal region of the abdomen. In the VD view (see Figs. 13–7 and 13–9 to 13–11), the ventriculus normally lies on the left of the bird's midline, with the cranial edge of the organ approximately at the level of the acetabula. In the lateral view (see Fig. 13–8), the ventriculus lies in the ventral abdomen, caudal to the liver and adjacent to the sternum. In pet and graminivorous species, the ventriculus often contains grit or other radiopaque material, making it a readily recognizable

landmark (see later, Figs. 13–24, 13–25, 13–27, 13–29). In raptors, the ventriculus may show the skeletal components of the bird's most recent meal (Fig. 13–17). The normal spleen is difficult to visualize and is typically visible only in medium- to large-sized species. The spleen is best imaged in the lateral view (see Fig. 13–8) at the junction of the proventriculus with the ventriculus. The liver normally lies under the ribs and does not extend caudal to the edge of the sternum. Birds lack a diaphragm, and the liver envelops the cardiac apex, producing the cardiohepatic angle on the VD view typical of most companion species (see Fig. 13–7) (see the section on the Cardiovascular System). On the VD view (see Figs. 13–7 and 13–9 to 13–11), the lateral edges of the liver are clearly defined by their contact with the air sacs, but the liver's caudal extent blends with the shadows of the ventriculus and intestines. The normal liver generally lies within the boundaries of bilateral lines extending from the humeral head to the femoral neck. On the lateral view (see Fig. 13–8), the liver lies in the ventral portion of the body cavity, bordered cranially by the heart, dorsally by the proventriculus, caudally by the ventriculus, and ventrally by the sternum. The regions of the intestines, including the ceca when present, are essentially indistinguishable from each other. However, in some individuals (particularly budgerigars), the duodenal loop may be separately imaged on the right of the midline near the body wall, overlying the caudal abdominal air sac. The intestinal loops occupy much of the abdomen caudal to the liver and to the right of the ventriculus. In the VD view (see Figs. 13–7 and 13–9 to 13–11), the loops lie between the ventriculus and the right caudal air sac, whereas in the lateral view (see Fig. 13–8) they lie dorsal to the ventriculus. The intestines in birds normally do not contain gas.

Urogenital System

Avian kidneys are difficult to evaluate radiographically because the middle and caudal divisions are recessed deeply in synsacral fossae, and are usually obscured by bone in the lateral view and by overlying viscera in the VD view. However, the cranial poles can usually be visualized in the lateral view (see Fig. 13–8) and occasionally in the VD view just ventral to the cranial part of the synsacrum. The

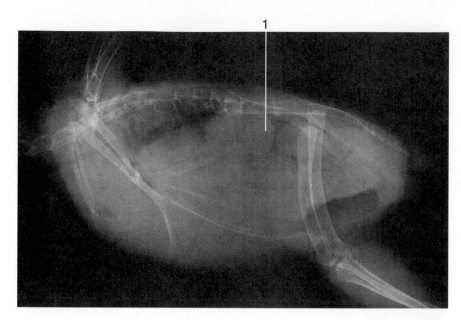

Figure 13–12

Lateral (Le-Rt) view of the body of a reproductively active female bobwhite quail. Multiple follicles are visible on the ovary, and the enlarged oviduct obscures most other abdominal detail. 1 = follicle on ovary.

cloaca should not be visible unless it contains air or an egg.

Because the reproductive organs of both sexes change dramatically in size and position in the various stages of the reproductive cycle, their radiographic appearance also varies widely. Gonads are generally not visible in reproductively inactive birds. As the gonads enlarge, they appear in the lateral and/or VD view as soft tissue densities ventral and slightly cranial to the cranial renal division. When reproductively active, follicles may be visible on the ovary (see Fig. 13–12). The active oviduct (see Fig. 13–12) occupies a large part of the caudal abdominal cavity but obscures much abdominal de-

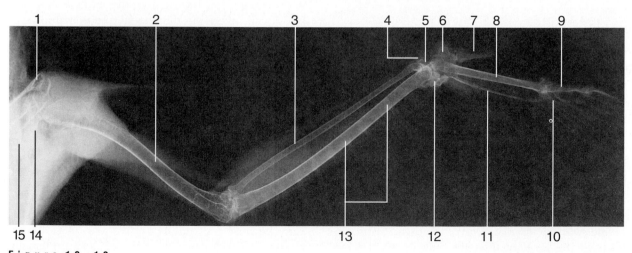

Figure 13–13

Ventrodorsal view of the wing of a red-tailed hawk. The additional bone of the carpal region (not a true carpal or sesamoid bone) is plainly imaged. Among species commonly presented to veterinarians, this bone is typical only of certain raptors. Note two phalanges in the major digit. 1 = clavicle, 2 = body of humerus, 3 = body of radius, 4 = additional bone of the carpal region, 5 = radial carpal bone, 6 = carpometacarpus, 7 = alular digit, 8 = major metacarpal bone, 9 = major digit (with 2 phalanges), 10 = minor digit, 11 = minor metacarpal bone, 12 = ulnar carpal bone, 13 = attachment sites of secondary flight feathers to body of ulna, 14 = scapula, 15 = coracoid bone.

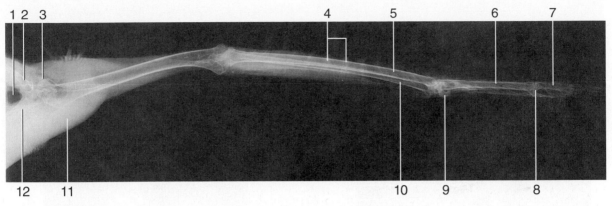

Figure 13-14

Craniocaudal view of the wing of a great horned owl. The pectoral muscles indicate the ventral body surface. The humeroscapular bone is a normal characteristic of many raptorial species, and must not be misinterpreted as an abnormality. Mineralization of the limb tendons (wing and pelvic limb, see Figs. 13–15 and 13–16) is typical of owls other than barn owls. 1 = clavicular air sac, 2 = scapula, 3 = humeroscapular bone, 4 = secondary flight feathers, 5 = ulna, 6 = superimposed major and minor metacarpal bones, 7 = major digit, 8 = minor digit, 9 = ulnar carpal bone, 10 = radius, 11 = pectoral muscles, 12 = coracoid bone.

tail and is difficult to distinguish from other abdominal soft tissue. The active testes or any part of the active female reproductive system can give the impression of an abdominal mass.

CONTRAST STUDIES

Gastrointestinal Series

Positive contrast radiography is particularly useful in examination of the gastrointestinal (GI) tract. Indications for contrast studies include regurgitation, persistent diarrhea, constipation, abnormal palpation, abdominal enlargement, or abnormalities observed on survey radiographs. Because of the risk of aspiration of contrast material, contrast study is contraindicated in comatose or laterally recumbent birds and in those with respiratory depression.

Contrast radiography should always be preceded by a complete physical examination and survey radiographs. In most cases, anesthesia should be avoided when possible, because of resultant alterations in GI motility and the danger of aspiration of contrast material. This is particularly true when a full contrast series is contemplated. However, in selected instances, as when dealing with an uncooperative or fractious individual, anesthesia may be judiciously used.

Iodine-containing agents should be used in sus-

pected cases of intestinal perforation because iodine is less likely than barium to cause peritonitis. However, the irritating and hygroscopic nature of iodine-containing compounds together with their potential for absorption through the intestinal wall make them unsatisfactory for the majority of cases. Barium sulfate is usually the contrast agent of choice, and it is used in a 25 to 35% solution by weight.

Contrast radiography gives best results when the GI tract is empty before the study. Lavage and/or aspiration of palpable material from the crop may be necessary prior to administration of the barium to facilitate adequate dosing, as well as to remove ingesta that would interfere with interpretation of the mucosa. Fasting before contrast radiography should not exceed 4 hours because of birds' high metabolic rate. The dose of barium varies with species, size, and presence or absence of the crop. The dose ranges from 0.025 to 0.05 ml/g body weight, with the lesser dose used in larger species and those lacking a crop. Examination for mucosal change requires a higher dose.

For administration of the contrast material, the bird is held in an upright position, the neck extended, and the mouth opened. A speculum may be necessary with larger species. The prominent glottis must be identified and avoided when passing the tube into the esophagus. An appropriate dose of barium is administered directly into the crop via

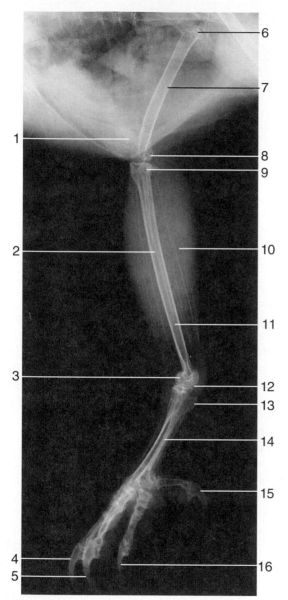

Figure 13–15

Mediolateral view of the pelvic limb of the great horned owl. Note the mineralized tendons of the limb musculature, typical of owls other than barn owls. (See also Figs. 13–14 and 13–16.) 1 = patella, 2 = body of tibiotarsus, 3 = condyles of tibiotarsus, 4 = digit II, 5 = digit III, 6 = head of femur, 7 = body of femur, 8 = condyle of femur, 9 = head of fibula, 10 = mineralized tendons of crural musculature, 11 = distal extremity of fibula, 12 = intertarsal joint, 13 = hypotarsus (calcaneus), 14 = body of tarsometatarsus, 15 = distal phalanx of digit I, 16 = distal phalanx of digit IV.

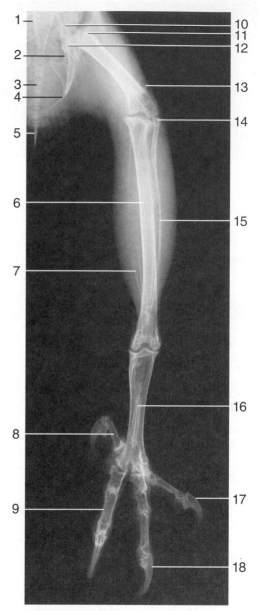

Figure 13–16

Craniocaudal view of the pelvic limb of the great horned owl. Note the mineralized tendons of the limb musculature, typical of owls other than barn owls. (See also Figs. 13–14 and 13–15.) 1 = synsacrum, 2 = ischium, 3 = free caudal vertebrae, 4 = pubis, 5 = pygostyle, 6 = body of tibiotarsus, 7 = mineralized tendons of crural musculature, 8 = digit I, proximal phalanx. In digit II, note the three phalanges. 10 = ilium, 11 = greater trochanter of femur, 12 = head of femur in acetabulum, 13 = patella, 14 = head of fibula, 15 = body of fibula, 16 = body of tarsometatarsus.

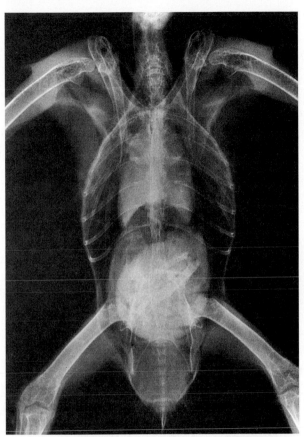

Figure 13–17

Gastric contents of a recently fed barn owl. The ventriculus contains the bones of a recently eaten prey item. Both the ventricular distension and the bony densities within it obscure other visceral detail. In raptors, this problem can be avoided by fasting the bird 12 to 24 hours prior to radiography.

to the region of interest. Care must be taken in this approach in that alterations in gut motility can distort typical transit times, which may result in missing the region of interest.

Typical contrast transit time of several species as described by Grimm and coworkers[10] is summarized in Table 13–1. Average transit time can be increased or decreased by alterations in gut motility induced by GI diseases. In addition to timing changes, films should be evaluated for obstruction, filling defects, masses, organ displacement, and altered mucosal pattern.

Contrast studies of the cloaca by enema are simple to perform but have little practical application because of the ease of direct visualization using endoscopy or an otoscope.

A double-contrast study using barium followed by air can be used to evaluate the thickness and condition of the wall of the crop, intestine, and cloaca. Unfortunately, the considerable variation in the intestinal mucosal pattern among individuals and species causes this procedure to be less informative than other forms of contrast study. The recommended volume of positive contrast medium for a double-contrast study is 25 to 50% of the volume recommended for a GI contrast study. Administration of the contrast material is followed with a double volume of air.

Excretory Urography

Contrast study of the urinary system is not commonly used in avian medicine, because gross and histologic characteristics of the kidney cause the resulting images to provide relatively little useful information. Nonetheless, the technique is established[11-13] and can be used to define renal dimensions or masses. Indications for excretory urography include polyuria/polydipsia, and, because of the passage of the lumbar and sciatic plexuses through the renal substance, nonspecific clinical signs of leg paresis or joint swelling. Warmed water-soluble iodinated contrast medium is administered intravenously into the brachial vein with iodine at a dose of 1.5 mg/g body weight. Radiographs are taken at 10 seconds (imaging the heart, aorta, and pulmonary artery), 60 seconds (imaging the kidneys and ureters), and 2 minutes (imaging the entire cloaca)

a rubber or ball-tipped metal feeding tube. Care must be taken during administration not to permit the barium to well up into the pharynx and cover the glottis. Chances of reflux can be reduced by placing a finger over the distal cervical esophagus just cranial to the crop while dosing, and by slow removal of the tube while avoiding pressure on the crop after dosing. The dose must be administered particularly slowly in species lacking a crop.

For a complete series in medium-sized birds, both VD and lateral views (Fig. 13–18) are taken at time intervals of 0, 15, and 30 minutes and 1, 2, 4, 8, and 24 hours after contrast administration. Practicality (as with highly stressed birds), or interest focused on a particular gut region may at times indicate a shorter series in which the exposure can be tailored

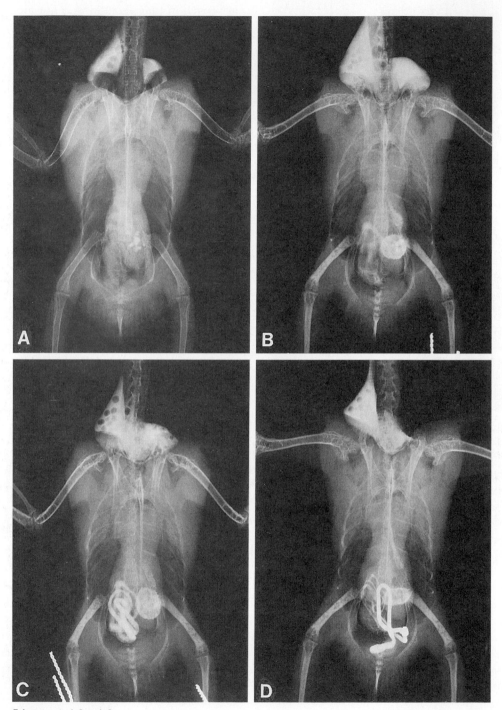

Figure 13–18

See legend on opposite page

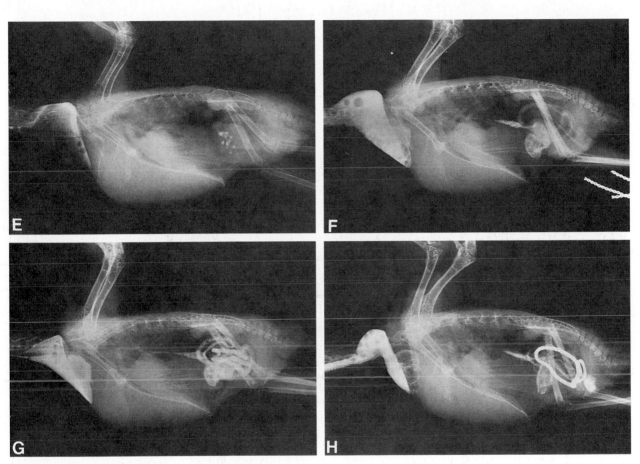

F i g u r e   1 3 – 1 8 *Continued*

Normal gastrointestinal contrast study of a cockatiel. These selected figures represent 0 minutes (*A* and *E*), 30 minutes (*B* and *F*), 2 hours (*C* and *G*), and 6 hours (*D* and *H*) after administration of barium. The retention of some barium in the crop in the later hours is related to the presence of ingesta in the crop.

Table 13–1

NORMAL AVERAGE TRANSIT TIMES OF BARIUM SULFATE IN COMMON AVIAN SPECIES

Time	Canaries	Budgerigars	Amazon Parrots	Hawks
0 min	Crop	Crop	Crop	Crop
10 min	Small intestine	Crop	Crop	Crop-stomach
15 min	Large intestine	Stomach	Stomach	Stomach
30 min	Cloaca	Stomach	Stomach	Small intestine
1 hr	Cloaca	Small intestine	Small intestine	Large intestine
1.5 hr	Empty	Small intestine	Small intestine	Large intestine
2 hr		Large intestine	Large intestine	Cloaca
3 hr		Cloaca	Cloaca	Cloaca
4 hr		Cloaca	Cloaca	Cloaca
8 hr		Empty	Empty	Empty

after contrast administration, and contrast material should be completely excreted in 5 to 7 minutes.

Miscellaneous Studies

Sinography may be indicated in cases of chronic rhinitis and sinusitis, suspected masses, and head trauma. A dose of 0.1 to 1.0 ml of a 15 to 20% organic iodine agent is directly injected into the infraorbital sinuses to image the sinus, periorbital region, and contralateral sinus, and to demonstrate the flow of contrast medium into the nasal cavity. Interpretation of sinography is complicated by the wide extent and overlap of the sinuses.

Other techniques of experimental interest include pneumocoelography, positive contrast peritoneography, nonselective angiography, tracheography, and bronchography, but these have little current use in avian medicine.

RADIOGRAPHIC SIGNS OF ABNORMAL CONDITIONS

Skeletal System

Radiographic examination is essential in evaluation of fractures. The radiographic signs of fractures as well as their classification, interpretation, and healing are similar in birds and mammals and do not require separate discussion here. However, special mention must be made of the possible development of airsacculitis following open fractures because diverticula of various air sacs fill the medullary cavity of many long bones.

Head trauma requires radiographic examination to rule out fractures of the facial or cranial region and of the scleral ring. In these cases, an oblique view of the head can be particularly helpful. Retrobulbar masses may also alter the position of the scleral ring.

The normally thin nature of avian cortical bone must be recalled when evaluating changes in bone density or when considering metabolic bone disease (Fig. 13–19). In such instances, bone density rather than cortical thickness should be evaluated, because bone disorders are characterized by decreased contrast between cortical bone and soft tissue. A normal change in bone density specific to birds occurs in osteomyelosclerosis (also called polyostotic hyperostosis), a hyperostotic change in the long bones associated with egg-laying in which the medullary cavity undergoes a diffuse or patchy increase in density (see Fig. 13–32). A similar but pathologic change occurs in cases of pathologic hyperestrogenism associated with ovarian disorders, but the opacities are more localized and more radiodense.

Many common mammalian disorders of bone are relatively rare in birds, although bone tumors (primary or metastatic) and arthritis are occasionally seen. Neoplasia is difficult to reliably distinguish from osteomyelitis radiographically, and additional studies such as biopsy or culture are best used to arrive at a definitive diagnosis. Arthritis usually results from infectious or traumatic etiology. Infectious arthritis is often associated with severe cases of *Salmonella* infection, tenosynovitis or infectious pododermatitis ("bumblefoot"). Because of the possibility of bone or joint involvement, birds with severe infectious pododermatitis require radio-

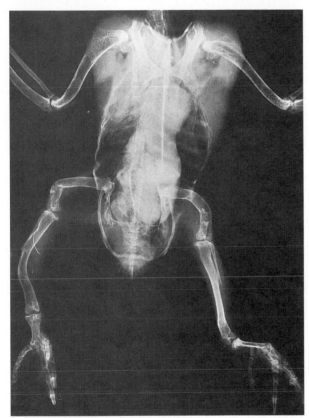

Metabolic bone disease in an African grey parrot. Multiple folding fractures and malunions are present in both femurs and right tibiotarsus. The overall decrease in skeletal density is also consistent with metabolic bone disease. (Courtesy of North Carolina State University College of Veterinary Medicine.)

graphic examination as a part of formation of prognosis as well as in evaluation of treatment. Degenerative osteoarthritis related to aging may also be seen in older psittacines (Fig. 13–20).

Respiratory System

The applicability of radiography in diagnosis of disorders of the upper airway is limited by the small size and complex structure of the avian skull. However, in severe cases of sinusitis, the infraorbital sinus may appear distorted. Presence of foreign bodies, obstruction of the trachea, and cervicocephalic air sac dilatation are also among the indications for radiographic evaluation of the respiratory system in the head and neck.

The lower respiratory system is frequently involved in clinical disease, but unfortunately it is difficult to evaluate radiographically. The extensiveness of the air sac system, the compact and relatively dense nature of the lungs, and extensive soft tissue overlap over all parts of the respiratory system render interpretation of subtle alterations challenging. Radiographs of exceptional positional and technical quality are required to evaluate this body system.

The lungs are difficult to evaluate radiographically because of their small size and the considerable soft tissue and bone overlap that is apparent on all views. Lesions in the cranial air sacs may appear to be in the lung because of the manner in which the air sacs overlap the lungs in both views. Nonetheless, primary lung lesions may still be discerned (Figs. 13–21, 13–22). Pulmonary neoplasia

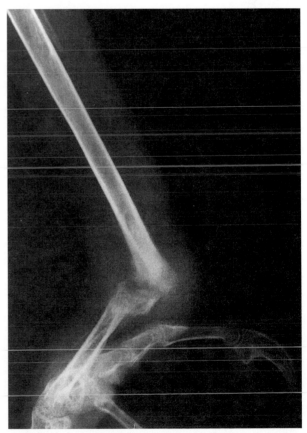

Degenerative arthritis of the intertarsal joint of a macaw. Note the soft tissue swelling and the degeneration of the articular surfaces. (Courtesy of R. Altman.)

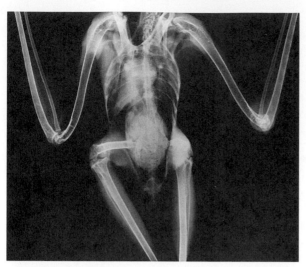

Traumatically induced consolidation of the right lung and luxation of the left elbow of a barn owl. The pulmonary lesion was consistent with hemorrhage.

is rare in birds, and changes in pulmonary density typically affect the reticular pattern of the lung. This pattern may either be accentuated, as in peribronchial infiltration, or decreased in prominence, as in luminal accumulation of fluid, exudate, or neoplastic or granulomatous infiltrations, resulting in lung consolidation.

Portions of certain air sacs can be evaluated radiographically. Because symmetry of the air sacs is an important radiographic feature, correct patient positioning is extremely important. Airsacculitis (Figs. 13–22, 13–23) may result from inflammation, hypovitaminosis A, or parasitism. Changes in air sac density resulting from airsacculitis may be subtle or profound and are related to the amount of fluid, exudate, or mural thickening present.

Comparison of the density of the air sacs with that of the surrounding air can be helpful, in that normal air sac density should approximate external air density. Subtle changes may be difficult to detect, owing in part to the difficulty of obtaining exclusively inspiratory films. Expiratory films can impart an impression of increased air sac density when none is present. Generalized airsacculitis produces an evenly distributed increase in density that may range from a faint, poorly defined haziness to frank consolidation of the air sac. On the lateral view, consolidated air sacs may show sinuous soft

tissue densities that somewhat obscure underlying thoracoabdominal viscera.

Other radiographically detectable abnormalities affecting the air sacs include mycotic infections, which produce patchy rather than diffuse increases in density, and granulomas of numerous etiologies, appearing as localized soft tissue densities. Rupture of the air sacs can produce pneumocoelom, reflected as an increase in the prominence of thoracoabdominal structures, elevation of the heart from the sternum, and increased visualization of the great vessels. Radiographic evidence of respiratory disease may also be reflected in the GI system, because birds in respiratory distress may experience aerophagia and may develop gas-filled bowel loops in the absence of GI disease.

Cardiovascular System

Cardiomegaly and microcardia are difficult to diagnose radiographically, although both pathologic en-

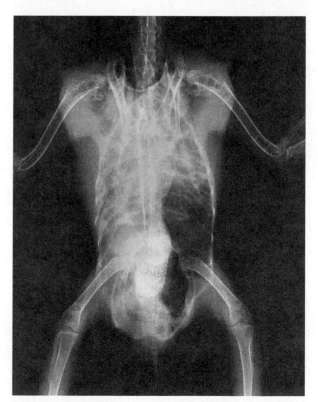

Asymmetrical airsacculitis in an Amazon parrot. The air sacs on the right are severely involved; in contrast, the air sacs on the left are moderately involved. Pulmonary infiltrates are also possibly present, but are difficult to evaluate. (Courtesy of K. Quesenberry.)

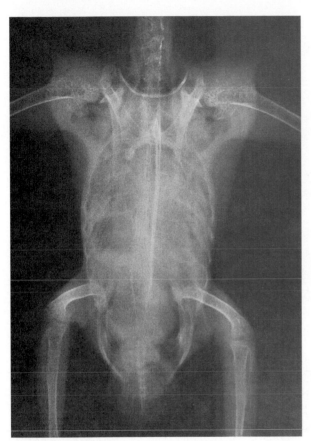

Figure 13–23

Severe airsacculitis in a parrot. The thoracic and abdominal air sacs are symmetrically involved to a degree resulting in general consolidation. (Courtesy of K. Quesenberry.)

largement and reduction of cardiac size have been reported in several avian species. Cardiomegaly[14–16] may widen or obliterate the cardiohepatic angle. Microcardia[17] is usually suggestive of an exigent state, often involving hypovolemia, and is an indication for immediate volume replacement therapy.

Gastrointestinal System

Radiographic evaluation of the crop and esophagus is generally limited to soft tissue mass (Fig. 13–24) or foreign body evaluation, or contrast study. Because of its ease of access, the crop is often better directly studied by endoscopy (see Chapter 45).

The proventriculus, being a dynamic organ, may require multiple films to properly characterize its condition. The proventriculus may present radiographic signs of foreign body, impaction, yeast infection, or tumors. Enlargement of the proventriculus may occur in overfed hand-reared juveniles. Pathologic proventricular dilatation (Fig. 13–25) in any species may occur as a result of loss of intestinal motility owing to infectious or toxic disorders. In addition, macaws (Fig. 13–26) and some other psittacine species develop neuropathic gastric dilatation with associated neurologic signs, which is usually fatal. This dilatation progresses from moderate in early stages of the disease to extreme in later phases. As with the normal proventriculus, evaluation of neuropathic gastric dilatation is best made from the lateral view, although in moderate-to-ad-

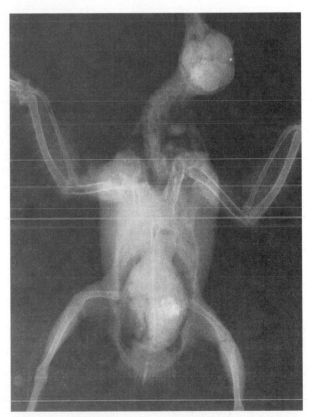

Figure 13–24

Candidiasis of the crop of a mourning dove. Multiple soft tissue densities are visible within the crop. A fracture of the right humeral shaft and hepatomegaly are also present. The encroachment of the enlarged liver into areas normally occupied by air sacs contributes to difficulty in evaluation of the remaining visible region of air sacs, which have an appearance consistent with either mild airsacculitis or a hazy increase in density imparted by obesity. The position of the ventriculus is clearly marked by the presence of radiopaque grit within it.

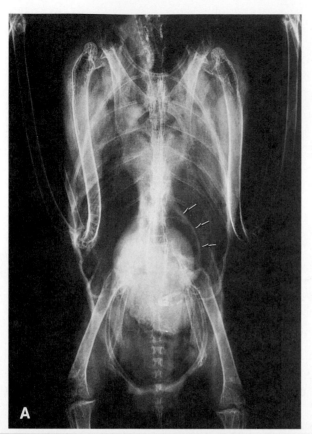

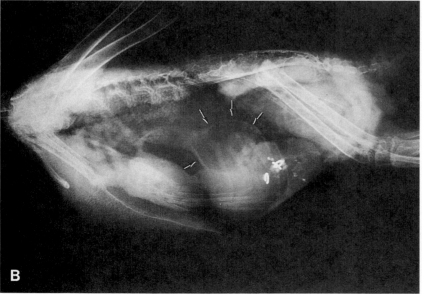

Figure 13–25

Gassy distension of the proventriculus and intestines in a cockatoo. Arrows indicate the proventricular borders. The gas accumulation is probably related to a toxic ileus caused by lead foreign bodies in the ventriculus. These figures demonstrate that proventricular dilatation can result from etiologies other than neuropathic gastric dilatation associated with psittacine birds. (Courtesy of North Carolina State University College of Veterinary Medicine.)

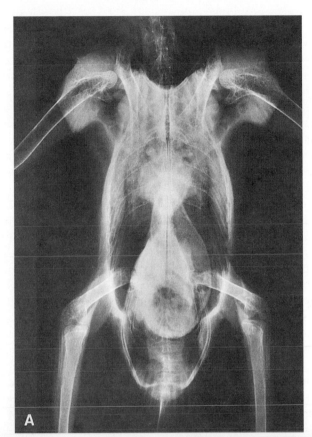

Figure 13–26

Severe proventricular dilatation in a blue and gold macaw. On the VD view *(A)*, the widely distended proventriculus contains material of a heterogeneous density. On the lateral view *(B)*, gas is visible within the proventriculus, and the spleen is clearly imaged against the gas density within the ventriculus. This patient suffered from neuropathic gastric dilatation. (Courtesy of K. Quesenberry.)

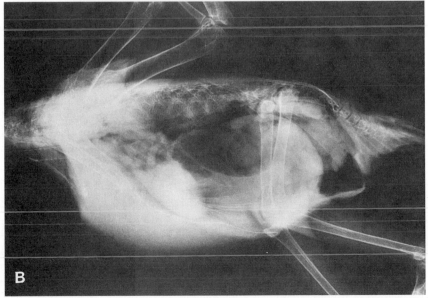

vanced cases of proventricular dilatation, the VD view also shows gross dilatation.

The ventriculus may become impacted or obstructed, which can occur when small caged birds are overfed grit. Foreign bodies, luminal masses, and accumulation of heavy metals (see Fig. 13–25) may also be apparent radiographically. The ventriculus may be displaced by abdominal masses (see Fig. 13–32), enlargement or tumor of other organs, or in relation to an abdominal hernia (see Fig. 13–33). The origin and size of the displacing mass dictate the direction and degree of ventricular displacement. For instance, gondal enlargement displaces the ventriculus caudoventrally, whereas hepatomegaly displaces it caudodorsally.

Splenomegaly frequently develops in birds with active systemic infection, and is best seen on the lateral view (Fig. 13–27). Particularly enlarged spleens appear on the VD view superimposed over the liver, to the right of and slightly cranial to the ventriculus. Infectious diseases generally produce smooth and even splenic enlargement, whereas splenic tumors tend to produce an irregular surface. It must be emphasized that although splenomegaly is commonly associated with psittacosis, it is not pathognomonic for this disease.

The liver is best evaluated on the VD view. Hepatomegaly commonly results from primary liver disease such as lipidosis, hepatitis, congestion, or tumors. Diagnosing hepatomegaly from a single film is unwise, because other unrelated factors such as displacement of the liver by abdominal masses or enlarged organs, peritonitis, and even poor positioning can convincingly mimic this condition. In a correctly positioned VD view (see Figs. 13–27, 13–31), hepatomegaly is indicated by widening or loss of the cardiohepatic angle, extension beyond normal lateral limits, and decreased size of the abdominal air sacs. Caudal displacement of the ventriculus may also be visible. Signs of hepatomegaly on the lateral view (see Fig. 13–27) are less consistent, but may include elevation of the proventriculus and ventriculus, and some decrease in the size of the triangular lucency of the thoracic air sacs. The lateral view is particularly helpful, however, in distinguishing the false sense of hepatomegaly that can be implied by peritonitis and ascites on the VD view. With peritonitis or ascites (see later, Fig. 13–32), the lungs are visible but most of the remainder of the thoracoabdominal cavity is a nondescript

haze, whereas in hepatomegaly, the thoracoabdominal organs are visible, although they may be displaced. Microhepatica and hepatic asymmetry occur less frequently than hepatomegaly but are also recognizable radiographically (Figs. 13–28, 13–29).

Radiographic signs of intestinal disease are generally similar to those seen in mammals. Both the VD and lateral views show the signs adequately. However, any gas in avian intestinal loops (Fig. 13–30; see also Fig. 13–25) is considered abnormal. Gas may accumulate in the loops from a number of causes, including enteritis, atony associated with neuropathic gastric dilatation, or toxicosis. Impaction and obstruction are rarer causes. Intestinal gas may also accumulate following anesthesia or aerophagia associated with primary respiratory disease. Uniformly distributed excessive fluid in the intestines may accumulate with enteritis, psychogenic polydipsia, or functional paralytic ileus resulting from a number of causes including bacterial or viral infections, septicemia, or toxicoses.

Radiographic evaluation of the gastrointestinal tract and other abdominal organs is greatly complicated in the obese bird (Fig. 13–31). Obesity can cause displacement of abdominal organs and a decrease in the size of the air sacs; it often convincingly mimics hepatomegaly. Great care should therefore be taken when evaluating body cavity films of obese birds.

Abdominal fluid accumulation resulting from peritonitis or ascites presents a general loss of visceral detail (Fig. 13–32). Visualization of gas-filled intestinal loops together with abdominal fluid is most consistent with enteritis. The lateral view is often particularly helpful in this diagnosis.

Abdominal hernias (Fig. 13–33) occur fairly frequently in female psittacine species, particularly in the budgerigar. The hernia is frequently associated with weakening of the abdominal musculature associated with egg-laying, egg-binding, or hyperestrogenism. Rarer causative factors of abdominal hernias applicable to either sex include trauma, straining, or abdominal masses. The lateral view is most helpful, showing loss of the integrity of the abdominal wall in association with a projecting soft tissue mass of varying size. Displacement of abdominal organs is evident, with displacement of the ventriculus being particularly characteristic. Contrast studies can be helpful in identifying contents of the hernial sac.

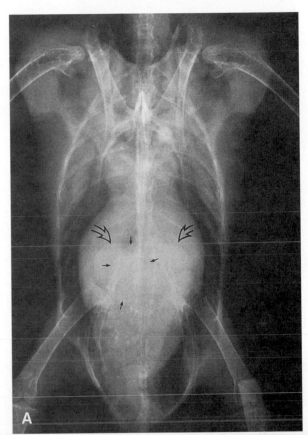

Figure 13-27

Hepatomegaly, splenomegaly, and reno-megaly in an Amazon parrot with psitta-cosis. The hepatomegaly is best seen on the VD view *(A)*, but is also appreciable on the lateral view *(B)* by the elevation of the proventriculus-ventriculus shadow. Solid arrows indicate splenic borders, open arrows indicate cranial division of the kidneys. (Courtesy of R. Altman.)

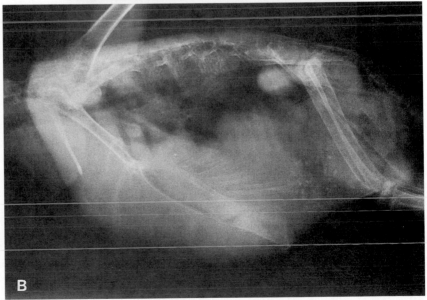

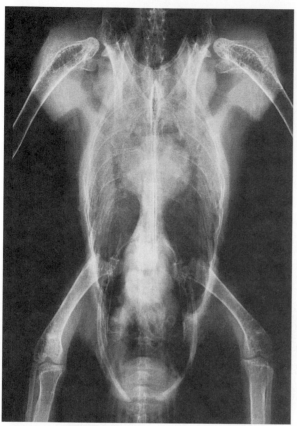

Figure 13–28

Microhepatica in a blue and gold macaw. The overall size of the liver is much smaller than normal. Consequently, more of the apical region of the heart is visible than normal, and the caudal air sacs present larger lucent areas than normal. (Courtesy of K. Quesenberry.)

Urogenital System

Radiology is of limited usefulness in examination of the avian urinary system because of the recessed position of the kidneys within the synsacrum and the close physical proximity of the gonads. Suspected renal change should be carefully evaluated, because distinction from gonadal change can be difficult. Nephritis or bolus fluid administration can produce a subtle increase in size of the kidneys with variable change in density. Dehydration and renal gout can produce increased renal density without enlargement. Renal tumors may occur in any species, and are particularly common in the budgerigar. Renal calcification (Fig. 13–34) may appear in various psittacine species, either associated with other renal disease or as an incidental finding

unassociated with clinical signs on films taken for other reasons.

Egg retention occurs commonly in many pet bird species, and presents a variable radiographic appearance (Fig. 13–35). Calcified eggs are readily visible at any point in the oviduct, but noncalcified eggs may also be retained. Noncalcified eggs are more difficult to visualize and must be carefully sought, because larger species frequently retain two eggs with one typically noncalcified. Egg yolk peritonitis, resulting from the escape of ova from the infundibulum or from rupture of the oviduct, occurs quite commonly but not exclusively in the budgerigar. The radiographic signs of this disorder are typical of peritonitis, including the presence of abdominal fluid.

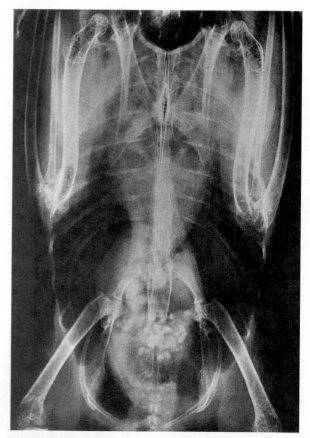

Figure 13–29

Asymmetrical liver in an Amazon parrot. The left side of the liver is markedly smaller than normal, and the right side is slightly enlarged. Note that this bird is well positioned, hence the abnormal shape of the liver is not a positional artifact. (Courtesy of North Carolina State University College of Veterinary Medicine.)

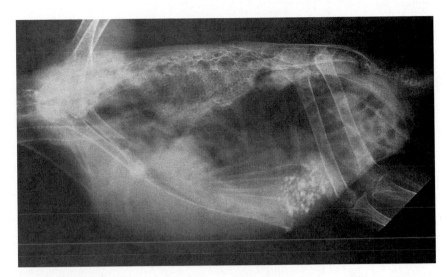

Figure 13 – 30

Intestinal gas in a parrot. The intestine contains gas throughout most of its length, clearly defining the course of the coils. This individual demonstrates an extreme degree of intestinal gas, but it should be kept in mind that any gas within the gut of birds is abnormal. This bird exhibited gut hypermotility and refractory diarrhea. (Courtesy of R. Altman.)

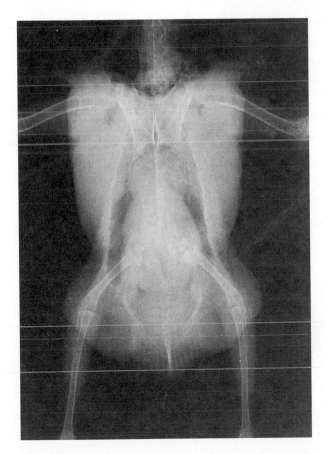

Figure 13 – 31

Obesity in a cockatiel. The liver shadow is enlarged and the cardiohepatic angle is nearly lost. Most abdominal detail is lost. The slightly increased density of the air sacs is difficult to interpret, because this appearance could result from either mild air sacculitis or increased soft tissue mass due to excessive body fat.

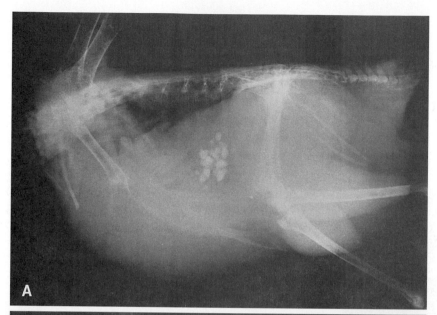

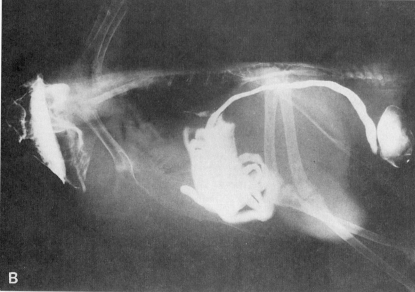

Figure 13–32

Abdominal mass, ascites, and osteo-myelosclerosis of all long bones of the limbs in a dove. Extreme care must be taken when handling birds with suspected ascites, and exact positioning must at times be sacrificed for the safety of the bird. The survey lateral view *(A)* shows diffuse fluid density throughout the abdominal cavity, with complete loss of visceral detail. The ventriculus is the sole recognizable organ, because of the radiopaque grit in its lumen. Ventricular displacement is evident on the survey film and is confirmed on the contrast film *(B)*. Contrast material within the digestive tract demonstrates marked cranioventral displacement of all gastro-intestinal organs other than the colon and cloaca. This pattern is consistent with a mass involving the oviduct. The patchy, hyperostotic densities within the medullary cavities of the long bones exemplify osteomyelosclerosis, associated with the bird's reproductively active state. (Courtesy of K. Quesenberry.)

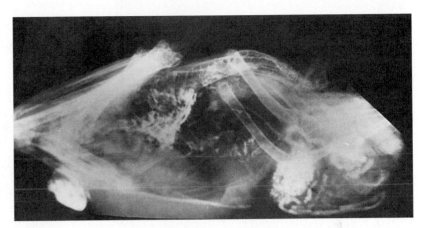

Figure 13–33

Abdominal hernia in a parrot. As shown in this film, contrast radiography can be helpful in identification of the contents of the hernial sac. Organ systems most commonly involved in herniation include the gastrointestinal and female reproductive tracts. In this instance, the ventriculus and part of the intestines occupy the hernial sac. (Courtesy of R. Altman.)

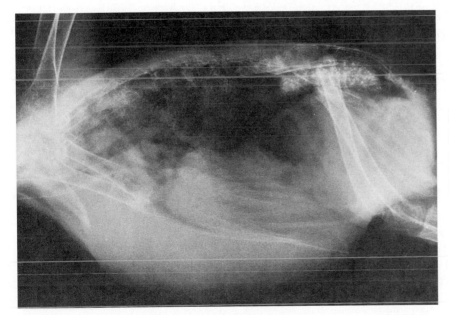

Figure 13–34

Nephrocalcinosis in an African grey parrot. The kidneys show calcification throughout their internal structure. The significance of this feature is unknown, and it is often considered an incidental finding. (Courtesy of K. Quesenberry.)

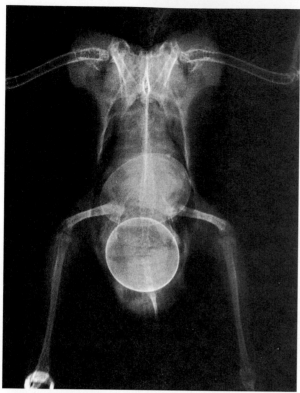

Figure 13–35

Egg retention in a cockatiel. Egg retention can involve multiple as well as single eggs. Note that the proximal egg is less calcified than the distal egg. Retained eggs do not necessarily, however, have such a typical appearance: they may be uncalcified and/or collapsed within the magnum of the oviduct. Also note the loss of general visceral detail caused by the physiologically enlarged active oviduct and physical displacement by the eggs. (Courtesy of K. Quesenberry.)

Tumors of the gonads are relatively common in psittacine species, again most commonly in the budgerigar, and must be carefully distinguished from less common renal tumors. Ovarian and testicular cysts are common in psittacine species, particularly the budgerigar. Apart from signs typical of a cystic organ, radiographic signs are nonspecific, in that displacement of surrounding organs is variable. For instance, the cystic gonad may displace the ventriculus either cranially or caudally. Once again, particular care must be taken to distinguish such lesions from similar ones involving the kidney.

References

1. Walsh MT: Radiology. In Harrison GL and LR Harrison (eds). Clinical Avian Medicine and Surgery. Philadelphia, WB Saunders, 1986, pp 201–233.

2. Smith SA, Smith BJ: Atlas of Avian Radiographic Anatomy. Philadelphia, WB Saunders, 1992.

3. Smallwood JE, Shively MJ, Rendano VT, Habel RE: A standardized nomenclature for radiographic projections used in veterinary medicine. Vet Radiol 26:2–9, 1985.

4. Wortman JA: Film/screen combinations for fine detail radiography. Vet Med Report 3:80–86. 1991.

5. McMillan MC. 1982. Radiology. In ML Petrak (ed): Diseases of Cage and Aviary Birds, ed 2. Philadelphia, Lea & Febiger, 1982.

6. Morgan JP, Silverman S: Techniques of Veterinary Radiography, Davis, CA, Veterinary Radiology Associates, 1982, pp 241–244.

7. Evans SM: Avian radiographic diagnosis. Comp Contin Ed Pract Vet 3:660–666, 1981.

8. Watters JW: Development of a technique chart for the veterinarian. Comp Contin Ed Pract Vet 11:568–571, 1980.

9. Altman RB: Radiography. Vet Clin North Am [Small Anim Pract] 3:165–173, 1973.

10. Grimm F, Kosters J, Wiesner H, et al: [Possible applications of contrast radiography to digestive tract of birds]. Proc Int Symp Erkrankungen Zoo Brno. Berlin, Akademie-Verlag, 1984.

11. McMillan MC: Imaging of avian urogenital disorders. Assoc Avian Vet Today 2:74–82, 1988.

12. Krautwald ME. Radiographic examination of the urinary tract in birds with organic iodinated contrast media. Proc Assoc Avian Vet 177–193, 1987.

13. McNeel SV, Zenoble RD: Avian Urography. J Am Vet Med Assoc 178:366–368, 1981.

14. Beehler BA, Montali RJ, Bush M: Mitral valve insufficiency with congestive heart failure in a Pukeko. J Vet Med Assoc 177:934–937, 1980.

15. Ensley PK, Hatkin J, Silverman S: Congestive heart failure in a greater mynah. J Vet Med Assoc 175:1010–1013, 1979.

16. McMillan MC: Radiology of avian respiratory disease. Comp Contin Ed Pract Vet 8:551–558, 1986.

17. McMillan MC: Imaging Techniques. In Ritchie BW, Harrison GJ, and Harrison LR (eds): Avian Medicine. Principles and Application. Lake Worth, FL, Wingers Publishing, 1994. pp 247–326.

Suggested Reading

Evans SM: Avian Radiography. In Thrall DE (ed): Textbook of Veterinary Diagnostic Radiology, Philadelphia, WB Saunders, pp 522–531.

Krautwald ME, Tellhelm B, Hummel GH, et al: Atlas of Radiographic Anatomy and Diagnosis of Cage Birds. Berlin and Hamburg, Paul Parey Scientific Publishers, 1992.

Lindley DM, Hathcock JT, Miller WW, DiPinto MN: Fractured scleral ossicles in a red-tailed hawk. Vet Radiol 29:209–212, 1988.

Liu S, Dolenszk EP, Tappe JP: Osteosarcoma with multiple metastases in a Panama boat-billed heron. J Am Vet Med Assoc 181:1396–1399, 1982.

McMillan MC: Radiographic diagnosis of avian abdominal disorders. Comp Contin Ed Pract Vet 8:616–632, 1986.

McMillan MC: Radiology of avian respiratory diseases. Comp Contin Ed Pract Vet 8:551–558, 1986.

McMillan MC: Avian gastrointestinal radiology. Comp Contin Ed Pract Vet 5:273–278, 1983.

McMillan MC: Avian Radiology. In Petrak ML (ed): Diseases of Cage and Aviary Birds. Philadelphia, Lea & Febiger, 1982, pp 329–360.

Montali RJ, Bush M, Thoen CO, Smith E: Tuberculosis in captive exotic birds. J Am Vet Med Assoc 169:920–927, 1967.

Morgan JP: Systematic radiographic interpretation of skeletal diseases in small animals. Vet Clin North Am 4:611–626, 1974.

Newton CD, Zeitlin S: Avian fracture healing. J Am Vet Med Assoc 170:620–625, 1977.

Paul-Murphy JR, Koblik PD, Stein G, Penninck DG: Psittacine skull radiography: Anatomy, Radiographic Technic and Patient Application. Vet Radiol 31:218–224, 1990.

Peavey GM, Silverman S, Howard EB, et al: Pulmonary tuberculosis in a sulfur crested cockatoo. J Am Vet Med Assoc 169:915–919, 1976.

Rubel GA, Isenbugel E, Wolvekamp P (eds): Atlas of Diagnostic Radiology of Exotic Pets. London, Schlutersche, Hannover, Wolfe Publishing Limited, and Philadelphia, WB Saunders, 1991.

Silverman S: Avian radiographic technique and interpretation. In Kirk RW (ed): Current Veterinary Therapy, VII. Philadelphia, WB Saunders, 1980.

Smith BJ, Smith SA, Flammer K, et al: The normal xeroradiographic and radiographic anatomy of the orange-winged Amazon parrot (*Amazona amazonica amazonica*). Vet Radiol 31:114–124, 1990.

Smith BJ, Smith SA, Spaulding KA, et al: The normal xeroradiographic and radiographic anatomy of the cockatiel (*Nymphicus hollandis*). Vet Radiol 31:226–234, 1990.

Smith SA, Smith BJ: The normal xeroradiographic and radiographic anatomy of the red-tailed hawk (*Buteo jamaicensis*), with reference to other diurnal raptors. Vet Radiol 31:301–312, 1990.

Smith SA, Smith BJ: Normal xeroradiographic and radiographic anatomy of the great horned owl (*Bubo virginianus*), with special reference to the barn owl (*Tyto alba*). Vet Radiol 32:6–16, 1991.

Smith BJ, Smith SA: Normal xeroradiographic and radiographic anatomy of the bobwhite quail (*Colinus virginianus*), with reference to other galliform species. Vet Radiol 32:127–134, 1991.

Smith BJ, Smith SA: Normal xeroradiographic and radiographic anatomy of the mallard duck (*Anas platyrhynchos*), with reference to other anserine species. Vet Radiol 32:87–95, 1991.

Stoskopf MK: Clinical imaging in zoological medicine: A review. J Zoo Wild Med 20:396–412, 1989.

Walsh MT, Mays MC: Clinical manifestations of cervicocephalic air sacs of psittacines. Comp Cont Ed Pract Vet 6:783–792, 1984.

Walsh MT: Radiology. In Harrison GL, Harrison LR (eds): Clinical Avian Medicine and Surgery, Philadelphia, WB Saunders, 1986, pp 201–233.

Maria E. Krautwald-Junghanns
Frank Enders

14

Ultrasonography

Diagnostic ultrasound as an imaging diagnostic technique has been used in veterinary medicine for approximately 20 years. One of the primary advantages of sonographic examination is in the diagnosis of soft tissue changes, because the inner structure of organs is demonstrated on the screen.

It was stated for a long time that sonography could not be applied to birds because of various anatomic peculiarities (particularly the air sac system). This is only partly true. Sonography in birds will certainly never acquire the same importance as it already enjoys in human medicine and will probably be attained in veterinary medicine only in work on mammals. Nevertheless, experience with ultrasonography in the past few years shows that there are various indications when sonographic examination in birds is a useful diagnostic technique.[1-6]

TECHNICAL EQUIPMENT

A computed ultrasound system with 64 gray scales is used for the sonographic examination. For documentation, the system is connected to a videorecorder and a videoprinter. The transducer the authors use is a mechanical sector scanner with a frequency of 7.5 MHz and a sector angle of 60°. The use of a transducer with a very small head size is necessary because the area of contact with the bird—in contrast to dogs and cats—is normally very limited. The scanner used in the authors' clinic has a working surface of 1.5 cm × 2.5 cm and was originally used for intraoperative sonography in humans (Fig. 14–1).

Various species of birds weighing from 40 g to 1 kg can be sonographically examined with this transducer. A stand-off consisting of semisolid gel (equal water equivalent material) is used for the examination of small birds. It is not possible to obtain a clear image of the superficial tissues without using the gel. For ultrasound examination, different sizes (depending on the patient's size) of a commercially available gel pad (Aquaflex ultrasound gel pad, Parker Laboratory, USA) are placed between the area of contact and the scanner.

PATIENT PREPARATION

The bird should be fasted for at least 3 hours or the food-filled gastrointestinal tract interposes between the transducer and other organs (e.g., parts of the liver). This period of fasting should be increased to 1 to 2 days for birds of prey to examine the gall bladder. As an alternative to fasting, liquid diets may be given in cachectic individuals. Food particles, especially bones in carnivorous species, may

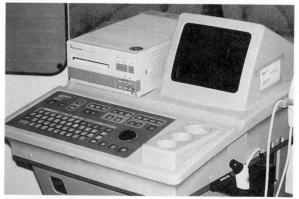

Figure 14–1

Ultrasound system with transducer and printer.

200

make it impossible for the sound beam to pass through.

For restraint, anesthesia is unnecessary. The birds are either held by an assistant or are fixed on a acrylic plate in dorsal or left lateral recumbency. Birds with severe circulatory problems should be examined in an upright position. The area of contact is quite small in most of the smaller species of birds and is situated between the processus xiphoideus of the sternum and the ossa pubis of the pelvis in the ventromedial approach. The lateral approach is done caudal to the last rib on the right side. The feathers are either parted in this area or plucked, depending on the species of bird. An acoustic gel is applied to the skin to enhance the offset-tissue interface (Fig. 14–2).

ORGANS AND ORGAN SYSTEMS

Examination of the Liver and Gall Bladder

Indications

The indications for sonography in birds and mammals are similar. Any clinical sign or laboratory finding hinting at abnormal liver function may be an indication for a sonographic examination of the liver.[1] Enlargement of the liver is frequently seen on radiographic examination. Often the liver has to be differentiated from the gastrointestinal tract by using a time-consuming contrast study. Further clarification by means of radiography is not possible. Ultrasound provides an excellent opportunity to obtain more information, especially on the internal structure of the organ. Radiologic evaluation of the internal organs, except for the air-containing lungs, is not possible if there is coelomic fluid. However, the fluid enhances sonographic detail, and examination of the liver is then easy.

Examination Technique

To examine the liver, the transducer is placed mediocaudally on the xiphoid in a craniodorsal direction. The organ is scanned systematically in transverse sections by sweeping from lateral to medial. The scanner is then turned through 90° and the longitudinal sections are checked.[2, 4]

Normal Appearance

The physiologic echotexture of the liver is homogeneous, delicately granulated, and of average echogenicity. The inner structure is interrupted by blood vessels passing transversely and longitudinally. These are seen as anechoic channels (Fig. 14–3).

Normally, locating the bird's livers is not difficult, but the digestive tract should be nearly empty, otherwise the food-filled gastrointestinal tract is interposed between the transducer and parts of the liver. Difficulties in ultrasonic examination may also occur if the liver is covered by other extremely enlarged organs. This is seen, for example, in psittacine birds with neuropathic gastric dilatation (macaw wasting disease). An exact liver puncture or biopsy, controlled by sonographic means, is possible (Fig. 14–4). This requires experience, and care must be taken.

The majority of birds usually examined in private practice—psittacines, pigeons, and passerines—do not have a gall bladder. To examine the gall bladder in species in which it is present, birds may have to fast for 1 to 2 days. A filled gall bladder is easily recognized sonographically as a round to oval structure caudal to the right liver lobe. The normal appearance is a smooth, clearly defined organ with thin echogenic walls and anechoic content. The phenomenon of acoustic enhancement is seen, as in other fluid-filled structures. Some large vessels,

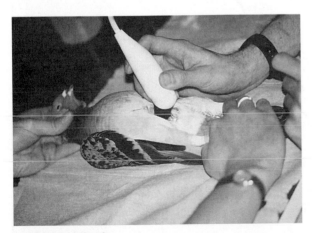

Figure 14–2

Patient position for sonography (ventromedial approach).

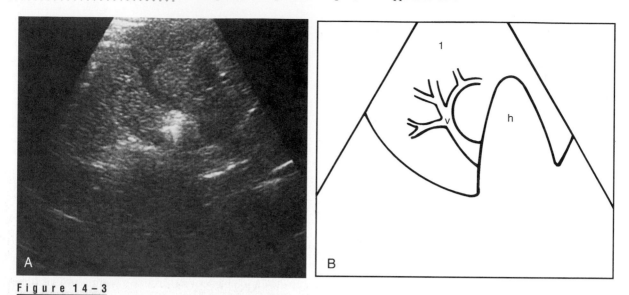

Figure 14–3

(*A* and *B*) Common buzzard *(Buteo buteo)*; normal appearance of the liver parenchyma (1) and liver veins (v) is demonstrated (h = heart).

such as the right portal vein, may be seen adjacent to the gall bladder.

Pathologic Changes of the Liver

One of the primary advantages of sonographic investigation of the liver is the ability to examine the liver parenchyma. The diagnosis is vastly improved in this area by the sonographic visibility of focal or diffuse alterations. Alterations of size and shape as well as changes in the liver vessels and gall bladder may also be differentiated sonographically.

An exact measurement of the liver is not possible because only parts of the liver are seen on one image. In most birds, a positive sign of hepatomegaly is, however, the existence of liver parenchyma caudally, distant from the xiphoid.

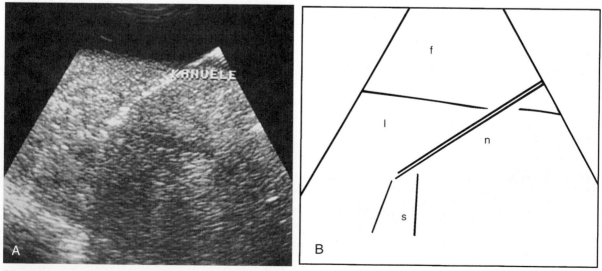

Figure 14–4

(*A* and *B*) Liver biopsy. The tip shadow (s) of the needle (n) is clearly visible (l = liver, f = fluid).

Because of incomplete visibility, it may be difficult to comment on the hepatic shape. The edges of the liver are clearly recognized when ascites is present. Nevertheless, parts of the liver's edge may be seen in most cases.

Abnormal liver vessels are often seen in connection with extreme hepatomegaly. Vascular diameter is increased, and the reflex intensity of the wall is enhanced.

Sonography is used in the authors' clinic primarily to diagnose liver disease, differentiate inflammatory processes from tumors, diagnose ascites (Fig. 14–5) or cysts, and estimate the extent of pathologic change as an aid to prognosis. The sonographic image of fatty liver degeneration, for example, is characterized by increased echogenicity and hepatomegaly. Hepatic neoplasms may be seen as obviously nonhomogeneous liver tissue. The parenchymal alterations can be focal or diffuse; diffuse necrosis may typically show a spotted nonhomogeneous pattern. Diffuse abscesses, granulomas, or necroses are sharply differentiated from the normal liver tissue (see Fig. 14–5). Depending on their content, these areas may occur as hypoechoic with corpuscular parts or as hyperechoic areas, partly separated into small cavernae. Hematomas are sometimes found in hypoechoic parts of the liver

and tend to organize after some days. This is associated with an increase of the reflex intensity.

Pathologic Changes of the Gall Bladder

Pathologic alterations of the gall bladder are rare in birds. Alterations in shape of the gall bladder are visible in birds with hepatomegaly. Abnormal content in the gall bladder is clearly seen. Apart from the anechoic bile, reflex-intense particles that can be stirred by moving the bird are visible in the lumen. On postmortem examination, these particles are usually identified as gall bladder concrements. Another possible sonographic diagnosis is neoplasia of the bladder wall or of the bile ducts.

Examination of the Spleen

Indications and Normal Appearance

Radiologic demonstrations of the normal spleen are difficult. The spleen in the ventrodorsal view is superimposed by other structures. In the lateral view, the spleen may occasionally be demonstrated in psittacines, but in other species, such as pigeons,

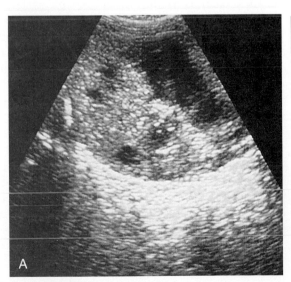 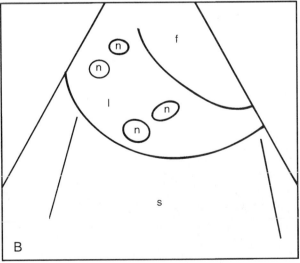

F i g u r e 1 4 – 5

(*A* and *B*) Mynah bird *(Gracula religiosa)* with ascites and focal liver necroses, especially on the left side. The liver parenchyma is of nonhomogeneous echogenicity with round hypoechoic areas (n = necrotic spots). Fluid (f) in the abdomen is seen as an anechoic area on the right side of the picture. In this case the ascites and the liver necroses were the result of a hemochromatosis (s = shadow enhancement).

it is not seen in this view. A contrast study is necessary in most cases of splenic enlargement to differentiate spleen from the gastrointestinal tract.

Although the normal spleen is very difficult to identify on sonography, an indication for sonographic examination is any case of suspected splenic disease when the radiologic diagnosis is inconclusive. Sonography may be helpful to differentiate inflammatory processes from tumors or a post-traumatic reaction.

Technique

The lateral approach is used for identification of the normal spleen. The size and shape of the spleen vary greatly between species. The spleen is slightly more echogenic, relative to the echogenicity of the liver. The parenchyma is of fine and dense granularity and of even texture throughout.

Pathologic Changes of the Spleen

With splenomegaly, the spleen is easily demonstrated from the ventromedial approach. It looks round to oval and has an average echogenicity. Homogeneous enlargement is seen with infection or trauma. Post-traumatic bleeding may be recognized as hypoechoic areas. Splenic tumors are usually of mixed echogenicity and may be seen as marked focal nonhomogeneous echotexture.

Examination of the Urogenital Tract

Kidneys

Indications

Sonographic examination of the kidneys is indicated when clinical signs of disease such as polydipsia, polyuria, abdominal swelling, and lameness is associated with nondiagnostic radiographs.

Normal Appearance

It is not possible to demonstrate the normal kidneys of birds sonographically because of the organs' position beside the vertebral column. In the ventromedial approach, the intestinal loops prevent visibility of the kidneys; in the lateral approach, the abdominal air sacs are interposed between the transducer and the organ.

Pathologic Changes of the Kidneys

A renal neoplasm is frequently accompanied by massive enlargement and parenchymal lesions. A neoplastic kidney is easily demonstrated by using the ventromedial approach to show a round nonhomogeneous structure (Fig. 14–6). Cysts may also be diagnosed sonographically. The characteristic appearance of a cyst is a clearly defined, rounded, anechoic structure with marked posterior acoustic enhancement.

Reproductive Tract

Indications

Sonography of the female reproductive tract is indicated in suspected egg-binding and abnormal egg production. In birds with abdominal swelling, sonography can help to identify cysts or tumors of the gonads.

Normal Appearance

The approach is ventromedial as well as lateral. The normal ovaries are difficult to identify in birds; inactive ovaries and testes cannot be demonstrated sonographically. The intestinal loops (ventromedial approach) and the abdominal air sacs (lateral approach) prevent examination. Determination of the bird's sex with intracloacal applied scanners has not met with success.

Developing follicles may be seen as round areas with anechoic content. The hyperechoic shell is easily differentiated from the surrounding tissue. The egg content is divided into two parts of differing echogenicity (hyperechoic yolk and surrounding hypoechoic albumen). In young chickens, the egg yolk is seen between the intestinal loops.

Pathologic Changes of the Reproductive Tract

It is easy to identify a shelled egg in an egg-bound bird by using the ventromedial and the lateral approaches. The demonstration of laminated eggs

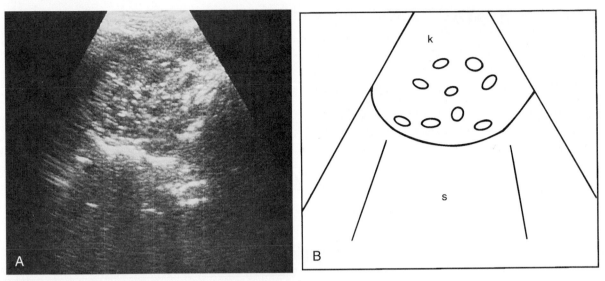

Figure 14–6

(*A* and *B*) Budgerigar *(Melopsittacus undulatus)* with renal adenocarcinoma. Massively enlarged kidney (k) with a nonhomogeneous parenchyma could be demonstrated from the ventromedial approach (s = shadow enhancement).

without shells is also possible by sonographic means. These appear as oval or round areas with different echogenicity and are easily differentiated from the surrounding tissue (Fig. 14–7).

Tumors of the ovary are clearly defined from the surrounding tissues as areas of increased echogeni-

city with a round or oval shape. Cystic ovaries show many round anechoic chambers in the whole parenchyma with distal enhancement (Fig. 14–8). Detecting abnormal follicular or egg development and monitoring the progress of the anomalies are possible uses of sonographic examination.

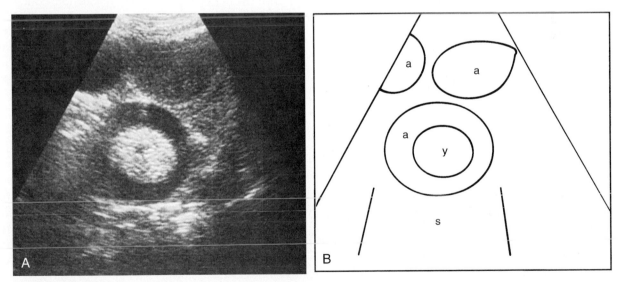

Figure 14–7

(*A* and *B*) Cockatiel *(Nymphicus hollandicus)* with a laminated egg. Because of the different densities of the egg content, this egg without a shell is seen as a round structure of different echogenicity (a = albumen, y = yolk, s = shadow enhancement).

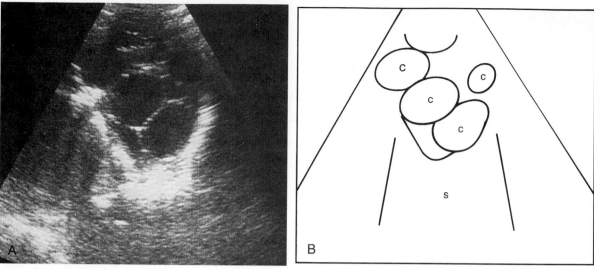

Figure 14–8

(*A* and *B*) Budgerigar *(Melopsittacus undulatus)* with ovarian cysts. Anechoic cysts (c) and distal shadow enhancement (s).

Examination of the Gastrointestinal Tract

Indications

Indications for a sonographic examination of the digestive tract are limited. A survey radiographic and radiographic contrast or double-contrast study of the gastrointestinal tract may provide sufficient information of pathologic alterations or functional disorders. However, sonography is sometimes useful in birds with diarrhea or internal papillomatosis.

Normal Appearance

The gastrointestinal tract can be difficult to examine sonographically. Examination is facilitated when the gastrointestinal tract is nearly empty and then filled with fluid for contrast purposes. Food particles, especially bones in carnivorous species, and gas content make it impossible for the sound beam to penetrate. The ventriculus of seedeaters is usually identified first, from either the ventromedial or the lateral approach. Grit may be easily seen as hyperechoic particles usually surrounded by a hypoechoic area (depending on the type of food ingested). The wall of the gizzard is seen as a round hypoechogenic margin. The proventriculus and the intestinal loops as well as the cloaca may be subsequently identified on the image (echogenic wall, hypoechoic content, typical shape). The motility of the intestinal loops is demonstrated clearly on the screen. The duodenal loop is especially easy to identify by its position and shape. A stand-off pad is necessary for the examination of the pancreas.[4] The cloaca is seen easily in the ventromedial approach (round echogenic wall, hypoechoic content) by sweeping the scanner caudally.

Pathologic Changes of the Gastrointestinal Tract

Dilatation of the proventriculus is seen in many noninfectious and infectious diseases such as neuropathic gastric dilatation and *Candida* infections. The massive dilatation is frequently accompanied by a thinning of the proventricular wall. Both changes may be clearly visualized in sonographic examination using the ventral as well as the lateral approach. A radiograph, however, may provide more information on gastrointestinal transit time (barium contrast study), alterations of the wall, or pathologic changes of the surrounding organs. Thickened intestinal walls may be seen in enteritis, tuberculosis, coligranulomatosis, or tumors. Thickened intestinal walls are identified quite clearly sonographically (Fig. 14–9), especially if accompanied by ascites.

Abnormal contents of the cloaca, such as uric acid concretions as well as cloacal dilatation in birds with spinal trauma may also be diagnosed by sonography. Examination of the cloaca is facilitated by retrograde application of fluid for contrast purposes. This technique may be necessary in birds with severe cloacal papillomatosis to obtain information of the extent and severity of the alterations in the cloacal wall.

Examination of the Heart

Indications

The diagnostic value of radiographic examination of the heart is limited. It is more appropriate in many instances to obtain information by using other diagnostic tools such as electrocardiography. Many techniques, however, are still insufficiently tested and evaluated. Many changes in the heart are difficult to diagnose, such as arrhythmias as a result of high heart rates, especially in small birds. Many cardiac alterations have probably not yet been described in the literature because of the lack of adequate methods of diagnosis in living birds.

Echocardiography has much to offer in avian cardiac evaluation. It is an excellent diagnostic tool for obtaining information on the heart's function or on pathologic alterations. A clinical sign that suggests the presence of cardiac insufficiency may justify sonographic examination. Other indications may be radiographic signs, such as alterations of the heart's size, shape, and radiographic density.

Normal Appearance

The heart is visible from the ventromedial approach in nearly all birds that the authors have examined. Exceptions occur when there are massive pathologic changes in the surrounding organs. The B-mode techniques may be used for sonographic examination of the heart.[5] A standardized schedule for routine echocardiography in birds has been described by Krautwald-Junghanns et al.[4] A definition has been given using the routine examination employed in human medicine—the apical four-chamber view as well as the apical two-chamber view from the ventromedial approach, and the right parasternal longitudinal views (four) and transverse views (four) from the right lateral approach.

With these views, the chambers, valves, great vessels, and motility of the heart and valves can be

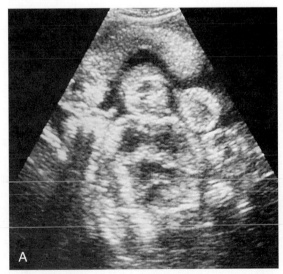
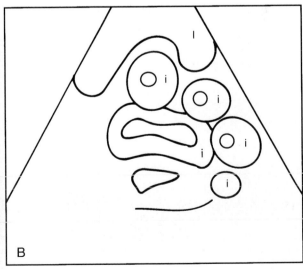

Figure 14–9

(*A* and *B*) Mynah bird *(Gracula religiosa)* with chronic enteritis, ascites. Massively enlarged intestinal loops (i) with hyperechoic wall and hypoechoic lumen, fluid in the abdomen, as well as a rounding of the liver's edge (l) were seen in this bird as a result of chronic generalized *Escherichia coli* infection.

identified sonographically. In the first parasternal longitudinal view, for instance, the left ventricle is differentiated clearly from the right by its larger size and by the thick wall (Fig. 14–10). The wedge-shaped right ventricle ends before the cardiac apex (Fig. 14–11). The interventricular septum extends cranially to the aorta, which is clearly differentiated in the third longitudinal parasternal view. Two valves of the aorta are seen. The right atrioventricular valve is seen as a relatively thick structure; one part of the right atrioventricular valve can be seen lying quite close to the septum. In most views the left atrium is visible as a round structure with a clear margin. For the evaluation of the right atrium, only the second longitudinal view and the apical four-chamber view may be used, whereas the vena cava caudalis is clearly shown just before it enters the right atrium in the fourth longitudinal view.

Pathologic Changes of the Heart

Many pathologic alterations of the heart are caused by secondary factors. For example, cardiac hypertrophy is often associated with chronic respiratory disease in mammals. However, this has not been documented in birds. An enlarged heart is easily

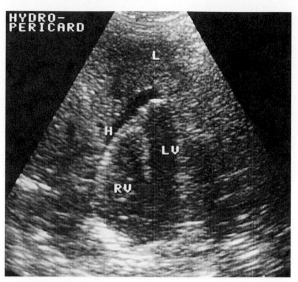

Figure 14–11

Grey parrot (*Psittacus erithacus erithacus*), ventromedial approach, apical four-chamber view, with pericardial effusion. Fluid (H = hydropericardium) is seen as an anechoic area between the liver parenchyma (L) and the heart (RV = right ventricle, LV = left ventricle).

recognized sonographically. A sonographic diagnosis of mitral valve regurgitation resulting in biatrial enlargement has been described in a mynah bird.[7]

Alterations of the pericardium, especially pericardial effusion, may be diagnosed in the sonographic examination. Ultrasound is the method of choice for differentiating pericardial effusion from cardiomegaly. The fluid is recognized as an anechoic band separating the epicardium and the pericardium (see Fig. 14–11).

There are no reports on the sonographic imaging of other possible pathology cardiac alterations in birds (e.g., congenital, metabolic, neoplastic disturbances). Various investigations on this subject are currently being undertaken.

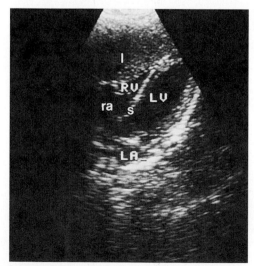

Figure 14–10

Pigeon *(Columba livia)* with normal appearance of the heart, right parasternal long axis view (LAX1) (RV = right ventricle, LV = left ventricle, LA = left atrium, ra = right atrium, s = septum, l = liver parenchyma).

References

1. Enders F, Krautwald-Junghanns M, Dühr D: Sonographic evaluation of liver diseases in birds. Proc 1993 European Conf Avian Med and Surg, 1993, pp 155–163.
2. Krautwald-Junghanns ME, Riedel U, Neumann W: Diagnostic use of ultrasonography in birds. Proc Assoc Avian Vet 269–275, 1991.
3. McMillan M: Imaging of avian urogenital disorders. Assoc Avian Vet Today 2(2):74–82, 1988.

4. Krautwald-Junghanns M-E, Schula M, Hagner D, et al: Transcoelomic two-dimensional echocardiography in the avian patient. J Avian Med Surg 9:19–31, 1995.

5. Schultz M: Echokardiographie am Taubenherzen, IX. München, DVG—Tagung über Vogelkrankheiten, 1994.

6. Silverman S: New frontiers in imaging avian and zoologic patients. Proc 1st Int Conf Zoo Avian Med 1987, 351–352.

7. Rosenthal K, Stamoulis M: Diagnosis of congestive heart failure in an Indian Hill mynah (*Gracula religiosa*). J Assoc Avian Vet 7(1):27–30, 1993.

15

Gerry M. Dorrestein

Avian Cytology

Cytology or examination of touch impressions, smears, and wet mounts of various lesions is extremely helpful for better disease definition. Cytology is a technique based on the morphologic study of individual cells. In disease, cytology can give information about pathophysiologic changes caused by the disease. Frequently, the agent causing the lesion can be identified.

The technique provides a simple and inexpensive method of diagnosis that can be performed in any veterinary practice. Because of the ease and rapidity of processing the samples, much information can be gathered in a short time.

The avian patient does not always lend itself to all of the diagnostic aids that are available for mammals. The small body size and blood volume of many birds, as well as the large number of different species, often limit the use of extensive biochemical and serodiagnostic evaluation techniques. Cytology can provide microscopic information about many different disease processes, which allows a more specific therapeutic approach. This is particularly true for external lesions, cysts, fluids, and biopsies. The cytologic examination of swellings, ocular and nasal discharges, wound smears, fluids, crop and cloacal swabs, and fecal smears can give much additional information about the nature and etiology of a process or symptom. The findings can also help to identify additional needed diagnostic tests such as microbiologic culture and/or histology.

At necropsy, cytology is an invaluable tool for defining the presumptive diagnosis so that initial treatment can be given to flock birds (Table 15–1). It gives rapid information about possible bacterial, mycotic, or yeast infections. The diagnosis of many protozoal infections, such as *Atoxoplasma* species

(see Color Fig. 15–1, Fig. 15–2), *Sarcosporidia* species (Fig. 15–3), and *Plasmodium* species, depends on demonstrating these organisms in impression smears from a selection of organs. For a quick differentiation between tumor and inflammation this technique is an invaluable aid.

The veterinarian should be aware of the limitations of diagnostic cytology. Cytology does not always provide a definitive diagnosis. It does not give histopathologic information concerning the architecture of the tissue (cells in the same smear may have originated from different areas of the organ or lesion), the size of the lesion, or the invasiveness of a malignant lesion. The cells observed may not necessarily represent the true nature of the lesion. An example of this is the imprinting of the ulcerated surface of a neoplastic mass that reveals the cytologic features of inflammation and infection only.

Cytologic evaluation is always an adjunct to other diagnostic procedures. A definitive diagnosis often requires a combined interpretation of the clinical history, physical examination, and evaluation of other diagnostic techniques, including radiographs, surgical investigations, microbiology, parasitology, histopathology, or even necropsy.

Cytopathology should not compete with histopathology; the two should complement each other in achieving the final diagnosis. Occasionally it is impossible to characterize the cells in a cytologic specimen, and a repeat smear or biopsy for histopathologic evaluation may be required to define the lesion.

SAMPLING TECHNIQUES AND SAMPLE PREPARATION

A successful cytologic examination[1-3] is possible when these four conditions are achieved: (1) a rep-

T a b l e 1 5 – 1

A LIST OF DISEASES IN WHICH CYTOLOGY GIVES IMPORTANT INFORMATION

Species	Disease	Organs to Be Examined
Bacterial Infections		
Canary/finch	Salmonellosis	Liver, spleen, lung, gut
	Yersiniosis	Liver, spleen, lung, gut
	Campylobacter	Gut (liver)
	Atypical tuberculosis	Liver, spleen, lung (gut)
	Staphylococci	Air sacs
	Duplococci	Lung, gut
	Megabacteria	Stomach, gut
Psittacine	Salmonellosis	Liver, spleen, lung, gut
	Pseudomonas	Lung, gut
	Clostridia	Gut
	Mycobacteria	All organs (tongue)
	Megabacteria	Stomach, gut
Pigeon	Salmonellosis	Joints (all organs)
	Streptococcus	Liver, spleen, lung, gut
Mycotic Infections		
Canary/finch	Candidiasis	Crop, gut
	Cryptosporidia	Stomach, gut
Psittacine	Candidiasis	Crop, gut
	Aspergillosis	Lung, air sac, syrinx
Pigeon	Yeasts	Gut
	Aspergillosis	Lung, air sac
Protozoa		
Canary	Flagellates	Esophagus, crop
	Atoxoplasmosis	Liver, spleen, lung (gut, brains)
	Toxoplasmosis	Lungs, brains
	Merozoites *(Isospora)*	Gut
Finch	*Trichomonas*	Esophagus, crop
	Cochlosoma	Gut
	Plasmodium	Blood, lung
Psittacine	*Plasmodium*	Blood, lung
	Haemoproteus	Blood, lung
	Trichomonas	Esophagus, crop
	Giardia	Duodenum
	Leucocytozoon	Muscle, heart
Lovebird	*Microsporidia*	Gut, brains, organs
Pigeon	*Trichomonas*	Esophagus, crop (liver)
	Hexamitiasis	Gut
	Merozoites	Gut
	Haemoproteus	Blood, lung
Miscellaneous		
Canary/finch	Anemia (red mites)	Blood, lung
	Septicemia	All organs
	Avian pox	Skin lesion
	Vacuolar degeneration	Liver
	Ornithosis	All organs
	Starch	Gut
Psittacine	Choking after forced feeding	Lung, air sac
	Metaplasia	Mucous glands, tongue, nostrils, syrinx
	Microfilaria	Blood, lung
	Chlamydiosis	All organs
	Herpesvirus	Liver
	Trypanosomes	Lung, liver
	Anthracosis	Lung
Mynah	Iron accumulation	Liver
Pigeon	Iron accumulation	Liver
	Crop milk	Crop
	Adenovirus	Liver

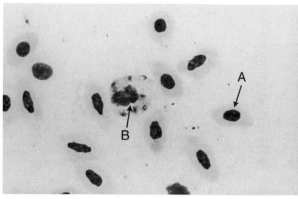

F i g u r e 1 5 – 2

Toxoplasma "pseudocyst" in a blue-crowned pigeon *(Goura c. cristata)*, lung. A, Mature erythrocyte with some postmortem changes; B, pseudocyst in erythrocyte.

resentative sample, (2) a good quality smear, (3) a good staining technique, and (4) a correct evaluation of the cytologic findings.[4]

The collection method used depends on the nature and consistency of the lesions being sampled. Before collection of the sample, the distribution, color, morphologic description, size, and odor (if present) of the lesion should be noted.[5]

For cutaneous lesions, scrapings can be collected with a cotton swab, glass slide, or spatula blade. A sample can be suspended in a small quantity of saline and a coverslip placed over the sample. Next, a "squash-prep" can be made by applying gentle pressure with a fingertip (in a twisting motion) to

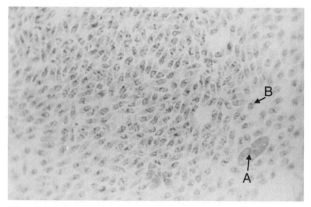

F i g u r e 1 5 – 3

Sarcosporidiosis in a blue-fronted parrot *(Amazona a. aestiva)*, muscle. A, Muscle cell nucleus, B, sporozoite.

the coverslip. This will help in revealing pathogens contained within keratinized material. Feathers need to be cut open to scrape the material from the shaft. Potassium hydroxide or chlorallactophenol can be used to digest keratinized material and improve visualization.[5] Exudates can be spread thinly.

Lesions containing fluid or purulent material can be sampled with a needle. If the lesion is cutaneous, it should be cleansed with a small amount of 70% alcohol and allowed to dry before sampling. In some cases, washes with sterile saline (e.g., for sinusitis, pneumonia, ingluvitis) provide a good technique to collect cellular material. Material collected can be used for both cytologic evaluation and microbial isolation attempts.

Conjunctiva or mucosa (beak, cloaca) is best sampled by touching the epithelia with a clean microscopic slide. The location of the sample often needs marking with a waterproof marker.

Fine-needle aspiration biopsy often provides a good cytologic sample from firm masses for a rapid presumptive diagnosis without radical tissue removal. This procedure can be performed in the examination room.

Aspirates should be examined first as wet mounts to enable the clinician to determine what additional preparations should be made. Some organisms, such as protozoa and nematode larvae, are better appreciated in a wet mount than in a stained preparation. Direct smears should be made from aspirated fluids with good cellularity (e.g., ascites or cyst contents). Smears can be made using the wedge method or the coverslip method commonly used for making blood smears. A "squash-prep" procedure should be used to make smears from thick tenacious fluid or from fluid that contains solid tissue fragments.

Fluids that have low cellularity require concentration methods to increase the smear cellularity. Sediment smears made after slow-speed centrifugation (500 rpm for 5 minutes) of the fluid or smear made with cytocentrifuge equipment usually provide adequate cytologic specimens.

Biopsy specimens and surgically removed masses can be evaluated cytologically, after cutting and scraping or touching with a microscope slide to make an impression smear.

At a standard necropsy, touch preparations should be made from the fresh-cut surfaces of liver, spleen, and lungs, and smears from a rectal scraping. All this material can be collected onto one slide. Extra impressions are to be made from macroscopically altered organs. It is important that cytologic specimens are from fresh sources, because cells degenerate rapidly following the death of the bird or after removal of the tissue.

Impressions of organs or tissues should be made from a freshly cut surface, which should be fairly dry and free of blood. This can be achieved by gently blotting the surface with a clean paper towel. Imprint slides can then be made by gently touching the glass or by touching the microscope slide onto the surface of the mass. It is important not to use too much pressure and to air-dry the sample quickly. Several imprints of the same organ should be made on each slide.

If the imprints show poor cellularity, more cells may be obtained by scraping the mass with a scalpel blade to improve exfoliation of the cells. The imprinting procedure can be repeated, or imprints can be made from the material remaining on the scalpel blade.

Fixation and Staining

Once a sample has been collected and a smear has been made, the specimen must be properly fixed to the slide. In case the preparations are to be sent to a diagnostic laboratory, they must be air-dried, well packed (broken sides are fairly common), and accompanied by distinct identification and case history.

The method of fixation depends upon which staining procedure is to be used. Fresh air-dried slides are adequate for Romanowsky stains (e.g., Giemsa stain and many quick stains).

A variety of stains and staining methods are used by cytologists, depending on the suspected disease or presence of pathogenic organisms. The classic and most common method used for initial evaluation of smears is Wright-Giemsa stain. Other stains are Ziehl-Neelson (*Mycobacterium* species), Giemsa (cells), Gram's (bacteria), methylene blue (fungi), modified Giminez (*Chlamydia* species), Stamp (*Chlamydia* species, see Color Fig. 15–4), and Sudan III (fat globules). Proper fixation must be applied if specific stains are used. For this information, telephone the diagnostic service.

The cytologic descriptions in this text are based

primarily on slides stained with a modified quick Wright's stain. The advantage of the quick stains is a short staining time (usually 20 sec), which allows rapid examination of the specimen and provides satisfactory staining quality. These stains are suitable for use in private veterinary practice where a simple staining procedure is desirable. Many quick stains also provide permanent reference smears for comparison with other cytologic specimens.

Common cytologic testing artifacts are[4]

1. Contamination of the slides with soap or formalin. This results in "exploded" erythrocytes ("smudge" cells).
2. A thick smear or impression.
3. Lysis of the cells because of thick or wet smears drying too slowly, too short fixation time in methanol, or collection of a needle biopsy with a wet needle.
4. Too much pressure by smearing, resulting in long deoxyribonucleic acid (DNA)/nuclear filaments by disruption of the cells and nucleus (see Color Fig. 15–5).

Stain precipitate on the smear should not be confused with bacteria or cellular inclusions. Stain precipitate varies in size and shape and is more refractive than bacteria or most cellular inclusions. The thickness of the smear affects the appearance of the cells and the quality of the smear. Thick areas do not allow the cells to expand on the slide, so they appear smaller and more dense when compared with the same cell type on thinner areas of the smear. Therefore, examination of the cells in thick smears should be avoided. Determination of the smear quality aids the cytologist in differentiating material that represents the true nature of the lesion from foreign material that was obtained by the collection technique or by contamination of the stain or microscopic slide.

Once the smears have been stained and dried, they are ready for microscopic examination. For a reliable evaluation of the cytologic changes in the sample, it is often necessary to consult a cytopathologist. Recognition of many etiologic agents is often simple and can give a presumptive diagnosis.

Scanning and low magnifications (objective 10× or 25×) are used initially to obtain a general impression of the smear quality. At these magnifications, the examiner is able to estimate the smear cellularity, identify tissue structures or large infectious agents (that is, microfilariae and fungal elements), and determine the best locations for cellular examination. Oil immersion (objective ×100) magnification is used to examine cell structure, bacteria, and other small objects.

In addition to viewing cellular structure, the cytologist should also determine background characteristics, the amount of blood or stain precipitation present, the thickness of different areas in the smear, and the distribution of the cells. The background characteristics may be useful in defining the nature of the material being examined. Protein aggregates create a granular background with the quick stains. Bacteria, crystals, nuclear material from ruptured cells, and exogenous material (for example, plant fibers, pollen, and talcum or starch crystals from examination gloves) may be seen in the noncellular background of the smear. Excessive blood contamination of a specimen dilutes and masks diagnostic cells, making interpretation difficult.

GENERAL PRINCIPLES OF CYTOLOGIC INTERPRETATION

The goal of cytology is to identify the cellular message and classify the cell response into one of the basic cytodiagnostic groups. These groups include inflammation, tissue hyperplasia or benign neoplasia, malignant neoplasia, and normal cellularity. The smears or impressions also give information about the possible etiology of the pathologic changes.

The cytologic appearance of many cells obtained from avian tissues and fluids is similar to those described for mammalian species. A cytologic classification divides body tissue into four groups: hemic, epithelial-glandular, connective, and nervous.

Hemic Tissue

Hemic tissue (blood and blood-forming tissue) is composed of cells that are found in the peripheral blood, bone marrow, and ectopic hematopoietic sites. Peripheral blood primarily contains the mature cells that are derived from cell lines located in the hematopoietic tissues. At necropsy, in impressions of the lungs, but also as a component of most cytologic preparations, blood cells are a common cell type. The following blood cells can be recognized: erythrocytes, thrombocytes, and leukocytes; granulocytes (heterophils or pseudoeosinophils, eosinophils, and basophils) and lymphocytes. (For the morphologic characteristics and pathophysiological conditions, see Chapter 11, Clinical Pathology.) Helpful references to the identification of avian leukocytes together with beautiful illustrations are found in more extensive handbooks.[2, 6] The common blood parasites are covered in the section on cytology of the lungs.

Epithelial Tissue Cells

Epithelial (including glandular) tissue cells tend to exfoliate in clumps or sheets. Epithelial cells (except mature squamous epithelium) are usually round or oval with abundant cytoplasm and have round or oval nuclei. The nuclear chromatin is generally smooth, and a prominent nucleolus may be visible. The cytoplasmic borders of epithelial cells are usually distinct, except for the liver. Normal epithelial cells are uniform in appearance.

Connective Tissue Cells

Connective tissue cells tend to exfoliate poorly and provide cytologic specimens with few cells. Often, traumatic exfoliation is required to obtain significant numbers of cells for evaluation. Depending on their origin, connective tissue cells tend to vary in the amount of cytoplasm and nuclear shape.

Nervous Tissue Cells

Nervous tissue cells are rarely seen on cytologic specimens, unless the specimens were made from central or peripheral nervous tissue. Nervous tissue cells may be present in smears from other tissues, but are of little significance.

CYTOLOGY OF INFLAMMATION

Inflammation may be caused by living agents (microorganisms) or nonliving agents (traumatic, thermal, toxic, or chemical agents). The cytology of inflammatory lesions may be classified into purulent and proliferative (including granulomatous) inflammatory reactions. Inflammatory cells include heterophils, eosinophils, macrophages, lymphocytes, plasma cells, and angiofibroblasts.

The *purulent reaction* is characterized by a predominance of heterophilic granulocytes. These cells will loose their granules and are called "toxic cells" (see Color Fig. 15–6). Overwhelming bacterial infections commonly cause degenerative changes to the heterophils (e.g., pyknosis, karyolysis, karyorrhexis, basophilic cytoplasm with phagocytic vacuolization). The agent may be phagocytized within the cytoplasm.

The cytology of *proliferative inflammation* shows many lymphocytes mixed with various numbers of plasma cells and macrophages. Occasionally, heterophils tend to be nondegenerate in appearance. This reaction becomes more granulomatous as evidenced by a predominance of mononuclear cells (macrophages and lymphocytes). A granulomatous reaction can also be represented by giant-cell formation or by macrophages coalescing into net-like sheets.

The inflammatory response can also be classified as either heterophilic (acute inflammatory response), mixed-cell (an established, active inflammation), or macrophagic inflammation (common in avian tuberculosis, chlamydiosis, foreign body reaction, mycotic infections, and cutaneous xanthomatosis).

CYTOLOGY OF MALIGNANT NEOPLASIA

For the cytologic diagnosis of neoplasia, certain criteria are required. In many cases, however, the differentiation between inflammation, hypertrophy, and neoplasia is not clearcut. The main cytopathologic criteria for the diagnosis of neoplasia can be divided into several categories: general cellular, nuclear, or cytoplasmic.

1. The general cellular features refer to the cell population on the smear. The neoplastic cells may appear related (have common origin) but can exhibit pleomorphism (variation in shape). Sometimes the nuclei are different from the nuclei of the normal tissue cells.

2. The changes in the nucleus include nuclear

hypertrophy, variations in size and shape of the nuclei and in the ratio of nuclei to cytoplasm (see Color Fig. 15–7), changes in the nucleoli, multinucleation, irregularity of the chromatin and nuclear membrane, and abnormal mitotic figures.

3. The cytoplasm can also be different (e.g., a different cytoplasmic volume; variations in the shape of the cytoplasmic borders; presence of basophilia, vacuolation, and inclusions bodies). Based on cytology only, it is very difficult and often impossible to classify the neoplasm as a carcinoma (epithelial), sarcoma (mesothelial, Fig. 15–8), or discrete cell (e.g., lymphoid leukosis) tumor. The presence of cell types that are foreign to the tissue being examined (ectopic cells) may indicate a metastatic neoplasm.

Clinically cytodiagnosis of swellings should differentiate between inflammation and neoplasms.

CYTOLOGY OF CONJUNCTIVA AND CORNEA

Samples can be obtained by using a sterile moist swab or a metal or plastic spatula to gently scrape the margins of the cornea or conjunctiva. Local ophthalmic anesthetics should not be used because they are toxic to cells. Normal conjunctival cytology shows a few epithelial cells occurring singly or in sheets, often with brown or black-pigmented granules in the cytoplasm. These granules should not be confused with bacteria. Corneal cells are nonkeratinized squamous epithelial cells with a central vesicular nucleus. A few extracellular bacteria are present on normal smears. Many inflammatory cells and much cell debris can be seen with bacterial conjunctivitis and corneal infections. Chlamydial or mycoplasmal infections of the eye may show inflammatory cells, cell debris, and epithelial cells and macrophages containing intracytoplasmic inclusions.

CYTOLOGY OF THE SKIN AND SUBCUTIS

The skin is composed of keratinized stratified squamous epithelium, and exfoliation produces primary cornified squamous epithelial cells. Bacterial infections are represented by large numbers of inflammatory cells, cell debris, and bacteria. Fungal infections may reveal fungal elements on cytologic examination. Foreign bodies produce granulomatous reactions with macrophages, giant cell formation, and a variable number of heterophils.

Cutaneous and subcutaneous masses should be examined cytologically. Pox lesions frequently produce cytologic features of inflammation and swollen epithelial cells with small, round, pale eosinophilic inclusions (Borrel and Bollinger bodies) when stained with Wright's stain. Subcutaneous lipomas are common in budgerigars, and a needle aspirate reveals numerous background fat droplets and a variable number of fat cells. Subcutaneous lymphosarcoma (lymphoid leukosis) is characterized by a marked number of immature lymphocytes with variable nuclear size.

CYTOLOGIC FEATURE OF FLUIDS

The accumulation of fluid in avian species is confined mainly to the abdominal cavity (ascites, peritonitis, hemoperitoneum), but is also encountered in isolated air sacs, in cysts, or as synovial fluid in the joints. Effusions can be classified as transudate, exudate, synovia, or hemorrhage.

The normal cytology of abdominal fluid, which is usually not present, occasionally shows mesothelial cells and macrophages. Mesothelial cells are round or oval and variable in size, and have a homogeneous basophilic cytoplasm and a centrally positioned round nucleus. Reactive mesothelial cells may show cytoplasmic vacuolization and eventually

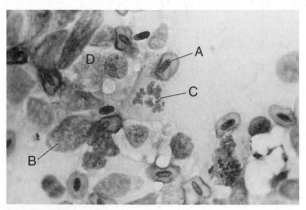

Figure 15–8

Sarcoma in a lovebird *(Agapornis* species), wing. A, Erythrocyte; B, undifferentiated tumor cells; C, mitotic figure; D, macrophage.

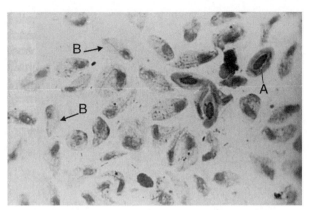

Figure 15–9

Trichomonas columbae in a pigeon *(Columba livia)*, crop. A, Erythrocyte; B, *Trichomonas* parasites. Notice the axostyle in each parasite.

may contain phagocytized material. It is difficult to differentiate transformed mesothelial cells, active histiocytes, and monocyte-derived macrophages.

Transudate fluids are characterized by low cellularity; exudate is characterized by high cellularity.

Purulent exudate may demonstrate bacteria or degenerated heterophils. Plasma cells frequently occur in chronic inflammatory lesions. They are lymphoid cells with an eccentric nucleus, dark blue cytoplasm, and a prominent Golgi apparatus. An egg-related peritonitis (yolk peritonitis) can be recognized by the presence of yolk drops, which are homogeneous, round, highly variable in size, and deeply basophilic in smears stained with quick stains. The same basophilic droplets can often be found in macrophages within the spleen, or in Kupffer cells and hepatocytes in the liver. Acute hemorrhagic effusions resemble peripheral blood smears.

Most normal avian joints contain a fluid volume that is too small for aspiration. Normal synovial fluid has poor cellularity; the majority of the cells are mononuclear. Septic joints usually have an increased synovial fluid volume. Cytologic examination reveals large numbers of heterophils and bacteria. In chronic *Salmonella* arthritis in pigeons, the smear demonstrates many polymorphonuclear heterophils, but bacteria are seldom seen. The eosinophilic granules often have disappeared. Chronic traumatic arthritis demonstrates many macrophages and erythrophagocytosis. Articular gout is often diagnosed by the gross appearance of the affected joint. The fluid is dense, white or yellow in color,

and cloudy. Large numbers of inflammatory cells are present. Urate crystals are birefringent needle-like crystals and are best seen under polarized light in a wet mount.

CYTOLOGY OF THE DIGESTIVE TRACT

Oral Cavity, Esophagus, and Crop

Examination of the oral cavity is part of the routine physical examination of a bird. White or yellow plaques, nodules, or ulcers may be found. Cytologic examination of these lesions aids in the diagnosis of candidiasis, trichomoniasis, poxvirus, bacterial infections, abscesses, and squamous metaplasia due to hypovitaminosis A.

Wet mounts aid in the identification of live *Trichomonas* species or other protozoa. At necropsy, these flagellate protozoa can be identified after staining by their undulating membrane, axostyle, and anterior flagellae (Fig. 15–9). Some other species of flagellates, without an axostyle or membrane, may also be present (Fig. 15–10).

The esophageal and crop lumina are lined by stratified squamous epithelium. These cells are polygonal with varying degrees of keratinization; they possess a condensed nucleus. Many extracellular bacteria (a variety of morphologic types) are visible and are often found in association with squamous cells. A rare *Candida*-like yeast may be present in normal crop fluid. Bacterial infections are indicated by leukocytes. Smears with a large num-

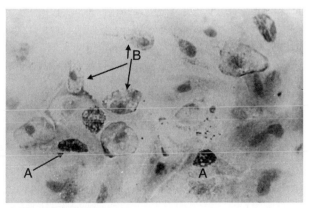

Figure 15–10

Flagellates in a canary *(Serinus canaria)*, crop. A, Squamous epithelial cell; B, flagellate without axostyle.

ber of bacteria of one morphologic type should be considered abnormal and an indication for bacterial culture. Candidiasis can be detected by demonstration of the oval, thin-walled yeasts (3–6 μm). They stain dark blue with quick stain and gram-positive with Gram's stain.

Cloaca

Cloacal cytology in a bird is indicated when inflammation, prolapse, or masses are detected. Wet mount preparations aid in the detection of worm eggs, coccidia, or protozoa.

Normal cloacal cytologic examination reveals a variable number of squamous cells that have varying degrees of keratinization, but most cells appear nonkeratinized and have a central vesicular nucleus. The normal mucosal cells of the intestinal lining are of the columnar type, often arranged in multicellular rows. In smears, the same changes may be found at necropsy.

At Necropsy: The Stomach, Intestinal Tract, and Cloaca

Stomach

In many species of birds a dilated ventriculus may be seen. In some species (e.g., canary, budgerigar, ostrich) this can be related to a "megabacterial" infection (Fig. 15–11). This organism can be demon-

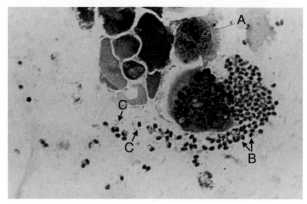

F i g u r e 1 5 – 1 2

Microsporidia and *Campylobacter* species in a star finch *(Bathilda ruficauda)*, duodenum. A, Epithelial cell; B, *Microsporidia*; C, *Campylobacter* species.

strated in a mucosal scraping. Candidiasis may be a cause of gastric ulceration.

Intestine and Cloaca

In most passerines (e.g., canaries and finches) and psittacines, bacterial flora is absent in the intestinal tract. At necropsy a mucosal scraping (mostly from the rectum) is prepared for cytologic evaluation. A variable amount of bacteria (rods, cocci, *Campylobacter* species [Fig. 15–12], *Vibrio* forms, "megabacteria," spores), fungi and yeasts, protozoa (coccidial schizonts, macro- and microgamonts [see Color Fig. 15–13], intra- and extracellular trophozoites, *Microsporidia* species [Fig. 15–12], flagellates), inflammatory cells, spermatozoa, starch or amylum particles, brown-black denatured hemoglobin (Fig. 15–14) and debris (plant material, chitin-skeletons of insects, urates) may be present. *Chlamydia* species may be demonstrated with a Stamp (see Color Fig. 15–15) or Macchiavellos stain, and *Mycobacterium* species with a Ziehl-Neelson stain.

CYTOLOGY OF THE RESPIRATORY TRACT

A sinus aspirate is indicated in avian patients with sinusitis. The left and right sinuses communicate in psittacine birds, but not in passerines and most other birds. Therefore, a single aspirate from one side in a parrot represents the sinus material from

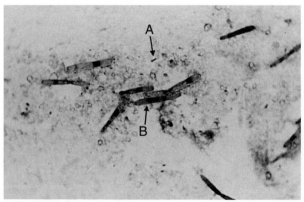

F i g u r e 1 5 – 1 1

"Megabacteria" in a lovebird *(Agapornis* species), rectum. A, Rodshaped bacterium; B, "megabacterium."

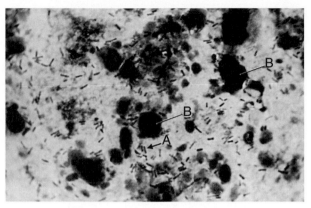

Figure 15–14

Hemorrhagic diathesis in a budgerigar *(Melopsittacus undulatus)*, rectum. A, Rod-shaped bacteria; B, denatured hemoglobin.

the bird is severely dyspneic. Tracheal swab samples can be obtained by passing a small cotton swab directly into the trachea.

The trachea and primary bronchi are lined by pseudostratified ciliated columnar epithelium with goblet cells, whereas the syrinx (located at the junction of the trachea and bronchi) consists of either bistratified squamous cells or columnar epithelial cells. Tracheal material exhibiting large numbers of heterophils and macrophages suggests tracheobronchitis, even in asymptomatic birds. Mycotic tracheal, bronchial, or syringeal lesions may be confirmed by the presence of fungal elements in a tracheal wash or postmortem scrapings (see Color Fig. 15–17).

Air sac samples can be obtained in a live bird by an endoscopic laparotomy technique, such as that used for surgical sexing of birds. At necropsy, scrapings can be made from the epithelial surface. The air sacs are lined by simple squamous epithelium. Airsacculitis is indicated by many inflammatory cells and a variable amount of background debris (Fig. 15–18). Intracellular bacteria indicate a bacterial etiology (Fig. 15–19), and fungal hyphae or elements confirm mycotic involvement. Special stains are required to confirm chlamydial infections.

both sides; in a canary the aspirate represents only one side. On cytologic examination, sinusitis is characterized by a moderate amount of background debris and a variable number of inflammatory cells, depending on the severity of the inflammation (Fig. 15–16). Sometimes the causitive agent is seen being phagocytized by leukocytes. An initial examination with an object lens 10× is essential to detect fungal elements.

Transtracheal aspiration is one method for evaluating upper respiratory disease in birds. The procedure is simple, but requires general anesthesia. A large-bore hypodermic needle can be inserted into an air sac to aid respiration during the procedure if

CYTOLOGY OF INTERNAL ORGANS

Lungs

At necropsy, the lungs are removed from the thoracic cavity and a freshly cut surface is blotted dry

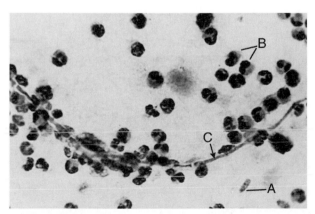

Figure 15–16

Mycotic sinusitis *(Aspergillus terreus)* in a red-fronted New Zealand parakeet *(Cyanoramphus novaezelandiae)*, sinus exudate. A, Erythrocyte; B, toxic heterophils; C, mycotic hyphae.

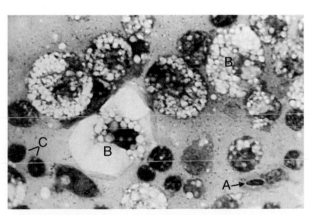

Figure 15–18

Activated macrophages in a Lady Gouldian finch *(Erythrura gouldiae)*, air sac. A, Erythrocyte; B, vacuolated macrophage; C, lymphocyte.

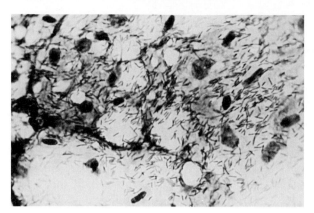

Figure 15–19

Pseudomonas sepsis, in a lovebird *(Agapornis* species), air sac.

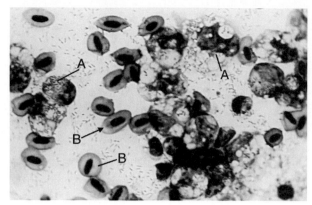

Figure 15–21

Rod-shaped bacterial pneumonia in a Lady Gouldian finch *(Erythrura gouldiae),* lung. A, Macrophage with rod-shaped bacteria; B, erythrocyte.

with a clean paper towel. Against this dried surface, an object slide is touched gently several times. The impression should be as thin as possible.

The impression smear of normal lung tissue consists mainly of blood cells mixed with columnar epithelial cells, ciliated cells, isolated cilia, pieces of striated muscle fibers, and an occasional macrophage or lymphocyte.

Pneumonia is characterized by the presence of many heterophils and vacuolated macrophages, often in an eosinophilic background because of edema and/or protein-containing fluids (exudate) in the respiratory tissue. The impression gives information on chlamydial, fungal, cryptococcal, and bacterial respiratory disorders (Figs. 15–20, 15–21). With severe anthracosis, macrophages may be

found with black phagocytized particles. This smear also gives an impression of the composition of the blood cells. In anemic birds, immature erythrocytes or their precursor cells may be recognized by the basophilic cytoplasm and the large round and vesiculated nuclei (see Color Fig. 15–22). Extracellular blood parasites (*Trypanosoma* species [Fig. 15–23], *Microfilaria* species) and intracellular schizonts (*Plasmodium* species) are easily seen under low-power magnification (see Color Fig. 15–24). Intracellular blood parasites (see Color Fig. 15–25) are found with high magnification in erythrocytes (*Plasmodium* species, *Haemoproteus* species [both with brown pigment], *Leucocytozoon* species [without

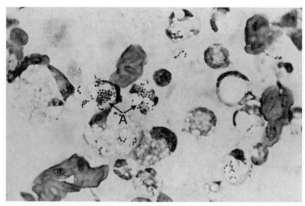

Figure 15–20

Cocci—pneumonia—in a hummingbird (Trochilidae), lung. A, Macrophage with cocci.

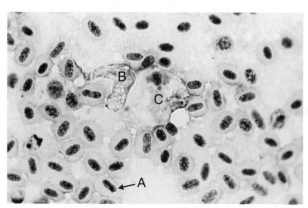

Figure 15–23

Trypanosoma avium in a sulphur-crested cockatoo *(Cacatua galerita),* liver. A, Erythrocyte; B, trypanosoma; C, Kupffer cell.

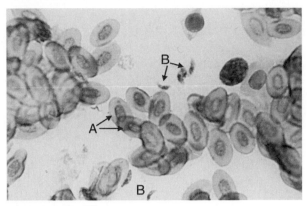

Figure 15–26

Toxoplasmosis in a canary *(Serinus canaria)*, lung. A, Erythrocyte; B, Trophozoites.

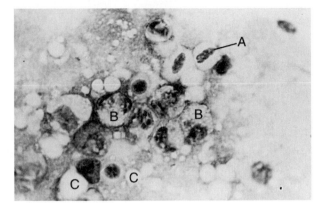

Figure 15–27

Activated macrophages (chlamydiosis) in a mealy Amazon *(A. farinosa)*, liver. A, Erythrocyte; B, macrophages; C, fat vacuoles caused by liver degeneration.

pigment]) and in leukocytes (*Leucocytozoon* species, *Atoxoplasma* species [see Fig. 15–1], *Toxoplasma* pseudocysts [see Figs. 15–2 and 15–26]).

Spleen

The avian spleen is a blood-forming and blood-destroying organ; it also contains lymphoid tissue. Impressions of the normal spleen show a significant amount of blood cells and heavy background cellular debris. Frequently, groups of lymphocytes in various stages of maturity can be seen. Macrophages showing varying degrees of erythrophago-

cytosis and iron accumulation are common. Cells with a variable amount of pale blue cytoplasm and indistinct cytoplasmic borders are present. These cells have an eccentric round or oval nucleus with coarse granular chromatin. They probably represent cells of the reticular stroma. Splenic impressions are good samples for the detection of bacterial infections, intra- and extracellular blood parasites, and chlamydial inclusions.

Liver

Cytologic examination of the liver can be done from smears or imprints made from aspiration or

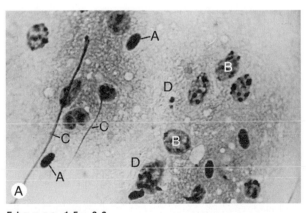

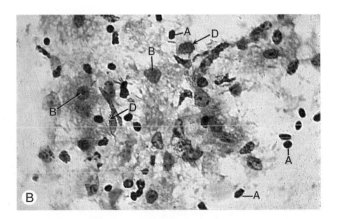

Figure 15–28

(A) Tuberculosis in an Old World kestrel *(Falco tinnunculus)*, liver (Hemacolor). A, Erythrocyte; B, liver cell nucleus with postmortem changes; C, nuclear filament; D, mycobacteria (nonstained rod-shaped bacteria). *(B)* Tuberculosis in an Old World kestrel *(Falco tinnunculus)*, liver (Ziehl-Neelson stain). A, Erythrocyte; B, liver cell nucleus with postmortem changes; D, mycobacteria (red, acid-fast stained rod-shaped bacteria).

excisional biopsy. At necropsy the freshly cut surface should be blotted very thoroughly until almost no cells are exfoliated. Liver specimens tend to provide a smear that is too cellular with an abundance of circulating blood cells. Background material is thick and basophilic (hepatocyte cytoplasm with many mitochondria) with a marked amount of cell fragments and free hepatocyte nuclei. Normal hepatocytes occur singly, in sheets, or in clusters. They are large and have abundant basophilic cytoplasm with coarse granulation (mitochondria). Fine eosinophilic granulation and iron particles can be detected in many cells. The nuclei are round or oval, are slightly eccentric in location, contain coarse chromatin, and have a single prominent nucleolus. The nuclei are uniform in appearance; an occasional binucleated cell can be seen. Occasionally, spindle-shaped stromal cells, lymphocytes, plasma cells, and macrophages are present.

Macrophages (Kupffer cells) often contain iron pigment or phagocytized material. Lymphoid aggregates may be found in most normal avian livers. These consist primarily of small mature lymphocytes. Reactive lymphoid aggregates contain a large number of plasma cells and often also heterophils. Large numbers of active macrophages can be seen with atoxoplasmosis or chlamydiosis (Fig. 15–27). Lymphoid neoplasia is indicated by large numbers of immature lymphocytes. Microfilarial larvae are sometimes found in liver cytology in birds without peripheral blood microfilarial infection. Mycobacterial species may be seen (sometimes even in birds without conspicuous macroscopic alterations) as empty, uncolored, rod-shaped ghosts, often grouped together in the basophilic background (Fig. 15–28*A*). An acid-fast staining technique confirms the diagnosis (Fig. 15–28*B*; see also Color Fig. 15–28*B*). Degenerated hepatocytes are seen with postmortem autolysis or hepatic disease.

Fatty livers show swollen hepatocytes with intracellular and extracellular lipid droplets. Inflammatory hepatic lesions are characterized by degenerate

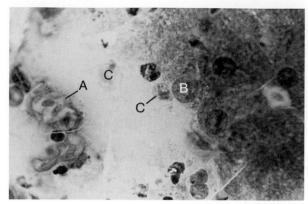

Figure 15–29

Trichomonas columbae in a pigeon *(Columba livia)*, liver. A, Erythrocyte; B, liver cell nucleus; C, *Trichomonas*. Notice flagella.

hepatocytes and marked inflammatory cell infiltration. Bacterial infections are recognized by intra- and/or extracellular bacteria; protozoal infection can be demonstrated (Fig. 15–29). Some viral infections may show intracytoplasmic or intranuclear inclusion bodies (see Color Fig. 15–30*A* and *B*). Neoplastic lesions contain cells with cytologic features of neoplasia.

References

1. Campbell TW: Avian Hematology and Cytology. Ames, Iowa State University Press, 1988.
2. Campbell TW: Cytology. In Ritchie BW, Harrison GJ, Harrison LR (eds): Avian Medicine: Principles and Application. Lake Worth, FL, Wingers Publishing, 1994, pp 199–222.
3. Fudge AM: Avian clinical cytology. Proc Assoc Avian Vet, Houston, 1988, pp 291–293.
4. Ingh TSGAM van den, Vos JH: Technical aspects of fine-needle aspiration cytology. Tijdsch Diergeneeskd 114:713, 1989.
5. Jacobson ER: Blood collection techniques in reptiles: Laboratory investigation. Cytodiagnostics. In Fowler ME (ed): Zoo and Wild Animal Medicine. Current Therapy 3. Philadelphia, WB Saunders, 1993, pp 148–149.
6. Lucas AJ, Jamroz C: Atlas of Avian Hematology. Washington DC, United States Department of Agriculture, Monograph 25, 1961.

Barbara L. Oglesbee

Differential Diagnosis

GASTROINTESTINAL SIGNS

Regurgitation

Behavioral/sexual

Crop: Intraluminal
Foreign body/ingluviolith

Neoplasia
Papilloma

Leiomyoma/leiomyosarcoma
Ingluvitis
Bacterial

Mycotic: Candidiasis, aspergillosis

Parasitic: Trichomoniasis
Extraluminal compression of crop
Neoplasia

Granuloma

Thyroid hyperplasia (goiter)
Esophageal stricture
In neonates

Overfeeding

Improper temperature/consistency of formula

Crop burn

Vomiting

Proventriculus/ventriculus
Foreign body
Small foreign bodies

Impaction
Grit

Food/seed
Neoplasia
Papilloma

Leiomyoma/leiomyosarcoma

Adenoma/adenocarcinoma

Fibroma/fibrosarcoma
Gastric ulcer

Neuropathic gastric dilatation (PDS)

Traumatic gastritis

Proventriculitis/ventriculitis
Bacterial: Gram-negative, megabacteria, *Mycobacterium avium*

Mycotic: Candidiasis, aspergillosis

Ingested chemical irritants
Intestines
Intestinal intussusception or volvulus

Intestinal obstruction
Neoplasia

Functional ileus resulting from generalized gastrointestinal disease
Liver disease

Pancreatitis

Peritonitis

Septicemia

Diabetes mellitus

Central nervous system (CNS) disorder

Infectious disease
Viral: Polyoma virus, herpes virus, hepato-

223

splenitis, pox virus, paramyxovirus, avian serositis virus

Chlamydiosis

Aspergillosis
Toxicity

Lead

Zinc

Organophosphate

Antibiotics
Trimethoprim-sulfa combinations

Doxycycline

Ketoconazole

Crop Stasis

Crop: Intraluminal
Foreign body/ingluviolith

Neoplasia

Ingluvitis
Bacterial

Mycotic (candidiasis)

Parasitic
Crop atony resulting from overstretching (neonates)

Trauma
Feeding tubes

Thermal burns
Crop: Extraluminal
Neoplasia

Thyroid hyperplasia (goiter)

Abscess

Crop rupture/perforation with subcutaneous sequestration of formula
Esophageal
Stricture

Abscess

Granuloma

Neoplasia

Proventriculus/ventriculus
Foreign body
Ingested foreign bodies

Impaction
Grit

Food/seed
Neoplasia

Granuloma

Internal papillomatosis

Gastrointestinal ulceration

Proventriculitis/ventriculitis
Bacterial

Mycotic

Toxic/chemical
Gastric dilatation
PDS, neuropathies, gastric dilatation

Other causes
Infections

Toxic

Mycotic

Degenerative or debilitative
Intestinal
Intussusception

Volvulus

Foreign body

Neoplasia

Functional ileus resulting from generalized gastrointestinal disease
Systemic disease
Viral
Polyoma virus, PDS, paramyxovirus, adenovirus
Bacterial sepsis

Sarcocystis infection

Metabolic
Dehydration

Hypokalemia

Liver disease/hepatic encephalopathy

Vitamin E/selenium deficiency

Toxic
 Heavy metal

 Organophosphate

 Hypervitaminosis D

 Hypercalcemia

Diarrhea

Infectious disease
 Chlamydiosis

 Mycotic: Gastrointestinal, candidiasis

 Viral: Polyoma virus, Pacheco's disease virus, reovirus, adenovirus, paramyxovirus

 Bacterial enteritis: *Escherichia coli, Enterobacter, Pseudomonas, Salmonella, Klebsiella, Campylobacter, M. avium, Mycoplasma* species; megabacteria

 Parasitic: Giardiasis, coccidiosis, cryptosporidiosis, hexamita, nematodes, trematodes, cestodes
Mechanical
 Intestinal intussusception

 Intestinal stricture/stenosis

 PDS

 Cloacolith
Dietary
 Dietary change
  Increased fruit/vegetable (fiber) content
 Food intolerance/allergy

 Ingested bacterial endotoxins

 Ingested abrasive foreign material
Toxic
 Heavy metal (lead, zinc)

 Antibiotic therapy

 Organophosphates

 Hypervitaminosis D

 Endogenous bacterial endotoxins
Metabolic disease
 Liver disease

 Renal disease

Pancreatitis

 Peritonitis
Abnormal microflora due to antibiotic therapy

Neoplasia

Papillomatosis: Intestinal, cloacal

Stress/excitement

Voluminous Stools, Undigested Food

Behavioral
 Nesting

 Housebreaking training
Malabsorption/maldigestion
 PDS

 Vitamin E/selenium deficiency

 Hepatic cirrhosis

 Enteritis
  Bacterial: Gram-negative, megabacteria, *M. avium*

  Mycotic *(Candida)*

  Parasitic (especially giardiasis)
 Exocrine pancreatic insufficiency
 Pancreatitis

  Pancreatic atrophy
 Intestinal neoplasia

Melena

Gastrointestinal ulceration

Neoplasia: Crop, esophagus, ventriculus, proventriculus, small intestine

Proventriculitis/ventriculitis

Hemorrhagic enteritis (HGE)
 Viral: Polyoma virus, reovirus, adenovirus, herpes virus
Intestinal papilloma

Gastrointestinal foreign body/traumatic gastritis/enteritis

Intussusception

Parasitic
  Coccidiosis

  Cryptosporidiosis
Coagulopathy

Starvation/anorexia

Bloody Droppings: Frank Blood

Cloacal papilloma

HGE
  Bacterial

  Heavy metal (lead)
Cloacal ulceration

Reproductive
  Egg binding

  Prolapse

Tenesmus

Gastrointestinal (GI) disease
  Enteritis

  GI parasitism
Cloacal disease
  Papilloma

  Cloacolith/cloacal impaction

  Cloacitis: Bacterial, candidiasis

  Cloacal prolapse

  Cloacal stricture (post injury/surgery)
Reproductive tract disease
  Egg-laying

  Egg binding/dystocia

  Uterine prolapse

Abdominal Distension

Obesity/lipoma/xanthoma

Abdominal wall hernia
  Estrogenic

Organomegaly
  Liver disease
    Inflammatory/infectious
      Chlamydiosis

      Bacterial hepatitis

      M. avium

      Viral hepatitis: Reovirus, polyoma virus, Pacheco's disease

      Mycotic: Aspergillosis

      Parasitic: Atoxoplasmosis, *Plasmodium* species, *Sarcocystis*
    Degenerative: Hemochromatosis (?), hepatic lipidosis

    Congestion: Congestive heart failure

    Hepatic neoplasia
  Proventriculus/ventriculus
    PDS

    Pyloric obstruction

    Neoplasia
  Small intestine
    Obstruction

    Neoplasia

    M. avium
  Large intestine
    Cloacolith

    Megacolon/neuropathic
  Renal neoplasia

Reproductive
  Testicular neoplasia

  Ovarian
    Ovarian neoplasia

    Cysts

    Hormonal (estrogen) add muscle weakness

    Oviduct/uterus
      Enlargement in egg-laying hen

      Egg binding/dystocia

      Metritis/salpingitis

      Cystic oviduct (?)

Ascites
  Modified transudate
    Liver disease

    Hypoalbuminemia

    Hemochromatosis

    Abdominal neoplasia

    Congestive heart failure

    Cystic (ovarian)

    Congenital circulatory/liver disorders
  Nonseptic inflammatory
    Avian viral serositis

    Yolk peritonitis

    Pancreatitis
  Septic inflammatory
    Ruptured intestine

    Ruptured abscess

    Yolk peritonitis

    Ruptured uterus

    Aspergillosis
  Hemorrhage (hemoperitoneum)

Polyuria/Polydypsia

Renal
  Inflammatory
    Glomerulonephritis resulting from other systemic or idiopathic disease

    Hypercalcemic nephropathy

    Renal gout

    Pyelonephritis (bacterial)

    Glomerulonephritis: Polyoma virus, paramyxovirus, pox virus, reovirus, adenovirus, aspergillosis
  Degenerative
    Hypovitaminosis A

    Obstructive uropathy: Urolith, cloacolith, neoplasia, egg binding
  Toxic
    Heavy metal

Drug-induced
    Aminoglycosides

    Allopurinol

    Sulfonamides

    Tetracyclines

    Cephalosporins
  Hypervitaminosis D
  Renal ischemia
    Hypoperfusion
      Dehydration

      Anesthesia

      Hypovolemia
  Neoplasia
    Adenocarcinoma

    Nephroblastoma
Systemic/metabolic
  Liver disease

  Pancreatitis

  Chlamydiosis

  Gastrointestinal disease

  Septicemia

  Localized abscess/salpingitis

  Neoplasia: Pituitary adenoma/adenocarcinoma

  Metabolic
    Diabetes mellitus

    Hypercalcemia
Dietary
  Increased water content of food (fruits, gruel)

  Breeding/feeding offspring

  Excess dietary sodium
Boredom, psychogenic polydypsia

Stress/excitement

RESPIRATORY SIGNS

Sneezing, Nasal Discharge

Nares/sinuses
  Hyperkeratosis resulting from hypovitaminosis A

Infectious causes
    Bacterial: *E. coli, Enterobacter, Klebsiella, Pseudomonas, Pasteurella, Bordetella, Salmonella, M. avium, Staphylococcus* species, *Streptococcus* species, spirochetes

    Chlamydia psittaci

    Mycoplasma species

    Viral: Pox virus, reovirus, paramyxovirus, polyoma virus

    Mycotic: *Aspergillus, Candida, Cryptococcus,* mucormycosis
Neoplasia

    Foreign body (seed hulls, etc)

    Rhinoliths

    Granuloma

    Congenital: Choanal atresia
Inhaled irritants (cigarette smoke, dust, perfumes, aerosols)

Trauma

Allergies

Iatrogenic
    Inhaled feeding formula

    Inhaled medications
Dry air, dehydration in winter

Dyspnea

Nares/sinuses
    Rhinoliths/plugged nares

    Neoplasia

    Choanal atresia

    Bacterial sinusitis

    Knemidokoptes species infection (?)
Glottis/trachea
    Mass
        Granuloma
            Foreign body
        Abscess

        Neoplasia

    Aspergillus

    Hyperkeratosis resulting from hypovitaminosis A
Infection
    Herpes virus (Amazon tracheitis)

    Pox virus
Parasitic
    Plaques resulting from trichomoniasis
Aspirated foreign body

Papilloma (obstruction of glottis)

Extraluminal compression
    Goiter

    Neoplasia
Lungs
    Bronchopneumonia
        C. psittaci

        Bacterial: Gram-negative, *Staphylococcus, Streptococcus, Mycoplasma, M. avium*

        Mycotic: *Aspergillus*

        Viral (pox, paramyxovirus, reovirus)

        Parasitic (sarcocystosis, trichomoniasis)
    Aspiration pneumonia

    Aerosolized toxins (Teflon)

    Congestive heart failure

    Chronic obstructive pulmonary disease
Air sacs
    Airsacculitis/air sac consolidation
        Aspergillus

        Bacterial

        Mycoplasmal

        Chlamydia

        Viral
    Extraluminal compression
        Obesity

        Ascites

        Hemocoelom

        Hepatomegaly

        Egg binding

        Neoplasia

FEATHER ABNORMALITIES

Feather Loss

Lack of feather regrowth
  Infection
    Psittacine beak and feather disease virus

    Polyoma virus
  Endocrinopathy: Hypothyroidism

  Follicular atrophy

  Delayed molt: Malnutrition, stress, debilitation

  Congenital baldness
Abnormal feather regrowth
  Infection
    Psittacine beak and feather disease virus

    Polyoma virus

    Polyfolliculitis
  Feather cysts

  Bacterial/mycotic folliculitis

  Nutritional deficiencies

  Endocrinopathy: Hypothyroidism

  Follicular trauma
Abnormal coloration of feathers
  Psittacine beak and feather disease virus

  Nutritional deficiencies

  Stress marks: Stress, disease, malnutrition

  Hepatopathy

  Thyroid supplementation

  Fungal growth on feathers

  Old feathers, wearing, delayed molt
Feather picking/self-mutilation
  Medical causes
    Systemic disease: Hepatopathy, intestinal
    disease, respiratory disease, abdominal ad-
    hesions, neoplasia, hypothyroidism

    Bacterial/mycotic folliculitis

    Malnutrition

    Cutaneous neoplasia, xanthomas

    Parasitic

    Endoparasites: Intestinal giardiasis, ascari-
    des, cestodes

    Ectoparasites: mites (scabies, myialges)
  Allergies

  Dry skin (environment)

  Environmental irritants (cigarette smoke)

  Cutaneous trauma
Behavioral causes
  Reproductive: Sexual frustration, nest build-
  ing, broodiness

  Overcrowding/territorial behavior

  Attention-getting device

  Boredom

  Insecurity: Lack of visual security or area to
  roost, harassment by people or other pets

  Change in routine/change in environment

  Anxiety/stress

  Habitual (in chronic cases)

INTEGUMENTARY LESIONS

Proliferative Dermatitis

Cutaneous papillomas

Viral
  Pox virus

  Herpes virus pododermatitis
Bacterial/mycotic dermatitis

Allergy: Insect bite hypersensitivity

Hyperkeratotic Dermatitis

Knemidokoptes mites (especially on face and
feet)

Malnutrition (hypovitaminosis A)

Bacterial/mycotic dermatitis

Cutaneous Mass

Mycobacteriosis

Neoplasia: Squamous cell carcinoma, melanoma, lymphoma, fibroma/fibrosarcoma

Lipomas, xanthomas

Abscess

Feather cysts

Gout

Ulcerative Lesions

Chronic or recurrent ulcerative dermatitis
  Bacterial (especially *Staphylococcus* species)

  Dermatitis

  Malnutrition

  Topical irritants

  Allergic

  Hormonal

  Intestinal giardiasis

  Metabolic disease

  Trauma/cellulitis

  Idiopathic
Pox virus

Thermal/chemical burns

Trauma/self-mutilation

NERVOUS SYSTEM

Seizures

Infectious (meningitis, meningoencephalitis)
  Newcastle disease virus, *C. psittaci*, bacterial,
  Sarcocystis
Head trauma

Toxicity
  Heavy metal

  Organophosphate

CNS neoplasia
Metabolic
  Hypocalcemia

  Hypoglycemia

  Hepatic encephalopathy
Idiopathic
  Epilepsy
Agonal

Ataxia

Infectious (meningitis, meningoencephalitis)
  Viral: Newcastle disease virus, polyoma virus,
  reovirus

  PDS

  C. psittaci

  Bacterial

  Toxoplasma
Toxicity
  Heavy metal

  Organophosphate
CNS neoplasia

Metabolic/nutritional
  Hypocalcemia

  Hypoglycemia

  Vitamin E/selenium deficiency

  Vitamin B_1 deficiency

  Hepatic encephalopathy

  Atherosclerosis

  Cerebral vascular accident
Spinal cord disease
  Vertebral fracture

  Vertebral subluxation

  Granuloma (aspergilloma, bacterial)

  Infarct

Paresis/Paralysis

Bilateral
  Infectious (meningitis, meningoencephalitis)

Viral
  Newcastle disease virus

  Polyoma virus

  Reovirus

  PDS
  C. psittaci

  Bacterial
Toxicity
  Heavy metal

  Organophosphate
CNS neoplasia

Metabolic/nutritional
  Hypocalcemia

  Hypoglycemia

  Vitamin E/selenium deficiency

  Vitamin B_1 deficiency

  Hepatic encephalopathy

  Atherosclerosis

  Cerebral vascular accident

Spinal cord disease
  Vertebral fracture

  Vertebral subluxation

  Granuloma (aspergilloma, bacterial)

  Neoplasia

  Infarct
Unilateral
  Spinal cord disease
    Granuloma

    Neoplasia

    Infarct
  Long bone fracture

  Sciatic nerve compression (rear limb)
    Renal neoplasia, renomegaly

    Testicular/ovarian neoplasia

    Granuloma

    Abscess

    Obturator paralysis
      Egg binding
  Brachial plexus avulsion (wing)

Jeffrey R. Jenkins

17

Hospital Techniques and Supportive Care

Hospital techniques and methods of treatment for the avian patient are often different from those used in other species. Similarly, techniques often vary from one group of birds to another. The following are descriptions of common techniques used in the author's practice. Each method presented is one way to perform a treatment or diagnostic test or collect a sample. The techniques apply to most avian species; exceptions are described when the variation is significant. Developing relationships with local pet shops and participation in local aviculture and species hobbyists clubs (falconry, pheasantry, pigeon fancy, etc.) build experience with various species. Experience helps in identifying individuals that are likely to strike, "foot," or bite.

BASIC EQUIPMENT

Much of the equipment needed to work on birds is available in the average small animal hospital. There are a few items that are important and worthy of mention here. An incubator, warmer, brooder, or intensive care bird cage, preferably oxygen (O_2) administration–compatible, maintained at 26 to 32°C (80–90°F) is needed. The ultimate bird incubator supplies radiant heat from the floor, is easy to clean and sterilize, and is inexpensive. Both the floor and air temperature should be monitored to ensure that the patient is not burned or overheated. A simple warming cage can be made using a glass aquarium, a heating pad, and a 60-watt bulb in a utility fixture. The temperature of the floor of the aquarium may

be further modified by layering towels between the heating pad and the glass. Many commercial warming units are available. Each has advantages and disadvantages. Because of the high number of diseases caused by airborne transmission in avian medicine, units that circulate air should be avoided unless they can be sterilized between patients.

A gram scale with an accuracy to plus or minus 1 g is necessary to calculate correct dosages and to monitor patient weight changes. Both mechanical (triple-beam) and electronic scales work well. Be careful to secure the scale so that it cannot be knocked to the floor by an excited patient. Velcro strips, which are available at most hardware stores, work well for this purpose.

A variety of syringes, small hypodermic needles, spinal needles, small butterfly catheters, feeding tubes, and small cuffed and Cole endotracheal tubes are needed. A 0.5 ml U-100 low-dose insulin syringe (Monoject, U-100 Low Dose Syringe, Sherwood Medical, St. Louis, MO) is calibrated and accurately delivers 0.01-ml increments. The attached 28-gauge 1/2-inch needle minimizes pain and is perfect for all but the largest patients. This syringe is readily available at a reasonable cost.

Bandage materials in small sizes should be prepared. Cotton felt cast padding (Webril Regular Finish Under Cast Padding, Kendall Healthcare Products Co, Mansfield, MA) works very well as a foundation for bandages and splints. The felt-like cotton forms well to the contours of the limb, is comfortable, and does not have the potential for fibers to pull tight and constrict the limb or bandaged area if picked by the patient, which may occur with Kling or brown gauze. Not-so-sticky tape, such as masking tape, paper skin tape, or the paper tape used to tape "pin curls" have proved satisfactory. In some situations a very sticky tape proves useful. Waterproof adhesive tape (Wet-Pruf, Kendall Healthcare Products Co, Mansfield, MA) stays in place for 4 to 6 weeks in a tape bandage but must be carefully applied. Nonstick (Telfa "Ouchless" Sterile Pad, Kendall Healthcare Products Co, Mansfield, MA), hydroactive (BioDres Biosynthetic Absorbent Wound Dressing, DVM, Dermatologics for Veterinary Medicine, Miami, FL), and semiocclusive (Tegaderm Transparent Dressing, 3M Medical Surgical Division, St. Paul, MN) bandages work well on avian skin and are recommended.

Plastic or metal speculums (Lafeber Co, Odell, IL) are necessary to open strong beaks. Alternatively, a speculum may be made by drilling a large hole in a plastic dog chew bone (Nylabone, Nylabone Products, Neptune, NJ).

Materials for collection of laboratory samples are needed. Some of these may be available from veterinary clinical laboratories. Swabs with modified Stewart's bacterial transport media are available in two sizes. Larger sizes (Culturette, Marion Laboratories, Kansas City, MO) work well for taking samples from most locations. Smaller swabs (Mini-Tip Culturette, Marion Laboratories) work well when sampling the choana, cloaca, and trachea of small species. Microhematocrit tubes, cover slips, and glass slides are necessary and are the same as those used with other animals. Micro–blood sampling tubes (Microtainer, Becton Dickinson, Rutherford, NJ) that collect 200 µl to 700 µl are available with a variety of anticoagulants, mixing beads, and inert gel serum separators. A very useful tube has a combination lithium heparin and gel barrier (Microtainer stat plasma separator, Becton Dickinson, Rutherford, NJ) that allows collection of a single tube for both hematologic and plasma chemistries.

Sterile rubber stoppered blood collection tubes (Monoject Blood Collection Tubes, Sherwood Medical, St. Louis, MO) are easy and economical containers in which to dispense small volumes of injectable medications. Larger volume sterile empty vials (Hollister-Stier, Miles, Inc., Spokane, WA) are available from allergy antigen suppliers in a variety of sizes for dispensing large volumes of injectable medication.

Silver nitrate sticks (Silver Nitrate Applicators,

Graham-Field, Inc., Hauppauge, NY), tissue cement (VetBond, Animal Care Products, 3M, St. Paul, MN), and ferric subsulfate styptic (ferric subsulfate, Mallinckrodt, Paris, KY) are needed as aids to stop hemorrhage. As described later, a syringe barrel with the tip removed works well to apply powdered styptic.

Towels and washcloths are needed for restraint. I prefer to use white towels that may be bleached when laundered for sanitation; they present a professional image to the client (Fig. 17–1). Other equipment that should be available in an avian practice includes an isoflurane vaporizer, Doppler monitoring equipment, electrosurgical or radiosurgical equipment, fine microsurgical equipment, surgical thermal support, magnification loupes or surgical microscope, and a fluid warmer.

VENIPUNCTURE AND CATHETERIZATION

Phlebotomy and Intravenous Injection

Blood samples must be obtained in a volume and quality that provide reliable results from the diagnostic laboratory. Two routes are commonly used—toenail clip and venipuncture. The choice of the site depends on the size and nature of the patient, volume of blood needed, and the experience of the person taking the sample. Volumes of 0.5 to 1.0% of the bird's body weight have proved safe (depending on the condition of the bird) and are in line with volumes that may be taken from

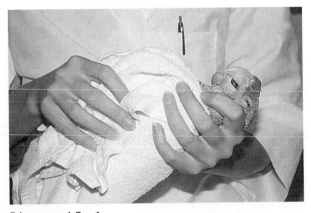

F i g u r e 1 7 – 1

Amazon parrot properly restrained in a towel.

other species[1] (see sections on body fluids, hypovolemia, and hypotension in Chapter 48). Clinicians should check with the laboratory that will be running the tests for their specific requirements prior to drawing a sample.

Three large peripheral veins are suitable for drawing blood samples: the jugular vein, basilic vein, and medial metatarsal vein. The jugular vein is the most accessible and the least prone to problems with extravasation of blood, making it the best choice for bleeding species weighing less than 1 kg. This vein may be used repeatedly for sampling or parenteral therapy if venipuncture is done carefully.

Species weighing less than 200 to 300 g may be restrained with the index and middle finger of the left hand holding and extending the head, while the ring finger and the little finger restrain the body. The thumb is free to manipulate the vein from its normal position under the edge of the esophagus and crop. The featherless area over the vein is lightly moistened with alcohol to better visualize the vein. The syringe, held in the right hand, may then be introduced from either direction, depending on personal preference. Venipuncture may be easier if the needle is slightly bent and placed bevel up.

Larger species usually require two persons. The assistant restrains the bird in a towel, in left lateral position with the head pointed toward the person drawing the sample. The wings and back of the bird are held firmly in the left hand while the bunched towel is held in the right. The person drawing the sample holds the bird's head (cautiously, so as not to be bitten in the left hand, with the little, ring, and middle fingers wrapped under the lower beak, and the thumb around the cranium (Fig. 17–2). This frees the index finger of the left hand to manipulate the vein. As before, the skin over the vein is moistened with alcohol and the feathers smoothed back. With the syringe in the right hand, the vein is approached cranial to caudal, with the needle bevel up. When the needle is withdrawn, the assistant moves the left hand so as to restrain the head and place light pressure on the jugular vein just cranial to the puncture site.

The basilic vein, located on the ventral aspect of the wing, can be used for sampling, but it is better used for injection. However, the basilic vein is routinely used for blood collection in pigeons, waterfowl, and raptors. For this technique, an assistant

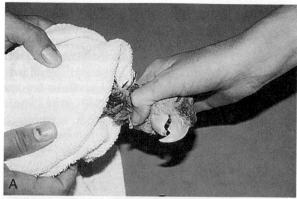

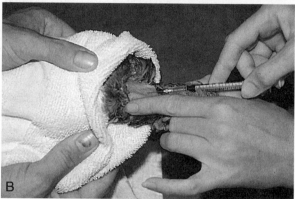

Figure 17–2

Jugular phlebotomy (or intravenous injection) in a large parrot. *(A)* An assistant restrains the bird in a towel in left lateral position with the head pointed toward the person drawing the blood. *(B)* The bird's head has been cautiously passed to the left hand with the second and ring finger under the mandible and the thumb over the crown. The index finger of the left hand is used to manipulate the crop and jugular vein. The vein is entered, cranial to caudal, with the syringe held in the right hand.

restrains the bird in a towel on a flat surface (Fig 17–3). The assistant may extend the wing; however, we prefer to have the person drawing the sample extend the wing and restrain it by placing light pressure on the antebrachium and primary feathers. The vein is entered distally to medially at a point just proximal to the elbow. One disadvantage to the use of this vein is hematoma formation. Digital pressure to the puncture site minimizes this problem.

Many species have a large medial metatarsal vein at the medial side of the intertarsal joint. The scaled skin of the lower leg covers the area, which helps to reduce hematoma formation, as does the skin held taut by the gastrocnemius muscle. The bird

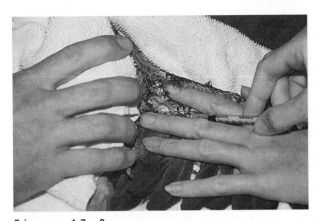

F i g u r e 1 7 – 3

Restraint and approach for intravenous injection or phlebotomy using the basilic vein.

must be restrained in a towel in dorsal recumbency (Fig. 17–4). The leg is extended by the person drawing the sample, and the vein is entered distal to proximal, with the bevel up. Two good locations to enter the vein are distal to the tibiotarsal-tarsometatarsal joint (best in Galliformes and Anseriformes) or just as the vein slips beneath the distal portions on the medial head of the gastrocnemius and the fibularis longus muscles. Pressure should be applied to the puncture site for several minutes after the needle is withdrawn. It is our experience that better samples and less hematoma problems arise if the veins are not held off during the sampling. Very large samples can be drawn, even from small veins, if aspiration is done slowly.

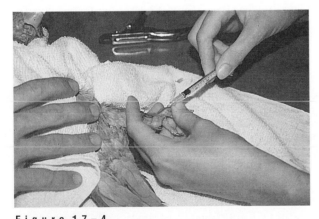

F i g u r e 1 7 – 4

Restraint and approach for intravenous injection or phlebotomy using the medial metatarsal vein.

If collecting the sample from a toenail, carefully clean several toenails and have a method of stopping the bleeding available. Blood may be collected by clipping the tip of one or more nails. removing just enough of the quick to let the blood flow freely into microhematocrit tubes (SP Microhematocrit capillary tubes, Scientific Products, McGaw Park, IL) or a microserum separator blood tube. Milking the blood from the toe causes lysis of cells and changes in both blood biochemical and hematologic results. Silver nitrate sticks, tissue cement, and ferric subsulfate work well for hemostasis. Tissue cement and silver nitrate are expensive and messy. We prefer the powdered form of ferric subsulfate packed into the barrel of a 1-ml tuberculin syringe with the Luer tip cut off, leaving an open barrel.

Blood Collection for Transfusion

Blood transfusions may be advantageous during surgery or postoperatively or in birds with blood loss or anemia resulting from disease or trauma. A single heterologous blood transfusion has been shown to be safe and anecdotally demonstrated to be efficacious.[2, 3] Investigators of chromium[51] Cr-labeled red blood cells administered as either homologous or heterologous transfusion in raptors have suggested that the half-life of the transfused cells is substantially shorter than previously thought.[4] Anticoagulant citrate dextrose (ACD) solution (ACD Solution, Formulation A, Baxter Healthcare Corp, Deerfield, IL) is used as an anticoagulant at a rate of 0.15 ml per milliliter of blood to be taken. Although no major studies have been performed on the effects of blood loss in psittacine species, it is generally agreed that a sample equal to 1% of the bird's blood volume may be safely taken, especially when that volume is replaced with crystalloid or colloid fluids.

The calculated volume of ACD is drawn into an appropriate-sized syringe through the butterfly catheter. In cases when the volume of ACD is very small, it is beneficial to dilute the buffer or add a small volume of saline to the syringe. This appears clinically to reduce the chance of thrombus formation during collection of the blood sample. Blood is most often taken from the right jugular vein. Isoflurane (AErrane, Ohmeda PPD, Inc., Liberty Corner, NJ) anesthesia is recommended, and a thorough sterile preparation of the site should be performed. The blood should be withdrawn slowly using a small-gauge butterfly catheter to minimize hemolysis and prevent a precipitous drop in blood pressure (Fig. 17–5). Following collection, one to three times the blood volume collected of saline or Ringer's solution or an equal volume of colloid fluids should be administered to the donor. The collection syringe is carefully removed from the butterfly catheter, and the fluids are administered through the same catheter over several minutes. The blood collected may be administered to the recipient through an interosseous catheter using a small disposable blood filter (Hemo-Nate filter, Gesco International, San Antonio, TX) or through the jugular or basilic vein, depending on the species.

Bone Marrow Aspiration Technique

Nonregenerative anemia, blood dyscrasia, thrombocytopenia, and neoplasia of the hematopoietic and reticuloendothelial systems are indications for bone marrow examination. Anesthesia is not required for this procedure but is recommended, especially if isoflurane is available. The proximal tibiotarsus and the sternum have proved to be good sites for collection.[5–8] The proximal tibiotarsus works best for most species, including those as small as a budgerigar. The sternal approach is reserved for those cases when the tibia is not available for some reason.

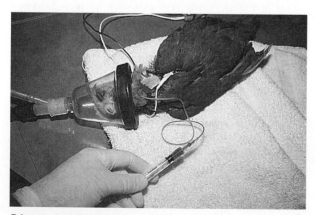

Figure 17–5

Red-lored Amazon parrot being used as a blood donor. The bird is anesthetized using isoflurane and the area of the jugular vein has been aseptically prepared.

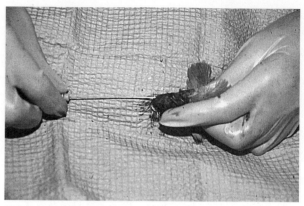

Figure 17–6

Position of the spinal needle for collection of bone marrow or placement of an intraosseous catheter in the tibiotarsus.

Spinal needles (Monoject 220 Spinal Needle, Diamond Point, Sherwood Medical Co, St. Louis, MO) are most useful to perform this procedure; however, pediatric Jamshedi needles (Kormed Corp, Minneapolis, MN) or disposable blood collection needles can be used. Other equipment needed is a scalpel blade and a 3- to 6-ml syringe.

The tibiotarsal technique is easily performed. First the bird is restrained in dorsal recumbency with the leg to be sampled extended and flexed at the stifle. The proximal end of the stifle is prepared for an aseptic procedure. Grasp the tibiotarsus in one hand using the thumb and index fingers to determine the position of the tibiotarsus. The biopsy needle is introduced into the cnemial crest through the insertion of the patellar tendon that is aligned with the diaphysis (Fig. 17–6). Gentle pressure is placed on the needle as it is carefully rotated. Take care not to allow the needle to wobble as it is turned. The needle is advanced to a point approximately one-third to one-half the length of the diaphysis. If a needle with a stylet is used, the stylet is removed. A 1- to 6-ml syringe is chosen based on the size of the patient. The syringe is firmly attached to the hub of the needle. Negative pressure is applied by pulling back quickly on the plunger of the syringe just until marrow appears in the hub of the needle or tip of the syringe. The needle is then removed and the marrow is spread on glass slides. Because of the fragility of avian cells, a cover slip technique is recommended.[8]

When collecting from the sternum, the bird is

placed in dorsal recumbency. An area over the widest part of the sternal right (keel) is aseptically prepared, and a small stab incision is made through the skin. The biopsy needle is held perpendicular to the sternum and advanced into the marrow by light pressure and rotation. Marrow is collected as with the specimen from the tibiotarsus. Complications include contamination of the sample with blood from overzealous aspiration. If no marrow appears in the syringe after three to four attempts, the needle may be plugged, and it should be removed and checked. There is often sufficient marrow in the shaft of the needle for cytology.

Intraosseous Catheterization

Intraosseous catheters provide a rapid, stable, and accessible route for fluid therapy. Either the tibiotarsus or ulna may be used, depending on the patient's clinical condition.[9] The use of an indwelling catheter in either the jugular vein[10] or basilic vein also has been advocated.[11] A major disadvantage to the intravenous technique is the instability of the catheter, requiring restraint or extensive bandaging.

The same approach used to collect bone marrow from the tibiotarsus may be used for placement of an intraosseous catheter and is our preferred site for small species or for short procedures (such as intraoperative fluid or blood administration) (Fig. 17–7). A 20- to 25-gauge spinal needle with a metal hub is used. The needle is placed as for bone marrow collection, then a tape "butterfly" is placed on the hub of the needle and sutured to the skin of the stifle. It is then capped with a prefilled male adapter plug (Male Adapter Plug-Short, Abbott Laboratories, North Chicago, IL) and flushed with a small volume of heparinized solution (500 IU heparin/L saline). When conscious, the patient will favor the leg with the catheter; however, signs of discomfort end with its removal.

Alternatively, an intraosseous catheter may be placed into the distal ulna (Fig. 17–8). With the bird anesthetized, the feathers are plucked from the area of the outer or lateral side of the distal ulna. This point is just proximal to the superficial ulnar artery and superficial digital flexor tendon, which may be seen through the skin.[12] The wing is supported in one hand while an appropriately sized spinal needle is positioned at the distal end of the ulna parallel

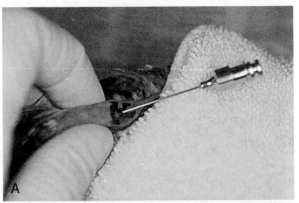

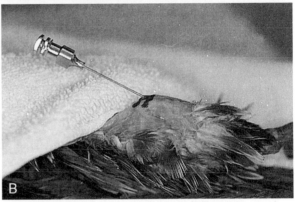

F i g u r e 1 7 – 7

(A and B) Placement of an intraosseous catheter into the tibiotarsus. The markings on the stifle joint outline the patella, patellar ligament, and cnemial crest.

to the diaphysis and then carefully driven into the medullary canal using firm pressure and a slight twisting motion. When the needle penetrates the cortex, it passes without resistance once in the marrow cavity. Aspiration of the syringe should produce a small amount of marrow in the hub of the needle. Resistance when driving the needle indicates that the needle is crossing another cortex and that the needle must be redirected. Once placed, the needle must be flushed with heparinized solution and secured, first with a "butterfly" of tape sutured to the skin and then with a light figure-eight bandage to immobilize the wing.[13]

Intravenous Catheterization

Intravenous catheterization may be preferred in some situations or by some practitioners. Indwelling

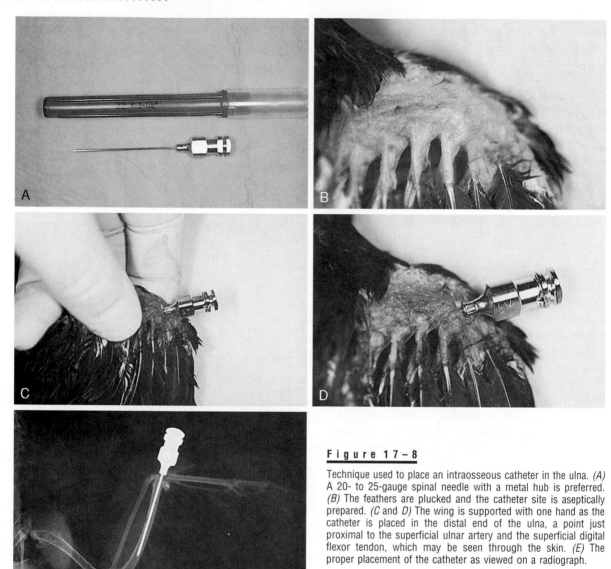

Figure 17–8

Technique used to place an intraosseous catheter in the ulna. *(A)* A 20- to 25-gauge spinal needle with a metal hub is preferred. *(B)* The feathers are plucked and the catheter site is aseptically prepared. *(C and D)* The wing is supported with one hand as the catheter is placed in the distal end of the ulna, a point just proximal to the superficial ulnar artery and the superficial digital flexor tendon, which may be seen through the skin. *(E)* The proper placement of the catheter as viewed on a radiograph.

Teflon catheters (Abbocath-T, Radiopaque FEB Teflon IV Catheter, Abbott Laboratories, North Chicago, IL) may be placed into either the basilic or jugular veins. For long-term catheterization, a vascular access device (VAD) or long-term catheterization of the jugular vein has been advocated.

For short procedures such as intraoperative fluid administration, a Teflon indwelling catheter may be placed into the basilic or jugular vein. Anesthesia is not required for these procedures; however, it does make the procedures much less stressful. When

using the basilic vein, the area around the vein is plucked and prepared as for sterile surgery, and a preflushed 24-gauge catheter is threaded into the vein (Fig. 17–9). A preflushed male adapter is placed in the catheter and a 1-×5-cm piece of adhesive tape (Zonas porous tape, Johnson and Johnson, New Brunswick, NJ) is placed in a wrapping fashion along the humerus, around the hub of the catheter so that it passes first over the more distal side of the catheter, then around the dorsal side, and exits on the proximal side where it is fastened to the propatagium of the wing. A tongue depressor is trimmed to a length 4 to 6 cm longer than the length of the humerus and is bandaged to the wing using cast padding or gauze and nonadhesive elastic bandage tape (Vetrap Bandaging Tape, 3M Animal Care Products, St. Paul, MN).[11]

When catheterizing the jugular vein the area is prepared as mentioned earlier. The vein is entered with a 18- to 24-gauge (most often 20-gauge) catheter of an appropriate length to reach the thoracic inlet. The feathers are plucked and the area overlying the jugular vein is prepared as described earlier.

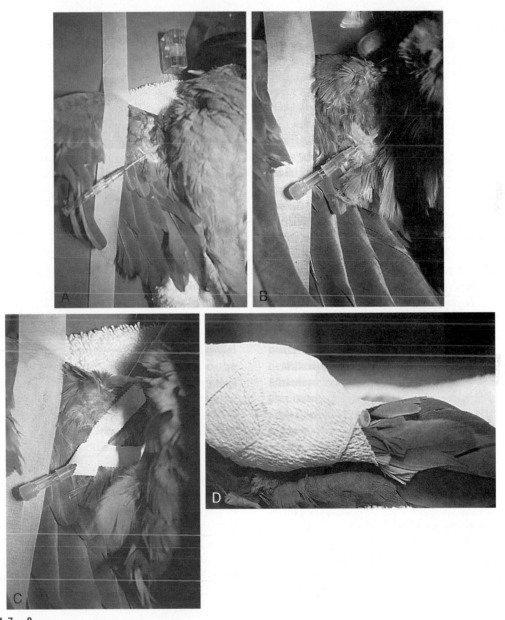

Figure 17–9

Steps involved in the placement of a an indwelling catheter in the basilic vein. *(A)* The bird is anesthetized or restrained and the area over the vein prepped. A preflushed 23- to 25-gauge catheter is introduced into the vein at the point where it crosses the antebrachium. *(B)* The catheter stylet is removed and the catheter capped using a preflushed male adapter plug. *(C)* A 1-×5-cm piece of adhesive tape is used to secure the catheter to the wing. *(D)* The male adapter is placed through the secondary feathers and the wing is wrapped with a figure-eight bandage incorporating a tongue depressor cut and padded to protect the catheter.

The vein is occluded to cause it to become distended. A point at about the caudal one-third is chosen for entry into the vein, with the needle stylus and the catheter threaded down the vein. The needle stylus is removed. Blood samples may then be drawn from the catheter. A preflushed male adapter is firmly attached to the catheter. The catheter should now be flushed to ensure patency and proper placement. Adhesive tape is attached to the catheter and male adapter, and the catheter is attached to the bird's neck by either suturing the tape to the skin or by incorporating the butterfly into a wrap around the neck.

If birds require long-term catheterization, a VAD or homemade central venous catheter using medical-grade polyethylene tubing may be placed into the left or right jugular vein. The specific details of using a VAD are beyond the scope of this chapter; however, the technique to place either of these catheters is similar and within the abilities of many avian practitioners.

The left, less dominant jugular vein is our preference for long-term catheterization. The anesthetized bird is placed in right lateral recumbency and the area over the left jugular vein is prepared for sterile surgery. A 2- to 3-cm incision is made parallel to the jugular vein, the vein is dissected, and the adventitia removed along 1 to 2 cm of its length. The center of a 15-cm piece of 6-0 braided absorbable suture is passed under the vein, then cut at its center to make two pieces. One is moved to the proximal extent of the dissected area of vein and the vein is tied off. A pair of mosquito hemostats attached to the suture aid in elevating the vein. A half hitch knot is placed in the other suture but not tightened.

Using magnification and a very sharp pair of iris scissors, a nick is made in the vein, and the catheter of the VAD, or a 6- to 10-cm piece of medical grade tubing, previously flushed with heparinized saline, is introduced into the vein and advanced to a point just below the thoracic inlet. The second suture is tied to secure the tubing in place. Hemostats or curved blunt Metzenbaum scissors are used to bluntly dissect a pocket for the VAD injection port, and the port is attached as directed by the manufacturer. If using tubing, a tunnel is made from the area of the jugular vein to a spot on the back of the neck where a hole is made in the skin. The tubing is passed through the hole, leaving adequate slack to allow for movement of the neck. The tubing is

sutured to the skin at the point of exit, trimmed to an appropriate length, and a blunt syringe needle or Luer stub adapter and a male adapter plug are attached. The VAD or catheter is flushed to ensure patency and the incision is sutured.[9] The VAD or catheter must be flushed regularly with heparinized saline solution to maintain patency.

CYTOLOGY AND MICROBIOLOGY SAMPLE COLLECTION

Samples are routinely taken from a number of locations for cytologic testing and bacterial culture. Because of the ease at which they are obtained, cloacal and choanal swabs are the most common samples. Samples collected from sinus aspirates, tracheal swabs and washings, and air sac washings are often neglected but may be of greater value.

Cloacal Swabs

Cloacal swabs are easily obtained and perhaps reflect the microbiologic flora of the digestive and urinary tract better than fecal swabs and culture. Commercial sterile swabs with modified Stewart's transport medium work well. The swab should be moistened with the transport medium prior to gently inserting it through the vent with a light rotary motion. The feathers surrounding the vent should not be allowed to contaminate the swab. The swab may then be rolled onto sterile glass slides, providing smears for cytology and a swab for culture.

Choanal Swabs

Choanal swabs provide information about both the oral pharynx and upper respiratory tract (important when evaluating the cytology and flora of this area). The swabs are easily obtained but require some method of controlling the beak or bill of the bird. Two methods used to hold the beak open are plastic or metal speculums and gauze loops. The advantage of the metal and plastic speculums is that they require only one or two persons to perform the procedure. The disadvantage is that the bird can damage the margins of its beak if the speculum is not carefully used.

With the bird in a towel, the assistant restrains the head in one hand and places the speculum with the other. To avoid injuring the bird, great care must be taken to ensure that metal speculums stay in the notch of the beak. With experience, one person may learn to hold the bird, place and hold the speculum with the hand that restrains the bird, and obtain the sample with the other. The gauze loop method is safer but usually requires an additional person for restraint. Gauze is looped over the upper and lower beak and pulled (requiring a surprising amount of effort) to open the bird's beak.

With the beak open, a moistened swab is used to collect the sample, gently rolling it across visible lesions in the oral cavity or at the most rostral aspect of the choanal opening. Caution must be taken when culturing abscesses in the palate of psittacines, because sometimes the abscess may erode into a palatine artery. If abscesses are opened carelessly, the resulting arterial bleeding may be very difficult to stop, even fatal, in a conscious, biting bird. It is best to work on these abscesses in an anesthetized bird.

Sinus Aspirates

Sinus aspirates may provide informative samples for evaluation of the upper respiratory tract. Two areas of the infraorbital sinus, rostral and ventral to the eye, can be aspirated (Fig. 17–10). When samples are required from the rostral area, the bird is either anesthetized and intubated or firmly restrained by an assistant. The bird's beak is held open using a speculum to increase the size (volume) of the sinus at the aspiration site. Using a 22- to 25-gauge needle and a 3- to 5-ml syringe, the needle is inserted at the commissure of the beak and directed vertically to a point between the eye and naris passing under the zygomatic bone. The needle should be held parallel to the skin, and the eye is carefully observed for movement. Misdirection of the needle can cause penetration of the globe. By carefully observing the eye during the procedure, motion of the eye may be seen before the globe is pierced.

The ventral aspect of the sinus may be approached from two directions. The needle can be introduced perpendicular to the skin at a point ventral to the zygomatic bone and just ventral to the eye. This is the best approach to collect material from ventral or retrobulbar lesions. Similar samples may be obtained by introducing the needle just caudal to the commissure of the mouth and directing it toward the point ventral to the globe at the zygomatic arch. Either approach should enable sample collection from the area of the sinus ventral to the eye.

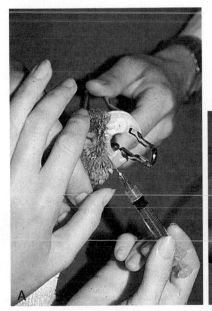
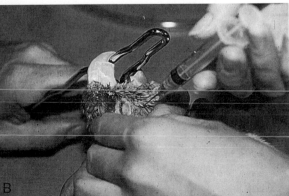

F i g u r e 1 7 – 1 0

Aspiration of the infraorbital sinus rostral *(A)* and ventral *(B)* to the eye.

Nasal Flushing

Nasal flushes may be used for both therapeutic and diagnostic purposes. There is often a marked clinical improvement in upper respiratory disease when treated with nasal flushes as an adjunct to systemic therapy. Both mechanical removal of accumulated discharges and the topical application of an antibiotic may contribute to improvement. A sterile solution, usually with an aliquot of antibiotics (if there is no intention to culture the collected material) is used for flushing. An aminoglycoside such as amikacin or gentamicin (50 mg/250 ml sterile water, saline, or Ringer's solution) or another antibiotic such as enrofloxacin (Baytril, Miles, Inc., Animal Health Products, Shawnee Mission, KS [100 mg/250 ml sterile water, saline, or Ringer's solution]) is added to the flush fluid. Recommended volumes are listed in Table 17–1.

Nasal flushing is simple and can be taught to clients. It has proved effective and safe in hundreds of flushes. For this procedure, the bird is restrained in a towel with the beak pointed downward, preferably over a sink or towel. The syringe is held against the naris so that it makes a tight seal with the butt end of the Luer tip. Solution is flushed into the nasal passage with light pressure, resulting in its expulsion from the opposite naris and the choanal opening (Fig. 17–11). With obstruction, fluid may flow from the lacrimal duct. This does not cause any damage and often flushes out large plugs of matter from the duct. With severe obstruction it may not be possible to flush any fluid through one or both of the nasal passages. In these cases it is sometimes possible to loosen the obstruction by flushing one side then the other for several tries. If the bird coughs or aspirates the fluid, its head should be released until it regains its normal respiratory pattern.

Tracheal Swabs and Washing

Miniature swabs work well for taking tracheal samples. Anesthesia is not necessary in most birds but may be helpful when working with dyspneic patients. The bird's mouth is restrained with a speculum or gauze loops and a moistened miniature swab is gently guided through the glottis at the base of the tongue, taking care to minimize contamina-

Table 17–1

NASAL FLUSH VOLUMES

Volume	Species
3–5 ml	Budgies, cockatiels
6–12 ml	Amazons, pionus, and grey parrots
12–20 ml	Large cockatoos and macaws

tion of the swab in the oral cavity. Most of the length of the trachea may be swabbed while rolling the swab between thumb and forefinger. The swab is removed, again taking care not to contaminate it. Smears are made by rolling the tip of the swab on sterile glass slides for cytology and Gram's stains, leaving the swab for culture.

Tracheal washing usually requires anesthesia. A sterile, soft catheter is passed through the glottis or through an endotracheal tube to the level of the syrinx. Sterile isotonic fluid is infused into the trachea and immediately aspirated back into a large syringe. Volumes of 1.0 to 2.0 ml/kg body weight are reported to be safe.[8] Recovery of 10 to 25% of the fluid is typical. Gas anesthesia can be maintained during the procedure by placing a catheter into the posterior thoracic air sac in severely dyspneic patients.

Air Sac Swabs and Washing

Sampling materials from the caudal thoracic and abdominal air sacs is easily performed in the avian

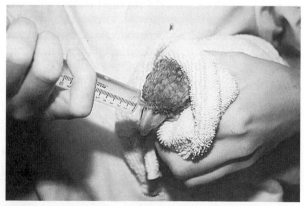

Figure 17–11

Nasal flushing of an Amazon parrot. The bird is restrained in a towel so that the beak is pointed downward, over a towel, sink, or collection bowl. The syringe is held against the naris so it makes a tight seal. Solution is flushed into the nasal passage with light pressure, resulting in its expulsion from the opposite naris and the choanal opening.

patient. The bird is anesthetized and restrained in right or left lateral recumbency as indicated by clinical signs, radiographs, or laparoscopy. The area over the last rib and thigh are prepared as for surgery. A nick incision is made in the skin caudal to the last rib and the muscles are bluntly separated using hemostats. A sterile endoscope with an operating channel (Karl Storz Veterinary Endoscopy, Goleta, CA) or otoscope cone of appropriate size on an operating otoscope is passed into the posterior thoracic or abdominal air sac. Lesions are easily identified and swabbed with a miniature swab, or a sterile soft catheter may be passed into the air sac to perform an air sac washing. Recovery of instilled fluid is maximized by positioning the bird with the head elevated so that the fluid stays in the air sac being examined. Care should be taken to avoid fluid entering the lungs of the bird.

TREATMENT TECHNIQUES

Crop Lavage

Lavage of the crop is indicated in birds with crop stasis or recent ingestion of toxic materials or poisons. Adult birds should be anesthetized and intubated. Baby birds usually can be lavaged without anesthesia. Baby birds are placed on a towel or other surface that provides good footing, and the head is held from the back and lifted to extend the neck. The tube is passed as in gavage feeding. Body temperature fluid (tap water works well) is infused into the crop, the crop is lightly massaged, and the fluid is aspirated or "siphoned" from the crop. Large-diameter tubes can be passed to aspirate particles of food or foreign material using a catheter-tipped syringe for aspiration. Siphoning works well to empty the crop, including large particulate material, without the tube becoming obstructed by the crop itself. It is accomplished by simply holding the tube lower than the crop once a flow of liquid has begun.[14]

Crop Foreign Body Recovery

It is not uncommon for pet birds to have foreign bodies in the crop. With luck, these may be removed blindly before they pass into the thoracic esophagus. When palpable in the crop, many foreign bodies may be retrieved through the oropharynx with a pair of alligator forceps. With the bird anesthetized, an endotracheal tube is placed. This is a very important step because retrieval of the foreign material may obstruct the glottal opening. A pair of blunt alligator forceps is carefully passed into the crop. The foreign body is palpated and held with one hand and "passed" into the open jaws of the forceps. Attention must be paid to the crop so as not to damage it in the procedure.

Foreign objects can sometimes be removed from the proventriculus or ventriculus through the oral cavity. Ferrous objects may often be retrieved using a small magnet attached to the end of a flexible catheter.[15] In large species, both flexible and rigid endoscopic equipment may be used to retrieve foreign bodies.

Air Sac Intubation

There are several situations in which intubation of an air sac may be advantageous. These include airway obstructions and procedures such as surgery or diagnostic tests involving the upper airway and surgery of the oral pharynx, where intubation of the glottis may interfere with the procedure. The tube is most often placed into the left abdominal air sac because of its relatively greater size, although right abdominal and cervical air sacs may be used.[16] The bird is positioned in dorsal or right lateral recumbency and the location for the tube is chosen so that it will not interfere with or be occluded by the legs, if the tube is to be left in place in the conscious bird. Most often the tube is placed just lateral to the ventriculus and medial to the thigh. This will place the tip of the tube in the left abdominal air sac. If the situation permits, the area is prepared for sterile surgery and a small skin incision is made at the location of the tube placement. Hemostats or blunt scissors are used to bluntly dissect through the body wall. A visual inspection is made of the area deep to the incision to ensure a clear area for placement of the tube. A sterile shortened endotracheal tube or modified soft rubber feeding tube is inserted through the hole, and the tube is checked for patency. A "butterfly" of tape is placed on the tube and sutures placed to attach the tube to the body wall. The tube is then attached to the anesthesia machine.

Tracheal Injections and Nebulization

Nebulization therapy is an important addition to the management of respiratory disease.[17] Small, disposable air- or oxygen-driven nebulizers are available at a reasonable cost (Acorn II Nebulizer, Marquest Medical, Englewood, CO). These units produce particles in the size range of 0.5 to 6 μm. Commercial humidifiers and vaporizers do not produce particles this small. Ultrasonic nebulizers are more expensive than air-driven nebulizers but can produce particles less than 0.5 μm in size (Ultra-Neb 99, DeVilbiss Health Care, Inc., Somerset, PA). The parabronchi of birds range between 0.5 and 2 mm in diameter and air capillaries vary from 3 to 10 μm in diameter.[18, 19] The effectiveness of nebulization therapy may be enhanced by minimizing the volume of the chamber holding the bird. This may be accomplished by placing the patient in a small container that is then placed inside a plastic bag.[17] As an alternative, a small nebulization or incubation chamber, anesthetic face mask, or 2-L plastic soda bottle works well as compared with the large chamber designed for dogs and cats.[20]

Another route for delivery of therapeutics to the lungs and airways of birds is intratracheal injection. The procedure may be done in the conscious bird. Volumes up to 2 ml/kg of water-soluble medications may be administered safely. I have administered numerous antibiotics, amphotericin B, and clotrimazole by this route. A small-diameter metal feeding needle is used to administer the drug. The bird is restrained in a towel and the beak is held open using a speculum or gauze loops. The medication is injected into the trachea with some degree of force. The bird is then released and allowed to cough and clear its throat.

NUTRITIONAL SUPPORT

Enteral Nutrition

When tube feeding the anorectic patient, attention must be paid to the nutritional needs of the patient. Supplying energy is of greatest importance. Birds

obtain all their energy from the metabolism of their diet. Energy is stored partly as glycogen in the liver and in muscle but mainly as fat. Free fatty acids increase in the circulation of birds in response to stress, much as glucose increases in the circulation of mammals. Lipids may be absorbed from the diet or synthesized via lipogenesis from carbohydrates and, to a limited extent, proteins. Dietary fats are hydrolyzed by lipase and absorbed throughout the length of the intestine and are then transported to the liver via the portal systems in the form of lipoproteins. Lipid synthesis occurs primarily in the liver; however, several other tissues, including adipose tissue, muscle, skin, and even bone, are sites of lipogenic activity. All carbohydrate metabolic pathways studied in mammals appear to be present in birds, although there are differences in the relative contribution of a given pathway to the overall energy requirements of a specific tissue or even to the animal as a whole. Avian carbohydrate metabolism is regulated much like that of mammals, and involves neural, hormonal, humoral, and nutrient components. Pancreatic hormones play a dominant role, with the insulin to glucagon ratio being the single most important factor. There is also a difference in the set points for biochemical reactions to occur. Blood glucose levels of carnivorous avian species remain stable during prolonged periods of fasting, unlike the fluctuating glucose levels observed in granivorous species (chickens). A comparison of liver enzyme activity from chickens and vultures indicates that vultures have much higher gluconeogenic levels than do chickens. During a prolonged fast, muscle glycogen in vultures is depleted markedly and the activity of critical gluconeogenic enzymes is increased 300 to 500%. As a result, hepatic glycogen depots are spared to a large extent.[21] Short-term fasting (1 to 8 days) in chickens does not decrease glucose use per unit of body weight as it does in fasted mammals. Rather it remains at about 10 to 13 mg/min/kg body weight over an 8-day fasting period, a level almost twice as high as that found in mammals.[21] Thus, it can be concluded that there is little glucose-sparing adaptation during short-term starvation in the chicken.

When birds are deprived of food, heat production, resting metabolic rate (MR), and body temperature diminish. Glycogen reserves are depleted in only a few to several hours after the onset of fasting. The respiratory quotient, an indication of the metabolism of glycogen, decreases and fat is preferentially metabolized. Next to fat, liver and muscle incur the greatest losses of weight during a fast (starvation). In one study, pigeons showed a loss of adipose tissue to 93%, spleen to 71%, pancreas to 64%, liver to 52%, heart to 45%, and muscle to 42% of respective initial weights during a fast.[22]

Supplying the energy needs of the avian patient is thus critical for successful treatment. Extrapolations of avian energy requirements may be made based on the resting MR and multipliers to calculate maintenance energy needs and the additional energy that may be required for disease or injury.[23] Calculation of the volume of feeding formula required may then be made, based on caloric needs of the patient divided by the caloric content of the feeding formula.

Calculation of Energy Required for the Avian Patient

The generally recognized formula for calculation of MR for a bird at rest is

$$MR \ (kcal) = K(W_{kg}^{0.75})$$

where MR is the resting or maintenance metabolic rate, W is the animal's body weight in kg, and K is a theoretical constant (for calculation of MR in kcal). For passerine birds K equals 129; in nonpasserine birds K equals 78. The exponent 0.75 represents the slope of the metabolic regression line that has been shown to correlate size and MR.

The metabolic rate of an active bird is somewhat greater than that of a resting bird. The difference between resting (inactive) and active birds has been reported to be between 1.24 to 1.23 and 1.1 to 1.4.[24] For simplicity we will use the value 1.5.

$$Active \ MR \ (kcal) = 1.5 \times MR \ (kcal)$$

An adjustment factor for growth, trauma, and disease is expressed as a multiple of MR.[25] (Table 17–2 lists adjustment factors for several conditions.) The energy requirement of the patient is

$$Energy \ requirement \ (kcal) = adjustment \ factor \\ \times \ active \ MR \ (kcal)$$

Table 17–2

ADJUSTMENT FACTORS TO METABOLIC RATE FOR SELECTED CONDITIONS

Condition	Adjustment
Starvation	0.5–0.7
Hypometabolism	0.5–0.9
Elective surgery	1.0–1.2
Mild trauma	1.0–1.2
Severe trauma	1.1–2.0
Growth	1.5–3.0
Sepsis	1.2–1.5
Burn	1.2–2.0
Head injury	1.0–2.0

To calculate the volume, in milliliters, of feeding formula required to meet patients' needs, we must divide the energy requirement by the caloric density of the feeding formula.

$$Vol(ml) = energy \ requirement \ (kcal) \\ \div \ caloric \ density \ of \ the \ feeding \ formula \ (kcal/ml)$$

This volume must then be divided into several feedings of reasonable volume and administered throughout the day.[23] The above process may be simplified by the use of computer software programs such as ZooDose. (Wildlife and Exotic Animal Teleconsultants, PO Box 10541, College Station, TX 77842, 800-659-8171.)

Many nutritional supplements may be used to supply the requirements of the anorectic avian patient. Considerations should be made to the digestibility and nutritive content of the formula. Products designed for mammals, including humans, may or may not meet these needs. Many of the available formulations are liquid. These products work well for a patient with a duodenal catheter. Liquids may be easily regurgitated or more often simply flow from the crop into the oral pharynx of weak or moribund patients, resulting in aspiration. Patients may be better served by a formulation that is more porridge-like or by having their nutritional needs met intravenously.

Oral Therapy and Alimentation

The most difficult task in avian medicine can be advancing medications past the beak of a large psittacine. Doing so even in small birds can be frustrating to the uninitiated. The procedures most often encountered are administration of oral medications to hospitalized birds and oral alimentation (tube feeding).

Curved metal feeding needles (Dosing Needles, Ejay International, Glendora, CA) or rubber feeding catheters (Sovereign Feeding Tube, Sherwood Medical, St. Louis, MO) may be used. Rigid tubes may risk damaging the crop but are safe if used cautiously. These tubes have a large ball at the tip for safety and are easier to use than soft rubber tubes, especially in small birds. Soft tubes are more difficult to pass and sometimes require a second person to hold a speculum in the bird's mouth.

When using a rigid tube the bird is restrained in a towel in the left hand and held against the handler's body. The tube, held in the right hand, is passed along the roof of the oral cavity from the left commissure toward the right side of the bird's oral pharynx. The ball tip of the catheter should be seen as it passes down the esophagus and into the crop to ensure proper placement; it may be felt with the thumb of the left hand as it passes through the cervical esophagus. An assistant may palpate the tube in the crop to confirm correct placement.

Soft tubes are passed in a similar manner; however, their use often requires a speculum. It is often easier to have an assistant restrain the bird and open its mouth with the speculum while passing the tube. Again, it is important to observe the tube passing into the esophagus and to palpate it in the crop prior to administering medication or other fluids. Soft tubes can be passed without a speculum in some birds. The tube is entered into the mouth at the left beak commissure and directed right and caudally into the esophagus. The tube is kept pressed against the fleshy beak commissure to prevent the bird from biting it with its beak.

Hold the bird with its head up and administer fluid through the tube slowly, allowing the crop time to expand. When the crop is full, the fluid fills the esophagus and can well up in the pharynx. If this occurs, the tube should be quickly removed and the bird released from restraint so that it may expel the excess. Adult birds have small crops and require tube feeding of small volumes at frequent intervals. As the crop adapts, larger volumes may be administered. (Table 17–3).

Catheter Duodenostomy

A technique for needle catheter duodenostomy and duodenal alimentation of birds has been de-

Table 17–3

SUGGESTED VOLUMES FOR TUBE FEEDING

Species of Bird	Volume (ml)
Budgerigar	1–3
Lovebird	2–3
Cockatiel	3–6
Conure (small)	4–12
Conure (large)	12–25
Parrot (Amazon, grey, etc.)	15–35
Cockatoo (medium to large)	20–40
Macaws (large)	35–60

scribed.[26] The bird is positioned in dorsal recumbency and prepared for sterile surgery. A 2- to 3-cm incision is made on the midline from the keel and extending caudally. The duodenal loop of intestine is identified by the presence of the duodenal arm of the pancreas between the descending and ascending segments. A 17- to 20-gauge needle-over-tubing type of indwelling jugular catheter is used. The needle is placed through the abdominal wall and then into the descending duodenum. The catheter is advanced into the ascending duodenum and the needle is withdrawn. One suture of 5-0 polypropylene is placed between the body wall and the duodenum at the point of catheter placement. A second suture is placed, securing the catheter to the outside of the abdomen, using a Chinese finger snare technique (a simple interrupted suture is placed, then the suture ends are tied around the catheter three or four more times). The catheter is flushed to ensure patency.

The catheter is routed behind the leg and wing and finally attached at the base of the neck with one or more sutures. If medical-grade tubing is used, it may be routed through a tunnel under the skin to emerge at the same location. The catheter is capped with a male adapter and flushed again. The catheter is removed by cutting the Chinese finger snare knot and applying gentle traction to the catheter.

Total Parenteral Nutrition

The nutritional needs of any patient are best met by an oral route; however, this route is not always available. Total parenteral nutrition (TPN) has been shown to be a feasible alternative and may offer an advantage in selected patients.[27–31]

Table 17–4 shows information to aid in the calculation of the nutritional requirements of the avian patient. The work sheet is for a TPN solution consisting of 20% lipid emulsion (Intralipid 20%, Kabi-Vitrum, Inc., Clayton, NC), 50% dextrose solution (dextrose 50% injection, USP, Abbott Laboratories, North Chicago, IL) and 8.5% crystalline amino acid solution with electrolytes (Travasol 8.5%, Baxter Healthcare Corp., Deerfield, IL). A multicomplex vitamin (M.V.I.–12, Astra Pharmaceutical Products Inc., Westborough, MA), 5 mEq of calcium gluconate (calcium gluconate injection, USP, 10%, LyphoMed Inc., Rosemont, MA), and 1 U heparin (heparin sodium, USP, 1000 U/ml, LyphoMed, Inc.) were added to the solution in the study by Degernes.[31] The lipid emulsion and dextrose solution are combined to equally supply the nonprotein ca-

loric requirements. Protein requirements are calculated at 6 g/kg and electrolytes supplied by the amino acid solution.

A yellow-nape Amazon parrot with sepsis and weighing 500 g may be used to illustrate the use of the work sheet.

Daily caloric needs $= 1.5_{\text{factor for sepsis}}$
$\times 1.5_{\text{factor for nonresting bird}}$
$\times (78_{K \text{ factor for nonpasserine bird}} \times 0.5 \text{ kg}^{0.75}_{\text{weight in kg}})$
$= 104$ kcal

Protein requirement $= 0.5$ kg $\times 6$ g/kg/day
$= 3$ g/day

Protein calories at 4 kcal/g $= 3$ g $\times 4$ kcal/g
$= 12$ kcal

Nonprotein calories $=$ daily energy needs $-$ protein calories $= 104$ kcal $- 12$ kcal $= 92$ kcal

---

Table 17–4

PARENTERAL NUTRITION WORK SHEET FOR PET BIRDS

Daily Energy Needs
Illness energy requirement $\times$ factor for active bird $\times$ ($78^*\times W_{kg}^{0.75}$) = _____ kcal/day
$^* =$ K, constant for nonpasserine bird.

Factor for active bird
    1.5 for normal bird (see energy needs, enteral nutrition)

Illness energy requirements
    1.0–3.0 depending on condition (see Table 17–2)

Protein Requirement
    6 g/kg/day for adult bird (use 1.5g or less in cases of renal disease)

    W(kg) $\times$ 6 g/kg/day = _____ kcal

Protein calories = 4 kcal/g:
    grams protein $\times$ 4 kcal/g = _____ kcal

Nonprotein calories = daily energy needs − protein calories = _____ kcal

Volume of Nutrient Solutions Required
(A) 8.5% amino acid solution = 85 mg protein/ml (0.085 g/ml = _____ ml

    _____ (from above) g/day ÷ 0.085 g/ml = _____ ml

(B) 20% lipid solution = 2 kcal/ml
    One-half of nonprotein calories (above) = _____ kcal ÷ 2 kcal/ml = _____ ml

(C) 50% dextrose solution = 1.7 kcal/ml
    One-half of nonprotein calories (above) = _____ kcal ÷ 1.7 kcal/ml = _____ ml
        (give ½ this volume first several doses then increase if glycosuria not a problem)

Total Daily Volume of TPN Solution
8.5% amino acid solution + 20% lipid solution + 50% dextrose solution = _____ ml

Electrolyte Requirement
Most are supplied by amino acid product with the exception of calcium gluconate at 5 mg/kg

Vitamins
Multivitamin additives, which provide all fat-soluble vitamins except vitamin K, are added to the TPN
Vitamin K is given SQ weekly.

Modified from Lippert AC and Armstrong PJ: Parenteral nutritional support. In Kirk RW (ed): Current Veterinary Therapy X. Philadelphia, WB Saunders, 1989, p 26.

Volume of nutrient solutions required:
(A) 8.5% amino acid solution = 85 mg protein/ml (0.085 g/ml).

    3 g/day ÷ 0.085 g/ml = 35 ml

(B) 20% lipid solution = 2 kcal/ml

    One-half of nonprotein calories = 46 kcal ÷ 2 kcal/ml = 23 ml

(C) 50% dextrose solution = 1.7 kcal/ml.

    One-half of nonprotein calories = 46 kcal ÷ 1.7 kcal/mL = 27 ml

Total daily volume of TPN solution = 35 ml + 23 ml + 27 ml = 85 ml

BANDAGING TECHNIQUES

Bandaging is a technique necessary for any clinician or technician working with birds. As with other animals, early attempts at bandaging are clumsy and unrewarding. The ability to wrap the bandaging material at a tension that stays in place and is not overly tight takes experience. Take special care to observe patients with bandages to ensure that the bandage does not restrict circulation from a limb or restrict respiration. I recommend use of isoflurane anesthesia when applying any bandage. Not only does anesthesia greatly reduce the stress to the avian patient but it also reduces the chance that the bird may be injured by physical restraint. Finally, using anesthesia results in a better bandage.

Most bandages used in birds incorporate three layers. The first layer is a soft conforming substance, such a smooth cotton cast padding (Webril Regular Finish Under Cast Padding, Kendall Healthcare Products Co., Mansfield, MA). The felt-like cotton forms well to the contours of the limb, is comfortable, and does not cause constriction if picked by the bird. The second layer is an nonadhesive elastic-type bandage (Vetrap Bandaging Tape, 3M Animal Care Products, St. Paul, MN). The second layer gives the bandage form, strength, and even pressure. Apply this type of product carefully; application of the tape too tightly interferes with circulation. With rare exceptions, the limb or part bandaged should be in a normal resting position and the tape applied so that no discomfort or reduction of circulation results. The third layer, or "chew layer," consists of an adhesive elastic bandage. I prefer a brand that is very strong but light in weight (Elastoplast elastic adhesive bandage, Beiersdorf Inc., Norwalk, CT).

This layer protects the bandage from destruction by all but the most aggressive bandage chewers. As with the second layer, great care must be taken not to apply this bandage material too tightly. An additional layer of nonadherent or other appropriate dressing must be used to cover an open wound or medicinal dressing under the bandage. In addition, materials may be added to a bandage or splint to increase its rigidity. Choice of materials depends on the bandage and its purpose. Bits of applicator stick or tongue depressor may be used for situations when the material does not need great strength and there is no need to conform to the shape or bend of a limb. Thermal plastics such as X-lite Orthopaedic Bandage (Runlite, Belgium), or thermoplastic splinting material (Veterinary Thermoplastic [VTP], Imex Veterinary, Inc., Longview, TX) work well for the latter purpose.

Bandage materials must be cut to an appropriate width for the bandage to "fit" the patient. Generally speaking, small species weighing less than 60 g require materials cut 1 cm wide (approx. ¼ inch); birds weighing up to 500 g require bandages 1 to 2 cm wide (approximately ¼–¾ inch); and larger species require bandages 2 to 4 cm wide (approx. ¾–1½ inch). If the materials are too wide the layers of the bandage do not lie smoothly and conform to the shape of the area bandaged, causing the bandage to be uncomfortable, clumsy, and more likely to fail.

Figure-Eight Bandage

Perhaps the most commonly applied bandage used on the wing is the figure-eight bandage. It can be used for purposes ranging from dressing wounds to splinting fractures. Many fractures of the wing, including those of the shoulder girdle and some humeral fractures, may be corrected using this bandage with or without a body wrap. Three layers are used when bandaging psittacines or other species that may chew or cause damage to the bandage. As with many techniques, there is no "correct" or "incorrect" method of applying this bandage. There are a few points that should be considered, however. If the bandage is wrapped so that it goes from medial to lateral as it passes across the front of the carpus, it will have a tendency to adduct the carpus and phalanges. If there is sufficient tension placed on the bandage, the adduction will be enough that the primary flight feathers (remiges) will not fold behind the secondaries. This position is uncomfortable to the patient, places abnormal forces on the joint, and may cause fractures to heal in an unnatural position. Therefore, there is some advantage to wrapping the materials in a lateral to medial direction as it passes across the carpus.

The bandage is started at the top of the "eight" by placing the free end of the bandage material under the fold of the carpus with the free end anterior (ventral) and the rolled remainder of the bandage posterior (dorsal) (Fig. 17–12). The free end is folded over the carpus and then covered with the first wrap of the bandage material, which is passed over the lateral surface of the wing (from the propatagium to the primary feathers) and around the carpus in a posterior to anterior and lateral to medial direction. If the primary feathers

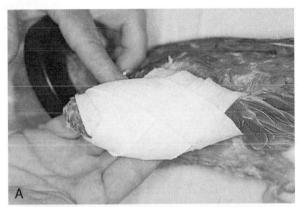

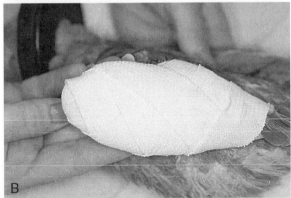

Figure 17–12

Application of a figure-eight bandage. *(A)* Initial layer of cotton felt is followed by elastic bandage (Vetrap) and tape to cover the carpus; *(B)* the final "chew layer" is of heavy adhesive elastic bandage.

have not been trimmed (most often wild birds) bandaging may be started by placing a turn of the bandage around carefully folded primary feathers then around the carpus, as described earlier. This completes the top of the "eight." The bandage is then passed on the medial side of the wing, under the axilla, including the long modified covert feathers of the humerus (tertiaries). The bandage is then passed up across the lateral surface of the wing and around the carpus, completing the bottom side of the "eight." Several wraps are added, each just overlapping the last farther down the wing. The wraps on the top of the "eight" overlap much more than those on the elbow (ventral to caudal) side. Do not wrap the propatagium to the extent that it may be damaged by the bandage. The second and third layers of the bandage are added in identical fashion (Fig. 17–12). If the wing is to be wrapped to the body, the figure eight is finished and then a wrap is added to immobilize the wing to the body just below the axilla of the opposite wing. Once again, three layers are recommended in psittacines. Only enough tension should be used to secure the limb in place. Care must be taken not the restrict the bird's breathing. If needed, a small margin of the sticky backing of the adhesive elastic bandage may be attached to the bird's feathers to hold the bandage in place.

Padded Bandages, Modified Robert Jones Bandages, Half Casts, and Spica Splints

A padded type is the most useful bandage when working with the legs of birds with body weights over 80 g. As with the figure-eight bandage, it is useful in several situations from tissue trauma to splinting fractures. With modification of the basic bandage to a spica-like splint to immobilize the hip, or an extension to incorporate the foot of the bird, it is possible to treat fractures from the proximal femur to the foot. The construction of the bandage is relatively simple. Three layers are incorporated as with the figure eight. The materials should be of proper width so that the bandage conforms to the shape of the leg without placing excessive force when wrapping the leg, and possibly compromising circulation.

Before bandaging, wounds should be covered with a nonadherent dressing. As alternatives, a hydroactive bandage or a semiocclusive bandage may be used. When splinting fractures, strips of adhesive tape placed on the limb and secured with adhesive tape encircling the limb may help in the reduction of the fractures while placing the bandage. With the bird in dorsal recumbency, a finger placed in the inguinal area of the bird while traction is placed on the leg at the distal end of the extremity reduces most fractures while the bandage is being constructed (Fig. 17–13).

All layers of the bandage are applied with little if any tension. The first layer is flat cotton cast padding. It is started at the tibiotarsal-tarsometatarsal joint and wrapped in partially overlapping layers progressing from the foot cranially. A second and third layer is added. More material may be added in convex areas. Care must be taken to ensure that the bandage material does not extend into the inguinal area so far that it places pressure on the vessels or nerves in this area. The second layer of nonadhesive elastic bandage is applied just tight enough that it stretches, but not so tight that all the wrinkle is removed from the bandage. This is so that circulation to the foot is not compromised. If the bandage must be rigid, a "half cast" of rigid

thermoplastic materials is made to fit the limb and is added after the first layer of elastic bandage and is covered with a second layer of nonadhesive elastic bandage. At this point the tape strips, if used, are incorporated into the bandage and secured by the second layer. To prevent the bird from turning its toes under, a stirrup of adhesive elastic bandage is placed under the foot. This stirrup should be the width of the weight-bearing portion of the bird's foot and long enough to extend to the middle of the tibiotarsal bone on either side of the foot. The center portion that will be under the foot of the bird should be covered with another piece of adhesive elastic bandage, to cover the sticky surface. Finally the third layer of adhesive elastic bandage is added to protect the bandage from damage (see Fig. 17–13).

Modifications to the padded bandage to immobilize the coxofemoral joint are made by extending the cotton cast padding and nonadhesive bandage over the hip and in figure-eight fashion around the body. The rigid thermoplastic material is then fabricated in a single piece to immobilize the leg and hip. It is covered with nonadhesive elastic bandage and then adhesive elastic bandage as de-

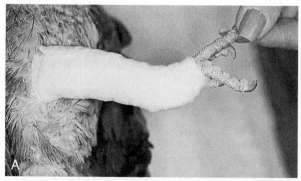
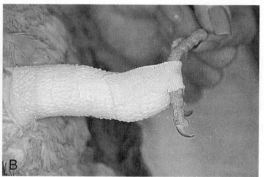
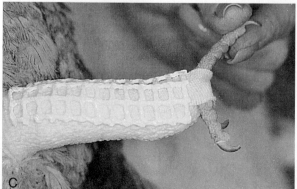

Figure 17–13

Method used to construct a modified padded bandage. *(A)* A layer of cotton felt followed by elastic bandage (Vetrap) and the application of a tape "stirrup" *(B)*; addition of thermoplastic splint molded to the shape of the leg to add strength *(C)*; a final "chew layer" of heavy adhesive elastic bandage is then added.

scribed earlier. The bandage may be extended to the foot and incorporated into a ball bandage or splint for the foot if the lesion involves the foot or digits.

Tape Bandages

The tape bandage was first described by Altman[32, 33] and works well as a splint for fractures of the legs and digits of small species (weighing less than 80 g). This simple splint consists of several layers of tape placed on either side of the limb and sealed anterior and posterior to form a rigid spine. The same principles that apply to any coaptive device used to splint a fracture apply to this splint. The joint above and below the fracture must be immobilized for the splint to be successful. In very small species (canaries and finches) a length of tape placed behind the limb then folded to cover the lateral surface provides the support needed to immobilize a fracture. Modifications to this simple idea are necessary for heavier species. Two tape "mats" made of three to five layers of waterproof adhesive tape cut to the limb's length and several inches wider than the limb are prepared. A scallop is cut into the center of one mat. This tape mat is attached to the medial side of the limb with the cutout area at the inguinal point of the limb. The limb is positioned so that the joints are slightly flexed and the fracture (if present) is reduced. The second tape mat is then attached to the lateral side of the limb. The bandage is trimmed so that approximately 1 cm extends on each side of the limb, and the two mats are firmly sealed together by clamping them with a hemostat or similar clamp. A stirrup, similar to that described for the padded bandage, is placed under the foot of the bird and covered with one last layer of adhesive tape. This bandage may be used to splint species weighing up to 600 g if a stiffener of thermoplastic bandage is added to the lateral side and incorporated into the layers of the bandage.

Thomas Splints

Thomas splints may be used as coaptive devices in the treatment of tibiotarsal and tarsometataral fractures of medium and larger species (weight greater than 80 g). The construction and techniques are very similar to those used in the construction of a splint for dogs or cats. Fourteen- to 18-gauge wire is chosen for most species. The loop of the wire frame is positioned vertically with the proximal bar bent away from the body at a 70° angle, then bent back ventrally to conform to the leg. The bars are positioned in the midsagittal plane and in an anterior and posterior position. The length of the splint must be long enough to completely cover the foot. The inguinal side is padded well so that the bird's weight is not positioned on the vessels in that area, compromising the circulation to the limb. The limb is isolated in the splint with narrow pieces of adhesive tape, and gentle traction is placed with tape stirrups attached to the bottom of the splint.

References

1. McGuill MW, Rowan AN: Biological effects of blood loss: Implications for sampling volumes and techniques. Institute of Laboratory Animal Resources (National Research Council) News 31(4):5–18, 1989.
2. Altman RB: Heterologous blood transfusions in avian species. Proc Assoc Avian Vet, San Diego, 1983, pp 28–32.
3. Altman R: Transfusions. Proc 13th Ann Vet Surg Forum, Semin 10, 1985, Avian Surgery, pp 22–23.
4. Sandmeir P, Stauber EH, Wardrop KJ, Washizuka A: Survival of pigeon red blood cells after transfusion into selected raptors. J Am Vet Med Assoc 204(3):427–429, 1994.
5. Campbell TW: Cytodiagnosis in avian medicine. Proc Int Conf Avian Med, 1984, pp 167–192.
6. VanderHeyden N: Bone marrow aspiration techniques in birds. Proc Assoc Avian Vet, 1986, pp 53–60.
7. Campbell TW: Basic principles of avian hematology and cytology. Proc Assoc Avian Vet, 1985, pp 267–276.
8. Campbell TW: Avian Hematology and Cytology. Ames, Iowa State University Press, 1988.
9. Jenkins JR: Advanced avian techniques. In Manual of Avian Laboratory Procedures. Proc. Assoc Avian Vet, 1992, pp 87–92.
10. Bond MW, Wolf S: Intravenous catheter therapy. Proc Assoc Avian Vet, *Nashville*, 1993, pp 8–14.
11. Bond MW: Intravenous catheter placement: IME. J Assoc Avian Vet 6(1):40, 1992.
12. Orosz S, Ensley P, Haynes C: Avian Surgical Anatomy, Thoracic and Pelvic Limbs. Philadelphia, WB Saunders, 1992.
13. Ritchie BW: In my experience: Intra-osseous fluid therapy. AAV Today 2(3):147–148, 1988.
14. Morris P, Personal communication, 1994.
15. Lumeij JT, Gootjes P, Wolvekamp WThC: A new instrument for removing gastric foreign bodies in birds. Proc Eur Conf Avian Med Surg, 1993, pp 91–98.
16. Rode JA, Bartholow BS, Ludders JW: Ventilation through an air sac cannula during tracheal obstruction in ducks. J Assoc Avian Vet 4(2):98–101, 1990.
17. Loudis BG, Southerland-Smith M: Methods used in the critical care of avian patients. In Fudge AM, Jenkins (eds): Semin Avian Exotic Pet Med 3(4):180–189, 1994.

18. King AS, McLelland J (eds): Birds: Their Structure and Function. London, Bailliere Tindall, 1984, pp 110–1144.
19. McLelland J: Anatomy of the lungs and air sacs. In King AS, McLelland J: Form and Function in Birds, vol 4. San Diego, Academic Press, pp 221–279, 1988.
20. Hetey P: In my experience. Alternate nebulization method. AAV Today 2:149, 1988.
21. Hazelwood RL: Carbohydrate metabolism. In Sturkie PD (ed): Avian Physiology. New York, Springer-Verlag, 1986, pp 303–325.
22. Wittrow GC: Energy metabolism. In Sturkie PD (ed): Avian Physiology. New York, Springer-Verlag, 1986, pp 253–268.
23. Quesenberry KE, Mauldin G, Hillyer E: Nutritional support of the avian patient. Proc Assoc Avian Vet, Seattle, 1989, pp 11–19.
24. Schmidt-Nelson K: Scaling: Why Is Animal Size So Important? Cambridge, Cambridge University Press, 1984.
25. Whittow GC: Regulation of body temperature. In Sturkie PD (ed): Avian Physiology, ed 4. New York, Springer-Verlag, 1986, pp 222–246.
26. Goring RL, Goldman A, Kaufman KJ, et al: Needle catheter duodenostomy: A technique for duodenal alimentation of birds. J Am Vet Med Assoc 189(9):1017–1019, 1986.
27. Janssen DL, Oosterhouis JE, Allen JL, et al: Lead poisoning in free-ranging California Condors. J Am Vet Med Assoc 189(9):1115–1117, 1986.
28. Lippert AC, Armstrong PJ: Parenteral nutrition support. In Kirk RW (ed): Current Veterinary Therapy X. Small Animal Practice. Philadelphia, WB Saunders, 1989, pp 25–30.
29. Harvey-Clark C: Clinical and research use of implantable vascular access ports in avian species. Proc Assoc Avian Vet, 1990, pp 191–209.
30. Degernes LA, Davidson GS, Kolmstetter C, et al: Preliminary report on the use of total parenteral nutrition in birds. Proc Assoc Avian Vet, New Orleans, 1992, pp 19–20.
31. Degemes LA, Davidson GS, Flammer K, et al: Administration of total parenteral nutrition in pigeons. Am J Vet Res 55(5):660–665, 1994.
32. Altman RB: Fractures of the extremities of birds. In Kirk RW (ed): Current Veterinary Therapy VI. Philadelphia, WB Saunders, 1977, pp 717–720.
33. Altman RB: Disorders of the skeletal system. In Petrak ML (ed): Diseases of Cage and Aviary Birds, ed 2. Philadelphia, Lea & Febiger, 1982, pp 382–394.

Infectious Diseases

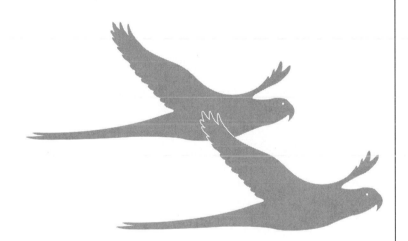

18 Gerry M. Dorrestein

Bacteriology

INTRODUCTION

Bacterial problems are considered common in avian practice, not only as a primary disease, but more often as a secondary infection or as a potential complicating factor. The result is a very common practice of using antimicrobials in avian medicine.

However, although at necropsy many different bacterial species are found and cultured, large-scale bacterial epidemics are uncommon in "normal" pet avian medicine. These are restricted to a few species (e.g., *Chlamydia psittaci*, *Mycobacterium* species, *Pasteurella multocida*, some *Salmonella* species, and *Yersinia pseudotuberculosis*). The *Chlamydia* species and *Mycoplasma* species and their medical problems are discussed in Chapters 23 and 24.

The interpretation of culture results is often difficult in a clinical setting. Bacterial culture and identification in veterinary practice are used for the identification of pathogens. This helps the practitioner to understand disease states and permits the selection of environmental changes or pharmacologic agents directed toward eradication of potential pathogens. Immunologically compromised adults or immature birds are more subject to microfloral overgrowth and infections by opportunistic bacteria than are adult, "healthy" counterparts.[111] Even nonpathogenic organisms like *Acinetobacter* species can infect the compromised host. At necropsy the bacteriologic findings do not always coincide with pathology.

So, how do we approach bacteriology and bacterial problems?

The most important factor to consider is whether a bird is clinically ill or if an aviary is experiencing problems. Each situation must be treated individually and with a good deal of contemplation, because no standards exist in avian bacteriology for processing, interpretation, and therapy.[67]

The therapeutic approach of bacterial problems is discussed briefly in this chapter; specific dosages are found in Chapter 40*B*, Formulary.

BACTERIOLOGY IN PRACTICE

In many practices a choanal and cloacal culture of all birds is recommended during their first or annual physical examination. However, interpretation of results indicating moderate to heavy growth of gram-negative bacteria is often confusing, especially in an otherwise healthy-appearing bird. Other practitioners recommend cultures only when a bird is sick or has some other problem.[79] Routine Gram's or DiffQuick stains can be very useful in picking up yeast infections, bacterial infections, and others.

Stained Smears or Cytology

Microbial cultures are essential for isolating, quantifying, and speciating bacteria and for antimicrobial sensitivity testing, but one cannot underestimate the value of direct microscopic examination of clinical material. Stained (Gram's stain or DiffQuick) and unstained (wet mount) slide preparations are relatively simple procedures that give immediate results with a minimum of equipment, time, materials, and expense. A direct examination may also be the only diagnostic method available when an organism cannot be cultured (e.g., megabacteria).[1] However, the method is much less sensitive than culture for the detection of small numbers of easily growing bacteria. A specimen must contain at least 10^5 organisms per milliliter before the organism can be detected on a smeared preparation. Negative results do not necessarily mean that bacteria are absent.[36] This technique lacks sufficient sensitivity when the clinician wants to rule out gram-negative organisms with higher pathogenic potential, such as *Pseudomonas* species.[45] See the chapter on cytology (Chapter 15) for information about staining and interpretation.

In general, using Quick stains can give information about the presence and morphology of the bacteria (cocci, rods, spore-forming bacteria, *Clostridium*-like, *Campylobacter* species, *Treponema* species, *Mycobacterium* species, filamentous bacteria, etc.) and other organisms like yeast, fungi, protozoa, flagellates, and others. Based on the results, combined with the clinical status of the patient, preliminary therapy can be initiated. In psittacines, 69 to 72% of the microorganisms isolated from organs at necropsy could also be found in direct smears of the feces.[31] This was not the case for *Staphylococcus* species and fungi. The stained smears may also show bacteria that do not grow at culture. To differentiate between gram-negative and gram-positive bacteria, Gram's staining is necessary. These methods give a general guide for interpretation of the microfloral balance of an individual, but they cannot be used to identify microorganisms.[68] Based on the collected information, sample sites and culture media should be selected to determine the species and antibiotic sensitivity of suspected pathogens. By using autoclaved, sterile glass slides, the media-moistened swab can, after careful insertion into the collection site, be "rolled" onto an area the size of a quarter on the sterile glass slide, and then replaced in the transport medium for possible culture submission.[45, 75]

Veterinary clinicians are often frustrated by the lack of correlation between Gram's stain results and aerobic bacterial culture. When the submitting veterinarian sees gram-negative rods on a Gram's stain and subsequently receives a report from the laboratory of "no gram-negative growth," there are three possible explanations[45]: (1) overdecolorization of the preparation of gram-positive bacteria; (2) visualization of fastidious or anaerobic gram-negative rods that will not grow in aerobic culture; (3) subsequent reswabbing of the patient for culture and collection of a sample different from the swab used for Gram's stain.

Inhouse Microbiology?

Some avian veterinarians conduct their own microbiology testing inhouse because of the number of cultures they collect. Individual cultures can be less expensive and the results can be obtained sooner. The main disadvantage of an inhouse bacteriology laboratory is the lack of experience of the laboratory personnel. Often it is the veterinarian or a technician who processes the samples. Years of training and experience are needed to become proficient in microbiology, even with the modern determination kits. Many mistakes can happen and possible pathogens can be missed with untrained personnel. In addition, many unnecessary treatments are started based on the isolation of contaminants or misinterpretations of the cultural results. The veterinarian must be aware of the increased possibility of error when using inhouse microbiology and weigh this against savings of time and cost.[67] Growing bacteria on plates without identifying the organisms and simply doing sensitivities on all organisms, pathogens or not, is malpractice! If the veterinarian has a large avian and exotic practice and wishes to establish a complete laboratory, the situation is different. Only when acceptable expertise can be developed that does justice to the clientele and the patient is a practice justified in doing routine avian and/or exotic laboratory work.

For small practices, most sampling kits and culture media can be obtained through the microbiological laboratory of a local hospital. Sterile swabs, several collection kits (aerobic, anaerobic, *Chlamydia*, *Campylobacter*, fungi, and yeasts), blood culture tubes (aerobic and anaerobic), Quick stain, (Gram's stain, methylene blue stain) are essential in any avian practice. For an inhouse laboratory necessary equipment includes an incubator, culture media for aerobic (blood-agar, selective *Enterobacter* agar [e.g., MacConkey], antibiotic sensitivity agar, and selective agar for fungi and yeasts), enrichment broth for *Salmonella* selection, sensitivity disks and tablets for each antibiotic tested against, and other materials.

Discussion of microbiologic techniques for the avian practitioner can be found elsewhere.[36, 47] The guide *Isolation and Identification of Avian Pathogens*, compiled for the American Association of Avian Pathologists, is invaluable. Care must be given to ensure proper results once the swab has been collected. The sample should be set up immediately if at all possible. If the swab must be transported to an outside laboratory it should be kept refrigerated in the appropriate transport medium and kept cool even during transport. Refrigeration and speed in processing reduce the likelihood that growth or death of certain species of microorganisms will occur. Another problem is overgrowth of the sample by contaminating bacteria.

A standard bacteriologic culture in our laboratory includes the inoculation of a blood agar plate and a selective medium (brilliant green agar or MacConkey). The swab is then placed into serum broth or, in the case of a cloacal swab into a *Salmonella* enrichment broth (tetrathionate). Incubation takes 24 to 48 hours at 37°C, aerobic and/or anaerobic, depending on the selected media. For anaerobic cultures, special containers are available that can chemically be made anaerobic (with gas packs), which allows incubation in normal incubators.

Interpretation of growth and isolation and identification of individual bacterial strains require training and experience. Identification is based on Gram's stain characteristics, colony morphology, and the use of biochemical tests. Several "dry"-chemical identification kits are commercially available (e.g., API-20E, Rapid E, N/F wheel, Rapid NFT Strip).

A common method used is to do a Gram's stain for each colony type and calculate the percentages of total blood agar bacterial growth for that type. Organisms growing on MacConkey plates are "identified" and reported as to the quantity of growth, and antibiotic sensitivity is determined as deemed necessary.[79] For final identification of suspected pathogens and to grow organisms that require special techniques (e.g., *Mycoplasma* species, *Campylobacter* species, anaerobes) outside laboratories are used.

SAMPLE COLLECTION

Proper sample collection technique is a prerequisite for the successful recovery of microorganisms re-sponsible for an infectious problem. The recovery of contaminants may result in improper or even harmful treatment. Factors essential for making a choice for a sampling technique, collection site, and transport or culturing medium include the clinical picture and history of the individual bird or aviary, impression smears, and the presumptive or differential diagnosis.

A variety of sterile swabs with associated transport media are commercially available for the isolation of aerobic bacteria. When the sample has been collected, the swab should be returned to its protective holder, placed in a sealed plastic bag, and sent to the laboratory as rapidly as possible. In extreme hot weather conditions, cooling or personal delivery may be indicated.

Aspirates and biopsy specimens can also be collected for microbial isolation attempts, including those for viruses, aerobic bacteria, and special organisms such as *Chlamydia psittaci*, *Mycoplasma* species, *Mycobacterium* species, and *Campylobacter* species, anaerobes, fastidious gram-negative organisms, yeasts, and fungi.

Although isolation of aerobic organisms is relatively inexpensive and fairly rapid to do, the other groups of pathogens listed earlier require isolation techniques that are far more specialized and costly.

Viruses, *Chlamydia*, and *Mycoplasma* species require special media and conditions for isolation. Most human and veterinary diagnostic laboratories have little experience with these pathogens in birds. The clinician needs to establish a special contact with either a university research laboratory or diagnostic laboratory to culture for these organisms. This author rarely performs a culture for viruses, *Mycoplasma*, *Chlamydia*, *Campylobacter* species, anaerobic organisms, or fungi unless cytology or (histo)pathology supports or suggests the presence of a member of one of these groups.

Fluids, aspirates, and biopsy specimens can be frozen on dry ice or in an ultrafreezer at −70°C until a decision is made on specific isolations that will be attempted. Most diagnostic laboratories have ultrafreezers for storage of biologic samples.[64]

Anaerobic bacteria play a minor role in avian disease. *Lactobacillus* species is a facultative anaerobe and therefore is commonly identified. Anaerobic microorganisms, as well as *Campylobacter* species, are frequently first identified on microscopic smears (DiffQuick or Gram's stain).

Samples submitted for anaerobic culture require special collection techniques to improve the success of recovery. For obligate anaerobes, anaerobic swab culturettes are available, and for biopsy specimens the samples should be delivered to the clinical pathology laboratory in an anaerobic pack system. These are available through various microbial and scientific supply companies. The specimens must be placed in the anaerobic transport system as soon as possible after collection.

Collect blood samples for culture in birds with suspected septicemia. The skin over the venipuncture collection site must be thoroughly cleansed before collection with three applications of both an organic iodine solution and 70% alcohol. Beware of inadvertent penetration of the esophagus with the needle prior to venipuncture of the jugular vein. This may result in a surprising growth of *Bacillus* species.[55] As large a volume of blood as is safe to collect is obtained in a syringe, and the sample is quickly added to the blood culture bottle containing the appropriate culture media. The top of the blood culture bottle must be cleansed several times with swabs of 70% alcohol before insertion of the needle. Sterile technique should be used throughout the collection process. Both aerobic and anaerobic bottles must be used. Blood culture bottles are commercially available from most microbiology or medical supply companies.

Collection Sites

The selection of the site of sampling is important; a cloacal culture seldom gives useful information for a pneumonia or crop stasis. Common collection sites, regardless of the method used, are the crop or esophagus in those species without a crop, the cloaca, and the choanal slit. Additional culture sites might include lesions, ears, and eyes.

It is good practice, before collecting samples for microbiologic culture, to prepare one or two (impression) smears and one wet mount from the same site for microscopic/cytologic and parasitologic examination. Based on the morphologic information of the agent present, a more directed microbiologic culture can be done. Take the smears as cleanly as possible, otherwise contaminations can interfere with future culture.

Digestive Tract

Cloacal Cultures

The most common site cultured is the cloaca. Swabs inserted in the cloaca should be moistened with sterile saline to decrease damage to the cloacal mucosa. Inadequate penetration into the proctodeum results in a decrease in the variety and concentration of microbial species cultured. An alternative is to culture feces immediately after the bird defecates.

Indication. Cloacal samples can be taken based on cytology results, when a bird is suffering from any disease, because secondary microbial imbalances are more the rule than the exception in birds without ceca (psittacines, passerines, pigeons). Comparing cytology smears from other members of a flock may alert the veterinarian that a possible microbial imbalance exists for the flock as a whole.

A bird suspected of having an intestinal disease or sepsis should have a cloacal culture taken after cytologic evaluation of a fresh fecal sample.

If a bird cannot be handled easily, a fresh fecal culture is sufficient.

In pigeons and flocks, collected fecal samples can be tested for the presence of *Salmonella* species using 1 g of feces in 10 ml enrichment broth (tetrathionate or selenite), which will be processed after 24 and 48 hours on a selective agar medium.

Crop Sampling

Crop cultures should be taken in birds with crop lesions, stasis, or impaction as indicated by a smear and a wet mount.

Proventriculus Samples

When there is an indication (e.g., a persistent filling defect with barium in the proventriculus), endoscopy can be used to sample mucus.[1] When sterile sampling is difficult, cytology and Gram's stain evaluation of the mucus can be performed.

Information from the proventriculus of small birds can also be collected by a proventricular gavage with sterile saline.[57]

Indication. Proventriculus samples are indicated

when there is suspicion of "megabacterium" infection.

Upper Respiratory Tract

These samples, especially sinus and trachea samples, are more easily taken when the bird is under gas anesthesia, preferably isoflurane.

Choana Samples

The choana can be sampled by holding the beak open with various restraining devices or a third person holding strips of gauze to force the beak open. Direct the swab dorsally into the choanal slit and then rostrally into the distal nasal cavity.[67] Choanal cultures taken from any location other than the most rostral choana should be interpreted carefully, because oral microflora and environmental organisms, such as those in food, are also present.

Indications. Choanal cultures are often indicated when a bird is showing either upper or lower respiratory signs. Choanal culture results are not a reflection of the lower respiratory tract flora. In case of suspected bacterial pneumonia, growth from the choana is not identical to culture of the trachea or lungs. It is possible that, among others, the agent of the pneumonia is isolated as well.

Nasal discharges are heavily contaminated with environmental organisms and culture should be avoided. It would be sensible to make a microscopic smear first.

Sinus Samples

A sinus aspirate is performed by infusing warm, sterile saline into the infraorbital sinus (nasal or paranasal flush) with a needle and syringe and then recovering as much of the infused fluid as possible. One particular approach is performed by directing the needle perpendicular to the skin just ventral and rostral to the orbit.[6]

In case of chronic infraorbital abscesses, sterile surgery may be needed to collect samples.[106]

Indications. The causative agent of a sinusitis may be isolated with a choanal culture but a sinus aspirate may be more revealing and easier to interpret. Again, cytology helps in selecting the right medium as well as in the interpretation of culture results.

Trachea Samples

Transglottal tracheal cultures and tracheal wash cultures can also be taken. Tracheal cultures are taken while the bird's beak is held open and a swab is placed in the upper trachea. Tracheal washes are performed by introducing a sterile catheter into the trachea, infusing sterile saline (approximately 1 ml for a large macaw), and recovering the infusion by suction with a syringe. This infused fluid can be difficult to recover, but mucus usually can be obtained.

Indications. Tracheal cultures or tracheal washes can be done for suspected lower respiratory infections, but they should be carefully interpreted.

Eye Samples

Eye discharges are often seen in avian respiratory disease. The conjunctival sac can be cultured by using a swab first dipped into sterile saline.[67]

Indications. Eyes should be cultured when any discharge or conjunctivitis is present and when bacteria are present inside macrophages on cytology test.

Skin and Adnexa

Skin lesions are often contaminated with environmental microorganisms, and it is difficult to differentiate between the "normal" permanent skin flora and a problem-inducing microorganism (e.g., *Staphylococcus aureus*). Skin defects should be cultured based on microscopic smears. Before sampling from subcutaneous lesions or the uropygial gland, the overlying skin should be thoroughly cleaned with iodine and 70% alcohol.

Feathers should be sampled by pulling them after cleaning the surrounding skin and collecting from the part of the sheath that is still inside the follicle. The "inside" of the feather is sampled after sterilizing the calamus and rachis and splitting these structures.

Internal Organs

Cultures of internal organs can be obtained during surgery or endoscopic laparotomy. The most common sites are lesions associated with liver, air sacs, and peritoneum.

Blood cultures can also be taken from larger birds using 1-ml blood and inoculating blood culture tubes. This technique may be a more useful diagnostic tool than currently accepted culture techniques in selected problems such as open or closed long bone fractures, soft tissue wounds, diarrhea (enteritis), suspected pneumonia, cachexia, polyuria, and nonspecific signs such as physical depression.[72] However, this application in avian medicine needs reevaluation.

Necropsy

If organs or lesions are to be cultured during necropsy, it is better to perform a sterile necropsy until all cultures are taken. This is in preference to searing the surface of organs, because many avian tissues are so small that searing may kill any possible pathogens. Samples routinely are taken from liver, cloaca, and any morphologically altered organ, after cytologic evaluation of the site. The lungs are very difficult organs for taking noncontaminated samples. These organs can only be reached adequately after the heart, stomach, and liver are removed. To do this, the esophagus must be cut with the risk of contaminating the lungs.

Carcasses older than 1 day may have contamination of internal tissues. This depends primarily on the method of storage (refrigerator) and shipment. In birds without ceca, postmortem contamination is less of a problem. However, blood collected by cardiac puncture is rarely contaminated.

APPROACH TO BACTERIAL PROBLEMS

Interpretation of Culture Results

The key factor to interpreting microbiology results is whether the bird is clinically ill or an aviary or flock is demonstrating clinical or subclinical signs, such as poor breeding success or disappointing racing results. If a baby bird is failing to thrive or has repeated crop stasis, a heavy growth of *E. coli* may be more suspicious than *E. coli* found in a normal juvenile. Adults can mask their physical signs well but blood values, behavior, a history of poor breeding performance, and physical examination reveal most abnormalities. If any of these tests is abnormal, heavy growths of yeasts and (gram-negative) bacteria from the cloacal swab will be even more significant.

The practitioner must also consider several other factors in deciding if the microorganisms cultured or not cultured are pathogenically significant.

A negative culture (no growth) has to be interpreted in view of the cytology, the clinical history, previous or concurrent administration of antimicrobial agents, and accepted validity and fallacies of the specific isolation method. A positive culture must be placed in the total diagnostic background and many issues should be considered.

Species of Bird

Different species of birds have different normal microflora. In Galliformes and other birds with well-developed ceca, a permanent intestinal flora including gram-negative bacteria is considered normal. The ostrich is a hindgut fermenter, as are many herbivorous mammals. When an ostrich is 3 weeks old, the microflora of the cecum and large intestine are like those of the rumen.[2]

In psittacines and passerines, a fixed or permanent gram-negative intestinal flora is considered to be absent. But cockatoos are known to have larger percentages of gram-negative bacteria in their cloacal swabs than most other psittacines, even when kept in the same environment.[44] Baby cockatoos also exhibit different "normal" microflora pictures from other psittacines fed on the same hand-feeding diet and housed in the same environment.[70]

Age of the Bird

The age of the bird is important. Hatchlings and older baby birds lack a fully developed immune system; therefore, the immune response mounted by these birds often is insufficient to provide an adequate response. Factors such as poor or inadequate nutrition, inappropriate environmental conditions, lack of cleanliness and hygiene in the nursery or nest box, concomitant disease states and agents, and stress of any nature are significant components of the manifestation and expression of bacterial overgrowth in the pediatric avian patient.[111] Cases involving the presence of gram-negative bacteria isolated or identified from healthy chicks should be considered on an individual basis. Many chicks thrive and prosper with abundant growth of members of the family Enterobacteriaceae if the chick is clinically healthy. Culture results from chicks often reflect more of a transient population of bacteria and yeast than may be encountered with similar cultures in adults.

Varied Diets and Environments

Often differences exist because of the varied diets and environments of birds. Birds kept on wire generally have less enteric bacteria than those kept in aviaries with access to ground or soil, and birds fed only on seed have less than those fed on soft foods. Birds of prey and a bird on a partial or completely carnivorous diet generally have more gram-negative bacteria than those on nonmeat diets. Waterfowl grow different bacteria than land birds as a result of the bacteria found in their aquatic environment.

Species of Bacteria

The species of bacteria is also important to consider. Not all gram-positive bacteria are nonpathogenic. *S. aureus*, *Listeria* species, and *Erysipelothrix* species are examples of primary pathogenic bacteria. *Staphylococcus* species can also be found in healthy birds. In the same instance, not all gram-negative bacteria in psittacines or Passeriformes are harmful. *E. coli*, *Enterobacter* species, and other bacteria in the family Enterobacteriaceae are often found in the crop and/or cloaca of healthy birds. The presence of *Klebsiella* species, especially resistant strains, is generally undesirable but can be difficult to eradicate in a healthy bird. A few colonies of *Klebsiella* isolated from the choanae of a healthy chick may be handled differently than heavy growth of the same organism from the cloaca, because the organism might be considered pathogenic in psittacine chicks in the choana

only.[111] *Pseudomonas* species, *Salmonella* species, and *Proteus* species are usually only found in birds that have some type of clinical illness, and thus treatment is indicated.

Amount of Bacteria

E. coli often grows in heavy amounts in healthy and clinically ill birds. This growth may be considered more significant if very little other normal flora is found. However, one should not assume that large numbers of gram-negative bacteria obtained from any site in the bird are abnormal. The causes of microbial population shifts are many and often are benign, but in clinically ill birds any microbial imbalance should be seriously considered.[67]

COMMON BACTERIAL PROBLEMS

The meaning and approach of bacterial isolates and problems will be first discussed by separation of problems based on the clinical presentation.

Clinically Normal, ''Normal'' Bacterial Presence

Normal birds and their environment can contain bacteria and fungi that in some instances are considered pathogenic for birds. In other situations these bacteria may be harmless and simply reflect normal microbial flora for that given bird.

All chicks should be born sterile, which essentially indicates that there are no culturable (an)aerobic bacteria present at birth. A population of "normal" bacteria is introduced usually through a first feeding from the parent bird (altricial species) or the hand-feeder, but also may be introduced by environmental contact (precocial and altricial birds) with any variety of organisms. Eyries have been shown to harbor anywhere between five and 13 identifiable bacterial species, and sometimes as many as 33.[3] In a study of the bacterial growth in nesting material of wild passerines, the whole scala of bacteria, which can be considered "normal flora," were found. Even nests with high numbers of gram-negative rods were successful in most instances; therefore, there was no proof that aerobic bacteria were responsible for problems in this wild population.[80]

The concept of normal microbial flora refers to the population of certain resident microorganisms that inhabit skin and mucous membranes of healthy birds. These residents can be fixed in that they are regularly found in a given location in the body at a given age. If this population of fixed residents is disturbed, it promptly reestablishes itself.

These residents can be transient, including both nonpathogenic and potentially pathogenic microorganisms that inhabit the body for various periods. These bacteria are received from the environment, do not produce disease, and do not establish themselves permanently in the bird. This transient flora varies, as we have seen earlier, depending on the species, environment, diet, and age of the bird.

In clinically normal passerines and psittacines, gram-positive bacteria (*Lactobacillus* species, *Corynebacterium* species, *S. epidermidis*, *Micrococcus* species, nonhemolytic *Streptococcus* and *Bacillus* species) can be isolated from the crop and cloaca and are probably fixed inhabitants, and gram-negative bacteria are either transient inhabitants or probable disease-causing agents. Recovery of gram-negative bacteria from birds defined as clinically normal ranges from under 10% of the total psittacine birds in the sample to around 60% of some species populations sampled.[44] In general, the microflora seen in wild psittacines are similar to those of captive species.[69] The results of a study of the microflora of a group of normal, healthy, adult, captive thick-billed parrots (*Rynchopsitta pachyrhyncha*) was largely similar to other psittacine species. A high prevalence of *Pasteurella* species (81%) in choanal culture was unusual, but not considered clinically significant based on the good general health status of the birds examined.[37]

E. coli was isolated from the crop or cloaca in 97 of 100 pigeons from 20 different pigeon lofts, indicating that the bacterium is a normal inhabitant of the intestinal tract in pigeons.[20] The involvement of *E. coli* in disease problems in pigeons indicates that *E. coli* is a facultative pathogenic bacterium in pigeons.

In wild psittacines, gram-positive bacteria were present in 100% of all cloacal and choanal cultures. Gram-negative bacteria were present in 90% of the choanal cultures and 70% in cloacal cultures.[69] *E. coli* is the most common bacterial organism in the raptor intestinal tract, followed by enterococci. However, as in other species, the intestinal tract harbors many of the organisms that can be isolated in bacterial disease in raptors, such as *E. coli*, *Salmonella* species, *Mycobacterium* species, *Clostridium* species, and *Pasteurella* species (fowl cholera). *Proteus* species is recognized as an opportunistic organism, but under the right conditions can also be a pathogen.[81]

It is often stated that in psittacines[50, 104, 107] and birds of prey,[66] under most circumstances, *Streptococcus* species, and most *Staphylococcus* species are normal bacterial flora in the respiratory tract. However, pure isolates of *Staphylococcus* species and *Streptococcus* species are associated with respiratory infections.[50] Other gram-positive nonpathogenic bacteria commonly isolated from the respiratory tract of psittacines include *Bacillus* species, *Corynebacterium* species, and *Lactobacillus* species.[50, 107] For birds of prey, also, the reference cited only discusses the nasal flora.[95] In Utrecht, we consider any growth in very low numbers from the trachea or deeper respiratory system as a temporary presence of inhaled bacteria that are not yet eliminated by the normal functioning defense mechanisms (acceptable). The isolation of low to fair numbers of the mentioned gram-positive bacteria are seen as contaminants from the choanae or aspirates from the pharynx or crop, indicating a possible problem with swallowing or crop emptying. Any significant numbers of bacteria, even without clinical symptoms, should be taken as abnormal. The choana is not a valid sample site for the deeper respiratory system.

The transient flora are of little significance as long as the normal resident flora remains intact. However, if the resident flora is disturbed, these transient organisms may proliferate and produce disease.

Whether thriving neonates or producing adults, birds can present with a relatively high percentage of gram-negative bacteria and fungi and still be clinically asymptomatic and have normal blood values.[67] Large numbers of different bacterial species indicate a hygiene and or management problem, and no antibiotic treatment should be given. It can be difficult to determine what treatment is necessary, if any, when culture reveals a heavy growth of a gram-negative, enteric bacteria. Consider if the bird is healthy or not, then look at the complete blood count (CBC) or other laboratory data for abnormalities. If none are found, treatment may not be indicated, unless there is something else in the history or physical examination that suggests antibiotics should be given.[79] Likewise, if the bird appears healthy but hematology results suggest an inflammatory or infectious process in addition to heavy growth of enteric bacteria, treatment is usually indicated.

Problems in interpretation regarding which bacteria are normal inhabitants and which are pathogens should be considered in the light of the fact that *most bacteria* do not produce disease, but rather achieve a balance with the host that ensures the survival, growth, and propagation of both bacteria and host. In addition, sometimes pathogenic bacteria are present in a bird, but the infection may remain latent and thus subclinical, resulting in increased difficulty with interpretation of their presence.

Bacteria as a Result of Other Problems

Heavy growth of potentially pathogenic organisms, or even bacteria that are normally considered nonpathogenic, may occur as a result of other problems the bird is having. These factors should be evaluated and corrected. These microbial imbalances, however, can be the eventual cause of death in a debilitated bird and should be addressed.[67]

Enterobacteriaceae and Other Gram-negative Bacteria

Gram-negative bacterial overgrowth is probably a major complication of illness in psittacines. Multiple body systems can be affected, including the respiratory, gastrointestinal, renal, and other systems. In choanal swab or sinus aspirate cultures, gram-negative bacterial growth is often considered abnormal and pathogenic. However, contamination from other oral surfaces or food material may affect these cultures, and sample collection techniques should preclude contamination. Large numbers of gram-negative bacteria are generally considered abnormal from any site in the bird, but interpretation and treatment should be related to clinical signs.

Hematologic changes associated with active gram-negative infections can include leukocytosis, heterophilia, and monocytosis. Morphologic changes can be seen in heterophils (toxic changes) and can indicate bacterial infection.[45]

In pediatric patients with bacterial complications, the clinical signs that can be noted are often vague and nonspecific. The majority of patients, however, usually fit into one of two categories—babies that fail to thrive and those that have digestive disturbance, which often results in slowed gut transit time.[15] In babies that fail to thrive, are weak and listless, and have slow-emptying crops and poor feeding responses, heavy (gram-negative) bacterial growth is common. These patients, however, may be affected simultaneously by a number of problem-causing agents, including inappropriate ambient environment (temperature and relative humidity), viral or yeast infections, and inadequate nutrition. The vast majority of babies with digestive disturbances have some degree of crop stasis, which actually may be an outward sign of gut stasis or may reflect a generalized systemic infection. The problems may be traced to other causative factors, but many of these problems are considered primarily to be caused by bacterial contamination.[111]

African greys, and other large parrots kept as pets or in quarantine, are frequently plagued with an inordinate amount of bacterial organisms that are difficult to treat. Chronic, necrotizing sinus conditions are often seen in practice. In these parrots, it is sometimes extremely difficult to eradicate gram-negative organisms, even with intensive therapy dictated by culture and sensitivity results. Gram-positive infections (e.g., *Bacillus* species) seem to occur more frequently in African greys than in other large psittacines.[97] The nutritional factors that contribute to avian bacterial infections cannot be overemphasized. Widespread malnutrition still damages the health of pet birds. In parrots, vitamin A deficiency, characterized by squamous metaplasia of salivary glands and other epithelial surfaces, is a common clinical finding in birds that were found to have active bacterial infections.[45]

In budgerigars and cockatiels, both gram-negative and gram-positive infections are common. Gram-negative organisms frequently isolated as contaminants or secondary pathogens include *Klebsiella* species, *Citrobacter freundii, E. coli, Salmonella* species, and *Pseudomonas* species.

Citrobacter freundii is the most common and most pathogenic of the *Citrobacter* species. This species is commonly seen in finches. Ostriches, particularly chicks and young birds, appear very susceptible to *Citrobacter* species. Antibodies against *Citrobacter* often crossreact in serologic tests with those to *Salmonella typhimurium. C. amalonaticus* is frequently recovered from the intestinal tract of normal psittaciformes.[50]

Klebsiella pneumoniae and *K. oxytoca* are frequently recovered from finches, in which the bacteria can function as primary pathogens. They can also be involved as opportunists in immunosuppressed or stressed patients. Often, infections are not detected until late in the disease process when respiratory signs occur. Systemic infections are common; local infections involve the sinuses, skin, oral cavity and crop, particularly in psittacines. These bacteria posses a mucoid capsule that may protect them from environmental extremes and many disinfectants. Heat and drying are the best methods of killing *Klebsiella* species.[50]

Primary or Secondary Local Bacterial Lesions of the Skin, Mucous Membranes, and the Upper Respiratory Tract

Bacteria can cause septicemic disease, or may be locally invasive. Clinical signs are many and varied, depending upon the location and the degree of infection.

The Skin

The prevalence of bacterial folliculitis as a cause of feather picking and pruritus in psittacines is reportedly low.[59, 76, 91] In one report, staphylococcal dermatitis, pyodermia, and pulpitis were diagnosed in 29 of 213 birds with feather loss and feather picking.[91] The propatagium appears to be the most susceptible area, and *Staphylococcus* species are the most commonly reported bacteria. Rosskopf and Woerpel[96] describe several birds with pruritic folliculitis from which *Aeromonas* species, *Pseudomonas* species, and *Serratia* species were isolated. In a case of progressive feather loss, dermatitis characterized by erythema, multiple pustules, and thickened skin on the back of the head, under the

mandibles, and on the shoulder and the back, a *Mycobacterium* species was demonstrated at necropsy.[35] Bacteria can secondarily infect wounds originating from trauma or self-mutilation.

Diagnosis is usually obtained by cytology, skin biopsy, and isolation of the organism.

Bumblefoot is a condition caused by improper perches or bruising and trauma of the plantar surface of the feet, especially in raptors. Pathogenic bacteria may be introduced at these sites and may lead to necrotizing abscess development.[17, 92] In birds of prey, *S. aureus* is an important pathogen of bumblefoot and can lead to septicemia.[50, 65] Bumblefoot is also seen in other birds. Although staphylococci are frequently isolated from these lesions, they are by no means the only bacteria that can be isolated from diseased tissue.

Amazons are frequently presented with self-traumatic lesions on the feet, caused by biting and chewing (pododermatitis). Cultures of these ulcerative lesions have yielded many different isolates, including *Staphylococcus, Pseudomonas, Klebsiella,* and *E. coli.* As an underlying cause, this problem has been associated with low circulating levels of thyroid hormone.[85] (See also Chapter 32.)

Antibacterial therapy aims to eliminate underlying pathogens, prior to a surgical approach. In all cases of suspected bacterial etiology, cultures and antibiotic therapy should be initiated immediately, followed by changes as needed in the treatment protocol, based upon antibiotic sensitivity and response to treatment.[17]

Pharynx and Cloaca

Enterobacteriaceae and some other gram-negative bacteria are commonly cultured from the pharynx and cloaca. In large psittacines, heavy growth of the gram-negative organisms in the pharynx occur with vitamin A deficiency resulting in a metaplasia of the salivary glands. In the cloaca, papillomas or an egg prolapse enhance the growth of gram-negative bacteria. Depending on several factors, they can develop to a septicemia with signs of diarrhea and other signs of gastroenteritis, polyuria, localized infections at various body sites, and generalized lethargy and inappetence. Isolation of one or more offending organisms from appropriate sample sites can narrow the diagnosis.[104] In chicks, a localized infection can become a systemic problem, with clinical signs including generalized lethargy, paleness, and dryness of the skin.[111]

Upper Respiratory Tract

Rhinitis, (chronic) sinus infection, (chronic) nasal discharge, and sneezing are common signs of upper respiratory tract problems that can be connected with Enterobacteriaceae infection. Infection with several other gram-negative bacteria (e.g., *Pseudomonas* species, *Aeromonas* species, *Pasteurella* species) and gram-positive organisms can also lead to rhinitis and (chronic) sinusitis, sometimes resulting in supraorbital abscesses.[106] In other cases it is restricted to a clear nasal discharge with mild to moderate sneezing and occasional erythrema of the nostrils. This condition is seen particularly in South American species.[6, 97] In ostriches, *Haemophilus* species and *Bordetella avium* are specifically mentioned in relation to respiratory problems like rhinitis/sinusitis, pneumonia, and air sacullitis.[58, 62]

Isolated from the nose of birds of prey, *Acinetobacter* species, *Moraxella* species, *Aeromonas* species, *Pseudomonas* species, and *Klebsiella* species are considered to be pathogens.[95]

Typical workups might include a microscopic smear, bacterial culture, and sensitivity (flush sample or choanal slit), a CBC, and a chlamydia test. Isolation of one or more offending organisms from appropriate sample sites can narrow the diagnosis.[6, 104]

Treatment include the use of antibiotics, nebulization, and in many cases sinus flushing and/or surgery.[106]

Specific Bacteria of the Respiratory Tract

Enterococcus faecalis. This organism was isolated from canaries with chronic respiratory problems with the predominant lesion being tracheitis. *E. faecalis* (formerly *Streptococcus faecalis*) is a well-known member of the intestinal flora of many mammals and poultry.

The typical symptoms and lesions were reproduced experimentally by subcutaneous and intraperitoneal inoculations. Attempts to cause infection by aerosolation were unsuccessful.[22] It is probable

that the infection spreads hematogenously after entering minor skin lesions.

There is no convincing evidence of successful therapy, especially in chronic cases. *E. faecalis* is notoriously resistant to many antibiotics.

Bordetella **Species.** *Bordetella avium* is a gram-negative, motile, strictly aerobic rod-shaped bacterium which grows readily on MacConkey's agar. *Bordetella* species, as its relative *Alcaligenes faecalis*, are considered opportunistic pathogens that potentiate viral and other bacterial infections.[50] *B. avium* has a strict trophism for ciliated epithelium of the upper respiratory tract. Bordetellosis, known as turkey coryza, is a highly contagious upper respiratory tract disease of young turkeys.[4] *Alcaligenes* infections are characterized by coalescent liver necrosis in addition to respiratory problems.

Infection with *Bordetella* species has been reported in psittacines and finches.[50] From several aviaries, *B. avium* was isolated from cockatiel chicks exhibiting nestling mortality, rhinitis, sinusitis, and temporomandibular rigidity ("lock jaw" syndrome). *Bordetella bronchiseptica* and *B. avium* was isolated from a group of ostrich chicks exhibiting stunting, tracheitis, impaction, and mortality.[16]

The diagnosis is based on the respiratory symptoms and isolation of the organism. Concurrent superinfections with other common gram-negative bacteria and yeast may overgrow the tiny colonies, and thus *Bordetella* can be easily overlooked. The potential for immunosuppression and resultant superinfection with other pathogens, including protozoa, should be considered.

Treatment of the cockatiel aviaries included the use of antibiotics, detection of carriers, eliminating positive birds, and disinfection and sanitization of the aviary. Antibiotic therapy alone was not effective in eliminating the infection in cockatiels. The ostrich chicks were treated successfully with oral oxytetracycline and intratracheal amikacin.[16]

Spirochaetaceae. Several reports of incidental findings of helical organisms in companion birds can be found. In some cases (pigeons, canaries, African greys) these organisms could be classified as a *Borrelia* species.[5] The infection, however, is more important as a tick-borne disease in poultry in (sub)tropical areas.

Helical bacteria have been seen in microscopic smears of the rectum at necropsy in waterfowl, ostriches, and Lady Gouldian finches with intestinal problems. These organisms reacted positively with fluorescent antibodies for *Treponema hyodysenteriae*.[28]

A necrotizing pseudomembranous typhlocolitis associated with a spirochete has been described from three separate flocks of rheas from the USA.[101] Lesions were severe and mortality was high. In one of the cases, in-contact ostriches and emus did not contract the disease.

In cockatiels, spirochetosis is frequently seen.[97] The organism can be demonstrated on the mucosa of the upper respiratory tract and pharynx. These findings are associated with clinical signs like depression and sneezing.[50]

The significance of these findings is unknown. Interference with the ciliary activity of the respiratory mucosa is conceivable.

Ears and Eyes

Ophthalmic diseases of bacterial origin are common in birds. Conjunctival swabs of 242 normal birds (42 different species out of eight orders) yielded 232 (95.9%) bacterial isolates with distinct dominance of the gram-positive bacteria, with Micrococcaceae and *Bacillus* species or Micrococcaceae and *Enterococcus* species as the most frequently isolated bacteria. Gram-negative isolates were less common and may be indicative of pathologic situations.[52]

Discharges from eyes and ears from which predominantly gram-negative bacteria are cultured are indicative of a treatable condition, but discharges can occur with no bacteria or fungi recovered or seen in cytology.

Conjunctivitis is frequently the result of a primary irritant, such as dust, food particles, or flies. Bacteria (e.g., *Staphylococcus* species or *Haemophilus* species), are often secondary invaders that further complicate the conjunctivitis. Treatment should be based on a cytologic examination and bacterial culture and sensitivity testing. Remember to test for *Chlamydia*.

Primary Bacterial Infections Restricted to a Particular Organ System (Lower Respiratory Tract and Intestinal System)

Intestinal System

Digestive disturbances are very common in birds. Heavy overgrowth of transient flora or even contaminants can occur as a complication of other causes and because of a compromised defense mechanism. This can result in more serious disease or death.

In (psittacine) chicks, many digestive disturbances, such as crop and intestinal stasis, are caused by a primary (gram-negative) bacterial infection or result in the development of a bacterial pathogenic invader. Additional digestive-related clinical signs include bloody or black stools, diarrhea, polyuria, intussusception, and regurgitation or vomiting. Straining to defecate and inability to pass fecal material or passage of only urates and urine also may be observed.[111]

There are, however, also primary pathogens that can attack a part of the digestive system. For the common bird species these are *Campylobacter* species, megabacteria, *Clostridium* species, and *Plesiomonas shigelloides*.

Campylobacter Species

Campylobacter species are gram-negative bacteria that may appear in different forms including short comma, S-shaped, long spiral, or even coccoid form. Growth is best on blood agar or selective media in a microaerobic environment after 72 to 96 hours at 37 to 42°C.

The most common avian species include *C. jejuni*, the most frequent, and probably also the most pathogenic. *C. coli*, which is considered to be nonpathogenic, is frequently confused with *C. jejuni*. *C. laridis* is isolated from gulls, and the pathogenicity is still not defined.

The host spectrum is large and includes poultry, waterfowl, gulls, crows, pigeons, rhea, ostrich, and many Passeriformes (especially Estrididae [40.8%] and canaries).[34] It is also found in Psittaciformes.

In many species clinical signs are associated with hepatitis and include lethargy, anorexia, diarrhea (frequently with yellowish-staining feces) and emaciation.[50] In ostriches, outbreaks are seen in 2-week to 4-month-old chicks.[87] In finches, a high mortality is seen especially among fledglings. In our experience, intestinal *Campylobacter* infections are becoming more common in association with mortality in nestlings and young birds of many different species, including ostriches.

The diagnosis is confirmed by demonstrating the faintly staining, curved rods in stained smears from the droppings, bile, or gut contents, and culturing the bacteria on special microaerophilic media.

At necropsy the liver is enlarged, pale or greenish, and congested. Coalescing necrotic hepatitis is a common histologic finding. In the finches, the intestine is filled with catarrhal contents containing parts of seeds and starch.

Treatment includes the use of antibiotics, but there is a discrepancy between the antibiogram and clinical recovery. Sanitation and disinfection of the aviary help.

Megabacteria

Megabacteria are large (20–50 μm), gram-positive, periodic acid-Schiff (PAS) positive, rod-shaped organisms that have some fungal characteristics and have been found in the proventriculus or droppings of several avian species.

Megabacteria infections were first described as a common problem in finches and small psittacines. It was the organism implicated for "going light," a wasting disease in budgerigars.[56] Nowadays it seems to emerge in many bird species (e.g., many large psittacines, ostriches,[63] quail, ibises). In Australia, megabacteria were demonstrated in many captive psittacines and passerines, as well as in wild-caught European goldfinches and wild-caught young sulphur-crested cockatoos.[41] Some authors suggest that the bacteria may be a component of the normal upper alimentary tract flora in budgerigars.[102]

Megabacteria have been associated with proventricular and ventricular disease, but the pathogenicity of megabacteria is unclear, and Koch's postulate has not been fulfilled.

Clinical signs include apathy, anorexia, regurgitation, and the passing of part or whole seeds in soft, watery, and dark green to brown-black feces. In 10-day to 6-week-old ostrich chicks, the behavior is apparently normal; the chicks peck at food, but do not ingest it. They cease to grow and lose weight.[62]

Birds progressively become emaciated and debilitated. Digestion is disturbed because of the decreased acid formation, which decreases enzyme activity and prevents hardening of the koilin layer.

The diagnosis is based on demonstrating the organism in wet mounts or stained microscopic smears. The bacterium seems to be a facultative anaerobe and exhibits its best growth on blood agar when incubated in air with 10% carbon dioxide at 37°C.[102]

At necropsy, the organism can be demonstrated in the mucus of the proventriculus. The proventriculus is mostly distended, and the mucosa is covered with a cloudy thick mucous layer, predominantly in the lower part of this organ. The wall of the proventriculus is thickened, often with small hemorrhages. The koilin layer may appear soft and devitalized.

Treatment includes acidification of the drinking water (hydrochloric or citric acid), easily digestible food, and extra nutritional support. In vitro studies have shown that the organism isolated from budgerigars and ostriches is sensitive to a number of antibiotics.[63, 102] Other studies indicate complete resistance to all common antibiotics.[49] Oral amphotericin B in budgerigars and oral nystatin in European finches were shown to be effective.[42]

Clostridium Species

Clostridial enteritides have been reported in poultry, waterfowl, and psittacine birds. Necrotic enteritis of the small intestine resulting in severe hemorrhagic diarrhea in poultry and waterfowl is caused by *Clostridium perfringens* types A and C.[40] *Clostridium* enterotoxemia has been reported from young ostriches on lucerne pastures. Birds became weak and sometimes had diarrhea. *C. perfringens* type A and D were isolated.[62] A similar disease, ulcerative enteritis, has been reported in young chickens, poults, and upland game birds (i.e., bobwhite quail [*Colinus virginianus*]) and is caused by *Clostridium colinum*.[9] In ostriches, also, an ulcerative gastritis has been reported.[103] It has been suggested that a change in diet, intestinal damage, intestinal stasis, and concurrent infection predispose to this disease. Raptors and birds with well-developed ceca such as Galliformes, Anseriformes, and Struthioformes may have clostridial organisms as part of the autochthonous flora.[50]

Clinical signs for *C. perfringens* in chickens are the result of enterotoxemia and include depression, dehydration, rapid mortality, diarrhea, hematochezia, polydipsia, emaciation, and death.

Postmortem lesions include darkened pectoral musculature, hepatomegaly, splenomegaly, and ballooning of the small intestine. The small intestine is often friable and may contain foul-smelling brown fluid. In advanced cases, small intestinal changes are most pronounced and may include a fibronecrotic or diphtheric enteritis ranging from a pinpoint focal erythromatous mucosal lesion to large, coalesced, perforating, necrotic ulcers of the jejunum, ileum (ceca), and rectum.

Similar postmortem lesions have been described in Psittaciformes from which a *Clostridium* species and *E. coli* were recovered. Lesions were observed in a Quaker parakeet (*Myopsitta monachus*), severe macaws (*A. severa*), and green-winged macaws (*A. chloroptera*). Other lesions included splenitis, pulmonary congestion, and pneumonia.[25] Hemorrhagic enteritis with *E. coli* and *C. perfringens* in a group of great-billed parrots (*Tanygnatus megalorynchos*) has been reported more recently.[100] In Australia, a severe form of necrotic enteritis has been described in lorikeets, both in the wild and in captivity. It was characterized by sudden death or necrotic tissue lining the intestine found on postmortem. It has been attributed to a clostridial organism, and ampicillins have stopped outbreaks.[51] *Clostridium* species have also been identified on numerous occasions through necropsy results on young Ramphastids (toucans) with a necrotic enteritis. Interestingly, none of the psittacines kept in close proximity were affected.[111] *Clostridium* species are also recognized as a potential pathogen in ostriches with necrotic enteritis.

The diagnosis is based ante mortem on the history, clinical signs, identification in cytology, and isolation of the organism from feces or cloaca. Postmortem diagnosis is by necropsy, histology, and anaerobic culture of liver and intestines and demonstration of serum toxins.[9, 50] As a quick aid in diagnosis, necrotic material (liver or intestine) can be crushed between two slides and stained with Diff-Quick and/or Gram's stain. Large, gram-positive rods, subterminal spores, and free spores can be seen.

Treatment and control includes antibiotics and laxatives. In a case of regular problems with *C. perfringens* infections in rheas, the annual administration of a multicomponent vaccine for small ruminants stopped the disease problems in this flock.[28] In South Africa, the present recommendation is to use the *C. perfringens* types B and D (lamb dysentery and pulpy kidney) vaccines at 1 week of age with repetition at 30 days of age.[62] The use by mistake of a *C. septicum* type D vaccine caused

sudden high mortality resulting from anaphylactic shock.

A paralytic-like disease in ostriches was associated with *C. chauvoei* infection.[78] At necropsy the lungs were hyperemic and edematous, and the intestines had prominent hemorrhages in their mucosa. The liver and kidney were enlarged, and the former also had necrotic foci. Smears taken from the hyperemic regions of the intestine and the necrotic foci of the liver were positive for *C. chauvoei* after staining with specific fluorescein-labeled antiserum.

Plesiomonas shigelloides

Plesiomonas shigelloides is a curved gram-negative, facultative anaerobic, oxidase-positive rod. It is a member of the family Vibrionaceae that is commonly found in surface water and seafood during summer months.

The organism is found in man, mammals, water-related birds (penguins, gulls, herons, etc.), reptiles, and fish. It can produce a mild to acute, self-limited diarrhea in man[46, 86] and birds.[30]

The microorganism destroys epithelial cells. In man bacteremia is reported, particularly in those who are immunocompromised.[38]

The organism is recovered using routine gram-negative selective media, but it prefers a shigelloides-selective agar.[30]

Bacteria in the Egg and Post-hatch Bacterial Infections

Bacteria can enter the egg as it passes through the oviduct or once it is laid, as the egg cools down. In chickens, both *E. coli* and *Mycoplasma* have been shown to enter eggs during passage through the oviduct. Embryonic deaths from infections with *Salmonella, E. coli, Staphylococcus*, and potentially *Chlamydia* have all been found.[82] Bacterial infection with other gram-negative organisms, including *Pseudomonas*, have been noted on occasion.

Eggs that have already been laid can be infected with these deadly microorganisms while in the incubator by contact with an infected egg or eggshell, or a contaminated cracked egg, or through contamination in an unclean incubator. In addition to exposure in an incubator, egg collection containers, hands, dirty nest boxes, or other fomites can be sources of contamination for a developing embryo.

In addition to causing embryonic death at any stage of development, bacterial infections can produce chicks that are small and weak at hatching. The majority of these chicks either die soon after hatching or survive for only a short time because of the overwhelming infection and the lack of adequate immunity.

Post-hatch bacterial infections also can be contracted through an exposed unretracted yolk sac or open umbilicus.[43] Common bacteria isolated from the yolk sac are the well-known gram-negative bacteria (e.g., *E. coli*, *Pseudomonas*, *Klebsiella*, *Proteus*, *Salmonella*), as well as the gram-positive bacteria *Staphylococcus* species. *Campylobacter jejuni* is also reported in ostrich chicks.[58]

Necropsy, including cytology and bacteriology, should always be recommended for chicks found dead in the shell, neonate deaths, and post-hatch deaths. Bacterial deaths in neonates in the early post-hatch state should have an environmental review included as part of the evaluation, because contaminated incubators and brooders may be the origin of the bacterial infection.[111]

Primary Bacterial Infections Resulting in Septicemia and Mortality in Infected Birds

Gram-negative Bacteria

E. Coli

E. coli is a gram-negative, rod-shaped, aerobic bacterium. It is the most common representative of the Enterobacteriaceae. In poultry, *E. coli* infections include colibacillosis, colisepticemia, coligranuloma, peritonitis, salpingitis, synovitis, omphalitis, air sac disease, and all other disease conditions caused entirely or partially by *E. coli*. The various serotypes are intestinal in all animals; therefore, their distribution is widespread. Among normal chickens, 10 to 15% of intestinal coliformes belong to potentially pathogenic serotypes.[53] Intestinal strains are not necessarily the same serotypes as those from the pericardial sac of the same bird. *E. coli* septicemia was diagnosed in 12% of pigeon necropsies. Clinical signs consisted of sudden death, vomiting, diarrhea, and weight loss.[20]

The various *E. coli* serotypes are classified according to antigenic structures, and some serotypes are considered more pathogenic than others. Neither endotoxins nor hemolysins are associated with disease-producing abilities of *E. coli* in birds. Pathogenic isolates are reported to differ from nonpathogenic isolates by their ability to bind Congo red.[10] Others, however, tried to determine pathogenicity of *E. coli* using Congo red unsuccessfully. Pathogenic *E. coli* grow in the presence of low concentrations of iron, and adhere to epithelial surfaces by means of pili. Exogenous iron increases pathogenicity.[11] Avian *E. coli* can produce enterotoxins that cause diarrhea by inducing hypersecretion of fluids into the intestinal lumen.[50]

E. coli–related air sacculitis and pericarditis in poultry may follow infections with adenoviruses, reoviruses, coronaviruses and infectious bursal disease viruses. There is evidence that this is also the case for *E. coli* and adenoviruses in racing pigeons.[33]

For pet birds the same situation occurs. Very few *E. coli* strains seem to be primary pathogens. However, it is difficult to classify an *E. coli* as a pathogen or not. The virulence is mostly based on the clinical and postmortem findings. There is no pathogenic serotyping available for avian *E. coli* strains other than those used in poultry.

The most common disease entities include colisepticemia (pericarditis, polyserositis, air sacculitis, pneumonia, arthritis), localized enteritis (catarrhal to pseudomembranous or ulcerative), coligranulomatosis (foci in liver, spleen, kidney, and/or intestinal subserosa), rhinitis, and fibrinous salpingitis or oophoritis.[50]

Lesions similar to those found as being caused by *E. coli* can also be caused by many other organisms. In psittacines and many other "pet" birds, these lesions may be caused by a myriad of gram-negatives such as *Pseudomonas* species, *Proteus* species, *Acinetobacter* species, *Enterobacter* species, *Klebsiella* species, and others.

Diagnosis is based on clinical signs, microscopic smears, isolation, and identification of the causative agent (and necropsy).

Treatment includes the use of antibiotics. Many *E. coli* strains are resistant to one or more drugs. Some authors include the administration of avian lactobacilli or lactulose in an effort to lower the intestinal tract pH and help to establish a proper autochthonous flora.[50] The value is still under discussion.

Vaccination is possible in poultry and waterfowl for certain strains. Essential are management of environmental factors, hygiene, and provision of a good diet to improve the physiology of the gastrointestinal tract.

Pseudomonas Species and *Aeromonas* Species

Pseudomonas and *Aeromonas* are gram-negative, rod-shaped, aerobic, quite vigorously growing bacteria that are taxonomically unrelated but clinically have many similarities. *Pseudomonas aeruginosa* and *Aeromonas hydrophila* are the most common avian pathogens from these large groups. They produce a variety of toxins and enzymes that may contribute to pathogenicity. Some biologic differences distinguish the species including types of toxins, pigment production, pathogenicity, and biochemical metabolism. *Pseudomonas* and *Aeromonas* isolates should be considered to have pathogenic potential even when isolated from "healthy" patients in low numbers.[45, 50] These infections remain a common and frustrating problem.

Both organisms are frequently found in aquatic environments like standing water in hoses or pipes, sprinklers and plant spray bottles, and other devices for increasing relative humidity. These are potential sources of infections. The use of cage litter such as corn cob bedding or walnut shell can predispose birds to *Pseudomonas* infections, particularly if the products are infrequently changed. These organisms are also found in fruits and vegetables that stay too long in the cage. *Pseudomonas* and *Aeromonas* can grow in solutions of minimal nutrient composition and have been isolated from a wide variety of environmental, clinical, and avicultural sites.

Clinical signs and/or recognizable changes in clinical pathology values characterize clinical gram-negative infections. Signs can include sneezing, wheezing, coughing, dyspnea, regurgitation, fluffing, sleeping, feather picking, diarrhea, or melena. Deaths resulting from *Pseudomonas* infection happen frequently with neonates, pediatric patients, and adult avian patients. Catarrhal to hemorrhagic enteritis with edema and fibrous inflammation of the serosal membranes are sometimes noted in nutritionally deficient or immunosuppressed patients.

Pseudomonas organisms can colonize bacterial lesions in which the primary etiologic agents have been killed with antibiotics and then serve as foci for hematogenous dissemination. Chronic and recurrent respiratory infections can be associated with *Pseudomonas* organisms that seem refractory to treatment.

In a survey of a diagnostic laboratory, the majority (78.7%) of *Pseudomonas* species were isolated from the upper respiratory or alimentary tract. The primary sites were the choanae or the general pharyngeal area.[45] Only 38.4% of the *Pseudomonas* cases were detectable before culture by identification of gram-negative organisms on a Gram's stain. The incidence was particularly high in Amazon and African grey parrots. There was a definite positive correlation between increased leucocyte count and *Pseudomonas* infection in psittacines; white blood cells; (WBC) 21,590/mm^3 (n = 170) for all *Pseudomonas* cases (23,700/mm^3 in sick birds and 18,700/mm^3 in healthy birds). The PCV was not affected.

In our experience, both *Pseudomonas* and *Aeromonas* are common isolates from the trachea, lung, and air sacs in young ostriches kept under wet and cold conditions.[28]

Treatment includes the use of antibiotics (enrofloxacin is the first-choice drug; trimethoprim/sulfamethoxazole is usually ineffective) for 10 to 14 days, topical drugs, and nebulization. But even for enrofloxacin, only about 50% of the isolated strains are sensitive in vitro.[26] The avian practitioner should also review the patient's nutritional history. The environment and feeding and drinking utensils should be adequately disinfected with hypochlorite, quaternary ammonium products, or glutaraldehyde-based disinfectants.

Pasteurella Species

Pasteurella multocida, is a gram-negative, rod-shaped bacterium. It stains bipolar in tissue smears when fixed in methanol and stained with methylene blue. *P. multocida* are differentiated into strains based on endotoxin production and capsule antigens. There is difference in virulence between different strains. Other commonly isolated but less pathogenic species include *P. pneumotropica* and *P. gallinarum*.

P. multocida is often isolated from pets or wild

birds that are attacked by cats.[73] This organism is common in the cat's mouth. Birds that are bitten by cats should receive prompt attention (antibiotics) because a fatal septicemia can develop rapidly. *P. multocida* frequently can be isolated from the upper respiratory tract of mammalian species such as cats, raccoons, pigs, cattle, and humans. Not all strains are pathogenic to birds. The final diagnosis is made at necropsy if therapy fails.

P. multocida is also the agent of avian cholera, a serious problem in migratory waterfowl. *Pasteurella* has been associated with disease in Galliformes, Anseriformes, Ciconiiformes, Psittaciformes, Columbiformes, and Passeriformes. Apparently normal birds may harbor virulent *P. multocida* in the choana.

Infections are usually transmitted via the upper respiratory tract and conjunctivae. *P. multocida* persist in the environment for up to 2 weeks after the removal of susceptible hosts.[93]

Immunity following infection usually prevents disease recurrence resulting from that strain, but birds remain carriers. They may be susceptible to disease from other strains, and under conditions of stress such as overcrowding, reduced nutrient intake, other diseases, egg-laying, heavy environmental contamination, and introduction of the organism into wounds (especially fight wounds), disease may occur.

Clinical signs of the acute form include cyanosis, dyspnea, and diarrhea followed by death. Survivors develop respiratory rales, sinusitis, conjunctivitis, or swelling of the infraorbital sinus. Granulomatous dermatitis has been noted in raptors, owls, and pigeons.

Postmortem lesions include petechiae or ecchymoses, exudative serositis, and necrotic foci in infected organs. In chronic cases, catarrhal to fibrinous changes can be seen in the upper and lower respiratory tract. Granulomatous lesions can be found in any organ, leading to arthritis, osteomyelitis, otitis media, dermatitis, and liver and spleen foci.

Diagnosis is based on clinical symptoms, cytology, necropsy, and isolation of the causative agent.

Treatment includes antibiotics, but treatment often fails. The production of vaccines from strains that persist in an aviary may provide successful long-term control.

In some birds without clinical symptoms *Pasteur-ella* species are present in the choana that differ from *P. multocida*. This occurs in thick-billed parrots[36] and in collared turtle-doves (*Streptopelia decaocto*).[28] The last isolate was closely related to *P. pneumotropica* based on Analytical Profile Index (API) determination, which is commonly isolated from the respiratory tract of mice. However, proper taxonomic classification is needed.

The family Pasteurellaceae also includes the genera *Actinobacillus* and *Haemophilus*, which can be pathogens in birds. *Actinobacillus* species can cause acute death in birds. Birds with a more chronic course typically develop joint lesions. The species causes chronic disease in goslings.[50] *Haemophilus* species probably serve as secondary invaders that sustain upper (rhinitis, sinusitis) and sometimes lower (pneumonia, air sacculitis) respiratory tract disease in species other than chickens.

Riemerella anatipestifer (*Pasteurella anatipestifer*)

In 15 unrelated cases, *Riemerella anatipestifer* strains were isolated from the upper and/or lower respiratory tract of domestic pigeons, most of them with a respiratory disease.[60] The main bacterial isolates from the conjunctivitis cases in lovebirds seen in our laboratory are identified as *Pasteurella anatipestifer*.[32]

Salmonella Species

Salmonella species are flagellated, gram-negative, rod-shaped bacteria that can infect many species of birds. They are ubiquitous and can, under suitable conditions, survive and multiply in the environment. Many animals can be subclinical carriers. Under certain conditions, infections with *Salmonella* species may be associated with disease; this is called *paratyphoid*.

In poultry, the number of *Salmonella* that establish themselves in the lower intestinal tract is affected by the presence of other bacteria that influence pH, produce volated fatty acids, and occupy adherence sites. The principle that underlies "competitive exclusion," is the situation whereby known enteric flora are introduced into young domestic fowls so that their intestines are an unfavorable environment for the multiplication of *Salmonella*. In birds without developed ceca (e.g., psittacines, passerines, pigeons, and doves) this principle is not likely to be effective, because enteric flora are not considered to be well developed. This might explain why these birds appear to be more susceptible to *Salmonella* infections (Table 18–1) than birds with fully functioning ceca.[50]

Pathogenicity may be associated with penetration of the mucosal membranes lining the alimentary tract. Infections may sometimes occur by inhalation. Localized infections are usually the result of transport in macrophages and deposition in areas of poor circulation. Fecal samples of experimentally infected doves showed some *Salmonella* within 24 hours post-infection, but then the feces stayed negative until clinical signs developed after 7 to 14 days, resulting in systemic lesions and large numbers of *Salmonella* in the feces.[28]

The incidence of various *Salmonella* species seems to vary with geographic location and the types of food consumed. Imported birds have often been found infected with *Salmonella* and may serve as reservoirs for nonindigenous species that can cause devasting outbreaks.[50] Although about 2000 different *Salmonella* species are recognized, only relatively few infect birds (see Table 18–1). Of the *Salmonella* isolated over a 25-year period in Utrecht, 67% of the psittacine isolates came from large parrots.[30] Some strains are host-adapted (such as *S. gallinarum-pullorum* to chickens and *S. typhi-*

murium var copenhagen to either pigeons or European finches (beware: two different biovars).

The different *Salmonella* species can be classified by serotype, phage type, antibiotic resistance patterns, plasmic profiles analysis, and biotype. These factors seem unrelated to virulence,[89] but they are very important for epidemiologic studies.

Six weeks after a *Salmonella* outbreak (*S. typhimurium ft506*) in a building with lorikeets and 2 weeks after the last mortality in that collection, there was a high mortality among young Mandarin ducks in another building. From these birds *S. typhimurium ft292* was isolated. These were two independent outbreaks. When in the following weeks *Salmonella* victims were found in other cages and buildings, including the building with the lorikeets, the isolation of *S.t. ft292* demonstrated a serious hygiene and management problem.[29]

In poultry and pigeons it is known that apparently healthy adult birds may harbor *Salmonella*, and eggs that are laid can have varying degrees of *Salmonella* contamination on their surface. These bacteria are motile and pass through pores in the shell. Some developing embryos may die from infection. If the chicks are subjected to environmental stress in the first few days of life, mortality due to systemic salmonellosis (i.e., paratyphoid) can be quite marked.[93]

A bird or a flock/group of birds may become

T a b l e   1 8 – 1

AN OVERVIEW OF THE SEROTYPING OF 766 DIFFERENT *SALMONELLA* STRAINS†

Species	Total	Psitt	Colum	Passe	Phasa	Anat	Others
S. typhimurium	82.6*	84.9	92.6	85.3	48.6	75.4	65.3
Non typhimurium	17.4	15.1	7.4	14.7	51.4	24.5	34.7
Total	766**	225[1]	188[2]	190[3]	35	53	75
*S. enteritidis***	35	17		3	6	1	8
S. dublin	5		1	1	1		2
S. agona	6			1	2	2	1
S. infantis	6		1	1	2	1	1
S. III (Arizona)	3			3			

Data from Dorrestein GM, Buitelaar MN: Results of bacteriological examination. Unpublished data, 1995.
Psitt = Psittaciformes; Colum = Columbiformes: Passe = Passeriformes; Phasa = Phasanidae; Anat = Anatidae
[1]Of which 78 African grey parrots, 51 amazons, 13 macaws, and 9 cockatoos (151 large parrots = 67.1%)
[2]Of which 160 homing pigeons (85.1%)
[3]Of which 86 canaries (45.2%)
*Percentages
**Absolute numbers
***List of possible zoonotic strains
†Isolated over a 25-year period at the Department of Veterinary Pathology, Utrecht University, from birds (other than commercial poultry)

infected with *Salmonella* by ingestion of contaminated food and or drinking water, contact with carriers (not necessarily of the same species), or vertical transmission. If the *Salmonella* species are pathogenic for that species, the appropriate predisposing factors are operative, and a sufficient number of organisms are introduced into the host, paratyphoid may occur.

Clinical signs vary from mild enteritis to a severely ill state with anorexia, lethargy, polydipsia, diarrhea, dehydration, and crop stasis. Acute death resulting from a systemic disease with polyserositis or petechial hemorrhages may be seen. In subacute to chronic cases central nervous system (CNS) signs, dyspnea, and indications of liver, spleen, kidney, or heart damage are common. Pigeons may have a localized infection such as meningitis, arthritis, tenosynovitis, or osteomyelitis. With high-dose infections, conjunctivitis, iridocyclitis, and panophthalmia may occur.[50] In nestlings during an outbreak, yolk sac infections can be found. Granulomatous dermatitis has been reported in several species.

Fecal culture may demonstrate the organism in living birds. At necropsy one or more of the following changes is found: muscle degeneration or necrosis, hepatomegaly, splenomegaly, air sacculitis, gastroenteritis (occasionally with ulcers and granulomas) and nephropathy, and the presence of bacteria in cytology. Numerous yellow necrotic foci are often present in organs. The diagnosis is confirmed by isolating the organisms.

Infection, especially in passerines and toucans, must be differentiated from *Yersinia pseudotuberculosis* infection by culture. Often *Salmonella typhimurium* can be isolated from the swollen joints in homing pigeons.

Elimination of infection is often very difficult and carriers can develop. This is partly explained by the occurrence of L-forms, which are resistant to common therapy and are thought to be the reason for vaccination failures. L-forms do not grow in routine cultures.[71]

Long-term (up to 3 weeks) antibiotic treatment is recommended, preferably based on an antibiogram. It is essential, especially in flock management, to address the contaminated environment, to trace carriers, remove subclinically infected breeders, and if possible to locate the vector (wild birds, rodents) or contaminated food and water supply.

There is considerable controversy concerning whether vaccination is effective for the prevention of salmonellosis in pigeons. Of seven vaccines tested, only two oil-adjuvanted vaccines gave some protective effect. The other vaccines had limited or no influence on the course of experimental salmonellosis. Vaccinations are advised in addition to antibiotics and culling of clinically affected pigeons in loft sanitation procedures after a clinical outbreak.[108]

The normal companion bird strains of *Salmonella* are not considered important human pathogens in healthy individuals, but they can cause problems in infants, geriatric patients, and those with immunosuppressive diseases. One of the human enteropathogens, *S. enteritidis*[38, 86] is commonly isolated from psittacines and other pet birds.[83] In Table 18–1 it can be seen that in the Netherlands *S. enteritidis* in companion birds is predominantly isolated from psittacines.[30] Although *S. typhimurium* can occasionally play a role in foodborne digestive disturbances, it is much less important than *S. enteritidis*.[86]

Humans carrying *Salmonella* can infect their companion birds. Such human-to-bird interactions have been shown to occur with the larger psittacine species.[50]

Yersinia pseudotuberculosis

Y. pseudotuberculosis is the most important pathogenic *Yersinia* species. This organism is gram-negative, forms ovoid-to-coccoid rods, and replicates at temperatures as low as 4°C in the environment. Five serovars are commonly found, but serovars 1 and 2 are most commonly isolated from birds (Table 18–2). This bacterium is indigenous to Northern and Middle Europe. Outbreaks are more common in the colder months.[12] In other parts of the world, including Canada, the US, Africa, and Australia, it is thought to have arisen from movements of European birds and rodents.

Many mammalian and bird species can become infected. Cuculiformes (turacos) and Piciformes (toucans, toucanets, aracaris, and barbets) are extremely susceptible and die peracutely with hemorrhagic to fibrinous pneumonia, hepatomegaly, and splenomegaly. In Fringillidae (finches), psittacines, and doves the course is more chronic with submiliary to miliary, sharply demarcated grayish foci in liver, spleen, and ceca. Pigeons are seldom infected.

Table 18-2

FREQUENCIES OF OCCURRENCE OF *YERSINIA PSEUDOTUBERCULOSIS* AND THE DISTRIBUTION OF SEROTYPES AMONG DIFFERENT ORDERS†

Species		Total	Passe[1]	Cuc/Pic[2]	Psitt[3]	Colum[4]	Others
serotype	1	57.9*	52.7	76.1	47.7	82.1	66.7
	2	38.5	43.8	22.8	44.2	17.9	30.8
	3	1.0	1.2	1.1			2.5
	4	0.7	0.6		2.3		
	5	1.9	1.8		5.8		
Total		579**	338	88	86	28	39

Data from Dorrestein GM, Buitelaar MN: Results of bacteriological examination. Unpublished data, 1995.
Passe = Passeriformes; Cuc = Cuculiformes; Pic = Piciformes: Psitt = Psittaciformes; Colum = Columbiformes
[1]Including 172 (50.9%) canaries (of which 63 [36.7%] serotype 1 and 104 [60.5%] serotype 2) and 49 (13.6%) mynahs and starlings
[2]Including 33 toucans, 19 touracos, 18 aracaris, and 12 barbets
[3]Only 1 amazon, 1 cockatiel, 1 lovebird, and 3 budgerigars; predominantly Australian parakeets
[4]Mostly doves, includes only 1 homing pigeon
*Percentages
**Absolute numbers
†Isolated over a 35-year period at the Department of Veterinary Pathology, Utrecht University, from birds (other than commercial poultry)

Clinical signs include lethargy, dehydration, diarrhea, and dyspnea. Emaciation, wasting, and flaccid paresis or paralysis are common with subacute or chronic cases.

The course of the disease, cytology, and (histo)pathology followed by isolation of the organism finalizes the diagnosis. Isolation of avian *Yersinia* strains can be difficult; therefore, "refrigerator enrichment" for 2 weeks may improve the isolation results.[48]

Treatment includes parenteral and oral administration of antibiotics and applying strict sanitary measures. Most experimental vaccines have proven to be ineffective after challenge. Some vaccines seem to give protection under practice circumstances.

Y. enterocolitica is a human pathogen, and is isolated as an incidental finding from wild birds.

Gram-positive Bacteria

Streptococcus and *Enterococcus*

Streptococcus and *Enterococcus* consist of numerous species that readily grow on common media. Differentiation between the species is based upon morphology and biochemical and serologic characteristics. The organisms are ubiquitous, and they are sensitive to most commonly used disinfectants.[50]

Both genera are considered part of the normal flora of skin and mucosa. Predisposing factors to disease include immunosuppression, concomitant infections, and exposure to a variety of toxins and pathogenicity factors that may be produced by some strains.

Clinical diseases include omphalitis in recent hatchlings, septicemia, joint lesions, and endocarditis.

Streptococcus pyogenes has been associated with bacteremia among others in several Psittaciformes. In the ostrich this organism together with *Corynebacterium pyogenes* can induce diphtheroid lesions in the mucosa of the beak cavity and the crop.

Septicemia in pigeons was often associated with *Streptococcus bovis*.[23] Most of these cases presented a history of hyperacute death in pigeons of all ages. In other birds, emaciation, polyuria, and green slimy droppings were present. Typical lesions found at necropsy were large, well-circumscribed areas of necrosis in the breast muscle, and tendinitis of the tendon of the deep pectoral muscle. Furthermore, arthritis and lesions that pointed to generalized septicemia were seen.[19, 21]

The organism was isolated from crop and cloaca samples in 40% of the Belgium racing pigeons as well as from 80% of the pooled fecal samples that were obtained from different pigeon lofts. Because clinical symptoms related to a *S. bovis* septicemia were observed in pigeons that already carried the bacterium in the intestinal tract for several months, it was concluded that *S. bovis* in pigeons is a facultative pathogenic agent.

Streptococcus suis is also associated with septicemic disease in small psittacines and finches.[24]

Enterococcus faecalis is frequently implicated as a cause of pneumonia in various birds, particularly Passeriformes, and primarily infects young birds. In acute cases, samples taken from the liver, heart, and brain are most diagnostic. Aggressive treatment with parenteral administration of antibiotics is recommended.

Staphylococcus

As mentioned earlier, most members of the genus *Staphylococcus* (apart from *S. aureus*) are commonly recovered from many avian species and are considered part of the normal flora. They are gram-positive cocci. When present in disease, they are generally considered to be secondary invaders.

S. aureus is very common in the environment and can frequently be isolated from the skin and mucosa of clinically normal birds. *S. aureus* can induce a wide range of clinical and pathologic lesions, including high embryonic mortality, yolk sac or umbilical inflammation, septicemia, arthritis-synovitis, osteomyelitis, vesicular dermatitis, gangrenous dermatitis, and bumblefoot.

Acute necrosis of the distal digits or adnexa of the head and neck is suggestive of a thrombi-inducing infection, which can be a sequela to *Staphylococcus* septicemia.[50] An acute onset of tremors, opisthotonos, and torticollis can often be linked to *Staphylococcus*-induced necrosis in the CNS. Chronic infections may result in valvular endocarditis.

The diagnosis is based on microscopic slides of the lesions and isolation and identification of the causative agent.

Avian Tuberculosis (*Mycobacterium* Species)

Mycobacterium infections have been reported from many pet birds. Susceptible psittacine species seem to be older Amazon parrots and *Brotogeris* species such as grey-cheeked parakeets at any age (as young as 4 months).[97] In general, this problem is uncommon in young birds, which does not mean that young birds are not infected.[14, 111]

It is endemic worldwide, especially in waterfowl, gallinaceous birds, Columbiformes, passerines, psittacines, and raptors. *M. avium* seems to be most often implicated. Recent development has re-

grouped this species around several subspecies. *M. intracellulare* has been designated as a distinct new species and is considered less pathogenic to birds than *M. avium*. It is, however, difficult to differentiate between the two species; therefore, they are routinely grouped together into the *M. avium-intracellulare* (MAI) complex. MAI complex strains are serologically different and have been divided into serovars.[50]

In some psittacine cases *M. tuberculosis*[14, 50] and *M. bovis*[50] have been found as the causative organism.

M. avium is very stable in the environment and difficult to eradicate from an infected premise. Transmission is through ingestion or aerosolation of feces. It is a zoonotic disease and often difficult to treat in humans (see Chapter 22). In 1995, using gene probes, *M. genavense* was identified from 17 out of 30 avian cultures.[61] This *Mycobacterium* causes disseminated infections in human acquired autoimmune disease (AIDS) patients and has only recently been identified as a pathogen. However, the pathogenicity of *M. genavense* in birds seems to be limited, because several birds kept in close contact with cage mates remained healthy.

In birds, three different types of lesions can be recognized: (1) the classical form with tubercles in many organs; (2) the paratuberculous form with typical lesions in the intestinal tract; (3) the nontuberculous form or atypical mycobacteriosis, which may be difficult to recognize at necropsy.[50]

Avian mycobacteriosis primarily involves the intestinal tract and presents as a chronic wasting disease, although acute deaths in well-fleshed birds can occur. Weight loss, depression, diarrhea, and polyuria that are poorly responsive to antibiotics are the most common client complaints. Poor feathering, cachexia, abdominal distention, lameness, and subcutaneous and conjunctival masses are typical physical findings. Dyspnea may be observed in birds with pulmonary involvement.[109]

In psittacines, the most common lesions are granulomatous lesions in the liver and spleen, but also gastrointestinal or lungs granulomas can be found. In combination with the other lesions, a dermatitis can occur.[35]

In some cases, especially macaws, granulomas are found in the bone marrow, which are visible on radiographs. In Falconiformes and Accipitriformes, arthritis or tubercle formation of the muscles of the thighs or tibiotarsus (shank) can be seen occasionally.[50]

In some psittacine species (*Amazona, Cacatua, Pionis, Brotogeris, Psittacula,* and *Eunymphicus*) distinct intestinal lesions can be found at necropsy comparable to that of paratuberculosis, with hypertrophic, clubbed villa in the small intestine.

In finches (canaries, hooded siskins, and Lady Gouldian finches) and small psittacines, atypical mycobacterial infections with no specific tuberculous lesions are common in some geographic areas, but are often incidental findings during necropsy. The most common finding at necropsy is hepatomegaly. The diagnosis is based on finding large numbers of acid-fast organisms in cytology and/or histology. This is referred to as atypical mycobacteriosis.[90, 94]

The definitive diagnosis is based on finding characteristic acid-fast rod-shaped organisms in feces, in cytologic smears, or histopathologic sections of chronic lesions from biopsy and necropsy specimens. The organisms can be seen in DiffQuick stained preparations as nonstaining, rod-shaped bacteria that are acid-fast using Ziehl-Neelson stain. Sometimes nonpathogenic acid-fast organisms can be found in the feces. These are passing bacteria and are always in very low numbers. Ante mortem diagnosis is based upon clinicopathologic findings, radiography, endoscopy, serology and culture or acid-fast stains of biopsy, bone-marrow, and fecal specimens.[88, 109] Numerous acid-fast organisms are present on cytologic examination of lesions caused by *M. avium*, in contrast to *M. bovis*, in which only a few acid-fast organisms are seen. The presence of acid-fast organisms in the stool is not diagnostic for mycobacterial-induced disease.

Unusual lesions associated with mycobacterial infection are chronic necrotizing ulceration of the tongue, and localized granulomatous lesions of the dermis around the nares and retro-orbital tissue primarily found in Amazon parrots. Isolation often yields *M. bovis* and occasionally *M. tuberculosis*. These infections have sometimes been traced back to the owner as the primary source.

Culture of *M. avium* is difficult and often requires human medical laboratories experienced in culturing *Mycobacterium*. Check with your laboratory for specific handling instructions. Newer diagnostic techniques include deoxyribonucleic acid–ribonucleic acid (DNA-RNA)–probe tests and polymerase chain reaction (PCR) tests; the latter can even be used for identifying *Mycobacterium* in tissue samples, particularly in paraffin-embedded sections. Identification of nonculturable mycobacteria from birds with an unspecific postmortem picture using molecular biologic methods revealed a large number of *M. genavense*.[61]

There are several reports of treatment regimens in psittacines. Treatment requires long-term therapy but is feasible in individual pets and is often successful.[99, 105, 109] Therapy is controversial because of resistance of the organism, the zoonotic nature of the disease, and the difficulty of successful treatment in humans.[50] The risk of transmission of *M. avium* to immunocompetent adults appears to be extremely small. However, the risk of transmission to children exists, and the risk to immunocompromised individuals may be quite significant. Therefore, humans undergoing steroid therapy, chemotherapy, or other immunosuppressing medication, and patients with human immunodeficiency virus infection or AIDS should carefully consider the wisdom of keeping a tuberculosis-positive bird.[98] The epidemiologic significance of the avian cases with *M. genavense* will remain obscure until the transmission is elucidated.

Euthanasia is often recommended. Contact birds should be removed from the contaminated area, quarantined for 2 years, and tested at regular intervals.[50] The area should be sterilized.

Nocardia Species

Nocardiosis has traditionally been considered an uncommon disease of the lungs and air sacs in birds. It has been reported in several psittacines[7, 13, 39, 77] and some other avian species.[8, 84]

In a recently reported case in a red-lored Amazon parrot, *Nocardia asteroides* caused a chronic sinusitis with a massive swelling and a gray-green exudate.[7]

Generally, the disease has occurred within the respiratory system, but it has also been observed as abscesses in the pectoral muscle in a macaw.[13] The abscesses or nodules had caseous contents within a capsule.

The diagnosis is based on demonstration and isolation of the *Nocardia* species. It is a branching, filamentous organism with silver- and gram-positive staining characteristics. It is partially acid-fast. The organism is present as a common soil saprophyte, but some forms are considered pathogenic. Routes of infection are thought to be via oral or respiratory routes. Variability in sensitivity and resistance to antibiotics has also been noted.

Erysipelothrix Species

Erysipelothrix rhusiopathiae is a gram-positive, rod-shaped bacterium. It is most common in waterfowl and fish-eating birds during cold weather when food is scarce and energy requirements are high. It is occasionally seen in other avian species including Psittaciformes.[54]

E. rhusiopathiae usually causes peracute death. If clinical signs occur, they may include lethargy, weakness, anorexia, and hyperemia or bruising of the featherless, nonpigmented skin.

The diagnosis is confirmed by isolating the organism.[50]

Listeria Species

Listeria monocytogenes is a gram-positive rod that causes beta-hemolysis on blood agar. *Listeria* species may infect a number of avian species, including Psittaciformes. Canaries appear to be more susceptible to infections than other birds.[50] *Listeria* species were isolated from feces from 11 (4.1%) of 270 pigeons in Germany. Three isolates were identified as *L. monocytogenes*, eight isolates as *L. innocus*, and one isolate as *L. seeligeri*. The last two strains are considered nonpathogenic soil inhabitants, found on plants and in rivers.[110]

Clinical disease is usually associated with sporadic death in a collection. Chronic infections can induce lesions in the heart, liver, and, rarely, the brain. If clinical signs are noted, they are generally associated with CNS signs and include blindness, torticollis, tremor, stupor, and paresis.[74]

At necropsy the presence of serofibrinous pericarditis and myocardial necrosis is considered suggestive of *Listeria*.

The diagnosis requires the isolation of *L. monocytogenes* from affected tissues. Appropriate transport media are necessary for proper shipment of samples.

Bacterial Toxins

Clostridium botulinum is a saprophyte and multiplies in decaying vegetable matter and animal carcasses. Spores of *Clostridium* species, including *C. botulinum*, survive for many years in the environment and germinate under suitable conditions. Botulinum toxins A to G, of which C is most commonly associated with disease in waterfowl and other avian species, are produced in particular circumstances. The toxin is relatively stable and is absorbed following ingestion. Toxin C can be isolated from the intestinal tract of maggots feeding on rotting carcasses. If this preformed toxin is ingested by a susceptible bird, it causes flaccid paralysis typical of *botulism* (limberneck). When these maggots are fed to insectivorous birds, clinical signs of botulism develop. Thus, botulism is not normally considered an infectious disease because it is caused by toxins produced by bacteria rather than by infection with the bacteria. *C. botulinum*, however, can sometimes colonize the ceca and produce toxins that are then absorbed by the host.

Botulism or "Western duck sickness" kills millions of waterfowl each year and there are occasional epizootics involving wading birds. Most major epizootics of botulism type C are associated with prolonged warm weather, an increased amount of stagnant shallow water, alkaline conditions, and accumulated rotting vegetation and dead aquatic vertebrates.[93]

THERAPEUTIC CONSIDERATIONS

The relationship between bacterial identification and the need for antibiotic therapy is a tenuous one. The identification and isolation of potential bacterial pathogens is not a "green light" for the recommendation of antibiotic administration. Rather, it should act as a signal that further consideration is necessary to reach a therapeutic plan if it is deemed necessary.[111]

Environmental evaluation and manipulation coupled with good hygiene, husbandry, and nutrition should always be considered as part of a therapeutic plan to aid in correcting a potential microbial problem.[45]

Disinfection Practices

The veterinary clinician should be vigilant about the disinfection practices of the pet owner, retailer, or aviculturist. A common misconception is that the use of chlorhexidine is effective as a therapeutic agent or disinfectant. In fact, chlorhexidine performs poorly against a number of gram-negative organisms, including *Pseudomonas*.[45] Disinfectants that are effective at recommended concentrations include sodium hypochlorite, quaternary ammonium products, and glutaraldehyde-based products.[43]

References

 1. Anderson NL: Candida/Megabacteria proventriculitis in a lesser sulphur-crested cockatoo (*Cacatua sulphurea sulphurea*). J Assoc Avian Vet 7:197–201, 1993.
 2. Angel R: Selected problems in ostriches and how they are affected by nutrition. Proc AOA Ostrich Med Conf, Las Vegas, 1992.
 3. Aphanius V, Evans RH, Walton BJ: Bacterial microflora of West Coast Peregrine Eyries. Minneapolis, MN, Raptor Research Foundation, 1988, pp 43–47.
 4. Arp LH, Skeeles JK: Bordetellosis (Turkey Coryza). In Calnek BW (ed): Diseases of Poultry, ed 9. Ames IA, Iowa State University Press, 1991, pp 277–288.
 5. Barnes HJ: Spirochetosis. In Calnek BW (ed): Diseases of Poultry, ed 9. Ames IA, Iowa State University Press, 1991, pp 304–319.
 6. Bauck L, Hillyer E, Hoefer H: Rhinitis: Case reports. Proc Assoc Avian Vet, New Orleans 1992, pp 134–139.
 7. Baumgartner R, Hoop RK, Widmer R: Atypical nocardiosis in a red-lored Amazon parrot (*Amazona autumnalis autumnalis*). J Assoc Avian Vet 8:125–127, 1994.
 8. Bergmann A, Schueppel KE, Kronberger H: [Nocardiose in a Turkish Bird] (*Cyanerpes cyaneus*). Proc. Int Symp Dis Zooanimals 10:293–296, 1973.
 9. Berkhoff HA: Ulcerative enteritis (quail disease). In Calnek BW (ed): Diseases of Poultry, ed 9. Ames, IA, Iowa State University Press, 1991, pp 258–263.
10. Berkhoff HA, Vinal AC: Congo red medium to distinguish between invasive and non-invasive *Escherichia coli* pathogenic for poultry. Avian Dis 30:117–121, 1986.
11. Bolin CA: Effects of exogenous iron on *Escherichia coli* septicemia in turkeys. Am J Vet Res 47:1813–1816, 1986.
12. Borst GHA, Buitelaar MN, Poelma FG, et al: Yersinia pseudotuberculosis in birds. Tijdschr Diergeneeskd 102:81–85, 1977.
13. Breadner S: Chronic *Nocardia* infection in a hyacinth macaw. Proc Assoc Avian Vet, Reno, 1994, pp 283–286.
14. Brown R: Sinus, articular and subcutaneous *Mycobacterium tuberculosis* infection in a juvenile red-lored amazon parrot. Proc Assoc Avian Vet, Phoenix, 1990, pp 305–308.
15. Clubb SL, Clubb KJ: Psittacine pediatrics. Miami, FL, Proc Assoc Avian Vet, 1986, pp 317–332.
16. Clubb SL, Homer BL, Pisani L, Head C: Outbreaks of bordetellosis in psittacines and ostriches. Proc Assoc Avian Vet, Reno, 1994, pp 63–68.
17. Degernes LA, Talbot BJ, Mueller LR: Raptor foot care. J Assoc Avian Vet 4:93–95, 1990.
18. De Herdt P, Desmidt M, Haesebrouck F, et al: *Streptococcus bovis* infections in pigeons: The disease under natural and experimental conditions. Proc 8th Conf Avian Dis, Munich, 1992, pp 239–244.
19. De Herdt P, Haesebrouck F, Devriese LA, et al: *Streptococcus bovis* infections in pigeons: Epidemiological studies. Proc 8th Conf Avian Dis, Munich 1992, pp 245–250.
20. De Herdt P, Van Ginneken C, Haesebrouck F, et al: *Escherichia coli* infections in pigeons: Characteristics of the disease and its etiological agent. Proc 9th Conf Avian Dis, Munich, 1994, pp 211–214.
21. Devriese LA, Ceyssens K, Uyttebroek E, Gevaerts D: Streptococcal infections in pigeons. Proc 2nd Eur Symp Avian Med Surg, Utrecht, 1989, pp 113–117.
22. Devriese LA, Uytenbroek E, Dueatelle R, et al: Tracheitis due to *Enterococcus faecalis* infection in canaries. J Assoc Avian Vet 2:113–116, 1990.
23. Devriese LA, Uyttebroek E, Geraert D, et al: *Streptococcus bovis* infections in pigeons. Avian Pathol 19:429–434, 1990.
24. Devriese LA, Haesebrouck F, De Hardt G, et al: *Streptococcus suis* infections in birds. Proc 9th Conf Avian Dis, Munich, 1994, pp 215–218.
25. Dhillon AS: An outbreak of enteritis in a psittacine flock. Proc Assoc Avian Vet, 1988, pp 185–188.
26. Dorrestein GM: Enrofloxacin in pet avian and exotic animal therapy. Proc Baytril Symp Bonn, 1992, pp 63–70.
27. Dorrestein GM: Infectious diseases and their therapy in passeriformes. In Antimicrobial Therapy in Caged and Exotic Pets. Int Symp, Trenton, NJ, Veterinary Learning Systems, 1995, pp 11–27.
28. Dorrestein GM: Unpublished data, 1995b.
29. Dorrestein GM, de Boer AM, Buitelaar MN, Schaftenaar W: The History of a Salmonella Problem in a Zoo. Proc 9th DVG Conf Avian Dis, Munich, 1994, pp 219–232.
30. Dorrestein GM, Buitelaar MN: Results of bacteriological examination. Unpublished data, 1995.
31. Dorrestein GM, Buitelaar MN, van der Hage MH, Zwart P: Evaluation of a bacteriological and mycological examination of psittacine birds. Avian Dis 29:951–962, 1985.
32. Dorrestein GM, van der Hage MH: Aviculture and veterinary problems in lovebirds. Proc Annual Meeting Assoc Avian Vet, Oahu, HI, 1987, pp 243–262.
33. Dorrestein GM, van der Hage MH: Adenovirus inclusion body hepatitis: A new pigeon disease? Proc 8th Symp Avian Dis, Munich, 1992, pp 2–14.
34. Dorrestein GM, van der Hage MH, Cornelissen JL: Campylobacter infections in cage birds—clinical, pathological and bacteriological aspects. Assoc Avian Vet Newsletter 5:89, 1984.
35. Drew ML, Ramsay E: Dermatitis associated with *Mycobacterium* spp. in a blue-fronted amazon parrot. Proc Assoc Avian Vet, Chicago, 1991, pp 252–254.
36. Drew ML, Joyner K, Lobingler R: Laboratory reference intervals for a group of captive thick-billed parrots (*Rhynchopsitta pachyrhyncha*). J Assoc Avian Vet 7:35–38, 1993.
37. Drewes LA, Flammer K: Clinical microbiology. In Harrison GJ, Harrison LR (eds): Clinical Avian Medicine and Surgery. Philadelphia, WB Saunders, 1986, pp 157–171.
38. DuPont HL: Enteropathogens. In Lederberg J (ed): Encyclopedia of Microbiology, vol 2. San Diego, Academic Press, vol 2, 1992, pp 63–68.
39. Ehrsam H, and Hauser B: [Nocardiose in a blue-winged king-parrot (*Alisterus amboinensis hypohonius*)]. Schweiz Archiv Tierheilk, 121:195–200, 1979.

40. Ficken MD: Necrotic enteritis. In Calnek BW (ed): Diseases of Poultry, ed 9. Ames, IA, Iowa State University Press. 1991, pp 264–267.

41. Filippich LJ, Parker MG: Megabacteria and proventricular/ventricular disease in psittacines and passerines. Proc Assoc Avian Vet, Reno, 1994, pp 287–293.

42. Filippich LJ, Perry RA: Drug trials against megabacteria in budgerigars (*Melopsittacus undulatus*). Aust Vet Pract 23:184–189, 1993.

43. Flammer K: Antimicrobial therapy. In Ritchie BW, Harrison GJ, Harrison LR (eds): Avian Medicine: Principles and Application. Lake Worth, FL, Winger Publishers, 1994, pp 434–456.

44. Flammer K, Drewes LA: Species-related differences in the incidence of gram-negative bacteria isolated from the cloaca of clinically normal psittacine birds. Avian Dis 32:79–83, 1988.

45. Fudge AM, Reavill DR, Rosskopf WJ: Clinical aspects of avian Pseudomonas infections: A retrospective study. Proc Assoc Avian Vet, New Orleans, 1992, pp 141–155.

46. Fung DYC: Foodborne illness. In Lederberg J (ed): Encyclopedia of Microbiology, vol 2. San Diego, Academic Press, 1992, pp 209–218.

47. Gaskin JM: Microbiologic techniques in avian medicine. In Jacobson ER, Kollias GV (eds): Exotic Animals. New York, Churchill Livingston, 1988, pp 159–176.

48. Gerlach H: [Diagnosis of Pseudotuberculosis in live birds]. Proc 1st Conf Avian Dis, Munich, 1979, pp 96–101.

49. Gerlach H: Resistance of megabacteria to treatment. J Assoc Avian Vet 4:205, 1990.

50. Gerlach H: Bacteria. In Ritchie BW, Harrison GJ, Harrison LR (eds): Avian Medicine: Principles and Application. Lake Worth, Winger Publishers, 1994, pp 948–983.

51. Gill J: Diseases of lorikeet. In Sindel S (ed): Australian Lorikeets. Chipping Norton, Surrey Beatty and Sons 1987, pp 23–27.

52. Goronczy P, Korbel R, Gerlach H, et al: A survey of the conjunctival flora of various clinically normal bird species. Proc 9th Conf Avian Dis, Munich, 1994, pp 202–210.

53. Gross WB: Colibacillosis. In Calnek BW (ed): Diseases of Poultry, ed 9. Ames, IA, Iowa State University Press, 1991, pp 138–144.

54. Gylstorff I: In Gylstorff I, Grim F (eds): Vogelkrankheiten. Stuttgard, Verlag Eugen Ulmer, 1987, p 316.

55. Harrison G: Bacteria in blood sample. IME, J Assoc Avian Vet 7:11, 1993.

56. Henderson GM, Gulland FM, Hawkley CM: Haematological findings in budgerigars with megabacterium and trichomonas infections associated with "going light." Vet Rec 123:492–494, 1988.

57. van Herck H, Duyser T, Zwart P, et al: A bacterial Proventriculitis in canaries (Serinus canaria). Avian Pathol 13:561–572, 1984.

58. Hicks KD: Ostrich pediatrics. Semin Avian Exotic Pet Med 2:136–141, 1993.

59. Hillyer EV, Quesenberry KE, Baer K: Basic avian dermatology. Proc Ann Conf Assoc Avian Vet, 1989, pp 101–121.

60. Hinz K-H, Ryll M, Glünder G: [*Riemerella anatipestifer*-like bacteria from pigeons with Respiratory Disease.] Proc 8th Conf Avian Dis, Munich, 1994, pp 245–248.

61. Hoop RK, Ossent P, Pfytter G: *Mycobacterium genavense*: A new cause of mycobacteriosis in pet birds? Proc 3th Eur Assoc Avian Vet Meeting, Jerusalem, 1995, pp 1–4.

62. Hüchzermeyer FW: Bacterial infection. In Ostrich Diseases. Onderstepoort, Agricultural Res Counsil, 1994, pp 15–25.

63. Hüchzermeyer FW, Henton MM, Keffen RH: High mortality associated with megabacteriosis of proventriculus and gizzard in ostrich chicks. Vet Rec 133:143–144, 1993.

64. Jacobson ER: Blood collection techniques in reptiles: Laboratory investigation. Pathologic evaluations. In Curr Ther Zoo Wild Animal Med, 3 Philadelphia, WB Saunders, 1993, 147–151.

65. Joseph V: Management and selected medical topics of raptors. Proc 100th Annual California Veterinary Medical Association Scientific Seminar, Anaheim CA, 1988, pp 411–423.

66. Joseph V: Raptor pediatrics. Semin Avian Exotic Pet Med 2:142–151, 1993.

67. Joyner KL: Practical approaches to diagnostics in avian medicine. Proc Assoc Avian Med Phoenix, 1990, pp 394–403.

68. Joyner KL: The use of gram stain results in avian medicine. Proc Assoc Avian Vet, Chicago, 1991, pp 78–97.

69. Joyner K, Berger de N, Lopez EH, et al: Health parameters of wild psittacines in Guatamala: A preliminary report. Proc Assoc Avian Vet, New Orleans, 1992, pp 287–303.

70. Joyner K, Swanson J: The use of a lactobacillus product in a psittacine hand-feeding diet: Its effect on normal aerobic microflora, early weight gain, and health. Proc Assoc Avian Vet, 1988, pp 127–137.

71. Kiessling D: [On the occurrence of bacterial L-forms in pigeons.] Proc 7th Conf Avian Dis, Munich, 1990, pp 159–170.

72. Kollias GV, Heard DJ, Martin H, Coburn GG: Principles, Techniques and Clinical Use of Blood Culture in Birds. Proc. 1st Int Conf Zool Avian Med, Oahu, HI, 1987, pp 167–168.

73. Korbel R: [Epizoology, clinic, and therapy of *Pasteurella multocida* in bird patients after cat bites]. Tierärzl Prax 18:365–376, 1990.

74. Korbel R: Ocular manifestations of systemic diseases in birds. Proc Eur Assoc Avian Vet, Vienna, 1991, pp 157–167.

75. Lane R: Use of gram's stain for bacterial screening. J Assoc Avian Vet 4:214–217, 1990.

76. Levine BS: Reviewing the integumentary syndromes common to captive birds. Vet Med 82:1155–1165, 1987.

77. Long P, Choi G, Silberman M: Nocardiosis in two Pesquet's parrots (*Psittrichas fulgides*). Avian Dis 27:855–859, 1983.

78. Lublin A, Mechani S, Horowitz, et al: A paralytic-like disease of the ostrich (*Struthio camelus masaicus*) associated with *Clostridium chauvoei* infection. Vet Rec 132:273–275, 1993.

79. McDonald SE: A selection of disease syndromes of psittacine birds. Proc 1st Conf Eur Assoc Avian Vet, Vienna, 1991, pp 46–73.

80. Mehmke U: Studies of the aerobic bacterial flora on the nesting material of singing birds. Proc 7th Conf Avian Dis, Munich, 1990, pp 309–320.

81. Needham JR: Bacterial flora of birds of prey. Recent Advances in the Study of Raptor Diseases. Keighley, England, Chiron Publications, 1980, pp 3–9.

82. Olsen GH: A review of some causes of death of avian embryos. Proc Assoc Avian Vet, Phoenix, 1990, pp 106–111.

83. Orosz SE, Altekruse S: *Salmonella enteritidis* infection in two species of psittaciformes. IME J Assoc Avian Vet 6:84, 1992.

84. Parnell MJ, Hubbard GB, Fletcher KC, Schmidt RE: Nocardia asteroides infection in a purple throated sunbird (*Nectarinia sperapa*). Vet Pathol 20:497–500, 1983.

85. Parrot T: Pododermatitis in three amazon parrots and treatment with L-Thyroxine. Proc Assoc Avian Vet, Chicago, 1991, pp 263–264.

86. Parsonnet J: Gastrointestinal microbiology. In Lederberg J (ed): Encyclopedia of Microbiology, vol 2. San Diego, Academic Press, 1992, pp 245–258.

87. Perelman B, Greiff M, Kuttin ES, Rogol M: Campylobacteriosis in ostriches. Isr J Vet Med 47:116–119, 1992.

88. Pieper K, Krautwald-Junghanns M-E, Kostka V: The diagnosis of tuberculosis in pet birds with the help of radiology—A contribution for the practitioner. Proc Eur Assoc Avian Vet, Vienna, 1991, pp 186–190.

89. Poppe C, Gyles CL: Relation of plasmids to virulence and other properties of salmonellae from avian sources. Avian Dis 31:844–854, 1987.

90. Rae MA, Rosskopf WJ: Mycobacteriosis in passerines. Proc Assoc Avian Vet, New Orleans 1992, pp 234–243.

91. Reavill DR, Schmidt RE, Fudge AM: Avian skin and feather disorders: A retrospective study. Proc Ann Conf Assoc Avian Vet, 1990, pp 248–255.

92. Redig PT: Health management of raptors trained for falconry. Proc Assoc Avian Vet, New Orleans, 1992, pp 258–264.

93. Reece RL: Avian pathogens: Their biology and methods of spread. In JE Cooper (ed): Disease and Threatened Birds. Cambridge, ICBP Technical Publication No 10, 1989, 1–23.

94. Remington KH: Atypical mycobacteriosis in a mixed collection of caged birds. Proc Assoc Avian Vet, Nashville, 1993, pp 256–262.

95. Richter T, Gerlach H: The bacterial flora of the nasal mucosa of birds of prey. Recent Advances in the Study of Raptor Diseases. Keighley, England, Chiron Publications, 1980, pp 11–14.

96. Rosskopf WJ, Woerpel RW: Treatment of feather folliculitis in a lovebird. Mod Vet Pract 64:923–924, 1983.

97. Rosskopf WJ, Woerpel RW: Psittacine conditions and syndromes. Proc Assoc Avian Vet, Phoenix, 1990, pp 432–459.

98. Rosskopf WJ, Woerpel RW (eds): Pet Avian Medicine. Vet Clin North Am Small Anim Pract 21:1223, 1991.

99. Rosskopf WJ, Woerpel RW, Asterino R: Successful treatment of avian tuberculosis in pet psittacines. Proc Assoc Avian Vet, Chicago 1991, pp 238–251.

100. Rupiper DJ: Hemorrhagic enteritis in a group of great-billed parrots (*Tanygnathus megalorynchos*). J Assoc Avian Vet 7:209–211, 1993.

101. Sagartz JE, Swayne DE, Eaton KA, et al: Necrotizing typhlocolitis associated with a spirochete in rheas (*Rhea americana*) Avian Dis 36:282–289, 1992.

102. Scanlan CM, Graham DL: Characterization of a gram-positive bacterium from the proventriculus of budgerigars (Melopsittacus undulatus). Avian Dis 34:779–786, 1990.

103. Smit JA: Necrotic enteritis and colitis in ratite birds. Proc 40th West Poult Dis Conf, 1991, pp 258–260.

104. Spenser EL: Common infectious diseases of psittacine birds seen in practice. Vet Clin North Am Small Anim Pract 21:1213–1230, 1991.

105. Stauber EH: Treatment of psittacine pet birds with avian mycobacteriosis—case reports. Proc 8th Conf Avian Dis, Munich, 1992, pp 231–238.

106. Tully TN Jr, Carter JD: Bilateral supraorbital abscesses associated with sinusitis in an orange-winged amazon parrot (*Amazona amazonica*). J Assoc Avian Vet 7:157–158, 1993.

107. Tully TN Jr, Harrison GJ: Pneumonology. In Ritchie BW, Harrison GJ, Harrison LR (eds): Avian Medicine: Principles and Application. Lake Worth, Winger Publishers, 1994, pp 556–581.

108. Uyttebroek E, Devriese LA, Gevaert D, et al: Protective effects of different salmonella vaccines in experimentally infected pigeons. Proc 7th Conf Avian Dis, Munich, 1990, pp 154–158.

109. Van Der Heyden N: Update on avian mycobacteriosis. Proc Assoc Avian Vet, Reno, 1994, pp 53–61.

110. Weber A, Potel J, Schäfer-Schmidt R: [Pigeons as Reservoir and Carrier of *Listeria*]. Proc 9th Conf Avian Dis, Munich, 1994, pp 241–244.

111. Worell AB: Pediatric bacterial diseases. Semin Avian Exotic Pet Med 2:116–124, 1993.

David N. Phalen

19

Viruses

Viral diseases of cage birds are common, often causing devastating losses of beloved pets and valued breeding stock. Because many of these viruses have a complex biology, their diagnosis and control is difficult. In addition, considerable substantiated and unsubstantiated information about these diseases has been widely disseminated in the scientific and lay literature. As a result, a tremendous amount of responsibility is placed on practitioners to recommend appropriate disease prevention strategies and minimize the consequences of disease outbreaks when they occur. The following chapter is designed to highlight the known material about documented viral diseases of cage birds and to discuss syndromes suspected to be caused by infectious agents.

DISEASE PREVENTION

The principles of disease prevention in cage birds are the same as those used in other traditional species:

1. Advanced planning on the number and species of animals to be acquired
2. Acquisition of stock from a reputable source with a known health history
3. Appropriate quarantine procedures
4. Pre- or post-purchase examinations with judicious use of testing
5. Proper management and nutrition
6. Good sanitation
7. Common sense

The first most important concept in disease prevention for the aviculturalist or pet owner is collection design. Ideally before birds are actually ac-

quired, some thought should be put into the pros and cons of keeping different species of birds. A basic rule that is rarely followed is to keep the collection as simple as possible. Many viral diseases are subclinical in some parrots but cause disease in others. This is particularly common when many parrot species from different geographic regions are combined. Recognition that parrots such as lovebirds (*Agapornis* species), cockatiels (*Nymphicus hollandicus*), budgerigars (*Melopsittacus undulatus*), and some conures have a high incidence of certain viral diseases is also important. An ideal aviary from a disease prevention perspective focuses on one species or group of similar species. Likewise, breeders or owners of expensive birds (e.g., cockatoos) should refrain from acquiring the less valuable high-risk birds, (e.g., budgerigars and lovebirds).

Often viral disease problems can be directly related to birds purchased on impulse or to the rapid acquisition of birds from multiple sources. It is very common for birds to be purchased at bird shows and sales, where the opportunity for disease transmission is highest. Birds are also commonly purchased from breeders or dealers before they are seen. Ideally, all new birds should come directly from reputable breeders. People in the market for a new bird should not be afraid to ask for references or to seek the endorsement of the aviculturalist's veterinarian. When possible, the breeder's facilities should be seen before a bird is purchased. A health certificate by the breeder's veterinarian and a reasonable guarantee of health by the breeder are other factors that suggest that the bird to be purchased is coming from a good source.

Quarantine procedures vary significantly with the

resources of the client. In large aviaries, a separate facility and staff may be designated to house and maintain quarantined birds. In a home, the new bird may be kept in a separate room and worked with only after the other birds are cared for. Separate feeding dishes and utensils should be maintained for the quarantined birds. In addition, even in private homes, foot baths or disposable shoe covers and separate clothing can be used to prevent movement of viruses from the quarantine area to other birds. Quarantine duration is a difficult subject. It needs to be long enough to be effective, but not so long that the client becomes frustrated and decides to abandon the process completely. A good compromise is 60 or 90 days, with the understanding that some diseases, (e.g., wasting disease and internal papillomatosis) may take years to become clinically apparent.

The veterinary examination is a critical part of disease prevention and should be done before or as soon as possible after a bird is purchased. In addition to the physical examination, each veterinarian has a preferred set of ancillary tests. A complete blood count, serum chemistry tests, Gram stains, and radiographs rarely identify a specific viral problem, but do give important insights into the general health of the bird. Additional diagnostic assays depend on the species of bird being examined and the nature of the home it will be entering. No matter how many tests are run, it must always be remembered that testing is not now and never will be the end-all to the control of viral diseases. No matter how good a test is, false positives and false negatives occur in a percentage of all samples.

The proper husbandry and diet for each species vary, but some general points need to be considered for all birds. Crowding and inadequate ventilation maximize disease transmission. Breeding multiple pairs in large flights is more conducive to disease transmission than individual cage breeding. Stress management is also important, and factors such as cage size, perch placement, nest box construction, visual barriers, climate control, and other species-specific considerations can all play an important role in minimizing stress.

Sanitation is another topic that is widely discussed among bird owners. For viral pathogens, excluding viruses is preferable to killing them with disinfectants. However, dilution effects can help reduce disease problems if the virus is there already.

Adequate spacing between cages and regular cleaning of facilities reduce virus concentrations. The importance of cleaning cannot be overemphasized. No matter what the virus or bacterial agent of concern, most of it is found in droppings, feather dander, and debris associated with captive birds. Routine removal of this material may be instrumental in reducing pathogen concentrations to below infective doses. Disinfection can only occur after the room or equipment to be disinfected is clean. Hand-feeding tools and seed and water cups are best disinfected after every use. Boiling them and soaking them in a disinfectant are both acceptable alternatives. Likewise, running them through a dishwasher, although not truly a sterilization process, may be more than adequate. Different viruses are susceptible to different disinfectants. Enveloped viruses are the most easily inactivated and are susceptible to chlorhexidine and quaternary ammonia products.[1] Nonenveloped viruses require phenolic compounds and sodium hypochloride (bleach), or stabilized chlorine dioxide, for inactivation, and even these may not always be adequate.[1-5]

Disinfection of entire facilities, especially those that contain large quantities of wood, may be very difficult. In the poultry industry, formaldehyde gas has been found to be an effective disinfectant. It is also a very dangerous agent and should be used only by qualified professionals. Local poultry extension agents should be contacted for more information on formaldehyde disinfection.

Common sense and animal ownership have never been synonymous, regardless of the species being discussed. Avian veterinarians need to spend as much time as possible educating their clients and the public at large about how they should go about protecting their animals. These efforts are practice builders and go a long way toward protecting our clients' valued animals.

DIAGNOSTIC PROCEDURES

Many diagnostic techniques are available for detecting virus infections in live birds and identifying viruses in tissues of necropsy specimens. Each of these techniques has its appropriate applications and limitations. Careful consideration of the biology of each virus and the limitations of available diagnostic tests is required for the practitioner to develop appropriate disease prevention programs and collect appropriate diagnostic samples.

Traditionally, serology has proved a useful tool in the diagnosis of viral infections. A positive antibody titer indicates that a bird has been or is currently infected with the virus for which the serum was assayed. Unfortunately, the presence or absence of antibodies to a specific virus does not always correlate with the presence or absence of virus shedding. Thus, a bird may be seropositive, yet may not be shedding virus. Likewise, a bird may be actively shedding virus, but because it is in the early stages of virus infection it may not have developed antibodies.

Several assays are available to detect antibody. Virus neutralization is a useful technique in that it can be used for serum from all species and it detects both immunoglobulins IgG and IgM. The limitation of a virus neutralization assay is that it often takes several days to run. A more rapid assay is the agar gel immunodiffusion assay. This assay is somewhat cumbersome and is less sensitive than the virus neutralization assay; therefore, it is not routinely used. Complement fixation assays are also used as a rapid means of detecting serum antibody. In birds, however, complement fixation tests may only detect IgG,[6] and occasionally anticomplementary substances in the serum invalidate the results. In addition, spurious results can be obtained if these assays are not carefully developed.[7] Another commonly used serologic assay is the enzyme-linked immunoassay or ELISA. This is a rapid and sensitive assay, but in general is prone to false positive results. Another major disadvantage to the ELISA is that it is dependent on the specificity of a secondary antibody. When an ELISA is going to be used for sera from multiple species of birds, the test needs to be validated for each species before the results can be adequately interpreted.

Genetic probes have been developed for several viruses and undoubtably will be available for others in the near future. In the live bird, deoxyribonucleic acid (DNA) or ribonucleic acid (RNA) is extracted from appropriate samples and the virus DNA or RNA, if present, is amplified to a detectable amount by a process called the *polymerase chain reaction* or PCR. PCR is an extremely sensitive technique and in some situations can detect a single virion. This degree of sensitivity is not always an advantage, because contamination of a sample, either in the field or in the laboratory, causes a false positive result. Again, the biology of the virus must be considered in interpreting the results of a PCR assay. If a bird is being assayed for virus shedding, but sheds virus only intermittently, a single negative PCR result is meaningless.

PCR can also be used to identify viruses in tissues. In some instances, however, the presence of a virus in the tissues does not mean conclusively that the virus was the cause of the bird's death. Therefore, PCR is best used in conjunction with histopathology examination, not independently. Genetic probes can also be used for in situ detection of virus. The routine use of these probes is limited to only a few viruses. Presently, diagnosis of these viral diseases in most situations can be done by histopathology examination, making their use unnecessary in most cases. In the future, development of probes for other viruses more difficult to detect by traditional light microscopy will greatly aid the pathologist.

Histopathology is still an extremely important diagnostic tool. However, the pathologist is at the mercy of the veterinarian. If the whole bird or a complete set of tissues is not submitted, critical diagnostic lesions will be missed. Many viral diseases leave few gross lesions yet affect many organs, and thus submitting a single piece of liver, kidney, or intestine often is a wasted effort. If the entire bird is submitted for necropsy, the pathologist has many options including electron microscopy, fluorescent antibody staining, and virus isolation.

Virus isolation is another time-honored method for virus diagnosis. For several virus diseases of birds, this is the only method of confirming a virus infection, and isolation may be necessary to determine the strain of the virus involved. Virus isolation, however, has many difficulties. Not all viruses can be recovered by routine methods. It is an expensive and time-consuming process, sometimes taking several weeks before the virus can be isolated and identified. Appropriately handled fresh tissues are required.

CIRCOVIRUSES

Clinical Presentations

A summary of clinical characteristics in common avian species is shown in Table 19–1.

T a b l e 1 9 – 1

CIRCOVIRUSES: CLINICAL PRESENTATIONS

Signs	Species Affected	Incidence
Feather dysplasia	Many parrot species	Common
Secondary *Aspergillus* and other infectious diseases	Juvenile African grey parrots and other parrot species	Uncommon
Polyomavirus in adult birds	Eclectus parrots	Common
	Other parrots	Uncommon
		Rare
Nestling mortality with prominence of the gall bladder	Canaries	Unknown

Psittacine Beak and Feather Disease

Psittacine beak and feather disease virus (PBFDV) infection has been documented in 42 parrot species[8] and probably is capable of infecting and causing disease in many others. Historically, cockatoos,[9–12] eclectus parrots *(Eclectus roratus)*,[13, 14] lovebirds,[9, 14, 15] budgerigars,[16, 17] and African grey parrots *(Psittacus erithacus)*[13, 14, 18, 19] have experienced a high incidence of this disease. PBFD has been recognized in several other Australian and southeast Asian parrots; a few African and southwest Asian parrots;[8] and in macaws,[14, 20] Amazon parrots,[14, 21] and a pionus parrot.[22]

There is some variation in the clinical presentation of this disease, which is in part because of the species affected, the age at which infection occurs, and other factors that are yet to be defined. In the cockatoo, PBFD occurs acutely in nestling and fledgling birds and as a chronic progressive disease in older birds.[9–12, 16, 23] The large majority of birds with the chronic form of PBFD first develop lesions between 6 months and 3 years of age.[24] Less often, birds up to 20 years old have presented with PDFD.[25] The first signs of PBFD are subtle. A lack of powder on the beak may be the first indication that powder down feathers are diseased (Fig. 19–1). Some birds present with a history of a delayed moult. Close inspection of these birds generally reveals at least a few dysplastic feathers. Both down and contour feathers are affected, but the disease may predominate in one or the other. Initially, diseased feathers are widely scattered and are associated with the pattern of moult. As the disease advances, all feather tracts become involved, generally in a somewhat symmetrical fashion (Fig. 19–2). In advanced cases, only down feathers, a few scattered contour feathers, or no feathers at all may remain.[8–11, 17, 22]

Affected feathers show varying degrees of dysplasia. Hyperkeratosis of the feather sheath is common, resulting in sheath thickening and retention. Growing feathers are short and may be pinched off either at their proximal ends or near their base (clubbing) (Fig. 19–3). Thinning of the rachis and recent and previous hemorrhage within the feather shaft are common. In some feathers there is so much disruption of feather growth that the sheath contains only a disorganized mass of keratin. Mildly affected feathers may show bowing, have transverse dystrophic lines, and fracture at any location along their length.[10, 11, 26]

Beak lesions are common in the sulphur-crested *(Cacatua galerita)*, Major Mitchell's *(C. leadbeateri)*, Moluccan *(C. moluccensis)* and umbrella cockatoos *(C. alba)*; little corella *(C. sanguinea)*; and galahs *(Eolophus roseicapillus)*. They are less frequent or entirely absent in other species.[10, 11, 13, 18] These lesions may occur at any stage of the disease,

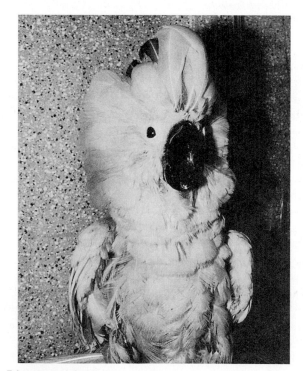

F i g u r e 1 9 – 1

Moluccan cockatoo with early lesions of psittacine beak and feather disease. The absence of powder on the beak of this bird is a result of virus-induced damage to the powder down feathers.

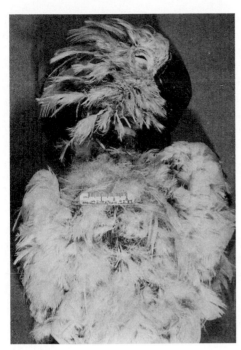

Figure 19-2

Advanced psittacine beak and feather disease in a Moluccan cockatoo. Dysplastic feathers are present in all feather tracts. (Photograph kindly provided by Dr. David Graham.)

but are most commonly seen in birds with advanced disease. Early changes in the beak are the result of hyperkeratosis of its superficial layer. These changes cause beak elongation and overgrowth (see Fig. 19–3). Longitudinal fissures develop subsequently. In the terminal stages of the disease the distal portion of the beak fractures, leaving underlying necrotic debris and bone. Necrosis of the palatine mucosa causes it to separate from the beak. The resulting space fills with caseous material. Beneath the caseous material is bone. These lesions are painful and birds may become partially or completely anorectic. Secondary infections of the beak and oral cavity are common. A pathologic process similar to the one occurring in the beak may also affect the nails of the feet. These lesions, however, are not generally a significant manifestation of PBFD.[9–11, 17, 22]

If beak lesions are not severe, birds can live with the PBFDV for many years. However, the vast majority of these birds die, either from their primary lesions or from secondary infectious diseases, within 6 to 12 months after the onset of the signs.[22]

Mounting evidence suggests that birds with PBFD have significant alterations in their immune function.[18, 22, 26, 27] As a result, infection from opportunistic pathogens including yeasts and other fungi, gram-positive and gram-negative bacteria, cryptosporidia, and avian polyomavirus, are common complications and often terminal manifestations of PBFD.[22]

Acute PBFD in nestling cockatoos may begin with nonspecific signs such as depression and regurgitation.[16, 23, 28, 29] Feather lesions develop rapidly and are extensive.[16, 23, 28, 29] These lesions may be identical to those seen in the chronic form of PBFD; more often, annular constricting bands near the base of the feather develop simultaneously in numerous feathers. These feathers break off easily and may bleed. They also tend to be loose in the follicles and are easily pulled out. An understated feature of this disease is the discomfort of the nestling. The damaged feathers are painful, and the birds do not want to be handled. Like the chronic form of PBFD, an early sign of infection is reduced powder on the beak. This sign is not specific, however, because young cockatoos do not always groom themselves as intensively as the adults and routinely have less powder on their beaks. Advanced beak lesions rarely have time to develop because the acute dis-

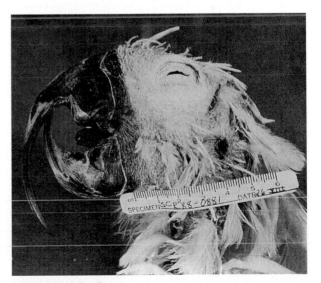

Figure 19-3

Advanced psittacine beak and feather disease in a sulfur-crested cockatoo. Note the prominent overgrowth of both the rhinotheca and gnathotheca and characteristic feather dysplasia. (Photograph kindly provided by Dr. David Graham.)

ease is often rapidly fatal. As with the older birds, however, the rate of disease progression can vary. Infection studies suggest that rapidly fatal disease is likely to occur in umbrella and sulphur-crested cockatoos, whereas a more chronic form of the disease can be expected in galahs.[23, 28, 29]

Acute PBFD also occurs in juvenile African grey parrots.[19, 29] In an experimentally infected bird, non-specific systemic signs preceded feather lesions.[29] Dystrophic feathers identical to those seen in cocka-toos also occur in African grey parrots. In addition, newly formed contour feathers that would normally be gray are sometimes red.[19] Red coloration of con-tour feathers, however, is not specific for PBFD. Not all African grey parrots with PBFD have demon-strable feather lesions. Schmidt reports that many juvenile African grey parrots dying with *Aspergillus* infections and systemic bacterial diseases also have beak and feather virus inclusions in their bursa.[18] This observation suggests that alterations of the im-mune system by the virus may predispose these birds to other diseases. Another disease linked to the PBFDV in African grey parrots is a progressive and fatal nonresponsive anemia.[13] Similar changes have also been observed in African grey parrots infected with a reovirus. Therefore, the pathogene-sis of this anemia remains to be determined.

In some populations of lovebirds, PBFD is com-mon.[14] Feather changes in lovebirds are less charac-teristic than in other species, and disease occurs most often in young adult birds. These birds appear unthrifty. They may shed feathers and not regrow them, or they may have a delayed molt. Dystrophic feathers may predominate, may be scattered, or may be absent entirely. Some of these birds survive for many months or years, and it is suggested that a small percentage spontaneously eliminate the vi-rus.[8]

PBFDV is enzootic in some budgerigar breeding facilities,[30] but it is not as widely disseminated as it is in the lovebird.[14] Most affected birds are fledg-lings. In the author's experience, diffuse feather changes similar to those seen in cockatoos are un-common. Instead, many of these birds have normal feathering except for the complete absence of pri-maries and secondaries. The owners refer to these birds as *runners* or *creepers,* and this form of the disease has been called *French moult*. These lesions are not specific for beak and feather disease, and identical feather abnormalities are caused by avian

polyomavirus infections. PBFDV and polyomavirus infections in budgerigars can also occur concur-rently.

PBFD in the eclectus parrot is very similar to that in the lovebird. Dystrophic feathers may or may not be present, but feather quality of clinically affected birds is poor. In the author's experience, fatal poly-omavirus infections in adult eclectus parrots have been correlated with concurrent PBFDV infections.

PBFDV infection in New World parrots is a recent discovery. Both subclinical[14] and clinical infec-tions[20, 21] have been documented. Clinically affected birds have feather lesions essentially identical to those of cockatoos.[20, 21] Like the cockatoos, disease has been seen in both adult and nestling birds. Resolution of the clinical signs has been docu-mented in some of these birds.[22]

Biology

The PBFDV is a nonenveloped, 14 to 17 nm, single-stranded, DNA virus.[31] It is a naturally occurring virus of wild Australian parrots where it causes disease in a high percentage of yearling cockatoos of several species.[9, 10, 32, 33] The exact route of trans-mission is not known, but has been postulated to be oral, via inhalation, or possibly by movement across the bursal follicular epithelium.[31, 34] Large quantities of the virus are shed in the feces[35] and feather dander.[34, 35] In addition, virus has been iden-tified in crop contents, suggesting that it can be transmitted to the offspring of infected birds by means of regurgitant feeding.[34] Vertical transmission has been postulated, because incubator-hatched chicks have developed disease.[22] Whether this was from viral incorporation into the egg, virus contami-nation of the shell, or some other environmental sources is not known. The role that vertical trans-mission plays in the dissemination of beak and feather infection remains uncertain. Susceptibility to infection may also be age-related. In budgerigars, experimental infection studies suggest that birds younger than 7 days of age are more susceptible to disease.[16] Similarly, adult galahs have been shown to be refractory to infection through the oral route.[23]

Virus replication occurs in a wide range of tis-sues, including the thymus, bursa of Fabricius, crop, esophagus, intestine, skin, and feathers.[27] Virus has also been identified in circulating leukocytes.[36]

Feather dysplasia results from virus-induced necrosis and disruption of the epidermal collar, intermediate and basal epidermis, and the feather pulp, and thrombosis and hemorrhage within the feather pulp.[10, 11] Damage to the germinal epithelium of the beak is similar, resulting in the observed gross changes. Necrosis of the bursa, thymus, and possibly circulating leukocytes may lead to immune suppression and secondary diseases.[22, 27]

Incubation periods may be as short as 3 to 4 weeks in nestling birds.[16, 23, 29] Prolonged incubation periods of months and possibly even years are more common. Virus can be detected in the blood before clinical signs are observed. In one report, virus could be detected in an experimentally infected bird 2 days after infection.[25] In the author's clinical experience, however, longer periods are required for naturally infected birds to become viremic.

The outcome of infection depends on the species infected and the individual bird. Transient viremias without the development of clinical signs appears to occur commonly.[14, 25] Virus elimination may depend on the timely development of circulating antiviral antibody.[35, 37] Most infections resulting in clinical disease are fatal. Uncommonly, clinical signs are only transient.

Diagnosis

In classic PBFD, clinical signs strongly support the diagnosis. In other cases, clinical signs may be absent or nonspecific. In both clinical and subclinical cases, a PCR-based diagnostic assay using whole blood has revolutionized the diagnosis of this disease.[14, 36] This assay directly detects viral DNA, and in carefully controlled studies it was found to be highly sensitive and specific.[14] In the field, careful sample handling is required to prevent both false positive and false negative results. Infected birds shed massive amounts of this virus, especially in feather dander, and contamination of the air and the environment readily occurs. Because of the sensitivity of this assay, contamination with even a single infected cell produces a false positive result. False-negative results may occur if the sample submitted contains excess heparin. A dilution of 0.01 of heparin (1:1000 U/ml) in 0.49 ml of blood is the recommended sampling procedure.[14]

Birds with clinical signs of PBFD that have posi-

tive PCR test results have a guarded prognosis. Uncommonly, some live many years with the disease. Uncommonly to rarely, clinical signs resolve and birds become virus-negative. If a bird has clinical signs and a negative result on the assay, it has been suggested that virus concentrations may either be so high as to interfere with the assay, or that birds are so leukopenic that little or no virus is present in the blood.[14] A third possibility is that the sample was improperly collected. Histopathologic examination of biopsies from PBFD birds can be used to confirm the clinical diagnosis.[38] Clinically normal birds with a positive test result represent birds in the early stages of infection, birds with a transient subclinical infection, or a sample that was contaminated at the time of collection. It has been recommended that all clinically normal birds with positive test results be retested in 90 days.[14]

Before the PCR-based assay was developed, diagnosis of PBFD was made by histopathologic examination of plucked growing feathers or biopsies of feathers and feather follicles.[10, 11, 38] Characteristic changes in the growing feather and its follicle and the presence of virus-induced intranuclear and intracytoplasmic inclusion bodies are considered diagnostic.[9–11, 26] Similar inclusion bodies are irregularly found in other tissues.[27] In the African grey and eclectus parrots, feather lesions may not be present.[13, 18, 30] In birds without feather lesions, PBFD is often not suspected by the clinician. Because inclusion bodies may only be found in the bursa, submission of a complete set of tissues is necessary for an accurate diagnosis. Immunohistochemical stains[39] and in situ hybridization[40] have been employed to increase the sensitivity and specificity of the histopathology examination. Although these are valuable tools for the study of PBFD, they are rarely necessary for routine diagnostic specimens.

Control

With the advent of a sensitive and specific diagnostic assay for PBFD, control of this disease has been greatly simplified. All new birds should be tested for the virus at the time of purchase. As an alternative, testing can be delayed a month so that if the bird was recently exposed it will have time to develop the viremic state. The most conservative method is to test initially after purchase and repeat the test in 30 days. Testing of new birds is of no avail unless all other birds in the aviary are also tested. Although expensive, testing all birds in valuable collections of at-risk species can avert future catastrophic losses. Birds with a positive test result should be removed immediately from the aviary because they potentially can shed massive amounts of virus.

Testing is not a panacea, and testing cannot be used as a substitute for sound management practices. Too often, breeders and pet store managers are willing to test the large valuable parrots, but not the smaller birds. Recent information suggests that in addition to lovebirds, budgerigars and cockatiels may also be important sources of this disease.[14] Breeders of large valuable species should be strongly discouraged from keeping the smaller species. Minimizing disease transmission in the pet store is not an easy task. Lovebirds, budgerigars, and cockatiels are important moneymakers for pet stores, and most pet store owners feel that economically they must carry them. In this case, efforts can be made to design facilities that keep these small species separate from the larger parrots. Special efforts should be made to isolate juvenile birds from all other birds in the store and to minimize their direct contact with the public. Another under-utilized approach to disease prevention is to have pet store owners purchase birds from disease-free suppliers. Appropriate testing of the parent flock and random sampling of the juvenile birds each year can be used to designate a flock free of specific pathogens. These breeders can use this information when advertizing their birds, and pet stores owners can do the same.

Private bird owners should be discouraged from handling other people's birds. They should also be warned about the risks posed by bird shows and encouraged to quarantine their birds after a show and retest these birds in 30 days. Movement of birds, especially nestlings, between aviaries should be strongly discouraged.

Routine hygiene methods and proper husbandry practices need to be consistently used. Cleaning is the best defense against pathogen buildup. The susceptibility of the PBFDV to disinfectants is not known. However, a similar virus, the chicken anemia virus, is highly resistant to all standard disinfectants.[3-5] Therefore, for this virus in particular, wash-

ing it away or filtering it out is a more important aspect of control than trying to disinfect the facilities.

Preliminary results suggest that an appropriate vaccination protects birds against disease.[23, 29] Because PBFDV has not been grown in cell culture, the development of a vaccine will have to depend on a breakthrough in the cultivation of the virus or in synthetic production of viral proteins.

Circovirus Infection in the Canary (*Serinus Canaria*)

A disease with high morbidity and mortality has been reported in nestling canaries. Affected birds have a distended abdomen and an enlarged gall bladder. Exudate in the air sacs has also been reported. The disease has been referred to as "black spot" by canary fanciers, because the enlarged gall bladder can be observed through the nestlings' skin. Lesions characteristic of circovirus infections in other birds are present in these canaries as are the characteristic intranuclear and cytoplasmic inclusion bodies. Diagnosis is most readily made in birds 10 to 20 days old. Preliminary studies suggest that this virus is genetically distinct from the PBFDV.[41]

AVIAN POLYOMAVIRUS

Clinical presentation in selected species is outlined in Table 19–2.

Disease Synopsis

Avian polyomavirus (APV) infection and disease was first recognized in budgerigars when it caused explosive outbreaks in commercial aviaries in the southern United States,[42, 43] and in Ontario, Canada.[44] Since then it has been found worldwide.[45–49] The first indication of APV in a budgerigar aviary is a sudden increase in nestlings mortality.[42–44, 46] Without intervention, disease persists in subsequent breeding seasons, although the mortality rate diminishes.[50] Affected birds are stunted, have dysplastic feathers, discolored skin, abdominal distension, ascites, hydropericardium, hepatomegaly with focal hepatic necrosis, and scattered petechial hemorrhages.[42–44, 46] Target organs vary from outbreak to

Table 19–2

AVIAN POLYOMAVIRUS: CLINICAL PRESENTATIONS

Signs	Species Affected	Incidence
Polyomavirus in Psittacines		
Nestling mortality at 10–20 days	Budgerigars	Common
Sudden death in 2- to 12-week-old nestlings	Macaws, conures, eclectus parrots, and ring-necked parrots	Common
	Cockatiels, lories, cockatoos, Amazon, and hawk-headed parrots	Uncommon
Short-term nonspecific disease and death in fledglings and young adults	Lovebirds	Common
Aplastic or dysplastic feathers, especially the primary wing and the tail feathers	Budgerigars	Common
	Other susceptible parrots	Rare
Sudden death in adult parrots	Eclectus parrots, cockatoos, and caiques	Uncommon
Polyomavirus in Passerines		
Sudden death in nestlings and young adults	Gouldian finches	Uncommon
	Other Australian finches	Unknown
	House sparrows, black-bellied seed crackers	
Unthriftiness and failure to thrive	Gouldian finches	Uncommon
	Black-bellied seed crackers	Unknown

outbreak; in at least one case, central nervous system signs were the predominate clinical finding.[51] In a variable percentage of infected nestlings the only sign of disease is feather dysplasia.[46, 52, 53] Affected feathers resemble those seen in the PBFD infection or they may fail to develop entirely. All feather tracts are susceptible, and generalized feather disease occurs. Most often, however, tail and primary wing feathers are excessively affected. If these birds are allowed to survive, normal feathers grow in with the next molt. APV disease (APVD) confined to feather changes has been called *French moult*. It should be noted that this term has also been applied to feather changes associated with the PBFDV, and that beak and feather virus-induced feather changes and APV-induced feather changes are virtually indistinguishable.

APVD in nonbudgerigar parrots is an acute rapidly fatal disease of hand-raised nestlings.[54–56] Macaws, conures, eclectus parrots, and ring-necked parakeets *(Psittacula krameri)* are at greatest risk. Less commonly, the disease is seen in Amazon parrots, lories, cockatoos, and hawk-headed parrots *(Deroptyus accipitrinus)*. Most affected birds die suddenly with little or no prodromal period. Clinical signs, when they do occur, last for less than 24 hours and include weakness, pallor, subcutaneous hemorrhage, prolonged bleeding times, anorexia, dehydration, inappetence, and crop stasis. Disease may occur in single birds or in numerous birds in the same facility. Disease occurs predominately in

birds 2 to 14 weeks old. Necropsy findings include generalized pallor with subcutaneous and subserosal hemorrhages. Hepatomegaly with or without mottling and splenomegaly are common but inconsistent signs (see Color Fig. 19–4). Infrequently, ascites and pericardial effusion are found.

APVD of adult birds has been noted.[57, 58] Although uncommon, this disease is characterized by the same signs and gross lesions as those seen in nestling parrots. In contrast to the nestling parrots, the only adult parrots reported with APVD have been eclectus parrots,[57, 58] cockatoos,[57] white-bellied caiques *(Pionites leucogaster),* and a single conure.[58]

APV is endemic in many lovebird collections. Signs are more often noted in fledglings and young adults, in which a nonspecific illness may proceed death. Mortality rates are variable but never reach the proportions observed in the budgerigar.[59, 60]

Polyomavirus-like infections and disease occur sporadically in passerines (Table 19–3).[30, 61–68] The precise relationship of this virus, or these viruses, to the avian polyomavirus that affects parrots is not known. Likewise, the host and disease spectrum of this virus still need to be defined. The author is aware of three Gouldian finch aviaries in which there was significant nestling mortality and/or loss of young adult birds. In these outbreaks, inclusion bodies characteristic for APV were identified in multiple tissues, and virus particles consistent with a polyomavirus were found. In one of these aviaries, surviving birds had serum antibody capable of neu-

T a b l e 1 9 – 3

PASSERINE SPECIES IN WHICH AVIAN POLYOMAVIRUS DISEASE IS SUSPECTED TO OCCUR

Tricolored nun *(Lonchura malacca)*[65]
Cordon bleu *(Uraeginthus bengalus)*[65]
Greenfinch *(Carduelis chloris)*[67]
Gouldian finch *(Erythrura gouldiae)*[30, 61, 66]
Painted finch *(Emblema picta)*[68]
Black-bellied seed crackers *(Pyrenestes ostrinus)*[62, 63]
Blue bill *(Spermophaga haematina)*[63]
House sparrow *(Passer domesticus)*[30]

tralizing a parrot APV isolate. In this particular outbreak, surviving birds were considered poor doers by the owner and were euthanitized. Histologically, splenic atrophy and glomerular sclerosis were identified. These lesions are consistent with previous APVD.

APVD in Gouldian finches has also been reported from Australia.[61, 66] In the aviaries described, virus inclusions and APV-like virions were found in fledgling and young adult birds. Hepatic necrosis was a predominate feature of this disease. In one of these reports,[66] high mortality of nestlings younger than 5 days of age was also observed. In addition, fledglings were unthrifty, had chronic candidiasis, and elongated narrowed mandibles. A cause-and-effect relationship between the nestling mortality and an APV infection was not shown because APV-like inclusions were demonstrated only in one fledgling and were not seen in the three nestlings examined.

APV infection has been studied in a closed colony of blue bills and seedcrackers.[62–64] The APV infection present in this colony was considered to be the primary cause of death in six birds. Subclinical persistent infections were common. This colony was experiencing many other infectious disease problems, and the relationship of the persistent APV infections to observed histologic lesions remains unclear. In situ hybridization studies suggest that this APV varies significantly from the psittacine APV.

Characteristic lesions of APVD have been observed in tissue sections from a house sparrow *(Passer domesticus)*, raising the possibility that an avian polyomavirus is endemic in wild birds in the US.[29]

Biology

APV is a 40 to 48 nm, nonenveloped, double-stranded DNA virus.[42–44, 69, 70] Although minor varia-

tions in the genetic code have been documented, the APV infecting parrots represents a single virus.[71, 72] Thus, a virus infecting one parrot species should be assumed capable of infecting others. Although the host range of APV is not known, it appears that APV can infect all parrots and possibly other nonpsittacine species.[71] A critical feature for understanding the control of APV is the concept of subclinical infection. Most APV infections of adult and nestling birds are subclinical, and only a small percentage result in disease.[50, 60, 73–75] The nature of disease, prevalence of disease, and the length of virus shedding in subclinical infections are all species-dependent.

In the budgerigar, within enzootic aviaries, nestling infections occur within the first few days after hatching, and the infection prevalence may reach 100%.[76] Virus is shed in the droppings and in feather and skin dander, and may be present in oral secretions.[50] Inhalation of aerosolized virus is a documented route of infection,[52] but other portals of entry are also possible. Characteristic APV-inclusion bodies were found in a day-old nestling budgerigar and have led to the speculation that vertical transmission may play a role in APV dissemination.[52, 77] In the author's experience, vertical transmission is not an important part of the epidemiology of this disease. Disease development is age-dependent. Infection studies in older budgerigars induced subclinical infection but not disease.[52] Infection studies in adult birds have not been done, but it is likely that adults are susceptible and that infection is also subclinical.

Following infection, APV replicates in a wide range of budgerigar tissues. Incubation periods in the budgerigar are very short, and virus neutralizing antibodies can be detected in nestlings as young as 9 days of age.[76] Virus-induced cytopathic effects appear to account for observed signs. For reasons yet to be determined, tissue virus concentrations may be very high in birds with no clinical signs and little histologic evidence of infection.[78] In both clinical and subclinical infections, high concentrations of virus are present in the serum.[78] Inapparently infected birds and those that survive the clinical disease shed virus in their feces and feather and skin dander until at least 6 months of age.[50] With the onset of breeding, virus levels within the tissues of these birds diminish and shedding may stop completely. Infection is maintained in the aviary through viral shedding of juvenile and young adult birds. Serologically, infected budgerigars maintain APV-neutralizing antibody titers for several years and possibly for life.[79]

How APV spreads so rapidly through commercial budgerigar aviaries is not known, but several management practices are suspected. In the past, it was a common practice for feed sacks to be recycled. Thus, feed sacks contaminated at one aviary may have distributed the virus to other aviaries. Bird buyers may have been and may continue to be another source of APV dissemination. These buyers go from aviary to aviary bringing the birds they have just purchased with them. The sale of birds from one aviary to another has been associated with disease outbreaks. The sale and exchange of birds and the mass movement of birds to and from bird shows probably accounts for the spread of virus among hobbyists' collections.

APV infection in nonbudgerigar parrots is common.[54–56] Epidemiologic study results suggest that most if not all parrot species of all ages are susceptible to infection. Most APV infections are asymptomatic. Disease occurs predominately in 2- to 14-week-old hand-raised nestlings of susceptible species.[54–56, 73] To date, experimental efforts to reproduce disease in nonbudgerigar parrots have failed,[80, 81] but inhalation of the virus is APV's likely means of entry. The target organs for virus replication are not known, but following infection, significant concentrations of the virus are shed in the droppings.[74] Precise incubation periods in nonbudgerigar parrots are also not known; however, disease typically follows 2 weeks after APV-free birds are introduced into a contaminated environment.[30] In adult birds and most nestlings, infection is asymptomatic.[60, 74, 75] These birds may shed virus for several days and possibly several weeks. In up to 15% of symptomatically infected birds, virus shedding at low concentrations continues indefinitely.[60] Infected birds develop neutralizing antibody titers that persist for months to years before declining to undetectable concentrations.[60, 75]

The pathogenesis of APVD in nonbudgerigar parrots is unclear. Intranuclear inclusion bodies characteristic of APV-infected cells are predominately found in mononuclear phagocytic cells.[54–56] The presence of high serum virus concentrations and of serum neutralizing antibody precedes the acute onset of disease.[73, 82] This author has postulated that

APV's cell specificity and the associated glomerular and vascular lesions are a manifestation of an immune-mediated disease.

Disease in adult birds is uncommon to rare.[57, 58] Given that the prevalence of subclinical infection is very high in adult birds, it remains unclear why certain individual birds should be susceptible to infection. One explanation, advanced by this author, is that APVD in adult birds is one manifestation of a concurrent APV and PBFDV infection. This outcome is rare and a second, more common, manifestation of concurrent APV and PBFDV infections is subclinical but active APV replication.[57] High concentrations of APV are found in the skin and feather follicles, making these PBFD-infected birds important sources of APV shedding.[30, 83]

The prevalence of both APV and PBFDV in lovebirds is high.[14] Because these birds often do not show signs of disease until they are young adults, they are a common source of disease for other species. Recent observations by this author and others suggest that the cockatiel is also an important source of virus dissemination.[84] Although APV disease in the cockatiel is nearly nonexistent, infection prevalence in one aviary was found to be high, and persistent virus shedding was identified in several individual birds.[60]

Dissemination of APV results from movement of recently infected and persistently shedding birds between aviaries, in and out of pet stores, and to and from bird shows and sales.

Diagnosis

Historic and gross necropsy findings are often sufficient to make the practitioner highly suspicious of APV infection. Confirmation requires histopathology examination.[42–44, 54–56] Histologically, the nuclei of APV-infected cells are enlarged and have marginated chromatin. Centrally their nucleus may be clear or may contain a finely granular basophilic to amphophilic inclusion. In the budgerigar, inclusions occur in multiple organs and tissue types including, but not limited to, liver, spleen, kidney (mesangial and tubule cells), feather follicles, skin, esophagus, brain, and heart.[42–44] In nonbudgerigar parrots, hepatic necrosis, although variable in degree, is consistently present. Karyomegalic changes with and without pannuclear inclusions are prominent in histiocytes within the perivascular sheaths in other splenic macrophages. Other cells of the macrophage mononuclear-phagocytic system, including Kupffer cells and glomerular mesangial cells, often demonstrate similar nuclear changes.[55–57] An immune-complex glomerulopathy may occur in up to two-thirds of these cases.[73, 82]

Given an adequate history and an appropriate selection of tissues, these lesions are pathognomonic. The presence of virus in the dead bird can be confirmed by electron microscopy, by immunofluorescent staining,[55] in situ hybridization techniques,[85] PCR of organ swabs,[36, 78] and inoculation of infected tissues into cell culture or eggs.[43, 55] Immunofluorescent staining can give the pathologist immediate confirmation of infection. PCR, although diagnostic for APV infection, does not prove that APV was the cause of the bird's death, and these results must be viewed in light of the histologic findings. In situ hybridization techniques are especially useful in the diagnosis of subclinical infection. Virus isolation is rarely used except as a research tool.

Control

PCR-based viral probes, serologic assays, prudent management strategies, and immunization are all tools that can used to prevent APV infection. Each of these tools has its limitations, and the proper combination of them is necessary to limit the threat of APV.

The PCR-based viral probe is the only test available that can detect virus shedding. In this assay, a cloacal swab is analyzed for the presence of viral DNA.[74] If the sample was not contaminated with airborne virus at collection, a positive result indicates active virus shedding at the time the sample was taken. This is a good test, but its results must be interpreted in light of the biology of the virus. If this test is used as a routine screening procedure, 95% or more of the birds examined will have negative results, with the exception of lovebirds and young budgerigars.[60] If birds are tested in an outbreak situation, the prevalence of virus shedding will be high.[60, 74] Most of these birds, however, only shed temporarily. Birds with a positive result on an initial swab should be retested at least once in 90 days. Birds with positive test results for shedding

on more than one sample should be considered persistent carriers.[60] Although many persistently shedding birds have positive results on repeated swabs, a small percentage of birds test positive only intermittently.[60] This means that a single negative sample does not rule out the possibility that the tested bird may be persistently infected. Repeated sampling of birds, although costly, is the only means to detect persistent infections.

Serologic testing is an important investigative tool for the practitioner when used properly. In the budgerigar, a high percentage of seropositive birds younger than 6 months old are shedding virus.[50] In nonbudgerigar parrots, the serologic status of the bird cannot be used to predict its virus shedding status.[74] Detectable antibody, however, does indicate previous virus infection, and this information may prove valuable in monitoring bird collections for APV activity.

Control of APV in budgerigar aviaries and in the hobbyist's collection requires strict biosecurity measures. Serologic testing can be used to determine if APV is already present in the aviary. If the budgerigar aviary is free of APV, all birds being introduced to the aviary should also be seronegative. Ideally, once an adequate number of breeding birds has been acquired or blood lines are established, the aviary should be closed to all new birds. All birds being taken to a show should be quarantined for 60 days and ideally should be found seronegative before being returned to the aviary. Both commercial breeders and hobbyists should minimize, or prohibit entirely, public access to their birds. Cages and all cage accessories should be thoroughly disinfected if they were used to house birds that were taken off the property. Serologic monitoring of a representative sampling of each year's offspring can be used to verify the aviaries' disease-free status.[86]

If APV is already present in the budgerigar aviary, proven management techniques can be used to eliminate it. Key to its elimination is the removal of birds that are shedding virus and aviary disinfection. The young adult and juvenile birds will be shedding virus. Therefore, breeding should be stopped and all birds with no previous breeding experience removed from the aviary. Items (e.g., plywood nest boxes) that cannot be disinfected should be replaced. The entire premises should be repeatedly cleaned and disinfected. Ideally, breeding facilities would be left unused for 3 to 6 months. After that interval, the experienced breeders may be reintroduced to the facilities. If the environment is adequately disinfected, offspring from these birds will be APV-free. Serologic testing of a selected cohort of the new birds can be used to verify that the infection cycle has been broken.[79]

Proper management decisions are prerequisite to the prevention of APVD in nonbudgerigar parrots. Because of the high incidence of APV in lovebirds, cockatiels, and budgerigars, and the high incidence of PBFDV in lovebirds, these birds must not be kept in the same facility that raises larger, more valuable species. Likewise, until the virus affecting passerines is identified, these birds should be kept from the aviary. Common sense management techniques emphasized at the beginning of this chapter must be adhered to precisely. Quarantine of new birds for as long as possible and repeated viral probes of cloacal swabs are indicated. Serologic testing has limited usefulness in this situation. There are many seropositive adult birds, and the vast majority of these are not shedding virus. On the other hand, detecting antibodies in a fledgling indicates that it was recently infected and that APV was active in the aviary or pet store from which it was acquired.

When an APV outbreak occurs in an aviary, the major objective is to stop the infection cycle between the asymptomatic but virus-shedding nestlings and new hatchlings or nestlings removed from their parents. Depending on the situation, several options exist. If breeding can be stopped, this is the best choice. If babies are still in the nest box, it is best to leave these birds with their parents. In nonbudgerigar parrots, excluding lovebirds, APVD rarely if ever occurs in parent-raised chicks. If the owner cannot or will not stop breeding the birds, the new chicks should be raised in an isolated facility by someone who is not in contact with the adults or the chicks. Testing all chicks and adults at the time of the outbreak is expensive, and the results can be predicted before the samples are even sent in. Many nestlings will be shedding virus, and if the virus is recently introduced to the aviary, many adults will be shedding virus as well. In the author's experience, testing should be delayed until mortality has stopped and the nestlings are weaned. At this point, nestlings should be tested at least twice, 1 month apart, before they are sold. Three months after the last death, adult birds can be tested

for virus shedding. Positive-testing birds can then be isolated and retested again.[60, 86]

To prevent APV infection and disease in subsequent years, careful evaluation of the aviary is required. Repeatedly, lovebirds are the source of virus, and if they are present in the aviary they must be eliminated.[60] PBFDV can play an important part in the onset of APV outbreaks and in the author's experience; testing for this virus is as important to control as is testing for APV virus shedding. Thorough cleaning and disinfection of the baby-raising areas must be done repeatedly. Phenolics, sodium hypochlorite, and stabilized chlorine dioxide are all proven disinfectants against APV.[2] If these precautionary measures are followed, APV infection and disease can be eliminated from the aviary in subsequently breeding seasons. To verify success, fledglings can be examined serologically. If multiple birds are tested and they are all seronegative, virus exposure was eliminated.

Control of APVD in the pet store is a challenge.[86] Birds coming into these facilities are often coming from multiple aviaries. Cockatiels, budgerigars, and lovebirds are generally present in these stores as well. Ideally all birds should be tested for serologic levels and for virus shedding before entering a store. Economically this is not feasible, especially for owners of the smaller species. In this situation, it can be recommended that the pet store not carry the smaller birds, or that they acquire only nestlings that are 14 weeks old or older. If these options are not acceptable, pet store owners should try to isolate their susceptible nestlings and have selected employees exclusively responsible for their care. Arrangements can be made with breeders so that their stock is evaluated for the presence of APV. If found negative and selected young are tested every year, pet store owners can feel confident that they are acquiring virus-free stock.

An unfortunate, but common, occurrence is the loss of nestlings in the pet store. This creates a delicate situation for the veterinarian, because often the breeder is being held accountable for the birds' death. Analysis of the pet store's situation and use of serologic testing can clarify the facts. If the bird died 2 weeks or longer after introduction to the store and lovebirds, budgerigars, and cockatiels are present in the store, APV infection probably occurred in the store. Serologic monitoring of the nestlings still in the owner's possession is also indicated. If all the nestlings examined are seronegative, APV is not present in the breeder's nestlings and the infection was acquired at the store.[86]

A commercial APV vaccine is now available. This vaccine produces virus neutralizing antibodies, and to date the reported complications of its use have been considered minor.[87, 88] The developers of this vaccine essentially recommend that all parrots be vaccinated. Initially, the vaccine is to be administered twice, 2 to 3 weeks apart. Birds are not considered protected until 2 weeks after the second vaccination. Because extremely young birds may not respond adequately to the vaccine, the first dose should not be administered until birds are 6 weeks of age or older. Even with vaccination, the vaccine's developer does not recommend that vaccinated birds be shipped to new facilities until they are past the age of susceptibility to APVD.

Although this vaccine apparently is safe and does produce a humoral immune response, much of the data regarding its testing is yet to be published. In addition, it has yet to be proven effective in infection trials where the traditional disease seen in field cases was produced in control birds. The practitioner should consider all aspects of APV infection and disease before endorsing this vaccine for all birds. In adult PBFDV-free birds the probability of birds ever developing APD disease is essentially none. Likewise, a closed aviary of breeding birds is not at risk for APVD. If it is to be truly effective, this vaccine is best used in high-risk situations, such as pet stores, aviaries where there is movement of birds in and out, and hobbyist's collections when birds being taken to shows could bring the infection back.

PAPILLOMAVIRUSES

Clinical presentation in common species is presented in Table 19–4.

Disease Synopsis

Cutaneous papillomas in parrots are uncommon to rare.[89] They have been reported in double yellow-head Amazon (*Amazona ochrocephala)*[89] and African grey parrots,[89, 90] budgerigars,[89, 91–93] a Quaker parrot (*Mylopsitta monachus),*[89] and a cockatiel.[89]

T a b l e 1 9 – 4

PAPILLOMAVIRUSES: CLINICAL PRESENTATIONS

Signs	Species Affected	Incidence
Locally extensive raised proliferative lesions of the face	African grey parrots Canaries	Rare Rare
Papilliferous lesions of the feet	Wild chaffinches and other Fringillidae	Common

Cutaneous papillomas of confirmed viral etiology have only been documented in an African grey parrot.[90, 94] This imported bird presented with papilliferous plaques of the commissures of the beak, eyelids, and face. The bird was followed for a year after presentation, during which time the lesions became more extensive.

In contrast, viral papillomas of European finches are common and have been recorded in both wild and aviary birds.[95–101] The chaffinch (*Fringilla coelebs),* brambling (*F. montifringilla),*[95, 96, 99] and bullfinch (*Pyrrhula pyrrhula)*[101] are most often affected. In these birds, papillomas predominate on the legs and feet; lesions of the face are rare. A single outbreak of papillomas of presumed viral origin was described in a flock of Belgium canaries.[101] Scattered focal raised lesions were present around the commissures of the beak and the eyelids, and on top of the head.

Biology, Diagnosis, and Treatment

Papillomaviruses are nonenveloped double-stranded DNA viruses that are approximately 45 nm in diameter. Except in complex systems, these viruses cannot be grown in vitro.[102] Two avian papillomaviruses have been identified. Both were derived from cutaneous lesions. Grossly, papillomas may resemble several other skin lesions, including those caused by poxviruses, fungal infections, and other neoplasms. Diagnosis can only be made by histologic examination. Proof of a virus etiology requires detection of virus particles by electron microscopy. Little information exists on specific treatment of papillomas. Localized growths have responded to surgical excision. Surgical excision of more extensive lesions is not practical. In humans and some mammals, cutaneous warts may spontaneously regress. Autogenous vaccines have proved useful in specific papillomavirus infections, but their value in the bird has not been investigated.[102]

ADENOVIRUSES

Clinical presentation in some species is presented in Table 19–5.

Disease Synopsis

Most practitioners first encounter adenovirus infections in psittacine birds as an incidental finding at necropsy in a bird that died from other causes. In the author's experience and from the literature, subclinical adenovirus infections are most common in lovebirds[103] and budgerigars.[104, 105] In both species, occasional characteristic intranuclear inclusion bodies (INIB) are found in the collecting ducts and tubules of the kidneys.[103–105] Adenoviruses may also be primary pathogens or may cause disease in conjunction with other virus infections. Typically, adenovirus-associated disease has been reported sporadically in individual birds or in isolated outbreaks and is uncommon to rare in pet and avicultural birds.

Adenoviruses have been most consistently associated with disease in lovebirds. Thirty percent mortality was reported in imported white-masked lovebirds *(A. personata)* with conjunctivitis.[106] In these birds, INIB were observed in the conjunctiva and the kidney. Acute necrotizing pancreatitis in a

peach-faced lovebird *(A. roseicollis),*[107] a multisystemic disease in Nyasa lovebirds *(A. lilianae),*[108] and hepatic necrosis in a black-masked lovebird[109] have all been attributed to adenovirus infections.

Hepatitis[109–114] or hepatitis and enteritis[113, 115, 116] have been reported from several psittacine species with adenovirus infections. In the late 1970s, several commercial budgerigar aviaries in Ontario experienced a high mortality rate in nestlings.[112] At necropsy these birds had enlarged livers and histologically there was a diffuse hepatitis with eosinophilic inclusion bodies. Adenolike virus particles were identified by electron microscopy. Subsequent outbreaks have not been reported. Bryant and Montali reported a mini-epizootic outbreak of inclusion body hepatitis in a mixed collection of waterfowl, shorebirds, and psittacine birds. In this outbreak, five Australian and South American parrots died.[110] Viruses morphologically similar to adenoviruses were identified by electron microscopy. Multifocal hepatic necrosis was attributed to an adenovirus infection in a single cockatiel that was found dead in a mixed collection of birds.[114] Adenovirus hepatitis and enteritis have also been reported in a Moluccan cockatoo, eclectus parrots,[113] and a double yellow-headed Amazon parrot.[115]

Adenovirus encephalitis in parrots is rare, and some of the evidence implicating adenoviruses to neurologic disease is circumstantial. Lowenstein[117] observed adenolike INIB in enterocytes in *Pionus* and *Neophema* species with persistent torticollis. Likewise, neurologic signs were prominent in outbreaks of disease in budgerigars that were characterized by a nonsuppurative encephalitis and hepatitis.[111] Two adenoviruses were isolated from the budgerigars. Experimental infection with these isolates reproduced the hepatic lesions but not the neurologic disease, suggesting the possibility that the neurologic lesions were induced by a concurrent virus infection, possibly a paramyxovirus. Perhaps the most convincing case of adenovirus encephalitis is described by Gerlach.[8] In this report, a Moluccan cockatoo showing progressive central nervous systems signs was found to have adenovirus-like inclusions within the brain.

Biology

Adenoviruses are nonenveloped, 65 to 90 nm double-stranded DNA viruses.[118, 119] Avian adenoviruses

Table 19–5

ADENOVIRUSES: CLINICAL PRESENTATIONS

Signs	Species Affected	Incidence
Hepatitis	Lovebirds	Uncommon
	Budgerigars	Rare
	Cockatiel	Rare
	Other psittacine birds	Rare
Pancreatitis	Lovebirds	Rare
Enteritis	Multiple psittacine birds	Rare
Conjunctivitis	Lovebirds	Rare
Encephalitis	Moluccan cockatoo	Rare
	Other species?	
Incidental finding at necropsy (renal and/or digestive system)	Lovebirds	Uncommon
	Budgerigars	Uncommon

have been best studied in poultry where they cause quail bronchitis,[120] hemorrhagic enteritis in turkeys,[121] and reduced egg production in chickens.[122] Adenoviruses have been implicated in a fading syndrome in ostrich *(Struthio camelus)* chicks[123] and as the causative agent of inclusion body hepatitis in pigeons.[124] In poultry, adenoviruses can be shed in the urine, feces, and respiratory secretions. Infection occurs through virus ingestion or inhalation. In addition, in chickens, vertical transmission is particularly important.[122] In general, adenoviruses often latently infect their host, resulting in either intermittent or low levels of virus shedding. Numerous stressors including other infectious agents can reactivate adenoviruses.

Essentially nothing is known of the biology of the adenoviruses affecting parrots. Given that adenovirus infection is generally an incidental finding, especially in lovebirds and budgerigars, low levels of virus shedding either through the urinary or digestive tracts may perpetuate the infection in these species. The role of vertical transmission in parrots is completely unknown.

Diagnosis and Control

Currently, the only diagnostic test for adenovirus infection in parrots is at necropsy. The presence of large intranuclear deeply basophilic inclusion bodies is characteristic of this disease, especially when seen in the liver, kidney, pancreas, or small intestine. Virus particles form characteristic paracrystalline arrays that can be viewed by electron microscopy. Likewise, individual virus particles can be demonstrated by negative stained preparations of homogenized tissues. A DNA probe for in situ hybridization was reported in 1994.[8] This technique, as well as virus isolation in cell culture,[122] can be used to verify adenovirus infection, but is rarely necessary. Conceivably, a genetic probe could be developed to detect parrot adenoviruses shedding, but there is little economic incentive to do this because the infection is so uncommon and results in few deaths.

With the current limited knowledge about this disease, general control measures outlined at the beginning of chapter are the best available means to reduce the threat adenoviruses might pose.

PACHECO'S DISEASE OR PARROT HERPESVIRUS

Clinical presentation in some species is outlined in Table 19–6.

Disease Synopsis

Pacheco's disease occurs almost exclusively in psittacine birds. Disease is most common in avicultural collections[125–131] and, in previous years, in imported birds housed in quarantine stations.[132] Outbreaks in pet stores and deaths in individual birds have also been reported.[132] The most common clinical presentation is a dead bird that died with little or no advanced evidence that it was ill. Other pertinent clinical information includes exposure to Patagonian *(Cyanoliseus patagonus),* nanday *(Nandayus nenday),* or mitred conures *(Aratinga mitrata).*[132, 133] A history of recent changes in the aviary, such as the addition of a new bird or birds being taken out of an aviary to a show and then returned, the onset of breeding, or surgical sexing, should also alert practitioners to the possibility that they are dealing with Pacheco's disease.[125, 132, 133] In a small percentage of birds, particularly macaws, clinical signs may precede death.[132, 134] Signs generally are nonspecific and include lethargy, depression, and anorexia. Profuse sulphur-colored (biliverdin-stained) urates are another nonspecific but consistently reported sign.[125–128, 131–133] Regurgitation, bloody diarrhea, and terminal central nervous system signs have been infrequently reported.[126, 132, 133, 135] Duration of clinical signs ranges from a few minutes to many days, possibly even several weeks. However, the vast majority of these birds die within a few hours to a few days of the onset of clinical signs. Only a few birds have been known to survive infection once

T a b l e 1 9 – 6

PACHECO'S DISEASE OR PARROT HERPESVIRUS: CLINICAL PRESENTATIONS

Signs	Species Affected	Incidence
Death with no premonitory signs	All parrots	Common
	Keel-billed toucan	Rare
Depression, lethargy, yellow urates, birds may survive several days	All parrots	Uncommon

signs have developed.[132, 135] Elevation in the serum aspartate aminotransferase concentrations[134, 136] and marked leukopenia have been reported in these birds.[134] Radiographically, hepatomegaly, spleno-megaly, and renal enlargement have also been documented.[134] The number of affected birds can vary from a single isolated case to hundreds.

Biology

The Pacheco's disease virus is a herpesvirus. It is enveloped, has double-stranded DNA, and is 180 to 200 nm in diameter.[129, 130, 137] In the acutely infected bird, virus is shed in feces and respiratory and ocular secretions.[131, 138] Ingestion and inhalation of the virus is suspected to be the most important means of transmission.[126, 139] Experimentally, the virus has been transmitted by nebulization, ingestion, and intraocular administration.[126] The incubation period typically ranges from 5 to 14 days[126, 129, 130, 132]; however, it has been suggested that in unusual cases the incubation period may take several weeks.[132] Virus replication probably occurs in a number of organs. Inclusion bodies are most often found in the liver and spleen, and to a lesser extent in the crop, small intestine, and pancreas.[125–127, 129–131, 135, 137, 139] Necrosis of the infected cells, particularly hepatocytes, accounts for the clinical signs.

Circumstantial evidence suggests that all psittacine birds are susceptible to Pacheco's virus infection. The prevalence of disease, however, is species-specific. Some conures (e.g., Patagonian, nanday, and mitred conures) appear relatively resistant to disease, whereas other conures like the half-moon conure (*Aratinga canicularis eburniostrum*) are very sensitive. Amazon, African grey, Senegal (*Poicephalus senegalus*), and Quaker parrots; budgerigars, and cockatiels are similarly highly susceptible to disease. Macaws show intermediate susceptibility, but death rates may still approach 80% in some outbreaks.[126, 132, 133, 139–141]

To the author's knowledge, the only documented naturally occurring case of Pacheco's disease in a nonpsittacine bird occurred in a keel-billed toucan (*Ramphastos sulfuratos*). Lesions in this bird and a second keel-billed toucan experimentally infected with Pacheco's virus were characteristic of the psittacine infection.[142] In another toucan (species not reported), a disease resembling Pacheco's disease

was described. Herpesvirus virions were identified in the tissues of this bird; however, fluorescent antibody staining of the tissues with a Pacheco's virus-specific antibody was negative.[143]

Subclinical infections in parrots are probably common. Antibody titers to Pacheco's virus isolates have been found in many apparently healthy birds.[29, 132, 135, 144] Like other herpesviruses, Pacheco's virus is believed to latently infect subclinically infected birds and birds that have recovered from disease.[132, 139] The percentage of birds that become latently infected is not known. Patagonian conures have been shown to shed virus and Patagonian, mitred, nanday, and possibly blue-crowned (*Aratinga acuticuadata*) and maroon-bellied (*Pyrrhura frontalis*) conures have been implicated as the source of disease outbreaks.[132, 142] Less commonly, Amazon parrots and macaws may also serve as virus reservoirs.[133]

The frequency of virus shedding in latently infected birds is not known, but is probably rare (once a year or longer) in the nonstressed bird.[142] Stress, such as surgery, transport, or the onset of breeding, may reactivate latent infections and initiate outbreaks.[132] Therefore, even closed aviaries may experience this disease years after they have purchased their last bird.

Although most isolates of the Pacheco's disease virus are serologically cross-reactive with the first US isolate, there is increasing evidence that Pacheco's disease is caused by a heterogeneous group of viruses. In Europe, three serologically unrelated viruses have been identified.[135, 145] Likewise, in the US States, four groups of herpesviruses have been identified by electrophoretic analysis of their proteins.[146] Histopathologic variations also suggest that more than one Pacheco's virus pathotype may exist.[142] These atypical pathotypes appear to have a greater affinity for the esophagus and intestines but less for the liver than the classic Pacheco's disease virus isolates.

Diagnosis

Although the clinical history and clinical appearance may suggest Pacheco's disease, confirmation of infection requires a necropsy, or in the rare birds that survive infection, isolation of the virus from feces or direct visualization of the virus in feces by electron microscopy. Grossly, these birds are generally well muscled and may have recently ingested food. Common gross lesions include hepatomegaly, splenomegaly, renal swelling, and serosal and epicardial hemorrhage. Uncommonly, the affected liver may be uniformly pale yellow, resembling the appearance of a diffuse lipidosis (see Color Fig. 19–5). In other birds the liver may have a diffuse mottling or have scattered, irregularly shaped discolored foci. In many or perhaps most cases, no liver lesions are observed grossly. Less commonly, submucosal hemorrhage with or without intraluminal blood may also be present.[125, 127, 130, 131, 135, 137, 139] Panigraphy and Grumbles[128] report the presence of air sacculitis in a sulfur-crested cockatoo with Pacheco's disease; if viral-induced, this feature of Pacheco's disease is uncommon. Because of the acute nature of this disease, gross lesions may be entirely absent in some birds.

Histologically, hepatic necrosis is present in the vast majority of the cases. Necrosis may be widely scattered but is generally extensive, and at times only the hepatocytes surrounding the central veins and portal triads are spared. Varying degrees of splenic lymphoid hyperplasia and necrosis, pancreatitis, and enteritis also occur. Eosinophilic and, less frequently, basophilic inclusion bodies are found in the liver, on the margins of the necrotic areas, and in bile duct epithelium. Inclusions sometimes are present in the spleen, intestinal epithelium, crop, and pancreas. Based on the clinical history and characteristic lesions, a histopathologic diagnosis of Pacheco's disease is readily made.[125, 129, 130, 135, 137, 139]

In laboratories with specific fluorescently labeled anti-Pacheco's virus antibody conjugates, diagnosis can be made on impression smears of liver or other affected organs.[142, 143] Biotinylated antibody conjugates have also been used to detect the virus in paraffin-embedded tissues.[138] The Pacheco's disease virus is readily grown in cell culture and in chicken eggs. Electron microscopy has been used to document the presence of a herpesvirus in some cases, but like virus isolation methods, it is primarily a research tool and is rarely necessary to make a diagnosis.[125, 128–130, 135]

Treatment

The approach to minimizing the effects of a Pacheco's virus outbreak is somewhat controversial.

Human traffic, movement of birds, or handling of birds is likely to help disseminate the virus. In contrast, others have found that mortality in Pacheco's virus outbreaks can be minimized by prophylactic use of acyclovir (Zovirax, Burroughs Wellcome). The potential efficacy of acyclovir was first suggested in a natural outbreak of Pacheco's disease in a private aviary.[131] Exposed birds were given an intramuscular injection of acyclovir 25 mg/kg once, and acyclovir was added to the drinking water (1 mg/ml) and food (400 mg/quart of seed) for 7 days. In this trial, seven of eight treated birds survived. In contrast, seven untreated birds died. Others have also found acyclovir effective in reducing mortality.[147–150] Norton and coworkers[147, 148] found that acyclovir gavaged at 80 mg/kg every 8 hours for 7 days reduced mortality in experimentally infected Quaker parakeets. Deaths still occurred after the treatments stopped, suggesting that longer treatment periods may be necessary. These investigators also found injectable acyclovir to be highly irritating, and felt that it is contraindicated to give the preparation either intramuscularly or subcutaneously. Obviously, capturing breeding pairs and injecting them or gavaging them every 8 hours maximizes the likelihood for movement of the virus from cage to cage. Therefore, the practitioner must balance the risk of medication with its possible benefits.

Additional control efforts may be beneficial. Barriers between cages can be erected, and cages can be moved farther apart. Again, the more movement of people and the more bird activity, the more likely the virus is to disseminate. Immunization in the face of an outbreak is of questionable benefit, because protective antibody titers are not expected for 2 weeks after vaccination. Fudge has suggested that vaccination not be initiated until 2 weeks after the last death.[151]

As with all viral diseases, the loss of birds to the virus may only be a portion of a breeder's problems. Reputations can be badly damaged when others find out about an outbreak. In addition, there is still no clear understanding of what to recommend to the breeder regarding the birds that survive. If birds are subclinically infected, they potentially can be a source of infection for other birds brought into the aviary. Thus, all birds in the aviary should be immunized. In the same manner, if they are sold, they could be a source of disease to other aviaries.

Until we have a means of detecting latently infected birds, this dilemma cannot be resolved.

Control

Control measures fall into three categories: savvy management practices, immunization, and testing. Given that some conure species have been repeatedly implicated in outbreaks of this disease, these birds should not be kept in a mixed collection. Domestically raised birds may have less exposure to Pacheco's virus as compared with wild-caught birds, but this has not been proven.[132] General practices such as a closed aviary, proper quarantine procedures, and acquisition of birds from reputable sources help to minimize the likelihood that Pacheco's virus is introduced to an aviary. Providing adequate spacing between cages and limiting human traffic in the aviary are also important preventative measures.

A single Pacheco's disease virus vaccine (Psittimune PDV, Biomune, 8906 Rosehill Road, Lenexa, KS 66215) is currently being marketed in the United States. This vaccine has not been universally accepted, in part because of uncommon complications linked to its use.[151–154] Documented complications have ranged from death in some smaller species immediately after injection to granulomas at the site of injection, particularly in cockatoos. To minimize risks of adverse effects of the vaccine, the manufacturer's recommendations should be followed precisely. Some authors recommend that the vaccine be given only subcutaneously, although it is approved for both subcutaneous or intramuscular injection in birds over 100 g.[153] Decisions on whether to use the vaccine can only be made on a case-by-case basis. Vaccination of an individually owned bird in a private home or birds in a closed breeding colony of cockatoos or macaws may have more risks than potential rewards. In contrast, a mixed collection of birds with questionable management is at high risk for this disease, and a vaccination program may prevent significant losses. It must be remembered that Pacheco's disease may be caused by a heterogeneous group of viruses, and the vaccine strain made may not protect against all of them.

Serologic testing has been used in a limited fashion to screen for previous virus exposure.[144] The belief is that if a bird is seropositive it may be latently infected and may shed the virus sometime in the future. Two problems exist with this concept. First, it is not known what percentage of seropositive birds shed virus. Second, antibody titers may not persist after infection, and antibody-negative birds have been found to be shedding virus.[142] To identify infected but serologically negative birds, it has been suggested that birds be vaccinated a few weeks before testing.[144] Birds with high antibody titers following vaccination presumably have been exposed to the virus before or were previously vaccinated, whereas birds with low titers are naive. In the author's opinion, additional carefully controlled research must be done before the value of serologic testing can be confirmed.

OTHER HERPESVIRUS DISEASES (PROVEN AND SUSPECTED)

Clinical presentation in some species is outlined in Table 19–7.

Cytomegalovirus in Australian Finches

A virus resembling a cytomegalovirus was described in a mixed collection of Gouldian and other Australian finches. These birds were housed out-of-doors. Both adult birds and nestlings were affected. Clinical signs included weight loss, anorexia, dyspenia, and severe conjunctivitis. Seventy percent of the Gouldian finches died. At necropsy, air sacculitis, intestinal serositis, and conjunctivitis were found. Inclusion bodies were found in the conjunctiva, respiratory epithelium, and liver.[155] Virus particles were identified by electron microscopy. In the

T a b l e 1 9 – 7

OTHER HERPESVIRUS DISEASES (PROVEN AND SUSPECTED): CLINICAL PRESENTATIONS

Signs	Species Affected	Incidence
Conjunctivitis	Australian finches	Uncommon
Reduced hatchability	English budgerigars	European report
Tracheitis	Amazon parrots	Rare
Papilliferous and plaque-like lesions of the foot	Cockatoos and macaws	Uncommon

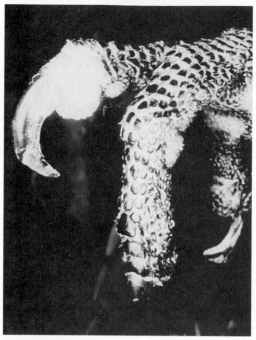

Figure 19–6

Discolored papilliferous lesion on the foot of a green-winged macaw. The presence of herpesvirus virions in similar lesions suggests that these lesions are of viral origin.

author's experience, this disease is uncommon to rare.

Budgerigar Herpesvirus

A herpesvirus has been isolated from English budgerigars in Europe. Its presence has been correlated with reduced hatchability and is believed to be transmitted vertically.[156] To the author's knowledge, this virus has not been recovered in North American budgerigars.

Amazon Tracheitis Virus

A virus believed to be a mutation of the infectious laryngotracheitis virus of chickens has been observed to cause a severe upper respiratory and tracheal disease in Amazon parrots and Bourke's parakeet *(Neophema bourkii)*.[157, 158] The duration of this disease is variable, but clinical signs have been reported to last up to 9 months. Although reported

to occur in the US, its prevalence in not known.[159] It should also be noted that similar lesions may be manifestations of other diseases.

Cutaneous Plaques and Papilliferous Lesions of the Foot

Lowenstein observed herpesvirus virions in proliferative lesions on the feet of macaws and cockatoos.[159, 160] These lesions show some species-specific variations. Lesions in cockatoos tend to be papilliferous, whereas those of macaws are raised depigmented plaques (Fig. 19–6).[134] These lesions have been reported to regress if treated topically with acyclovir.[134] To date, this herpesvirus has not been characterized and nothing is known of its incidence or biology.

POXVIRUSES

Clinical presentation in some species is presented in Table 19–8.

Disease Synopsis

Poxvirus infections occur in many avian species; however, the practitioner is only likely to see this disease in canaries *(Serinus canarius)*,[8, 161–163] recently imported wild-caught birds,[164–167] and indigenous wild birds.[163, 168, 169] Birds of any age can be

Table 19–8

POXVIRUSES: CLINICAL PRESENTATIONS

Signs	Species Affected	Incidence
Diphtheritic lesions of the mouth or crusty,	Canaries housed out-of-doors	Common
ulcerated, often nodular lesions of the head,	Imported Amazon and pionus parrots	Common
legs, and feet	Wild birds	Common
Mild crusty, often nodular, lesions of feet and face	Psittacines housed out-of-doors	Uncommon
Nonspecific systemic signs with or without cyanosis	Canaries housed out-of-doors	Uncommon
Nodular or large neoplastic-like lesions of the face, head, legs, feet, and body	Various nonpsittacine species	Uncommon

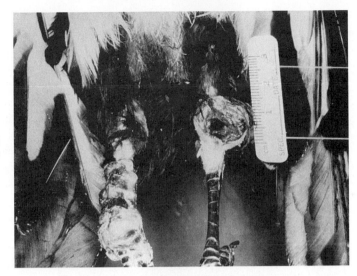

Figure 19–7

Cutaneous pox lesions on the legs and foot of a black-billed magpie *(Pica pica)*. (Photograph kindly provided by Dr. Lucio Filippich.)

affected, but the incidence of disease is highest in juveniles.[8, 163] Poxviruses produce lesions of the skin and the mucous membranes of the oral and respiratory cavity, and less commonly cause a systemic disease.

The cutaneous, or dry form, of the disease occurs in several avian species including some passerines and other land birds.[8, 163, 165] Affected birds develop rapidly enlarging neoplastic-like masses of the face, featherless areas of the body, and the feet (Figs. 19–7, 19–8). Lesions of the face and feet are most common. Lesions on the face predominate around the eyes and commissures of the beak. The number

and size of the lesions may vary from one or more small scabbed-over nodules to multiple large extensive masses that interfere with vision and prehension. Necrosis and ulceration of the overlying skin develop as the disease progresses. Lesions generally disseminate and enlarge over a period of 1 to 2 weeks. Regression may not begin until 4 to 6 weeks after the signs first begin. In rare cases, lesions may persist for months.[169] Regression, once it begins, results in a rapid resolution of the disease, often with few permanent effects.

A mild form of dry pox occurs in some adult birds introduced to outdoor aviaries in the southern US. The source of this infection may be either indigenous species or wild breeding populations of introduced parrots.

The mucosal or wet form of pox is common in canaries raised out-of-doors[162] and in imported nestling blue-fronted Amazon parrots *(Amazona aestiva aestiva)* and pionus parrots,[164, 166, 170] mynahs *(Gracula* species),[166] and lovebirds.[171] Unilateral or bilateral blepharitis, chemosis, and conjunctivitis mark the early stage of this disease.[162, 167] As the disease worsens, it is characterized by diphtheritic lesions of the oral cavity and trachea and crusty erosive lesions of the eyelids (Fig. 19–9).[162, 164, 167, 170] These lesions pose a serious threat to life, because affected birds stop eating and secondary bacterial and fungal infections of the damaged tissue are common.[170] Extensive oral and tracheal lesions can obstruct airflow, resulting in dyspnea and asphyxiation. Scabs often seal the eyelids shut, and second-

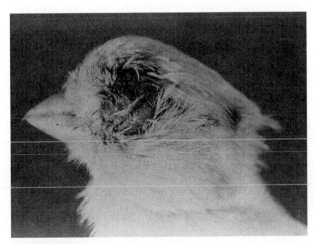

Figure 19–8

Ocular lesions of cutaneous or "dry" pox in a canary. (Photograph kindly provided by Dr. David Graham.)

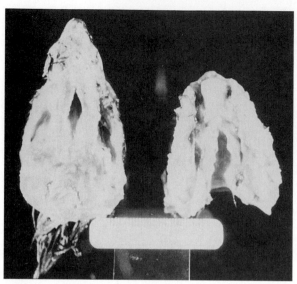

Figure 19-9

Mucosal or "wet" pox in a nestling Amazon parrot. (Photograph kindly provided by Dr. David Graham.)

ary conjunctivitis, keratitis, corneal ulceration, and corneal perforation may follow.[170] If untreated, many of these birds die. Surviving birds often have long-term ocular complications. Mild lesions of little consequence included slight deformation and depigmentation of lids and the deposition of subepithelial crystals in the cornea. More serious sequelae include obstruction of the nasal lacrimal duct, chronic conjunctivitis and corneal erosion, corneal neovascularization, symblepharon, cataracts, and enlargement or collapse of the eye.[170] In some birds, cutaneous pox may also accompany the mucosal form.

Systemic pox presents as an acute onset disease in canaries. Affected birds have chemosis of the eyelids; they are depressed and dyspneic; they stop eating; and most die within 2 to 3 days. Cutaneous lesions only develop in birds that survive the acute phase of the disease. On necropsy, these birds have extensive air sac lesions and pneumonia. Marked proliferation of bronchial and parabronchial epithelium is noted on histopathology examination.[8, 162]

Biology

Poxviruses are large, (250–350 nm) enveloped DNA viruses. There are numerous poxviruses, and indi-

vidual poxviruses have differing host specificities. Some infect only a single species, whereas others infect several. The relationship between different poxviruses is complex and has been examined serologically, through infection studies, and by comparison of virus proteins and DNA sequences. The canary poxvirus infects only canaries and canaries hybridized to other species. The range of the parrot poxvirus appears to be confined to South American parrots.[8, 163] A mynah poxvirus has been isolated that may infect only mynahs. However, at least one species of mynah may also be susceptible to the starling poxvirus.[163]

It is generally accepted that poxviruses cannot penetrate healthy mucous membranes or skin. Thus, they require an open wound or an insect vector for transmission. Disease in canaries is exclusively a disease of birds raised out-of-doors and exposed to mosquitoes. In contrast, disease in nestling parrots may be transmitted on hand-feeding utensils. Abrasions of the mouth, the result of aggressive feeding behavior in these birds, are believed to be the portals of entry for the virus. Although less common, aerosolized virus in feces or feather dander may directly infect respiratory epithelium.[163]

Pox lesions may be localized to the area of infection, or the virus may become systemic, resulting in a disseminated disease.[8, 163] Poxviruses grow best in replicating cells. They produce a hormone analogous to epidermal growth factor. This hormone induces cell division and results in the observed proliferative lesions. Following infection, several weeks may pass before the body mounts an effective immune response. When it does, the lesions regress rapidly. Following infection, immunity is believed to be life-long. The infection cycle is maintained by virus in the environment and by latent infections. Virus in dried scabs is very resistant to the environment and has been shown to survive outside the bird for more than a year. Latent infections in chickens have been reactivated experimentally, but it is unclear what the role of latency is in the course of the natural disease.[163]

Diagnosis

Characteristic clinical signs in susceptible species are highly suggestive of poxvirus infections. In some birds, pox lesions, however, may resemble those of several other diseases. Pox infections can be confirmed either at necropsy or with cytologic examination. Poxviruses replicate in the cytoplasm and form large eosinophilic intracytoplasmic inclusions (Bollinger bodies) (Fig. 19–10). The presence of these inclusions in fixed stained tissues, scrapings, or aspirates is pathognomonic. Inclusion bodies are generally common, but in the mucosal form of the disease, especially in advanced lesions, they may be rare. Characteristic proliferative lesions are also found in poxvirus infections, but these can be lost with the development of secondary bacterial or fungal disease. Virus isolation or experimental infection can be used to confirm a diagnosis, but these techniques are predominately research tools.[163, 164, 167]

Treatment

Treatment, when necessary, is predominately supportive, and is designed to keep the animal alive until its own immune system can eliminate the virus. In parrots, vitamin A (10,000 to 25,000 IU/300 g, intramuscularly, once) has been suggested to be efficacious. Antibiotics and antifungals are indicated when secondary infections complicate the disease. Fluid therapy and tube feeding may be necessary in the anorectic bird. Intensive management of ocular lesions in nestling parrots is felt to limit complications. In one report, affected eyes were washed daily with Johnson's baby shampoo and rinsed with 1 ounce of 2% merbromin (Mercurochrome) and 4 ounces of balanced saline solution (Collyrium) daily. Topical chloramphenicol ointment was also applied. Scabs were allowed to fall off without assistance because manual removal appeared to result in more lid damage.[170] Although tempting, surgical removal of large tumor-like pox lesions is not indicated, because masses regrow.[165]

Control

In canaries, screening in outdoor aviaries eliminates mosquitoes and stops transmission of the disease. If this is impractical, a commercial modified live canary pox vaccine (Poximune-C, Biomune, Lenexa, KS) is available. Field studies reported by the manufacturer of this vaccine suggest that immunization in the face of an outbreak is efficacious.[172] The efficacy of this vaccine in other species against other poxviruses has not been tested. Given the divergence of poxviruses and the variable response of different avian species to attenuated viruses, the practitioner should use this vaccine only in canaries.

Control in imported hand-fed parrots requires proper hygiene. Each bird needs to be fed with its own hand-feeding implement, affected birds need to be isolated and fed last, and handlers must wash their hands frequently. Vaccination trials with a killed pox vaccine suggested that early vaccination

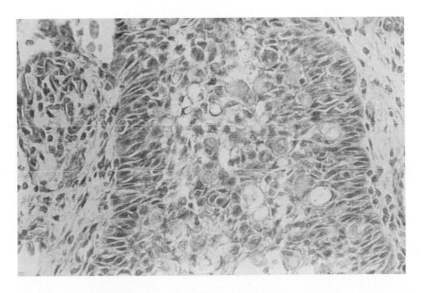

Figure 19–10

Hematoxylin- and eosin-stained section of a cutaneous pox lesion. Cells containing intracytoplasmic eosinophilic inclusion bodies are numerous. The inclusions are so massive as to obscure the remaining cellular structures.

of parrots in the country of origin immediately after capture would significantly reduce mortality.[173, 174]

PARAMYXOVIRUSES

Clinical presentations are listed in Table 19–9.

Disease Synopsis

Exotic Newcastle disease or velogenic viscerotropic Newcastle disease (VVND) is a reportable disease that continues to be a major threat to the poultry industry. In the US, since the imposition of quarantine procedures for all imported birds, outbreaks of this disease have all originated from smuggled parrots[175, 176] or fighting cocks.[175] Mexican and Central American parrots, in particular juvenile yellow-naped (*Amazona ochracephala auropalliata*)[175] and double-yellow headed Amazon parrots,[176] are most commonly implicated as sources of these outbreaks.

Manifestations of VVND include depression, anorexia, weight loss, and diarrhea.[176–178] Respiratory signs are intermittently seen. Neurologic signs are inconsistently present and are found predominantly in birds that survive the first several days of infection. They include ataxia, torticollis, opisthotonos, dilatation of the pupils, head bobbing, unilateral or bilateral paralysis of the wings or legs, and chorea. Morbidity and mortality are species-dependent. In one study of experimentally infected birds, 55% of the orange-fronted conures died, whereas only 29% of the double yellow-headed Amazon parrots and 22% of the budgerigars died. Other parrot species may be even less susceptible to disease. Birds that survive infection or that are inapparently infected may shed virus from 3 weeks to over 1 year.[177]

Paramyxovirus-2 (PMV-2) is a virus whose reservoir appears to be wild passerine birds.[179, 180] The virus has a worldwide distribution. Many, possibly most, infections result in a transient respiratory disease or are entirely asymptomatic.[179, 181] Many virus isolates have come from asymptomatic birds, suggesting that persistently infected birds may serve to potentiate virus spread. PMV-2 is believed to have caused a fatal disease in an African grey parrot.[181] At necropsy, the bird was cachectic and had tracheitis and pneumonia. Alexander reports that PMV-2 parrot isolates are predominately derived from birds that were housed with imported finches.[179]

PMV-3 is more pathogenic than PMV-2. Infection and disease occur predominately in psittacine birds, but may spill over into in contact passerine species.[179, 182–187] PMV-3 has been recognized in Japan, Europe, Britain, and the US.[179] It is most often associated with recently imported birds, although

Table 19–9

PARAMYXOVIRUSES: CLINICAL PRESENTATIONS

Signs	Species Affected	Incidence
Exotic Newcastle Disease Virus (Paramyxovirus-1 [PMV-1])		
Nonspecific, systemic signs with variable mortality, central nervous system disease, conjunctivitis, and respiratory disease	Many parrot species are susceptible In the US, most often found in smuggled Mexican and Central American parrots	Sporadic
Paramyxovirus-2 (PMV-2)		
Pneumonia, tracheitis, and death	Imported parrots exposed to finches	Uncommon to rare
Inapparent infection or upper respiratory signs	Wild and imported passerines	Common
Paramyxovirus-3 (PMV-3)		
Central nervous system signs: torticollis, circling, inability to fly, variable mortality	Numerous parrots, especially *Neophema* species	Moderately common, mostly imported birds
	Canaries and finches	Uncommon, mostly imported birds
Neurologic signs with myocarditis at necropsy	Cockatiels	One report
Paramyxovirus 5 (PMV-5)		
Not reported, other than high mortality	Budgerigar	Multiple outbreaks in Japan in the early 1970s

outbreaks in an outdoor aviary of cockatiels has also been documented.[188] *Neophema* species, *Agapornis* species, *Amazona* species, cockatiels, and budgerigars are most susceptible to disease. In these birds, neurologic signs and signs of pancreatic insufficiency predominate.[182, 187] Initially birds go off feed and "fluff up." Death may follow in as little as 1 to 2 days. If the disease is prolonged, central nervous system signs inseparable from those described for velogenic viscerotropic Newcastle disease (VVND) develop. PMV-3 also targets the pancreas, and some birds have voluminous stools containing undigested starch and fat.[182] Mortality rates are variable. In one reported outbreak in lovebirds, several hundred birds died. Others report high morbidity but low mortality.

VanDerHeyden and Reed describe an unusual form of PMV-3 in cockatiels.[188] These birds were held in an outdoor aviary. Infection was confined to nestlings. Affected birds had classic neurologic signs but were also dyspneic. At necropsy, a lymphoplasmacytic myocarditis resulting in cardiomegaly and pericardial effusion was the predominant finding.

In PMV-3 infections in finches, nonspecific signs including diarrhea, dysphagia, dyspnea, and conjunctivitis have been reported.[186, 187] Death follows in a few days, or birds survive with clinical signs for 2 weeks and then recover.

PMV-5 has been isolated only from budgerigars. In the early 1970s, outbreaks of disease caused by this virus resulted in high mortality rates in many Japanese budgerigar collections.[189] Since then, PMV-5 has not been isolated.[179]

Biology

Paramyxoviruses are enveloped single-stranded RNA viruses.[190] They hemagglutinate red blood cells, and this property is extremely useful diagnostically. There are nine PMV serotypes. Only serotypes 1, 2, 3, and 5 cause disease in psittacine birds. Within serotypes, there may be considerable variation in pathogenicity. Although PMV-2 and PMV-3 are capable of causing disease in parrots and passerines, they are relatively minor pathogens. PMV-5, at least for now, has disappeared entirely.

Numerous strains of PMV-1 exist. Strains are classified according to their ability to cause disease in chickens, and according to the type of disease that the virus causes (Table 19–10).[191] Low virulent strains of PMV-1 are enzootic in wild bird populations throughout the world. During the 20th century, epizootic outbreaks of highly virulent (exotic) PMV-1 or VVND have caused devastating losses to the poultry industry. Most countries control this disease through immunization programs.[190] In the US, the disease has been eradicated, and strict regulations on the importation of birds are enforced to prevent its re-entry. All birds entering the US are quarantined for 30 days. Birds dying in the first 15 days are cultured for VVND, and cloacal swabs are obtained from a subset of the live birds for virus isolation. If VVND is found, the birds are refused entry into the country.[192] Small outbreaks of VVND continue in the US almost on a yearly basis and have been traced back to smuggled parrots and fighting cocks.[175, 176]

Infected birds shed large quantities of virus in

Table 19–10

STRAINS OF PARAMYXOVIRUS-1 ACCORDING TO PATHOGENICITY IN CHICKENS

Strain		Pathogenicity	Target Organs	Time to Death in Inoculated Eggs (Hours)
Velogenic*				
	Viscerotropic	Highly	Digestive	<60
	Neurotrophic	Highly	Respiratory Central nervous system	<60
Mesogenic		Moderately	Respiratory Central nervous system	60–90
Lentogenic		Mildly	Respiratory	>90
Inapparent		Not pathogenic	Intestinal	

*Exotic Newcastle disease

their feces and respiratory secretions. Both inhalation and ingestion of virus result in infection. Persistent virus shedding from inapparently infected or recovered birds may last for months to more than 1 year. Movement of these birds, or movement of contaminated material (e.g., by vehicles, clothing, and cages) can further disseminate the virus.[190]

Diagnosis

Ultimately, the diagnosis of VVND or any other paramyxovirus infection can be made only by virus isolation. Clinical signs and historic information can, however, alert practitioners to the possibility that they are dealing with this disease. Young Mexican and Central American parrots, particularly the yellow-naped and double-yellow headed Amazon parrots, are most often implicated in VVND outbreaks.[175–177] These birds should be viewed with suspicion if they were acquired in large numbers or acquired at a below-market-value price, do not have leg bands or have loose-fitting closed bands, are generally unhealthy, or originate in states bordering on Mexico. The loss of multiple birds and the development of neurologic disease should also alert practitioners to the possibility of this disease.[176] Ancillary tests are of limited value for diagnosis. Complete blood count results have been reported to be normal. Hypoglycemia, hyponatremia, and hyperkalemia may be present, along with mild elevations in serum creatine phosphokinase, alkaline phosphatase, and aspartate aminotransferase concentrations.[176–178] Findings at necropsy are generally nonspecific. Gross lesions may be entirely absent or may consist of serosal hemorrhages and mucosal necrosis of the gastrointestinal tract.[177] The trachea, lung, liver, and spleen should be shipped on ice, not frozen for virus isolation.[8] Histologically, vascular, lymphoid, and respiratory lesions are variably present.[190] A nonsuppurative encephalomyelitis may be the only indication of VVND infection.[193]

If this disease is suspected, it should be immediately reported to the appropriate government authorities. In the US, facilities believed to house VVND-infected or -exposed birds are quarantined. All birds are swabbed cloacally three times, 7 to 10 days apart. If VVND is identified in a collection, all the birds are destroyed.[176]

Preventative health measures outlined in the be-

Table 19–11
AVIAN INFLUENZA: CLINICAL PRESENTATION

Signs	Species Affected	Incidence
Variable, but may include central nervous system signs	Several parrot species reported	Rare

ginning of this chapter provide the aviculturalist and pet bird owner with considerable protection from this disease.

AVIAN INFLUENZA

Clinical presentations are listed in Table 19–11.

Disease Synopsis and Biology

Avian influenza (AI) viruses are orthomyxoviruses. They are enveloped viruses with a segmented RNA genome. AI viruses are classified on the basis of the antigenic relationship of their hemagglutinating antigens (HA) and neuraminidase antigens (NA). Thirteen HAs and nine NAs have been identified. There is considerable variability in the pathogenicity of influenza viruses. Most infections result in few or no signs. However, virulent strains have caused devastating losses in flocks of wild birds, wild and domestic waterfowl, and poultry. In the early 1980s an outbreak of AI in Pennsylvania cost over $60 million to eradicate. The most important reservoirs of infection are wild birds.[194]

Although isolated from several passerine and psittacine species, AI in cage and aviary birds is rare, and most isolations have been from birds dying in quarantine.[195–198] In parrots, reported signs were strain-dependent and ranged from ataxia and torticollis to depression, diarrhea, and rough plumage.[198] Mortality rates were also strain-dependent.[8] Diagnosis of AI is dependent on isolation of the virus. Virus is most readily recovered from the cloaca or trachea. Swabs of these organs from necropsy specimens or live birds can be submitted for virus isolation.[194]

EASTERN EQUINE ENCEPHALITIS (EEE)

Clinical presentation in some species is outlined in Table 19–12.

Table 19-12

EASTERN EQUINE ENCEPHALITIS: CLINICAL PRESENTATIONS

Signs	Species Affected	Incidence
Respiratory distress, paraparesis, and death	Gouldian finch	One reported outbreak
Abdominal distension, polyserositis, and death	Macaws Others?	One confirmed outbreak

Disease Synopsis, Biology, and Diagnosis

EEE is an alphavirus of the family Togaviridae.[199] It is a mosquito-borne virus that is endemic in wild birds in the eastern and southeastern US.[199–201] Several mosquito species and possibly other biting insects are responsible for virus transmission and may serve as reservoirs of infection.[200] EEE infections in wild birds are often asymptomatic, whereas infections in horses, man, and some domestic avian species result in a severe, often fatal disease in which neurologic signs predominate.[199–201] Sporadic outbreaks of disease in humans and horses are most common in the late summer and fall when insect vectors are abundant. Bird-to-bird transmission also occurs through cannibalism, although this is thought to play a minor role in the dissemination of EEE.[200]

EEE has been isolated from two Florida aviaries where it was believed to cause significant mortality. In the first outbreak, Gouldian finches housed out-of-doors consistently experienced respiratory signs and paraparesis followed by death. Twenty one of 25 birds died. EEE was recovered from the only bird for which virus isolation was attempted. Histologically, a multifocal bronchopneumonia was identified; nervous tissue was not examined.[202]

The second aviary lost four macaws ranging in age from 7 to 12 weeks.[203, 204] Clinical signs varied from sudden death to decreased appetite with abdominal distension. Grossly, serositis with extensive abdominal fluid was found in three birds (Fig. 19–9). Histologically, in addition to the serosal lesions, hepatic disease, interstitial pneumonia, and lymphocytic proventriculitis were consistent findings. EEE was isolated from an inoculum of pooled tissues from two of the birds.[205] Infection studies in chickens reproduced many of the same lesions seen

in the parrots. A fifth macaw from the same aviary also died immediately preceding this outbreak. Histologically, it was diagnosed with psittacine proventricular dilatation syndrome (PPDS).

This report of EEE in parrots raises many questions. With the exception of the bird dying with PPDS, all the other birds were incubator-raised and would have had little opportunity for mosquito exposure. How the virus was transmitted to them is not known. In this aviary, also, many birds both before and after the apparent EEE outbreak developed PPDS. Whether this was a coincidental occurrence or whether it represents a cause-and-effect relationship is also not known.

Because so little is known about this disease in cage birds, few suggestions for control can be made. Practitioners in the southern and eastern portions of the US may suspect EEE if neurologic signs occur in birds housed out-of-doors during the late summer and fall. Although histologic evidence may suggest this disease, proof of EEE infection requires virus isolation. Brain, spleen, liver, or blood should be submitted for virus isolation.[200] They should be sent on ice, but not frozen.[203, 204] Indoor housing or screening would be expected to reduce exposure to insect vectors.

REOVIRUS

Clinical presentation is listed in Table 19–13.

Disease Synopsis

The vast majority of psittacine reovirus isolates have been from recently imported birds.[206–212] Reported outbreaks of disease for which a reovirus has been attributed began in quarantine or within a few

Table 19-13

REOVIRUS: CLINICAL PRESENTATIONS

Signs	Species Affected	Incidence
Depression, weakness, weight loss, diarrhea, paralysis, yellow pigmentation of the urates, and edema of legs and head	Recently imported Old World parrots, especially African grey parrots	Common
	Imported New World and aviary parrots	Uncommon

weeks following quarantine.[206] Disease outbreaks were initially described in imported lots of African grey parrots,[206–208] but epornitic outbreaks of this disease have since been described in other African, Indian, and Australian parrots.[206–208, 210] Less commonly, New World parrots may also be susceptible to infection and disease.[206–208, 210]

Experimentally, clinical signs are those of an acute systemic disease.[208, 209] They include lethargy, anorexia, and yellow-orange staining of the urates. In naturally occurring outbreaks, nasal discharge, dyspnea, dilated pupils with intraocular hemorrhage, cachexia, edema of the head and legs, and paralysis have all been observed.[206, 213] Many experimental and naturally occurring infections are fatal, with death following as early as a day after the onset of clinical signs.[209] Numerous birds may die suddenly in a few days, or low daily death rates extending over several weeks may occur.[206–208]

In experimentally infected birds, within 2 days inoculated birds had a demonstrable decrease in serum albumen and a concurrent increase in gamma globulins.[208] In naturally occurring infections, heterophilia followed by a marked heteropenia and anemia have been described.[207] Elevations in serum lactate dehydrogenase and aspartate aminotransferase levels have also been documented.[207, 208]

Some natural outbreaks of reovirus disease are complicated by multiple other infectious agents such as *Salmonella* species, *Aspergillus* species, and avian PMV-3 infections.[206–208, 210] Each of these pathogens contributes to the clinical picture, making it difficult to know if observed clinical signs are from a reovirus infection alone, a combination of reovirus infection with other infectious agents, or the result of another pathogen entirely. Likewise, it is not known if reovirus infections may predispose birds to other secondary infections, or if the conditions for outbreaks of reovirus disease are also favorable for these other diseases.

Biology

Reoviruses are nonenveloped, approximately 75 nm, double-stranded RNA viruses with a segmented genome.[209, 214] They are highly refractory to many disinfectants.[214] Reoviruses are not always pathogenic, and they have been routinely isolated from apparently healthy poultry.[214] They have been regularly isolated from shipments of imported birds. At first, reoviruses were not correlated with disease[211, 212]; subsequently, however, clinical and experimental evidence demonstrated conclusively that reoviruses can be primary pathogens.[108, 206–210] In poultry, ingestion of the virus is believed to be the most common means of infection, although inhaled virus may also be infectious.[214] Experimentally, parrots have been infected orally, intramuscularly,[208, 209] and intrathecally.[208] Clinical evidence of disease can be observed as early as 4 days after infection.[207] Death occurs within 6 to 18 days.[208, 209] Not all birds develop signs, and not all birds with signs die.[208] Clubb states that New World parrots are less likely to die with reovirus infections.[207]

Symptomatically infected birds and birds recovering from disease may potentially be carriers. The long-term shedding of reovirus has not been documented in parrots. Circumstantial evidence, however, has suggested that survivors of a previous reovirus outbreak were the source of a second.[208] In poultry, transmission of reovirus occurs in a small percentage of eggs.[214] The role that vertical transmission may play in disseminating this disease in parrots is not known.

Diagnosis

Reovirus should be suspected in sudden or slowly progressive outbreaks of disease in recently imported birds. Gross necropsy findings are nonspecific. Hepatosplenomegaly and focal depressed discolorations of the hepatic capsular and cut surfaces are the most common lesions described.[108, 206, 207, 209, 213, 215, 216] Less commonly, serosal hemorrhages, enteritis, renal enlargement, and air sacculitis have been found.[206, 207, 209, 210] Lesions from concurrent diseases (e.g., aspergillosis, salmonellosis, and psittacosis) have also been present.[206, 207, 210] Multifocal coagulative hepatic necrosis was a nonspecific but nearly uniform finding.[108, 209, 213, 215, 216] Splenic and bone marrow necrosis also occurs. Focal mononuclear cell infiltrates, another nonspecific finding, have also been reported in the liver, kidney, and lamina propria of the intestine.[209] Intravascular thrombi may account for the head and limb edema seen in some birds.[207, 209]

Confirmation of reovirus infection can be made

by fluorescence antibody staining of impression smears, electron microscopy of crushed tissue preparations or fixed sections, and virus isolation in chicken eggs and cells. The lung, liver, spleen, and intestines should be submitted for virus isolation.[209, 210] An immunodiffusion assay has been found to be beneficial in detecting antibodies in birds surviving infection.[208]

Prevention and Control

Generally, reovirus infections are associated with imported wild-caught birds. As a result, the prevalence of reovirus infection and disease has declined dramatically with the decline in the number of wild-caught birds imported each year. For the typical hobbyist or aviculturalist, reoviruses pose only a very limited threat, and standard disease prevention measures should go a long way to reducing any danger this virus might pose. In contrast, newly imported birds should be quarantined for prolonged periods (at least 60 days) before being introduced into a collection.

In the face of an outbreak, the use of chlorhexidine in the drinking water has been suggested to reduce mortality. Likewise, an experimental vaccine given early in an outbreak appeared to reduce mortality.[207]

MISCELLANEOUS VIRAL DISEASES

This section briefly mentions viruses that have been reported only once or whose detection or isolation is of unknown significance.

An entero-like virus was identified in wild-caught, 7 to 10-week-old galahs and sulphur-crested cockatoos in Australia. Ten to 20% of the birds studied developed a green to green-yellow mucoid diarrhea within a week of capture. Accompanying signs included depression and reduced food consumption. All birds died or were euthanized within 4 weeks of the onset of signs. Histologically, blunting and fusion of the duodenal and jejunal villi were observed. Virus particles could also be identified in some enterocytes.[217]

An organism thought to be a coronavirus was isolated from three parrots originating from two pet shops.[218, 219] Clinical signs were not reported, but

experimental infections produced hepatic and splenic lesions in chicks and adult budgerigars. Unlike the day-old chicks, the adult budgerigars did not die. Detailed characterization of this agent was never completed, and its identity remains unknown.

Gough and coworkers describe a short-lived disease in a lovebird, species not reported, in which the bird had rapid weight loss and paralysis of the left leg. On histopathology examination, few lesions were found to account for clinical signs. A rotavirus was isolated from this bird, but its relation to the observed disease remains unknown.[220]

A small virus resembling a parvovirus was identified in cockatoos with beak and feather virus infections and a diarrheal disease.[37] Further characterization of this virus has not been undertaken, and its relationship to the observed clinical signs remains unknown.

DISEASES THOUGHT TO BE CAUSED BY INFECTIOUS AGENTS

Internal Papillomatosis of Parrots

Clinical presentation in some species is outlined in Table 19–14.

Disease Synopsis

Internal papillomatosis of parrots (IPP) is a disease of New World parrots. Macaws; hawk-headed, pionus, and Amazon parrots; and conures are susceptible.[221–225] Susceptibility is at least somewhat species-specific and disease is especially common in hawk-headed parrots and green-winged *(Ara chlo-*

T a b l e 1 9 – 1 4

INTERNAL PAPILLOMATOSIS OF PARROTS: CLINICAL PRESENTATION

Signs	Species Affected	Incidence
Papilliferous lesions of the oral cavity, esophagus, lacrimal duct, conjunctiva, and vent	Macaws, hawk-headed and Amazon parrots	Common
	Conures	Moderately common
	Pionus parrots and caiques	Uncommon
Bile and/or pancreatic duct carcinoma	Macaws, Amazon parrots	Moderately common

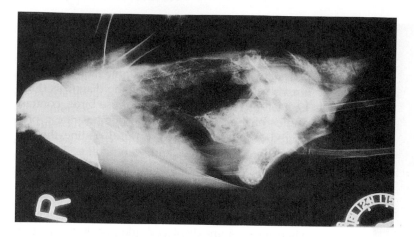

Figure 19–15

Contrast study of the blue and gold macaw shown in Figure 19–13, lateral view. Contrast material is present in the dilated lumina of the proventriculus and ventriculus.

tion of PPDS from one affected aviary to another through the movement of birds suggests, however, that PPDS is caused by an infectious agent.[233, 234, 239, 247] The presence of intranuclear inclusion bodies and virus particles in nerve[251, 252] and proventricular mucosal cells[248] have also fueled speculation that this disease is caused by a virus.

If virally induced, the onset of disease following infection must vary tremendously. After exposure to affected birds, new cases may not develop for weeks to more than 1 year. The explanation for such a prolonged incubation period is not known. It has been postulated that these lesions may reflect an immune-mediated disease triggered by an initial virus infection.[108] If this proves to be the case, variable and often prolonged periods between the onset of infection and the development of disease should be expected.

Diagnosis

Common clinical signs, described earlier, should increase practitioners' suspicions that they are dealing with PPDS. Other diseases, however, can cause similar signs. Diffuse internal papillomatosis of the crop, proventriculus, and ventriculus; proventricular and ventricular tumors; foreign bodies; lead poisoning; mycobacterial infections; and diseases resulting in the disruption of the ventricular koilin layer are but a few diseases that can mimic PPDS.[235, 245, 247, 254, 255]

Radiography with and without contrast media is an important diagnostic tool. A presumptive diagno-

sis can be reached if the proventriculus or ventriculus is massively dilated. Many times, however, radiographic changes of PPDS are subtle. Delayed passage of contrast media and loss of the normal narrowing of the proventricular-ventricular junction may be the only radiographic findings. Overinterpretation of radiographic findings can also result in a misdiagnosis of PPDS. Care must be taken in evaluating the proventriculus, because there is considerable species variation in size and shape. In addition, hand-fed nestlings routinely have some dilation of the proventriculus.[247]

Most PPDS-affected birds die after a short course of disease and diagnosis is made at necropsy. In the classic case, the proventriculus is massively distended with ingesta, and its walls are so thin as to be transparent (Fig. 19–16).[233, 234, 238, 240, 242] Ventricular dilatation and atrophy of the muscularis is less frequent. In a small percentage of cases the small intestines are dilated.[243, 248, 249] Frequently, gross lesions of the digestive system are not definitive, and diagnosis is dependent on histopathology examination. Histologically, a lymphoplasmacytic infiltration of the intrinsic and extrinsic nerves of the proventriculus, ventriculus, crop, and intestine is found.[108, 236, 241, 242, 252] The degenerative changes found in these nerves account for the gastrointestinal signs. Lesions are not always generalized, and thus it is best to submit the entire alimentary tract, or at least multiple transverse sections through the crop, proventriculus, ventriculus, and intestine to the pathologist. A nonsuppurative encephalomyelitis is another manifestation of PPDS. Because these lesions may be widely scattered, but have an increased frequency in the brainstem,[236, 241, 246, 249, 252] the entire brain and at least some of the spinal cord should be submitted for histopathology examination.

In cases of PPDS when proventricular and ventricular distension is absent or minimal, diagnosis can be confirmed only by biopsy of the proventriculus,[256] ventriculus[243, 247] or crop.[235] Biopsy of the crop is the least risky. PPDS-specific lesions of the crop, however, are variably present[235, 236] and when they are present are not always diffuse.[235] In contrast, PPDS-specific lesions were detected in the proventriculus and ventriculus in 100% of the cases reported in one study.[236] Biopsy techniques for these organs are described.[247, 256] Both techniques impart some risk to the bird, especially if it is already compromised by advanced disease. Because disease is not found in all nerves, and because not all biopsy specimens contain nerves, PPDS cannot be ruled out with a negative biopsy report.

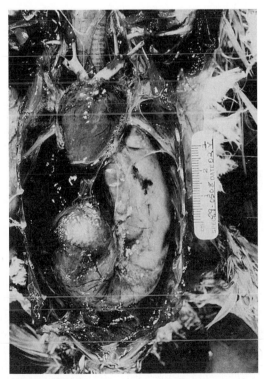

Figure 19–16

Blue and gold macaw with psittacine proventricular dilatation syndrome. The proventriculus is massively distended with seeds. (Photograph kindly provided by Dr. David Graham.)

Treatment

There is no treatment for the primary disease. In most cases, clinical signs progress rapidly and the birds die. In others, disease progression may take weeks to months and the birds may have a reasonably good quality of life during this time. Liquid or soft diets may prolong the life of birds with impaired gastrointestinal motility.

NEOPLASIA

Neoplasia is a common diagnosis in cage birds and poultry. Details of avian neoplastic diseases are presented elsewhere in this book, and readers are referred to an excellent review of lymphoid neoplasia in pet birds by Coleman.[257] Marek's disease, a herpesvirus, and several retroviruses are the etiologic agent of most of the tumors observed in poultry.[258–260] The role viruses may play in neoplastic disorders of cage birds remains unknown. Of the cage birds, the incidence of neoplastic disease is perhaps the highest in the budgerigar. Increasingly, evidence suggests that an oncogenic retrovirus may play a role in the development of these tumors. In one study, 47.3% of budgerigars with renal tumors had group-specific antigens for the avian leukosis virus in their sera.[261] In a second study, retrovirus sequences were found in six of eight budgerigar tumors.[262] More detailed studies must be completed before a cause-and-effect relationship can be proven.

Canaries are another species in which neoplasia, particularly lymphoid neoplasia, is common.[257, 263] To date, nothing has been published verifying a virus etiology for these tumors. However, the frequency of this disease, as well as its tendency to occur in multiple birds within the same aviary, suggests that a virus may be involved.

Multifocal Tumors Involving the Lungs in Cockatiels

The author is aware of several cockatiel aviaries in which there has been an unusually high incidence of neoplasia involving the lungs.[264] Clinically, birds present with a history of increasing exercise intolerance and dyspnea. By the time the owner recog-

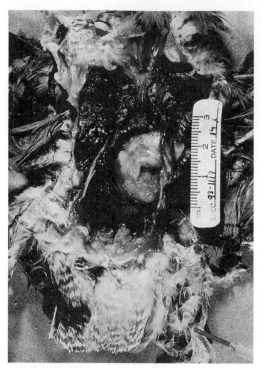

Figure 19–17

Large thoracic mass in a cockatiel presenting with severe dyspnea. Several other cockatiels in the same small aviary developed similar tumors.

nizes the disease, birds may be in severe respiratory distress. Infrequently, paresis or paralysis of the legs may be another presenting sign. These tumors are rapidly growing and highly invasive. Multiple tumors are generally found in the lung. As these tumors grow they compress and collapse adjacent lung parenchyma and air sacs. Dyspnea develops most often as the tumors extend into the thoracic inlet and collapse the trachea. Neurologic signs develop when the tumor invades the vertebral column and compresses the spinal cord. Radiographically, one or more masses of soft tissue density is visible in birds with clinical signs.

At necropsy, these tumors are light tan to yellow (Fig. 19–17). A single pulmonary mass may be present, but multiple masses are more common. Histologically, neoplastic cells are found in multiple organs. The histologic appearance of these tumors is variable. However, a fairly consistent finding is histiocytic-like cells with marked enlargement of their nuclei reminiscent of cytopathic effects induced by the avian APV. To date, APV DNA has not been detected in these tumors using multiple virus specific probes. In addition, anti-APV antibodies have not been detected in the serum of several affected birds examined. The possible role that a virus may play in this disease awaits additional investigation.

References

1. Scott FW: Feline infectious diseases - practical virucidal disinfectants. Proc AAHA 46th Ann Meeting, 1979, p 804.
2. Ritchie BW, Prichard N, Pesti D, et al: Susceptibility of avian polyomavirus to inactivation. J Assoc Avian Vet 7:193–195, 1994.
3. Goryo M, Sugimura H, Matsumotto S: Isolation of an agent inducing chicken anaemia. Avian Pathol 14:483–496, 1989.
4. Taylor SP: The effect of acetone on the viability of chicken anemia agent. Avian Dis 36:753–754, 1992.
5. Urlings HAP, DeBoer GF, van Roozelaar DJ, Koch G: Inactivation of chicken anemia virus in chickens by heating and fermentation. Vet Q 15:85–88, 1993.
6. Grimes JE, Phalen DN, Arizmendi F: Chlamydia latex agglutination antigen and protocol improvement and psittacine bird anti-chlamydial immunoglobulin reactivity. Avian Dis 37:817–824, 1993.
7. Grimes JE: Personal communication, 1995.
8. Gerlach H: Viruses. In Ritchie BW, Harrison GJ, Harrison LR (eds): Avian Medicine: Principles and Application. Lake Worth, FL, Wingers Publishing, 1994, pp 862–948.
9. McOrist S, Black SG, Pass DA, et al: Beak and feather dystrophy in wild sulphur-crested cockatoos (*Cackatua galerita*). J Wildl Dis 20:120–124, 1984.
10. Pass DA, Perry RA: The pathology of psittacine beak and feather disease. Aust Vet J 61:69–74, 1984.
11. Pass DA, Perry RA: The pathogenesis of psittacine beak and feather disease. Proc Int Conf Avian Med, Toronto, 1984, pp 113–119.
12. Smith R: PB and FD: A cluster of cases in a cockatoo breeding facility. Proc Assoc Avian Vet, 1986, Miami, pp 17–20.
13. Speer B: In my experience: Unusual expression of PBFD. J Assoc Avian Vet 4:19, 1990.
14. Dahlhausen B, Radabaugh S. Update on psittacine beak and feather disease and avian polyomavirus testing. Proc Assoc Avian Vet, Nashville, 1993, pp 5–7.
15. Ritchie BW, Niagro FD, Latimer KS, et al: Ultrastructural, protein composition and antigenic comparison of psittacine beak and feather disease virus recovered from four genera of psittacine birds. J Wildl Dis 26:196–203, 1990.
16. Wylie SL, Pass DA: Experimental reproduction of psittacine beak and feather disease/french moult. Avian Pathol 16:269–281, 1987.
17. Ritchie BW, Niagro FD, Lukert PD, et al: A review of psittacine beak and feather disease. J Assoc Avian Vet 3:143–149, 1989.
18. Schmidt R: In my experience: Pathologist's view of PBFD in African greys. J Assoc Avian Vet 4:19, 1990.
19. Allen SK: In my experience: Psittacine beak and feather disease in an African grey parrot. J Assoc Avian Vet 4:18–19, 1990.
20. Greenacre CB, Latimer KS, Niagro FD, et al: Psittacine beak

and feather disease in a scarlet macaw *(Ara macao)*. J Assoc Avian Vet 6:95–98, 1992.

21. Huff DG, Schmidt RE, Fudge AM: Psittacine beak and feather syndrome in a blue-fronted Amazon *(Amazona aestiva)*. AAV Today 2:84–86, 1988.

22. Latimer KS, Rakich PM, Niagro FD, et al: An updated review of psittacine beak and feather disease. J Assoc Avian Vet 5:211–220, 1991.

23. Raidal SR, Firth GA, Cross GM: Vaccination and challenge studies with psittacine beak and feather disease virus. Aust Vet J 70:437–441, 1993.

24. Graham DL: Feather and beak disease: Its biology, management, and an experiment in its eradication from a breeding aviary. Proc Assoc Avian Vet, Phoenix, 1990, pp 8–11.

25. Ritchie BW, Latimer KS, Lukert PD, et al: Preventing psittacine beak and feather virus infections. Proc Joint Conf Am Assoc Zoo Vet and Am Assoc Wildl Vet, East Lansing, 1995, pp 193–198.

26. Jacobson ER, Clubb S, Simpson C, et al: Feather and beak dystrophy and necrosis in cockatoos: Clinicopathologic evaluations. J Am Vet Med Assoc 189:999–1005, 1986.

27. Latimer KS, Rakich PM, Kircher IM, et al: Extracutaneous viral inclusions in psittacine beak and feather disease. J Vet Diagn Invest 2:204–207, 1991.

28. Ritchie BW, Latimer KS, Niagro FD, et al: Experimental reproduction of psittacine beak and feather disease. Proc Assoc Avian Vet, Houston, 1988, pp 5–6.

29. Ritchie BW, Niagro FD, Latimer KS, et al: Antibody response to and maternal immunity from an experimental psittacine beak and feather disease vaccine. Am J Vet Res 53:1512–1518, 1992.

30. Phalen, DN: Unpublished observation, 1990.

31. Ritchie BW, Niagro FD, Lukert PD: Characterization of a new virus from cockatoos with psittacine beak and feather disease. Virology 171:83–88, 1989.

32. Marshall R, Crowley A: A field study for the control of PBFD virus in wild-caught cockatoos. Proc Assoc Avian Vet, Chicago, 1992, pp 37–41.

33. Raidal SR, McElnea CL, Cross GM: Seroprevalence of psittacine beak and feather disease in wild psittacine birds in New South Wales. Aust Vet J 70:137–139, 1992.

34. Ritchie BW, Niagro FD, Latimer KS, et al: Routes and prevalence of shedding of psittacine beak and feather disease virus. Am J Vet Res 52:1804–1809, 1991.

35. Raidal SR, Sabine M, Cross GM: Laboratory diagnosis of psittacine beak and feather disease by hemagglutination and hemagglutination inhibition. Aust Vet J 70:133–137, 1993.

36. Niagro FD, Ritchie BW, Latimer KS, et al: Polymerase chain reaction detection of PBFD and BFD virus in suspect birds. Proc Assoc Avian Vet, Phoenix, 1990, pp 25–37.

37. Ritchie BW, Niagro FD, Latimer KS, et al: Hemagglutination by psittacine beak and feather disease virus and use of hemagglutination-inhibition for detection of antibodies against the virus. Am J Vet Res 52:1810–1815, 1991.

38. Latimer KS, Niagro FD, Rakich PM, et al: Comparison of DNA dot-blot hybridization, immunoperoxidase staining and routine histopathology in the diagnosis of psittacine beak and feather disease in paraffin-embedded cutaneous tissues. J Assoc Avian Vet 6:165–168, 1992.

39. Latimer KS, Rakich PM, Steffens WL, et al: A novel DNA virus associated with feather inclusions in psittacine beak and feather disease. Vet Pathol 28:300–304, 1991.

40. Ramis A, Latimer KS, Niagro FD, et al: Diagnosis of psittacine beak and feather disease (PBFD) viral infection, avian polyomavirus infection, adenovirus infection and herpesvi-

rus infection in psittacine tissues using DNA *in situ* hybridization. Avian Pathol 23:643–657, 1994.

41. Goldsmith TL: Documentation of passerine circoviral infection. Proc Assoc Avian Vet, Philadelphia, 1995, p 349.

42. Bozeman LH, Davis RB, Gaudry D, et al: Characterization of a papovavirus isolated from fledgling budgerigars. Avian Dis 25:972–980, 1981.

43. Davis RB, Bozeman LH, Gaudry D, et al: A viral disease of fledgling budgerigars. Avian Dis 25:179–183, 1981.

44. Bernier G, Morin M, Marsolais G: A generalized inclusion body disease in the budgerigar *(Melopsittacus ungulatus)* caused by a papovavirus-like agent. Avian Dis 25:1083–1092, 1981.

45. Hirai K, Nonaka H, Fukushi H, et al: Isolation of a papovavirus-like agent from young budgerigars with feather abnormalities. Jpn J Vet Sci 46:577–582, 1984.

46. Müller H, Nitschke R: A polyoma-like virus associated with an acute disease of fledgling budgerigars *(Melopsittacus undulatus)*. Med Microbiol Immunol 175:1–13, 1986.

47. Randall CJ, Less S, Inglis DM: Papovavirus-like infection in budgerigars *(Melopsittacus undulatus)*. Avian Pathol 16:623–633, 1987.

48. Pascucci S, Maestrini N, Misciattelli N, Giovannetti L: Malattia da virus papova-simile nel papagllino ondulato *(Melopsittacus undulatus)*. Clin Vet (Milan) 106:38–41, 1983.

49. Sztojkov V, Saghy E, Meder M, et al: A hullamos papagaj *(Melopsittacus undulatus)* papovavirus okozta megbetegedesenek hazai megallapsitasa. Magy Allatorv Lapja 40:59–63, 1985.

50. Phalen DN, Wilson VG, Graham DL: Organ distribution of avian polyomavirus DNA and virus-neutralizing antibody titers in healthy adult budgerigars. Am J Vet Res 54:2040–2047, 1993.

51. Mathey WJ, Cho BR: Tremors of nestling budgerigars with BFD. Proc 33rd West Poult Dis Conf, Davis, CA 1984, pp 102.

52. Bernier G, Morin M, Marsolais G: Papovavirus induced feather abnormalities and skin lesions in the budgerigar: Clinical and pathological findings. Can Vet J 25:307–310, 1984.

53. Krautwald M-E, Kaleta EF: Relationship(s) of French moult and early virus induced mortality in nestling budgerigars. Proc 8th Int Congress World Vet Poult Assoc, Jerusalem, 1985, pp 115.

54. Clubb SL, Davis RB: Outbreak of a papova-like infection in a psittacine nursery—a retrospective view. Proc Int Conf Avian Med, Toronto, 1984, pp 121–130.

55. Graham DL, Calnek BW: Papovavirus infection in hand-fed parrots: Virus isolation and pathology. Avian Dis 31:398–410, 1987.

56. Jacobson ER, Hines SA, Quesenberry K, et al: Epornitic of papova-like virus associated disease in a psittacine nursery. J Am Vet Med Assoc 185:1337–1341, 1984.

57. Phalen DN, Wilson VG, Graham DL: Epidemiology and diagnosis of avian polyomavirus infection. Proc Assoc Avian Vet, Chicago, 1991, pp 27–31.

58. Ritchie BW, Niagro FD, Latimer KS, et al: Polyomavirus infections in adult psittacine birds. J Assoc Avian Vet 5:202–206, 1991.

59. Pass DA: A papova-like virus infection of lovebirds *(Agapornis sp.)*. Aust Vet J 62:318–319, 1985.

60. Phalen DN, Wilson VG, Graham DL: Long-term virus neutralizing antibody and virus shedding in avian polyomavirus infected parrots. Submitted for publication.

61. Forshaw D, Wyle SL, Pass DA: Infection with a virus resembling papovavirus in Gouldian finches. Aust Vet J 65:26–28, 1988.

62. Garcia A, Latimer KS, Niagro FD et al: Avian polyomavirus infection in three black-bellied seedcrackers *(Pyrenestes ostrinus).* J Assoc Avian Vet 7:79–82, 1993.

63. Garcia A, Latimer KS, Niagro FD, et al: Diagnosis of polyomavirus infection in seedcrackers *(Pyrenestes sp.)* and blue bills *(Spermophaga haematina)* using DNA *in situ* hybridization. Avian Pathol 23:525–537, 1994.

64. Howerth EW, Harmon BG, Latimer KS, et al: Necropsy finding in 111 black-bellied seedcrackers *(Pyrenestes ostrinus)* from the Riverbanks Zoological Park, 1989–1994. Proc Joint Conf Am Assoc Zoo Vet/Wildlife Disease Association/ American Association of Wildlife Vets, Ann Arbor, 1995, pp 212–215.

65. Johnston KM, Riddell C: Intranuclear inclusion bodies in finches. Can Vet J 27:432–434, 1986.

66. Marshall R: Papova-like virus in a finch aviary. Proc Assoc Avian Vet, Seattle, 1989, pp 203–207.

67. Sironi G, Rampin T: Papovavirus like splenohepatic infection in green finches *(Carduelis chloris).* Clin Vet 110:79–82, 1987.

68. Woods L: Case report: Papova-like virus in a painted finch. Proc Assoc Avian Vet, Seattle, 1989, pp 218–219.

69. Lehn H, Müller HL: Cloning and characterization of budgerigar fledgling disease virus, an avian polyomavirus. Virology 151:362–370, 1986.

70. Rott O, Kroger M, Müller HL, Hobom G: The genome of budgerigar fledgling disease virus, an avian polyomavirus. Virology 165:74–86, 1988.

71. Stoll R, Luo D, Kouwehoven B, et al: Molecular and biological characteristics of avian polyomaviruses: Isolates from different species of birds indicate that avian polyomaviruses form a distinct subgenus within the polyomavirus genus. J Gen Virol 74:229–237, 1993.

72. Phalen DN, Wilson VG, Derr J, et al: Phylogenetic analysis of variants of avian polyomaviruses derived from parrots. Submitted for publication.

73. Phalen DN, Wilson VG, Graham DL: Avian polyomavirus infection and disease: A complex phenomenon. Proc Assoc Avian Vet, New Orleans, 1992, pp 5–10.

74. Niagro FD, Ritchie BW, Lukert PD, et al: Avian polyomavirus: Discordance between neutralizing antibody titers and viral shedding in an aviary. Proc Assoc Avian Vet, Chicago, 1991, pp 22–26.

75. Wainwright PO, Lukert PD, Davis RD, Villegas P: Serological evaluation of *Psittaformes* for budgerigar fledgling disease virus. Avian Dis 31:673–676, 1987.

76. Phalen DN, Wilson VG, Graham DL: Avian polyomavirus biology and its clinical applications. Eur Conf Avian Med Surg, Utrecht, 1993, pp 200–216.

77. Davis RB: Budgerigar fledgling disease (BFD). Proc 32nd Western Poultry Dis Conf, Davis, 1983, pp 104.

78. Phalen DN, Wilson VG, Graham DL: Polymerase chain reaction assay for avian polyomavirus. J Clin Microbiol 29:1030–1037, 1991.

79. Phalen DN, Wilson VG, Graham DL: Production of avian polyomavirus seronegative budgerigars *(Melopsittacus undulatus)* from seropositive adults. Avian Dis 39:897–899, 1995.

80. Ritchie BW, Niagro FD, Latimer KS, et al: A polyomavirus overview and evaluation of an experimental polyomavirus vaccine. Proc Assoc Avian Vet, New Orleans, 1992, pp 1–4.

81. Ritchie BW, Niagro FD, Latimer KS, et al: Efficacy of an inactivated polyomavirus vaccine. J Assoc Avian Vet 7:187–192, 1993.

82. Phalen DN, Wilson VG, Graham DL: Characterization of avian polyomavirus-associated glomerulopathy of nestling parrots. Avian Dis 40:140–149, 1996.

83. Latimer KS, Niagro FD, Campagnoli R, et al: Diagnosis of concurrent avian polyomavirus and psittacine beak and feather virus infections using DNA probes. J Assoc Avian Vet 7:141–146, 1993.

84. Hunter B: Personal communication, 1995.

85. Garcia A, Latimer KS, Niagro FD, et al: Diagnosis of polyomavirus-induced hepatic necrosis in psittacine birds using DNA probes. J Vet Diagn Invest 6:308–314, 1994.

86. Phalen DN, Wilson VG, Graham DL: A practitioner's guide to avian polyomavirus testing and disease. Proc Assoc Avian Vet, Reno, 1994, pp 251–258.

87. Ritchie BW, Niagro FD, Latimer KS, et al: Antibody response and local reactions to adjuvanted avian polyomavirus vaccine in psittacine birds. J Assoc Avian Vet 8:21–26, 1994.

88. Ritchie BW, Latimer KS, Lukert PD, et al: Prevention of avian polyomavirus infections through vaccination. Proc Assoc Avian Vet, Philadelphia, 1995, pp 3–11.

89. Petrak ML, Gilmore CE: Neoplasms. In Petrak ML (ed): Diseases of Cage and Aviary Birds, ed 2. Philadelphia, Lea & Febiger, 1982, pp 606–637.

90. Jacobson ER, Mladinich CR, Clubb S, et al: Papilloma-like virus infection in an African gray parrot. J Am Vet Med Assoc 183:1307–1308, 1983.

91. Beach JE: Disease of budgerigars and other cage birds. A survey of *post-mortem* findings. Vet Rec 74:10–15, 63–68, 134–140, 1962.

92. Arnall L: Further experiences with cage birds. Vet Rec 73:1146–1154, 1961.

93. Blackmore DK: The pathology and incidence of neoplasia in cage birds. J Small Anim Prac 6:217–233, 1965.

94. O'Banion MK, Jacobson ER, Sundberg JP: Molecular cloning and partial characterization of a parrot papillomavirus. Intervirology 33:91–96, 1992.

95. Jennings AR: Tumors of free-living wild mammals and birds in Great Britain. Symp Zool Soc Lond 24:273–287, 1968.

96. Lina PHC, van Noord MJ, de Groot FG: Detection of virus in squamous papillomas of the wild bird species *Fringilia coelebs.* J Natl Cancer Inst 50:567–571, 1973.

97. Moreno-Lopez J, Ahola H, Stenlund A, et al: Genome of an avian papillomavirus. J Virol 51:872–875, 1984.

98. Blackmore DK, Keymer IF: Cutaneous diseases of wild birds in Britain. Br Birds 62:316–331, 1969.

99. Osterhaus ADME, Ellens DJ, Horzinek MC: Identification and characterization of a papillomavirus from birds (Fringillidae). Intervirology 8:351–359, 1977.

100. Sironi G, Gallazi D: Papillomavirus infection in green finches *(Carduelis chloris).* J Vet Med B 39:454–458, 1992.

101. Dom P, Ducatelle R, Charlier G, De Herdt P: Papilloma-like virus infections in canaries *(Serenius canaria).* Eur Conf Avian Med Surg, Utrecht, 1993, pp 224–231.

102. Shah KV, Howley PM: Papillomaviruses. In Field BN, Knipe DM (eds): Fields Virology, ed 9, vol 2. New York, Raven Press, 1990, pp 1651–1676.

103. Lowenstine LJ, et al: Adenovirus-like particles associated with intranuclear inclusion bodies in the renal tubules of lovebirds *(Agapornis* spp.) and a common murre *(Uria aalgae).* Proc 33rd West Poult Dis Conf, Davis, 1984, pp 105–107.

104. Mori F, Touchi A, Suwa T, et al: Inclusion bodies containing adenovirus-like particles in the kidneys of psittacine birds. Avian Pathol 18:197–202, 1989.

105. Tsai SS, Park JH, Iqbal BM, et al: Histopathological study on dual infections of adenovirus and papovavirus in budgerigars *(Melopsittacus undulatus).* Avian Pathol 23:481–487, 1994.

106. Jacobson ER, Gardiner C, Clubb S: Adenovirus-like infec-

tion in white-masked lovebirds (*Agapornis personata*). J Assoc Avian Vet 1:22–34, 1989.

107. Wallner-Pendleton E, Helfer DH, Schmitz JA, et al: An inclusion-body pancreatitis in *Agapornis*. Proc 32nd West Poult Dis Conf, Davis, CA, 1983, p 99.

108. Graham DL: An update on selected pet bird virus infections or reovirus, papovavirus, and adenovirus infections and ruminations on the etiology of infiltrative splanchnic neuropathy (of the "wasting macaw" complex) of lympho- and myeloproliferative disease, and of feather and beak dyskeratogenesis. Proc Assoc Avian Vet, Toronto, 1984, pp 267–280.

109. Pass DA: Inclusion bodies and hepatopathies in psittacines. Avian Pathol 16:581–597, 1987.

110. Bryant WM, Montali RJ: Outbreak of a fatal inclusion body hepatitis in zoo psittacines. Proc 1st Int Conf Zoo Avian Med, Oahu, 1987, p 473.

111. Gassmann R, Monreal G, Bayer G: Isolierung von Adenoviren bei Wellensittichen mit zentralnevosen Ausfallserscheinungen. II. DVG-Tagung. Vogelkrankht 1981, München, pp 44–47.

112. Hunter B, Gagnon A, Onderka D, Goltz J, Holmes B: Viral hepatitis in budgerigars in Southern Ontario. Can Vet J 20:176, 1979.

113. Ramis AJ, Marlasca MJ, Majo N, et al: Inclusion body hepatitis (IBH) in a group of *Eclectus roratus*. Proc Eur Assoc Avian Vet, 1991, pp 444–446.

114. Scott PC, Condron RJ, Reece RL: Inclusion body hepatitis associated with adenovirus-like particles in a cockatiel (Psittaciformes; *Nymphicus hollandicus*). Aust Vet J 63:337–338, 1986.

115. Gómez-Villamandos JC, Mozos E, Sierra MA, Pérez J, Mendez A: Inclusion bodies containing adeno-like particles in the intestine of a psittacine bird affected by inclusion body hepatitis. J Wildl Dis 28:319–322, 1992.

116. McFerran JB, Connor TJ, McCracken RM: Isolation of adenoviruses and reoviruses from avian species other than domestic fowl. Avian Dis 20:519–524, 1976.

117. Lowenstine LJ: A potpourri of interesting avian cases. Proc 1st Int Conf Zoo Avian Med, Oahu, 1987, pp 105–107.

118. Horwitz MS: Adenoviridae and their replication. In Fields BN, Knipe DM (eds): Field's Virology, ed 2, vol 1. New York, Raven Press, 1990, pp 1679–1721.

119. McFerran JB: Adenovirus (group I) infections of chickens. In Calnek BW (ed): Diseases of Poultry, ed 9. Ames, Iowa State University Press, 1991, pp 553–563.

120. Winterfield RW, DuBose RT: Quail bronchitis. In Calnek BW (ed): Diseases of Poultry, ed 9. Ames, Iowa State University Press, 1991, pp 564–566.

121. Domermuth CH, Gross WB: Hemorrhagic enteritis and related infections. In Calnek BW (ed): Diseases of Poultry, ed 9. Ames, Iowa State University Press, 1991, pp 567–572.

122. McFerran JB: Egg drop syndrome. In Calnek BW (ed): Diseases of Poultry, ed 9. Ames, Iowa State University Press, 1991, pp 573–582.

123. Raines AM, Kocan A, Schmidt R: Pathogenicity of adenovirus in the ostrich (*Struthio camelus*). Proc Assoc Avian Vet, Philadelphia, 1995, pp 241–245.

124. Goodwin MA, Davis JF: Adenovirus particles and inclusion body hepatitis in pigeons. J Assoc Avian Vet 6:37–39, 1992.

125. Arnold ID: An outbreak of psittacine herpesvirus in rosellas. Proc Assoc Avian Vet, Phoenix, 1990, pp 283–241.

126. Gaskin JM, Robbins CM: An explosive outbreak of Pacheco's parrot disease and preliminary experimental findings. Proc Am Assoc Zoo Vet, Knoxville, 1978, pp 241–253.

127. McCluggage DM: Pacheco's parrot disease in a psittacine breeding aviary. Proc Assoc Avian Vet, Boulder, 1985, pp 115–119.

128. Panigrahy B, Grumbles LC: Pacheco's disease in psittacine birds. Avian Dis 28:808–812, 1984.

129. Simpson CF, Hanley JE, Gaskin JM: Psittacine herpesvirus infection resembling Pacheco's parrot disease. J Infect Dis 131:390–396, 1975.

130. Simpson CF, Hanley JE: Pacheco's parrot disease of psittacine birds. Avian Dis 21:209–219, 1977.

131. Smith GC: In my experience: Use of acyclovir in an outbreak of Pacheco's parrot disease. AAV Today 1:55–56, 1987.

132. Gaskin J, Raphael B, Major A, Hall G: Pacheco's disease: The search for the elusive carrier bird. Proc Am Assoc Zoo Vet, Seattle, 1981, pp 24–28.

133. Gaskin JM: Considerations in the diagnosis and control of psittacine viral infections. Proc 1st Int Conf Zoo Avian Med, Oahu, 1987, pp 1–14.

134. Rosskopf WJ, Woerpel RW: Avian viral diseases: Clinical presentation, treatment, and environmental implications. Proc Assoc Avian Vet, Phoenix, 1990, pp 506–523.

135. Krautwald M-E, Kaleta EF, Forester S, et al: Heterogenicity of Pacheco's disease and its causative agents. Proc Assoc Avian Vet, Houston, 1988, pp 11–21.

136. Godwin JS, Jacobson ER, Gaskin JM. Effects of Pacheco's parrot disease virus on hematologic and blood chemistry values of Quaker parrots (*Myopsitta monachus*). J Zoo Anim Med 13:127–132, 1982.

137. Cho BR, McDonald TL: Isolation and characterization of a herpesvirus of Pacheco's parrot disease. Avian Dis 24:268–277, 1980.

138. Ramis A, Tarrés J, Majó N, Ferrer L: Immunocytochemical diagnosis of Pacheco's parrot disease. Proc Eur Conf Avian Med Surg, Utrecht, 1993, pp 253–259.

139. Graham DL: Acute avian herpesvirus infections. In Kirk RW (ed): Current Veterinary Therapy VII, Small Animal Practice. Philadelphia, WB Saunders, 1980, pp 704–706.

140. Gaskin JM: The serodiagnosis of psittacine viral infections. Proc Assoc Avian Vet, Houston, 1988, pp 7–10.

141. Gaskin JM: Psittacine viral diseases: A perspective. J Zoo Wildl Med 20:249–264, 1989.

142. Graham DL: Personal communication, 1995.

143. Charlton BR, Barr BC, Castro AE, et al: Herpes viral hepatitis in a toucan. Avian Dis 34:787–790, 1990.

144. Angulo AB: Personal communication, 1995.

145. Tritt S: Serotyping of psittacine herpesviruses. Proc Eur Conf Avian Med Surg, 1993, Utrecht, pp 241–252.

146. Baig M, Graham DL: Personal communication, 1994.

147. Norton TM, Kollias GV, Gaskin JM, et al: Acyclovir (Zovirax) pharmacokinetics and the efficacy of acyclovir against Pacheco's parrot disease in quaker parrots. Proc Assoc Avian Vet, Oahu, 1989, pp 3–5.

148. Norton TM, Gaskin J, Kollias GV, Homer B, et al: Efficacy of acyclovir against herpesvirus infection in Quaker parakeets. Am J Vet Res 52:2007–2009, 1991.

149. Parrot T: New clinical trials using acyclovir. Proc Assoc Avian Vet, Phoenix, 1990, pp 237–238.

150. Rosskopf Jr WJ: Clinical use of acyclovir. AAV Today 1:56, 1987.

151. Fudge AM: Psittacine vaccines. Proc Assoc Avian Vet, Phoenix, 1990, pp 292–300.

152. Curtis-Velasco M: In my experience: Vaccination reaction in umbrella cockatoos. J Assoc Avian Vet 4:206, 1990.

153. Curtis-Velasco M, Schmidt RE, Fudge AM, et al: In my experience: Open forum on use of Pacheco's disease vaccine in psittacines. J Assoc Avian Vet 5:10–14, 1991.

154. Multiple authors: In my experience: Open forum on use of Pacheco's disease vaccines in psittacines. J Assoc Avian Vet 5:10–14, 1991.

155. Desmidt M, Ducatelle R, Uyttebroeck E, et al: Cytomegalovirus-like conjunctivitis in Australian finches. J Assoc Avian Vet 5:132–136, 1991.

156. Winterroll G: Herpesvirusinfektionen bei Psittaciden. Prakt Tierarzt 5:321–322, 1977.

157. Helfer DN: A new viral respiratory infection in parakeets. Avian Dis 24:781–783, 1980.

158. Winteroll G, Gylstorff I: Schwere durch herpesvirus verusachte erkrankung des repirationsapparates bei Amazonen. Berl Munch Tierarztl Wochenschr 92:277–280, 1979.

159. Lowenstein LJ: Emerging viral diseases of psittacine birds. In Kirk RW (ed): Current Veterinary Therapy IX, Small Animal Practice. Philadelphia, WB Saunders, 1986, pp 705–709.

160. Lowenstein LJ: Diseases of psittacines differing morphologically from Pacheco's disease, but associated with herpesvirus-like particles. Proc 31st West Poult Dis Conf, 1982, pp 141–142.

161. Hartig F, Frese K: Tumorförmige tauben—und kanarienpocken. ZB1 Vet Med B, 20:153–160, 1973.

162. Johnson BJ, Castro AE: Canary pox causing high mortality in an aviary. J Am Vet Med Assoc 189:1345–1347, 1986.

163. Tripathy DN: Pox. In Calnek BW (ed): Diseases of Poultry, ed 9. Ames, Iowa State University Press, 1991, pp 583–596.

164. Boosinger TR, Winterfield RW, Feldman DS, Dhillon AS: Psittacine pox virus: Virus isolation and identification, transmission, and cross-challenge studies in parrots and chickens. Avian Dis 26:437–444, 1982.

165. Dorrestein GM, van der Hage MH, Grinwis G: A tumour-like pox-lesion in masked bull finches (*Pyrrhula erythaca*). Proc Eur Conf Avian Med Surg, Utrecht, 1993, pp 232–240.

166. Karpinski LB, Clubb SL: An outbreak of pox in imported mynahs. Proc Assoc Avian Vet, Miami, 1986, pp 35–38.

167. McDonald SE, Lowenstine LJ, Ardans AA: Avian pox in blue-fronted Amazon parrots. J Am Vet Med Assoc 179:1218–1222, 1981.

168. Kirmse P: New wild bird hosts for pox viruses. Bull Wildl Dis Assoc 2:30–33, 1966.

169. Kirmse P: Host specificity and long persistence of pox infection in the flicker (*Colaptes auratus*). Bull Wildl Dis Assoc 3:14–20, 1967.

170. Karpinski LG, Clubb SL: Post pox ocular problems in blue-fronted Amazon and blue-headed pionus parrots. Proc Assoc Avian Vet, Boulder, 1985, pp 91–100.

171. Dorrestein GM, van der Hage MH: Aviculture and veterinary problems in lovebirds. Proc 1st Int Conf Zoo Avian Med, Oahu, 1987, pp 243–262.

172. Biomune: Technical bulletin: Canary pox vaccine efficacy and safety.

173. Winterfield RW, Clubb SL, Schrader D: Immunization against psittacine pox. Avian Dis 29:886–890, 1985.

174. Clubb SL, Esklund KH: Field trials with a killed psittacine pox vaccine. Proc Assoc Avian Vet, Houston, 1988, pp 145–152.

175. Grass EE: Viscerotropic velogenic Newcastle disease. Proc 59th NE Conf Avian Dis and 8th Mid-Atlantic States Avian Med Semin, Atlantic City, 1987, p 70.

176. VanDerHeyden N: Velogenic viscerotropic Newcastle disease in three Amazon chicks. Proc Assoc Avian Vet, New Orleans, 1992, pp 158–161.

177. Erickson GA, Mare CJ, Gustafson A, et al: Interactions between viscerotropic velogenic Newcastle disease virus and pet birds of six species. I. Clinical and serologic responses and viral excretion. Avian Dis 21:642–654, 1977.

178. Rosskopf WJ: V.V.N.D. Viscerotropic velogenic Newcastle disease. Proc 59th NE Conf Avian Dis and 8th Mid-Atlantic States Avian Med Semin, Atlantic City, 1987, pp 71–75.

179. Alexander DJ: Avian paramyxoviruses. Proc 34th West Poult Dis Conf, Davis, CA, 1985, pp 121–126.

180. Goodman BB and Hanson RP: Isolation of avian paramyxovirus-2 from domestic and wild birds in Costa Rica. Avian Dis 32:713–717, 1988.

181. Collins DF, Fitton J, Alexander DJ, et al: Preliminary characterization of a paramyxovirus isolated from a parrot. Res Vet Sci 19:219–221, 1975.

182. Crosta L: Paramyxovirus serotype 3 infection in neophema parakeets. Proc Eur Conf Avian Med Surg, Utrecht, 1993, pp 269–274.

183. Hitchner SB, Hirai K: Isolation and growth characteristics of psittacine viruses in chicken embryos. Avian Dis 23:139–147, 1979.

184. Hirai K, Hitchner SB, Calnek BW: Characterization of paramyxo-, herpes-, and orbiviruses isolated from psittacine birds. Avian Dis 23:148–163, 1979.

185. Leach MW, Higgins RJ, Lowenstine LJ, Shor B: Paramyxovirus infection in a Moluccan cockatoo (*Cacatua moluccensis*) with neurologic signs. AAV Today 2:87–90, 1988.

186. Schemera B, Toro H, Kaleta EF, Herbst W: A paramyxovirus of serotype 3 isolated from African and Australian finches. Avian Dis 31:921–925, 1987.

187. Smit T, Rondhuis PR: Studies on a virus isolated from the brain of a parakeet (*Neophema* sp). Avian Pathol 5:21–30, 1976.

188. VanDerHeyden N, Reed WM: In my experience: Paramyxovirus group 3 infection in cockatiels. AAV Today 1:53–54, 1987.

189. Nerome K, Nakayama M, Ishida M, Fukumi H: Isolation of a new avian paramyxovirus from budgerigars (*Melopsittacus undulatus*). J Gen Virol 38:293–301, 1978.

190. Alexander DJ: Paramyxoviruses. In Calnek BW (ed): Diseases of Poultry, ed 9. Ames, Iowa State University Press, 1991, pp 496–519.

191. Alexander DJ. Newcastle disease. In Purchase HG, Arp LH, Domermuth CH, Pearson JE (eds): A Laboratory Manual for the Isolation and Identification of Avian Pathogens, ed 3. Dubuque, Kendall/Hunt Publishing Company, 1989, pp 114–120.

192. Walker JW, Heron BR, Mixson MA: Exotic Newcastle disease eradication program in the United States. Avian Dis 17:486–503, 1973.

193. Kouwenhoven B: Newcastle disease. In McFerran JB, McNulty MS (ed): Virus Infections of Birds. New York, Elsevier Science Publishers BV, 1993, pp 341–362.

194. Easterday BC, Hinshaw VS: Influenza. In Calnek BW (ed): Diseases of Poultry, ed 9. Ames, Iowa State University Press, 1991, pp 532–551.

195. Senne DA, Pearson JE, Miller DL, Gustafson GA: Virus isolations from pet birds submitted for importation into the United States. Avian Dis 27:731–744, 1983.

196. Slemons RD, Cooper RS, Orsborn JS: Isolation of type-A influenza viruses from imported exotic birds. Avian Dis 17:746–751, 1973.

197. Alexander DJ: Influenza A isolations from exotic caged birds. Vet Rec 123:442, 1988.

198. Shivaprasad HL, Woolcock PR, Sakas PS: Avian influenza in psittacines and a passerine. Proc Assoc Avian Vet, Reno, 1994, pp 259–260.

199. Peters CJ, Dalrymple JM: Alphaviruses. In Fields BD, Knipe DM (eds): Fields Virology, ed 2, vol 1. New York, Raven Press, 1990, pp 713–761.

200. Ianconescu M: Arbovirus infections. In Calnek BW (ed): Diseases of Poultry, ed 9. Ames, Iowa State University Press, 1991, pp 674–679.
201. Ritchie BW: Avian Viruses Function and Control. Lake Worth, FL, Winger's Publishing, 1995.
202. Curtis-Velasco M: Eastern equine encephalomyelitis virus in a lady Gouldian finch. J Assoc Avian Vet 6:227–228, 1992.
203. Gaskin JM, Homer BL, Eskelund KH: Preliminary findings in avian viral serositis: A newly recognized syndrome of psittacine birds. J Assoc Avian Vet 5:27–34, 1991.
204. Gaskin JM, Homer BL, Eskelund KH: Some unofficial thoughts on avian viral serositis. Proc Assoc Avian Vet, Chicago, 1991, pp 38–42.
205. Gaskin JM: Personal communication, 1994.
206. Clubb SL: A multifactorial disease syndrome in African grey parrots *(Psittacus erithacus)* imported from Ghana. Proc Int Conf Avian Med, Toronto, 1984, pp 135–149.
207. Clubb SL, Gaskin J: Psittacine reovirus: An update including a clinical description and vaccination. Proc Assoc Avian Vet, Boulder, 1985, pp 83–90.
208. Gaskin JM: Considerations in the diagnosis and control of psittacine viral infections. Proc 1st Int Conf Zoo Avian Med, Oahu, 1987, pp 1–14.
209. Graham DL: Characterization of a reo-like virus and its isolation from and pathogenicity for parrots. Avian Dis 31:411–419, 1986.
210. Meulemans G, Dekegel D, Charlier G, et al: Isolation of orthoreoviruses from psittacine birds. J Comp Pathol 93:127–134, 1983.
211. Rigby CE, Pettit JR, Papp-Vid G, et al: The isolation of salmonellae, Newcastle disease virus and other infectious agents from quarantined imported birds in Canada. Can J Comp Med 45:366–370, 1981.
212. Senne DA, Pearson JE, Miller LD, Gustafson GA: Viral isolations from pet birds submitted for importation into the United States. Avian Dis 27:731–744, 1983.
213. Mohan R: Clinical and laboratory observations of reovirus infection in a cockatoo and a grey-cheek parrot. Proc Int Conf Avian Med, Toronto, 1984, pp 29–33.
214. Rosenberger JK, Olson NO: Reovirus infections. In Calnek BW (ed): Diseases of Poultry, ed 9. Ames, Iowa State University Press, 1991, pp 639–647.
215. Ashton WL, Randall GC, Dagless MD, Eaton TM: Suspected reovirus-associated hepatitis in parrots. Vet Rec 114:467–477, 1984.
216. Wilson RB, Holscher M, Hodges JR, Thomas S: Necrotizing hepatitis associated with a reo-like virus infection in a parrot. Avian Dis 29:568–571, 1985.
217. McOrst S, Madill D, Adamson M, Philip C: Viral enteritis in cockatoos *(Cacatua* sp.). Avian Pathol 20:531–539, 1991.
218. Hitchner SB, Hirai K: Isolation and growth characteristics of psittacine viruses in chicken embryos. Avian Dis 23:139–147, 1979.
219. Hirai K, Hitchner SB, Calnek BW: Characterization of a new corona-like agent isolation from parrots. Avian Dis 23:515–521, 1979.
220. Gough RE, Collins MS, Wood GW, Lister SA: Isolation of a chicken embryo-lethal rotavirus from a lovebird *(Agapornis* species). Vet Rec 122:363–364, 1988.
221. Cribb PH: Cloacal papilloma in an Amazon parrot. Proc Int Conf Avian Med, Toronto, 1984, pp 35–37.
222. Graham DL: Internal papillomatous disease. Proc Assoc Avian Vet, Houston, 1988, p 31.
223. Graham DL: Internal papillomatous disease—a pathologist's view of cloacal papillomas—and then some! Proc Assoc Avian Vet, Chicago, 1991, pp 141–143.
224. McDonald SE: Clinical experiences with cloacal papillomas. Proc Assoc Avian Vet, Houston, 1988, pp 27–30.
225. VanDerHeyden N: Psittacine papillomas. Proc Assoc Avian Vet Houston, 1988, pp 23–26.
226. Bond MW, Downs D, Wolf S: Utilizing papilloma infected blue and gold macaws *(Ara ararauna)* in a breeding collection. Proc Assoc Avian Vet, Philadelphia, 1995, pp 469–471.
227. Hillyer EV, Moroff S, Hoefer H, Quesenberry KE: Bile duct carcinoma in two out of ten Amazon parrots with cloacal papillomas. J Assoc Avian Vet 5:91–95, 1991.
228. Coleman CW: Bile duct carcinoma and cloacal prolapse in an orange-winged Amazon parrot *(Amazona amazonica).* J Assoc Avian Vet 5:87–89, 1991.
229. Sundberg JP, Junge RE, O'Banion MK, et al: Cloacal papillomas in psittacines. Am J Vet Res 4:928–932, 1986.
230. Goodwin M, McGee ED: Herpes-like virus associated with a cloacal papilloma in an orange-fronted conure *(Aratinga canicularis).* J Assoc Avian Vet 7:23–25, 1993.
231. Greenwood AG, Storm J: Laser surgery of psittacine internal papilloma. Proc Eur Conf Avian Med Surg, Utrecht, 1993, pp 217–223.
232. Rosskopf WJ Jr: Vaccine therapy for papillomas. AAV Today 1:202, 1987.
233. Woerpel RW, Rosskopf WJ: Clinical and pathological features of Macaw Wasting Syndrome. Proc 33rd West Poult Dis Conf, Davis, CA, 1984, pp 89–90.
234. Woerpel RW, Rosskopf WJ: Proventricular dilatation and wasting syndrome: Myenteric ganglioneuritis and encephalomyelitis of psittacines: An update. Proc Int Conf Avian Med, Toronto, 1984, pp 25–28.
235. Doolan M: Crop biopsy—a low risk diagnosis for neuropathic gastric dilatation. Proc Assoc Avian Vet, Reno, 1994, pp 193–196.
236. Graham DL: Wasting/proventricular dilatation disease: A pathologist's view. Proc Assoc Avian Vet, Chicago, 1991, pp 43–44.
237. Gregory CR, Latimer KS, Niagro FD, et al: A review of proventricular dilatation syndrome. J Assoc Avian Vet 8:69–75, 1994.
238. Ridgeway RA, Gallerstein GA: Proventricular dilatation in psittacines. Proc Assoc Avian Vet, San Diego, 1983, pp 228–230.
239. Phalen DN: An outbreak of psittacine proventricular dilatation syndrome (PPDS) in a private collection of birds and an atypical form of PPDS in a nanday conure. Proc Assoc Avian Vet, Miami, 1986, pp 27–34.
240. Clark FD: Proventricular dilatation syndrome in large psittacine birds. Avian Dis 28:813–816, 1984.
241. Hughes PE: The pathology of myenteric ganglioneuritis, psittacine encephalomyelitis, proventricular dilatation of psittacines, and macaw wasting syndrome. Proc 33rd West Poult Dis Conf, Davis, CA, 1984, pp 85–87.
242. Turner R: Macaw fading or wasting syndrome. Proc 33rd West Poult Dis Conf, Davis, CA, 1984, pp 87–88.
243. Degerness L, Flammer K, Fisher P: Proventricular dilatation syndrome in a green-winged macaw. Proc Assoc Avian Vet, Chicago, 1991, pp 45–49.
244. Lutz ME, Wilson RB: Psittacine proventricular syndrome in an umbrella cockatoo. J Am Vet Med Assoc 198:1962–1963, 1991.
245. Rich GA: Classic and atypical cases of proventricular dilatation disease. Proc Assoc Avian Vet, New Orleans, 1992, pp 119–125.
246. Shivaprasad HL, Barr BC, Woods LW, et al: Spectrum of lesions (pathology) of proventricular dilation syndrome. Proc Assoc Avian Vet, Philadelphia, 1995, pp 505–506.

247. Bond MW, Downs D, Wolf S: Screening for psittacine proventricular dilatation syndrome. Proc Assoc Avian Vet, Nashville, 1993, pp 92–97.

248. Suedemeyer WK: Diagnosis and clinical progression of three cases of proventricular dilatation syndrome. J Assoc Avian Vet 6:159–163, 1992.

249. Joyner KL, Kock N, Styles D. Encephalitis, proventricular and ventricular myositis, and myenteric ganglioneuritis in an umbrella cockatoo. Avian Dis 33:379–381, 1989.

250. Malley DM: Case report: A case study of a Moluccan cockatoo with proventricular dilatation. Proc Ann Conf Eur Assoc Avian Vet, 1991, pp 271–272.

251. Mannl A, Gerlach H, Leipold R: Neuropathic gastric dilation in Psittaciformes. Avian Dis 31:214–221, 1987.

252. Gerlach H: Update of the macaw wasting syndrome. Proc Assoc Avian Vet, Miami, 1986, pp 21–25.

253. Graham DL: Surprises at necropsy: Failure of differential diagnosis. Proc Assoc Avian Vet, Houston, 1988, pp 177–178.

254. Ingram IA: Proventricular foreign body mimicking proventricular dilatation in an umbrella cockatoo. Proc Assoc Avian Vet, Phoenix, 1990, pp 314–315.

255. Graham DL: Infiltrative splanchnic neuropathy, a component of the "wasting macaw" complex. Proc Int Conf Avian Med, Toronto, 1984, p 275.

256. McCluggage DL: Proventriculotomy: A study of select cases. Proc Assoc Avian Vet, New Orleans, 1992, pp 195–200.

257. Coleman CW: Lymphoid neoplasia in pet birds: A review. J Avian Med Surg 9:3–7, 1995.

258. Calnek BW, Witter RL: Marek's disease. In Calnek BW (ed): Diseases of Poultry, ed 9. Ames, Iowa State University Press, 1991, pp 343–385.

259. Payne LN, Purchase HG: Leukosis/Sarcoma group. In Calnek BW (ed): Diseases of Poultry, ed 9. Ames, Iowa State University Press, 1991, pp 386–439.

260. Witter RL: Reticuloendotheliosis. In Calnek BW (ed): Diseases of Poultry, ed 9. Ames, Iowa State University Press, 1991, pp 439–456.

261. Neumann U, Kummerfeld N: Neoplasms in budgerigars *(Melopsittacus undulatus):* Clinical, pathological, and serological findings with special consideration of kidney tumors. Avian Pathol 12:353–362, 1983.

262. Gould WJ, O'Connell PH, Shivaprassad HL, et al: Detection of retrovirus sequences in budgerigars with tumors. Avian Pathol 22:33–45, 1993.

263. Dorrestein GM, van der Hage MH, Zwart P: Disease of passerines, especially canaries and finches. Proc Assoc Avian Vet, Boulder, 1985, pp 53–70.

264. Graham DL, Phalen DN: Unpublished observation, 1994.

Barbara L. Oglesbee

20

Mycotic Diseases

ASPERGILLOSIS

Aspergillosis is an infectious, noncontagious disease of pet and wild birds caused by the ubiquitous soil saprophyte, *Aspergillus* species. The most common species isolated in diseased birds is *Aspergillus fumigatus*; the forms *A. flavus, A. niger,* and others play a lesser role. Infection generally occurs via inhalation of airborne spores. The organism may then penetrate respiratory tissues, reproducing by simple division of tubular hyphae to form mycelia. Tissue invasion incites an inflammatory response, with heterophils, lymphocytes, and monocytes infiltrating the lesion.

Aspergillosis is an opportunistic infection, causing disease only under conditions of immunosuppression or exposure to overwhelming numbers of organisms. Following inhalation of spores, phagocytic cells and normal respiratory microbial clearance mechanisms are responsible for controlling infections. If intrapulmonary defense mechanisms are adequate and the numbers of spores inhaled are kept to a minimum, the organism is eliminated from the host, or colonization may be limited to the site of primary infection, causing little or no harm to the bird.

Many factors may contribute to immunosuppression and increased susceptibility to aspergillosis. Stress, as may occur in shipping, quarantine, or capture of wild birds, is frequently implicated as a predisposing factor.[31, 34] Aspergillosis often occurs following a prolonged illness, or following a traumatic event such as an injury or smoke inhalation.[24, 37] The use of immunosuppressive doses of corticosteroids favors fungal infection. Malnutrition or vitamin deficiencies, especially hypovitaminosis A,

often seen in birds on diets consisting of seed only, also contribute to disease susceptibility.[30] Prolonged antibiotic use may also play a role in disease susceptibility.[6] For example, aspergillosis may occur following treatment for chlamydiosis due to the immunosuppressive effects of tetracycline in conjunction with the debilitated state of the diseased bird.

Environmental factors play a significant role in the development of this disease by increasing the burden of fungus to which birds are exposed. *Aspergillus* grows readily in damp litter, especially corn cob litter and eucalyptus bark, soiled with feces.[18, 25] Poor sanitation, which occurs when nest boxes and incubators are inadequately cleaned or when bird feces and seed hulls are allowed to accumulate in cages, may also promote growth of the organism. Poor ventilation and dusty environments in conjunction with these factors increase the likelihood of inhalation of airborne spores.

Two forms of the disease, acute and chronic, are recognized.[23, 30, 33, 37] The acute form, seen most often in wild birds or psittacines under poor sanitary conditions, occurs following inhalation of an overwhelming number of spores.[17, 34] In this form of the disease, massive, rapid colonization of the lungs occurs, and the lungs become diffusely infiltrated with miliary granulomas.[30, 34] Severe dyspnea is often seen, with rapid progression to death, because treatment is usually ineffective. Diagnosis is made at necropsy, where these pulmonic nodules are visible grossly. Histologically, multiple foci containing fungal hyphae and rimmed by hemorrhage and heterophilic, mononuclear, and multinuclear cell infiltrates are seen.

The most commonly encountered form of Aspergillosis is the chronic form. This form, seen most often in psittacines, follows a stressful event or immunosuppression. Under these circumstances, the bird is unable to effectively eliminate or contain even small numbers of *Aspergillus* organisms, and fungal colonization of respiratory tissues ensues.[7] Initial lesions are most often found in areas of high oxygen tension and low blood supply, such as in the thoracic and abdominal air sacs and in the large airways, especially the syrinx (Fig. 20–1).[25, 30, 31] Radiating hyphae often form loosely attached plaques, over which a connective tissue plaque may be formed. Fungal plaques and necrotic debris may cause partial or complete obstruction of the trachea or bronchi, or may completely fill the air sac. In some cases, sporulation may occur after a period of growth, with colonies of fruiting bodies grossly visible within the respiratory tract.

Hematogenous dissemination to other organ systems may occur as a result of colony extension into blood vessels. Dissemination may also result from direct extension into pneumatic bone, the peritoneal cavity, and surrounding structures. The extent of fungal colonization is dependent upon the integrity of the host's immune system. Clinical signs are often inapparent until fungal colonization is exten-

sive, because this disease is often insidious in onset and slowly progressive.[6, 25, 30, 34, 37]

In some cases, fungal colonization may be limited to a localized point of entry, such as the mouth, gastrointestinal tract, eye, central nervous system (CNS), kidney, or bone.[4, 7, 8, 22, 25, 37] *Aspergillus* species has been reported as a cause of rhinitis and sinusitis in psittacines.[1, 42]

Clinical Signs

Clinical signs of the acute form may include inappetence, polydipsia, polyuria, anorexia, dyspnea, and cyanosis. Sudden death may occur without premonitory signs.

In the chronic form, clinical signs vary with the location of the infection. Because the respiratory tract is the most common site of primary colonization, problems related to the respiratory system are frequently the presenting complaint. The type of respiratory signs seen depend on the extent and location of colonization. A change in voice, reluctance to talk, or a respiratory click can be heard when lesions involve the main airways, especially the syrinx. Severe dyspnea is often seen if the lesion becomes large enough to occlude the trachea or mainstem bronchi. Often, colonization is limited to these locations only.[30, 37] If the lungs or sacs are involved, dyspnea, tachypnea, or exercise intolerance may be seen. The first respiratory sign often noted is a prolonged respiratory recovery rate following handling or flight.[30, 34] If a main airway is not occluded, respiratory signs may be completely absent, even when extensive lesions are present.

In a large number of cases, nonspecific signs, such as weight loss, muscle wasting, inappetence, diarrhea, polyuria, depression, or lethargy are the only clinical signs present. Green discoloration of the urates (biliverdinuria) and hepatomegaly are seen with hepatic involvement. Ataxia, torticollis, or seizures may indicate CNS involvement, usually as a result of the space-occupying effects of fungal granulomas.[30] Extension of fungal granulomas from the caudal air sacs into the spinal cord or sacral plexus causing unilateral or bilateral rear limb paresis or paralysis has been reported.[20]

If fungal colonization is limited to the upper respiratory tract, such as the periorbital sinus and nasal cavity, unilateral or bilateral mucoid to mucopuru-

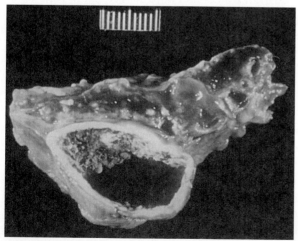

F i g u r e   2 0 – 1

Chronic granulomatous airsacculitis and pneumonia caused by *Aspergillus fumigatus*. This cross section of lung and air sac illustrates the extreme thickening of the air sac caused by chronic inflammation and fibrosis, associated with luminal plaques formed by fungal hyphae and the associated inflammatory infiltrates. Granulomatous foci are also observed throughout the pulmonary parenchyma.

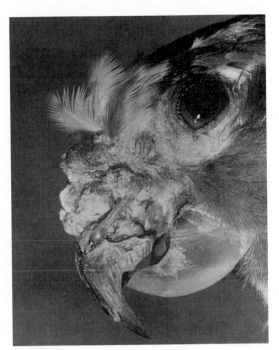

Figure 20–2

Beak deformation caused by chronic *Aspergillus* infection in a Meyer parrot. Granulomatous inflammation, initiated within the nares, has spread along the base of the beak, leading to exuberant granulation tissue formation, a hyperkeratotic scale, and severe erosion of the beak.

lent nasal discharge may be present.[1, 42] The nostrils may become plugged with inspissated exudate. If extension into the beak or periorbital bone occurs, destruction of normal architecture may become severe, causing beak malformation and nasal or periorbital swelling (Fig. 20–2).

Diagnosis

Ante mortem diagnosis of aspergillosis may be difficult, particularly in chronic cases. Signs are often nonspecific, and fungal mycelia are usually intimately associated with tissues, making them rarely visible in body fluids or exudates.[10] A careful history may reveal the presence of an underlying environmental or immunosuppressive factor, or a history of chronic debility, weight loss, voice change, or exercise intolerance. Aspergillosis should be strongly suspected in cases when debilitated animals are nonresponsive to or worsen with antibiotic treatment.

A severe leukocytosis of 20,000 to greater than 100,000 white blood cells per microliter is usually present with aspergillosis. The differential count usually reveals a heterophilia with a left shift, monocytosis, and lymphopenia. With chronic infection, a nonregenerative anemia and increased serum total protein with an increased globulin portion may be present. Increases in serum aspartate aminotransferase and bile acids may occur with hepatic involvement.

Endoscopy is an invaluable tool in the diagnosis of aspergillosis. With episodes of severe dyspnea, tracheal endoscopy may reveal a single lesion occluding the trachea or syrinx. Tracheal endoscopy may be facilitated by administering oxygen and gas anesthetics via a breathing tube into the caudal thoracic or abdominal air sac. A thick white discharge or plaque may be seen within the tracheal lumen, a sample of which should be taken for cytologic examination and culture. Endoscopy of the abdominal air sacs may reveal a diffuse cloudiness or the presence of white or yellow plaques. These plaques may be covered with a green-gray pigmented mold. Samples may be obtained directly with biopsy forceps or via air sac lavage for culture and cytology.

Radiographic changes may not be visible in early cases; however, with advanced disease radiographic abnormalities can include a prominent parabronchial pattern, loss of definition of the air sacs, asymmetry of the air sacs because of air sac consolidation or hyperinflation, or focal densities within the lungs or air sacs (Fig. 20–3).[30] Hepatomegaly or renomegaly may be visible radiographically with involvement of these organ systems.

Definitive diagnosis is based on identification of the organism on cytologic or histopathologic examination of lesions, and by culture of the organism from the site of infection. It should be noted that isolation of *Aspergillus* species on culture alone does not constitute a definitive diagnosis, because this organism is ubiquitous and contamination is common. Microscopically, mycelia of *Aspergillus* species are composed of slender, tubular septate hyphae of uniform width, which periodically branch at a 45° angle (Fig. 20–4). Occasionally, fruiting bodies may be seen with elongated spores resembling a "holy water sprinkler" (*Aspergillus*) from which the organism derives its name.[10] The organism may be seen in histopathologic samples stained with hematoxylin-eosin, periodic acid-Schiff, or

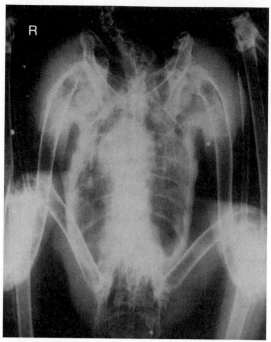

Figure 20-3

Ventrodorsal radiograph of a red-tailed hawk with aspergillosis. Note the asymmetry in the generalized increased opacity of the air sacs (right more severe than left). Irregular confluent opacities also appear throughout the lungs. (Photograph courtesy of Patrick Redig.)

Grocott's stain. Molds of *Aspergillus* species grow readily at room temperature on Sabouraud dextrose agar or blood agar. The white colonies of *A. fumigatus* turn green after a few days when sporulation occurs. Microscopic identification may be achieved by staining of smears from these colonies with lactophenol blue or new methylene blue stain.

Treatment

Treatment of aspergillosis is often difficult. The disease generally carries a poor to grave prognosis when tissue colonization is extensive. Because infections caused by *Aspergillus* species tend to become walled-off by the bird's inflammatory response and therefore isolated from the bloodstream, the prognosis is poorer if one must rely on systemic administration of antifungal agents alone.[16] The best prognosis for treatment success exists when granulomatous lesions are debrided, and when topical therapy can be administered in conjunction with

early, aggressive systemic antifungal therapy. Topical therapy may be achieved by nebulization, nasal or air sac flushing, or surgical irrigation of abdominal cavities.

Antifungal agents commonly employed against *Aspergillus* species include amphotericin B (Fungizone, Squibb), flucytosine (Ancobon, Hoffman-La Roche), ketoconazole (Nizoral, Janssen) and itraconazole (Sporanox, Janssen). Amphotericin B is generally accepted as the drug of choice for initial treatment of severe infections.[1, 16, 24, 34, 35, 37] It is fungicidal, and resistance by strains of *Aspergillus* species rarely occurs. In severe cases of respiratory aspergillosis, amphotericin B may be given intravenously, by intrathecal injection and nebulization simultaneously, along with flucytosine or one of the azole antifungals. Treatment is initiated by intravenous injection of amphotericin B at a dosage of 1.5 mg/kg every 8 hours for 3 to 5 days.[34] If the main airways are involved, a solution of amphotericin B diluted with 0.9% saline may also be given by intratracheal injection using a tom cat urinary catheter (Sherwood Medical, St. Louis, MO).[16, 25, 34, 36] A dosage of 1 mg/kg every 8 to 12 hours has been recommended when used in this manner.[1] Amphotericin B may also be used for nebulization by making a 1 mg/ml solution with 0.9% saline, which is nebulized for 15 minutes every 12 hours.[1] A solution of 0.05 mg/ml (50 mg/L 0.9% saline) has been recommended for irrigation.[34] Amphotericin B is potentially nephrotoxic, and a possible toxicity resulting from crystal deposition in soft tissues surrounding the sinuses has been reported.[42]

Flucytosine (Ancobon, Hoffman-La Roche) may be given orally at 20 to 60 mg/kg every 12 hours in conjunction with and following amphotericin B treatment. It is fungistatic, and therefore must be administered for prolonged periods of time, in most cases for up to 6 months or longer. It is widely distributed to tissues, including the CNS. Most fungi rapidly develop resistance to flucytosine.[16] It therefore should not be used alone as a primary treatment of severe *Aspergillus* infections, but in conjunction with amphotericin B or one of the azole antifungals. Periodic monitoring of the complete blood count (CBC) is recommended, because flucytosine is potentially toxic to the bone marrow.

Ketoconazole has been given orally at 20 to 30 mg/kg every 12 hours for 2 to 6 weeks or in conjunction with other antifungal agents as a treat-

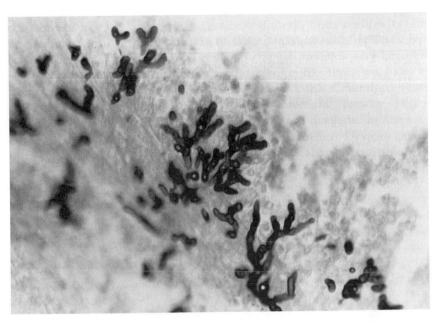

Figure 20–4

Histologic appearance of an *Aspergillus* plaque growing within the lumen of an air sac of an Amazon parrot (Grocott's stain, 40× magnification). Note the dichotomous branching of the septate hyphae characteristic of this genus of fungi.

ment for aspergillosis.[1, 16, 35, 37] Of all of the azole antifungal agents, however, itraconazole has greater specificity against *Aspergillus* species.[1, 16, 17, 22] Itraconazole has been administered orally with a high-fat meal (to enhance absorption) at a dosage of 5 to 10 mg/kg every 12 hours and appears to be very effective.[1, 16, 17, 22, 38] It has, however, been reported to cause profound anorexia in African grey parrots, and should be used with caution until its safety in psittacines is established.[1] Several days are required to reach steady-state serum levels of the azole antifungal agents. Therefore, in severe cases, treatment should first be initiated with intravenous amphotericin B in conjunction with the azole antifungal administration.[16, 22] Long-term treatment, in most cases for several months following the resolution of clinical signs, has been recommended.[16, 17, 38]

Most birds with chronic aspergillosis have severe immunocompromise, and thus supportive care consisting of fluid therapy, forced alimentation, and a heated environment are imperative to successful treatment. Antibiotic treatment based on culture and susceptibility testing may be necessary if a secondary bacterial infection is present.

Prevention

Aspergillus is an opportunistic pathogen; therefore, every attempt should be made to reduce predisposing immunosuppressive factors such as stress and malnutrition. To avoid inhalation of a large number of spores, birds should be housed in a well-ventilated area, with the bedding changed daily. When treating other illnesses, the benefits of long-term or repeated antibiotic usage, or the use of immunosuppressive doses of corticosteroids, must be weighed against the possibility of opportunistic deep mycotic infections. Both flucytosine and itraconazole have been used prophylactically in birds deemed to be at high risk for the development of aspergillosis.

CANDIDIASIS

Avian candidiasis is an opportunistic disease of birds, most often affecting the gastrointestinal tract. Disease is seen commonly in young or immunosuppressed birds and often occurs following prolonged treatment with antibiotics. The organism most often responsible for disease in pet birds is *Candida albicans*, although *C. parapsilosis* has been reported as a cause of systemic infection.[19]

C. albicans can be a normal inhabitant of the avian gastrointestinal tract. Disease occurs when innocuous superficial colonization progresses to deep tissue invasion, depending largely on dwindling host resistance factors.[10] The normal bacterial flora of oral and gastrointestinal mucosal surfaces have an inhibitory effect on the growth of *Candida* species. Therefore, suppression of this normal flora by antibiotic use (especially tetracyclines), or changes in pH may allow superficial fungal propagation. Deep tissue invasion may extend from superficial lesions when host defenses are compromised, either locally or from systemic immunosuppression. If left unchecked, dissemination may then follow.

Predisposing immunosuppressive factors in the development of candidiasis are similar to those discussed for aspergillosis. In addition, candidiasis frequently occurs as a secondary invader following bacterial or viral infections, or from lesions caused by hypovitaminosis A. Mycotic ingluvitis caused by *Candida* species is common in young birds, because of their incompetent immune status and immature development of normal gastrointestinal microflora. Husbandry factors, such as poor hygiene within the nursery and cross-contamination of feeding formulas and implements, contribute to disease outbreaks.

Candidiasis occurs most commonly in the gastrointestinal tract, especially in the small intestine, mouth, crop, esophagus, proventriculus, and ventriculus.[6, 23] Lesions have also been reported in the cloaca, respiratory tract, skin, uropygial gland, beak, and eye.[2, 12, 22, 28]

Clinical Signs

Clinical signs referable to the gastrointestinal tract are most commonly encountered. Infection of the crop mucosa (ingluvitis) may cause inappetence, regurgitation, or delayed crop emptying. With deep infection, this may progress to complete crop stasis and palpable crop thickening. Symptoms are especially common in neonates, and this condition is commonly referred to as "sour crop" by aviculturists. With infection of the proventriculus and lower gastrointestinal tract, vomiting, malaise, weight loss, and diarrhea may also be seen. Malnutrition because of decreased gastrointestinal motility and decreased absorption of nutrients is often encountered in cases of chronic enteric candidiasis. Infection of the crop, proventriculus, and lower gastrointestinal tract may occur simultaneously.

Local infection of the mouth or beak may cause halitosis, mucoid exudates, or the presence of white, caseous lesions within the oral cavity. If colo-nization by *Candida* species occurs within the respiratory tract, clinical signs similar to those described for rhinitis or main airway obstruction caused by aspergillosis may be seen. Ocular, dermal, venereal, and uropygial gland infections have been reported in nonpsittacine species.

Diagnosis

Because *C. albicans* is considered to be a normal inhabitant of the avian gastrointestinal tract, a positive culture or identification of yeasts on Gram's stained specimens alone is insufficient for definitive diagnosis.[26, 27] Diagnosis is based on a history of underlying disease or immunosuppressed state, clinical signs, visualization of lesions, the identification of large numbers of yeasts on cytologic samples, positive cultures, and/or the identification of pseudohyphae in tissue samples.[5]

If mycotic ingluvitis is suspected, the crop may be visualized directly via insufflation and endoscopic examination. With superficial infections, the crop may appear hyperemic and covered with mucoid exudate. Samples of this exudate should be obtained for cytologic examination and culture. With deep infections, the crop mucosa may appear roughened and coated with a mucoid to catarrhal exudate. With progressive severity, creamy white plaques may appear, progressing to the formation of a diphtheritic membrane, or a characteristic "turkish towel" appearance to the mucosa.[6, 7] If the infection lies in the proventriculus and the crop appears normal, similar lesions may be visualized within the proventriculus via flexible endoscopy in birds weighing over 500 g. In smaller birds, the proventriculus may be visualized via a rigid endoscope inserted through an incision into the crop.

Dry-mounted samples obtained for cytologic examination from the site of infection may be stained with Dif-Quick, Gram's, or new methylene blue stains. The presence of pseudohyphae, which appear as slender, nonbranching chains of tubular cells, indicates tissue invasion (Fig. 20–5). Blastospores, appearing as oval, thin-walled yeasts with a 3 to 6 μm diameter with broad-based budding may also be seen (see Fig. 20–5, insert). High numbers of yeasts seen in stained samples from the crop, mouth, or feces support a diagnosis of candidiasis. *Candida* species grow well on Sabouraud

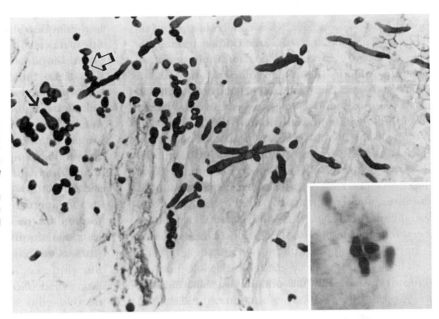

Figure 20-5

Histologic appearance of granulomatous ingluvietis caused by *Candida albicans* in a cockatiel (Grocott's stain, 40× magnification). Note the nonbranching pseudohyphae formed by chains of fungal cells *(open arrow)*. Budding yeasts are also observed in histologic section *(solid arrow)*, although the broad-based budding typical of these blastospores may be more evident following Gram's staining of crop washes *(inset)*.

dextrose agar, forming even, creamy colonies within 1 to 3 days.

Treatment

Superficial infections limited to the gastrointestinal tract generally respond well to oral nystatin (Mycostatin, Squibb) at 300,000 units/kg every 8 hours.[35] Nystatin is safe and effective, but is not absorbed systemically, making direct contact with infected tissues necessary. Flucytosine given orally at 20 to 60 mg/kg every 12 hours may also be used to treat candidiasis; however, it is common for yeasts to rapidly develop resistance to this drug.[16]

Deep or resistant infections may be treated with ketoconazole or fluconazole. Ketoconazole tablets can be crushed and mixed with an acidic liquid (such as orange juice) and given by mouth at 20 to 30 mg/kg every 12 hours. Fluconazole is considered to be the most effective antifungal agent available against tissue-based yeasts, and is the drug of choice for resistant yeast infections and ocular and CNS infections.[16] Fluconazole has been empirically given at 2 to 5 mg/kg every 24 hours.[32] Regurgitation may be seen in some birds, especially cockatoos and cockatiels. Many birds with candidiasis have immunosuppression, and thus supportive care and the elimination of underlying infections are essential to successful therapy.

In addition to systemic antifungals, topical treatment for cutaneous or oral lesions consists of debridement and application of 3% amphotericin B ointment. Ocular lesions have also been treated with 3% amphotericin B ointment or subconjunctival injections of a solution of 25 mg amphotericin B per milliliter of sterile water.[12] Rhinitis caused by *Candida* species may be treated as described for aspergillosis.

Prevention

Candidiasis is generally considered to be an opportunistic, secondary invader. The reduction of stress and provision of a clean environment aid in preventing infection. In the nursery, utensils should be thoroughly disinfected after feeding baby birds. Leftover hand-rearing formulas should be discarded beyond one feeding. If a nursery has a history of recurrent *Candida* infections, nystatin may be added to hand-rearing formulas at a rate of 100,000 units/50 ml of formula.

If prolonged antibiotic therapy is expected, nystatin has been used prophylactically at the same dosages listed for treatment. Chlorhexidine (Nolvasan, Fort Dodge) given in the drinking water (20 ml of 2% solution per gallon water) may be used to control, but not to treat infections.[16]

CRYPTOCOCCOSIS

Cryptococcosis in avian species is a relatively uncommon mycotic disease caused by the saprophytic fungus, *Cryptococcus neoformans*. Although *C. neoformans* is commonly isolated in the feces of pigeons, canaries, and psittacine birds, naturally occurring disease caused by this fungus is rare.[14, 21] Birds were believed to be naturally resistant to infection because of their relatively high body temperatures, and by the inhibitory effects of their normal intestinal flora.[9] *C. neoformans* is unable to grow in vitro or in chicken embryos in vivo at temperatures at or above 40°C, the core temperature of most birds.[14, 21]

Despite this, naturally occurring disease caused by *C. neoformans* has been reported in Columbiformes and in a Moluccan cockatoo, a thick-billed parrot, an African grey parrot, and in green-winged macaws.[9, 14, 15, 21, 36] In all but one of these reports, initial colonization appears to have occurred within the respiratory tract, with subsequent dissemination. It has been suggested that the upper respiratory tract may be more susceptible to initial colonization because of its lower temperature.[14] Dissemination to the meninges, brain, intraocular and periocular tissues, tongue, and bone marrow were reported.

Clinical Signs

Nonspecific signs such as weakness, listlessness, anorexia, and diarrhea are commonly reported in birds diagnosed with cryptococcosis. Soft tissue swelling in the region of the sinuses and periorbital tissues and nasal discharge have been reported with ocular and upper respiratory system involvement. Neurologic signs, such as weakness, progressive paralysis, and limberness of the jaw and neck may occur with brain and meningeal involvement. With lower respiratory tract colonization, moderate to severe dyspnea is seen.

Diagnosis

Diagnosis of cryptococcosis is based on clinical signs, the identification of the organism on cytologic or histologic examination of samples, and by isolation on culture. Grossly, a mucoid exudate may be observed, which represents relatively pure colonies of the yeast, the myxomatous consistency of these lesions reflecting the abundant mucopolysaccharide-rich capsules characteristic of this organism. Fine needle aspirates or impression smears may be stained with India ink, new methylene blue, or Gram's stain. Tissue specimens may be stained with hematoxylin and eosin, periodic acid-Schiff, mucicarmine, or silver stains. *C. neoformans* appears as large, oval budding yeasts (4–7 μm) surrounded by a mucopolysaccharide capsule two to four times the diameter of the cell body. Surrounding inflammatory response is usually minimal, consisting of epithelioid macrophages or multinucleated giant cell and heterophils.[14, 15, 35] *C. neoformans* grows well on Sabouraud-dextrose agar.

Treatment

Therapeutic success in the treatment of deep mycotic infections is dependant on early diagnosis and aggressive treatment. As with treatment for aspergillosis, a combination of amphotericin B and itraconazole or fluconazole is the therapeutic regimen of choice. Of the azole antifungals available, fluconazole is most effective against tissue-based yeasts, is widely distributed to the extracellular space, and is the drug of choice for mycotic infections of the eye, cerebral spinal fluid, and other privileged sites.[16] In the majority of avian *Cryptococcus* cases published, treatment was not attempted, and diagnosis was based on postmortem examination. In one case, intralesional injections of amphotericin B were somewhat successful.[14]

UNUSUAL MYCOTIC INFECTIONS

Deep infections by normally saprophytic fungi are uncommon, but may occur with unsanitary husbandry practices or under conditions leading to systemic immunosuppression. Reports of less common deep mycotic infections are sporadically found in the literature. In pet birds, these include mucormycosis, rhinosporidiosis, trichosporosis, and penicilliosis. Mycotic infections of the air sac, kidneys, and tongue caused by *Mucor* species have been reported in African grey parrots.[3, 13] Weight loss and polyuria were reported in a green-winged macaw with granulomatous inflammation of the liver, lung, and myocardium caused by *Trichosporon beigelii*.[40]

Reports of superficial mycoses or dermatomycoses are also quite rare. *Trichophyton* species, *Microsporum gypseum*, and *Candida* species have been reported as a cause of dermatomycoses in birds.[25, 28] In one report, several genera of fungi were cultured from pigeons and various species of psittacines.[41] These fungi were believed to be the cause of feather plucking as a result of the response to treatment with antifungal agents. Clinical manifestations of dermatomycoses included feather loss, pruritus, self-mutilation, skin thickening, and brittle feathers. Treatment with a biweekly application of a salicylic acid solution or a 1:2000 dilution of copper sulfate was used.[41]

References

1. Bauck L, Hillyer E, Hoefer H: Rhinitis: Case reports. Proc Assoc Avian, Vet, 134–139, 1992.
2. Beemer AM, Kuttin ES, Kantz Z: Epidemic venereal disease due to *Candida albicans* in geese in Israel. Avian Dis 14:212–217, 1973.
3. Burr EW, Huchzermeyer FW, Made VD: Mucormycosis in a parrot. Mod Vet Pract 63(12):961–962, 1982.
4. Bygrave AC: Leg paralysis in pheasant poults (*Phasianus colchicus*) due to spinal aspergillosis. Vet Rec 109:516, 1981.
5. Campbell TW: Disorders of the avian crop. Comp Contin Educ Pract Vet 5(10):813–824, 1983.
6. Campbell TW: Mycotic diseases. In Harrison GJ, Harrison LR (eds): Clinical Avian Medicine and Surgery. Philadelphia, WB Saunders, 1986, pp 464–472.
7. Chute HL: Fungal infections. In Hofstad MS (ed): Disease of Poultry. Ames, The Iowa State University Press, 1972, pp 458–462.
8. Chute HL, O'Meara DC: Diagnosis of unusual cases of avian mycosis. Can Vet J 10:385–387, 1961.
9. Clipsham RC, Britt JO: Disseminated cryptococcosis in a macaw. J Am Vet Med Assoc 183(11):1303–1305, 1977.
10. Cotran RS, Kumar V, Robbins S: Fungal protozoal and helminthic diseases and sarcoidosis. In Robbins S (ed): Pathologic Basis of Disease, 4th ed. Philadelphia, WB Saunders, 1989, pp 385–433.
11. Courtney CH, Forrester DJ, White FH: Rhinosporidiosis in a wood duck. J Am Vet Med Assoc 171(9):989–990, 1977.
12. Crispin SM, Barnett KC: Ocular candidiasis in ornamental ducks. Avian Pathol 7:49–59, 1978.
13. Dawson CO, Wheeldon EB, McNeil PE: Air sac and renal mucormycosis in an African gray parrot (*Psittacus erithacus*). Avian Dis 20(3):593–600, 1976.
14. Ensley PK, Anderson MP, Fletcher KC: Cryptococcosis in a male Becarri's crowned pigeon. J Am Vet Med Assoc 175(9):992–994, 1979.
15. Fenwick B, Takeshita K, Wong A: A Moluccan cockatoo with disseminated cryptococcosis. J Am Vet Med Assoc 187(11):1218–1219, 1985.
16. Flammer K: An overview of antifungal therapy in birds. Proc Assoc Avian Vet, 1–4, 1993.
17. Forbes NA: Diagnosis of avian aspergillosis and treatment with itraconazole. Vet Rec 130:519–520, 1992.
18. Fudge AM, Reavill DR: Bird litter and aspergillosis warning. J Assoc Avian Vet 7(1):15, 1993.
19. Goodman GJ, Widenmeyer JC: Systemic *Candida parapsilosis* in a 20 year old Blue-fronted Amazon. Proc Assoc Avian Vet 105–119, 1986.
20. Greenacre CB, Latimer KS, Ritchie BW: Leg paresis in a black palm cockatoo (*Probosciger aterrimus*) caused by aspergillosis. J Zoo Wildl Med 23(1):122–126, 1992.
21. Grinder LA, Walch HA; Cryptococcosis in Columbiformes at the San Diego Zoo. J Wildl Dis 14:389–394, 1978.
22. Hines RS, Sharket P, Friday RB: Itraconazole treatment of pulmonary, ocular, and uropygeal aspergillosis and candidiasis in birds. Proc Am Assoc Zoo Vet, 322–326, 1990.
23. Hubbard GB, Schmidt RE, et al: Fungal infections of ventriculi in captive birds. J Wildl Dis 21(1):25–28, 1985.
24. Jenkins J: Aspergillosis. Proc Assoc Av Vet, 328–330, 1991.
25. Keymer IF: Mycoses. In Petrak ML (ed): Diseases of Cage and Aviary Birds. Philadelphia, Lea & Febiger, 1982, pp 599–605.
26. Kocan RM, Hasenclever, HF: Normal yeast flora of the upper digestive tract of some wild columbids. J Wildl Dis 8:365–368, 1972.
27. Kocan RM, Hasenclever HF: Seasonal variation of the upper digestive tract yeast flora of feral pigeons. J Wildl Dis 10:263–266, 1974.
28. Kuttin ES, Beemer AM, Meroz M: Chicken dermatitis and loss of feathers from *Candida albicans*. Avian Dis 20(1):216–218, 1975.
29. Long P, Choi G, Silberman M: Nocardiosis in two Pesquet's Parrots (*Psittrichas fulgidus*). Avian Dis 27(3):855–859, 1983.
30. McMillan MC, Petrak ML: Retrospective study of aspergillosis in pet birds. J Assoc Avian Vet 3(4):211–215, 1989.
31. Migaki G: Mycotic diseases in captive animals—mycopathologic overview. In Montali RJ, Migaki G (eds): The Comparative Pathology of Zoo Animals. Washington, DC, Smithsonian Institution Press, 1980, pp 267–275.
32. Parrot T: Clinical treatment regimes with fluconazole. Proc Assoc Avian Vet pp 15–19, 1991.
33. Quesenberry K, et al: Roundtable discussion: Clinical therapy. J Assoc Avian Vet 5(4):196–191, 1992.
34. Redig PT: Aspergillosis. In Kirk RW (ed): Current Veterinary Therapy, VII. Small Animal Practice. Philadelphia, WB Saunders, 1983, pp 611–613.
35. Ritchie BW: Avian therapeutics. Proc Assoc Avian Vet, Phoenix, 1990, pp 415–430.
36. Rosskopf WJ, Woerpel RW: Cryptococcosis in a Thick-billed parrot. Avian/Exotic Pract 1(4):14–18, 1984.
37. Rosskopf WJ, Woerpel RW: Successful treatment of aspergillosis in two psittacine birds. Proc Assoc Avian Vet 119–128, 1985.
38. Shannon D: Treatment with itraconazole of penguins suffering from aspergillosis. Vet Rec 130:479, 1992.
39. Stroud RK, Duncan RM: Aspergillosis in a red-crowned crane. J Am Vet Med Assoc 183(11):297–298, 1983.
40. Taylor M: Systemic trichosporonosis in a green-winged macaw. Proc Assoc Avian Vet 219–220, 1988.
41. Tudor DC: Mycotic infections of feathers as a cause of feather pulling in pigeons and psittacine birds. Vet Med Sm Anim Clin 78(2):249–253, 1983.
42. Van der Mast H, Dorrestein GM, Westerhof J: A fatal treatment of sinusitis in an African grey parrot. J Assoc Avian Vet 4(3):189, 1990.

21

Parasitology

Parasites of birds are as diversified in their adaptations to their way of life as are their avian hosts. Avian parasite communities select compartments within their avian hosts to enhance resource utilization, just as the birds have radiated into new habitats and niches in their environments. The sites of development of the adults of these parasites include most organ systems. Although some are generalists in their habitat selection, others are specialists and live only in certain portions of a particular organ. Parasite size ranges from tiny intracellular protozoans to easily visualized helminths and arthropods. The protozoan or single-celled forms inhabit a variety of organs, some living within cells and others as extracellular forms. The helminths may reside in tissues, cavities, in the lumen of tubular organs, or on the surface of the eyes. Arthropods reside usually on the surface of birds, but mites may move into the quill shafts, nasal passages, choana, and respiratory airways.

Parasites may cause severe damage to their vertebrate hosts in a variety of ways, or they may cause little or no damage. If they are of sufficient size in relation to the lumen of the organ they live in, they may cause mechanical obstruction, such as *Ascaridia* species do. They may invade cells and destroy their temporary homes, as do the coccidians. They may steal nutrition from the host, as do the tapeworms, which have evolved highly competitive body surfaces to compete with the host's intestinal mucosa. They may cause marked anemia through blood sucking, as do some nematodes, some mites, and most flies that are pests of birds. Biting flies, which are only temporary parasites, may carry infective stages of protozoa or filarial worms that are inoculated when the fly feeds. Some arthropod pests may cause breaks in the avian integument and allow secondary infections of bacteria or fungi to become established, or they may allow entry of larval flies that develop into myiasis.

Although it has not been documented for birds, some parasites in other hosts release chemicals that adversely affect the host. Other parasites induce tumor formation. We do not know the significance of most parasites that occur in birds, and there is much to be learned. Avian veterinarians and managers of aviaries can contribute to our knowledge by being alert to apparently new parasites and seeking the assistance of parasitologists.

RECOGNITION OF MAIN GROUPS OF PARASITES

The development and implementation of modern antiparasitic drugs do not help unless they are used on parasites that they were designed to control. Thus, proper identification of parasites is very important in their control. Use of antiparasitic agents is covered in the formulary. Potential drugs for each group of parasites will be given as an indication of what could be used. The formulary then provides specific regimens.

Nematodes

If worms are cylindrical in shape, they are probably nematodes, commonly called roundworms. They vary in length from several millimeters to several centimeters. An exception is the female of *Tetrameres* species, which in the gravid state appears grossly more like a flatworm. Upon microscopic examination, a complete intestinal tract is seen, indicating that it is a nematode.

Nematodes may be found in nearly any part of the bird, from the surface of the eye to any portion of the intestinal tract, subcutaneously, between the meninges, and in the blood vessels and body cavity. Fenbendazole and ivermectin are the two most commonly used anthelmintics for nematodes. Hygienic procedures such as reducing the buildup of feces are important to reduce the development of infective stages or the availability to intermediate hosts of the stages infective to them. Desiccation is very important for controlling many nematodes, but some nematodes have very resistant eggs, which reduces the potential for the larvae drying out.

Trematodes

Flukes (trematodes) are unsegmented flatworms that range in size in birds from slender forms, 5 mm in length, to heavier bodied types that may be up to 2 cm in length. The avian flukes all have at least an oral sucker, and most have a ventral sucker as well.

Trematodes reside in many sites including the surface of eyes, the proventriculus, small intestine, liver, gall bladder, kidney, and blood vessels. The main anthelmintics used for flukes are praziquantel and clorsulon. Because all fluke life cycles are indirect and require a gastropod as the first or only intermediate host, habitat modification may be used for controlling these parasites. Birds maintained inside rarely become infected with flukes, but those in outdoor exhibits or propagation programs are at risk. Modifying the aquatic portions in outdoor exhibits may be useful to control aquatic snails. Keeping birds in elevated cages helps with many fluke problems, but some of these parasites use an arthropod as a second intermediate host, and in these circumstances, screening may be necessary to reduce the potential of infection.

Cestodes

Tapeworms (cestodes) are segmented flatworms that are composed of a holdfast organ (the scolex) and a series of sections (proglottids). It is important to remove the entire tapeworm including the scolex if it is to be identified to genus or species. Praziquantel and epsiprantel are two good anthelmintics for tapeworms, and fenbendazole has some activity against some cestodes. All avian tapeworms have an indirect life cycle, and arthropods are usually the intermediate hosts. Reducing fecal buildup reduces the chance of intermediate hosts becoming infected and being eaten by the birds.

Acanthocephalans (Thorny-headed Worms)

Thorny-headed worms (acanthocephalans) are present in some groups of birds such as raptors and waterfowl. They have a spiny proboscis. Their bodies are cylindric, but when found at necropsy, they are firmly attached to the mucosa of the small intestine (the only site for adults). They can be removed from the mucosa by carefully using dissecting needles to tease the host tissue away from the attachment site of the worm. If the body wall is ruptured, the spiny proboscis inverts into the body, because it is everted through hydraulic action. It cannot be identified further if this happens. Sometimes, if the bird has been dead for a period prior to necropsy, the proboscis inverts into the flaccid body, the body becomes wrinkled, and the worms resemble stout-bodied tapeworms. To induce the proboscis to evert, the worms are placed in tap water in the refrigerator overnight. Osmotic pressure reinflates the intact acanthocephalan body.

All acanthocephalans have indirect life cycles and use arthropods as their intermediate hosts and sometimes paratenic hosts (an alternate route into the final host). Unfortunately, there are no anthelmintics effective against the spiny-headed worms, and the cycle must be broken by elimination of the feces if possible and reducing contact with infected intermediate hosts.

Coccidians

Coccidians are a diversified group of protozoan parasites in which part of the life cycle occurs in the epithelial cells lining the intestines or ceca (some are in kidneys in birds). These cycles may be direct, involving a single host, or they may be indirect and rely in part upon a predator-prey relationship to infect the definitive host (one in which the sexually mature forms develop). Their entire development in their hosts is intracellular. Some of the more complex cycles have the potential for the parasite to develop in nearly any tissue, as does *Toxoplasma gondii,* whereas others are more specific in the use of endothelial cells and muscles of their intermediate host (species in which asexual reproduction occurs or in which the infective stage for the definitive host develops), as do *Sarcocystis* species.

Drugs used to prevent coccidiosis through prophylactic or therapeutic therapy are decoquinate, amprolium, and a combination of pyrimethamine and sulfaquinoxaline.

No proven therapy has been developed for *Cryptosporidium* species. Feces must be removed to eliminate spread of a coccidian to related species or to noninfected members of the same avian species within an aviary. If an indirect cycle is used, feces of the definitive host must be kept away from the birds to help break the cycle. A good example of how this may be done is provided by *Sarcocystis falcatula,* a coccidian that uses North American opossums as the definitive host and usually cycles through cowbirds and grackles, which do not seem to be affected. However, when the infective stages in the opossum feces (sporocysts) are eaten by psittacine birds, the birds are usually devastated by the infection.[1, 2] Using electric fences around aviaries keeps opossums far enough away to break the cycle.[3]

Malarial Parasites

Malarial parasites are protozoans that are transmitted by blood-sucking flies. Infections in birds are seen in a variety of reticuloendothelial system tissues as exoerythrocytic forms and circulating cells of erythroid or leucocytic series. All stages in birds develop intracellularly. Gametocytes are acquired when the appropriate vector feeds on a parasitemic bird. After a short development period, the fly inoculates the infective forms into the next avian host.

Drugs used for therapy include chloroquine and primaquine. Screening of cages to preclude entrance of vectors is another means of breaking the cycle. Penguins in captivity need to be separated from mosquitoes either by being housed indoors

or in mosquito-proof enclosures outdoors, because penguins are highly susceptible to avian malaria.

Flagellated Protozoans

Flagellated protozoans in the digestive tract move with the assistance of flagella. These parasites are lumen-dwellers and have a direct life cycle. Their infective stages are passed in the feces, and thus elimination of fecal accumulation helps in their control. Drugs for these parasites include metronidazole and carnidazole.

Arthropods

Arthropods are jointed-legged animals with an exoskeleton. Parasitic forms include mites and ticks, which have eight legs as adults and nymphs (immature forms that resemble the adults), and fleas, lice, and biting flies, which have six legs. Fleas are laterally compressed and have long hind legs suited for jumping. Biting lice are dorsoventrally flattened and have chewing mouthparts. Biting flies have wings and come in a variety of body sizes. For true ectoparasites, ivermectin and pyrethrins are used for treatment. Biting flies can be controlled by using screens and habitat modification to eliminate or reduce breeding sites.

RANGE OF TYPES OF PARASITES SEEN IN BIRDS

This section is not intended to cover every parasite seen in birds, but includes the genera most likely to be encountered by veterinarians. The examples give an indication of the parasite diversity in some organs and an indication of the differences that may occur between related genera. To be safe, it is advisable to submit properly prepared specimens (see Diagnosis section) to a qualified parasitologist.

Protozoa

Coccidians are generally identified by the morphology of the fully developed (sporulated) oocyst (resistant stage passed in the feces). The genus *Ei-*

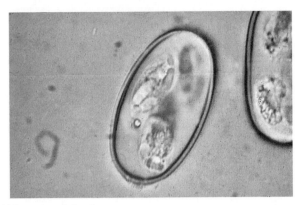

Figure 21-1

Sporulated oocyst of *Eimeria* species from a blue-fronted Amazon, 44×22 μm.

meria produces an oocyst that is subdivided into four sporocysts, each of which contains two sporozoites (Fig. 21–1). The genus *Caryospora* has one sporocyst and eight sporozoites. The genus *Cryptosporidium* has four naked sporozoites in the oocyst and no sporocysts. Because the sporozoites are so small, they are visible only by transmission electron microscopy. Four other genera *Isospora, Sarcocystis, Toxoplasma,* and *Atoxoplasma,* have two sporocysts each with four sporozoites (Fig. 21–2).[4] *Sarcocystis* sporocysts are normally released from the oocysts and are formed only in the definitive hosts, which may be predaceous birds. Oocysts of *Toxoplasma* are produced only in felids, never birds. *Atoxoplasma*[5] oocysts are indistinguishable from those of *Isospora,* and one study indicated that

the species in canaries, which was called *Atoxoplasma,* was *Isospora serini.*[6]

Species of *Eimeria, Isospora, Cryptosporidium,* and *Atoxoplasma* gain entrance to the bird through ingestion of oocysts. The first three of these develop in cells lining the intestines[7] or ceca of their avian host, as does *Atoxoplasma,* which also has stages in circulating monocytic phagocytes. Stages in peripheral blood are very rare and therefore *Atoxoplasma* is seldom diagnosed in blood smears.

Species of *Cryptosporidium* appear as tiny knobs attached to enterocytes, but in reality they are just inside the limiting membrane of the enterocytes. *Sarcocystis* has stages that undergo asexual reproduction in endothelial cells, then form macroscopic cysts in the muscles in birds that are intermediate hosts, or they undergo production of oocysts in the enterocytes in birds that are definitive hosts. When birds are clinically affected by this genus, it is the asexual phase in the endothelium that causes the damage. Asexually multiplying forms of *Toxoplasma* occur within a variety of avian tissues, and the only source of infection for nonpredaceous birds is the oocyst produced by felids. Predaceous birds may acquire the infection by eating prey species that carry the same tissue stages that develop in the avian host.[8, 9] Identification of the tissue-inhabiting forms is difficult and best left to qualified parasitologists.

Malarial parasites include species of *Plasmodium, Haemoproteus,* and *Leucocytozoon. Plasmodium* species are usually seen on blood films as schizonts and gametocytes with golden or black refractile pigment granules in the parasite cytoplasm (Fig. 21–3). Schizonts are multinucleate bodies resulting from asexual reproduction, and gametocytes (Fig. 21–4) contain a single nucleus per parasite occurring in mature erythrocytes or sometimes in erythroblasts. Species of *Haemoproteus* only have pigmented gametocytes in erythrocytes (Fig. 21–5). *Leucocytozoon* species only have unpigmented gametocytes (Fig. 21–6) in altered circulating blood cells. The host cell type cannot be determined, but they are in erythrocytes in some cases and in leucocytes in others.

Different families of flies transmit different genera of malarial parasites. Mosquitoes are vectors of *Plasmodium* species, black flies are vectors for *Leucocytozoon* species (an exception in the Orient are biting midges, which transmit *Leucocytozoon caulleryi*

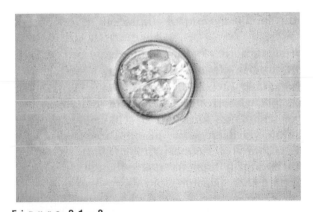

Figure 21-2

Sporulated oocysts of *Isospora puella* from a fairy bluebird, 23×22 μm.

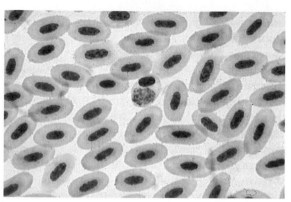

Figure 21–3

Schizont of *Plasmodium relictum* from a mourning dove.

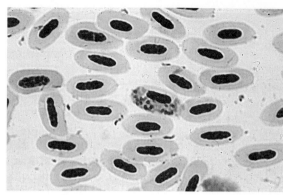

Figure 21–5

Gametocyte of *Haemoproteus columbae* from a mourning dove.

to chickens), and biting midges or no-see-ums and louse flies transmit *Haemoproteus* species.

The only genus of piroplasm recognized in birds is *Babesia*. This genus develops in the erythrocyte cytoplasm and appears as small bluish bodies, each with a tiny magenta nucleus. The piroplasms multiply to a maximum of four merozoites per erythrocyte. Unlike erythrocytic schizonts of *Plasmodium*, these lack pigment. *Babesia* species are transmitted by ticks.

Microsporidians are complex protozoans of the genus *Encephalitozoon* that are rarely found in birds, but are most often reported from lovebirds. This parasite has been reported to kill large numbers of lovebirds.[10] The spores are intracellular and appear as tiny (<2 μm) dark-staining ellipsoid bodies with most stains. Their identity can only be determined

by transmission electron microscopy, with which the coiled polar filament becomes apparent. Little has been done with this parasite in birds, and they are most often found in cells of renal tubules, liver, and intestinal epithelium. The means of transmission is not proven, but it has been suggested that the spores are passed in feces or urine,[10] which presumably makes them available for oral ingestion.

Gut flagellates of birds include *Giardia*, *Hexamita*, *Trichomonas*, *Histomonas*, and *Cochlosoma*. The arrangement of the flagella is useful for identification, but this is difficult to ascertain. *Giardia*[11, 12] trophozoites are smooth swimmers. As they roll over, the large concave suckers on the anterior ends are seen. *Cochlosoma* species also have a sucking disc,[13] but they are smaller than trophozoites of *Giardia* species and are most commonly found in

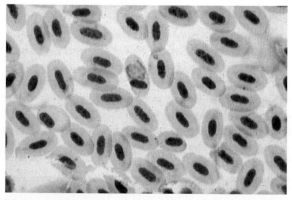

Figure 21–4

Gametocyte of *Plasmodium relictum* from a mourning dove.

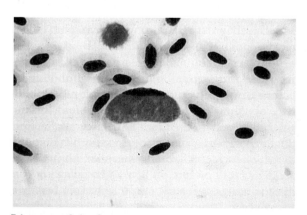

Figure 21–6

Gametocyte of *Leuococytozoon toddi* from a red-tailed hawk.

anatids. These parasites (cochlosoma species) are an important problem in Australian finches as well, especially Estrilidae. *Trichomonas* species have a tuft of anteriorly positioned flagella, a supportive rod (the axostyle) that runs the length of the cell, and an undulating membrane that appears as a wave passing along the cell edge in living specimens. They move in a jerky manner. *Histomonas* species have a single flagellum when it is in the lumen of the ceca, but is amoeboid after it enters the cecal wall.

Giardia species and *Hexamita* species reside in the lumen of the small intestine. *Histomonas* species live in the lumen and wall of the ceca and in the parenchyma of the liver.[14] *Trichomonas gallinae* lives in the oropharyngeal region. *Cochlosoma* species dwell in the ceca and cloaca. Some of these (*Giardia* and *Hexamita* species) have cysts. The cysts are the infective stage and are passed in the feces. *Trichomonas* species are passed to new hosts when the hosts drink water containing the trophozoites, via pigeon milk to squabs, and through eating infected prey. *Histomonas* species are transmitted by becoming incorporated in the eggs of *Heterakis* species and usually occur in gallinaceous birds, but a *Histomonas*-like organism was a cause of death in transplanted trumpeter swans.* In severe outbreaks it may be ingested directly from the soil. *Cochlosoma* species presumably are ingested as trophozoites.

Helminths

Roundworms may reside in many parts of the avian host. They are one of the most varied groups of internal parasites of birds. The mature ascaroids are heavy-bodied nematodes with three large lips, and they usually live in the intestines. They enter the host when the larvated eggs are eaten. *Porrocaecum* species and *Contracaecum* species can be separated by the presence of dentigerous ridges on the lips on *Porrocaecum* species. *Ascaridia* species are one of the most common nematodes in birds. Males have a prominent precloacal sucker[15] (Fig. 21–7). *Heterakis* males also have a precloacal sucker, but they have a large posterior bulb in the

---

*Dr. Lynn Creekmore, personal communication.

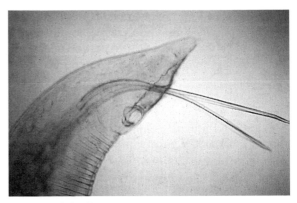

Figure 21–7

Ascaridia species, posterior end of male showing precloacal sucker, from the small intestine of a quaker parakeet.

esophagus, and the posterior ends are drawn out like pinworms. They also reside in the ceca.

Eustrongylides species are large worms found in the ventriculus of wading birds, and they lack the three large lips. A fish is the second intermediate host and it is eaten by the avian host.[16] The strongylate nematodes (males have a copulatory bursa at the posterior end) live in the small intestine, ventriculus, and respiratory system (Fig. 21–8). Most of these have direct life cycles in which the third larval stage is eaten.

Syngamus species live in the trachea, have a large mouth cavity, and are found in pairs with the male permanently attached to the female in permanent copula. *Cyathostoma* species also reside in the tra-

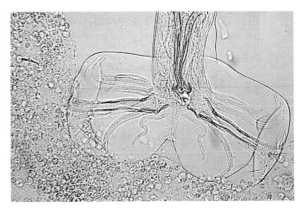

Figure 21–8

Ornithostrongylus species, copulatory bursa on a male from the small intestine of a pigeon.

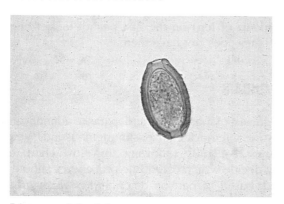

Figure 21–14

Capillaria species from a pigeon, 54×32 μm.

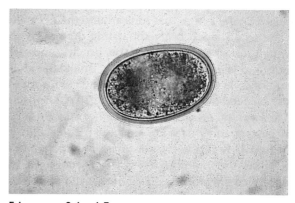

Figure 21–17

Ascaridia species from a macaw, 78×50 μm.

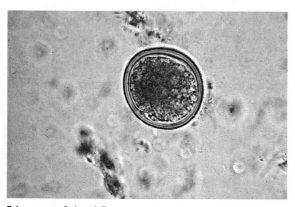

Figure 21–15

Contracaecum species from a pelican, 63×53 μm.

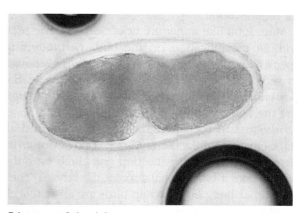

Figure 21–18

Deletrocephalus species from a rhea, 163×74 μm.

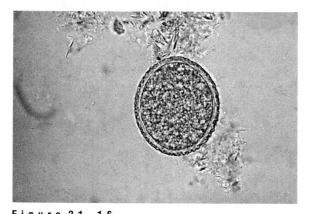

Figure 21–16

Porrocaecum species from a bald eagle, 66×56 μm.

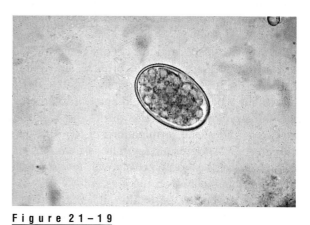

Figure 21–19

Codiostomum species from an ostrich, 55×35 μm.

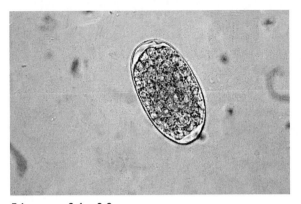

F i g u r e   2 1 – 2 0

Ornithostrongylus species from a pigeon, 75 × 38 μm.

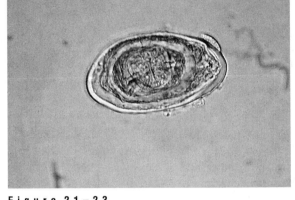

F i g u r e   2 1 – 2 3

Cestode egg from a Lady Gouldian finch, 93 × 50 μm.

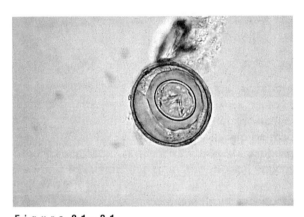

F i g u r e   2 1 – 2 1

Hymenolepis species from a chicken, 58 × 48 μm.

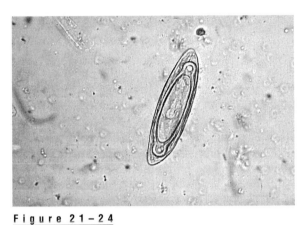

F i g u r e   2 1 – 2 4

Centrorhynchus species from a bald eagle, 80 × 22 μm.

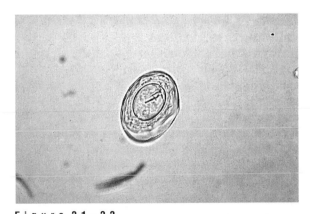

F i g u r e   2 1 – 2 2

Cestode egg from a barred owl, 50 × 32 μm.

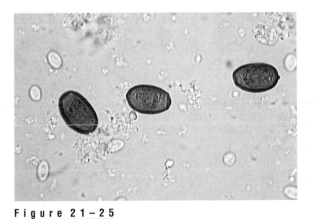

F i g u r e   2 1 – 2 5

Platynosomum species from a cockatoo, 31 × 20 μm.

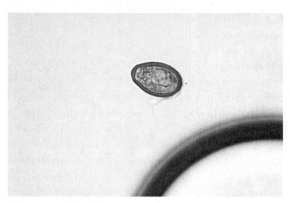

Figure 21–26

Dicrocoelid fluke egg from a vasa parrot, 36 × 23 μm.

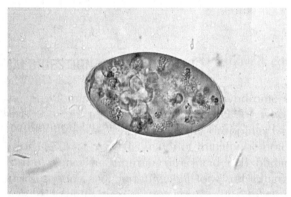

Figure 21–27

Strigeid fluke egg from a red-shouldered hawk, 94 × 55 μm.

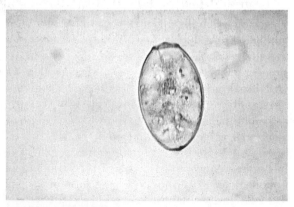

Figure 21–28

Orchipedum from a sandhill crane, 72 × 44 μm.

about 1 g feces in sodium nitrate (568 g/1000 ml water). Pass it through a tea strainer to eliminate large debris. Fill a tube with the mixture until a slight positive meniscus is formed. Add a coverslip to the top and allow to stand in vertical position for 10 to 15 minutes. The coverslip is then placed on a slide and systematically examined until the entire coverslip has been viewed under 100× total magnification.

Sedimentations are used to detect eggs of trematodes, which do not float under normal conditions. This method concentrates the eggs, but be aware that anything that floats on a flotation will become part of the sediment, along with the fluke eggs. Mix feces with a 0.5% soapy water solution (use inexpensive liquid dish soap), place in a 50-ml centrifuge tube and allow to stand for 5 minutes. Decant the solution, being careful not to pour off the sediment, because this is where the eggs are. Repeat this process until the solution remains clear and then examine the sediment for eggs, viewing under 100× total magnification.

Blood smears are used to detect infection with parasites that have stages in the blood (see Fig. 21–12). The smear is fixed in methanol, stained with Giemsa or Wright's stain, and examined under oil immersion.

Biopsies may be taken to make impression smears (Wright's/Giemsa stain) or fixed and processed for histologic sections. The impressions and tissue sections are viewed microscopically to detect the stages possibly present.

Ectoparasite examination may include brushing the feathers for lice and larger mites, picking macroscopic parasites off the host, and scraping skin for tissue-inhabiting forms (see Fig. 21–12).

Methods for necropsy include the same procedures in addition to examining the host for helminths and internal mites. The surface of the eyes should be examined and may need to be placed in normal saline to facilitate finding helminths. The mouth should be opened and visually examined for flukes and then the choanal slit should be opened with a moist, cotton-tipped swab to look for mites. The swab is then placed into a dish with saline. The viscera are removed from the body cavity and each organ (crop, esophagus, proventriculus, ventriculus, small intestine, ceca [if present], large intestine, liver with gall bladder, heart, lungs, spleen, and kidneys) is placed into a separate Petri dish in saline. The body cavity and air sacs should be searched for helminths and mites. The cranium may then be opened to examine the meninges for adult filarial worms. Slit open the nasal passages or flush with water to remove the nasal mites. The filarioid nematodes under the skin may be found by removing the skin and looking for nematodes. Collect a fecal sample from the large intestine if a fresh one has not been produced in the cage, and then do the fecal examinations.

You are now ready to examine the organs. Remember to collect and formalin-fix representative tissues for histologic examination. Tubular organs (gut and trachea) are slit open lengthwise, and the contents and mucosal scrapings are examined for helminths. Nematodes in the trachea should be apparent before scraping the mucosa. The proventriculus may need to be squeezed or teased apart to release those worms embedded in the wall. The koilon of the ventriculus needs to be stripped free from the muscles and examined for the nematodes that might reside there. The gut contents of large birds such as ratites may be placed in a #50 standard sieve and washed to remove the soluble material and fine particulate material to facilitate seeing the worms. Solid organs may be teased apart in saline to release any helminths present. The gall bladder must be opened to find flukes present there. Parasites recovered should be processed as suggested (see Fig. 21–12).

The testing solutions are prepared with the following recipes. Glycerin alcohol is 90 ml 70% ethanol and 10 ml glycerine. The alcohol:formalin:acetic acid (AFA) fixative is 85 ml 85% ethanol, 10 ml commercial formalin, and 5 ml of glacial acetic acid. Lactophenol is two parts glycerine, one part distilled water, one part melted phenol crystals, and one part liquid lactic acid. Hoyer's mounting medium is 30 g gum arabic, 200 g chloral hydrate, 20 ml glycerol, and 50 ml distilled water. Normal saline is 0.85 g sodium chloride in 100 ml of water.

CLINICALLY SIGNIFICANT PARASITISM

A summary of the ill effects of some of the parasites presented in earlier sections follows. One must remember that little or nothing is known about the clinical impact of many of the parasites found in birds. The extent of the damage is usually a reflection of the number of parasites present. Realize also that there are many species of birds for which little is known about their parasites. Do not hesitate to make contact with a parasitologist who is willing to render assistance, because identifying parasites can be very difficult.

The oropharyngeal region of birds may contain pathogenic *Trichomonas gallinae*. Pathogenic strains of *T. gallinae* may be found in birds raised in captivity[19] or free-ranging birds.[20] Avian trichomoniasis causes morbidity and mortality. It induces caseation necrosis of the mouth and pharynx that leads to partial blockage of the esophagus and trachea, and sometimes lesions extend into the lungs or liver.[21] The birds may become weak, emaciated, depressed, dehydrated, and dyspneic and they may regurgitate.[19, 21]

Adult *Tetrameres* (= *Microtetrameres*) *nestoris* in the ducts of the proventricular glands of a parrot causes destruction of secretory cells and thickening and some necrosis of the epithelium. At least 280 adult worms were recovered from a bird, but no history was provided other than that the bird was dead.[22]

Pigeons infected with *Capillaria columbae* become emaciated, listless, and have diarrhea. Where the adults attach to the small intestine mucosa, necrosis occurs. In heavy infections, the entire mucosa may be sloughed off. This debris may block the large intestine, resulting in stasis of fluid in the lower small intestine. Death may result.[23] This genus can also be important in parrots and toucans.

Giardiasis has been reported to cause mortalities of 20 to 50% in pet birds.[24] Diarrhea is a common consequence of giardiasis, and *Giardia* is often found with concurrent bacterial or chlamidial infections. Other signs include hyperproteinemia, eosinophilia, anorexia, depression, and in some species feather picking. Feather picking, best recognized in cockatiels, begins on the legs and may extend to wings, sometimes leading to bleeding from self-trauma. Shifting-leg lameness has also been found associated with giardiasis in cockatiels and budgerigars.[12]

While hexamitiasis has been known in poultry and pigeons for a long time, it has been recognized only recently in pet birds. Cockatiels and a splendid grass parakeet were diagnosed with this disease. Signs included weariness and emaciation; upon necropsy, the duodenum was dilated and gross de-

2. Bicknese EJ: Review of avian sarcocystosis. Proc Assoc Avian Vet 1993, pp 52–58.

3. Clubb SL, Frenkel JK: *Sarcocystis falcatula* of opossums: Transmission by cockroaches with fatal pulmonary disease in psitticine birds. J Parasitol 78:116–124, 1992.

4. Swayne DE, Getzy D, Siemons RD, et al: Coccidiosis as a cause of transmural lymphocytic enteritis and mortality in captive Nashville warblers (*Vermivora ruficapilla*). J Wildl Dis 27:615–620, 1991.

5. Partington CJ, Gardiner CH, Fritz D, et al: Atoxoplasmosis in Bali Mynahs (*Leucopsar rothschildi*). J Wildl Zoo Med 20:328–335, 1989.

6. Box ED: Life cycles of two *Isospora* species in the canary, *Serinus canarius* Linnaeus. J Protozool 24:57–67, 1977.

7. Hooimeijer J: Coccidiosis in lorikeets infectious for budgerigar. Proc Assoc Avian Vet, 1993, pp 59–61.

8. Howerth EW, Rich G, Dubey JP, Yogasundram K: Fatal toxoplasmosis in a red lory (*Eos bornea*). Avian Dis 35:642–646, 1991.

9. Hartley WJ, Dubey JP: Fatal toxoplasmosis in some native Australian birds. J Vet Diagn Invest 3:167–169, 1991.

10. Randall CJ, Lees S, Higgins RJ, Harcourt-Brown NH: Microsporidian infection in lovebirds (*Agapornis* spp.). Avian Pathol 15:223–231, 1986.

11. Box ED: Observations on *Giardia* of budgerigars. J Protozool 28:491–494, 1981.

12. Fudge AM, McEntee L: Avian giardiasis: Syndromes, diagnosis, and therapy. Proc Assoc Avian Vet, 1986, pp 155–164.

13. Watkins RA, O'Dell WD, Pinter AJ: Redescription of flagellar arrangement in the duck intestinal flagellate, *Cochlosoma anatis* and description of a new species, *Cochlosoma siricis* n. sp. from shrews. J Protozool 36:527–531, 1989.

14. Douglass EM: Histomoniasis in zoo birds. Vet Med/Sm Anim Clin 76:1013–1014, 1981.

15. Mines JJ, Green PE: Experimental *Ascaridia columbae* infections in budgerigars. Aust Vet J 60:278–280, 1983.

16. Spalding MG, Forrester DJ: Pathogenesis of *Eustrongylides ignotus* (Nematoda: Dioctophymoidea) in Ciconiiformes. J Wildl Dis 29:250–260, 1993.

17. Bartlett CM, Anderson RC: *Lemdana wernaarti* n. sp. and other filarioid nematodes from *Bubo virginianus* and *Asio otus* (Strigiformes) in Ontario, Canada, with a revision of *Lemdana* and a key to avian filarioid genera. Can J Zool 65:1100–1109, 1987.

18. Atyeo WT, Gaud J: Feather mites (Acarina) of the parakeet, *Melopsittacus undulatus* (Shaw) (Aves: Psittacidae). J Parasitol 73:203–206, 1987.

19. Murphy J: Psittacine trichomoniasis. Proc Assoc Avian Vet, 1992, pp 21–24.

20. Greiner EC, Baxter WL: A localized epizootic of trichomoniasis in mourning doves. J Wildl Dis 10:104–106, 1974.

21. Garner MM, Sturtevant FC: Trichomoniasis in a blue-fronted Amazon parrot (*Amazona aestiva*). J Assoc Avian Vet 6:17–20, 1992.

22. Clark WC, Black H, Rutherford DM: *Microtetrameres nestoris* n. sp. (Nematoda: Spirurida), a parasite of the North Island kaka, *Nestor meridionalis septentrionalis* (Aves: Psittaciformes). N Z J Zool 6:1–5, 1979.

23. Wehr EE: Studies on the development of the pigeon capillarid, *Capillaria columbae*. USDA Tech Bull #679, 1939.

24. Panigraphy B, Elissalde G, Grumbles LC, and Hall CF: *Giardia* infection in parakeets. Avian Dis 22:815–818, 1978.

25. Harper FDW: *Hexamita* species present in some avian species in South Wales. Vet Rec 128:130, 1991.

26. Goodwin MA: Cryptosporidiosis in birds—a review. Avian Pathol 18:365–384, 1984.

27. Gardiner CH, Imes GD: *Cryptosporidium* sp. in the kidneys of a black-throated finch. JAVMA 185:1401–1402, 1984.

28. Mason RW, Hartley WJ: Respiratory cryptosporidiosis in a peacock chick. Avian Dis 24:771–776, 1980.

29. Gajadhar AA: *Cryptosporidium* species in imported ostriches and consideration of possible implications for birds in Canada. Can Vet J 34:115–116, 1993.

30. Box ED, Smith JH: The intermediate host spectrum in a *Sarcocystis* species in birds. J Parasitol 68:668–673, 1982.

31. Smith JH, Meier JL, Neill PJG, Box ED: Pathogenesis of *Sarcocystis falcatula* in the budgerigar. II. Pulmonary pathology. Lab Invest 56:72–84, 1987.

32. Jacobson ER, Gardiner CH, Nicholson A, Page CD: *Sarcosytis* encephalitis in a cockatiel. J Am Vet Med Assoc 185:904–905, 1984.

33. Smith JH, Neill PJG, Box ED: Pathogenesis of *Sarcocystis falcatula* (Apicomplexa: Sarcocystidae) in the budgerigar (*Melopsittacus undulatus*). III. Pathologic and quantitative parasitologic analysis of extrapulmonary disease. J Parasitol 75:270–287, 1989.

34. Levine ND: The genus *Atoxoplasma* (Protozoa, Apicomplexa). J Parasitol 68:719–723, 1982.

35. Poelma F, Zwart P, Strik WJ: *Lankesterella* (*Atoxoplasma* Garnham, 1950) infections in birds in the Netherlands. Neth J Vet Sci 4:43–50, 1971.

36. Khan RA, Desser SS: Avian *Lankesterella* infections in Algonquin Park, Ontario. Can J Zool 49:1105–1110, 1971.

37. Fix AS, Waterhouse C, Greiner EC, Stoskopf MK: *Plasmodium relictum* as a cause of avian malaria in wild-caught Magellanic penguins (*Spheniscus magellanicus*). J Wildl Dis 24:610–619, 1988.

38. Quesenberry KE, Tappe JP, Greiner EC, et al: Hepatic trematodiasis in five cockatoos. J Am Vet Med Assoc 189:1103–1105, 1986.

39. Kock MD, Duhamel GE: Hepatic distomiasis in a sulphur-crested cockatoo. J Am Vet Med Assoc 18:1388–1389, 1982.

40. Ackerman N, Isaza R, Greiner E, Berry CR: Pneumocoelom associated with *Serratospiculum amaculata* in a bald eagle. Vet Radiol Ultrasound 33:351–355, 1992.

41. Bigland CH, Liu SK, Perry ML: Five cases of *Serratospiculum amaculata* (Nematoda: Filarioidea) infection in prairie falcons (*Falco mexicanus*). Avian Dis 8:412–419, 1964.

42. Tidemann SC, McOrist S, Woinarski JCZ, and Freeland WJ: Parasitism of wild Gouldian finches (*Erythrura gouldiae*) by the air-sac mite *Sternostoma tracheocolum*. J Wildl Dis 28:80–84, 1992.

43. Greve JH, Graham DL, Nye RR: Tenosynovitis caused by *Pelecitus calamiformis* (Nematoda: Filarioidea) in the legs of a parrot. Avian Dis 26:431–436, 1982.

44. Allen JL, Kollias GV, Greiner EC, Boyce W: Subcutaneous filariasis (*Pelecitus* sp.) in a yellow-collared macaw (*Ara auricollis*). Avian Dis 29:891–893, 1985.

45. Bartlett CM, and Greiner EC: A revision of *Pelecitus* Railliet & Henry, 1910 (Filarioidea, Dirofilariinae) and evidence for the "capture" by mammals of filarioids of birds. Bull Mus Natn Hist Nat Paris (Sect. A, 4e ser.) 8:47–99, 1986.

46. Brooks DE, Greiner EC, Walsh MT: Conjunctivitis caused by *Thelazia* sp. in a Senegal parrot. JAVMA 183:1305–1306, 1983.

47. Schmidt RE, Toft JD II: Ophthalmic lesions in animals from a zoological collection. J Wildl Dis 17:267–275, 1981.

48. Toft JD II, Schmidt RE, Hartfiel DA: *Philophthalmus gralli* in zoo waterfowl. In Montali RJ, Migaki G (eds): The Comparative Pathology of Zoo Animals. Symposium of the National Zoological Park, 1980, pp 395–399.

49. Blue-McLendon A, Graham DL, Ambrus SI, Craig TM: Cere-

brospinal nematodiasis in emus. Proc Assoc Avian Vet 1992, pp 326–327.

50. Smith DA, Kwiecien JM, Smith-Maxie L: Encephalitis in emus resulting from migration of *Baylisascaris* sp. Proc Assoc Avian Vet, 1993, pp 301–303.

51. Armstrong DL, Montali RJ, Kazacos KR, Doster AR: Cerebrospinal nematodiasis in blue and gold macaws and scarlet macaws associated with *Baylisascaris procyonis*. Proc 1st Int Conf Zool Avian Med, 1987, pp 489–490.

52. Evans RE, Tangredi B: Cerebrospinal nematodiasis in free-ranging birds. J Am Vet Med Assoc 187:1213–1214, 1985.

53. Shane SM, Stewart TB, Confer AW, Pirie GJ: *Knemidokoptes pilae* infestation in the palm cockatoo. Avian Exotic Pract 2(2):21–25, 1985.

James W. Carpenter
Edward J. Gentz

22

Zoonotic Diseases of Avian Origin

Man's interactions with birds, especially companion birds, has increased dramatically in recent years. In fact, companion birds are increasing in numbers more rapidly than any other group of warm-blooded animals.[1] In addition, birds are frequently used in animal-facilitated therapy with special populations such as the elderly or those who are physically or mentally impaired. Because of the increased interactions between humans and birds, the opportunities and potential for diseases being transmitted from bird to humans are increasing. There has been an increased prevalence of zoonotic disease in the US, and this increase has paralleled the rise in cases of acquired immunodeficiency syndrome (AIDS).[2] Fortunately, however, pet birds pose a low risk to immunocompromised persons.[3] But, because of the increased number of patients with AIDS and other immunocompromising diseases, elderly people, and bird breeders who are at greater risk for acquiring zoonotic diseases of avian origin, it is important that the veterinary profession become knowledgeable about these health risks and develop strategies (i.e., appropriate sanitation, hygiene, and veterinary care) to better manage our captive birds to prevent the spread of potential diseases to humans.

Although there are many diseases that may be transmitted from birds to humans, the practical importance of most of these diseases to the general population is very small (Table 22–1). Probably the most commonly encountered avian zoonotic diseases are chlamydiosis, salmonellosis, and allergic alveolitis. Even *Mycobacterium avium* is only of minor significance, and one report states that *M.*

avium infection in human beings has not been shown to be pet-associated.[2] There are, however, other diseases that are potentially zoonotic and/or indirectly associated with birds, such as histoplasmosis associated with pigeon droppings, but the majority of these diseases are largely of academic interest (see Table 22–1).

DISEASES OF REASONABLE SIGNIFICANCE

Chlamydiosis

Chlamydia psittaci is the causative organism of chlamydiosis, also referred to as psittacosis in psittacine birds and ornithosis in other avian species. *C. psittaci* is a nonmotile, obligate, intracellular, bacterial parasite with two morphologically distinct forms. The smaller elementary body (0.2–0.3 μm) is the infectious form, whereas the larger reticulate body (0.6–0.8 μm) is the intracellular, metabolically active form.[4] Chapter 23 provides information on the clinical signs, diagnosis, and treatment of chlamydiosis in birds.

Chlamydiosis is a reportable disease in 47 of 50 states. Between 1975 to 1984 and 1982 to 1991, 1136 cases (with eight deaths) and 1344 cases (with six deaths) of human chlamydiosis were reported to the Centers for Disease Control (CDC), respectively.[5, 6] People most at risk of contracting chlamydiosis are owners of pet birds, pet store employees, and pigeon fanciers. Other people at risk include farmers, laboratory workers, poultry processing plant employees, quarantine station workers, ren-

Table 22–1

ZOONOTIC DISEASES, DIRECTLY, INDIRECTLY, OR POTENTIALLY ASSOCIATED WITH BIRDS

Disease and Status	Agent
Diseases of Reasonable Significance	
Chlamydiosis	*Chlamydia psittaci*
Salmonellosis	*Salmonella* spp.
Campylobacteriosis	*Campylobacter jejuni*
Yersiniosis (pseudotuberculosis)	*Yersinia pseudotuberculosis, Y. enterocolitica*
Newcastle disease	Newcastle disease virus (paramyxovirus)
Allergic alveolitis	Antigens of avian origin
Infrequent, Rare, or Potential Diseases	
Mycobacteriosis (avian tuberculosis)	*Mycobacterium avium*
Colibacillosis	*Escherichia coli*
Erysipelas	*Erysipelothrix rhusiopathiae*
Listeriosis	*Listeria monocytogenes*
Influenza	Influenza A virus (orthomyxovirus)
Rabies	*Lyssavirus* (rhabdovirus)
Toxoplasmosis	*Toxoplasma gondii*
Cryptosporidiosis	*Cryptosporidium* spp.
Giardiasis	*Giardia* spp.
Lung cancer (?)	Inhalation of avian antigens
Other diseases	*Pasteurella* spp., *Pseudomonas* spp., *Vibrio* spp., ringworm (*Trichophyton* spp.)
Infrequent or Potential Diseases Indirectly Associated With Birds	
Staphylococcal food poisoning	*Staphylococcus* spp. toxin
Clostridium perfringens food poisoning	*Clostridium perfringens* toxin
Bacillus cereus food poisoning	*Bacillus cereus* toxin
West Nile fever	Flavivirus
Mosquito-borne encephalitides	Alphavirus, flavivirus, bunyavirus
Aspergillosis	*Aspergillus fumigatus*
Histoplasmosis	*Histoplasma capsulatum*
Cryptococcosis	*Cryptococcus neoformans*

dering plant employees, veterinarians, veterinary technicians, wildlife handlers and rehabilitators, and zoo employees.[5, 6] Human infections generally result from the inhalation of an infective aerosol. The incubation period varies from 5 to 14 days.

Veterinarians are ethically responsible for the notification of potentially exposed employees and the owners of infected birds concerning the potential health consequences of exposure to chlamydiosis.[7] Practitioners should also institute appropriate measures to prevent the possible dissemination of chlamydiosis. Veterinarians performing necropsy of birds suspected to be infected with *C. psittaci* should take adequate precautions to prevent infection, not only of themselves, but of others around them.[8]

No symptoms are pathognomonic for chlamydiosis in humans. The most common symptoms include chills, cough, fever, headache, malaise, and myalgia. Others may include anorexia, diaphoresis, nausea, photophobia, thoracic pain, and vomiting.

Pneumonia frequently develops, leading to such differential diagnoses as brucellosis, coccidiomycosis, histoplasmosis, influenza, Legionnaires' disease, mycoplasmosis, Q fever, tuberculosis, and tularemia.[5, 6] Hospitalization is required in 87% of people with chlamydiosis. Fatality is less than 1% in properly treated patients. Immunocompromised, immunodeficient, and immunosuppressed persons are at greater risk.[1, 9]

Chlamydiosis has been documented in a total of 159 avian host species, nearly a quarter of which are psittacines. New World parrots are more susceptible to chlamydial infection than either Australian or African psittacines. Chlamydiosis has been reported in 114 species of free-living wild birds,[10] including raptors.[11] The avian families most commonly represented by these species include Charadriiformes (23%), Passeriformes (22%), and Anseriformes (16%). When the source of infection was known, the vast majority (70%) of human cases of chlamydiosis were the result of exposure to pet caged birds. Other common avian sources of human infection included turkeys (16%) and either domestic or wild pigeons (10%).[7]

Salmonellosis

Salmonellosis is the most important zoonosis in developed countries, and it is perhaps the most widespread zoonosis in the world. *Salmonella* was first isolated from a human source in 1880 and initially from an animal source in 1885.[12] The total number of human cases in the US annually may be as high as 5 million.[13] *Salmonella,* a member of the Enterobacteriaceae, is a gram-negative, aerobic, nonspore-forming rod. Salmonellae are not highly resistant to physical or chemical agents and are readily destroyed by standard cooking and pasteurization procedures. *Salmonella* organisms, however, are able to survive over 4 months in stagnant water and longer in soil.[14]

There are approximately 2000 different serotypes of *Salmonella,* all of which have variable pathogenicity in birds. *S. typhimurium* is the most commonly encountered serotype in poultry, although *S. gallinarum* and *S. pullorum* also commonly infect fowl. These latter species are not very pathogenic for humans, but have caused disease in children.[13] *S. typhimurium* is the most common isolate from both wild birds[15, 16] and pet birds.[17] Chapter 18 provides information on the clinical signs, diagnosis, and treatment of salmonellosis in birds.

Salmonella infection has been documented in such diverse avian species as blackbirds, canaries, cowbirds, finches, herons, ostriches, penguins, seagulls, sparrows, and starlings.[18] Domestic, wild, and zoo birds are all equally susceptible.[19] Feral pigeons may have an incidence rate of well over 20%. Human cases of salmonellosis have involved phage types found in wild birds.[15] Easter chicks and ducklings may be a source of infection for people, especially children.[12] Salmonellosis is transmitted to humans via contaminated food and fomites. Wild birds can be an important part of the "*Salmonella* cycle" by contracting salmonellosis from contaminated feed or feces and then contaminating new environments. Herring gulls are carriers of a range of *Salmonella* serotypes similar to that causing infection in man, and they likely ingest these serotypes at

untreated sewage outfalls.[20] The incidence of salmonellosis may be increasing in psittacine birds.[21]

In humans, gastroenteritis is the most common clinical syndrome caused by *Salmonella*. Those most seriously affected are infants, children, and the elderly.[12] The incubation period is 6 to 72 hours. Abdominal cramping, diarrhea, and vomiting are commonly accompanied by fever and headache. Recovery generally occurs within 2 to 4 days. Differential diagnoses include gastroenteritis caused by shigellosis, *Clostridium perfringens, Escherichia coli,* enteroviruses, and gastrointestinal parasites. Case fatality rate averages 1 to 2%. Enteric fever, or septic syndrome, may follow gastroenteritis or may be seen as a separate clinical syndrome.[18]

Human salmonellosis usually results from the ingestion of contaminated food or water.[22] Human infections with *S. enteritidis* have been associated with egg consumption.[23] An infective dose of 400,000 to 16 million *Salmonella* organisms must enter a person's gastrointestinal tract for infection to occur. In addition, it is possible for any organ or body tissue to be affected by inflammation or abscess formation resulting from *Salmonella*. Arthritis, bronchopneumonia, endocarditis, meningitis, osteomyelitis, and pyelonephritis can be caused by *Salmonella* infection. Antibiotics are generally contraindicated for human salmonellosis, except in cases of prolonged fever or septicemia, because they may prolong the carrier period and cause antibiotic-sensitive strains to emerge.[18]

Campylobacteriosis

Formerly known as vibrionic enteritis, campylobacteriosis is caused by *Campylobacter jejuni,* now recognized as a distinct species separate from *C. fetus*.[24] *C. jejuni* is a gram-negative, nonspore-forming, motile, curved or V-shaped rod with a single polar flagellum. With a worldwide distribution, *C. jejuni* is a principal cause of enteritis in humans. In some of the developed countries, the prevalence may equal or exceed salmonellosis as a cause of bacterial diarrhea. The number of *Campylobacter* organisms (500) necessary to cause disease in people is significantly less than the number of salmonellae required to produce a similar enteritis.[25]

Campylobacteriosis in humans is an acute illness with an incubation period of 2 to 5 days. Predisposing factors include debilitation, stress including pregnancy, and impaired immune response. Principal symptoms are abdominal pain that precedes diarrhea, fever, and vomiting, which are often accompanied by arthralgia, backache, headache, malaise, and myalgia.[25] The principal sites of disease in humans are the jejunum and ileum, but the colon may also be involved. Generally, recovery is spontaneous in 7 to 10 days. Differential diagnoses may include appendicitis, salmonellosis, and ulcerative colitis. Although complications are rare, septicemia has occurred. Sequelae can include arthritis, endocarditis, hepatitis, pericarditis, placentitis, pneumonitis, purulent meningitis, and thrombophlebitis. Case fatality can reach 50% in infants. Prognosis is good in older children and adults if uncomplicated by underlying disease. Between 5 and 14% of all diarrhea cases in Australia, Canada, the Netherlands, Sweden, the United Kingdom, and the USA are caused by *C. jejuni*.[13]

Infection with *C. jejuni* in poultry has been described as avian infectious hepatitis and avian vibrionic hepatitis. Healthy birds of many species, particularly poultry, have a high rate of intestinal infection with *C. jejuni*. The high carrier rate in many different avian species represents a health hazard for people. The prevalence rate of *C. jejuni* in herbivorous birds, however, is considerably lower than in scavengers such as crows and gulls.[26] Out of the wide range of suitable animal hosts for *C. jejuni,* the greatest similarity to human clinical isolates are poultry strains, followed by strains from wild birds.[27]

Free-living birds may act as significant reservoirs for the maintenance and dissemination of *C. jejuni* in nature.[26] *C. jejuni* has been isolated from such wild species as blackbirds, pigeons, sparrows, and starlings in Virginia.[28] In Norway, high rates of infection were found in crows, gulls, and puffins.[22] *C. jejuni* was also isolated in a large percentage of crows, pigeons, and starlings in Japan, as well as magpies and bulbuls.[26] Although one study found that 35% of migratory waterfowl cultured harbored *C. jejuni,*[29] none of the birds exhibited gross lesions of the liver or gut and were apparently healthy when the samples were collected. *C. jejuni* has been isolated from zoo birds such as the flamingo and motmot.[30] Prevalence rates of *C. jejuni* have been reported to be 25% in Galliformes and 8% in Columbiformes. An extremely low prevalence rate

of *C. jejuni* in psittacines represents a low risk of human infection from these species.[31]

The best method of diagnosis is demonstration of rising antibody titer. Alternatively, the organism can be directly identified from diarrheic feces using dark-field microscopy.[25] Serologic techniques used to diagnose campylobacteriosis include complement fixation (CF), enzyme-linked immunosorbent assay (ELISA), fluorescent antibody (FA), and indirect hemagglutination.

Yersiniosis (Pseudotuberculosis)

Yersinia pseudotuberculosis and *Y. enterocolitica* are gram-negative coccobacilli belonging to the Enterobacteriaceae family. *Y. enterocolitica* is the causative agent of yersiniosis, whereas *Y. pseudotuberculosis* causes pseudotuberculosis. *Y. enterocolitica* has a worldwide distribution, with human disease reported in more than 30 countries on five continents. Incidence rates are highest in Scandinavia, Belgium, Eastern Europe, Japan, South Africa, and Canada.[13] *Y. pseudotuberculosis* also has a worldwide distribution, with the greatest concentration of cases occurring in Europe and the eastern part of the former Soviet Union, and only sporadically in the Americas. Infection with *Y. enterocolitica* is less common in wild animals but more common in humans than infection with *Y. pseudotuberculosis*.[32]

Pseudotuberculosis was first reported in canaries in 1884.[33] Early cases were also reported in yellow buntings and pigeons. The disease was first reported in turkeys in 1924. The first report of pseudotuberculosis in birds in North America was in canaries in 1906, and later reported in a blackbird in New Jersey in 1940[34] and in turkeys in the USA in 1944. Although outbreaks have occurred in chickens, they appear to be largely resistant to virulent canary or turkey strains of *Y. pseudotuberculosis*.

Yersiniosis is of much greater importance in birds than mammals. Sporadic infection has been recorded in more than 50 species of wild and domestic birds.[32] Pigeons and doves appear to be the most common sylvatic avian reservoir hosts. Outbreaks have been reported in these species in Denmark, England, France, Germany, and the USA.[33] Feed contaminated with the feces of wild pigeons has been the source of *Yersinia* infection in zoo animals.[35] Outbreaks have been reported in buntings in England, Denmark, and Germany. Infections in gallinaceous birds have been reported in Denmark, England, France, and Sweden.[33] Single disease episodes have been reported in such miscellaneous species as crows and purple martins (Canada),[36] grackles (USA),[37] owls (Sweden), swans (France), and waxwings (Denmark).[33] Epizootics in wild avian populations can lead to human infection through massive environmental contamination via intense fecal shedding.

Mortality has approached 100% in epizootics in commercial aviaries, including canaries, finches, and rarely, budgerigars. From 1969 to 1974 in zoos in England, pseudotuberculosis was the second most frequent bacterial cause of death in birds, ranking behind only avian tuberculosis.[33] Zoo birds that appear to be particularly susceptible to *Y. pseudotuberculosis* include canaries and toucans.[38]

Y. enterocolitica has been found much less frequently in avian hosts. Isolations have been reported from two pigeons in Canada,[39] budgerigars in England,[40] two owls, a bunting, a gull, and a tern in Norway,[22] a canary and goldfinch in Belgium, and a Canada goose and Pekin robin in Ontario.[36] *Y. enterocolitica* may be overlooked as a cause of enteritis in birds because when cultured, it is easily overgrown by *E. coli.*

The majority of animal strains of *Y. pseudotuberculosis* and the strain found most frequently in humans are both serologic type I. *Y. pseudotuberculosis* was cultured from both the feces of a man with clinical pseudotuberculosis and his pet canary.[34] The clinical manifestations in humans of both *Y. pseudotuberculosis* and *Y. enterocolitica* are similar.[35] Incubation period is variable, ranging from 7 to 21 days. The most common form, acute mesenteric lymphadenitis, presents as an acute pseudoappendicitis. Erythema nodosum can occur either as a separate clinical entity or in association with mesenteric lymphadenitis. Mesenteric lymph node enlargement is less common with *Y. enterocolitica* infection, in which the characteristic lesion is inflammation of the terminal ileum. Enteritis is a common manifestation of *Y. enterocolitica* infection but is rarely encountered with *Y. pseudotuberculosis.* Hepatomegaly occurs in roughly three-quarters and icterus in approximately one-half of all cases. Septicemia is rare. Diagnosis is via isolation of the organism from blood, feces, liver, spleen, or affected lymph nodes. This normally sporadic disease generally runs a benign course in people, although up to 50% mortality can be seen in septicemia cases, even with the use of antibiotics.[33]

Newcastle Disease

Newcastle disease, also known as avian distemper and avian pneumoencephalitis among other names, is caused by a single-stranded ribonucleic acid (RNA) paramyxovirus. There are four pathotypes of varying severity: lentogenic, mesogenic, neurotropic velogenic, and viscerotropic velogenic. Viscerotropic velogenic Newcastle disease (VVND) has been eliminated from the US since its last outbreak in 1974, which was caused by imported parrots,[41] and did not become established in wild bird populations.[42] The virus is resistant to sunlight and is stable over wide ranges of pH.

Newcastle disease has been reported in at least 236 species of birds.[43] Highly susceptible species include ostriches, pigeons, psittacines, and domestic poultry. Moderately susceptible species include passerines, penguins, raptors, and storks. Waterfowl appear to be among the least susceptible avian species, although the occurrence of the virus in migratory ducks reflects a potential source for the spread of Newcastle disease over considerable geographic distances.[42] Mynah birds may be as efficient viral carriers as parrots. Canaries are relatively refractory to infection with the virus.[44] Outbreaks of Newcastle disease have occurred in exotic bird parks, quarantine facilities, private bird collections, and zoologic gardens.[43]

Approximately 37 cases of human infection with Newcastle disease were reported in the literature from 1943 to 1971.[45] More than 100 descriptions of human reaction to Newcastle disease virus currently appear in the literature.[46] Human infection with Newcastle disease is not a reportable disease in the US, although avian VVND is. People primarily at risk include poultry farmers, poultry processing plant workers, and veterinarians handling diseased birds or vaccines. Live vaccines are pathogenic for humans. Human populations in close contact with poultry have higher titers to Newcastle disease virus than those with more limited poultry contact. The virus does not appear to be transmitted between people. Quarantine or isolation of human patients is not required.

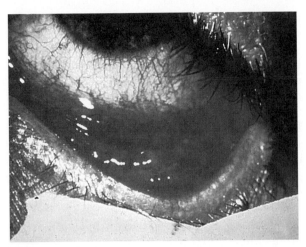

Figure 22-1

Acute phase of conjunctivitis in humans caused by the Newcastle disease virus usually lasts 3 to 4 days. Scleral, conjunctival, and subconjunctival tissues are swollen and inflamed. Recovery is spontaneous and complete in 1 to 2 weeks, usually without permanent damage. (From Donham KJ, Mutel CF: Poultry Zoonoses, Rural Health Series, Institute of Agricultural Medicine, The University of Iowa, Iowa City, IA.)

The incubation period in people is 1 to 2 days. The most common manifestation of human disease is conjunctivitis, either unilateral or bilateral, without corneal involvement (Fig. 22–1). Eye washings from these cases are the most successful source for virus isolation. Virus isolation has also been successful from blood, saliva, and urine. Immune response produces low levels of neutralizing antibodies, which do not prevent the reoccurrence of ocular inflammation. Other symptoms can include chills, fever, headache, malaise, pharyngitis, and possibly, encephalitis and hemolytic anemia.[45] The multiplication of Newcastle disease virus in human hosts is limited.[46] Recovery is spontaneous, following a course of infection ranging from 3 days to 3 weeks.

Allergic Alveolitis

Allergic alveolitis, also called hypersensitivity pneumonitis, bronchiolitis, allergic interstitial pneumonitis, parakeet dander pneumoconiosis, and pigeon lung disease, is a respiratory disease of humans induced by hypersensitivity to avian antigens including serum, feathers, feather dust, and fecal material.[1] Most reports seem to be associated with budgerigars and pigeons. Clinical signs in humans vary, and may include malaise, chills, fever, shortness of breath, myalgia, and coughing.[47–49] The disease is a cell-mediated (type IV) immune response with serum immunoglobulin G (IgG) and surface immunoglobulin A (IgA), which is atypical of reactions to inhaled antigens.[1] Clinical signs result from a reduction of vital lung capacity and impairment of alveolar-capillary diffusion.

The disease may be acute, subacute, or chronic.[1] The acute form occurs 4 to 8 hours after exposure to a heavy load of avian antigen. Coughing, dyspnea, fever, and chills occur. The subacute form results from long-term exposure to moderate antigen load and is characterized by a dry cough and progressive dyspnea. A skin test is a useful diagnostic tool in both conditions. If further exposure to avian antigens can be prevented, the prognosis is good. The disease is often unrecognized in the subacute stages because it mimics influenza or a variety of other mild respiratory infections.[1]

The chronic form of allergic alveolitis is irreversible and results from low-dose exposure to avian antigen over a long time. Clinical signs include progressive dyspnea, nonproductive cough, weight loss, and inspiratory rales. The lungs undergo interstitial granulomatous and inflammatory changes in the alveoli accompanied by pulmonary fibrosis.[1] To prevent further deterioration, an individual must prevent any further exposure to avian antigens. Patient history and a skin test result are important for diagnosis. The chronic form is most common in clients with companion birds.[1]

INFREQUENT, RARE, AND POTENTIAL ZOONOTIC DISEASES

Mycobacteriosis (Avian Tuberculosis)

The *Mycobacterium avium* complex consists of *M. avium, M. intracellulare,* and *M. scrofulaceum.* These acid-fast bacilli cannot be differentiated by culture or biochemical methods, and are thus most reliably identified by serotyping via seroagglutination. Although the *M. avium* complex has over 20 distinct serotypes, only serovars 1, 2, and 3 commonly cause disease in birds.[50] These first three serovars represent the *M. avium* serovars pathogenic for birds. Serotype 1 is most frequently reported in the US, whereas serotype 2 is most commonly reported in Europe. Serotype 3 is only sporadically isolated from birds and has only been reported from Europe. Serotypes 2 and 3 are more highly pathogenic than serotype 1.[51] The serovars isolated most frequently from human beings are 1, 4, and 8. Additionally, serovars 4 and 8, which are commonly isolated from tuberculous swine, are commonly isolated from humans affected with AIDS.[52]

Avian tuberculosis occurs most frequently in north temperate–zone birds. It has been reported in a wide array of birds of all kinds, including domestic fowl, passerines, shorebirds, raptors, and waterfowl.[53] The natural hosts of avian tuberculosis, both poultry and wild birds, are able to act as reservoirs for human infection.[54] Zoo birds are commonly affected; 137 birds died of avian tuberculosis at the National Zoo between 1969 and 1975.[50] Those least affected included ratites and psittacines, although avian tuberculosis has been reported in numerous psittacine species.[51] *M. avium* has also been isolated as an environmental contaminant in house dust, soil, and water.[52] *Mycobacterium* are able to survive for years in bird facilities. Chapter 18 gives further information on tuberculosis in birds.

A 1938 literature review found 13 confirmed reports of human infection with *M. avium,* and a subsequent literature review revealed 57 additional human cases reported between 1946 and 1968 in Great Britain, Czechoslovakia, Denmark, the US, Australia, and Canada.[55] Between 1955 and 1975, 98 human cases were reported in Western Germany.[54] The number of human cases of avian tuberculosis in Massachusetts increased fivefold from 1972 to 1983.[56] Although people with AIDS, congenital severe combined immunodeficiency disease, or leukemia are at a higher risk to become infected with *M. avium,*[52] this increased risk is not documented.[3] As a matter of fact, pet birds are an unlikely source of *M. avium* infections in human beings because *M. avium* isolates from birds differ in antibiotic susceptibility, serovars, and genetic sequencing from human isolates.[3] Nevertheless, persons with impaired immune function probably should not have contact with pet birds with clinical *M. avium* infections.[3]

Several different clinical manifestations of avian tuberculosis occur in human patients. Pulmonary localization of chronic cavitary tuberculosis usually occurs in males over 40 years of age. Cervical lymphadenitis occurs in young children. Systemic lymphogenic disease also occurs.[57] Treatment of avian tuberculosis in humans is generally unsuccessful, largely because *M. avium* is quite resistant to antituberculosis agents. Pulmonary and extrapulmonary infections are often progressive and fatal. Diagnosis is via fecal acid-fast stains and blood culture.[52] Cervical lymphadenopathy in children carries the most promising prognosis when treated via surgical excision.[55]

Colibacillosis

Colibacillosis is an infectious disease of humans and animals caused by *Escherichia coli*. Clinical signs generally include enteritis and diarrhea. Although pathogenic strains of *E. coli* have been isolated from birds, the majority of the Psittaciformes do not harbor this bacteria in their digestive, respiratory, or reproductive tracts.[1] Although it is difficult to differentiate pathogenic from nonpathogenic strains of *E. coli* or to document whether avian *E. coli* actually infects humans, there is at least one report of direct transmission of this bacteria from poultry to humans.[58] The potential for human infection is exposure from infected birds with strains virulent for humans.[1]

Erysipelas

Occurring worldwide, erysipelas is an infection of humans, terrestrial mammals, wild and domestic birds, and aquatic animals caused by *Erysipelothrix rhusiopathiae*.[1] Turkeys are the most common species involved, and swine and rodents serve as reservoir hosts. The infection in humans occurs in food processing workers of poultry, pork, and seafood.

Listeriosis

Listeriosis is a bacterial disease caused by *Listeria monocytogenes* and is usually manifested at the extremes of age, during pregnancy, or among immunocompromised individuals as an acute meningoencephalitis with or without associated septicemia, less frequently with septicemia only.[59] Although domestic animals, wild animals, canaries, fowl, and other birds including Psittaciformes are susceptible hosts, listeriosis is unlikely to occur in companion birds and has rarely been reported in humans as being bird-transmitted.[1] Conjunctivitis in humans as a result of contact with *L. monocytogenes*–infected birds, though, has been reported.[60] The organism is frequently found free-living in water and mud.

Influenza

The influenza viruses belong to the group Orthomyxovirus and consist of three types, categorized as A, B, and C, differentiated on the basis of proteins in the nucleoprotein and the matrix protein. Type A influenza viruses are the most important zoonotic agents and have been associated with recent widespread epidemics and pandemics; type B has been associated with regional or widespread epidemics; and type C has been associated with sporadic cases and minor localized outbreaks.[59] Influenza A viruses are worldwide in distribution, and only type A viruses have been isolated from birds. In humans, influenza affects mainly the respiratory system and is temporarily incapacitating; mortality is usually low, except during major epidemics.

Avian influenzas are contagious infections of birds caused by a variety of type A influenza viruses. There is some serologic evidence of human infection by avian influenza viruses and at least one documented isolation of an avian influenza virus (fowl plague) from a human patient.[61] Although direct animal-to-human transmission of influenza is rare, there is evidence that suggests that the pandemic strains of influenza A viruses in China originated from the domestic duck and were transmitted to humans via the domestic pig, which acted as a "mixing vessel" for two-way transmissions of the viruses.[62] In one case in the Ukraine, it was concluded that poultry farm workers had actually introduced influenza virus type A into their poultry flocks.[63]

Infected birds can shed the virus via respiratory secretions, conjunctiva, and feces. Clinically affected free-ranging birds have been known to infect domesticated birds. Birds may serve as reservoirs for human and mammalian influenza A infections,

and, theoretically, humans may also be able to infect their companion birds.[64]

Many avian influenza A viruses have been isolated that contain human hemagglutinin and neuraminidase surface antigens, and reports suggest that spread of influenza from people to avian species and the reverse may occur.[61] There is also evidence that recombination occurs between avian and mammalian influenza viruses; some of these viruses may have resulted by recombination during infection either by avian viruses in mammals or mammalian viruses in birds. Therefore, there is potential for development of new strains of influenza virus in wild birds that could be infectious for human beings, and there are many opportunities for human beings to become exposed to such influenza viruses, to which they would have little or no immunity.

Many strains of influenza viruses have been recovered from wild birds of many species, including waterfowl, and are widespread in geographical range. In North America, infection rates among migrating birds sampled in the US range from 5% among southern migrating birds sampled in the US to as high as 30% among fledgling birds in Canadian breeding areas.[65] Many avian species, particularly large congregations of migrating birds, may serve as main reservoirs for virus recombination.[64]

In addition to poultry, the turkey, duck, tern, finch, parakeet, mynah, weaver, owlet, bluebird, oriole, Amazon parrot, pittas, peckers, thrush, tanager, hoopee, and cockatoo have all been shown to be naturally infected with a large variety of influenza A strains and may be important reservoirs for viral activity.[66] With a few exceptions, most avian viral isolates have been from asymptomatic birds or from those with other disease entities producing clinical signs.

Rabies

Rabies is a disease of the central nervous system of warm-blooded animals and man caused by a rhabdovirus of the genus *Lyssavirus*. Although most, if not all, warm-blooded animals are susceptible to infection with rabies virus, rabies generally is not regarded as a disease of avian species.

In most cases when rabies has been observed in birds, it was experimentally induced.[67] The disease has been experimentally induced in birds including owls, hawks, falcons, ravens, songbirds, pigeons, geese, ducks, chickens, and peafowl.[67] In an experiment with a great horned owl that was allowed to feed on a rabid skunk, the owl developed antibodies to the rabies virus, but did not develop clinical signs. In controlled studies, birds were more resistant to infection than were most other warm-blooded animals. In a survey of 343 wild birds, 23 (6.7%) had low passive hemagglutination titers for rabies, with the majority of the positive samples being from birds of prey.[67]

Theoretically, therefore, a raptor feeding on a rabid animal carcass, given the proper time frame, could transmit the rabies virus on its talons or in its mouth to man. This may have implications for rehabilitators and veterinarians working with birds of prey. To date, however, there has been no evidence of rabies transmission from birds to man.

Toxoplasmosis

Toxoplasmosis is caused by *Toxoplasma gondii,* a coccidian protozoan belonging to the Sporozoa. It is obligately intracellular and exists in a number of different stages in its various hosts.[68] The form of the parasite found during acute infection of the host is a slender, arc-shaped trophozoite ($\approx$ 2–4 μm $\times$ 4–7 μm) with one end more tapered than the other.

In man, the primary infection frequently is asymptomatic; acute disease may occur with fever, lymphadenopathy, and lymphocytosis.[59] Rare manifestations include cerebral signs, pneumonia, generalized skeletal muscle involvement, myocarditis, a maculopapular rash, and death. A primary infection during early pregnancy may lead to a variety of fetal infections. Toxoplasmosis is especially a problem in immunosuppressed patients. The disease is worldwide in mammals, birds (pigeons and chickens), and humans. Rodents, swine, cattle, sheep, goats, chickens, and birds are intermediate hosts of *T. gondii.* Cats acquire the infection as a feces-borne infection from other cats, or by eating infected mammals (especially rodents) or birds. The sexual cycle of the parasite occurs only in cats. Although transplacental infections in humans may occur, most infections are acquired by eating raw or undercooked infected meat (generally pork or mutton) containing cysts, or by ingestion of infective oocysts in food, water, or dust contaminated with feline feces.[59]

There is a relatively high prevalence of *T. gondii* infections in chickens and pigeons, and sporadic outbreaks of toxoplasmosis have been described in many other species.[68] Although *T. gondii* cysts may be found in edible tissues of chickens in the USA, poultry probably is not important in the transmission of human toxoplasmosis because poultry usually is frozen and well-cooked to avoid contamination by other organisms.[69]

Cryptosporidiosis

Cryptosporidium species, a coccidian protozoan, is an enteropathogen producing clinical disease in numerous host species including humans; cryptosporidiosis is now regarded as a newly emergent zoonosis.[70] Known avian hosts of cryptosporidia include chickens, turkeys, quail, pheasants, peafowl, geese, ducks, parrots, budgerigars, canaries, and finches.[70, 71] Clinical infections in humans may result in persistent diarrhea, malabsorption, abdominal pain, fever, and vomiting, and immunosuppressed individuals are the most susceptible. The life cycle of *Cryptosporidium* is generally similar to that of other enteric coccidia requiring ingestion of infective sporulated oocysts.

Results of some transmission studies suggest that *Cryptosporidium* may be a single-species genus, making the zoonotic potential of this disease greater than previously envisioned. However, other studies have shown that isolation from quail and pheasant were only transmissible to other avian hosts and not to mammalian hosts; conversely, isolates from humans were found to be infective only to other mammals and not to birds.[70]

Although there have been no reports of cryptosporidia of avian origin infecting man, infections in domestic animals and pets may be regarded as potential reservoirs of infection for susceptible humans because the parasite can cross at least some host barriers. Even if avian cryptosporidiosis was shown to be zoonotic, cryptosporidial infections in avian species tend to be subclinical, and to have shedding rates so low that cryptosporidia would still pose little threat to humans, especially immunologically competent individuals.

Giardiasis

Giardia species are among the most widely distributed of the intestinal protozoan parasites of animals, and in the US they account for the largest percentage of human intestinal parasitism. In humans, diarrhea and malabsorption are the primary effects observed in clinical giardiasis. The life cycle of this protozoan is direct, with infection in a suitable host requiring ingestion of the organism in the cyst stage. Transmission of *Giardia* among humans occurs in crowded, unsanitary conditions and by drinking water contaminated with cysts; food-borne transmission has also been documented.[72]

Avian species reported with giardiasis include herons, turkey vultures, house sparrows, bitterns, egrets, avocets, western meadowlarks, redbacked shrikes, cockatiels, budgerigars, conures, Amazon parrots, cockatoos, and macaws.[73, 74] However, there appears to be no documentation of *Giardia* of avian origin infecting humans. Therefore, the public health implications of *Giardia* of avian origin are unknown. Evidence suggests that direct transmission of *Giardia* from other companion animals to humans may occur, and *Giardia* from wild animals is know to be capable of infecting humans.[72]

Lung Cancer (?)

In a 1992 published retrospective study, it was concluded that pet birds are associated with increased risk of developing primary lung cancer in human beings.[75] However, some authors question the validity of the study and the interpretations of the results, and conclude that the potential association between pet bird ownership and lung cancer merits additional epidemiologic investigation.[76]

Other Diseases

Other bacteria in birds including *Pasteurella* species, *Pseudomonas* species, and *Vibrio* species may have zoonotic potential, and ringworm (*Trichophyton* species) of avian origin has also been reported to occur in humans.

INFREQUENT AND POTENTIAL DISEASES INDIRECTLY ASSOCIATED WITH BIRDS

Diseases in this group are not zoonotic in the strictest sense of the word, but they may indirectly be associated with human disease. That is, birds may be a reservoir for arthropod-borne diseases and a source of food-borne illnesses, and their droppings may provide a medium for mycotic organisms.

Staphylococcal Food Poisoning

Staphylococcal food poisoning is caused by an enterotoxin produced by *Staphylococcus* species (generally *S. aureus*) and can produce a gastroenteritis in man. Although the disease is not commonly transmitted from birds to man, human contact occurs via handling contaminated egg contents or birds with surface lesions.[1]

Clostridium perfringens Food Poisoning

Toxins produced by several strains of *Clostridium perfringens* can result in an intestinal disorder in humans characterized by sudden onset of colic followed by diarrhea; nausea is common.[59] The disease is usually mild, of short duration, and rarely fatal in healthy persons. The disease is widespread and relatively frequent in countries with cooking practices that favor multiplication of *Clostridium* to high levels. Reservoirs for the organism are the soil and, occasionally, the gastrointestinal tracts of humans and animals, including poultry. Almost all outbreaks are associated with inadequately heated or reheated meats, usually stews, meat pies, or gravies made of beef, turkey, or chicken.[59] Spores survive normal cooking temperatures, and germinate and multiply during slow cooling, storage at ambient temperature, or inadequate rewarming. Heavy bacterial contamination is usually required for clinical disease.

Bacillus cereus Food Poisoning

Food poisoning can be caused by *Bacillus cereus*, an aerobic spore former. Clinical signs in humans are associated with the production of enterotoxins and include nausea and vomiting in some, and colic and diarrhea in others. The reservoir for this food-borne disease is the soil, although the organism is also commonly found in raw, dried, and processed food.[59] The disease is transmitted through ingestion of food that has been kept at ambient temperatures after cooking, permitting multiplication of the organisms.

West Nile Fever

West Nile Fever is a mosquito-borne viral (flavivirus) disease of humans in Egypt, Israel, India, France, and is probably widespread in parts of Africa, the Northern Mediterranean area, and Asia.[59] The disease involves a vertebrate-mosquito cycle, with birds being a source of the mosquito infection. The disease causes fever, headache, malaise, arthralgia or myalgia, rashes, and occasionally nausea, vomiting, and meningoencephalitis.

Mosquito-borne Encephalitides

Eastern, Western, St. Louis, and Venezuela encephalitis and other less common encephalitides are a group of acute inflammatory diseases of short duration involving parts of the brain, spinal cord, and meninges.[59] They are caused by neurotropic viruses (alphavirus, flavivirus, or bunyavirus). Birds are important in the ecology of the arboviruses. Disease syndromes appear depending on environmental conditions, virus prevalence in the avian reservoir, and presence of the appropriate bird-to-man mosquito vector. Humans are considered to be accidental hosts for both viruses and play no role in the transmission cycle. Natural or experimental infections with eastern equine encephalitis have been described in 51 native species of birds from Canada, North America, and the Caribbean,[77] with pigeons, chickens, pheasants, prairie chickens, ducks, and geese especially posing as a potential source of disease for humans.[1] Specific isolation studies of encephalitis viruses from commonly maintained pet bird species could not be found.[66]

Aspergillosis

Aspergillosis is a fungal infection of humans, animals, and birds caused by the saprophytic fungus *Aspergillus fumigatus* and occasionally by other species. The disease is transmitted via airborne spores of the fungus. The source of infection is the environment (i.e., moldy straw and fodder), not transmission from one animal to another.[1] *Aspergillus* is a potential problem for immunocompromised populations and for patients with chronic disease, and may be contracted by humans performing necropsies on infected birds.[1]

Histoplasmosis

Histoplasmosis is basically a disease of the pulmonary system caused by the imperfect dimorphous fungus *Histoplasma capsulatum*. It is not a contagious disease but is generally spread by the inhalation of airborne spores of *H. capsulatum*. The principal habitat of *H. capsulatum* is soil enriched with the feces of gregarious birds such as blackbirds and chickens and, to a lesser extent, pigeons; bat habitats, such as attics and caves where their guano has accumulated, are also potential sources of the fungus.[78] Old chicken coops, bell and church towers inhabited by pigeons, and starling and blackbird roosts are frequently the point source of outbreaks of histoplasmosis.[78] In the US, the disease in humans is found primarily in the lowlands of the Ohio, Mississippi, and Missouri River valleys (Arkansas, Texas, Tennessee, Missouri, and Kansas).

Histoplasmosis is not a clinical problem in birds. Because the body temperature of most birds is too high to support the growth of this mycotic organism, their primary role is as a mechanical vector to transport the fungi from place to place.[79]

Although approximately 90% of human infections are asymptomatic, the other 10% who have symptoms may have acute pulmonary histoplasmosis, disseminated histoplasmosis, or rarely, chronic cavitary histoplasmosis (Fig. 22–2).[78] In the acute or common form of the disease, the patient develops influenza-like symptoms (nonproductive cough, chest pains, and dyspnea) and, if severe, develops fever, night sweats, weight loss, and hemoptysis. Prevention includes avoiding the classical habitats of *H. capsulatum*.

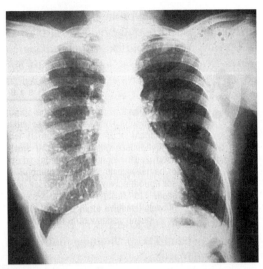

Figure 22-2

Chest radiograph of a man infected with *Histoplasma capsulatum*. Note the multiple small, radiodense nodules scattered throughout the lungs. (From Donham KJ, Mutel CF: Poultry Zoonoses, Rural Health Series, Institute of Agricultural Medicine, The University of Iowa, Iowa City, IA.)

Cryptococcosis

Cryptococcosis is caused by the yeast-like fungus *Cryptococcus neoformans*. The disease occurs worldwide and affects humans and a great diversity of mammals, including domestic animals, lower primates, bats, and a variety of exotic animals.[78] Because the disease is not reportable, accurate data on its incidence and prevalence are not available. The disease generally has pulmonary manifestations, although occasionally it may disseminate to the viscera, skin, bones, or central nervous system.

The fungus is commonly found in soil contaminated with pigeon excreta and in accumulations of pigeon excreta in old nests and under roosting sites.[78] Humans and animals become infected either through inhalation of the yeast or, less commonly, by direct inoculation of the skin. Pigeons are resistant to infection by the fungus, although their excreta provide a suitable substrate for growth of *C. neoformans*. The multiplication of *C. neoformans* in pigeon excreta has been attributed to the fact that creatinine, which is abundant in pigeon excreta, is assimilated by *C. neoformans* but not by other species of yeast.[78] *C. neoformans* also occurs in the dried droppings of starlings or other avian species

and has been isolated from the roosts of canaries and psittacines.[66, 80] Prevention of the disease should include limiting exposure to an accumulation of pigeon droppings. Pet birds, therefore, are an unlikely source of *Cryptococcus* infection for human beings.[3]

Birds, including companion species, are susceptible to cryptococcosis, although they are more resistant to the infection than mammals because of their high core body temperature.[66] Clinical signs include depression, weakness, anorexia, weight loss, acute diarrhea, incoordination, blindness, dyspnea, nasal exudates, oral masses, and death.[66]

References

1. Harris JM: Zoonotic diseases of birds. Vet Clin North Am (Sm Anim Pract) 21:1289–1298, 1991.
2. Gill DM, Stone DM: The veterinarian's role in the AIDS crisis. J Am Vet Med Assoc 210(11):1683–1684, 1992.
3. Angulo FJ, Glaser CA, Juranek DD, et al: Caring for pets of immunocompromised persons. J Am Vet Med Assoc 205(12):1711–1718, 1994.
4. Wyrick PB, Richmond SJ: Biology of chlamydiae. J Am Vet Med Assoc 195:1507–1512, 1989.
5. Williams LP Jr: Review of the epidemiology of chlamydiosis in the United States. J Am Vet Med Assoc 195:1518–1521, 1989.
6. Satalowich FT, Barrett L, Sinclair C, et al: Compendium of chlamydiosis (psittacosis) control, 1994. J Am Vet Med Assoc 203:1673–1680, 1993.
7. Garbe JL: Legal aspects of chlamydiosis in birds. J Am Vet Med Assoc 195:1574–1576, 1989.
8. Graham DL: A color atlas of avian chlamydiosis. Semin Avian Exotic Pet Med 2:184–189, 1993.
9. Harris JM: Avian companions and the human-animal bond. J Am Vet Med Assoc 195:1517–1518, 1989.
10. Brand CJ: Chlamydial infections in free-living birds. J Am Vet Med Assoc 195:1531–1535, 1989.
11. Fowler ME, Schultz T, Ardans A, et al: Chlamydiosis in captive raptors. Avian Dis 34:657–662, 1990.
12. Steele JH: Salmonellosis: A major zoonosis. Arch Environ Health 19:871–875, 1969.
13. Acha PN, Szyfres B: Zoonoses and Communicable Diseases Common to Man and Animals, ed 2. Washington DC, World Health Association, 1987.
14. Meier JE: Salmonellosis and other bacterial enteritides in birds. In Kirk RW (ed): Current Veterinary Therapy VIII. Philadelphia, WB Saunders, 1983.
15. MacDonald JW, Brown DD: *Salmonella* infection in wild birds in Britain. Vet Rec 94:321–322, 1974.
16. Tizzard IR, Fish NA, Harmeson J: Free-flying sparrows as carriers of salmonellosis. Can Vet J 20:143–144, 1979.
17. Mohan R: *Salmonella* infection in pet birds. Proc Ann Mtg Assoc Avian Vet, 1983, pp 78–82.
18. Williams LP Jr: Salmonellosis. In Steele JH (ed): CRC Handbook Series in Zoonoses, vol. II (Section A). Boca Raton, CRC Press, 1980.
19. Komorowski RA, Hensley GT: Epizootic salmonellosis in an open zoo aviary. Arch Environ Health 27:110–111, 1974.
20. Butterfield J, Coulson JC, Kearsey SU, et al: The herring gull

Larus argentatus as a carrier of salmonella. J Hyg (Camb) 91:429–436, 1983.

21. Panigrahy B, Grimes JE, Rideout MI, et al: Zoonotic diseases in psittacine birds: Apparent increased occurrence of chlamydiosis (psittacosis), salmonellosis, and giardiasis. J Am Vet Med Assoc 175:359–361, 1979.

22. Kapperud G, Rosef O: Avian wildlife reservoir of *Campylobacter fetus* subsp. *jejuni, Yersinia* spp., and *Salmonella* spp. in Norway. Appl Environ Microbiol 45:375–380, 1983.

23. Ebel ED, Mason J, Thomas LA, et al: Occurrence of *Salmonella enteritidis* in unpasteurized liquid egg in the United States. Avian Dis 37:135–142, 1993.

24. Shane SM, Montrose MS: The occurrence and significance of *Campylobacter jejuni* in man and animal. Vet Res Comm 9:167–198, 1985.

25. Prescott JF, Munroe DL: *Campylobacter jejuni* enteritis in man and domestic animals. J Am Vet Med Assoc 181:1524–1530, 1982.

26. Ito K, Kubokura Y, Kaneko K, et al: Occurrence of *Campylobacter jejuni* in free-living wild birds from Japan. J Wildl Dis 24:467–470, 1988.

27. Rosef O, Kapperud G, Lauwers S, Gondrosen B: Serotyping of *Campylobacter jejuni, Campylobacter coli,* and *Campylobacter laridis* from domestic and wild animals. Appl Environ Microbiol 49:1507–1510, 1985.

28. Smibert RM: *Vibrio fetus* var. *intestinalis* isolated from the intestinal content of birds. Am J Vet Res 30:1437–1442, 1969.

29. Luechtefeld NA, Blaser MJ, Reller LB, Wang WL: Isolation of *Campylobacter fetus* subsp. *jejuni* from migratory waterfowl. J Clin Microbiol 12:406–408, 1980.

30. Luechtefeld NA, Cambre RC, Wang WL: Isolation of *Campylobacter fetus* subsp. *jejuni* from zoo animals. J Am Vet Med Assoc 179:1119–1122, 1981.

31. Yogasundram K, Shane SM, Harrington KS: Prevalence of *Campylobacter jejuni* in selected domestic and wild birds in Louisiana. Avian Dis 33:664–667, 1989.

32. Mair NS: Yersiniosis in wildlife and its public health implications. J Wildl Dis 9:64–71, 1973.

33. Stovell PL: Pseudotubercular yersiniosis. In Steele JH (ed): CRC Handbook Series in Zoonoses, vol II (Section A). Boca Raton, CRC Press, 1980.

34. Beaudette FR: A case of pseudotuberculosis in a blackbird. J Am Vet Med Assoc 97:151–157, 1940.

35. Baskin GB, Montali RJ, Bush M, et al: Yersiniosis in captive exotic mammals. J Am Vet Med Assoc 171:908–912, 1977.

36. Hacking MA, Sileo L: *Yersinia enterocolitica* and *Yersinia pseudotuberculosis* from wildlife in Ontario. J Wildl Dis 10:452–457, 1974.

37. Clark GM, Locke LN: Case report: Observations on pseudotuberculosis in common grackles. Avian Dis 6:506–510, 1962.

38. Borst GHA, Buitelaar M, Poelma FG, et al: *Yersinia pseudotuberculosis* in birds. Vet Bull 47:507–509, 1977.

39. Langford EV: *Yersinia enterocolitica* isolated from animals in the Fraser Valley of British Columbia. Can Vet J 13:109–113, 1972.

40. Giles N, Carter MJ: *Yersinia enterocolitica* in budgerigars. Vet Rec 100:362–363, 1980.

41. Walker JW, Heron BR, Mixson MA: Exotic Newcastle disease eradication program in the United States. Avian Dis 17:486–503, 1973.

42. Pearson GL, McCann MK: The role of indigenous wild, semidomestic, and exotic birds in the epizootiology of velogenic viscerotropic Newcastle disease in southern California, 1972–1973. J Am Vet Med Assoc 167:610–614, 1975.

43. Kaleta EF, Baldauf C: Newcastle disease in free-living and pet birds. In Alexander DJ (ed): Newcastle Disease. Boston, Kluwer Academic Publishers, 1988.

44. Erickson GA, Mare CJ, Beran GW, Carbrey EA: Epizootiologic aspects of viscerotropic velogenic Newcastle disease in six pet bird species. Am J Vet Res 39:105–107, 1978.

45. Chang PW: Newcastle disease. In Steele JH (ed): CRC Handbook Series in Zoonoses, vol II (Section B). Boca Raton, CRC Press, 1981.

46. Pedersden KA, Sadasiv EC, Chang PW, Yates VJ: Detection of antibody to avian viruses in human populations. Epidemiol Infect 104:519–525, 1990.

47. Reed CE, Sosman A, Barbec RA: Pigeon-breeders lung. J Am Med Assoc 193:81–85, 1965.

48. Warren WP: Hypersensitivity pneumonitis due to exposure to budgerigars. Chest 62:170–174, 1972.

49. Hargreave FE, Pepys J, Longbottom JL, Wruith DG: Bird breeders (fanciers) lung. Lancet 1:446, 1966.

50. Montali RJ, Bush M, Thoen CO, Smith E: Tuberculosis in captive exotic birds. J Am Vet Med Assoc 169:920–927, 1976.

51. Forster F, Gerlach H: Mycobacteria in Psittaciformes. Proc First Int Conf Zoo Avian Med, 1987, pp. 39–56.

52. Kiehn TE, Edwards FF, Brannon P, et al: Infections caused by *Mycobacterium avium* complex in immunocompromised patients: Diagnosis by blood culture and fecal examination, antimicrobial susceptibility tests, and morphological and seroagglutination characteristics. J Clin Microbiol 21:168–173, 1985.

53. Gale NB: Tuberculosis. In Davis JW, Anderson RC, Karstad L, Trainer DO (eds): Infectious and Parasitic Diseases of Wild Birds. Ames, Iowa State University Press, 1981.

54. Meissner G, Anz W: Sources of *Mycobacterium avium* complex infection resulting in human diseases. Am Rev Resp Dis 116:1057–1064, 1977.

55. Falk GA, Hadley SJ, Sharkey FE, et al: *Mycobacterium avium* infections in man. Am J Med 54:801–810, 1973.

56. du Moulin GC, Sherman IH, Hoaglin DC, Stottmeier KD: *Mycobacterium avium* complex, an emerging pathogen in Massachusetts. J Clin Microbiol 22:9–12, 1985.

57. Kubin M, Kruml J, Horak Z, et al: Pulmonary and nonpulmonary disease in humans due to avian mycobacteria. I. Clinical and epidemiologic analysis of nine cases observed in Czechoslovakia. Am Rev Resp Dis 94:20–31, 1966.

58. Ojeniyi AA: Direct transmissions of *Escherichia coli* from poultry to humans. Epidem Inf 103:513–522, 1989.

59. Benenson AS (ed): Control of Communicable Diseases in Man, ed 15. Washington DC, The American Public Health Association, 1990.

60. Gerlach H: Bacteria. In Ritchie B, Harrison G, Harrison L (eds): Avian Medicine: Principles and Application. Lake Worth, FL, Wingers Publishing, 1994.

61. Campbell CH, Butterfield WK: Influenza of domestic fowl. In Steele JH (ed): CRC Handbook in Zoonoses, vol II (Section B). Boca Raton, CRC Press, 1981.

62. Shortridge KF: Pandemic influenza: A zoonosis? Semin Resp Infect 7(1):11–25, 1992.

63. Shablovskaya EA, Voronenko SG, D'yachenko AP: Circulation of influenzavirus within poultry farms. Voprosy-Virusologii 3:308–310, 1985.

64. Gerlach H: Viruses. In Ritchie B, Harrison G, Harrison L (eds): Avian Medicine: Principles and Application. Lake Worth, FL, Wingers Publishing, 1994.

65. Easterday BC: Influenza virus infections of wild birds. In Steele JH (ed): CRC Handbook in Zoonoses, vol II (Section B). Boca Raton, CRC Press, 1981.

66. Ritchie BW, Dreesen DW: Avian zoonoses: Proven and potential diseases. Part II. Viral, fungal, and miscellaneous diseases. Compend Collection 10(6):26–31, 1988.

67. Gough PM, Jorgenson RD: Rabies antibodies in sera of wild birds. J Wildl Dis 12:392–397, 1976.

68. Jacobs L, Frenkel JK: Toxoplasmosis. In Steele JH (ed): CRC Handbook Series in Zoonoses, vol I (Section C). Boca Raton, CRC Press, 1982.
69. Dubey JP: Toxoplasmosis. J Am Vet Med Assoc 189(12):166–170, 1986.
70. O'Donoghue PJ: *Cryptosporidium* infections in man, animals, birds and fish. Aust Vet J 62:253–258, 1985.
71. Barnes JH: Parasites. In Harrison GL, Harrison LR (eds): Clinical Avian Medicine and Surgery. Philadelphia, WB Saunders, 1986.
72. Kirkpatrick CE, Farrell JP: Giardiasis. Compend Contin Educ Pract Vet 4(5):367–376, 1982.
73. Ritchie BW, Dreesen DW: Avian zoonoses: Proven and potential diseases. Part I. Bacterial and parasitic diseases. Compend Collection 10(4):18–25, 1988.
74. Meyer EA, Jarroll EL: Giardiasis. CRC Handbook Series in Zoonoses, vol I (Section C). Boca Raton, CRC Press, 1982.
75. Kohlmeier L, Arminger G, Bartolomycik S, et al: Pet birds as an independent risk factor for lung cancer: Case-control study. Br Med J 305:986–989, 1992.
76. Angulo FJ, Millikan RC, Malmgren R: Question link between human lung cancer and pet bird exposure (letter). J Am Vet Med Assoc 202(9):1345, 1993.
77. Dardiri AH, Yates VJ, Chang PW, et al: The isolation of eastern equine encephalomyelitis virus from brains of sparrows. J Am Vet Med Assoc 130:409–410, 1957.
78. Ajello L, Kaplan W, Padhye A: Mycotic and actinomycotic zoonoses. In Steele JH (ed): CRC Handbook Series in Zoonoses, vol II (Section A). Boca Raton, CRC Press, 1980.
79. Wolf AM: Systemic mycoses. J Am Vet Med Assoc 194(9):1192–1196, 1989.
80. Bauck L: Mycoses. In Ritchie B, Harrison G, Harrison L (eds): Avian Medicine: Principles and Application. Lake Worth, FL, Wingers Publishing, 1994.

Keven Flammer

23

Chlamydia

hlamydiosis in birds is caused by *Chlamydia psittaci* and is also known as psittacosis, ornithosis, and parrot fever. Chlamydiosis has been reported in more than 100 species of birds, but avian infection is most frequently reported in psittacines, pigeons, and turkeys.[1] It is relatively common in caged birds where it presents a challenge for the avian practitioner because chlamydiosis is difficult to diagnose, difficult to treat, and potentially transmissible to people.

Total eradication of *Chlamydia* from all pet and aviculture birds is probably an unattainable goal. However, the clinical significance of this disease can be greatly reduced if the biology of the organism is understood and a "commonsense" approach is used toward its control. Clinical disease occurs when birds are exposed to new strains and where poor husbandry, overcrowding, poor nutrition, or concurrent diseases render the bird more susceptible to infection. If birds are well cared for, protected from exposure to new birds harboring new *Chlamydia* strains, and endemic *Chlamydia* is eliminated or reduced by appropriate treatment, *C. psittaci* seldom causes problems.

STRAINS AND SPECIES OF *CHLAMYDIA*

Three species of *Chlamydia* are of medical importance—*C. trachomatis, C. pneumoniae,* and *C. psittaci. C. trachomatis* and *C. pneumoniae* infect only humans, causing reproductive tract/ocular and pulmonary infections, respectively. Control of *C. trachomatis* is an area of active research and there is enough similarity with *C. psittaci* that some of the advances made for diagnosing and treating

this disease agent can be adapted to the control of *C. psittaci.*[2]

C. psittaci can infect a wide variety of animals, including mammals, birds, reptiles, insects, and humans. It is an important pathogen in birds, cats, ruminants, swine.[2] Although *C. psittaci* is currently classified as a single species, a variety of techniques have demonstrated significant differences between the strains infecting various animals. It is likely that with further refinement, *C. psittaci* will be divided into subspecies demonstrating particular host affinity. Transmission of *Chlamydia* between diverse animal species is possible but it is unlikely that this is a frequent occurrence.

The strains affecting birds have been divided into four to five serovars (psittacine, duck, turkey, and pigeon 1 and 2), based on various research methods.[3, 4, 5] The avian strains have been labeled after the host where they were found, but transmission between these hosts occurs, and thus the significance of this classification is unknown. Some investigators believe that it will be possible to differentiate pathogenic and nonpathogenic strains with use of deoxyribonucleic acid (DNA) probes and polymerase chain reaction (PCR) testing.[6] Others investigators believe that the factors determining virulence for a particular strain are altered by host-to-host transmission, making designation of a pathogenic or nonpathogenic strain meaningless because pathogenicity cannot be predicted for a new host.[3, 7]

CLINICALLY SIGNIFICANT ASPECTS OF THE BIOLOGY OF CHLAMYDIOSIS

The biology of this unique organism partially explains why definitive diagnosis and treatment are so challenging. *Chlamydia* are obligate intracellular bacterial parasites and possess a cell envelope similar to that of gram-negative bacteria. They contain both ribonucleic acid (RNA) and DNA and are capable of synthesizing most of their needs but are incapable of generating high-energy phosphate bonds and are therefore dependent on the host cell for energy.[8]

Chlamydia have a biphasic life cycle and exist in two forms as elementary and reticulate bodies.[8] Elementary bodies are small particles that can exist outside of the host and are infectious but do not multiply. Elementary bodies are shed from infected birds in the feces and urine and in ocular and respiratory exudates. They are ingested or inhaled by a new host and enter epithelial cells where they form a cytoplasmic endosome. The elementary bodies then transform into reticulate bodies that become metabolically active and reproduce by binary fission. This forms a large intracytoplasmic inclusion filled with many daughter reticulate bodies. The reticulate bodies then condense into elementary bodies that are passed on to daughter cells if the cell divides or released if the host cell undergoes lysis. Released elementary bodies may infect other host cells, including macrophages, or may be released into the environment if the lysed cell borders the respiratory, ocular, or digestive tract.

Chlamydia are highly adept at evading the host's immune system. Endosomes formed by bacteria other than *Chlamydia* are usually fused with lysosomes and destroyed by the host cell. *Chlamydia* endosomes somehow evade this process, and their intracellular location helps protect them from detection by the systemic immune system. Infected cells may also reproduce, passing *Chlamydia* to daughter cells and perpetuating the infection without systemic release of immunogenic elementary bodies.[8]

By evading the host's immune system, *Chlamydia* strains of low virulence produce persistent latent infections. Latently infected birds shed *Chlamydia* intermittently and pose a danger because the chlamydial strain they shed may be more virulent for other avian species or people.[3] Latent infections can also become symptomatic and threaten the host bird if stress or concurrent disease reactivates a latent infection. There are anecdotal reports of asymptomatic birds living in a single-bird, isolated household for years and then suddenly exhibiting clinical signs of chlamydiosis.[9]

The biology of *Chlamydia* also explains why treatment is difficult and not always successful. The elementary bodies are metabolically inert and therefore not susceptible to antibiotics. *Chlamydia* are only susceptible to antibiotics when they are metabolically active or reproducing in the reticulate body stage. Because *Chlamydia* can remain dormant in cells for long periods of time, prolonged treatment periods of approximately 45 days are recommended.[10] There is nothing magical about this length of treatment; the rationale is to treat the bird until *Chlamydia* become metabolically active (and therefore susceptible to the antibiotic) or the host cell dies. However, because dormant *Chlamydia* can be passed to daughter cells, infection can persist even with prolonged antibiotic treatment. In most cases, 45 days of treatment is successful, but anecdotal reports reveal that *some* birds may not be cleared of infection with treatment periods greater than 45 days.[3]

Sparse research on the avian immune response to *Chlamydia* indicates that host immunity is primarily mediated by T-lymphocyte response.[10, 11] The role of antibody in protection is unclear. It is known that elevated immunoglobulin G (IgG) and IgM antibody titers detected by complement fixation tests are not protective, nor will inoculation of immune serum convey protection. It is important to note that immunity to infection is short-lived, and treated birds are susceptible to reinfection shortly after treatment ends.[1]

It is unlikely that a vaccine will be available for avian chlamydiosis in the near future. There is antigenic variation in the different strains of avian *C. psittaci* and substantial variation in the avian host response to chlamydia.[13] This poses difficulty for proving safety and efficacy in many species of birds that would need to be vaccinated. Experimental vaccines made from killed suspensions of infected yolk sac material provided some protection from clinical signs following challenge, but the birds still became infected and shed the organism. Birds vaccinated with live vaccines of attenuated organisms established persistent infections and shed the vaccine organism. Thus far, a vaccine that will prevent persistent infection and provide long-lasting immunity has not been developed for any species, including humans. Research is being targeted at producing a subunit vaccine that will block one of the metabolic processes unique to the chlamydia genus.[1]

TRANSMISSION AND PATHOGENESIS

Infectious elementary bodies are shed in digestive contents, feces, urine, saliva, and ocular, nasal, and respiratory exudates. Aerosols of infectious material spread *Chlamydia* through the air, and new hosts are infected when elementary bodies are ingested or inhaled. Nestling birds can be infected when fed by the parents, or possibly by vertical transmission through the egg. Avian caretakers can spread the disease by tracking feces into neighboring cages or contaminating food or water supplies. Arthropod vectors can also spread *Chlamydia,* but it is unlikely that this is a major mode of transmission in captive bird collections. All birds sharing the same air space with an infected bird should be considered exposed to *Chlamydia,* although not all exposed birds develop infection.

Chlamydia elementary bodies are unstable if exposed to heat, sunlight, or adverse environmental conditions. However, they can remain infectious for months if protected by dried fecal material. They are susceptible to numerous disinfectants, including quaternary ammonium products, benzalkonium chloride (e.g., Roccal), 70% ethanol, and 3% hydrogen peroxide.

CLINICAL SIGNS

Chlamydiosis is frequently diagnosed in psittacine and columbiform birds. The highest incidence is seen in birds recently purchased from commercial sources (e.g., import stations, wholesalers, and pet stores), but disease also occurs in domestic collections. Especially high rates of infection are seen in budgerigars and cockatiels.

The severity of clinical signs of chlamydiosis depends on the virulence of the particular *Chlamydia* strain and the immune status and condition of the host. Strains that cause no signs in one host may be pathogenic for a different bird.[3] Clinical signs vary dramatically from totally asymptomatic carriers to severe infections with a high flock mortality. Asymptomatic carriers are common and may carry the organism for years and then emerge with clini-

cal signs following some stressful episode (e.g., change in surroundings or start of breeding season, cold weather). In the author's experience, asymptomatic carriers are the most common, followed by birds with chronic manifestations of the disease. Chlamydiosis should be included in the differential diagnosis of any ill psittacine bird.

Clinically ill birds manifest signs that are similar to those of many infectious diseases.[1,3,9,14,15,16] There are no pathognomonic signs of avian chlamydiosis, and the disease is easily confused with common bacterial and viral infections. The signs observed depend on the organ systems that are affected. Depression, anorexia, weight loss, and ruffled feathers are common signs. Systemic infection of the liver, kidneys, and digestive tract cause diarrhea and watery green urine (biliverdinuria). Infection of the respiratory tract can cause keratoconjunctivitis, rhinitis, sinusitis, dyspnea, and rales. Central nervous system signs are less common and can include convulsions, tremors, head tilt, and posterior paresis. Concurrent infections with other organisms may also contribute to clinical signs.

Chlamydiosis may be overlooked in breeding collections infected with strains of low pathogenicity because the only signs may be reduced production and nestling mortality. Other diseases frequently accompany chlamydiosis that are easier to identify (e.g., microbial and parasitic infections) and may be blamed for the production losses and the *Chlamydia* missed. Some flocks prophylactically treated with antichlamydial drugs have seen an increase in production following treatment.

In addition to the classic signs of chlamydiosis described earlier, certain syndromes are common among some groups of birds. Reduced egg production, low hatchability, and nestling mortality are common complaints in avicultural collections of cockatiels and budgerigars. Chlamydiosis in lovebirds is often associated with a high death rate in adults as well as in their offspring. Sporadic mortality and conjunctivitis (with or without other clinical signs) may be seen in Australian parakeets. Amazon parrots frequently have green-stained urine, indicative of biliverdinuria due to hepatic dysfunction. Macaws may show only lower respiratory signs, characterized by severe dyspnea. Cockatoos may show chronic wasting and other general signs, but they also commonly become asymptomatic shedders of the disease.

Chlamydia also infects nonpsittacine birds. As with psittacines, the signs are usually nonspecific. Morbidity and mortality are highest in young birds. The clinical signs in pigeons are similar to those of psittacines, with conjunctivitis and rhinitis being common signs.[17] Conjunctivitis is a predominant sign in adult geese and ducks, and systemic infection with moderate to high morbidity and mortality is seen in ducklings.[18] Pheasants and chickens are relatively resistant to infection, and clinical signs of generalized illness are usually seen only in young birds.[1] Adult ratites infected with *Chlamydia* displayed only nonspecific signs of general illness, but high mortality was noted in the chicks.[3] *Chlamydia* occasionally causes outbreaks in zoologic collections, and the signs are similar to those observed in other birds.

COMMON LABORATORY TESTING AND NECROPSY RESULTS

Changes in routine diagnostic data, such as history, physical examination data, clinical pathology test results, and radiography, may guide a clinician toward a tentative diagnosis of chlamydiosis, but confirmation requires specific laboratory testing. Some clinicians diagnose infection based on a response to therapy following treatment with antichlamydial drugs; however, many bacterial diseases cause the same clinical picture as chlamydiosis and may also respond to treatment with these drugs.

Alterations in routine diagnostic tests depend on the severity of the disease process and the organs that are affected. Asymptomatic birds usually show no changes. Sick birds are frequently anemic, and have a leukocytosis characterized by heterophilia and possibly monocytosis. Elevation in aspartate aminotransferase (AST), lactate dehydrogenase (LDH), plasma bile acids, and occasionally uric acid may occur. Hepatomegaly, splenomegaly, and opacity and thickening of the air sacs may be seen radiographically or laparoscopically.

Classic gross necropsy appearance may include any combination of the following: enlarged, swollen, congested, and mottled liver and spleen; thickened air sacs with diffuse cloudiness and fibrinous deposits; fibrinous pericarditis; bronchopneumonia; nephrosis; enteritis; conjunctivitis; and keratitis.[19] Unfortunately, not all birds that die from chlamyd-

iosis show the classic signs. It has been estimated that only 50% of the cockatiels diagnosed at necropsy with chlamydiosis had hepatomegaly.[20]

Chlamydiosis is difficult to diagnose from routine histopathology examination. Changes are nonspecific, host- and chlamydial strain–dependent, and may include focal necrosis in multiple organs including the liver, spleen, and kidney characterized by proliferation of monocytes; epithelioid granulomas in the liver and lung; bronchopneumonia; fibrinous air sacculitis, peritonitis, and pericarditis; and orchitis. Nonsuppurative meningitis may be seen in birds displaying central nervous system (CNS) signs. Suspect organ sections should be stained with an immunofluorescent or vital stains that will demonstrate *Chlamydia* inclusions. Inclusions are most easily demonstrated in serosal membranes, liver, spleen, and affected air sacs.

DIAGNOSIS

The clinical and pathologic features of avian chlamydiosis are variable and similar to other diseases, and thus confirmation of infection requires use of a specific chlamydia test. Serologic, antigen capture, culture, and cytologic tests are available, each with its own advantages and disadvantages. Infected birds showing clinical signs are most easily identified because ill birds frequently shed the organism and develop antibody titers. Asymptomatic carriers are more difficult to identify, and despite recent advances in diagnosing avian chlamydiosis, there is no test or combination of tests that reliably determines that a bird is free of *Chlamydia*. It is important to convey this information to bird owners. Negative test results reduce the chance that a bird is infected, but there is always some risk that the bird may test positive in the future.

Despite the limitations of *Chlamydia* testing, it is still desirable to routinely test birds because many *Chlamydia*-positive birds will be identified, and negative test results reduce the probability that the bird has *Chlamydia*. A combination of negative tests and/or repeated test results further reduces those odds. It is also desirable to test birds rather than simply treat all birds suspected of infection because treatment is difficult and it may be necessary to document the infection for legal reasons. Samples for diagnostic testing must be taken before initiating therapy with antibiotics that have antichlamydial activity (tetracyclines, macrolides, fluoroquinolones, and chloramphenicol). These drugs can interfere with diagnostic tests by reducing antibody production, reducing antigen shedding, and reducing the viability of *Chlamydia*.

Research on *Chlamydia* testing has been hindered because there is no "gold standard" test that can be used to unequivocally determine if a bird is *Chlamydia*-free, and hence determine if a particular test is accurate. Tests are compared only with each other and described in terms of relative sensitivity and specificity. Some tests are also limited by availability. Important factors to consider for each test are:

- The incidence of suspected false-positive results (bird not infected but a positive test) and false-negative results (bird infected, negative test)
- The reliability of identifying clinically ill birds
- The reliability of identifying asymptomatic birds with latent infections
- How public health officials may interpret positive test results

Serologic Tests

A positive serologic test result indicates only that the bird has been exposed to *Chlamydia* and has mounted an antibody response. Because titers can persist for long periods after infection (and treatment), a positive titer does not necessarily indicate that a bird is actively infected. However, a persistently infected bird presumably mounts a greater antibody response, and thus a single, greatly elevated titer is presumptive evidence of infection. To confirm infection serologically, paired sera should demonstrate a rising titer, but the appropriate collection interval has not been determined for the many avian species seen by avian veterinarians.[21] Birds with positive titers should receive a general health workup (complete blood count, chemistry panel, and bile acid test) to look for additional signs of illness, should be tested with another method (antigen capture or culture), should be treated to reduce the possibility of infection, or should be isolated and retested at a later date.

A negative titer does not guarantee that a bird is free of infection. Measurable titers may not be present in early infections, in young or immunosuppressed birds incapable of mounting an antibody response, and in some species of birds when titers remain low despite infection. Treatment with antichlamydial antibiotics may also depress antibody titers.

Direct Complement Fixation (DCF)

Elevated titers can persist for months after infection has presumably resolved. False-negative results are common in certain species (cockatiels, African grey parrots, budgerigars).[21–25]

Latex Agglutination (LA)

High (≥640) or rising titers usually indicate that the bird is actively infected. False-negative results are relatively common in asymptomatic carriers. Limited observations on the persistence of titers indicate that following treatment, the titer may initially rise but should eventually decline. Followup titers, weeks to months after treatment can be used to investigate if treatment is effective. A negative titer following treatment is a good sign, but does not guarantee that treatment was effective. A positive titer following treatment is difficult to interpret because positive titers may persist for months to years in treated birds.[22–25]

Grimes suggests that combining DCF and LA titers provides the most information and suggests the following for interpretation.[25]

1. Current infection likely if LA titer low to moderate (20–320), DCF titer negative low or LA four times greater than DCF
2. Recent past chlamydial infection: LA < 160, DCF 320 to 5210
3. Difficult to interpret: Equally high LA and DCF titers

Blocking Antibody Enzyme-linked Immunosorbent Assay Test

This test (BELISA) was developed in Germany and is currently unavailable in the US.[26] The significance of a positive test result was difficult to interpret because approximately 60 to 70% of the asymptomatic birds tested were positive. Either this test is extremely sensitive and identified birds with minute amounts of antibody (indicating past exposure or current infection), or it resulted in numerous false-positive results. Because there is no gold standard with which to compare results, there is no way to confirm the accuracy of this test. It was suggested that positive titers may indicate persistent chlamydial infections that were missed by other methods.[27] Birds with positive titers should be tested with other methods and monitored closely for health problems. False-negative results occur due to low antibody production.

Antigen Detection Tests

A number of new antigen-capture enzyme-linked immunosorbent assay (ELISA) tests have been developed for diagnosing *C. trachomatis* infection in people. Because *C. psittaci* and *C. trachomatis* share some common antigens, some of these tests may be useful in birds. Antigen capture tests do not require that the organism be viable, and this is an advantage when compared with culture. These tests require careful attention to detail; results may be influenced by collection methods.

By mid-1995, none of the available ELISA tests have been extensively validated for use in birds, and thus (as with all chlamydia tests) the results should be interpreted with care. These procedures have been developed for testing human urethral and cervical samples and may give false results when used in testing samples contaminated with bacteria and other debris, such as avian fecal samples. Transport media and the type of swabs and surfaces from which samples are collected may all influence results. Clinicians should use the materials supplied by the manufacturer or laboratory and follow instructions carefully. Pooling of samples is not recommended to avoid reducing sensitivity of the test.

Four tests have been evaluated in birds, including Clearview Chlamydia, the IDIEA Chlamydia test, the Chlamydiazyme test, and the Kodak Surecell Kit.[3, 27–29] The Clearview and Surecell tests can be performed in most veterinary practices; the other tests require some specialized equipment. False-

positive results resulting from cross-reactivity with bacteria are possible with all four of these tests but appear to be most common with the Clearview and Chlamydiazyme test. *Staphylococcus aureus* and *S. hyicus, Actinobacillus salpingitidis, Acinetobacter calcoaceticus,* and other bacteria may cause false-positive reactions. For this reason, cloacal swabs, rather than fecal samples, are recommended for use with antigen tests.

The sensitivity of these tests also varies. None are as sensitive as culture, which can presumably detect *Chlamydia* in samples containing as few as 20 elementary bodies. The number of elementary bodies detected by the four tests are: SureCell (70), Clearview (170), IDIEA (600), and Chlamydiazyme (4800).[3] These tests are most useful for screening cloacal swabs or tissue samples from ill birds that would presumably be shedding large amounts of *Chlamydia*. If used as a screening test for asymptomatic birds, negative results should be interpreted with caution because these tests miss intermittent shedders and may not detect samples with low numbers of *Chlamydia*.

Cytology Testing

Intracytoplasmic chlamydial inclusions can be identified in smears or tissue impressions stained with dyes (Gimenez and Macchiavello's stain)[14] or, preferably, with immunofluorescent antibody (IFA) stains. Samples containing large amounts of cells provide the greatest chance of finding *Chlamydia*. Direct smears can be made from feces, cloacal swabs, and ocular and nasal exudates, but infections may be missed unless the bird is showing marked clinical signs and shedding large numbers of *Chlamydia*. Nonspecific staining is also a problem. More reliable results are obtained from impression smears from the liver, spleen, and air sacs, especially if IFA stains are used.

The reliability of results depends on the method used and the expertise of the pathologist/cytologist. Results are most reliable for IFA-stained tissue sections and are unreliable for vital staining of feces or exudates.[3] At best, cytology should be used as a screening method, and outcome of culture or antigen tests used to confirm negative results.

Culture

Isolation of *Chlamydia* in cell culture or embryonated eggs is currently used as basis of comparison for all other diagnostic tests; however, even this test is not completely reliable. False-positive results are rare. False-negative results can occur because birds shed *Chlamydia* intermittently, because low numbers of viable *Chlamydia* are present in the sample, because viable *Chlamydia* are lost during transport, or because of concurrent treatment with antichlamydial drugs. Feces or cloacal swabs are most frequently selected for culture, although ocular and nasal exudates, choanal slit cultures, and biopsy specimens from the liver or kidney can also be collected.

Sample handling is important to maintain viability of the *Chlamydia*. Fresh material should be collected with Dacron swabs and placed in a *Chlamydia* transport medium that inhibits the growth of bacteria. Samples should be refrigerated but not frozen until shipment on ice to the laboratory by overnight mail. Few laboratories provide culture testing, and the individual laboratory should be contacted to obtain transport media and instructions for sample collection. Concurrent drug treatment may also invalidate culture tests. Drugs that interfere with *Chlamydia* culture results include tetracyclines, macrolides, chloramphenicol, and fluoroquinolones.

Identification of intermittent shedders can be improved if multiple tests are performed or if samples are collected over a period of several days and pooled into a *Chlamydia* transport medium. A practical suggestion is to collect samples daily for 5 to 7 days. This will improve results but not identify every shedding bird. For example, the author cultured fecal samples collected daily from an asymptomatic scarlet macaw for 29 days and found *Chlamydia* in only three samples. To screen large avian collections, fecal samples from several birds can be pooled into a single sample for isolation. Then, if positive results are found, birds in that sample group can be tested individually to determine which are truly positive. Pooling samples does have limitations because positive samples with low numbers of *Chlamydia* may be further diluted by negative material.

In situations when a confirmed diagnosis is required (e.g., when human illness has occurred, there is potential legal action, or treatment may be particularly difficult) culture is the preferred test because positive results are difficult to dispute.

Polymerase Chain Reaction Testing

PCR testing is currently in the experimental stages. The test can be used to amplify the production of highly specific DNA fragments of the *Chlamydia* genome and is therefore both highly sensitive and highly specific.[6, 30–32] By amplifying specific portions of the genome in combination with an avian probe, it may be possible to identify specific *Chlamydia* strains isolated from patients.[6] This may aid in determining if the strain is pathogenic. The major disadvantage of this method is its extreme sensitivity, which can result in false-positive results if the laboratory or sample is contaminated by minute amounts of *Chlamydia* in the environment. PCR methodology is encouraging and may eventually provide a test that will accurately determine if a bird is free of infection.

PRE- AND POST-TREATMENT CONSIDERATIONS

An organized approach to treatment reduces complications.[33] Local public health regulations should be determined and followed. To reduce the incidence of side effects, both the bird owner and supervising veterinarian must be prepared to reduce stress in the flock, monitor the health status of the birds, and maximize husbandry to reduce exposure to environmental sources of bacteria and yeast that may cause secondary microbial infections. During treatment, the aviary must be disinfected to reduce the chance of re-exposure to chlamydia, and the birds must be monitored to mitigate the effects of treatment.

If a single bird in a collection tests positive for chlamydiosis it can be assumed that all birds sharing that bird's air space or having any form of contact are exposed to chlamydiosis. Although not all exposed birds become infected, it is safest to recommend that all exposed birds be treated. This recommendation can be modified if the owner is willing to isolate and repeatedly test individual birds to prove that they are not infected. For example, an owner may want to avoid treatment in certain birds if they know that treatment will be difficult (e.g., hyacinth macaws). The risk of this approach is that testing is never 100% accurate, and a single shedding bird might reinfect the flock when treatment ends.

The bird owner and avian caretakers should take precautions to avoid human infection and spread of infection to unexposed birds. The caretaker should wear protective clothing and shoes that stay with the quarantined group of birds. Wearing a face mask reduces potential inhalation of infectious particles. Exposed birds should be serviced last, and the caretaker should wash or shower immediately afterward. Infectious waste should be carefully bagged and disinfected before discarding. Precautions are most important at the start of treatment. It is thought that shedding of infectious *Chlamydia* probably ends in the first 2 weeks of treatment. More extensive recommendations for minimizing human exposure have been published.[34]

Stress should be minimized by making sure that the birds are sheltered from adverse climatic conditions, removed from exhibit or areas with heavy traffic, and breeding stopped. If a large number of asymptomatic birds are to be treated, it may be better to quarantine the birds and delay treatment until it can be done properly than rush in and treat too quickly. If a diet change is required, adapting the birds to an unmedicated version of the food is often helpful in increasing acceptance. Eliminating concurrent diseases such as bacterial and yeast infections also aids treatment.

All birds should be weighed and examined before treatment to establish baseline information. Subclinical infections by gram-negative bacteria and yeast are common in psittacine birds, and these can be identified by culturing cloacal swabs. Because these pathogens are often resistant to tetracyclines, asymptomatic infections may become symptomatic when the birds are treated and normal alimentary tract flora are reduced. Microbial infections should be eliminated prior to tetracycline treatment or treated concurrently.

Birds should be carefully monitored during treatment to ensure that they are eating adequate amounts of food and that secondary microbial infections do not occur. They should be weighed and examined at the start of treatment, day 3, and then weekly if no other problems are encountered. The droppings should be examined daily for bile staining, which indicates inadequate food consumption, and diarrhea, which may indicate a secondary infection.

Ill birds and those refusing treatment or losing too much weight should be tube-fed, provided good supportive care, and treated with oral or parenteral drugs. When their condition is stable, treatment with medicated food can be tried again if this is more convenient. If a bird becomes ill during treatment, the following problems should be investigated: starvation, secondary infection by another pathogen (especially gram-negative bacteria or yeast in the alimentary tract), and treatment failure.

Husbandry should be maximized to reduce exposure to microbial pathogens from environmental sources. If used, cooked mash should be made fresh daily. Spilled food should be promptly removed. The water bowls and cage should be kept scrupulously clean. Nest boxes should be removed or thoroughly cleaned to reduce the chance of fungal infections (especially aspergillosis). Birds do not develop long-term immunity to chlamydiosis, and the aviary or cage should be thoroughly cleaned and disinfected prior to the end of treatment to remove *Chlamydia* from the environment. All items that cannot be disinfected (e.g., nest material) should be carefully bagged and discarded.

Following treatment, the birds should be rested and readapted to their routine diet. Calcium should be supplemented to permit the birds to restore depleted stores. It may be wise to culture cloacal swabs and examine Gram-stained fecal smears to diagnose potential microbial infections. When an aviary has been treated for chlamydiosis, new birds should be tested or prophylactically treated to prevent reintroduction of *Chlamydia* into the aviary.

DRUG SELECTION

Disclaimer: No drugs have been adequately tested in psittacine birds, and thus all of the recommendations should be viewed as experimental. The author assumes no responsibility for the safety or efficacy of any of the suggested treatment regimens.

A number of drugs inhibit the growth of *Chlamydia,* including tetracyclines, macrolides, chloramphenicol, and the fluoroquinolones. At concentrations achievable in birds, most of the agents tested so far are bacteriostatic and presumably effective only when *Chlamydia* are metabolically active or dividing. Because *Chlamydia* can remain dormant in cells, extended treatment periods of approximately 45 days are thought necessary to eliminate the parasites from the host. Historically, chlortetracycline (CTC)-medicated food is the treatment regimen most commonly recommended or mandated by animal and public health regulatory agencies.[14, 34] Newer regimens using doxycycline, and to a lesser degree, enrofloxacin, have been proposed to solve some of the problems experienced when CTC regimens are employed.

Treatment failures are possible with any treatment regimen. It has even been suggested that some birds are never completely cleared of infection. It is difficult to determine if birds are permanently infected because of the insensitivity of current testing methods. However, the author believes that there is good historic evidence to support treating infected birds and exposed flocks. It is rare to see clinical evidence of chlamydiosis in bird collections if treatment is completed, husbandry improved, and new birds carefully screened for chlamydiosis.

Treatment regimens with at least some experimental evidence to support their use include:

- CTC-medicated mash and pelleted diets
- Intramuscularly administered doxycycline hyclate (Vibravenos)
- Orally administered doxycycline
- Subcutaneously administered long-acting oxytetracycline
- Doxycycline-medicated mash
- Enrofloxacin-medicated feed and water

All regimens except CTC-medicated food are considered experimental and may not be permitted by public health regulatory officials in some parts of the US. This is despite the fact that treatment failures occur with CTC and that doxycycline regimens may be therapeutically superior and safer for the birds. The data supporting use of enrofloxacin-medicated feed and water is promising but currently too limited to recommend for widespread use.

General Considerations When Selecting a Treatment Regimen

The selection of treatment method depends on applicable public health regulations, those drugs and formulations that are available, the abilities of the bird owner to deliver the drug, and finally, that which the birds will accept. Multiple bird collections can be treated with medicated feed. CTC pellets can be purchased commercially or a medicated mash diet can be prepared. Individual birds, birds that are ill, and those refusing medicated feed can be treated by direct (oral or parenteral) administration of doxycycline or oxytetracycline.

Each method has advantages and disadvantages. Feeding a medicated diet reduces labor but requires a stressful change in diet that may be poorly accepted by the birds. Oral administration of doxycycline quickly establishes therapeutic concentrations and precludes the need for a change in diet; however, this method requires daily capture to deliver the drug. In some countries an intramuscular formulation of doxycycline (Vibravenos, Pfizer, West Germany) can be administered every 5 to 7 days. This regimen is effective and reduces the labor and stress associated with daily capture. Unfortunately, this intramuscular formulation of doxycycline is expensive and is not currently available in all countries, including the US. Long-acting oxytetracycline is more readily available but causes greater tissue irritation, must be administered every 2 to 3 days, and has less experimental data to guide its use. Greater information on each regimen is provided in the sections to follow.

Often a combination of methods may be required. If a bird is clinically ill with chlamydiosis, oral or intramuscular administration of doxycycline or subcutaneous (sc) oxytetracycline should be used to quickly establish therapeutic concentrations. When the bird's condition is stable, a medicated diet can be tried or treatment continued with doxycycline.

It is important to recognize that any treatment regimen may have adverse effects on the birds. The most common problems are weight loss and secondary microbial infections that occur because of the stress of a diet change or repeated capture for drug administration, and because long-term treatment alters normal alimentary tract flora. To reduce the incidence of side effects, both the bird owner and supervising veterinarian must be prepared to monitor the health status of the birds, reduce stress, and maximize husbandry to reduce exposure to environmental sources of bacteria and yeast that may cause secondary microbial infections.

Chlortetracycline-medicated Food

Historically, CTC medicated diets have been most often recommended for treating avian chlamydiosis.[14] The goal of therapy is to maintain CTC blood concentrations above 1 µg/ml for the duration of the treatment period. This standard is based on limited experimental studies correlating treatment efficacy with maintenance of CTC blood concentrations above 1 µg/ml for 30 to 45 days.[35–38] However, maintenance of blood concentrations as low as 0.1 µg/ml and treatment periods as short as 3 weeks were effective in eliminating infection from experimentally infected Amazon parrots.[39] The relationships between the blood concentrations maintained by specific therapeutic regimens and therapeutic efficacy in various species of psittacine birds are currently ill-defined.

Chlortetracycline is usually delivered via medicated food because direct oral or parenteral administration is impractical because of the drug's short elimination half-life (3–4 hours in pigeons)[40] and because medicated water fails to maintain adequate CTC blood concentrations. To achieve the recommended blood concentrations, medicated diets must be fed as the sole source of food. Dietary calcium interferes with the absorption of tetracycline and should be reduced to 0.7% or less of the diet.[14]

Chlamydiosis in small birds (budgerigars, canaries, and finches) can be treated with a medicated millet seed diet (Keet Life, Hartz Mountain) or 0.5% CTC-medicated mash or pellets for 30 days.[14] Other birds require greater dietary CTC concentrations, and food containing 0.5 to 1% CTC is recommended for larger psittacines. Medicated pelleted feeds are commercially available in many countries, or the bird owner can prepare a cooked mash or nectar diet and add CTC powder after cooking.

Composition of the base diet influences treatment success.[41] Achievement of adequate antibiotic concentrations is determined by the amount of diet consumed, the amount of antibiotic available for absorption, and the concentration of antibiotic included in the diet. The amount of diet consumed is determined primarily by the energy content and the palatability of the diet. Less antibiotic is consumed if the energy content is high (because birds eat primarily to meet energy requirements) or if the diet is unpalatable. Divalent cations (e.g., calcium) and certain proteins can bind tetracycline antibiotics and render them unavailable for absorption. Therefore, a diet can have the adequate amount of antibiotic but still produce inadequate plasma concentrations because of binding by these items. High concentrations of antibiotic may actually decrease palatability and may result in lower plasma antibiotic concentrations than would be achieved with a diet containing less antibiotic.

The interactions between palatability, energy content, and potential binding agents in the diet are complex, and the pharmacologic efficacy of a particular medicated diet cannot be predicted without feeding it to birds and actually measuring the concentrations of antibiotic maintained in the blood or plasma. It should be noted that pelleted diets can be marketed in the US for treatment of chlamydiosis if they meet only two criteria—they must contain 1% CTC and less than 0.7% calcium. Palatability, energy content, and the presence of agents that might bind the antibiotic are not evaluated. Very few of the pelleted diets currently on the market have been evaluated to determine if they maintain adequate antibiotic concentrations in any psittacine bird, and thus treatment with a medicated pellet is no guarantee of treatment success. The same is true if homemade medicated mash diets are used.

Treatment of small birds with the medicated seed diet is relatively uncomplicated because the treatment ration is familiar and readily accepted. In larger psittacine birds, poor acceptance of the treatment diet is frequently encountered because cooked mashes and pellets are perceived as foreign food by birds that are usually fed seed and fruit diets.[42] Even birds that are accustomed to pelleted diets may refuse medicated pellets because of the bitter taste of the CTC. This results in low antibiotic consumption, treatment failure, and continued shedding of *Chlamydia*. Affected birds, already suffering the effects of chlamydiosis, may starve and die. Some bird owners, faced with the debilitating effects of treatment on their birds, suspend treatment and are often reluctant to have birds tested for chlamydiosis in the future. The fear of the adverse effects of treatment and lack of bird owner compliance with treatment recommendations contributes to the high numbers of *Chlamydia*-positive birds found in the pet trade.

The adverse effects of CTC treatment can be mitigated by careful planning. If the birds are asymptomatic and treatment can be delayed, food acceptance can be increased by gradually switching the birds to an unmedicated form of the treatment diet and then starting medication when the diet is accepted. Birds refusing to eat medicated diets can be tube-fed a blenderized version of the treatment diet or treated with oral or intramuscular administration of doxycycline until diet consumption improves.

Doxycycline

Doxycycline is a semisynthetic tetracycline derivative with numerous pharmacologic advantages when compared with CTC. It is more lipophilic, more completely absorbed from the gastrointestinal tract, has fewer adverse effects on normal alimentary tract flora, achieves greater tissue concentrations, and has a longer elimination half-life than other tetracyclines.[43] Several treatment regimens using doxycycline have been developed in an attempt to solve some of the problems encountered when using CTC-medicated diets.

Orally Administered Doxycycline

The prolonged elimination half-life of doxycycline makes it possible to maintain therapeutic concentrations in birds dosed orally once or twice daily. Doxycycline can be administered directly into the mouth or delivered into the crop via a tube.

Preliminary pharmacologic investigations using oral doxycycline have demonstrated that therapeutic concentrations can be maintained with once-daily oral administration in several psittacine species.[44] Once-daily administration requires high doses that may cause regurgitation in some individuals (especially macaws) and may not be suitable for all individuals. The elimination half-life varies with the species. At oral doses of 50 mg/kg, the half-life averages 4 to 10 hours in cockatiels and Amazon parrots, and greater than 20 hours in cockatoos and macaws.* Based on these studies, preliminary

---

*Flammer K, unpublished studies.

dosage guidelines for treating chlamydiosis with orally administered doxycycline can be made. Cockatiels and blue-fronted and orange-winged Amazon parrots maintain therapeutic plasma concentrations when treated with 40 to 50 mg/kg once a day (sid). African grey parrots, Goffin's cockatoos, blue and gold macaws, and green-winged macaws maintained adequate plasma concentrations when treated with 20 to 25 mg/kg sid. In untested species it is impossible to precisely extrapolate dosages; however, 25 mg/kg sid is the recommended starting dose in cockatoos and macaws, and 25 to 50 mg/kg is recommended in other species. All birds should be monitored carefully and the dose reduced or treatment suspended if signs of hepatotoxicity occur. If regurgitation occurs, another form of therapy should be selected.

Intramuscularly Administered Doxycycline

A specific doxycycline formulation, Vibravenos, that is appropriate for intramuscular (IM) administration is available for treating avian chlamydiosis in Europe; in Canada and some other countries it is also available. Blood concentrations exceeding 1 μg/ml are maintained for 4 to 7 days when large doses (75–100 mg/kg) are injected into the pectoral muscles. Dosage regimens requiring only 8 to 10 injections in a 45-day period have proved efficacious in a variety of psittacine species.[45-53] This regimen is practical for treating both individuals and groups of birds. Negative aspects of this treatment regimen include expense, the large injection volume that must be administered, and irritation and necrosis at the site of injection.

A labeled formulation of doxycycline appropriate for IM administration is not currently available in the US. The injectable labeled formulations that are available should not be used because they cause extensive muscle necrosis and possible death. These formulations can be given intravenously to severely ill patients. Research to develop a pharmacist-compounded IM formulation is proceeding, and a suitable product may be available in the future.

Doxycycline-medicated Feed

The pharmacologic advantages of doxycycline also make it useful to medicate feed. Because doxycycline is eliminated more slowly than CTC, less drug is required, and the palatability of the ration is improved. Published information on use of doxycycline-medicated diets is sparse. The author has completed preliminary trials with three different doxycycline-medicated diets in four species of psittacine birds.[41, 54] The results of these trials illustrate the difficulties of extrapolating information from different diets or different species to others.

African grey and blue-fronted Amazon parrots maintained adequate doxycycline plasma concentrations (>1 μg/ml) when fed a rice, corn, bean, and oatmeal mash medicated at 0.1% doxycycline (one-tenth the concentration used for CTC rations).[41] Goffin's cockatoos fed the identical ration established higher doxycycline concentrations.* These species differences are most likely related to the longer elimination half-life demonstrated by Goffin's cockatoos in previous trials with orally administered doxycycline.

The base diet can also affect the drug concentrations achieved. African grey parrots treated with pellets medicated with 0.5% doxycycline maintained lower plasma doxycycline concentrations than those treated with the 0.1% doxycycline-medicated mash mentioned earlier.† The differences in these diets is probably related to energy content. The pellets contained greater energy than the mash so the birds ate less, and therefore consumed less drug. Goffin's cockatoos fed a corn/soybean mash medicated with 0.1% doxycycline developed toxic concentrations of doxycycline (sometimes exceeding 10 μg/ml).‡ Several birds became anorectic and demonstrated elevated AST and LDH levels. They returned to normal 2 days after treatment was stopped. The corn/soybean diet had even lower energy content than the mash described earlier, and the birds consumed huge amounts of food. Doxycycline-medicated food can be used to treat chlamydiosis, but the base diet is important and birds treated with a regimen untested in that species should be monitored closely.

For treatment of smaller birds, Dorrestein reported that effective blood concentrations (mean 1.02 μg/ml) were maintained in parakeets fed seed (90% hulled millet, 10% cracked wheat, $\pm$5% hulled

sunflower seeds) impregnated with 240 ppm doxycycline.[55]

Oxytetracycline

Trials with injectable oxytetracycline were conducted to provide an alternative to the injectable doxycycline regimens not available in the US. In Goffin's cockatoos, adequate plasma concentrations (>1 μg/ml) were maintained when long-acting oxytetracycline (LA 200, Pfizer) was administered subcutaneously at 50 to 100 mg/kg every 2 to 3 days.[56] Similar results were found in four other avian species (African grey parrots, blue and gold macaws, orange-winged Amazon parrots, and pigeons).* IM administration causes severe tissue irritation and is not recommended. SC administration causes localized irritation at sites of repeated injection; however, injection sites on the back of the neck and between the shoulders are well tolerated. Injecting the wingweb or sites where local irritation may inflame nerves, vessels, or tendons should be avoided. Although most larger birds tolerate treatment for the full 45-day period, injectable long-acting oxytetracycline is most suitable for initiating treatment and then switching to medicated feed.

Fluoroquinolones

The fluoroquinolone antibiotics have been extensively investigated for activity against *C. trachomatis* in humans. Thus far, several compounds have demonstrated good in vitro activity,[57, 58] but none has been more efficacious than doxycycline in clinical comparison trials. It is not known whether these data can be extrapolated to *C. psittaci* treatment in birds. If effective against chlamydiosis, the fluoroquinolones could offer a number of exciting advantages. They are bacteriocidal and may require shorter treatment periods. Unlike the tetracyclines, fluoroquinolones have extensive activity against gram-negative bacteria and could be used to treat simultaneous infections. Use of fluoroquinolones may also prevent some of the secondary microbial infections that occur with CTC or doxycycline use.

Enrofloxacin, the most readily available veteri-

---

*Flammer K, unpublished studies.
†Flammer K, unpublished studies.
‡Prus SE, Flammer K, unpublished studies.

*Flammer K, unpublished data.

nary fluoroquinolone, has antichlamydial activity. The in vitro minimum inhibitory concentration (MIC) of enrofloxacin for chlamydia is 0.125 µg/ml, the minimal bacteriocidal concentration is 50 to 75 µg/ml. Concentrations of 0.5 to 1.0 µg/ml caused irreversible damage to *C. psittaci* in cell culture.[59] It is difficult to extrapolate from in vitro susceptibility tests to efficacy in live birds, and these concentrations can at best be used as a guide. As indicated later, it is possible to achieve plasma or blood concentrations of 0.5 to 1 µg/ml with several routes of administration, and thus it is possible that enrofloxacin could be an effective treatment. However, despite this promising pharmacologic information, anecdotal information from US avian practitioners indicates that enrofloxacin alleviates clinical signs but seldom clears birds of *Chlamydia* infection. More information is needed before enrofloxacin can be recommended as a sole treatment for chlamydiosis.

The pharmacokinetics of enrofloxacin has been investigated in several avian species. As with other drugs, the plasma or blood concentrations attained depend on the route of administration and age and species of bird tested. Therapeutic concentrations (>0.5 mg/L) were maintained in pigeons treated with 5 mg/kg sid-bid or 100 to 200 mg/L drinking water.[60] IM or oral administration at doses of 7.5 to 15 mg/kg twice daily maintain plasma concentrations that are effective for most gram-negative bacteria in African grey parrots.[61] Similar results were found in Goffin's cockatoos and blue-fronted and orange-winged Amazon parrots.* For ease of administration, the IM formulation can also be administered orally. In trials with multiple psittacine species food medicated with 250 to 1000 ppm attained serum concentrations of 0.3 to 0.8 µg/ml,[59] and 0.66 to 4.10 µg/ml with 500 ppm.[62]

Trials with medicated drinking water have provided conflicting results. In one study, African grey parrots achieved low plasma concentrations (0.1–0.2 mg/L), despite providing high doses (190–3000 mg/L).[63] In Germany, concentrations therapeutic for most gram-negative bacteria (>0.5 mg/L) were achieved in Patagonian conures, African grey parrots, and Senegal parrots treated with drinking water containing 500 mg/L enrofloxacin.[59]

The side effects of long-term enrofloxacin admin-

---

*Flammer K, unpublished studies.

istration have been reported only in pigeons. The drug was well tolerated in adults, but reduced egg hatchability was seen in adults receiving 800 mg/L for 225 days and growth abnormalities were seen in some nestlings that received an estimated dose of 200 mg/kg/day from medicated parents.[64, 65]

Future Treatment Regimens

Newly developed macrolide antibiotics (e.g., azithromycin and clarithromycin) have produced promising results in humans.[66, 67] These drugs achieve high and prolonged tissue concentrations with a single oral dose. Treatment with five doses of azithromycin in a 14-day period was as effective as 14 doses of doxycycline in people infected with *C. trachomatis*. These compounds have not yet been investigated in birds.

In the US, trials with a micronized suspension of doxycycline maintained therapeutic concentrations for 72 hours in pigeons injected with 100 mg/kg body weight.[68] This suspension may provide a product for US veterinarians that will achieve the effectiveness and safety of the Vibravenos product.

PUBLIC HEALTH AND LEGAL CONCERNS

C. psittaci infection in people is called "psittacosis" or "ornithosis" and causes an influenza-like syndrome characterized by fever, headaches, and muscle aches. Atypical pneumonia commonly develops, and the disease may progress to cause meningitis, neuritis, or cardiac complications. Chronic psittacosis can result in valvular endocarditis and thrombophlebitis.[69–73] The signs are nonspecific and, as in birds, disease can only be diagnosed by testing specifically for the disease. People experiencing illness should advise their physician and request testing. In the authors' experience, physicians are often reluctant to test for psittacosis and sometimes must be strongly encouraged to look for this disease. Initial diagnostic samples should be collected before treatment begins. Treatment with doxycycline for 3 weeks is usually successful, and the response within the first few days of drug administration is often dramatic.

The reported incidence of psittacosis in people is low. Approximately 140 cases per year were reported to the US Centers for Disease Control during 1978–1987. Because psittacosis is difficult to diagnose, the actual number of cases is probably underreported. People in contact with caged birds (bird owners, veterinarians and their staff, pet shop workers, etc.) and turkey processing plant workers are at greatest risk. *C. psittaci* in people is most often acquired from birds; strains from mammals are seldom reported. Bird owners should be advised that transmission from an infected bird is unlikely but possible.

Avian chlamydiosis is a reportable disease in most states in the US, and veterinarians should fulfill their legal obligations by reporting confirmed infections to the state public health veterinarian, state department of agriculture or other appropriate agency. It is usually up to local public officials (often at a county level) to decide if there is a threat to public health and if they need to intervene. In most states, regulatory authorities seldom intervene if there are no human infections. In some cases, local officials quarantine exposed birds and mandate the method of treatment (usually CTC-medicated food). Local public health officials may or may not be physicians or be familiar with chlamydiosis. Their job is to guard public health. They often welcome the expertise of an avian veterinarian if approached with a cooperative attitude. In an attempt to standardize recommendations for *Chlamydia* control, a document has been published by the US National Association of State Public Health Veterinarians[34]; this document is updated on a regular basis.

Avian veterinarians working with pet stores, zoos, and other establishments with birds exposed to the public should determine the attitude of their local officials and develop preemptive plans to deal with a positive chlamydiosis case, should it occur. Housing for birds, employee traffic patterns, and other factors can influence how many birds must be treated if an outbreak occurs. Pet stores in particular face economic hardship if their birds are quarantined and are not available for sale. The number of exposed birds can be reduced if groups of birds are housed in separate areas of the pet store and new arrivals are quarantined for at least 14 days prior to mixing with the sale stock.

References

1. Grimes JE, Wyrick PE: Chlamydiosis (Ornithosis). In Calnek CW (ed): Diseases of Poultry. Ames, Iowa State University Press, 1991, pp 311–325.
2. Schacter J: Chlamydial infections—past, present, future. J Am Vet Med 195:1501–1506, 1989.
3. Gerlach H: Chlamydia. In Ritchie BW, Harrison GJ, Harrison LR (eds): Avian Medicine, Principles and Application. Lake Worth, FL, Wingers Publishing, 1994, pp 984–996.
4. Anderson AA, Tappe JP: Genetic, immunologic, and pathologic characterization of avian chlamydial strains. J Am Vet Med 195:1512–1516, 1989.
5. Anderson AA: Comparison of avian Chlamydia psittaci isolates by restriction endonuclease analysis and serovar-specific monoclonal antibodies. J Clin Microbiol 29:244–249, 1991.
6. Dorrestein GM: PCR diagnostic testing for Chlamydia psittaci. Semin Avian Exotic Pet Med 2:171–174, 1993.
7. Glystorff I: Chlamydiales. In Glystorff I, Grimm F: Vogelkrankheiten Verlag Eugen Ulmer. Stuttgart, 1987, pp 317–322.
8. Wyrick PB, Richmond SJ: Biology of chlamydiae. Reports from the Symposium on Avian Chlamydiosis. J Am Vet Med 195:1507–1512, 1989.
9. Fudge AM: Update on chlamydiosis. Vet Clin North Am Sm Anim Pract 14:201–221, 1984.
10. Arnstein P, Buchanan WG, Eddie B, Meyer KF: Control of psittacosis by group chemotherapy of infected parrots. Am J Vet Res 11:2213–2227, 1968.
11. Page LA: Studies on immunity to chlamydiosis in birds, with particular reference to turkeys. Am J Vet Res 36:597–600, 1975.
12. Page LA: Stimulation of cell-mediated immunity to chlamydiosis in turkeys by inoculation of chlamydial bacterin. Am J Vet Res 39:473–480, 1978.
13. Schnorr KL: Chlamydial vaccines. J Am Vet Med Assoc 195:1548–1561, 1989.
14. Cooper R: Psittacosis—An ever-present problem in caged birds. In Kirk RW (ed): Current Veterinary Therapy VII. Philadelphia, WB Saunders, 1980, pp 677–686.
15. Gerlach H: Chlamydia. In Harrison GJ, Harrison LR, (eds): Clinical Avian Medicine and Surgery. WB Saunders, Philadelphia, 1986, pp 457–463.
16. Harrison GJ: A practitioner's view of the problem of avian chlamydiosis. J Am Vet Med Assoc 195:1525–1528, 1989.
17. Tudor DC: Pigeon Health and Disease. Ames, Iowa State University Press, 1991.
18. Strauss J: Microbiologic and epidemiologic aspects of duck ornithosis in Czechoslovakia. Am J Ophthalmol 63:1246–1259, 1967.
19. Graham DL: Histopathologic lesions associated with chlamydiosis in psittacine birds. J Am Vet Med Assoc 195:1571–1573, 1989.
20. Graham DL: Surprises at necropsy: Failure of differential diagnosis. Proc Assoc Avian Vet, 1988, pp 177–178.
21. Grimes JE: Direct complement fixation and isolation attempts for detecting Chlamydia psittaci infections of psittacine birds. Avian Dis 29:873–877, 1984.
22. Grimes JE: Enigmatic psittacine chlamydiosis: Results of serotesting and isolation attempts, 1978 through 1983, and considerations for the future. J Am Vet Med Assoc 186:1075–1079, 1985.
23. Grimes JE: Chlamydia psittaci latex agglutination antigen for rapid detection of antibody activity in avian sera: Comparison with direct complement fixation and isolation results. Avian Dis 30:60–66, 1986.
24. Grimes JE: Serodiagnosis of avian chlamydia infections. J Am Vet Med Assoc 195:1561–1564, 1989.
25. Grimes JE: Interpretation of avian host chlamydial titers using various serologic methods. Semin Avian Exotic Pet Med 2:161–166, 1993.

26. Geberman H, Janeczek F, Gerlach H, Kosters J: Infections with Chlamydia psittaci: Alternative for diagnosis and control. Proc Assoc Avian Vet, 1988, pp 69–78.

27. Fudge AM: Blocking antibody ELISA testing of pet birds: Implication for chronic infections. Semin Avian Exotic Pet Med 2:167–171, 1993.

28. Fudge AM: ELISA testing for avian chlamydiosis. Vet Clin North Am Small Anim Pract 21:1181–1188, 1991.

29. Kingston RS: Evaluation of the Kodak SureCell chlamydia test kit in companion birds. J Assoc Avian Vet 6:155–157, 1992.

30. Hewinson RG, Griffiths PC, Rankin SES, et al: Towards a differential polymerase chain reaction test for Chlamydia psittaci. Vet Rec 128:381–382, 1991.

31. Hewinson RG, Rankin SES, Bevan BJ, et al: Detection of Chlamydia psittaci from avian field samples using PCR. Vet Rec 128:129–130, 1991.

32. Kaltenboeck B, Kousoulas KG, Storz J: Detection and strain differentiation of Chlamydia psittaci mediated by a two-step polymerase chain reaction. J Clin Microbiol 29:1969–1975, 1991.

33. Flammer K: An update on the diagnosis and treatment of avian chlamydiosis. In Kirk RW, Bonagura JD (eds): Current Veterinary Therapy XI. Philadelphia, WB Saunders, 1992, pp 1150–1153.

34. National Association of State Public Health Veterinarians: Compendium of chlamydiosis (psittacosis) control, 1994. J Am Vet Med Assoc 206:1874–1879, 1995.

35. Arnstein P, Buchanan WG, Eddie B, Meyer KF: Control of psittacosis by group chemotherapy of infected parrots. Am J Vet Res 11:2213–2227, 1968.

36. Arnstein P, Buchanan WG, Eddie B, Myer KF: Chlortetracycline chemotherapy for nectar-feeding psittacine birds. J Am Vet Med Assoc 154:190–191, 1969.

37. Wachendorfer JG: Epidemiology and control of psittacosis. J Am Vet Med Assoc 162:298–303, 1973.

38. Wachendorfer G, Burski B: Further studies on improving oral prevention and treatment of psittacosis in lovebirds, cockatiels and other medium-sized parakeets with medicated feed. Tierarztl Wschr 97:18–21, 1984.

39. Glystorff J, Jakoby R, Gerbermann H: [Investigations of the efficacy of different medicated feed to parrots infected with Chlamydia psittaci]. Tierarztl Wschr 97:91–99, 1984.

40. Dorrestein GM: Studies on pharmacokinetics for some antibacterial agents in homing pigeons (Columba livia) (thesis). State University of Utrecht, 1986.

41. Flammer K, Aucoin DP, Whitt D: Preliminary report on the use of doxycycline-medicated feed in psittacine birds. Proc Assoc Avian Vet, 1991, pp 1–5.

42. Flammer K: Treatment of chlamydiosis in psittacine birds in the United States. J Am Vet Med Assoc 195:1537–1540, 1989.

43. Sande MA, Mandell GL: Antimicrobial agents: tetracyclines, chloramphenicol, erythromycin, and miscellaneous antibacterial agents. In Goodman LS, Gillman A (eds): The Pharmacological Basis of Therapeutics, ed 6. New York, Macmillan, 1982, pp 1170–1186.

44. Flammer K: Avian chlamydiosis—Observations on diagnostic techniques and use of oral doxycycline for treatment. Proc First Intl Conf Zool Avian Med, Turtle Bay, Hawaii, September, 1987, pp 149–158.

45. Jakoby JR: Prophylaxis of psittacosis in Agaporides by intramuscular application of doxycycline. Praktische Tierarztl 59:206–208, 1978.

46. Jakoby JR: Prevention and treatment of psittacosis with doxycycline (tetracycline) in parrots and parakeets. Tierarztl Wschr 92:91–95, 1979.

47. Jakoby JR: [Doxycycline for treatment and prophylaxis of psittacosis]. In Krankerheiten der Vogel. Tagung der Fachgruppe Geflugelkrankheiten (der DVG), 7–8 Marz 1979 in Munchen. Giessen-Lahn, German Federal Republic 43–61, 1979.

48. Luthgen W, Schulz W, Hauser KW: [Parenteral administration of doxycycline to cockatoos, with reference to prevention and treatment of psittacosis]. Praktische Tierarztl 60:233–236, 1979.

49. Jakoby JR: Prevention and treatment of psittacosis with doxycycline (tetracycline) in parrots and parakeets. Tierarztl Wschr 92:91–95, 1979.

50. Henning K, Krauss H: Field studies on development of resistance to tetracycline in Chlamydia psittaci. Tierarztl Wschr 99:381–382, 1986.

51. Gylsdorff I: The treatment of chlamydiosis in psittacine birds. Isr J Vet Med 43:11–19, 1987.

52. Dorrestein GM: Update in avian chemotherapy. Proc Assoc Avian Vet, 1988, pp 119–122.

53. Dorrestein GM: Chlamydiosis: A new approach in diagnosis and therapy. Proc Assoc Avian Vet, 1989, pp 29–34.

54. Prus SE, Clubb SL, Flammer K: Plasma concentrations of doxycycline achieved by feeding a medicated diet in macaws. Avian Dis 36:480–483, 1992.

55. Dorrestein GM: Chlamydiosis: A new approach in diagnosis and therapy. Proc Assoc Avian Vet, 1989, pp 29–34.

56. Flammer K, Aucoin DP, Whitt DA, Styles DK: Potential use of long-acting oxytetracycline for the treatment of chlamydiosis in Goffin's cockatoos. Avian Dis 34:228–234,

57. How SJ, Hobson D, Hart CA, et al: A comparison of the in vitro activity of antimicrobials against Chlamydia trachomatis examined by giemsa and a fluorescent antibody stain. J Antimicrob Chemother 15:399–404, 1985.

58. Bowie WR: In vitro and in vivo efficacy of antimicrobials to Chlamydia trachomatis. Infection 10[Suppl 1]:S46–S52, 1982.

59. Lindenstruth H: Field trial of the efficacy and acceptability of Baytril in imported psittacines in relation to the state program of prophylaxis and therapy of psittacosis (thesis). Vet Med Dis 1992.

60. Dorrestein GM: Pharmacokinetics of Baytril in homing pigeons after different administration routes. Proc Fourth Symp Avian Dis, Munich, 1988, pp 226–228.

61. Flammer K, Aucoin DP, Whitt DA: Intramuscular and oral disposition of enrofloxacin in African grey parrots following single and multiple doses. Vet Pharmacol Ther 14:359–366, 1991.

62. Jung C: Study of acceptance, pharmacokinetics, and adverse reactions of enrofloxacin in psittacines, as well as efficacy after an experimental infection with Chlamydia psittaci (thesis). Vet Med Dis 1992.

63. Flammer K, Aucoin DP, Whitt DA, Prus SA: Plasma concentrations of enrofloxacin in African grey parrots treated with medicated water. Avian Dis 34:1017–1022, 1990.

64. Krautwald ME, Pieper K, Rullof R, et al: Further experience with the use of Baytril in pet birds. Proc Assoc Avian Vet, 1990, pp 226–236.

65. Rullof R: Study of toxicity of Baytril (enrofloxacin) in healthy homing pigeons (Columba livia domestica) with particular emphasis on fertility and feather formation. Vet Med Dis 1991.

66. Johnson RB: The role of azalide antibiotics in the treatment of Chlamydia. Am J Obstet Gynecol 164:1794–1796, 1991.

67. Jones RB: New treatments for Chlamydia trachomatis. Am J Obstet Gynecol 164:1789–1793, 1991.

68. Doolen M, et al: Determination of blood levels of a new doxycycline after intramuscular injection in the domestic pigeon. Proc Eur Conf Avian Med Surg 1993, pp 111–115.

69. Centers for Disease Control: Psittacosis surveillance, 1975–1984, issued 1987. Atlanta, GA. Department of Heath and Human Services, Centers for Disease Control.
70. Yung AP, Grayson ML: Psittacosis—a review of 135 cases. Med J Aust 148:228–233, 1988.
71. Filstein MR, Ley AB, Veron MS, et al: Epidemic of Psittacosis in a college of veterinary medicine. J Am Vet Med Assoc 179:569–572, 1981.
72. Schacter J, Sugg N, Sung M: Psittacosis: The reservoir persists. J Infect Dis 127:44–49, 1978.
73. Fowler ME: Psittacosis in a veterinary hospital. Proc Am Assoc Zoo Vet, 1982, pp 20–21.

Mary B. Brown
Martha L. Ewing

24

Mycoplasmal Infections

Mycoplasmas have long been recognized as important respiratory pathogens in the commercial poultry industry.[15] However, little attention has been given to the role that these microorganisms may play in respiratory disease in pet birds. The majority of reports are limited to case reports,[1, 8, 13] although several recent experimental infection studies[4, 5, 7] have confirmed the pathogenic potential of mycoplasmas in budgerigars. In addition, mycoplasma species have been isolated from racing pigeons with evidence of respiratory disease.[10, 11]

Mycoplasmal respiratory disease is often chronic and clinically silent. When present, clinical signs of disease in poultry include rales, sneezing, nasal exudate, sinusitis, air sacculitis, and conjunctivitis.[15] Similar signs have been reported in naturally infected budgerigars,[1] yellow-naped Amazon parrots,[4] racing pigeons,[10, 11] severe macaws,[8] and cockatiels (unpublished data). However, with the exception of the isolate from yellow-naped Amazon parrots,[4] no attempts have been made to confirm the pathogenic potential of the mycoplasmal strains in live birds. Adler did demonstrate that the mycoplasmal isolate from budgerigars could propagate in chicken embryos but did not cause mortality.[1]

CLINICAL SIGNS

In domestic poultry, *Mycoplasma gallisepticum, M. synoviae,* and *M. meleagridis* are important agents of chronic respiratory disease. *Mycoplasma iowae* is a less common cause of respiratory disease. Additionally, arthritic manifestations are observed with *M. synoviae.* The most common clinical manifestations in domestic poultry are air sacculitis, sinusitis,

decreased egg production and/or hatchability, and in some cases synovitis.[15] Although morbidity is frequently high, mortality usually is associated with secondary infections, especially from viral agents or *Escherichia coli.*[15]

Unfortunately, little information is available on clinical signs in natural infections of exotic or pet birds. Various mycoplasmas have been isolated from caged birds with signs of rhinitis and conjunctivitis, but no clear causal association has been demonstrated. An outbreak of respiratory disease in a flock of over 1000 yellow-naped Amazon parrots resulted in mortality rates of less than 20%.[4] Birds submitted for necropsy were observed to have ruffled feathers, sinusitis, rales, and blepharoconjunctivitis. Extensive air sacculitis with caseous exudates and purulent exudate in the sinus cavity was noted. A variety of gram-negative bacteria as well as *M. gallisepticum* and *M. iowae* were isolated from the sinus and trachea. The observed mortality rates are consistent with synergistic infections observed in poultry. A contributory role for mycoplasmas in this outbreak was strengthened by the experimental induction of air sacculitis in budgerigars infected with the parrot isolate.[4] Although experimentally infected chickens did not develop air sacculitis, the birds were colonized by the parrot isolate.

Similar clinical signs were observed in 20 racing pigeons from flocks experiencing weight loss, decreased performance, and severe respiratory distress following activity.[10, 11] Clinical evaluation and necropsy confirmed respiratory distress, conjunctivitis, excessive mucous exudate in the trachea, and thickened air sacs. Both bacterial and mycoplasmal species were isolated. The most common mycoplasmal isolates were *M. columbinum* and *M. columborale*. Some birds did respond to antimicrobial therapy.

DIAGNOSIS

Much effort has gone into the development of serologic screening protocols to ensure that commercial poultry flocks are mycoplasma-free. Most of these protocols are based on a preliminary screening plate agglutination test followed by a second confirmatory test (usually hemagglutination inhibition or enzyme-linked immunosorbent assay [ELISA]). Although the presence of specific antibody is a common method for determination of exposure to *M. gallisepticum* and *M. synoviae* in poultry, serology testing has not been applied to exotic birds. Although commercial ELISA tests are currently available for use with poultry, the lack of species-specific antibodies that recognize immunoglobulins from exotic species limits their usefulness. We have successfully used a monoclonal antibody prepared against immunoglobulins from blue and gold macaws that cross-reacted with immunoglobulin from a range of conure species in conjunction with a commercial ELISA. The test was used to screen for the presence of specific antibody to both *M. gallisepticum* and *M. synoviae*. The results of the study are summarized in Table 24–1. Specific antibody to *M. gallisepticum* was found in 20% of the golden conures tested, suggesting that these birds had prior exposure to the pathogen. Fewer birds (8%) had antibody to *M. synoviae*. Although antibody to *M. gallisepticum* and *M. synoviae* was not detected in other conure species, this may be a reflection of the low numbers of birds in the other groups rather than an indication of lack of exposure in these species. These data suggest that commercial ELISA tests can be applied to screening of birds other than poultry if appropriate second antibodies are available. Such screens would be most valuable in breeding operations or in aviaries with large collections. For individual birds, such tests might be appropriate as a confirmatory test of mycoplasmosis.

Deoxyribonucleic acid (DNA) based tests using the polymerase chain reaction (PCR) have been applied with success to the avian mycoplasmas. These tests are especially appropriate for microorganisms that are fastidious or require long incubation periods for growth. Both genus-specific and species-specific primers have been published for *M. gallisepticum* and *M. synoviae*. Although these tests are not commercially available, most university laboratories and many clinical diagnostic laboratories routinely perform PCR testing for other pathogens and could adapt the procedures to detect avian mycoplasmas using published primers.

Traditional culture of mycoplasmas is also an option for diagnosis.[9] However, most of the avian pathogens grow slowly, and cultures may often become overgrown with contaminants or more rapidly growing commensal flora. Commercial media (SP4 and A7) are now available for isolation of mycoplasmas and ureaplasmas. Incubation times for primary isolation may be long (2–4 weeks). If a mycoplasma is isolated, the species identity may be determined by reaction with specific typing antiserum by tests such as immunofluorescence, growth

T a b l e 2 4 – 1

PRESENCE OF SPECIFIC ANTIBODY TO *MYCOPLASMA GALLISEPTICUM* AND *MYCOPLASMA SYNOVIAE* IN THE SERUM OF CONURE SPECIES

Conure Species (N)	Number (N) of Birds With Specific Antibody To		
	M. Gallisepticum	*M. Synoviae*	*Both*
Golden (39) *(Aratinga guarouba)*	8	3	2
Sun (4) *(Aratinga solstitialis)*	0	0	0
Mitred (3) *(Aratinga mitrata)*	0	0	0
Gold cap (2) *(Aratinga auricapilla)*	0	0	0
Jandaya (9) *(Aratinga jandaya)*	0	0	0
Patagonian (4) *(Cyanoliseus patagonus)*	0	0	0
Painted (1) *(Pyrrhura picta)*	0	0	0
Red-throated (4) *(Aratinga holochlora rubritorquis)*	0	0	0
Finches (2) *(Aratinga finschi)*	0	0	0

inhibition, or immunobinding. DNA-based tests such as 16S rRNA sequence, hybridization with species-specific DNA probes, or restriction fragment length polymorphism (RFLP) may be used to differentiate species.

EXPERIMENTAL INFECTION

Budgerigars have been experimentally infected with *M. gallisepticum* and *M. synoviae*.[4, 5, 7] Mycoplasmas were able to colonize and induce air sac lesions in these trials, suggesting that budgerigars are susceptible to respiratory mycoplasmosis. Furthermore, the budgerigars were more sensitive than chickens to *M. gallisepticum* isolated from parrots.[4] Some experimental infection data suggest that, unlike observations in poultry, mycoplasmas may not persist in infections of budgerigars. However, some care must be taken in interpretation of this observation because the strains used in the infection studies were not obtained from natural infections of budgerigars but from those of either parrots or chickens. The development of clinical signs and lesions in budgerigars experimentally exposed to avian mycoplasmas suggests that budgerigars may be an appropriate model to determine pathogenic potential of avian mycoplasma species, especially those isolated from sources other than poultry.

ANTIBIOTIC TREATMENT

Appropriate antibiotic therapy may alleviate clinical signs of disease but does not eradicate the mycoplasma from the host.[3, 6] Because mycoplasmas lack a cell wall, penicillin and other cell-wall–active antibiotics are inappropriate and may actually exacerbate clinical disease.[5] Antibiotics that target protein synthesis (tetracyclines, macrolide-lincosamide-streptogramin B group, aminoglycosides) or DNA replication (fluoroquinolones) are appropriate for treatment of mycoplasmosis.

Effective antibiotics and development of antibiotic resistance in mycoplasmas have been extensively reviewed.[6, 12] Although the majority of information available concerns mycoplasmas of human origin, data are available for some veterinary isolates. Commonly used antibiotics that are effective in alleviation of clinical signs of disease and reduc-

tion of clinical lesions caused by mycoplasmas (but that do not necessarily eradicate mycoplasmas) include erythromycin, tylosin, tiamulin, gentamicin, tetracyclines, streptomycin, spiromycin, lincomycin, and spectinomycin.

The choice of antibiotics and route of administration are dependent upon the assessment of the clinician. Antibiotics are most commonly administered in drinking water, but may also be given in food or by injection. For example, chlortetracycline has been administered in both food and water with success in poultry.[14] Lincomycin and spectinomycin act synergistically when administered in drinking water. Inhalant products that can be administered via humidifiers or aerosol may also be effective in alleviation of clinical signs but do not affect or lessen lesion severity.[5]

VACCINATION

No completely effective vaccine is available for any mycoplasmal species to date. However, vaccines are available for use in poultry that provide some efficacy in prevention of air sacculitis and egg loss.[2] None of these vaccines has been tested in avian species other than poultry. Vaccines are one of two types: (1) killed vaccines with adjuvants, or (2) live attenuated vaccines. Both types of vaccines elicit a strong immune response; live vaccines also act to colonize the respiratory tract and thus compete for the ecologic niche when field strains are encountered.

SUMMARY

Despite the importance of respiratory mycoplasmosis in domestic poultry, there is little documentation on the importance of mycoplasmal disease in exotic and caged birds. However, experimental infection studies and case reports suggest that mycoplasmosis should be considered as part of a differential diagnosis, particularly in birds with chronic respiratory infection. Antibiotic therapy may alleviate clinical signs but should not be expected to eradicate the microorganism. Serologic and DNA-based diagnostic tests may be applicable in certain instances. Isolation requires more time than is required for other organisms and may be difficult as a result of the fastidious nature of the avian pathogens.

Acknowledgment

The authors acknowledge Morris Animal Foundation for financial support.

References

1. Adler HE: Isolation of a pleuropneumonia-like organism from the air sac of a parakeet. J Am Vet Med Assoc 130:408–409, 1957.
2. Barile MF: Vaccinations against mycoplasma infections. In Razin S, Barile MF (eds). The Mycoplasmas, vol IV. New York, Academic Press, 1985, pp 452–492.
3. Barile MF, Bove JM, Bradbury JM, et al: Current status on control of mycoplasmal diseases of man, animals, and insects. Bull Inst Pasteur 83:339–373, 1985.
4. Bozeman LH, Kleven SH, Davis RB: Mycoplasma challenge studies in budgerigars *(Melopsittacus undulatus)* and chickens. Avian Dis 28:426–434, 1983.
5. Brown MB, Butcher GD: *Mycoplasma gallisepticum* as a model to assess efficacy of inhalant therapy in budgerigars *(Melopsittacus undulatus).* J Clin Microbiol 35:834–839, 1991.
6. Brunner H, Laber G: Chemotherapy of mycoplasma infections. In The Mycoplasmas, vol IV. Razin S, Barile MF (eds): New York, Academic Press, 1985, pp 403–450.
7. Butcher GD, Brown MB: Reduction of clinical signs in budgerigars experimentally infected with *Mycoplasma gallisepticum.* J Assoc Avian Vet 4:227–230, 1990.
8. Gaskin JM, Jacobson ER: A mycoplasma associated epornitic in Severe Macaws *(Ara severa severa).* Proc Am Assoc Zoo Vet, 1979, pp 59–61.
9. Jordan FTW: Avian mycoplasmas. In Tully JG, Whitcomb RF (eds): The Mycoplasmas, vol II. New York, Academic Press, 1979, pp 1–48.
10. Keymer IF, Leach RH, Clarke RA, et al: Isolation of *Mycoplasma* spp. from racing pigeons *(Columba livia).* Avian Pathol 13:65–74, 1984.
11. Reece RL, Ireland L, Scott PC: Mycoplasmosis in racing pigeons. Aust Vet J 63:166–167, 1986.
12. Roberts MC: Antibiotic resistance. In Mycoplasmas: Molecular Biology and Pathogenesis. Maniloff J, McElhaney RN, Finch LR, Baseman JB (eds): Washington, DC, American Society for Microbiology, 1992, pp 513–524.
13. Spenser EL: Common infectious diseases of psittacine birds seen in practice. Vet Clin North Am Small Anim Pract 21:1213–1230, 1991.
14. Timms LM, Marshall RN, Breslin MF: Evaluation of the efficacy of chlortetracycline for the control of chronic respiratory disease caused by *Escherichia coli* and *Mycoplasma gallisepticum.* Res Vet Sci 47:377–382, 1989.
15. Yoder HW Jr: *Mycoplasma gallisepticum* infection. In Hofstad MS, Calnek BW, Helmboldt CF, et al (eds): Diseases of Poultry. Ames, Iowa State University Press, 1984, pp 236–250.

Noninfectious Diseases

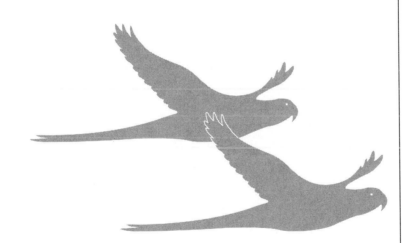

Elizabeth V. Hillyer
Susan Orosz
Gerry M. Dorrestein

25

Respiratory System

Anatomy of the Respiratory System

Susan Orosz

The cere is the area around the most dorsal surface of the maxillary rhamphotheca or upper bill that may be feathered or unfeathered in various species of psittacines. In adult male budgerigars, the cere is usually blue; in adult females it is usually brownish-pink. Changes in the cere's normal color pattern are suggestive of gonad tumors in this species.

The nares or nostrils are located dorsally within the area of the cere in psittacines. The openings may be shaped abnormally as a result of chronic upper respiratory infection and should be noted on the physical examination. Air moves through the nares into the nasal cavity. In Amazon parrots and Galliformes, a rounded, keratinized structure called the operculum is found in the rostral-most extent of the nasal cavity. It acts as a baffle to deflect and prevent inhalation of foreign bodies.

The nasal cavity in most species is divided by a nasal septum. Within the lateral walls of the cavity are highly vascularized nasal conchae. Most birds have three conchae—the rostral, middle, and caudal nasal conchae. The middle concha is the largest of the three. A clinically important anatomic feature is the relationship of the conchae to the openings of the infraorbital sinus—the only true paranasal sinus of birds (Fig. 25–1). This sinus opens dorsally into both the middle and caudal nasal conchae. The caudal nasal concha drains only into the nasal cavity by its dorsal opening into the infraorbital sinus (Fig. 25–2). As a result, the only passageway for drainage of mucopurulent material in the infraorbital sinus is the caudal nasal concha up through the dorsal opening, or over the middle nasal concha, into the nasal cavity.

The infraorbital sinus is located ventromedial to the orbit and has numerous diverticuli (Fig. 25–1). A rostral diverticulum extends into the maxillary rostrum or bill; a preorbital diverticulum lies rostral to the orbit; a postorbital diverticulum may be subdivided to surround the opening of the ear; and a mandibular diverticulum extends into the mandibular rostrum. In addition to its communication with the nasal conchae, the infraorbital sinus also communicates with the cervicocephalic air sac at its caudal-most extent. Knowledge of the relationship of this sinus and air sac with the bones of the skull is important during examination of the upper respiratory system and during irrigation and surgical drainage procedures.

The larynx is composed of four almost fully ossified cartilages with an overlying mucosa or laryngeal mound. The larynx is not involved in sound production in birds. The rima glottis represents the laryngeal opening into the trachea and is not covered by an epiglottis as it is in mammals. The rima glottis and trachea are larger in diameter on a per weight basis than they are in mammals. This principle provides one reason why it is easier to intubate birds than mammals. This increased diameter directly reflects one physiologic adaptation of birds—the use of their beaks for the manipulation of objects. The increased length of the trachea is part of an adaptation in birds whereby the increased

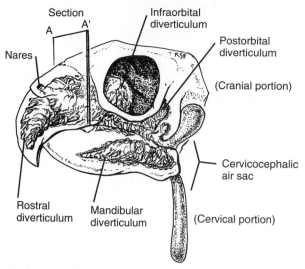

F i g u r e   2 5 – 1

Schematic representation of the extent of the intraorbital sinus in the skull of a parrot. The laminae of bone are separated by trabeculae of bone and the diverticula extend into those spaces.

length of their necks allows use of their beak to manipulate objects. However, the increase in length causes an increased air resistance. A wider rima glottis, as well as a wider trachea, is necessary to reduce this resistance. To compensate for the wider

and longer trachea and its corresponding increase in deadspace, the respiratory rate of birds is less than that of mammals, with a larger tidal volume. These anatomic and physiologic differences are important when selecting endotracheal tubes for anesthetic procedures. In addition, the tracheal rings of birds are complete. They are shaped like a signet ring and overlap to form a more rigid trachea than that of a comparably sized mammal. These two facts are important to reduce the possibility of tracheal kinking when moving the neck. Overinflation of a cuffed endotracheal tube is potentially easier in a bird because of the less expansive nature of the trachea. Overinflation can lead to mucosal edema and difficulty breathing. Whenever possible, uncuffed endotracheal tubes should be used. (See Chapter 46, Avian Anesthesia and Analgesia.)

The trachea often bifurcates immediately after entering the thoracic inlet. At this bifurcation is the syrinx, which represents the voice box of birds. It is highly variable among species but represents a number of cartilages, which may be ossified, and syringeal muscles and membranes. Most syringeal muscles are external to the tracheal bifurcation. Depending on the species, birds may also have internal syringeal muscles within the space of the trachea and/or bronchi. This narrowed internal

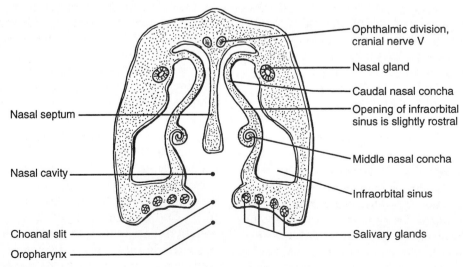

F i g u r e   2 5 – 2

Coronal section of the head (section A of Figure 25–1) just rostral to the eye. The infraorbital sinus is continuous with the caudal concha but not with the more cranial nasal part of the nasal cavity. The sinus has two openings. Both are dorsal. One is depicted here with the caudal nasal conchae; the other is slightly more rostral, over the dorsal extent of the middle nasal concha. This dorsal arrangement makes drainage of pus difficult.

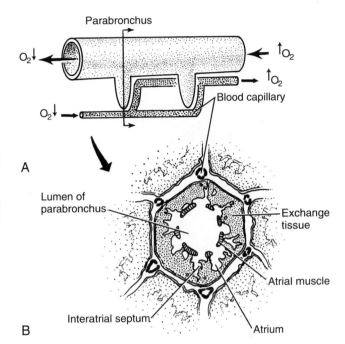

Figure 25–3

Diagram of the parabronchus. *(A)* Longitudinal section demonstrating air flow in the parabronchus cross current to the blood flow. *(B)* Transverse section of the parabronchus *(arrow, A)*. Air moves from its lumen through the infundibula into the air capillary, which functionally is like a mammalian alveolus. The air–capillary exchange surface is more efficient in birds than in mammals.

diameter of the syrinx is a common site for tracheal granulomas and foreign bodies.

The lungs are paired and attached firmly to the ribs and dorsal body wall. They appear spongy on radiographs and are best visualized using a lateral view. The mainstem bronchi divide into secondary bronchi. These bronchi subsequently divide into parabronchi. All parabronchi anastomose freely with other parabronchi and have expansions within their walls, called atria, that allow for gas exchange (Fig. 25–3). Parabronchi maintain a constant mean diameter within a species.

The mediodorsal and medioventral secondary bronchi connect to form a functional unit. These bronchi terminate at the cranial pulmonary air sacs and form the basis of the paleopulmonic respiratory system. The parabronchi of the lateroventral secondary bronchi connect with the laterodorsal secondary bronchi, and they in turn are connected to the mediodorsal secondary bronchi. The cranial pulmonary air sacs are expandable sacs that are connected to the lungs by these bronchial arrangements and include the cervical, clavicular, and cranial thoracic air sacs. The lateroventral bronchi are connected with the caudal pulmonary air sacs of the lungs. These caudal air sacs are the caudal thoracic and abdominal air sacs. This latter arrangement represents the neopulmonic respiratory system. Air sacs,

in general, are similar histologically to a peritoneum, with squamous to columnar epithelium, a basement membrane, and an underlying connective tissue support. Only in the area immediately surrounding an opening of a parabronchus does the tissue change to ciliated columnar epithelium. The paleopulmonic and neopulmonic systems are best defined physiologically rather than anatomically.

Birds do not have a diaphragm and rely on the pressure changes in the air sacs relative to the atmospheric pressure to move air through a nonexpansible lung. The pressure changes within the air sacs are the result of volume changes in the thoracoabdominal cavity. On inspiration, the ribs move cranioventrally, thereby increasing the thoracoabdominal space. This results in a lowering of the pressure in the air sacs (Fig. 25–4). On expiration, the ribs move caudodorsally, thereby reducing the space in the "chest" and increasing the pressure in the air sacs. Expiration is an active process requiring skeletal muscle contraction. For this reason, it is extremely important when holding a bird that the sternum be allowed to move freely or the bird will suffocate. Alternatively, to ventilate an apneic bird the sternum can be compressed and then allowed to recoil into its resting position.

Gas exchange occurs in the walls of the parabronchi, the atria, and more importantly in the air

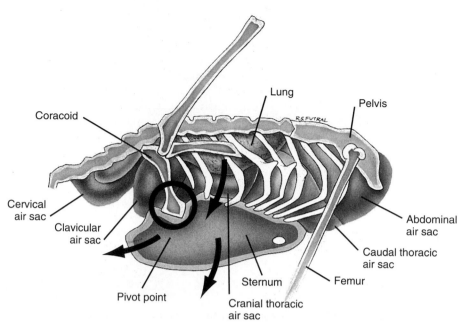

Coracoid

Lung

Pelvis

R.S.FUTRAL

Cervical air sac

Clavicular air sac

Abdominal air sac

Caudal thoracic air sac

Pivot point

Sternum

Femur

Cranial thoracic air sac

F i g u r e 2 5 – 4

Schematic of a longitudinal section of the body of a bird depicting the pulmonary air sacs. The volume of the coelom expands on inspiration because of the ventral cranial rotation of the sternum. This action is likened to that of a bellows. The pivot point is at the coracoid sternal junction.

capillaries, which are the avian equivalent of alveoli. The blood-gas barrier of birds is similar to that of mammals in that it consists of an endothelial capillary cell, a common basal lamina, and an air capillary epithelium of squamous cells. The difference is that the blood-gas barrier is much thinner in birds than in mammals. The diameter of the air capillaries of birds is much smaller than that of an alveolus of mammals, allowing for a much larger number of air capillaries in a given space when compared with mammals.

Because of the unidirectional continuous flow of air of the paleopulmonic system, birds are more efficient than mammals in capturing oxygen (O_2) and removing carbon dioxide (CO_2). The nonoxygenated blood enters at an approximately 90° angle from the parabronchus. This cross-current gas exchange also enhances the ability to oxygenate the blood.

The epithelial cells of the lung act as fixed macrophages and transfer engulfed material to interstitial macrophages. Air that enters the caudal air sacs is filtered less than that of the cranial air sacs, making the caudal air sacs more susceptible to disease.

Gerry M. Dorrestein

Physiology of Avian Respiration

The avian respiratory system is different in both structure and function from the mammalian respiratory system. Four anatomic features—the nostrils, tracheal system, lungs, and air sacs—transport air between the atmosphere and the circulatory system of a bird.

Birds lack a diaphragm. Most birds inhale by lowering the sternum, which enlarges the chest cavity and expands the air sacs. On exhalation, contrac-tion of the muscles of the sternum and ribs compresses the air sacs and pushes fresh air from them through the lungs and caudal air sacs or the trachea and cranial air sacs. During flight, wing and breathing movements are independent.[1]

If a bird is unable to move its ribs, it rapidly suffocates. This can occur with overly aggressive restraint or by surgeons resting their hands on the body cavity during surgery. Bandages that encompass the body cavity can also interfere with breathing, particularly if they are wrapped tightly around the caudal portion of the sternum or ribs.[2]

With each breath, a bird replaces 50% of the air in its lungs. Because no residual air is left in the lungs during the ventilation cycle of birds, as it is in mammals, birds transfer more oxygen during each breath. Two respiration cycles are necessary for the one-half volume of air that enters the air sacs to move totally through the avian respiratory tract. This process appears to be relatively inefficient, but fresh air is always entering the lungs both on inspiration and expiration. Thus, overall, birds have a more efficient rate of gas exchange than do mammals.[1]

The rates of breathing decrease with increased size of a bird. When not flying, a 2-g hummingbird breathes about 143 times a minute, whereas a 10-kg turkey breathes only seven times a minute. In flight, birds meet the increased oxygen demand by increasing their respiratory rates to 12 to 20 times their normal resting rates.[3]

Most birds inhale through their nostrils (or nares) at the base of their bill. Air passes through the external nares into complex, paired nasal chambers separated by a nasal septum. Each chamber has elaborate folds called conchae that increase the epithelial surface area over which air flows. The conchae cleanse and heat the air before it enters the respiratory tract. Olfactory tubercles sample its chemistry (smell). The conchae are well supplied with nerves and a network of blood vessels, called the rete mirabile, that help to control the rate of water and heat loss from the body.[3]

The rapid influx of inspired air into the caudal air sacs and the similarity of this air to environmental air have been used to explain the apparent prevalence of air sac infections and pathology in the caudal air sacs versus cranial air sacs. However, it should be noted that half of the inspired air enters the lungs. The prevalence of caudal air sacculitis may be a reflection of the air layering that occurs in this location.[2]

Avian sinuses are restricted laterally by the skin and subcutaneous tissues of the face. The infraorbital sinuses in some birds (e.g., psittacines and waterfowl) communicate.

The interconnection of the nasal cavity, infraorbital sinuses, and the porous calvaria creates a situation in which inflammatory reactions in the sinus or nasal passage can involve most anatomic structures of the head.[2]

The trachea consists of complete cartilaginous rings in most avian species. In some birds, like the whooping crane and helmet curassow, the trachea makes extra bends in or outside the sternum before connecting to the syrinx. In some birds (e.g., penguins and petrels) a median septum divides the trachea into right and left channels over the length beginning shortly distal to the larynx.

The avian larynx, located at the top of the trachea, at the back of the oral cavity, serves only to open and close the glottis and thereby keep water and food out of the respiratory tract; it does not include vocal cords. All songs and calls come from the syrinx, which is located in the body cavity at the junction of the trachea and the two primary bronchi.

In contrast to mammalian lungs, which are large, inflatable, bag-like structures that hang in the chest cavity, avian lungs are small, compact, spongy structures molded among the ribs on either side of the spine in the chest cavity. Avian lungs weigh as much as the lungs of mammals of equal body weight, but because avian lungs have much greater tissue density they occupy only about one-half the volume.[3] Healthy bird lungs are well vascularized and light pink in color.

The internal structure of the mammalian lung resembles a bush, with many subdividing bronchial stems and branches. The bronchial branching patterns and connections in bird lungs closely resemble the plumbing of a steam engine.[3] Branching from each of the two primary bronchi that traverse the entire lung are about 11 secondary bronchi, four of which (the craniomedial bronchi) service the anterior and lower parts of the lung. Most of the lung tissue comprises roughly 1800 smaller interconnecting tertiary bronchi (parabronchi); these lead into tiny air capillaries that intertwine with blood capillaries, where gases are exchanged.

Surfactant in the parabronchi functions to keep fluids from entering the air capillary area and prevents transudation. Dilation and contraction of the bronchi and ostium are controlled by smooth muscles.

The air sac system is an integral part of the avian respiratory system. Air sacs are thin-walled structures (only one to two cell layers thick) that extend throughout the body cavity and into the wing and leg bones. The number of air sacs varies from six to at least 12 in different species. Most birds, however, have nine air sacs: the cervical sacs (two), anterior thoracic sacs (two), large posterior thoracic sacs (two), large abdominal sacs (two), and a single interclavicular sac. The abdominal air sacs also carry air to leg and pelvic bones; the interclavicular sac branches into the wing bones, sternum, and syrinx. Pressure in the syrinx from the interclavicular sac is essential for vocal sound production.[4]

Pathology involving the syrinx is best diagnosed and treated when signs of disease are first recognized. If a bird stops talking or has a voice change it should be evaluated immediately for lesions developing in the perisyringeal area (frequently aspergillosis).[2]

The air sacs connect directly to the primary and secondary bronchi and in some species connect indirectly to some tertiary bronchi.[3] The air sacs make possible a continuous, unidirectional, efficient flow of air through the lungs. They not only help

to deliver the huge quantities of oxygen needed, but also help to remove the potentially lethal body heat produced during flight. Internal air sacs also protect the delicate internal organs during flight.

In most birds, cervicocephalic air sacs are present and are divided into cephalic and cervical portions. They connect to caudal aspects of the infraorbital sinus. These air sacs may function as insulating air layers for retention of heat, to control buoyancy, to reduce the force of impact with the water in fish-eating birds, and to support the head during sleep or flight.[1]

Avian respiration maximizes contact of fresh air with the respiratory surface of the lung. Air flows to the avian lung through one set of bronchi to enter the gas-exchange areas and exits through another set. Fifty percent of the inhaled air during the first inhalation in the cycle passes through the primary bronchi to the posterior air sacs (Fig. 25–5). During the exhalation phase of the first breath, the

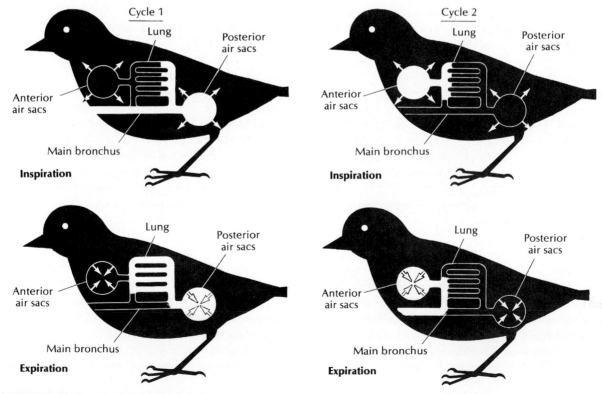

Figure 25–5

The unidirectional movement of a single inhaled volume of air *(white)* through the avian respiratory system. Two full respiratory cycles (inspiration, expiration, inspiration, expiration) are required to move the gas through its complete path. (From Gill FB: Ornithology, ed 2. New York, WH Freeman and Co, 1995, p 121.)

inhaled air moves from the posterior air sacs into the lungs where it flows through the air-capillary system—the primary site of O_2 and CO_2 exchange. The next time the bird inhales, this O_2-depleted air moves into the anterior air sacs. During second exhalation, the CO_2-rich air is then expelled from the anterior air sacs, bronchi, and trachea back into the atmosphere. The continuous airflow through the avian lung allows more efficient extraction of oxygen than occurs in the mammalian lung.

All birds have a paleopulmonic system of bronchi and parabronchi in the medioventral-mediodorsal lung. In addition, most pet species have a neopulmonic system in the ventrolateral part of the lung. A current of parallel tubes of air moves in one direction counter to pulmonic vessels in the paleopulmonic system, allowing gas exchange to occur with greater efficiency than in the neopulmonic system. In the neopulmonic system, air moves in both directions in the parabronchi, mixing oxygenated air with air having a higher partial pressure of CO_2. These physiologic and anatomic adaptations account for a 20% increase in the diffusion capacity for oxygen in birds when compared with that of mammals.[1]

SOUND PRODUCTION BY THE SYRINX

The vocal virtuosity of birds stems from the structure of their unusual and powerful vocal apparatus, the syrinx. Contraction of thoracic and abdominal muscles forces air from the main air sacs through the bronchi to the syrinx. On each side of the syrinx is a thin, glass-clear membrane (m. tympaniformis interna). Sound is caused by the vibration of the air column as air passes through the narrow (syringeal) passageways, which are bounded on opposite sides by corresponding projections called the internal labium and external labium (Fig. 25–6). Vibration of the internal tympaniform membrane, regulated by its mass, internal tension, and protrusion into the adjacent air column, determines the sound charac-

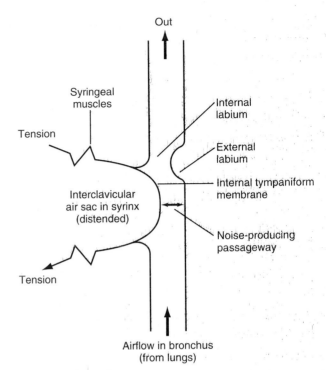

Figure 25–6

Sound production in the syrinx depends on the tension of the internal tympaniform membrane, which is controlled by pressure in the interclavicular sac, contraction of the syringeal muscles, and the diameter of the air passageway. (From Gill FB: Ornithology, ed 2. New York, WH Freeman and Co, 1995, p 238.)

teristics. Pressure in the interclavicular air sac pushes the thin membrane into the bronchial air space, into position for vibration and creation of sounds. Many birds can stimulate the two sides of the syrinx independently and thus can sing two songs simultaneously.

A needle puncture of the interclavicular air sac prevents buildup of the pressure needed to move the tympaniform membranes, thereby rendering a bird voiceless. Syringeal muscles control the details of syrinx action and change the tension of the tympaniform membrane as a bird sings.[4, 5] These muscles are especially well developed in passerines and psittacines.

Elizabeth V. Hillyer

Clinical Manifestations of Respiratory Disorders

GENERAL PRINCIPLES OF THE PHYSICAL EXAMINATION

The capability of flight, particularly at high altitudes, is a remarkable feat that is made possible in part because the avian lung has the most efficient gas exchange system of the air-breathing vertebrates.[1] Many other unique anatomic and physiologic adaptations of the avian respiratory system make it probably the most divergent of the body systems from those of mammals. The avian practitioner must be aware of the normal features of avian respiratory anatomy and how these influence the choice of diagnostic and treatment techniques for respiratory tract disease.

Respiratory problems are seen commonly in pet bird clinical practice. Birds are susceptible to a variety of respiratory pathogens and to a variety of noninfectious causes of respiratory problems. Early signs of respiratory problems are often not recognized and, as a result, birds with chronic respiratory disease are seen commonly in practice. These patients represent some of the most interesting therapeutic and diagnostic challenges encountered by the avian practitioner.

Observe the bird for overall attitude and nature of respirations. The respirations should be hardly noticeable in a normal, calm bird. With the stress of being in the examination room, however, even normal birds develop an increase in respiratory effort and may even begin open-mouth breathing or panting. Therefore, to evaluate a bird's true respiratory status at rest, it may be necessary to leave the bird in a dark, quiet place for a few minutes or to observe it from the opposite side of the room. Determine whether there is excessive respiratory effort, manifested by a tail bob, pronounced excursions of the sternum, or open-mouth breathing. If the bird can withstand the stress of manual restraint, perform a complete physical examinations, first determining the bird's overall condition, body weight, and level of hydration (see Chapter 10, Physical Examination).

Inspect the shape of the nares and cere; they should be bilaterally symmetrical and free of evidence of discharge. In the center of each naris is the operculum, which is normally keratinized and smooth and dry in appearance. In birds with chronic rhinitis, the operculum may be hidden under dried discharge or partially eroded by the inflammatory process. Always be aware of its presence when cleaning discharge from the nares; clean gently around the periphery of the nares, rather than directly in the center. The eyes and shape of the face should also be bilaterally symmetrical; facial or periorbital swellings can result from sinusitis. Perform a thorough oral examination with particular attention to the choanal slit and larynx. The choanal slit should be moist, clean, and bordered by slender, tapered papillae. Discharge in the choana is seen with rhinitis, sinusitis, and choanal abscesses. Blunting with or without abscesses of the choanal papillae is seen most commonly with hypovitaminosis A and infections, including bacterial, fungal, and chlamydial infections. The laryngeal mound should be symmetrical and covered with normal, smooth mucous membrane.

Palpate the neck and the trachea, which usually runs along the right side of the neck. Transillumination of the trachea may be useful to identify intraluminal lesions or parasites, such as tracheal mites, *Sternostoma tracheacolum.*

Auscultation of the respiratory tract in birds is not as useful as in mammals because of differences in airway anatomy. Fluid noises and clicks associated with respiration in birds are usually indicative of severe respiratory disease and are often audible with the naked ear held against the bird's body. Lower respiratory tract infection may result in harsh respiratory sounds, particularly on inspiration. Isolated air sac disease often does not result in audible changes. Arrhythmias and murmurs, although uncommon, are abnormal on cardiac auscultation.

GENERAL PRINCIPLES OF DIAGNOSIS AND TREATMENT

Clinical signs associated with the most common respiratory conditions are described in Table 25–1.

T a b l e   2 5 – 1

COMMON CLINICAL SIGNS AND PHYSICAL ABNORMALITIES ASSOCIATED WITH RESPIRATORY DISEASE

Upper Respiratory Disease

Rhinitis, Nasal Irritation

Nasal discharge
Sneezing
Staining of or dried discharge in the feathers around the nares
Scratching, rubbing, self-trauma around the nares with or without feather loss
Frequent head shaking or yawning to dislodge discharge
Discharge in the choana (with or without nasal discharge)
Swollen cere
Plugged nares
Open-mouth breathing
Epiphora, conjunctivitis
With chronic rhinitis: vertical grooves in the beak under each naris
Seen in conjunction with sinusitis; therefore see signs for sinusitis

Sinusitis

Periorbital swellings (fluctuant, soft, or firm)
On oral examination: swelling(s) of lateral oropharynx
Self-trauma around cere and eyes
Chronic or recurrent rhinitis; see signs for rhinitis
Sunken eye(s) in macaws with chronic sinusitis

Lower Respiratory Disease

Tracheitis, Tracheal Disease

Usually seen in conjunction with upper respiratory disease or other lower respiratory disease
Cough
Tachypnea, dyspnea, open-mouth breathing if tracheal lumen size affected
Voice change

Pneumonia, Air Sacculitis

Decreased stamina, exercise intolerance
Increased recovery time after exercise or stress
Chronic "poor doer," cachexia
Cough
Tail bob
Tachypnea
Dyspnea, open-mouth breathing

False signs that could be mistaken for evidence of respiratory disease are listed in Table 25–2.

Factors Predisposing to Respiratory Disease

Infectious causes are probably more common than noninfectious causes of respiratory disease. However, several factors are important in predisposing birds to respiratory tract infection; these must be identified and corrected if antimicrobial therapy is to be effective. Most predisposing factors are management-related, particularly inadequate nutrition and environmental problems.

T a b l e   2 5 – 2

NORMAL NOISES THAT COULD BE MISTAKEN FOR SIGNS OF RESPIRATORY DISEASE

Avian Species	Normal Noise
African grey parrot	Growl
Many cockatoo species	Hiss
Pionus parrots	Moist respiratory sound when excited
Many species	Cough or sneeze noise mimicking human
Baby Amazon parrots (begging for food)	"Ack-ack" sound

Proper nutrition is basic to avian health and the health of the immune system. Vitamin A (or β carotene) intake is essential to maintain epithelial integrity. Hypovitaminosis A is manifested as an increased susceptibility to infection and, when severe, results in squamous metaplasia of mucosal and glandular epithelium and ultimately hyperkeratotic granulomas, which can occur in a number of sites in the upper respiratory tract, including the sinuses and choanal region. If a bird with respiratory disease has been receiving or eating a marginal diet, administer one dose of parenteral vitamin A (see Formulary, Chapter 39B) and develop a plan with the owner to feed the bird a better diet. Educate the owner about foods that contain high levels of β-carotene, such as carrots, red peppers, green leafy vegetables, cantaloupe, mangoes, and peaches. Provide supplemental oral minerals and vitamins if needed.

A well-ventilated, dust- and toxin-free environment is fundamental to avian respiratory health. Birds should not be exposed to cigarette smoke, strong odors or sprays, or aerosols of any kind. Blue and gold macaws seem to be particularly susceptible to respiratory irritants and must be housed in well-ventilated environments. The importance of aeroallergens as agents of disease in birds is uncertain; however, the clinical impression of many avian

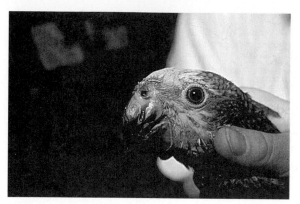

Figure 25–7

Mucoid rhinitis in a blue-fronted Amazon parrot.

practitioners is that birds can develop respiratory allergies.

Free-standing air filters can be used to reduce airborne particulates. The most effective mechanical filters are high-efficiency particulate air (HEPA) filters, whereas the most effective electric filters are electrostatic precipitators. Standard vacuum cleaners tend to mobilize dust and allergens; therefore, warn clients against vacuuming with susceptible birds in the room. Vacuums with a HEPA filter or central vacuums with the collecting bag outside the house are effective at reducing levels of dust.[6]

APPROACH TO COMMON PRESENTING PROBLEMS

Nasal Discharge

In normal birds, water may be seen at the nares soon after the bird drinks or bathes. However, any persistent discharge at the nares is abnormal and can range from clear, serous fluid to opaque, yellow mucus (Fig. 25–7) to firm caseous material.

Nasal discharge is an indication of rhinitis, typically infectious or irritant, and is seen with a variety of conditions (Table 25–3). Nasal discharge can be the sole presenting sign in an otherwise healthy bird; can occur in conjunction with conjunctivitis, sinusitis, or lower respiratory tract infection; or can be one aspect of a multisystemic disease, such as chlamydiosis.

Bacterial infection is probably the most common cause of rhinitis in psittacine birds; however, as previously discussed, poor nutrition and environmental factors often are underlying causes. Gram-negative bacteria are the most common bacterial pathogens. Other infectious agents causing nasal discharge include reovirus in Amazon parrots; Amazon tracheitis virus (a herpesvirus); *Chlamydia psittaci*, and fungal organisms, particularly *Aspergillus* species (Fig. 25–8).[7–9] *Mycobacterium avium* is an uncommon cause of rhinitis. In the author's experience, viral infections are uncommon. The presence of a foreign body in the nasal cavity or choana may elicit nasal discharge. The diagnostic and therapeutic approach to nasal discharge varies according to the historic and clinical findings.

History and Physical Examination

Important questions regarding a bird with nasal discharge pertain to the nature of the illness, possible exposure to other birds, and details about the bird's environment that could identify predisposing factors. Ascertain how long the nasal discharge has

---

Table 25–3

DIFFERENTIAL DIAGNOSIS FOR NASAL DISCHARGE

Infectious Disease	Other Factors
Bacterial infection, particularly gram-negative organisms	Neoplasia
Viral infection, e.g., reovirus[8]	Choanal atresia
Fungal infection, particularly with *Aspergillus* species	Allergy?*
Infection with *Chlamydia psittaci*	Important predisposing factors
Respiratory Irritants	Low humidity (native tropical species, Amazon parrots, macaws, etc.)
Dust, foreign body	Malnutrition, particularly hypovitaminosis A
Cigarette, cigar, pipe, or marijuana smoke; cooking fumes	
Powder from other birds (especially cockatoos, cockatiels, and African grey parrots)	

*The existence of allergies has not been documented in birds.

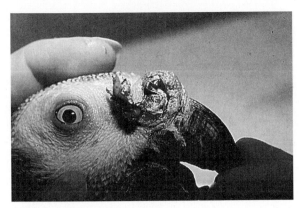

Figure 25–8

Nasal aspergilloma in an African grey parrot.

been present and whether the bird is sneezing, coughing, or showing other signs of respiratory disease. Does the bird show a decrease in activity or appetite? Determine whether it has been recently exposed to other birds or to humans who spend time around other birds. What diet is the bird offered and what does it actually eat? Malnutrition, particularly hypovitaminosis A, is a common predisposing factor in rhinitis.

Environmental factors that predispose to or cause rhinitis include low humidity and airborne respiratory irritants. Birds from moist, tropical climates in particular, such as Amazon parrots and macaws, tend to have problems with low humidity during the winter months in homes heated without humidifying systems. If the owner uses a humidifier, record the type. Is it a steam vaporizer, a cold air ultrasonic humidifier, or a hot air ultrasonic unit? The unit should be cleaned regularly. Obtain details about the bird's environment. Potential problems include exposure to cooking fumes; to cigarette, cigar, pipe, or marijuana smoke; or to an avian species that produces an abundance of powder, such as a cockatoo, cockatiel, or African grey parrot. Are ongoing construction and renovation projects producing dust? Are the respiratory problems associated with a particular season or type of weather?

On physical examination, check the nares, choana, and larynx. Determine whether either naris is plugged with discharge or whether the discharge is free-flowing. Record the nature of the discharge. Check the cere for evidence of inflammation and the feathers above the cere for evidence of dried

nasal discharge (Fig. 25–9). With chronic rhinitis, the nares may become larger, smaller, or asymmetrically eroded; a groove may become evident in the beak under the naris with chronic discharge. Check for evidence of other upper or lower respiratory tract disease.

Diagnostic Testing

The minimal data base for a bird with nasal discharge comprises complete history, physical examination, and results of fecal Gram's stains. Bacterial culture and, ideally, a Gram's stain and cytologic examination of nasal aspirate or flush are also indicated (see Chapter 17, Hospital Techniques and Supportive Care), particularly if the discharge is tenacious or caseous or if the rhinitis is long-standing. Baseline culture and cytology test results are invaluable in the event of treatment failure. An aspirate of nasal discharge or a carefully obtained culture from the cranial end of the choana can provide useful information; however, cultures from these sites may be contaminated with the normal flora and must therefore be interpreted judiciously.

Mycoplasmas are difficult to isolate, and although they have been recovered from psittacine and passerine species, there is no proof of their pathogenicity in caged birds.[10]

Perform a complete blood count (CBC) and blood biochemistry panel to evaluate the bird systemically if the rhinitis is severe or chronic or if the bird is showing signs of systemic illness. Plasma

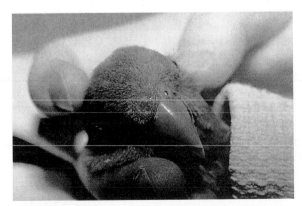

Figure 25–9

Unilateral rhinitis with swelling of the cere in a crimson-winged parakeet.

protein electrophoresis, *Chlamydia* testing, or a fungal culture may be indicated depending on history and other clinical signs. Plasma protein electrophoresis is helpful in establishing whether blood proteins reflect an inflammatory response, which is supportive of an infectious etiology. An enzyme-linked immunosorbent assay (ELISA) test for detection of antibodies to *Aspergillus* shows promise for use in psittacine birds[11]; the ELISA appears capable of detecting antibodies in psittacines. However, test results must be interpreted in conjunction with other clinical findings; because aspergillosis is often a disease of immunosuppressed birds, infected birds may not exhibit seroconversion.*

Treatment—General Principles

Base selection of a treatment regimen on the preliminary diagnosis and according to the severity of rhinitis and other clinical signs. Specific treatment for rhinitis can be local or systemic or both. In addition, environmental and dietary modifications, such as increased humidity and an improved diet, are necessary for most affected birds.

Local therapy for rhinitis comprises cleaning the nares, flushing the nares as necessary one or more times, and topical medication. Techniques for cleaning and flushing the nares are covered in Chapter 17, Hospital Techniques and Supportive Care. Sterile flush solution introduced into the naris normally drains out through the choana into the mouth and possibly out of the ipsilateral eye. In birds with chronic rhinitis, discharge may obstruct the normal channels and cause the flush solution to exit from the ipsilateral eye or from the contralateral naris if the nasal septum is eroded by inflammation.

Choose the appropriate topical medication based on clinical and laboratory results. For topical antibiotic therapy, ophthalmic solutions are ideal because they are convenient and safe to apply in close proximity to the eyes. If a particular antibiotic is not available as a veterinary preparation, many human ophthalmic antibiotic preparations are available by prescription. Avoid solutions containing corticosteroids, which are unnecessary and potentially dangerous to birds.

---

*For further information regarding submission of samples for aspergillosis ELISA testing, contact The Raptor Center, 1920 Fitch Avenue, St. Paul, MN 55108; (612) 624–3013.

The choice of systemic antibacterial, antifungal, or other therapy depends on diagnostic findings.

Nasal Plugs Without Discharge

Psittacine birds that are fed a marginal diet, housed in a dry environment, and denied access to baths or showers often accumulate dust, debris, and exfoliated epithelial cells in the nares that can become solid plugs of foreign material. Affected birds sound like they have a nasal obstruction and make a nasal snuffling noise when excited or winded. On expiration, the infraorbital sinuses may puff out in the region between the beak and eyes. (With unilateral obstruction, asymmetrical enlargement of the cere can be seen.)

If these plugs are not removed, they can, in addition to causing obstruction, serve as a nidus for infection. The strands or plugs of debris can be removed by moistening them first with wet cotton swabs and then gently cleaning the nares with a small bone or earwax curet. Very firm impactions need to be softened with several drops of saline flushed into the nares 3 to 5 minutes before curettage. Clean around the periphery of each naris, taking care not to damage the central operculum. Consider flushing the nares with sterile saline to ascertain or establish proper drainage into the choana.

Recommend an improved diet, frequent bathing, and other management changes to prevent recurrence of the nasal plugs. Administer one injection of vitamin A (see Formulary, Chapter 39B). If infection is suspected based on the appearance of the debris or the presence of mucoid or other discharge, proceed with diagnostic tests and treatment as for rhinitis.

Mild to Moderate Rhinitis Without Systemic Illness

If the bird is strong, active, and eating well but has a slight serous nasal discharge with or without associated sneezing, start with a conservative treatment regimen, namely management changes, while a nasal culture result is pending. Make sure the nares and choana are clean and unobstructed. Carefully clean dirt or debris out of the nares with a wet cotton swab or small bone curet. Some of these birds require no treatment other than improvements in management and diet (see later).

A bird with mucoid or copious nasal discharge that is not showing signs of systemic illness can be treated by the owner at home while results of cultures and other diagnostic tests are pending. Based on the results of cytologic examination of a smear, this can be a local antibiotic treatment. If the nares are obstructed with debris or discharge, clean them gently with a small curet, wet cotton swabs, and a sterile saline flush. For birds that are active and eating well, topical therapy is usually effective. This author and others believe that systemic therapy is not necessary for these otherwise "healthy" birds.[12, 13]

Teach the owner how to hold the bird and administer one or two drops of an ophthalmic solution into each nostril and then send the owner home with this medication to administer two to three times daily for 7 to 14 days, depending on the bird's clinical condition. Until culture results are available, choose an antibiotic with a predominantly gram-negative spectrum, such as gentamicin or tobramycin, a broad-spectrum antibiotic such as ciprofloxacin or chloramphenicol, or an antimycotic formulation.

Make dietary recommendations and administer one dose of parenteral multivitamins if it is suspected that the bird is nutritionally deficient. Advocate environmental modifications including increased humidity and elimination of exposure to dust and smoke. To expose the bird to steam at least once daily, the owner can bring the bird into the bathroom when showering. For native tropical psittacines in northern climates, a high-quality humidifier should be placed in the room with the bird during the winter. The safest and most effective humidifiers are probably cool air evaporative units because they produce very fine water droplets and are self-sterilizing. The author has worked with several birds that suffered from recurrent rhinitis in winter until this management change was made.

Eliminating exposure to dust and smoke is done on a case-by-case basis, possibly by moving the bird to a new location, moving smokers to other parts of the house, and installing air filtration systems in the room where the bird is housed.

Severe Rhinitis

Systemic treatment, in addition to topical medication, is indicated in birds that have tenacious nasal discharge or are showing even mild signs of systemic illness. Based on cytologic test results of the discharge, a broad-spectrum antibiotic can be administered while culture results are pending. If chlamydiosis is suspected based on results of a Macchiavellos stain, select the antibiotic accordingly. If bacteria or elementary bodies are not seen on cytology, a mycotic infection or a primary vitamin deficiency is a more likely cause. In addition, make the dietary and environmental recommendations outlined earlier.

Birds with tenacious nasal discharge often benefit from regular flushing of the nares with sterile saline. Have the owner bring the bird for daily nasal flushing or admit the bird to the hospital for several days of nasal flushing two to three times daily. Alternatively, in birds with moderate discharge, the owner can administer pediatric saline nose drops (Ayr nasal drops, Ascher, Lenexa, KS) at home.

Recurrent and Nonresponsive Nasal Discharge

Further diagnostic testing is necessary if nasal discharge does not resolve with therapy or if it recurs when therapy is discontinued. It is particularly important to pursue further diagnostic procedures if the appropriate management changes have been made and more than one antibiotic has already been administered. Overmedicating with antibiotics will change the normal microbial flora of the gastrointestinal tract and predispose the bird to gastrointestinal candidal overgrowth.

Lack of response to an antibiotic occurs if the pathogen is resistant to the specific antibiotic chosen. Even if the choice of therapy is appropriate, nasal discharge recurs if a nidus of infection remains in a site, such as the infraorbital sinuses or an abscess pocket, not readily penetrated by the medication.

Therefore, the first step in evaluating recurrent and nonresponsive rhinitis is twofold: (1) identify the etiologic agent and (2) determine whether the bird has sinusitis, a choanal abscess, or another nidus of infection. Take the bird off medication for 1 week to optimize culture results. If a systemic evaluation has not been done, take whole body radiographs and submit blood samples for a CBC and serum biochemistry profile. Then, ideally under anesthesia, perform a thorough oral, nasal, and choanal examination. A small endoscope can be used to examine the choanal region in medium-sized to large birds. Perform skull radiographs to evaluate the bony sinuses. If available, computed tomography (CT) scanning has proven to be a valuable technique for evaluation of the nasal passages and sinuses for evidence of bony involvement or soft tissue masses (granulomas) (Fig. 25–10). If there is radiographic or CT evidence of sinus involvement or if sinus involvement is suspected, even when imaging techniques are nondiagnostic, schedule a sinus exploratory procedure (trephination) to evaluate the region, collect diagnostic samples, and remove discharge as necessary.

To identify the causative agent, the best approach is to submit samples for culture and cytologic testing or tissue biopsy. Diagnostic samples may include aseptically obtained nasal or sinus aspirates or flushes, abscess or abscess wall material, and sinus epithelium. If the lower respiratory tract is also involved, a tracheal wash may provide useful information. Submit specimens for bacterial and fungal cultures.

A smear stained with DiffQuick gives information about involvement of bacteria (cocci, rods, acid-fast) or yeasts, fungi, or none of these. In addition, the smear provides information about the cell types involved. Special stains to consider for cytology and biopsy specimens include Macchiavellos (*Chlamydia*) and periodic acid-Schiff (PAS) stains.

Treatment of recurrent or chronic rhinitis depends on the results of diagnostic testing. The approach to choanal abscesses is covered later. For

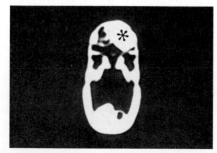

F i g u r e 2 5 – 1 0

Computed tomographic scan of the head of an African grey parrot. A large opaque area *(asterisk)* suggestive of a granuloma is present in the nasal cavity.

birds with sinusitis, see the discussion in Periorbital Swelling.

Sneezing

Sneezing in the absence of nasal discharge is normal. Birds often sneeze several times during the course of a day, and, similar to humans, may sneeze once or multiple times. If a bird's nares and choana are clean and dry but the owner still complains of excessive sneezing, make recommendations on how to increase humidity and decrease dust in the environment. Daily bathing may also help to reduce sneezing.

If discharge is present in the nares, proceed as described earlier for nasal discharge.

Choanal Discharge and Abscesses

Discharge within the choana is seen commonly in birds with rhinitis. In some birds with rhinitis, particularly those with very thick mucoid or caseous secretions, the nares are dry but secretions are evident within the choanal opening. Alternatively, some birds show chronic nasal discharge resulting from an abscess or foreign body within the choana.

Choanal discharge or abscess usually is evident during the oral examination as glistening or pale to yellow matter within the choana. The choanal slit may be asymmetrical and, with an abscess, the palatal area may bulge. Mucoid discharge can often be dislodged simply by flushing the nares. If the discharge is not easily dislodged or appears to be caseous, examine the area more closely with the bird under sedation or anesthesia. Use moist cotton swabs to explore within the choana. If caseous material is found, remove it using cotton swabs or a curet in conjunction with saline flushes of choana and nares. Choanal abscesses can be quite large, with a diameter of up to 2 to 3 cm in a medium-sized psittacine. Aseptically collect specimens for culture and cytology or biopsy testing.

Treatment for choanal discharge from rhinitis is the same as for nasal discharge. Treatment for choanal abscess includes local debridement, flushing, and both local and systemic medication based on results of cultures and cytologic testing.

Abnormalities of the Glottis

Swelling and erythema of the laryngeal mound can occur secondary to infection, neoplasia, or trauma, such as that from a feeding tube. Infectious agents affecting this area include bacteria, viruses such as Amazon tracheitis virus or poxvirus, fungi such as *Candida*, and parasites such as *Trichomonas*. In New World psittacines, papillomas may occur on the rim of the glottis or hidden under the rim, where they can be visualized only with the bird under anesthesia.[14]

Periorbital Swelling

The most common causes of periorbital swelling are conditions that affect the infraorbital sinuses, particularly sinusitis and hyperkeratotic sinus granulomas caused by hypovitaminosis A. Sinusitis in caged birds is caused by bacterial, fungal, mycobacterial (rare), or chlamydial organisms (uncommon). Other causes of periorbital swelling include trauma, orbital infection or masses, neoplasia, and subcutaneous emphysema (Table 25–4). In the author's experience, sinusitis in psittacines tends to occur as an individual problem, whereas sinusitis in passerines, such as canaries, can occur either as an individual problem or as an outbreak affecting many birds.

History and Physical Examination

Question the owner about the onset (slow vs. sudden) and duration of the periorbital swelling and whether the bird is showing other respiratory signs, such as sneezing, nasal discharge, coughing, tail bob, or reduced activity or vocalizations. Has there

Table 25–4

DIFFERENTIAL DIAGNOSIS FOR PERIORBITAL SWELLING

Sinusitis: bacterial, fungal, mycobacterial
Subcutaneous emphysema
Trauma
Subcutaneous hemorrhage
Neoplasia
Orbital mass
Granuloma due to hypovitaminosis A

been recent exposure to other birds? Has there been recent trauma? Obtain specific details about the bird's diet and environment. Malnutrition, particularly hypovitaminosis A, can predispose the bird to sinusitis. A bleeding disorder can result in hemorrhage, which can cause periorbital swelling.

Observe the bird for signs of respiratory compromise. Perform a complete physical examination, with special attention to structures of the head and neck. Examine the eyes and orbital region for evidence of ophthalmic or orbital abnormalities. Bruising and abrasions in the periorbital region are usually indicative of trauma; however, birds with sinusitis may scratch or rub the area, causing similar signs. Palpate the skull and bony orbit for possible fractures.

In birds with sinusitis, periorbital swelling may be unilateral or bilateral and is often most prominent ventral to the eye. Alternatively, the swelling may be restricted to the supraorbital region. Swellings can be fluctuant, soft, or firm on palpation depending on the nature of the secretions. Periorbital swelling may be the sole presenting sign with sinusitis or may occur in conjunction with other respiratory tract abnormalities, most commonly nasal and choanal discharge. Other possible concomitant physical abnormalities include conjunctivitis, oropharyngeal swellings, and swellings lateral to the oral commissures. The author has seen one bird with severe *Aspergillus* sinusitis that eroded through the frontal bone with resultant swelling caudal to the cere. Chronic, untreated sinusitis can cause severe disruption of normal anatomy (Fig. 25–11) or can cause an abscess and skin necrosis, with rupture and discharge through the side of the face.[16]

Diagnostic Testing

The initial diagnostic approach to birds with periorbital swelling varies depending on physical examination results. A full ophthalmologic examination is indicated for suspected abnormalities of the globe or orbit (see Chapter 33, Disorders of the Special Senses). Skull radiographs are indicated for suspected sinusitis or fractures of the skull or orbit, particularly in medium-sized to larger species. CT scanning, if available, is a more sensitive diagnostic technique (see Fig. 25–10). However, radiographs may be financially impractical or not useful for

respiratory compromise can often be visualized, particularly in medium-sized to larger birds. However, a study comparing radiography with CT in birds with respiratory disease found that, in the early stages of disease, lesions may not be evident and misinterpretation is common. Moreover, the severity of disease may not correlate with radiographic findings.[22] Nonetheless, radiographs are an integral part of the data base in evaluating birds with respiratory disease.

Anesthetize tachypneic or dyspneic birds with isoflurane, rather than positioning birds with physical restraint, both to minimize stress and to obtain well-positioned films, which are essential for respiratory tract evaluation. While the bird is anesthetized, carefully examine the oral cavity, choana, and nares, and collect blood for CBC, blood biochemistry panel, and other laboratory tests as indicated by the specific circumstances. Other tests could include plasma protein electrophoresis and *Chlamydia* testing. An air sac tube may be indicated for oxygen and anesthetic administration in birds requiring work around the head, neck, or trachea.[23]

The choice of further testing depends on the results of preliminary tests. If there is evidence of tracheal disease, such as a change in tracheal diameter or a suspected tracheal mass, consider a tracheal wash to obtain samples for culture and cytologic testing or tracheoscopy to visualize the abnormality, obtain a biopsy, or remove the mass. If pulmonary or air sac densities are present, consider laparoscopy to better visualize the abnormal area and obtain biopsies for culture and histopathologic examination.

Goiter is the most common cause of tachypnea and tail bob in budgerigars. Therefore, if the dietary history, clinical signs, and physical examination findings are compatible with goiter, and the bird's condition seems to be stable, a therapeutic trial with iodine is often the most practical step instead of pursuing diagnostic testing. If the bird does not respond to treatment for goiter, continue as outlined earlier.

Handling the Dyspneic Bird

The differential diagnosis (see Table 25–6), diagnostic tests, and basic treatment regimens for dyspneic birds are the same as for birds with tachypnea and tail bob. The difference in clinical approach to tachypneic versus dyspneic birds is in patient handling techniques. Dyspneic birds die from even minimal stress; they do not tolerate physical restraint.

Hospitalize the dyspneic patient in an incubator with oxygen and anesthetic ports, and maintain the bird in oxygen. To perform diagnostic or treatment procedures, anesthetize the bird with isoflurane gas, which gives rapid induction, relatively safe anesthesia, and rapid recovery. Place an air sac tube if upper airway disease is suspected. If the bird has diffuse pneumonia or air sacculitis, an air sac tube is unlikely to be beneficial. As discussed above, radiographs are the most informative preliminary tests to guide further therapy and diagnosis.

Treatment

Administer initial treatment in dyspneic birds while the bird is still under anesthesia. There is no specific treatment for respiratory toxins, although one dose of a rapidly acting corticosteroid (e.g., dexamethasone sodium phosphate 6–8 mg/kg intravenously [IV]) may be beneficial. Therapy for sarcocystosis is often unsuccessful; however, some birds respond to a trimethoprim-sulfa combination (30 mg/kg intramuscularly [IM] or orally [PO] twice daily [bid]) given in conjunction with pyrimethamine (Daraprim 0.5 mg/kg PO bid for 30 days).[24] Good supportive care, including fluids and vitamin therapy, is important for all dyspneic birds. Tube-feeding into the crop is risky because of possible aspiration. Instead, concentrate on offering tempting foods to encourage the bird to eat voluntarily. If the bird remains anorectic, tube feedings can be given, but the procedure must be done quickly with small volumes of formula. Alternatively, enteral nutrition can be given by a surgically placed proventricular or duodenal feeding tube. In addition, parenteral nutrition can be administered through an intravenous or intraosseous catheter.

Small Birds, Diagnostic Tests Not Possible

Diagnostic testing may not be possible for some birds with tachypnea, tail bob, or dyspnea because of limitations related to the small size or debilitated state of the patient. When dealing with breeding flocks, a diagnostic postmortem examination may complete or even replace the clinical examination. (See Chapter 49, Passerines).

In small passerine species, such as finches and canaries, reproductive problems such as egg binding commonly cause tachypnea and tail bob; these are usually detectable on physical examination. Treatment can be tailored accordingly. Other nonrespiratory diseases causing respiratory signs in these species are listed in Table 25–6. For canaries and finches without evidence of abdominal or other nonrespiratory disease, important differentials for tachypnea include air sac mites and bacterial infection of lungs or air sacs or both. Canary poxvirus causes outbreaks of respiratory disease with high mortality in canaries. In one canary population, poxvirus, air sac mites (*Sternostoma* species), and *Enterococcus faecalis* tracheitis were the most common necropsy findings in birds with dyspnea.[25]

Financial constraints may limit diagnostic options for canaries and finches, and treatment is often based only on physical examination findings, particularly for individual pets. In a flock situation, a thorough necropsy of one or more birds is indicated. For suspected canary pox, separate affected birds into a quarantine area and vaccinate the rest of the flock; these two procedures may stem the outbreak.

For individual pet canaries and finches, nonspecific treatment for tachypnea and tail bob may be necessary. The author uses the following: (1) one small drop of 1% ivermectin (Ivomec, Merck & Co., Rahway, NJ) on the skin over the right jugular vein to treat air sac mites (repeat again in 10 to 14 days); and (2) broad-spectrum antibiotic therapy. A trimethoprim-sulfa combination or enrofloxacin is a good first-line choice for therapy. Ideally, the antibiotic should be administered orally or parenterally. However, many owners cannot capture or restrain their birds; therefore, the medication must be given in the food and water. Enrofloxacin can be administered in water; however, the bird must be monitored carefully because some birds do not drink medicated water. A possibility for antibiotic therapy is weekly injection of a long-acting doxycycline preparation (Vibravenös, Pfizer, Inc., Zürich) (not available in the USA). Nebulization is another means of administering medication to birds with respiratory disease (see Chapter 17, Hospital Techniques and Supportive Care). For home treatment,

however, nebulization may not be practical because equipment must usually be rented from medical supply stores.

Tracheal Disease

Infectious etiologies of tracheal disease in psittacines include aspergillosis, bacteria, and viruses, all of which may be associated with disease in the lower airways. Ideally, treatment should be both local and systemic. Administer the appropriate antibiotic or antifungal medication by the oral or parenteral route. In addition, administer antibiotics, if indicated, by nebulization (see Chapter 17, Hospital Techniques and Supportive Care). Amphotericin B can be diluted and administered intratracheally or by nebulization.[26]

If tracheoscopy is unsuccessful in retrieving a tracheal foreign body, a tracheotomy may be necessary.[27] Tracheal aspergillomas are best treated with surgical debridement via endoscopy or tracheotomy in conjunction with intratracheal and systemic antifungal agents.[18]

Pneumonia and Air Sacculitis

Nebulization therapy is the most effective clinical treatment for lower airway disease. Begin nebulization with an antibiotic if bacterial pneumonia or air sacculitis is suspected. Administer other medications parenterally while the bird is hospitalized in conjunction with good supportive care, including fluid therapy and nutritional support. Oxygenating these birds before handling is beneficial.

Surgical removal of localized air sac granulomas caused by *Aspergillus* infection is an option,[28] but the procedure is difficult and carries considerable risk.

Acute Onset of Respiratory Distress

Sudden onset of dyspnea is a true emergency requiring immediate medical attention. Hospitalize affected birds and place them in oxygen while the diagnostic and treatment plan is developed. The most common differential diagnoses for acute dyspnea are listed in Table 25–6. Question the owner about possible exposure to respiratory toxins, including vapors from overheated nonstick cooking pots or ovens in self-cleaning mode. Cockatiels can aspirate millet seeds; suspect this if the bird was eating when it became dyspneic.

If you suspect tracheal obstruction or foreign body aspiration, anesthetize the bird with isoflurane gas and place an air sac tube, which is both diagnostic and therapeutic. Birds with upper airway obstruction become markedly improved once the tube is in place, allowing tracheoscopy or other procedures to be performed to diagnose or alleviate the obstruction (see previous section). The improvement after air sac tube placement is less dramatic in birds with diffuse pulmonary or air sac disease.

Subcutaneous Emphysema

Subcutaneous emphysema typically takes two forms in birds: (1) multilocular, crepitant air pockets and (2) focal pockets of air resulting in discrete swellings, which are sometimes very large. The latter condition is thought to occur as the result of air sac rupture and is easily diagnosed clinically (see later). The former condition is typically the result of trauma or infection with gas-producing bacteria such as *Clostridia* and is not discussed further here.

NONINFECTIOUS CAUSES OF RESPIRATORY DISEASE

Respiratory Toxins

Exposure to fumes from overheated or burning nonstick cookware coatings made of polytetrafluoroethylene (for example, Teflon) causes respiratory distress with high mortality in birds. (See Chapter 35, Toxicities.) The most common presentation is sudden death with or without a history of acute dyspnea preceding death; however, affected birds may show wheezing, dyspnea, weakness, ataxia, and terminal convulsions. Gross necropsy findings include pulmonary hemorrhage and congestion.[29, 30] Sudden death has also been reported in psittacines exposed to fumes from an oven in self-cleaning mode. These birds suddenly show signs of choking, fluid regurgitation, trembling, and ataxia shortly be-

fore death. The most significant necropsy findings are in the respiratory tract and include diffuse pulmonary edema and congestion with multifocal pulmonary hemorrhage.[31]

There is no specific treatment for birds exposed to respiratory toxins, and the prognosis is poor. Administer one dose of a rapid-acting corticosteroid, such as dexamethasone sodium phosphate (6–8 mg/kg IV) and place the bird in oxygen. Administer supportive care as necessary. Prevention is important. Warn bird owners of the danger of nonstick coatings and self-cleaning ovens. Birds should not be housed in the kitchen.

Tracheal Lacerations and Rupture

Tracheal lacerations are typically the result of trauma, particularly attack by a predator. Affected birds may show a head tilt as a compensatory mechanism to seal the tracheal wound. Respiratory distress and subcutaneous emphysema are other possible clinical findings. The diagnosis is based on radiographic evidence, and treatment is with surgical repair.[28]

A complete tracheal rupture suspected to be the result of trauma has been reported in a mallard duck. The duck presented for acute onset of dyspnea, and neck palpation revealed an abnormality in the ventral midcervical region with subcutaneous emphysema. The diagnosis was made with positive radiographic examination, and the trachea was surgically anastomosed.[32]

Focal Subcutaneous Emphysema (Air Sac Rupture)

Focal subcutaneous pockets of air are thought to be caused by air sac rupture; however, the precise etiology is rarely established clinically. This condition occurs almost exclusively in psittacines, particularly Amazon parrots, macaws, and cockatiels. Air-filled swellings usually occur around the head, on the dorsal cervical region, and on the flanks. Swellings can be small and localized or diffuse. These air-filled swellings are very fluctuant on palpation, and the diagnosis is easily confirmed with examination of a fine-needle aspirate.

Air sac rupture has commonly been attributed to

trauma; however, a traumatic event is rarely identifiable. One author feels that preexisting air sac infections are the most common cause.[12] When possible, perform a systemic evaluation of affected birds, including CBC, blood biochemistry, plasma protein electrophoresis, and whole body radiographs.

Specific treatment for air sac rupture entails making a drainage site that will remain open for several days to weeks. Needle aspiration empties the swelling, but most swellings rapidly fill with air again. The choice of technique for drainage depends on the size of the bird and the size and chronicity of the swelling. In small birds, a 5- to 10-mm opening made with a disposable ophthalmic cautery unit (Storz Sure Temp Surgical Cautery, Storz Instrument Co., St. Louis, MO) is often effective. In larger birds, a larger opening is often necessary. Cautery is useful because of slower rate of wound closure compared with a scalpel incision. An opening created by cautery heals spontaneously, removing the pressure of the trapped air and allowing time for healing of the ruptured membranes. Use of an indwelling Teflon dermal stent has been described to treat chronic subcutaneous emphysema in larger psittacines.[33]

Aspiration Pneumonia

Aspiration of food can occur with improper feeding techniques for baby birds and adults or with improper tube-feeding of a bird that is too weak or sedated for the procedure. Iatrogenic administration of barium into the trachea may also occur. The diagnosis is based on a history of possible aspiration, coupled with compatible physical examination findings, which include gradually worsening respiratory distress. Radiographic results are usually normal initially, although radiographic evidence of focal pneumonia or focal pulmonary abscess may develop with time. Some birds survive the initial event showing minimal clinical signs, but present later as "poor doers" with persistent leukocytosis with or without respiratory signs.

There is no specific treatment for aspiration. Hospitalize the bird if necessary to provide supportive care and oxygen therapy. Administer a broad-spectrum antibiotic to prevent or minimize bacterial infection. The prognosis is variable and depends on host factors and on the amount and type of aspirated material. Give the owner a guarded prognosis and recommend a wait-and-see approach. Some birds survive aspiration; however, persistent, localized abscess formation is possible.

Hypovitaminosis A

Nutritional deficiencies, particularly hypovitaminosis A, play an important role in predisposing birds to respiratory tract infection. In addition, birds with hypovitaminosis A may develop focal keratinaceous granulomas in areas of the respiratory tract, such as the choana and sinuses. Always realize that hypovitaminosis A occurs in combination with multiple nutrient deficiencies.

Neoplasms

Respiratory tract neoplasms are rare in birds. In one report that included a literature review and a survey of pathology records at a university hospital, seven respiratory neoplasms were identified in caged bird species.[34] These comprised a fibrosarcoma of the air sac in a double yellow-headed Amazon parrot; a laryngeal papilloma in a yellow-headed Amazon; and five pulmonary neoplasms, including an adenoma and a mixed epithelial and connective tissue tumor in two macaws, adenomas in a peach-faced lovebird and a musky lorikeet, and a fibrosarcoma in a cockatiel.

A recent report describes a malignant melanoma in an 8-year-old African grey parrot that appeared to have arisen from the nasal cavity and subsequently metastasized to the oropharynx, internal carotid artery, and abdominal organs.[35] The bird had been initially presented with the complaints of left infraorbital and maxillary beak swelling and bilateral serous nasal discharge. The tumor grew rapidly, ultimately causing deformation of the maxillary beak, palate, and choanal slit.

Respiratory Disease of Blue and Gold Macaws

Blue and gold macaws appear to be more susceptible than other common caged bird species to airborne irritants and may develop chronic, progressive respiratory disease if housed in poorly ventilated areas, particularly if placed with other species that produce an abundance of powder, such as cockatiels, African grey parrots, and cockatoos. The term "pulmonary hypersensitivity syndrome" has been coined for this condition.[12] Affected birds present with signs of chronic respiratory disease, including wheezing with excitement, exertional inspiratory and expiratory dyspnea, facial skin cyanosis, and a dry cough. Polycythemia is a common laboratory abnormality and is thought to be a response to hypoxia.[36, 37] Possible radiographic changes include thickening of bronchiolar walls on the lateral view, great vessel enlargement, right-sided cardiomegaly, and hyperinflation of the air sacs.[12] Lung biopsy is diagnostic; histopathologic changes at necropsy include pulmonary interstitial cellular and fibrous tissue infiltrates and pulmonary atrial smooth muscle hyperplasia.[37]

Pulmonary disease is often advanced at the time of diagnosis. Affected birds should be moved to an environment with good ventilation. There is no proven pharmacologic treatment for this syndrome.

Pulmonary Silicosis

Pulmonary silicosis has been reported in a 6-year-old blue and gold macaw that suffered from bouts of dyspnea with handling over a 6-month period.[38] At necropsy, there were several poorly defined, unencapsulated pyogranulomatous nodules in and around the parabronchi. At the center of these nodules was a crystalline material that was identified as aluminum silicate. The source was determined to be peat moss used as bedding material in the aviary, which was poorly ventilated. Pulmonary silicosis resulting from inhalation of fine particulates from a sand substrate has been reported in ring-necked pheasants.[39]

Choanal Atresia

Choanal atresia, a congenital absence of the choanae, has been reported in two psittacine birds—a 4-month-old African grey parrot showing bilateral, serous nasal discharge since 4 days of age, and a 4-year-old umbrella cockatoo showing chronic, copious, serous to purulent, bilateral ocular discharge

with episodic nasal discharge.[40] Oral examination was normal for the African grey parrot; however, the cockatoo lacked a choanal slit. The diagnosis of choanal atresia was made in both birds using rhinography, which showed blockage of contrast material at or dorsal to the level of the palate. The contrast material flowed normally into both infraorbital sinuses. Endoscopy in the African grey parrot revealed the presence of a persistent membrane covering the choanae.[40]

References

1. King AS, McLelland J: Form and Function of Birds. vol 4. San Diego, Academic Press, 1989.
2. Tully Jr TN, Harrison GJ: Pneumonology. In Ritchie BW, Harrison GJ, Harrison LR (eds): Avian Medicine: Principles and Application. Lake Worth, FL, Wingers Publishing, 1994, pp 556–581.
3. Gill FB: Ornithology, ed 2. New York, WH Freeman and Company, 1994.
4. Greenewalt CH: Bird Song: Acoustics and Physiology. Washington, DC, Smithsonian Institution Press, 1968.
5. Gaunt AS, Gaunt SLL: Syringeal structure and avian phonation. Curr Ornithol 2:213–245, 1985.
6. National Asthma Education Program: Executive summary: Guidelines for the management of asthma. Bethesda, MD, US Department of Health and Human Services, Public Health Service, National Institutes of Health, Publication No. 91–3042A, 1991.
7. Gerlach H: Viruses. In Ritchie BW, Harrison GH, Harrison LR (eds): Avian Medicine: Principles and Application. Lake Worth, FL, Wingers Publishing, 1994, pp 862–948.
8. Wainwright PO, Pritchard NG, Fletcher OJ, et al: Identification of viruses from Amazon parrots with a hemorrhagic syndrome and a chronic respiratory disease. Proc 1st Intl Conf Zool Avian Med, Oahu, September 6–11, 1987, pp 15–19.
9. Bauck L, Hillyer E, Hoefer H: Rhinitis: Case reports. Proc Assoc Avian Vet, New Orleans, September 1–5, 1992, pp 134–139.
10. Gaskin JM: Mycoplasmosis of caged birds. Proc 1st Intl Conf Zool Avian Med, Oahu, September 6–11, 1987, pp 57–60.
11. Brown PA, Redig PT: Aspergillus ELISA—a tool for detection and management. Proc Assoc Avian Vet, Reno, September 27–October 1, 1994, pp 295–300.
12. Fudge AM, Reavill DR, Rosskopf WJ, Jr: Diagnosis and management of avian dyspnea: a review. Proc Assoc Avian Vet, Nashville, August 31–September 4, 1993, pp 187–195.
13. Oglesbee BL: Case Reports. Vet Clin North Am Small Anim Med 21(6):1299–1306, 1991.
14. VanDerHeyden N: Psittacine papillomas. Proc Assoc Avian Vet, Houston, September 27–October 1, 1988, pp 23–25.
15. Tully TN Jr, Carter JD: Bilateral supraorbital abscesses associated with sinusitis in an orange-winged Amazon parrot (Amazona amazonica). J Assoc Avian Vet 7(3):157–158, 1993.
16. Bennett RA, Harrison GJ: Soft tissue surgery. In Ritchie BW, Harrison GH, Harrison R, Harrison L (eds): Avian Medicine: Principles and Application. Lake Worth, FL, Wingers Publishing, 1994, pp 1096–1136.
17. van der Mast H, Dorrestein GM, Westerhof J: In my experi-

ence: a fatal treatment of sinusitis in an African grey. J Assoc Avian Vet 4(3):189, 1990.

18. McDonald SE, Messenger GA: Successful treatment of mycotic tracheitis in a raven. Proc Assoc Avian Vet 1984, pp 155–163.

19. McMillan MC, Petrak ML: Retrospective study of aspergillosis in birds. J Assoc Avian Vet 3(4):211–215, 1989.

20. Rosenthal K, Stamoulis M: Diagnosis of congestive heart failure in an Indian Hill mynah bird (Gracula religiosa). J Assoc Avian Vet 7(1):27–30, 1993.

21. Garner MM: Trichomoniasis in a blue-fronted Amazon parrot (*Amazona aestiva*). J Assoc Avian Vet 6(1):17–20, 1992.

22. Krautwald-Junghanns M-E, Schumacher F, Tellhelm B: Evaluation of the lower respiratory tract in psittacines using radiology and computed tomography. Vet Radiol 34(6):382–390, 1993.

23. Rode JA, Bartholow S, Ludders JW: Ventilation through an air sac cannula during tracheal obstruction in ducks. J Assoc Avian Vet 4(2):98–102, 1990.

24. Page CD, Schmidt RE, English JH, et al: Antemortem diagnosis and treatment of sarcocystosis in two species of psittacines. J Zoo Wildl Med 23(1):77–85, 1992.

25. Devriese LA, Uyttebroek E, Ducatelle R, et al: Tracheitis due to *Enterococcus faecalis* infection in canaries. J Assoc Avian Vet 4(2):113–116, 1990.

26. Prus SE: Avian antifungal therapy. Semin Avian Exotic Pet Med 2(1):30–32, 1993.

27. Howard PE, Dein FJ, Langenberg JA, et al: Surgical removal of a tracheal foreign body from a whooping crane (*Grus americana*). J Zoo Wild Med 22(3):359–363, 1991.

28. Dustin LR: Surgery of the avian respiratory system. Semin Avian Exotic Pet Med 2(2):83–90, 1993.

29. Wells RE: Fatal toxicosis in pet birds caused by an overheated cooking pan lined with polytetrafluoroethylene. J Am Vet Med Assoc 182(11):1248–1250, 1983.

30. Wells RE, Slocombe RF, Trapp AL: Acute toxicosis of budgerigars (*Melopsittacus undulatus*) caused by pyrolysis products from heated polytetrafluoroethylene. Clinical study. Am J Vet Res 43(7):1238–1242, 1982.

31. Stoltz JH, Galey F, Johnson B: Sudden death in ten psittacine birds associated with the operation of a self-cleaning oven. Vet Human Toxicol 34(5):420–421, 1992.

32. Crystal MA, Clark G: What is your diagnosis? J Am Vet Med Assoc 200(10):1547–1548, 1992.

33. Harris JM: Teflon dermal stent for the correction of subcutaneous emphysema. Proc Assoc Avian Vet, Chicago, September 23–28, 1991, pp 20–21.

34. Leach MW: A survey of neoplasia in pet birds. Semin Avian Exotic Pet Med 1(2):52–64, 1992.

35. André JP, Delverdier M, Cabanié P, Bartel G: Malignant melanoma in an African grey parrot (*Psittacus erithacus erithacus*). J Assoc Avian Vet 7(2):83–85, 1993.

36. Taylor M: Polycythemia in the blue and gold macaw—a report of three cases. Proc 1st Intl Conf Zool Avian Med, Oahu, September 6–11, 1987.

37. Taylor M, Hunter B: In my experience: a chronic obstructive pulmonary disease of blue and gold macaws. J Assoc Avian Vet 5(2):71, 1991.

38. Rae MA, Duimstra JR, Snyder SP: Pulmonary silicosis in a blue and gold macaw (*Ara ararauna*). Proc Assoc Avian Vet, Chicago, September 23–28, 1991, pp 260–261.

39. Fitzgerald SD, Reed WM: Diagnostic exercise: Sudden death in captive ring-necked pheasants. Lab Anim Sci 41(3):279–280, 1991.

40. Greenacre CB, Watson E, Ritchie BW: Choanal atresia in an African grey parrot (*Psittacus erithacus erithacus*) and an umbrella cockatoo (*Cacatua alba*). J Assoc Avian Vet 7(1):19–22, 1993.

41. Desmidt M, Ducatelle R, Uyttebroek E, et al: Respiratory adenovirus-like infection in a rose-ringed parakeet (*Psittacula krameri*). Avian Dis 35(4):1001–1006, 1991.

42. Curtis-Velasco M: Eastern equine encephalomyelitis virus in a Lady Gouldian finch. J Assoc Avian Vet 6(4):227–228, 1992.

43. Hillyer EV, Anderson MP, Greiner EC, et al: An outbreak of *Sarcocystis* in a collection of psittacines. J Zoo Wildl Med 22(4):434–445, 1991.

Heidi L. Hoefer
Susan Orosz
Gerry M. Dorrestein

26

The Gastrointestinal Tract

Susan Orosz

Anatomy of the Digestive System

The soft palate is absent in birds. Instead, birds have an incomplete hard palate with a median choanal slit (Fig. 26–1). The mucous membranes of the palate on its oral surface have caudally directed choanal papillae in psittacines and Galliformes. Blunting of the choanal papillae is associated with hypovitaminosis A and chronic upper respiratory infections. Caudal to the choanal slit is the infundibular cleft, which represents the opening of the right and left eustachian tubes. In birds that need to make rapid altitude adjustments, the short, broad structure of the eustachian tubes and the location of the tube openings directly into the oropharynx

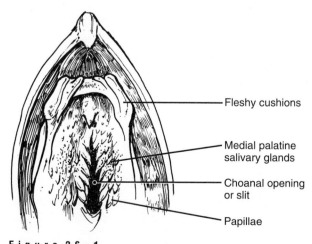

Figure 26–1

The roof of the oropharynx of a psittacine. The choanal papillae are directed caudally, and the ends should be pointed in healthy birds. There are numerous small collections of salivary glands scattered throughout this area with microscopic multiple openings.

are important for equalizing pressure changes, in comparison with the small but long eustachian tubes in mammals.

The tongue is supported by a hyoid apparatus, and its structure is dependent on the functions of the individual species. In woodpeckers and nectar eaters, the tongue is long, narrow, and protrusible to allow its use as a probe, brush, or a capillary tube. In parrots, finches, and raptors, tongues are adapted for manipulating their food items. This function is particularly well developed in psittacines, the only birds with intrinsic tongue muscles.

Tongue movement in the other orders of birds is the result of the great mobility of the hyoid apparatus. An additional adaptation for swallowing food is the caudally directed choanal papilla. These papillae may also be found on the laryngeal mound that surrounds the opening of the larynx.

Salivary glands are most developed in birds with relatively dry diets, and least developed in fish eaters. Birds do not have the large well-defined salivary glands of mammals, but instead have multiple small collections of glandular tissue in the roof and floor (maxillary, palatine, and sphenopterygoid) of the oropharynx and at the angle of the mouth (mandibular, cricoarytenoid salivary glands). These glands predominantly secrete mucus but may also secrete some amylase. The epithelium of the oropharynx is a stratified squamous type, which can be keratinized in regions where abrasions occur, particularly in birds with hard, seed-type diets.

The esophagus is often thin-walled. The cervical esophagus is found on the right side of the neck in

Figure labels:
- Fleshy cushions
- Medial palatine salivary glands
- Choanal opening or slit
- Papillae

comparison with the left side in mammals. A number of species, including psittacines, Galliformes, and Columbiformes, have a crop or ingluvies that acts as a food storage organ. The crop may be oriented horizontally or transversely. It may be absent (gulls and penguins) or may be a fusiform widening as in raptors. Contractions of the crop and the opposing esophageal wall push food distally into the thoracic esophagus and then into the stomach.

The stomach of birds lies in the left craniodorsal thoracoabdominal cavity and is covered by other abdominal organs and the posthepatic septum. It is subdivided into three parts. The most rostral portion is the proventriculus or the true glandular stomach. This is followed by the second portion, termed the intermediate zone, and the third portion, the ventriculus or gizzard, which is used for grinding and mixing. The pylorus connects the ventriculus to the cranial duodenum.

The varying diets of the species are reflected in the differing anatomic types of stomachs (Fig. 26–2). The storage form of the stomach is associated with piscivores and carnivores, which feed on soft food items. It is thin and sac-like, making it difficult to identify each portion or component of the stomach externally. The stomach that is designed for grinding is associated with insectivores, herbivores, and granivores. These birds eat foods that are relatively indigestible and thereby require a thick, muscular gizzard for grinding foodstuffs. It is relatively easy to distinguish the proventriculus from the ventriculus externally in birds with this stomach type. An intermediate stomach type between the two described is associated with frugivores and testacivores.

The proventriculus generally lacks the longitudinal folds of the thoracic esophagus. There may be folds internally in both the storage and intermediate stomach types. The cells of the gastric glands secrete both pepsinogen and hydrochloric acid (HCl). Additionally, there are mucin-secreting cells. The gastric glands usually open at the tips of the papillae.

The ventriculus of the grinding-type stomach has four muscular bands that attach by extensive aponeuroses. These are derived from the original circular smooth muscle layer and are arranged asymmetrically to provide rotatory and crushing movements (Fig. 26–3). The ventriculus acts as a unit with the proventriculus to chemically and physically digest the foodstuffs. The epithelium of the ventriculus is

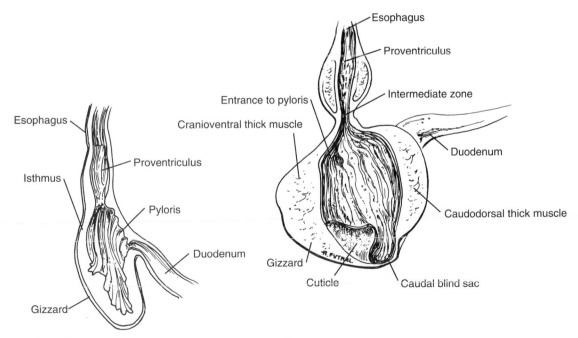

F i g u r e   2 6 – 2

Comparison of the stomach compartments of a granivorous bird with those of a carnivorous bird. The stomach compartments include the proventriculus, the ventriculus, and the isthmus which separates the first two compartments.

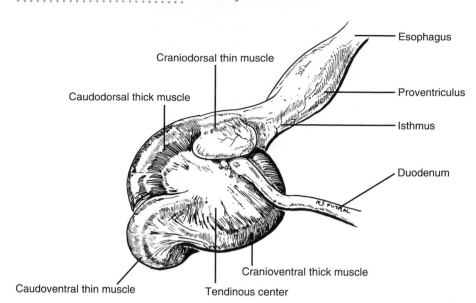

Craniodorsal thin muscle

Caudodorsal thick muscle

Esophagus

Proventriculus

Isthmus

Duodenum

Caudoventral thin muscle

Tendinous center

Cranioventral thick muscle

Figure 26-3

The stomach of a granivorous bird. The stomach consists of a proventriculus, isthmus, and ventriculus. The esophagus grossly appears to be continuous with the proventriculus, the glandular portion. Mixing occurs between the proventriculus and ventriculus in a rotatory manner.

a simple columnar type with crypts. These crypts are the site for the opening of tubular glands, which are composed of protein-secreting chief cells. Endocrine cells present in the epithelium are also thought to play a role in the metabolism of foodstuffs and the regulation of the movement of ingesta.

In the grinding type of stomach, a carbohydrate protein complex, termed the "koilin" or "cuticle," rests on the epithelium of the ventriculus. Previously thought to be keratin, it helps to protect the epithelium during the grinding process.

The intestinal tract continues with the U-shaped duodenum, ileum, jejunum, and a large intestine (Fig. 26–4). The two limbs (descending and ascending) of the duodenum are joined by a ventral mesentery. Although birds do not have Brunner's glands as in mammals, mucus is secreted by goblet cells.

The bile (common hepatoenteric duct or cystoenteric) and pancreatic ducts numbering one to three open in close proximity to each other at the distal end of the ascending duodenum. Mixing of ingesta occurs between the compartments of the stomach and the duodenum through a defined sequence. This gastroduodenal sequence is initiated and coordinated by an intrinsic neuronal network. It is influenced by the chemical nature and the volume of the duodenal contents.

The jejunum and ileum of most birds are composed of a number of U-shaped loops attached to a dorsal mesentery. The vitelline (Meckel's) diverticulum is the remnant of the attachment of the yolk sac to the intestine and demarcates the jejunum proximally from the ileum distally. The supraduodenal loop of the intestine sits cranial to the duodenum in situ. This loop represents the distal-most portion of the ileum. There is a supracecal loop of intestine in falcons and penguins.

The large intestine begins with the outpouchings of the ceca and includes a short, straight segment of intestine along the dorsal body wall. The presence and structure of ceca vary with the species of bird. Ceca are absent in psittacines, sacculated and large in ostriches, expanded distally in owls, small in passerines, and large in Galliformes.

The folds and villi of the intestinal tracts of various bird species differ greatly. The intestinal epithelium has three primary cell types, including chief cells for the absorption of nutrients, goblet cells for the secretion of mucus, and endocrine cells, which help regulate motility and metabolism of the foodstuffs. Digestion and absorption of nutrients occur in the small intestine, as in mammals.

The pancreas is a pale, lobulated organ that lies mostly within the two limbs of the duodenum. It consists of ventral, dorsal, and splenic lobes. These lobes are variable amongst species, but in fowl, the majority of the pancreatic islets are found in the splenic lobe. The exocrine portion of the pancreas

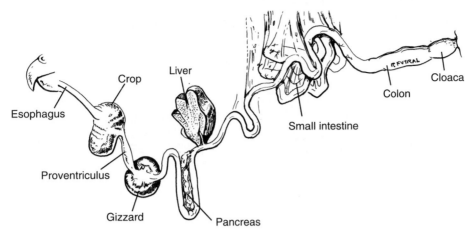

Figure 26–4

Overview of the avian gastrointestinal tract. Some birds may have a supraduodenal loop that occurs as a loop at the distal end of the ileum. A supracecal loop occurs in some species. Psittacine birds do not have a ceca, as shown in this diagram.

consists of compound tubuloacinar glands that secrete amylase, lipase, a variety of proteases, and bicarbonate. These glands are drained by one to three pancreatic ducts into the distal portion of the ascending colon.

The liver is composed of right and left lobes with a variable number of intermediate processes. The main lobes may be subdivided. If a gall bladder is present, it is usually associated with the right lobe. A gall bladder is not found in most parrots, pigeons, and ostriches. In birds without a gall bladder, each lobe is drained by a separate hepatoenteric bile duct into the duodenum. In birds with a gall bladder, the hepatocystic duct drains bile from the right lobe into the gall bladder, and the cystoenteric duct drains bile from the gall bladder into the intestine. The common hepatoenteric bile duct drains bile from both lobes into the small intestine. At the microscopic level, the classic lobule of mammals is difficult to distinguish in birds, although the cell types and their basic functions are similar.

Physiology of Digestion | Gerry M. Dorrestein

Because birds expend energy at a tremendous rate, they must feed frequently to refuel themselves.[1] Adaptations for feeding are a conspicuous feature of avian evolution. These adaptations include not only the mode of locomotion birds use while feeding but also anatomic specializations of the bill and tongue, legs and feet, crop, stomach, and intestines.

Seeds sustain many of the common pet birds. Pigeons, doves, and fowl swallow seeds whole and grind them in the gizzard. Most passerines and psittacines that specialize in eating seeds crack and shuck the seed husks with powerful bills. These birds extract seed kernels by either crushing or cutting the seed hull. In the crushing method, the seed, held by one or both margins of the bill, is pressed against a central ridge in the horny roof of the mouth to pop the kernel from the shell. In the cutting method, a bird uses its tongue to lodge the seed in furrows of the hard palate and then cuts the husk with rapid forward and backward movements of the sharp edges of the jaws. In both cases, the cut husks fall out of the mouth, and the clean kernel is swallowed.

AVIAN DIGESTIVE SYSTEM

Because birds lack teeth that chew food before swallowing, the avian digestive system is specialized to process unmasticated food. The major parts of this system, the oral cavity, esophagus, crop, two-chambered stomach (proventriculus and gizzard), liver, pancreas, intestine, and cloaca, are further specialized to accommodate particular types of diets and feeding practices. Linked to the development of flight and high metabolic rates, the digestive system of most birds extracts nutrients and energy with high efficiency from small volumes of rapidly processed food.

Oral Cavity

The oral cavity (oropharynx) houses taste buds, salivary glands, and a tongue that is often specialized. The taste buds in the soft palate aid in food selection. Three major sets of salivary glands and a variety of smaller ones provide lubrication, essential for the passage of food toward the esophagus. In some species the saliva contains amylase.

Some birds produce salivary secretions for other uses as well—sticky secretions to catch insects, glue for attaching nests to the wall, to build nests, to form boluses for winter food supply, and others.

The tongue aids in the gathering and swallowing of food. Extremely sensitive structures, bird tongues are filled with tactile sensory corpuscles, especially at the tip. These corpuscles are best developed in the spoon-tipped tongues of seedeating songbirds, which manipulate tiny seeds, and in the strong, club-shaped, muscular tongue of parrots.[1]

Esophagus

In most birds, food passes from the oral cavity to the stomach through the esophagus, a muscular structure lined with more or less developed lubricating mucous glands. Swallowing involves a rapid rostrocaudal movement of the tongue and the larynx, assisted by sticky saliva and caudally directed papilla on the tongue. During swallowing, the choana, infundibulum cleft, and glottis are closed.[2]

The crop, an expanded esophageal section found in most birds, stores and softens food and regulates the flow through the digestive tract. The crop of pigeons produces a nutritious product, called pigeon or crop milk, for their young during the first week after hatching. Prolactin controls the production of crop milk, which consists of desquamating cells of the proliferating stratified squamous epithelium of the crop. Crop milk physically resembles mammalian milk and contains a high concentration of fat (6.9–12.7%) and protein (13.3–18.6%), but lacks carbohydrates, casein, lactose, and calcium. The crop of psittacines and passerines may also produce some secretions that are regurgitated and fed to neonates.[3, 4]

In some birds, including budgerigars, newly hatched birds are fed on a secretion from the hen's proventriculus (rather than the crop) that is often incorrectly called crop milk. This fluid has a particularly high protein content, essential for the young, rapidly developing bird.[5]

Contractions of the crop and gizzard seem to be coordinated, and the stomach may influence crop activity. Distension of the crop increases in the proventriculus acid secretion and may inhibit gizzard contractions.[2]

Stomach

Shapes and morphologic structures of the stomach in birds differ more than any other internal organ, reflecting the dietary habits of different species. The proventriculus, most developed in fish-eating birds and raptors, secretes acidic gastric juices (pH 0.2–1.2) from its glandular walls, thereby creating a favorable chemical environment for digestion. The avian gizzard, the functional analogue of mammalian molars, is a strong, muscular structure used primarily for grinding and digesting tough food.

The polymerization of koilin, the tough, water-resistant polymerized polysaccharide-protein–complex layer that lines the internal grinding surface of the gizzard, is induced by the pH of the contents in the lumen of the gizzard. In cases of gastric disturbances that disrupt the production of gastric acid (HCl) the pH can be increased, and hence the hardening of the koilin layer is not complete. This layer stays soft and gelatinous. A common example is an infection with megabacteria, in which the measured pH can be as high as 7.0 to 7.3.

The gizzard can also contain large quantities of grit and stone, which help to grind food.

There is discussion about the need for grit in normal, healthy psittacine or passerine birds. It is said to be required only by birds that consume whole, intact seeds, like pigeons, doves, free-ranging gallinaceous species, and ratites. Psittacines and passerines normally remove the fibrous hull, allowing the ingested portion to be easily acted upon by the digestive enzymes.

There have been numerous reports of birds, especially with health problems and depraved appetites, consuming copious quantities of grit and developing crop or gastrointestinal impactions. Considering the small change of benefit and the potential risk, ad libitum feeding of grit should be avoided.[6] Others have shown that addition of some grit may increase digestibility of a diet.[2]

The gizzard is not as muscular in birds that eat softer foods such as meat, insects, or fruit; in raptors and fish-eating birds it may take the form of a thin-walled sac.

Contractions of the gizzard, proventriculus, and duodenum are normally totally coordinated in a sequence. In birds there is also a unique normal gastroduodenal motility called "intestinal refluxes." During the reflux period gastric motility is inhibited. In many species, especially carnivores, one other unique gastric function occurs, egestion (oral expulsion) of pellets of indigestible material.

In mammals, inhibition of the gastric emptying begins in the duodenum, with involvement of regulatory receptors specific for osmolarity, acidity, fats, and the amino acid tryptophan.[7]

Liver

The liver, the hub of the body's metabolic activities, is an indispensable component of the body's homeostatic system. In the embryo and shortly after hatching, the liver plays an important role in the synthesis of blood cells. After birth, its primary role as the body's central metabolic unit develops along with its specialized functions of bile acid formation and excretion of the byproducts of metabolism. In mammals the liver is also an endocrine organ involved in regulating growth by producing somatomedin.[7]

The core of liver activity is metabolic processing of the incoming nutrients and compensating for the impacts of the competing demands by the various tissues of the body for maintenance, growth, egg production, and reproduction. The liver acts as an excretory organ, like the kidneys, for xenobiotics (dyes, drugs, and toxins), for the byproducts of heme metabolism, and for certain other metabolites via the bile. This concurrent excretion includes the formation of important components for protecting the body (by oxidation and conjugation) from hazardous substances that may have been absorbed; however, a few agents may be made more toxic.

Several of the numerous metabolic functions of the liver include the following:

1. The formation of bile salts and their recycling, both necessary for digestion of lipids (emulsifying lipids and pancreatic enzyme activation). In the racing pigeon plasma bile concentrations are the single most useful, available test for determining liver dysfunction.[4]

2. The excretion of pigment biliverdin issued from the hemoglobin of erythrocytes that have lived out their lifespan. Green-colored urates are suggestive of liver disease. Icterus or jaundice, which is caused by a hyperbilirubinemia, is seen very infrequently in birds.[4]

3. The filtration and limited storage of blood draining the intestine through a venous portal system before it flows from the liver into the systemic circulation.

4. Some metabolic transformations of nutrients (e.g., vitamin D3, carbohydrate, lipid, protein) induced by resident enzymes.

5. Synthesis of plasma proteins to help repair wear and tear of tissues, and of clotting factors to correct effraction or breakage in the wall of blood vessels.

Selective storage functions, which can be drawn from an examination of the hepatocyte structure, are that of iron as ferritin, especially at the level of macrophages (Kupffer's cells) and that of vitamins (liposoluble A and D; water-soluble B_{12}).

In many bird species (e.g., mynah birds, toucans, birds of paradise) a "low iron threshold" leads to iron storage disease (hemochromatosis), wherein high levels of iron are stored in hepatocytes.

Intestine

The length of a bird's intestinal tract averages 8.6 times the length of its body but varies from three times body length to 20 times body length in the ostrich. The intestine tends to be short in species that feed on fruit, meat, and insects and long in species that feed on seeds, plants, and fish. The detailed histology and patterns of relief of the absorption surfaces also vary according to the diet.[1]

Transit time of food through the digestive tract varies from less than $\frac{1}{2}$ hour in the case of berries ingested by thrushes to $\frac{1}{2}$ day or more for less easily digested food.

Assimilation of digested food through the intestinal walls depends on the nature of the food digested. Hummingbirds assimilate 97 to 99% of the energy in nectar, which consists primarily of simple sugars and water. Other foods are less easily assimilated. Raptors assimilate 66 to 88% of the energy contained in ingested meat and fish. Herbivores assimilate as much as 60 to 70% of the energy contained in the young plants they ingest but only 30 to 40% of the energy in ingested mature foliage.

Most birds cannot digest lactose, and many passerine songbirds cannot digest sucrose because they lack the respective enzymes. Ingestion of lactose and/or sucrose can cause sickness resulting from malabsorption.

Ceca aid in the digestion of plant foods. They are most prominent in fowl and ostriches, in which they functionally resemble the cecum of horses. They also tend to be larger in young birds than in adults. The precise role of ceca in digestion remains unclear, but it appears that bacteria in the ceca further digest and ferment partially digested foods into usable biochemical compounds that are absorbed through the cecal walls. Ceca may also function to separate the nutrient-rich fluid in partially digested food from the fibrous portion, which is eventually eliminated. Ceca are poorly developed or nonexistent in most arboreal birds, perhaps because of the unacceptable weight of the watery, partially digested food in the intestine and the large structures required to handle it. Indeed, well-developed cecal fermentation is restricted to ground-dwelling and flightless birds and is much more common in mammals than in birds.

The last part of the digestive tract, rectum and cloaca, are primarily involved in excretion and mineral and water balance.

PHYSIOLOGY OF THE DIGESTIVE TRACT

In general, birds prefer familiar food. In the wild, the preference for familiar foods lessens the number of unpleasant, poisonous, or otherwise dangerous prey. Familiar food also can be found more readily than unfamiliar food if the foraging bird uses a specific "search image," as we do when we look for a friend in a crowd or for a jigsaw puzzle piece with a particular shape.

The young bird must learn what is food and what is not, and which "food" is potentially harmful.

Psittacines, in particular, have individual preferences for food based on previous experience (or habit), food placement (position in the cage), particle size, fat content, texture, shape, color and taste. These preferences can be strong, and this limited feeding pattern can result in severe nutrient deficiencies if the selected food is not nutrient-complete and balanced.[6]

Little is known about the degree to which the diets and foraging behavior of wild birds are directed toward nutrition. It is usually assumed that birds passively obtain adequate nutrition in the course of their daily foraging to meet their energy needs and rarely suffer malnutrition or nutritional stress.[8] However, given the opportunity, some birds are able to actively select concentrations of certain amino acids (namely, valine and lysine) in synthetic diets which satisfies their amino acid requirements.[9]

Ideally, intake and expenditure of energy are roughly equal so that the bird neither gains nor loses much weight. The amount of time a bird must feed each day depends on its total energy requirements and achieved rate of energy intake. Low forage time allows birds to build up energy reserves or undertake energy-expensive activities such as moulting and breeding, and allows more time to establish dominance and property rights over other individuals, court mates, and rear young. Birds vary their foraging time and effort in relation to their energy requirements and foraging success.

Studies with poultry have shown that if the energy content of the diet is increased, for example, by increasing the proportion of fat, birds decrease intake to compensate for this. If no changes are made to the other nutrients, eventually deficiencies develop. Conversely, when the dietary energy density is diluted, intake of the energy increases so that the bird meets its energy requirement for maintenance. However, if the diet is excessively dilute, the ability to adjust intake may be overridden because gastrointestinal capacity becomes a limiting factor.

Most birds maintain minimal fat reserves, probably because the survival benefits of large energy reserves do not offset the costs of carrying excess weight. In general, large birds can store more fat and can fast longer than smaller birds. Fasting birds draw first on their glycogen deposits, then on lipids. Only the lipid reserves of cardiac muscle are exempt from normal use, and as a last resort, body tissues can be metabolized after fat deposits are exhausted. Pectoral muscles begin to atrophy during periods of food stress; even gonadal tissues may be sacrificed.

Obtaining adequate nutrition for the moult is probably not a major problem for birds in the wild. Muscle tissues can be broken down as needed for most of the amino acids required. Keratin synthesis, however, requires disproportionately high proportions of sulphur-containing amino acids, especially cysteine. To have cysteine available in amounts to continue feather growth overnight when birds fast, they store extra reserves in the liver during the day, when possible, feeding selectively on foods containing such amino acids if needed; the stored cysteine is liberated for use at night.[9]

Diseases of the Gastrointestinal Tract

Heidi L. Hoefer

GENERAL CONSIDERATIONS

Diseases of the gastrointestinal tract are common in clinical avian practice. Part of this stems from the improper management and handling of birds associated with the pet trade, and poor husbandry techniques. Malnutrition, dietary indiscretion, indiscriminant use of antibiotics, stress, and overcrowding predispose many birds to disease. With this in mind, it is important to recognize and correct the initiating factors as well as provide symptomatic therapy.

Clinical signs of gastrointestinal disease are nonspecific but most often include abnormal droppings, vomiting or regurgitation, weight loss, and inappetence or anorexia. In this chapter, the common causes of avian gastrointestinal tract disease are reviewed and briefly discussed. Hepatobiliary diseases are presented as a separate section in the second half of this chapter. Emphasis is on the disorders typically encountered in a clinical avian practice. More detailed information on specific disease entities can be found in other section of this book.

THE AVIAN BEAK

The horny bill (rhamphotheca) is a hard, keratinized structure that covers the rostral aspect of the upper and lower jaw bones. Lips and teeth are lacking in all species of birds and are functionally replaced by the cutting edge of the beak.[10] The beak can take a variety of shapes, depending on the natural diet. Because the forelimbs of the bird have evolved into instruments of flight, the beak has adapted to many manipulative procedures that include prehension, nest building, and locomotion in the parrot.

The horny tissue of the beak is worn down by the normal activity of the bird and is continually replaced. In pet birds, the beak is not subjected to normal wearing and may need periodic trims. The tip of the beak contains an abundant blood supply and profuse sensory nerve endings. Injury to the beak can be very painful; be careful when performing beak trims on pet birds. In adult poultry, the beak is cut back to prevent cannibalism; this procedure is associated with a reduction of food intake and body weight that can last more than 6 weeks.[11] It is not unusual for a bird to become reluctant to crack seeds following trauma to the tip of the beak. Include an examination of the beak in any bird that presents for anorexia or dysphagia.

Diseases of the beak are frequently encountered in clinical avian practice. Perforations and cracks are common sequelae to fighting in psittacines and Galliformes, who often use the bill for defense. Congenital anomalies of the bill are not uncommon and may result in twisting and malalignment. Trauma, malnutrition, infection, neoplasia, and metabolic conditions can also affect the beak. Diseases of the beak are covered in more detail in other sections of this book. (See Chapter 32, Avian Dermatology.)

THE OROPHARYNX

Oropharyngeal lesions are frequently diagnosed in clinical avian practice (Table 26–1). Clinical signs are variable but may include dysphagia, gaping or "yawning," inappetence, and anorexia. Affected individuals may appear clinically normal, and oropharyngeal lesions may be incidentally discovered during examination.

Examination

A cursory examination of the oropharynx may be possible during routine physical examinations in some species. Use sedation if necessary to fully examine the oral cavity for lesions and to take samples. The use of a speculum aids in visualization of the oral cavity. However, be careful when using metal devices because they can damage the beak and the commissures of the mouth in the struggling bird. Gauze strips may be safer; apply the strips to the upper and lower beak (Fig. 26–5).

Inspect the oral mucosa and tongue. Normal epithelium is slightly moist, smooth, and, depending on the species, may be pink or darkly pigmented.

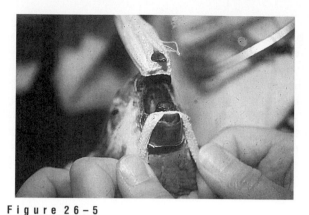

Figure 26–5

Gauze strips can be applied to the upper and lower beak to facilitate oral examination.

Abnormal mucosa may contain white plaques, ulcerations, swellings, depigmentation, and the absence or blunting of the oral papillae (Fig. 26–6). The accumulation of dried mucus or food can be seen in some sick birds. Most birds have a neutral odor to the mouth, although some parrots (Amazon parrots and cockatoos) have a slightly musty smell that is normal for the species. A foul smell to the oropharynx may indicate a crop infection or gastroenteritis.

Table 26–1
COMMON OROPHARYNGEAL LESIONS

- Exudative/proliferative lesions
    Pox virus (especially Amazon parrots)
    Trichomoniasis
    Candidiasis
    Bacterial plaques (especially gram-negative)
    Hypovitaminosis A
    Sinusitis (choanal lesion)
- Neoplasia
    Papilloma
    Squamous cell carcinoma
    Adenocarcinoma
    Fibrosarcoma
- Trauma
    Cagemate fights
    Foreign body ingestion (toys, wood, sharp objects)
    Electric cord bites

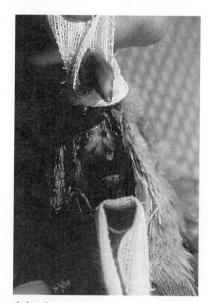

Figure 26–6

Oral examination of an Amazon parrot with hypovitaminosis A. Close inspection reveals a pale swelling adjacent to the choana.

Check the choana for abnormalities. The blunting or absence of choanal papillae can be seen in hypovitaminosis A. Because the nasal cavity communicates directly with the choanal opening, disorders within the sinuses may be accompanied by oral lesions. Accumulation of mucus and purulent debris within the choana may be associated with drainage from a sinus infection. The cranial edge of the choanal opening may appear swollen; gentle pressure on the area with a cotton swab will often produce necrotic debris.

Oropharyngeal Lesions

Hypovitaminosis A

Hypovitaminosis A can result in the formation of swellings in the mucosa and the production of copious amounts of thick, tenacious mucus that is difficult to remove. This is most commonly seen in parrots on an all-seed diet without adequate vitamin supplementation. Discrete swellings or nodules form along the sides of the tongue, on the margins of the choanal opening, and in the intermandibular space as viewed from the external surface (see Fig. 26–6). The swellings represent squamous metaplasia of the salivary and mucous glands and hyperkeratosis resulting from chronic hypovitaminosis A. There may be a secondary bacterial component in some cases. Aspiration of the lesions produces a thick, white caseous material. Cytology of the sample typically shows cornified squamous epithelial cells without inflammation.[12] Mild cases respond to vitamin supplementation, but in advanced cases, the swellings interfere with normal alimentation.

Lance and debride the lesions under sedation. Administer parenteral vitamin A and recommend diet changes to prevent recurrence of these lesions. In general, prognosis is good.

Avian Pox

Avian pox infection (*Avipoxvirus*) in the "wet form" or the diphtheroid form results in lesions in the oropharyngeal cavity. Exudative lesions of the oral mucosa form initially. These lesions often become secondarily infected and appear as caseous plugs and swellings or plaques in the choana and through-

out the oropharynx. Affected birds may have concurrent involvement of the unfeathered skin around the eyes and beak. Amazon parrots are particularly susceptible to the diphtheritic form of pox virus infection, especially recently imported birds.[13, 14] These birds often present with dysphagia and can be dyspneic if the larynx becomes affected. Base the diagnosis on history, clinical signs, and biopsy of affected tissues. Presence of intracytoplasmic inclusion bodies called "Bollinger bodies" is characteristic of pox virus.[15]

Treatment for pox is supportive and symptomatic; consider antibiotics for secondary infections, supplemental vitamin A, and topical treatment. Severely affected individuals may succumb despite therapy. Virus shedding is associated with active lesions; isolate all affected birds during treatment. Because mosquitoes are the primary means of carrier transmission, vector control is important in the prevention of psittacine pox. Vaccinate susceptible individuals.[16, 17] Important differential diagnosis for the oral pox lesions includes bacterial infections, hypovitaminosis A, candidiasis, and trichomoniasis. Consider Amazon tracheitis virus (herpes virus) in Amazon parrots that also have dyspnea.[18]

Candidiasis

Candidiasis, caused by *Candida albicans,* can form plaques or thickened, exudative mucosal lesions. The plaques adhere to the mucosal surfaces and are difficult to remove with a cotton swab. Young birds are most susceptible to yeast infections; however, certain conditions can predispose adult birds to gastrointestinal candidiasis. Prolonged antibiotic therapy, malnutrition, poor sanitation, and concurrent illness predispose to overgrowth of *Candida.*

Swab the lesions and do a Gram's stain to obtain a preliminary diagnosis; submit affected tissue for biopsy and culture. Initiate treatment immediately. There are several antifungal agents effective against *Candida.* (See Chapter 20, Mycotic Diseases.) Diluted chlorhexidine (Nolvasan, Fort Dodge, 0.5 ml/ 8 oz drinking water) is useful in the drinking water in very mild infections or as a preventive measure in susceptible individuals.[19] Nystatin is usually effective and nontoxic but it must come in contact with the yeast to be effective and is not absorbed from the gastrointestinal tract. An oral suspension is available (Mycostatin, Apothecon) but it is a large dose (1 ml/300 g body weight) and distasteful; consider using another antifungal in the larger species. The author prepares a concentrated ketoconazole suspension (50 mg/ml) by crushing the tablets (Nizoral, Janssen) into a buffered microcrystalline cellulose suspending agent (Ora-Plus, Paddock Laboratories) that can be readily dosed in smaller volumes (15–25 mg/kg orally twice daily). Fluconazole (Diflucan, Roerig; 2–5 mg/kg orally twice daily)[20] or flucytosine (Ancoban, Roche; 50–75 mg/kg PO q 12 hours) can be used in resistant infections. Be careful when using the azole drugs or flucytosine because of their potential toxicity.

Abscesses and Granulomas

Abscesses and granulomas can form in the oropharyngeal cavity. These are usually the result of hypovitaminosis A or pox virus infections (see Fig. 26–6). Gram-negative bacteria are most common; however, gram-positive organisms and anaerobes can play a role. *Mycobacterium* species can result in oral granulomas.[21] Caseous plugs in the cranial aspect of the choanal opening are usually associated with chronic sinusitis and may be of bacterial or fungal (*Candida* species or *Aspergillus* species) origin. Obtain samples from these lesions for cytologic evaluation and culture and sensitivity testing. Request acid-fast stains (Ziehl-Neelsen) if mycobacteriosis is suspected.

Trichomoniasis

Trichomonas gallinae infection occurs in psittacine birds, including budgerigars, cockatiels, and Amazon parrots.[22–26] It is a common problem in pigeons, doves, and raptors ("frounce"). *T. gallinae* is a flagellated protozoan that affects the upper gastrointestinal tract and upper respiratory system. Oral lesions consist of white or yellow plaques, exudates, or nodules in the oropharynx. Infection also involves the esophagus and crop in some birds and can result in crop thickening and stasis. Regurgitation, dysphagia, and poor weight gains are a result. Dyspnea occurs with laryngeal or tracheal involvement.

Diagnosis is straightforward; make a direct wet mount immediately after sampling to check for protozoal motility. Perform a Gram's stain on the sample to identify concurrent bacterial and fungal overgrowth. Culture and sensitivity testing are recommended for all lesions. Treat with antiprotozoal agents; metronidazole suspensions (Flagyl, Searle, 10–30 mg/kg orally twice daily) can be prepared for oral use or carnidazole tablets (Spartrix, Wildlife Laboratories) can be used in pigeons or raptors.

Capillaria Infections

Oropharyngeal lesions are sometimes caused by *Capillaria* species, which are thread-like nematodes that burrow into the mucosa of the oropharynx, the esophagus, and the crop. Diphtheritic lesions may result from severe infection in the gallinaceous birds. Capillariasis is rarely a problem in domestically raised companion species.

Neoplasias

Neoplasia of the oropharyngeal cavity is uncommon. Sporadic reports include a fibrosarcoma in the oral cavity of a budgerigar[27] and primary squamous cell carcinoma of the tongue and pharynx in Galliformes.[28, 29] Choanal lymphosarcoma was seen in an Amazon parrot in the author's practice. Papillomas can occur throughout the gastrointestinal tract of psittacines, including the oropharyngeal cavity.[30, 31] South American parrots (Amazons and macaws) are particularly susceptible to these benign growths. Biopsy any unusual lesion or growth for a definitive diagnosis.

Trauma

Trauma to the oropharynx can occur from defective toys, foreign body ingestion, cagemate fighting, and the consumption of very hot foods or chemical toxins. Unsupervised psittacines may suffer electric burns from chewing on electric cords, often associated with charred or blackened facial feathers. Strings can be found wrapped around the lower beak or tongues in Galliformes or Columbiformes. Clinical signs of oral trauma include beak rubbing, scratching at the mouth, gaping or "yawning," and dysphagia. Tongue lacerations tend to bleed profusely. Treatment of traumatic oral lesions includes suturing of tongue lacerations, wound debridement, and supportive care.

The approach to oropharyngeal lesions is relatively straightforward. The most important differentials include candidiasis, hypovitaminosis A, trichomoniasis, pox virus, and bacterial infections (Table 26–1). Biopsy all lesions and submit samples for culture and sensitivity testing. Make slides for special staining and cytologic examination. On initial presentation, take a sample for a direct wet mount and a Gram's stain and consider a quick stain (Diff-Quik, American Scientific Products). Initiate therapy based on these findings while awaiting laboratory results. A fresh wet mounted specimen must be viewed immediately to check for flagellate motility associated with trichomoniasis. In severe cases, hospitalize the bird for daily debridement, parenteral antibiotics, and supportive care (gavage feeding and fluids as needed).

DISORDERS OF THE ESOPHAGUS AND CROP

The primary function of the crop is food storage, and, in some species, the softening and swelling of food. Crop problems are common in clinical avian practice (Tables 26–2 and 26–3). Clinical signs almost always include regurgitation, anorexia, gaping ("yawning"), and dysphagia. Some birds are dyspneic from aspiration of crop contents. Crop disor-

Table 26–2

MAJOR CAUSES OF CROP STASIS IN NEONATES

- Improper formula preparation
    Improper consistency (too thick or thin)
    Improper temperature
- Crop burns (microwave)
- Improper ambient temperature
- Substrate ingestion (wood shavings, corn cobs)
- Bacterial overgrowth (especially gram-negative)
- Candidiasis
- Trichomoniasis
- Acute viral diseases
    Polyomavirus
    Herpes virus (Pacheco's disease)
- Systemic disease
    Sepsis
    Viremia
    Renal or hepatic failure

Table 26–3

MAJOR CAUSES OF CROP STASIS IN ADULT BIRDS

- Goiter in budgerigars
- Trichomoniasis
- Candidiasis
- Bacterial ingluvitis (gram-negative)
- Lead poisoning
- Proventricular dilatation syndrome
- Outflow obstruction
    Neoplasia
    Foreign body
    Ingluvolith
- Systemic disease
    Renal failure
    Hepatic failure
    Peritonitis
    Sepsis
    Viremia
    Pancreatitis

ders can be primary or secondary. Although more common in juveniles, they can occur in birds of all ages.

Crop Stasis

The impairment of the normal motility of the crop results in crop stasis. The crop area may be visibly enlarged or may be obscured by the thick feathering surrounding the neck. It is important to palpate and visualize the crop to rule out a ruptured cervicocephalic air sac or lipomatous deposit, that can resemble an enlarged crop. The static crop may contain a variety of material from ingested food or foreign bodies to an accumulation of fluid and mucus.

Part the feathers and swab the skin with an alcohol-soaked cotton ball to view the external crop. Transillumination with a bright penlight reveals crop contents (Fig. 26–7). Be careful during manipulation of a bird with crop stasis; palpation of a fluid-filled crop can result in regurgitation during the examination and can increase the risk of aspiration of crop contents. Minimize handling of any bird actively regurgitating or vomiting.

Neonates

Crop stasis in neonates is common in psittacines and is related to improper management, infection,

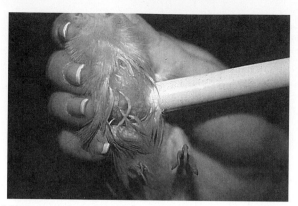

Figure 26-7

Transillumination of an enlarged crop with a bright penlight in this budgerigar reveals seeds and fluid.

dehydration, or metabolic imbalances (see chapters on pediatrics and hand-raising). In healthy baby birds, the crop empties regularly; however, improper preparation and administration of formula can result in delayed emptying of the crop. The crop of these birds remains visibly and palpably distended for prolonged periods. Regurgitation is common. Foods that are too cool, too high in fat, or too thick may result in slow crop transit time. Formula that remains in the crop for prolonged periods becomes rancid from fungal and bacterial overgrowth and results in "sour crop" and eventually complete crop stasis. Affected birds become dehydrated, and what begins as a primary mechanical crop disorder can very quickly result in serious systemic disease.

Crop impaction can occur with hand-feeding formulas, especially those too rich in particulate matter or not prepared with adequate amounts of water. The thin or liquid portion of the formula passes readily from the crop, leaving behind a very thick and doughy material that remains in the crop. Warm water crop gavages and gentle massaging can restore crop motility and may help to prevent secondary ingluvitis and dehydration.

Chicks kept on wood shavings or corn cob bedding materials are susceptible to substrate ingestion. Ingested bedding material can result in partial blockage of the crop and delayed emptying of crop contents. Transilluminate the crop with a bright light source to reveal the foreign material for identification. Some small particles may pass through the digestive tract without assistance. To remove a large

foreign body, manipulate the object back up the esophagus and retrieve it with a forceps. If it is not retrievable, perform an ingluvotomy for surgical removal (see Chapter 41, Soft Tissue Surgery).

Delayed crop emptying time and crop stasis are nonspecific signs in the very young bird and do not indicate the extent or severity of disease. In some acute viral infections (e.g., polyoma virus and herpes virus [Pacheco's disease]), crop stasis may be the only clinical sign noted prior to death. The clinician must therefore distinguish between management error and infectious disease in birds that are hand-fed. Obtain a detailed history from the owner or breeder including specifics regarding formula preparation and feeding intervals.

Bacterial and Mycotic Infections

Bacterial and mycotic ingluvitis often occur concurrently and may be primary or secondary. Crop stasis often results in the overgrowth of gram-negative bacteria and yeast (*Candida* species). Severe infection can lead to dehydration, anorexia, and systemic disease. Evaluate the crop for microbial overgrowth by culture and sensitivity testing and Gram's stains of swabs or fluid taken from the crop. Budding yeast bodies are easy to identify on a Gram's stain; hyphae formation indicates tissue invasion and the need for systemic antifungal therapy (see Color Fig. 26–8).[3]

Trichomonas Infection

Trichomoniasis can result in crop stasis, especially in Columbiformes, raptors, budgerigars, and cockatiels.[12, 22, 23, 25, 32] Juvenile and adult birds can be affected, although infections tend to be more extensive in the immune-incompetent young. Exudative lesions can form in the oropharyngeal cavity as well as in the esophagus, crop, and respiratory system. Direct wet mounts and microscopic examination of a crop swab or aspirate readily reveal the motile flagellates.

Thyroid Gland Enlargements

Thyroid gland enlargements can result in crop emptying disorders in mature budgerigars. A low iodine diet predisposes the bird to the development of goiter or thyroid gland hyperplasia. This can result in the accumulation of thick, mucoid liquid in the crop with subsequent crop distension, stasis, and regurgitation (Fig. 26–9). Goiter has been reported in cockatiels but is generally uncommon in other psittacine species.[33] Thyroid adenomas and adeno-carcinoma are uncommon but can occur.[27] Diagnosis is most often made based on clinical signs and signalment (i.e., a middle-age budgerigar on an unsupplemented seed diet presents with crop stasis and regurgitation). Thyroid gland enlargement cannot be palpated and can rarely be seen radiographically. Treatment consists of iodine supplementation and crop management. (See Management of Crop Stasis.)

Lead Poisoning

Lead intoxication impairs gastrointestinal motility and can result in crop stasis. Lead poisoning is a common toxicity reported in both caged and wild birds.[34–38] High levels of ingested lead can lead to crop stasis, regurgitation, anorexia, hemoglobinuria (Amazon parrots and cockatiels especially), polyuria, and variable neurologic effects. Diagnosis is based on a history of foreign body ingestion and elevated blood lead levels (>20 μg/dl). Radiographs can be helpful if the ingested metal is still in the gastrointestinal tract.

Begin chelation therapy with injectable agents (calcium ethylenediamine tetraacetic acid [EDTA],

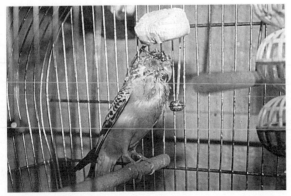

F i g u r e 2 6 – 9

The feathers around the head and neck are matted together from regurgitated fluid in this budgerigar with crop stasis.

30 mg/kg subcutaneously [SC] every 12 hours) and administer supportive care immediately while awaiting the return of laboratory blood results. Acute lead poisoning is an emergency; affected birds are in critical condition and can deteriorate quickly. Polyuria, regurgitation, and crop stasis result in rapid dehydration, and aggressive fluid therapy is indicated. Although potentially toxic, EDTA therapy is relatively benign except for the associated painful injection. Oral chelation therapy with D-penicillamine twice daily or dimercaptosuccinic acid (DMSA) can be used when the bird's condition is stabilized and normal gastrointestinal motility resumes. (See Chapter 35, Toxic Diseases.)

Proventricular Dilatation Syndrome

Proventricular dilatation syndrome (PDS) describes a condition that results in myenteric ganglioneuritis and the subsequent disruption of gastric motility (see later). Although it is essentially a disease of the proventriculus, affected birds may develop crop stasis. Clinical signs of PDS may mimic those of lead poisoning. Diagnosis is based on clinical signs, radiographic findings, proventricular or ventricular biopsy, and lack of significant response to treatment.

Foreign Bodies

Foreign bodies can result in crop stasis or impaction. Foreign body ingestion occurs in uncaged psittacines and Galliformes most commonly. Ingluvioliths can form in the crop of companion birds; the cause for this formation is speculative.[39, 40] Remove foreign matter surgically by ingluvotomy.

Tumors

Tumors of the crop and esophagus are uncommon. Papillomatous lesions can occur throughout the gastrointestinal mucosa, including the crop and esophagus. Internal papillomas occur most frequently in macaws and Amazon parrots.[31] Leiomyosarcoma[27] and squamous cell carcinoma have been reported in psittacines.[41, 42] Clinical signs include intermittent regurgitation, difficulty swallowing, and poor weight gain. Affected birds do not always have obvious clinical signs or palpable tumors and may require contrast radiographs or endoscopy to diagnose an intraluminal lesion.[41, 43] Biopsy is required for definitive diagnosis.

Extraluminal neoplasms can be seen in the area of the crop. Complete obstruction of the crop is rare, but it is important to recognize the occurrence of masses that may initially appear to be intraluminal. The author has had a case of a thymic branchial cyst in a lovebird and another incidence in a parrot of lymphosarcoma that appeared to be within the crop on initial presentation.

Management of Crop Stasis

Crop stasis and impactions require hospitalization for crop management and supportive care. Affected birds can be very debilitated and must be handled carefully. Be especially cautious during jugular venipuncture; these birds are at a risk for regurgitation and aspiration when excessively manipulated. Actively regurgitating birds should not be handled.

Therapy involves treatment of the crop while treating or correcting the initiating factors. Remove crop contents by gentle gavage with warm water with a soft feeding tube or metal gavage needle. Congealed or curdled formula can be broken up with gentle external massage of the crop and multiple flushings. Be careful not to aspirate too aggressively; the mucosal lining of the crop can be damaged from excessive suction along the crop wall. Culture crop contents and make slides for further evaluation. Examine a fresh wet mounted specimen to check for flagellate activity and a Gram's stain to assess bacterial populations and candidal overgrowth. When the crop is empty, it is much easier and safer to perform jugular venipuncture. The minimal data base consists of a hemogram and a plasma biochemistry profile; consider ancillary diagnostics such as chlamydial testing, blood lead analysis, and polyomavirus antigen testing (Avian Research Associates, Milford, OH). Radiographs are sometimes indicated. Contrast radiography can help to evaluate the gastrointestinal tract for lesions, obstructions, foreign bodies and to access gastrointestinal transit time.

Administer oral antibiotics and antifungals into the empty crop for local effects on microbial overgrowths. Nystatin oral suspension is effective for most mild cases of candidiasis and can be safely used for prolonged periods. Consider using a ketoconazole or fluconazole suspension in more extensive fungal infections (see Candidiasis, earlier). Parenteral antibiotics must be administered if the crop is static; choose a broad-spectrum drug with good activity against gram-negative bacteria. Carnidazole or a metronidazole suspension can be used for flagellates. Fluids are usually administered subcutaneously, but they can also be given intraosseously with a butterfly catheter in small chicks or an indwelling catheter in larger birds. Administer oral fluids if the crop is moving. Tube-feed small, frequent amounts of a diluted, balanced, low-residue, lactose-free liquid diet (Deliver, Mead Johnson). Intestinal motility stimulants can be a useful adjunct to therapy. Parenteral metoclopramide (Reglan, A.H. Robins, 0.5 mg/kg intramuscularly every 8–12 hours), although associated with potential side effects, has been safely used in neonates and adults with some success.

Refractory cases of crop stasis can be managed with the surgical placement of a proventricular or duodenal feeding tube (see Chapter 41, Soft Tissue Surgery).[44] Total parenteral nutrition should be considered in protracted cases; however, very little research has been done in this area in pet avian species.[45, 46]

CROP AND ESOPHAGEAL TRAUMA

Most cases of crop or esophageal traumatic injuries involve hand-fed juvenile psittacines. Punctures and burns are often the result of improper hand-feeding techniques. Foreign bodies can also potentially result in perforations if not retrieved in a timely manner. Poultry tend to pick up metal objects, fishing hooks are a problem in waterfowl, and raptors are susceptible to perforating bones. Puncture wounds of the crop and esophagus can occur from dog or cat bites. Lacerations are sometimes seen in racing pigeons that collide with inanimate objects (antennae, wires). Diagnosis is relatively straightforward; gently pluck or cut back some of the surrounding feathers to reveal the full extent of the trauma.

Punctures

Pharyngeal and esophageal punctures are most common in baby birds fed by a syringe or a feeding tube. Some species of birds (e.g., macaws) are vigorous feeders that actively "pump" their heads and necks during a feeding response. Catheter-tipped syringes can puncture the pharyngeal wall in the back of the mouth, and formula may be deposited into the soft tissues surrounding the neck. Feeding tubes can puncture the esophagus or crop or be swallowed by the bird. Perforating pharyngeal and esophageal injuries can result in extensive soft tissue damage. Affected birds may develop swelling, erythema, and edema of the neck and crop area. If a large amount of food is deposited outside the alimentary tract, immediate surgical intervention is required to flush out affected areas and control cellulitis and infection. Unsuspecting owners may not initially realize the severity of the injury until the bird becomes depressed and anorectic. Prognosis depends on the severity of the puncture, the amount of food involved, and the length of time prior to surgical repair. The presence of extensive cellulitis, edema, adhesions, and congealed formula greatly obscures normal anatomy, and surgery can be quite difficult in some birds.

Burns

Thermal burns of the esophagus and crop are common in baby birds. This is a direct result of overheating the formula or from "hot spots" in microwaved formula that is not thoroughly mixed. Damage to the crop mucosa results in delayed emptying of crop contents. With mild burns, edema and erythema may form over the external crop surface and resolve spontaneously. Severe burns result in crop fistulas. Birds often present for discolored feathers over the crop from formula leakage onto the neck feathers. A scab usually forms over the crop burn. When the scab is displaced or removed, formula leaks from the fistula and onto the feathers. Surgery is necessary when the fistula is open and leaking. These cases are not considered emergencies, but surgical repair of the crop is necessary to prevent slow weight gains, prolonged weaning times, and secondary crop infections.

Prognosis depends on the severity and extent of damage to the crop. Acute burns are difficult to assess and need to be observed until healthy tissue can be readily delineated from devitalized areas. Surgical intervention is indicated. Some burns are so extensive that very little viable crop tissue is available for surgical repair, and prognosis in these cases is poor.

REGURGITATION

Regurgitation is defined as the expulsion of material from the mouth or esophagus, and, in avian species, from the crop. Vomiting is the expulsion of material from the stomach (proventriculus and ventriculus) and/or intestines. Regurgitation can be normal or it can signal the onset of crop or systemic disease. It is ideal to be able to differentiate between regurgitation and vomiting, but this is not always clinically possible in birds. Many avian clinicians use these two terms interchangeably. For the purpose of clinically evaluating an avian patient, it seems impractical to approach regurgitation and vomiting as two separate diseases.

The first step in the workup of the regurgitating bird is to first establish that a problem exists. Behavioral regurgitation is common in many avian species (Tables 26–4, 26–5). Some birds regurgitate to their owners, toys, or cagemates as a sign of courtship. Others may regurgitate from the stress of traveling, excess handling, or excitement. Birds of prey typically regurgitate or "cast up" the undigestible components of a recent meal. Pigeons and doves produce a "crop milk" that is regurgitated to their

---

Table 26–4

CAUSES OF REGURGITATION IN JUVENILE BIRDS

- Fear and excitement
- Overfilling of crop
- Shrinkage of crop during weaning
- Improper formula temperature
- Improper formula consistency
- Crop burns
- Crop stasis (see Table 26–3)
- Candidiasis
- Trichomoniasis
- Bacterial ingluvitis
- Foreign matter ingestion (substrate)
- Acute viremia
    Polyoma virus
    Herpes virus (Pacheco's disease)

Table 26–5

CAUSES OF REGURGITATION IN ADULT BIRDS

- Behavioral
    - Fear and excitement
    - Courtship behavior
    - Crop milk in pigeons
    - Cast formation in raptors
- Dietary indiscretion
    - Toxins
    - Plants
    - Spoiled food
    - Foreign material
- Motion sickness
- Goiter in budgerigars
- Food allergy
- Proventricular dilatation syndrome
- Lead poisoning
- Crop stasis (see Table 26–3)
- Gastroenteritis
    - Protozoa (coccidians, flagellates)
    - Megabacterium (budgies; canaries)
    - Candidiasis (*C. albicans*)
    - Bacteria (gram-negative)
- Medications (especially sulfa drugs, doxycycline, ketoconazole)
- Gastrointestinal obstruction
    - Stricture
    - Grit impaction
    - Enterolith
    - Neoplasia
    - Parasites
    - Intussusception
    - Torsion/volvulus
    - Koilin degeneration
    - Paralytic ileus
    - Foreign body
- Systemic/metabolic disease
    - Hyperuricemia
    - Pancreatitis
    - Peritonitis
    - Hepatopathy
    - Egg-binding
    - Sepsis

young. Baby birds may regurgitate if overfed or during weaning as the crop size begins to decrease. Signalment and a detailed history can determine if there is a behavioral pattern associated with episodes of regurgitation.

Crop and Esophageal Disorders

Crop and esophageal disorders often result in regurgitation (see earlier and Tables 26–2, 26–3). When behavioral causes have been ruled out, the next step is to thoroughly evaluate the crop as the source of the problem. Any factor that results in crop irritation or dysfunction can lead to regurgitation. Some birds may regurgitate from the administration of oral medications (e.g., macaws on doxycycline, sulfa drugs, and ketoconazole.)[47, 48] Food allergy, although poorly documented, is a potential cause of regurgitation. Dietary indiscretion, foreign body ingestion, ingluvitis, crop impaction, and crop stasis often present with regurgitation. Neoplasia or papillomas of the oropharyngeal cavity, esophagus, and crop may result in intermittent episodes of regurgitation. Goiter in budgerigars is a common cause of chronic regurgitation in this species. Free-flighted psittacines are at a higher risk for foreign body ingestion with subsequent regurgitation and dysphagia. An esophageal stricture has been reported

to cause chronic regurgitation in a macaw.[49] Helminths (e.g., *Capillaria*) must be considered in non-psittacine species.

Gastric Disorders

Gastric disorders can lead to regurgitation and vomiting (see later). Any condition that results in the decreased motility of the proventriculus or ventriculus can, in turn, result in crop and esophageal motility disorders. An example is the motility dysfunction that occurs with proventricular dilatation syndrome. Lead intoxication can also result in a static gut with secondary crop involvement. Gastric disorders are commonly caused by gram-negative overgrowth, megabacteria in budgerigars and canaries, viral infection, toxin or plant ingestion, heavy metal intoxication, candidiasis, protozoal infection, and neoplasia. Outflow obstructions caused by neoplasia, foreign material, grit impaction, and enteroliths are possible. A localized proventricular lesion can be difficult to diagnose and identify as the source of the problem. Radiographs can determine luminal obstructions, dilatation, or gas in the proventriculus. Surgical biopsies of the proventriculus or ventriculus can be performed for a definitive diagnosis if primary gastric lesions are suspected.

Metabolic Disorders

Metabolic disorders can cause regurgitation. Hyperuricemia, hepatopathies, pancreatitis, peritonitis, and reproductive tract dysfunctions are important differential diagnoses in the regurgitating bird. It is important to screen for systemic diseases when evaluating the regurgitating bird, especially in chronic cases or debilitated patients.

Management of Regurgitation

The initial diagnosis of regurgitation is based on history and physical examination. A detailed history should include possible foreign body exposure (is the bird out of the cage unattended?), inappropriate food (avocado? plants?), and the administration of medication or supplements (grit or over-the-counter medications?). During the physical examination, the crop must be carefully palpated. It may feel normal or may be thickened or distended, or may contain ingested matter. The presence of food in the crop does not indicate disease unless the bird has been anorexic. Transillumination of the crop with a bright light source can reveal crop contents for identification (see Fig. 26–7). Chronically regurgitating birds often have dried material pasted to the head and facial feathers. It is typical to see, for example, the budgerigar with goiter with the head feathers matted together from regurgitated crop fluid (see Fig. 26–9). The bird may appear healthy or may be thin from chronic disease.

The crop can be evaluated through cytologic examination of crop contents or a swab of the crop mucosa. If there is fluid in the crop, use a metal feeding needle or a soft red rubber tube to aspirate the fluid for analysis and empty the crop. Place a drop of crop aspirate on a glass slide for immediate microscopic examination for flagellates (*Trichomonas* specie). Another slide can be examined with Gram's stain to check for bacterial overgrowths and yeast infections (*Candida* species). Submit abnormal crop fluid for culture and sensitivity testing. If fluid cannot be palpated in the crop, flush the crop using a small volume of sterile water or saline to obtain samples. The crop mucosa can be swabbed with a cotton-tipped swab for most medium-sized birds. In small birds, a smaller tipped cotton swab can be used (Mini-tip Culturette, Becton-Dickin-

son). Use a speculum during a crop swab or flush in larger birds to prevent chewing on the swab or feeding tube.

Full-body radiographs are recommended for the regurgitating bird. Empty the crop before radiographs are taken to avoid the possibility of aspiration. These birds must also be carefully monitored for regurgitation when recumbent or sedated for radiographic positioning. The administration of contrast (barium or iohexol) can help to delineate the gastrointestinal tract, evaluate for intraluminal or mural lesions, and assess transit time. Always take survey radiographs first to evaluate for ingested foreign material. It may be difficult to detect subtle mural lesions radiographically. A rigid or flexible endoscope can be used for further examination of the crop and proventriculus in larger species.

Whenever possible, laboratory testing should be done to rule out metabolic or systemic disease. Screening tests include a hemogram and plasma biochemistry analysis. Consider ancillary diagnostic tests such as blood lead levels, plasma bile acids, plasma electrophoresis, urinalysis, and *Chlamydia* testing.

Treatment of regurgitation disorders depends on the general condition of the bird and initial diagnosis. Acute regurgitation in an otherwise healthy bird can be managed on an outpatient basis in most cases. Chronically regurgitating birds are hospitalized for tests and supportive care. Crop stasis or impaction is often accompanied by dehydration and debilitation. These birds must be handled carefully. Always keep in mind that an ill bird may not initially appear "sick" and it may be better to hospitalize than to send home a critical case. One or two episodes of regurgitation may signal the onset of severe systemic disease; the condition of some of these birds can deteriorate quickly.

GASTRIC DISORDERS—THE PROVENTRICULUS AND VENTRICULUS

The avian stomach consists of two parts: the glandular stomach or proventriculus, and the caudal ventriculus (gizzard) or muscular stomach. The proventriculus is continuous with the esophagus and is the site of gastric juice secretion. The koilin, or cuticle, is a hardened membrane that covers the surface epithelium of the gizzard. It is a carbohydrate-protein complex that is constantly wearing away and being replaced. The stomach of the bird varies according to diet; carnivores and piscivores or soft food eaters differ anatomically and physiologically from herbivores and granivores (seedeaters) that feed on relatively indigestible matter.[10] Baby birds on formula feeds, fruit and nectar eaters, and anorexic birds on tube feedings may have a slightly dilated proventriculus as a result of the diet. This distinction becomes important when evaluating a particular species for gastric disorders, (e.g., radiographically these two groups differ significantly, and what might appear to be pathologic for one species may be normal for another). In general, most of the pet bird species are granivorous, including psittacines, passerines, Columbiformes, and Galliformes. Lories and lorikeets are nectar-eating species.

Clinical signs of gastric disorders vary. Birds can present with mild inappetence or anorexia; weight loss is common. Vomiting is often a feature of gastric disorders, especially when motility disruptions or outflow obstructions occur. Gastric ulceration can lead to melena and anemia. Occasionally, a mild malaise may be followed by sudden death if gastric bleeding is acute and extensive. Diarrhea and maldigestion may be seen. It is difficult to isolate a specific gastric condition based on clinical evaluation because of the complexity of the avian two-part stomach, the likelihood of concurrent disease, and the ability of birds to mask signs of illness. There are, however, several diseases of clinical importance that affect the avian stomach, and these are discussed later and in other sections of this book.

Proventricular Dilatation Syndrome

This syndrome, also called neuropathic gastric dilatation, myenteric ganglioneuritis, and splanchnic neuropathy, is a relatively common disease seen in psittacine birds. PDS results in the dilatation and progressive dysfunction of the proventriculus of affected birds. It is characterized by regurgitation, progressive weight loss ("wasting"), weakness, passage of improperly digested food (seeds) in the feces, and lack of response to therapy. Some birds have concurrent neurologic signs that include limb weakness, ataxia, and difficulty perching.[50-52] Histo-

logically, birds suffer from mononuclear (plasmacytic and lymphocytic) infiltration of the splanchnic nerves of the muscular tunics of the proventriculus, ventriculus, and sometimes the crop or duodenum.[31, 50-54] Nonsuppurative encephalitis, myelitis, and radiculoneuritis can also occur concurrently or, in some cases, prior to the onset of gastrointestinal signs.

The cause of the syndrome is unknown but speculated to be viral in origin; evidence suggestive of a paramyxovirus[52, 55] or togavirus[56] have been reported. One report suggests the possibility of a relationship between PDS and a recently recognized disease of neonates and juvenile psittacines, avian viral serositis.[56] Repeated attempts to identify and confirm an infectious agent have failed. The etiology of PDS is still unclear, but histologic and epidemiologic evidence exists to suggest the possibility of an infectious agent. Aviary outbreaks have been reported,[57] but these are usually sporadic and not all exposed birds develop the disease.

Although most commonly reported in cockatoos and macaws, many different psittacine species have been reported with the disease, and all psittacines should be considered at risk.[50, 52-54, 57] Although more commonly seen in young birds in the author's practice, birds of any age can be affected. Initial clinical signs can be weight loss, or birds can present with the classic signs of regurgitation, undigested seeds in the droppings, and variable neurologic signs. Some birds have neurologic signs before gastrointestinal disease is evident. Other conditions can mimic PDS (e.g., foreign body ingestion, lead or zinc poisoning, gastric neoplasia, bacterial or fungal proventriculitis, grit impaction, and koilin defects). Plasma biochemistry panels and hemogram results are often unremarkable.

The presumptive diagnosis of PDS is based on history, clinical signs, and radiographs. Survey radiographs may show a dilated proventriculus and ventriculus with variable amounts of gas and fluid. (See Fig. 13–26, Chapter 13, Radiology.) Contrast radiographs are often needed to delineate the proventriculus, rule out foreign bodies, and assess transit time. Early in the course of the disease, the proventriculus may appear radiographically normal; a prolonged transit time may be the first indication of a problem. Keep in mind that a dilated proventriculus can occur with other conditions and these must be ruled out. Baby birds on formula feedings

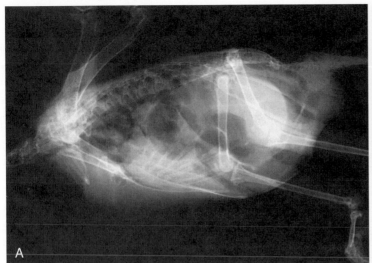

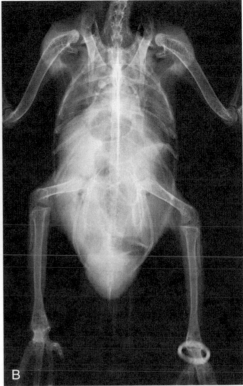

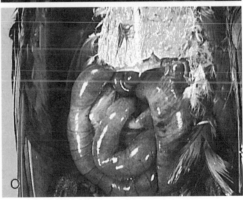

Figure 26–10

(*A* and *B*) Radiographs of a macaw with a generalized ileus. There is a large amount of gastrointestinal gas throughout the abdomen. *(C)* Necropsy of the macaw revealed distended, gas-filled intestines. The suspected cause was viral enteritis.

have a larger proventriculus than mature birds. Chronic dilatation may be related to generalized ileus secondary to infection or toxicosis (Fig. 26–10).[58] However, PDS is the main differential in a bird with typical clinical signs, relatively normal blood tests, and a lack of response to symptomatic treatment. Definitive ante mortem diagnosis can usually be made with proventricular or ventricular biopsy; however, this is not a benign procedure. The proventricular wall can be very thin, friable, and difficult to suture; postsurgical complications are common.[59] Full-thickness crop biopsy may show the characteristic lesions in some affected birds and poses fewer surgical risks.[61]

Prognosis is poor with PDS. Most birds exhibit a progressive, irreversible deterioration after clinical signs are noted. Supportive care includes fluids; metoclopramide or cisapride; parenteral antibiotics; oral antifungal agents; and small, frequent formula feedings. Duodenal or ventricular feeding tubes, which bypass the proventriculus, are sometimes used with variable success. The use of corticosteroids for the treatment of PDS is controversial and should only be considered after a definitive diagnosis has been made.

Neoplasia

Primary gastric neoplasia is sporadically reported in companion birds (see Chapter 34, Neoplasia). Proventricular or ventricular adenocarcinomas are the most commonly described malignancy, with lesions occurring most often at the isthmus or junction between the proventriculus and gizzard.[61] Most cases in the literature report its occurrence in psittacine species, with an unusually high rate of occurrence in the grey-cheeked parakeet (*Brotogeris pyrrhopterus*).[42, 58, 61–65]

Clinical signs of gastric neoplasia are variable. Neoplastic infiltration results in mucosal ulceration and blood vessel erosion. Anemia and weakness can be seen with chronic gastric bleeding. Sudden death from acute hemorrhage may be the only clinical sign. Chronic weight loss, vomiting, maldigestion (seeds in droppings), and melena are also possible. The lesions are not always grossly visible at necropsy, and histologic examination is necessary to distinguish neoplasia from inflammatory lesions.

Bacterial Infection

Bacterial proventriculitis can be primary or secondary. The normal alimentary tract flora of psittacines consists predominately of gram-positive rods and cocci, to include *Streptococcus, Lactobacillus, Bacillus,* and *Corynebacterium.*[66–68] Disruption of the normal alimentary tract flora by stress or disease can result in opportunistic bacterial overgrowth and secondary infections. The organisms most often implicated are the gram-negative bacteria of the Enterobacteriaceae (*Escherichia coli, Klebsiella, Salmonella, Enterobacter*) and the Pseudomonaceae (*Pseudomonas*).[69–73] Poor sanitation and hygiene, contaminated water and food supplies, use of wood or corn cob bedding, and exposure to other animals (such as rodents) can introduce bacterial contaminants into the environment. Stress, age, concurrent disease, and malnutrition can result in suppression of the immune system and can predispose an individual to infection.

Megabacteria infection of the proventriculus has been reported in budgerigars and canaries.[22, 66, 74] Inflammatory proventriculitis is caused by a very large rod-shaped gram-positive bacterium presently classified as megabacterium. Although very little information is available on its involvement in disease, it is considered an avian pathogen. Vomiting, chronic weight loss, and melena occur in affected birds. Ante mortem diagnosis is difficult, and response to treatment is poor.

Mycobacteriosis (*M. avium*) can affect the alimentary tract of birds. Although more typically seen in the intestines, proventricular lesions are possible.[75]

Koilin Disorders

Koilin erosions and dysgenesis can result in maldigestion, ulcerations or perforations, and outflow obstructions. In some species (e.g., magpies and starlings), it is normal for the koilin layer to be massively shed periodically in one piece. In the majority of birds, the koilin is worn away and continually replaced. Infectious, parasitic, and toxic agents can cause ulceration and deformation of the ventricular lining. Mycotic infections can result in degeneration of the koilin layer.[76] Exposure to high levels of zinc or copper is erosive to the gizzard and can cause necrosis and sloughing of the koilin layer.[77, 78] Zinc toxicosis in a macaw resulted in gastric outflow obstruction from ulceration and sloughing of the koilin.[79] Birds that are enclosed in poorly galvanized zinc cages are at a risk for zinc toxicosis ("new wire disease").[80, 81]

The definitive diagnosis of gastric disorders in birds can be difficult ante mortem. Radiographs are helpful in localizing a lesion within the gastrointestinal tract; in larger birds, endoscopy and biopsy are possible. Exploratory surgery can be performed if the bird's condition and size do not preclude a safe surgical approach. Although it is very difficult to ascertain the presence of a localized proventricular infection, the alimentary tract flora of an individual can be evaluated by culture and sensitivity of both crop and cloacal samples. Broad-spectrum antibiotics with activity against most enteric pathogens are used until the results of sensitivity testing are received.

DIARRHEA

Diarrhea is excessive water in the feces. Typically, in mammals, it is useful to classify diarrhea into small and large bowel types, depending on the origin of the problem. Although both small and large intestinal disorders occur in birds, it is impossible to make this distinction clinically and is probably of little significance therapeutically. Diarrhea may be best approached in avian species by dividing it into acute and chronic problems, and by evaluation of concurrent clinical signs. Even this type of classification can be problematic because multibird caging, aviary housing, and unobservant owners can obscure the onset of clinical signs.

The clinician must first establish that diarrhea is truly a problem. What many bird owners call "diarrhea" may actually be polyuria. Excess fruit or water-laden vegetables can result in a physiologic excess of urine in the droppings. Gout, diabetes mellitus, and other diseases can also result in polyuria, and any bird with watery droppings should be examined. One way to differentiate polyuria from diarrhea when speaking to concerned owners over the phone is to have them withhold fruit and vegetables for 2 days. If the problem persists, the bird must be seen.

Diarrhea has many causes in birds (Table 26–6) and it can take on a variety of appearances. Some simple causes to rule out include the use of medications, abrupt diet changes, plant or toxin ingestion, excitement or stress, and egg-laying. During the course of a day, a particular bird may normally have several different types of droppings. Most birds presented to the veterinarian for a clinical examination have some degree of diarrhea from excitement and travel to the clinic. Therefore, it is recommended that a sample of droppings from the cage bottom at home be brought along during a clinical evaluation. A detailed history is important to rule out management-related enteric disturbances.

Dietary Causes

Dietary indiscretion is a common cause of acute diarrhea in captive species. Free-flighted house pets, especially psittacines, are at a high risk of foreign object ingestion. Unsupervised birds may eat houseplants, painted walls, and human medications. Some "bonded" owners offer chocolate and alcohol to their birds. Backyard poultry flocks may pick up objects around the yard, especially metals and rocks. Heavy metal (lead and zinc) poisoning is common in birds and is often accompanied by diarrhea and other gastrointestinal signs. Overeating grit supplements can be a problem in some birds, especially in nutritionally compromised individuals that develop pica. It is important to obtain a thorough history that includes details on environment,

---

T a b l e 2 6 – 6

COMMON CAUSES OF DIARRHEA

• Excitement/stress	• Protozoal parasites
• Diet	*Giardia*
Food allergy	*Cryptosporidium*
Malnutrition	Coccidia
Rapid diet change	• Parasitic
Poor quality food	Nematodes
Dietary indiscretion	Flukes
• Bacterial diseases	Tapeworms
Gram-negative bacteria	• Pancreatitis
Mycobacteriosis (*M. avium*)	• Hepatitis
Chlamydiosis (*C. psittaci*)	• Renal disease
Megabacteria	• Foreign bodies
• Viral infections	• Gastrointestinal obstruction
Polyoma virus	• Ileus (paralytic)
Herpes virus	• Proventricular dilatation syndrome
Reovirus	• Lead poisoning
Paramyxovirus	• Toxin ingestion
• Candidiasis (*C. albicans*)	• Impending egg-laying
• Neoplasia	

housing, behavior, and supervision. Diagnosis is based on history, radiographs, and endoscopy in larger birds.

Bacterial Enteritis

The most common cause of diarrhea in pet avian species is bacterial infection. Most enteric pathogens belong to the gram-negative family Enterobacteriaceae. These bacteria are ubiquitous and are considered to be part of the normal gastrointestinal flora of humans, mammals, and even some species of birds. Other bacteria of clinical importance include *Pseudomonas* species, *Aeromonas* species, *Bordetella* species, and megabacterium. (See Chapter 18, Bacteriology.) *Clostridium* is an important intestinal pathogen and can result in ulcerative enteritis. Flock outbreaks have been reported.[66, 82] Salmonella infections are widespread in both captive and free-ranging avian populations. It is especially a problem in Galliformes, pigeons, and lories and lorikeets.[83] Some pathogens have zoonotic potential (e.g., *Chlamydia, Mycobacterium, Salmonella,* and *Yersinia*) and care must be taken in handling the feces of affected birds.

Enterobacteriaceae can function as primary or secondary pathogens; it is important to try to make this distinction clinically. Stress, malnutrition, poor hygiene, and concurrent disease often predispose birds to opportunistic bacterial overgrowth. Hypovitaminosis A may initiate a defect in the epithelial integrity of the gastrointestinal tract and favor conditions for opportunistic bacteria and yeast.

The diagnosis of bacterial diarrhea is based on culture and sensitivity testing and clinical evaluation of the bird. A fecal Gram's stain is useful for identifying bacterial populations and the presence of yeast. A Gram's stain does not always correlate with culture results and should not be done *in lieu* of culture and sensitivity testing. Although most gram-negative rods are potential pathogens, the presence of gram-negative bacteria on a fecal culture or Gram's stain is not always synonymous with disease. Certain bacteria can be cultured in the feces and may be of little or no significance in one bird but may cause disease in another (e.g., *E. coli, Enterobacter cloacae,* and *E. agglomerans*).[73, 84] Results of laboratory testing used in conjunction with the overall health assessment of the patient are important in deciding when and how aggressively to treat.

Mycobacteriosis

Mycobacteriosis is a disease of the alimentary tract of avian species. Transmission occurs primarily through the fecal-oral route. Because the main portal of entry is through the intestines, colonization occurs in the intestines and the viscera.[66] Clinical disease varies but typically consists of a chronic wasting disease despite a good appetite. It is often accompanied by diarrhea. Other clinical signs may include shifting leg lameness. Tubercle formation within the intestinal wall intermittently sheds the acid-fast organisms into the intestinal lumen. Fecal acid-fast staining has been suggested as a means of diagnosing mycobacteriosis[66, 85] but is unreliable because fecal shedding is intermittent.

Certain laboratory parameters can place avian mycobacteriosis high on a differential list; these include leukocytosis with monocytosis; elevated liver enzymes and bile acids; and anemia, with negative testing for chlamydiosis. Radiographic abnormalities are common and include hepatomegaly, splenomegaly, and/or a thickened intestinal wall. Diagnosis is based on the demonstration of acid-fast rods in tissue biopsies or in cytologic preparations; samples can be submitted for culture and typing of the organism. Touch preparations of tissue biopsies stained with DiffQuik may reveal numerous, clear, and almost refractile rod-shaped bacteria that do not take up stain properly ("ghosts"). Perform acid-fast staining (Ziehl-Neelsen) on all samples. Successful treatment has been reported[85, 86] but may not be recommended in some cases because of the zoonotic potential.

Chlamydia Infection

Chlamydiosis often results in yellow-green diarrhea (see Color Fig. 26–11D). *Chlamydia psittaci* is an obligate intracellular bacterial parasite that has a wide host spectrum among birds. It has zoonotic potential in humans. The acute systemic disease in birds is accompanied by anorexia, depression, watery droppings, and upper and lower respiratory tract infection. Subacute and protracted disease occurs with some less virulent strains and may result in progressive weight loss and chronic diarrhea. The chlamydial organism propagates within the epithelial cells at the site of entry, typically lung and air sacs or intestines. High numbers of organisms can be shed in the feces of affected birds; be careful when handling the droppings in suspect cases.

Candida Infection

Candidiasis is a common problem in birds. *Candida albicans* is an opportunistic organism that may be a normal inhabitant of the digestive tract. Infections most commonly involve the upper alimentary tract (oral cavity, crop, and esophagus), but gastrointestinal infection can also occur. Candidiasis often accompanies gastrointestinal flora upsets and is seen in birds with poor immune response, malnutrition, and concurrent disease. Diets high in carbohydrates or refined sugars (breads, cookies, crackers) may also predispose an otherwise healthy bird to candidal overgrowth. Overuse of antibiotics predisposes to candidiasis, especially in immature birds.

Diagnosis is made by demonstration of the budding organism on a fecal Gram's stain, and fecal mycotic culture. Monitor susceptible individuals with periodic Gram's stains. Administer prophylactic antifungal agents during antibiotic administration in juveniles or during long-term antibiotic therapy in mature birds.

Several therapeutic agents are available for the treatment of candidiasis. The choice of antifungal agent depends on the size and tractability of the bird as well as the severity of the infection. Nystatin suspension works well in hand-fed juvenile birds. It acts locally by direct contact and should be given prior to feeding when the crop is empty. Because nystatin is not absorbed, it is not recommended for use in systemic infections. Ketoconazole is an effective systemic antifungal agent with low toxicity; fluconazole or flucytosine is also effective. It is important to identify and correct the predisposing factors to prevent recurrence.

Protozoan Infections

Gastrointestinal protozoans are a common cause of diarrhea in many avian species. *Giardia* is the most important flagellate in the lower gastrointestinal tract of psittacines. Although many species of birds are at risk, incidence seems to be the highest in toucans and the smaller psittacines (e.g., budgerigars, lovebirds, and cockatiels).[87–91] The trophozoites inhabit the small intestine of affected birds and may result in the production of mucoid diarrhea. Some birds remain asymptomatic carriers and may intermittently shed the organism without showing clinical signs. Giardiasis can result in poor growth and high mortality in some budgerigar and cockatiel neonates. Feather picking has also been associated with intestinal infections in small psittacines.

Diagnosis of *Giardia* can sometimes be difficult. Demonstration of the cyst or trophozoite form on a direct fecal smear or on mucosal scrapings at necropsy is possible. Zinc sulfate fecal floats, enzyme-linked immunosorbent assay (ELISA) testing, and various staining techniques have been used in the detection of *Giardia* (see Chapter 21, Parasitology). Treatment with antiprotozoals is not always effective; resistance and reinfection are possible.

Cryptosporidium is a small intracellular coccidian that is a parasite of the gastrointestinal tract. Although uncommonly identified in clinical avian practice, gastrointestinal cryptosporidiosis has been reported in many species of pet birds including cockatiels, budgerigars, cockatoos, and finches.[92–96] *Cryptosporidium* can infect the salivary glands, proventriculus, small intestine, cecum, colon, and cloacal epithelium of birds.[93] Intestinal infection is associated with small intestinal villous atrophy, resulting in malassimilation and the production of osmotic diarrhea. Diarrhea may be acute and severe. Some birds show chronic weight loss without diarrhea. Diagnosis is made by demonstration of the organism in intestinal epithelium or the infective cysts in a fecal flotation. Modified acid-fast stains are useful for the detection of the oocysts in fecal samples.[97] Treatment is considered ineffective.

Other protozoan parasites can cause enteritis and diarrhea. Coccidiosis is common in canaries, finches, mynahs, toucans, lories, pigeons, and Galliformes.[98] *Isospora, Eimeria, Cryptosporidium,* and *Atoxoplasma* are the genera most often implicated in gastrointestinal disease in birds. Infections may result in severe disease or can be subclinical. Coccidian parasites are not as commonly identified in domestic psittacine birds.

Parasitic Infection

Gastrointestinal helminths are uncommon in domestic hand-raised pet psittacines. Helminths are more of a problem in Gallinaceous species, wild birds, imported birds, and birds maintained in outdoor enclosures. Infection can be subclinical or may result in diarrhea, poor weight gain, and mortality. Ascarids and *Capillaria* species are an important problem in imported macaws and, when present in high numbers, can lead to diarrhea, vomiting, and chronic weight loss.[98] Tapeworms are most commonly found in finches and Old World psittacines (African grey parrots, cockatoos, and eclectus parrots).[99] Tapeworm infections are relatively nonpathogenic but in high numbers can result in diarrhea, an unthrifty appearance, and impaction. Flukes are most commonly found in imported Old World psittacines, especially cockatoos. Hepatic trematodiasis may be associated with hepatomegaly, weight loss, diarrhea, and death.[89, 100, 101]

Parasitic infections can be diagnosed by fecal evaluation in the live bird or on postmortem evaluation. The identification of parasites in a fecal sample is not always indicative of disease; laboratory findings should correlate with clinical signs and concurrent problems should be identified. Treatment is recommended but not always effective.

Ileus

Ileus refers to the generalized impairment of intestinal motility and may be caused by inflammatory disorder, such as peritonitis or enteritis, or by neurogenic factors. The passage of feces is abnormal; there may be diarrhea or no feces at all. Vomiting is sometimes present. Neurogenic (paralytic) ileus results from motor impairment and can be seen with PDS or lead poisoning. Obstructive segmental ileus can result from foreign matter ingestion, enteroliths, mural lesions like granulomas or neoplasia, intussusception, and parasites.

Birds with ileus are in a crisis; the pooling of fluid into the intestines leads to rapid dehydration. Gram-negative bacterial overgrowth results in endotoxin release, shock, and depression. Ileus is not a common clinical entity in most pet bird species; however, it must be recognized early and appropriately managed. Rapid diagnosis and aggressive supportive therapy are important. Diagnosis can be made with survey radiographs (see Fig. 26–10); contrast films can outline a blockage and allow assessment of motility. Surgical correction of the obstruction may be indicated in some birds; these birds must first be rehydrated and their condition stabilized. Prognosis is poor in most cases.

Diagnostic Approach to Diarrhea

The first step in the diagnosis of a gastrointestinal problem is to obtain a very detailed and pointed history. Does the bird have free range? Does it have access to grit? Is the problem acute or chronic? Has the diet recently been changed? Is the bird acting sick? Is this a flock problem? Was this bird imported? Has she been laying eggs? Remember that most inexperienced bird owners do not always know what information is pertinent to the problem at hand. It is important to take a holistic approach with the avian patient; try to focus on the "big picture" by correlating other clinical signs with the history. A thin, scruffy bird with poor feathering on an all-seed diet is suffering from more than just diarrhea. Malnutrition, especially hypovitaminosis A, can predispose the bird to gastrointestinal upsets. Because the onset of diarrhea may indicate an underlying systemic or metabolic disease, it should not be overlooked as a simple problem until proved otherwise.

Feces Sampling

Evaluation of the feces is first in the workup of diarrhea. Visual examination is important; check dropping color, consistency (diarrhea or polyuria?), and texture (undigested seeds? grit?). Examine a direct wet mounted specimen immediately on a fresh sample to check for flagellate motility. If *Giardia* infection is suspected, use a drop of iodine on the slide to help elucidate the organism or collect several samples to submit for zinc sulfate flotation or ELISA testing. Perform a fecal Gram's stain on any bird with diarrhea. Culture and sensitivity testing is recommended in most cases, even if the Gram's stain appears normal. Fecal flotation can be done if parasites are suspected. Fecal acid-fast stains have reportedly been useful as an adjunct test in the workup of mycobacteriosis,[85] but the test is unreliable because of the intermittent shedding of the organism in the feces. This is also true with fecal antigen testing for *Chlamydia* and polyoma virus; these tests are simple to perform but not always reliable because of intermittent shedding of the organism.

Laboratory Testing

Laboratory testing is recommended even in acute diarrhea or in birds that do not appear "sick." Establish a minimum data base with a hemogram and plasma biochemistry analysis. Leukocytosis with monocytosis and heterophilia is typical of granulomatous diseases like chlamydiosis or mycobacteriosis. Eosinophilia is sometimes seen with *Giardia* infections or infection with other parasites. The evaluation of uric acid levels and liver enzymes is particularly important in the workup of watery droppings. Perform other diagnostic blood tests as needed; consider serology for *Chlamydia,* plasma electrophoresis, lead testing, and bile acids tests. Perform serologic titers for paramyxovirus (PMV-1) in pigeons with chronic diarrhea. (See Chapter 50, Columbiformes.) Evaluate concurrent problems as potentiating factors in the development of diarrhea. For example, psittacine beak and feather disease (circovirus) results in immune suppression and can predispose the affected individual to other infections like gastrointestinal cryptosporidiosis.[94] Several tests are available for the diagnosis of circovirus.

Radiographic Examination

Radiographs are especially important in cases of dietary indiscretion, obstruction, or organomegaly. Take survey films first to check for gastrointestinal foreign bodies; consider contrast studies to evaluate luminal contents, mural lesions, and transit time. Contrast radiographs are also helpful in the diagnosis of nonalimentary tract disease (e.g., renal neoplasia or egg yolk peritonitis). If possible, perform endoscopy or laparoscopy to obtain biopsies if a lesion is detected on radiographs.

Management of Diarrhea

Treatment of diarrhea is based on severity of disease, the overall health status of the patient, and the primary cause of illness. Acute, mild diarrhea in an otherwise healthy individual, without recent exposure to other birds, can be treated on an outpatient basis. If a fecal direct and Gram's stain is normal, and a bacterial enteritis is suspected, use a broad-spectrum antibiotic pending the results of fecal culture. If the bird's condition is stable, consider withholding medication until at least hematology and biochemistry profile results are available. Administer parenteral vitamin A to any bird on an inadequate diet (Injacom, Hoffman LaRoche). Supplement with *Lactobacillus* products (Aviguard, Pet Med Tech) if gastrointestinal flora upsets are suspected. Treat mild candidiasis with oral antifungal agents.

Hospitalization is recommended for birds with moderate or severe diarrhea and for those with a history of depression, anorexia, or lethargy. Many frightened birds look alert and "healthy" on physical examination; credence should be given in these cases to an owner's assessment of illness in the home environment. Sick birds require supportive care to include subcutaneous fluids, parenteral antibiotics, gavage feedings, and a quiet, warm environment. If acute lead poisoning is suspected, begin chelation therapy with calcium EDTA immediately. If the bird has a history of recent egg-laying, consider parenteral calcium. Give parenteral vitamin A and D_3 to a sick bird on a deficient diet. Take full-body radiographs when the bird's condition is stable.

BLOODY DROPPINGS

Bloody droppings have many possible etiologies in birds (Table 26-7). Because the cloaca represents a common opening, the source of the bleeding can be from the gastrointestinal, reproductive, or urinary tract. The majority of cases seen in clinical pet avian practice involves cloacal prolapses or cloacal lesions. Acute lead poisoning in some psittacine species (Amazon parrots, cockatiels) can cause the urates to appear "bloody" from hemoglobinuria (see Color Fig. 26-11B). Hepatic disease with con-

T a b l e   2 6 – 7

COMMON CAUSES OF BLOODY DROPPINGS

- Cloacal papillomas
- Cloacal neoplasia
- Cloacitis
- Egg-laying
- Prolapsed cloaca
- Prolapsed oviduct
- Hemorrhagic gastroenteritis
- Viral disease
    Herpes virus (Pacheco's disease)
    Polyoma virus
- Coagulopathies
    "Conure bleeding syndrome"
    Hepatopathy
    Disseminated intravascular coagulation (DIC)
- Lead poisoning
- Foreign body ingestion
- Renal neoplasia (uncommon)

current coagulopathy can result in indiscriminant hemorrhage.

"Conure bleeding syndrome" is thought to be a coagulation disorder that frequently appears in the acute onset of frank blood in the droppings. Hemorrhagic gastroenteritis is not commonly seen but when it occurs, *Salmonella* and *Clostridium* infections may be considered. Occasionally, "bloody droppings" are related to dietary pigments from foods like beets or cranberries. The presence of uncontrolled or abnormal bleeding in any bird should always be considered an emergency.

Prolapse of the Cloaca

Cloacal prolapses can involve intestines, cloaca, or oviduct. Increased abdominal pressure and cloacal irritation results in tenesmus and prolapse. Oviduct prolapse occurs in egg-laying hens and may be associated with deficient diets or abnormal eggs (See Chapter 36, Urogenital Disorders.) This is especially common in the smaller species (cockatiels, budgerigars, lovebirds) that lay multiple eggs in a clutch. Excessive sexual behavior can result in irritation and prolapse. Cockatoos sometimes develop chronic, intermittent cloacal prolapse from idiopathic straining.

Prolapses appear pink and shiny or may become hemorrhagic and edematous from exposure and self-trauma. There may be blood in the droppings or on the tip of the beak (see Fig. 26–10C). Straining

and constipation may occur and some birds may vocalize.

Treatment involves the identification and correction of the primary cause. A thorough cloacal examination is the initial diagnostic step. Consider further examination under sedation to fully evaluate the deeper structures for lesions. Take radiographs to evaluate the abdomen for space-occupying masses. A barium enema may be performed but can be difficult to interpret.

Prolapses must be reduced to prevent further trauma to the cloaca and to alleviate discomfort. For temporary treatment, place pursestring sutures to tighten the cloacal opening. Chronic recurrent cases require surgical intervention; consider a cloacopexy or a hysterectomy if egg-laying is a problem. The author has used a thin Silastic strip as a "subcutaneous pursestring" to tighten the cloacal sphincter with variable success in larger birds with apparent cloacal laxity (Fig. 26–12). Egg-bound birds need heat, parenteral calcium, and vitamin D_3.

Papillomas

Papillomas are the most commonly reported cloacal mass in pet birds. They usually occur in New World psittacines (Amazon parrots, macaws, and conures), although other species may be affected. They can intermittently "pop out" of the vent and are commonly mistaken for prolapses. Bleeding is sometimes associated with cloacal papillomas. Papillo-

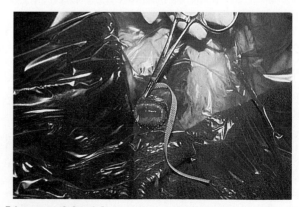

F i g u r e   2 6 – 1 2

The use of a Silastic implant to improve cloacal tone and reduce prolapse and straining in an umbrella cockatoo. A thin Silastic strip is placed subcutaneously and functions like a pursestring.

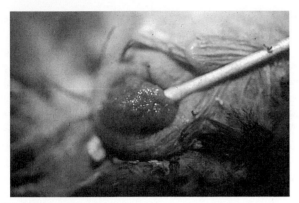

Figure 26–13

Cloacal papilloma in an Amazon parrot. Note the raspberry-like irregularity to the mucosal surface.

mas are mucosal lesions and may be focal or may develop 360° around the cloacal wall. Usually the lesions are located at the mucocutaneous junction of the cloaca but can sometimes occur deeper in the cloacal vault and may be difficult to initially identify. The cause is unknown but is suspected to be viral; the condition may be contagious to actively breeding birds. Presumptive diagnosis can be made from the identification of the roughened, raspberry-appearing lesion arising from the cloacal mucosa (Fig. 26–13).

The application of acetic acid (vinegar) to the papilloma turns the area white and can be helpful in identifying some of the smaller and more obscure lesions. Biopsy the lesion to obtain a definitive diagnosis. There is a high correlation between papillomatosis and cholangiocarcinoma in Amazon parrots.[31, 102–105] Perform a biochemistry profile on any bird with a cloacal papilloma or prolapse and consider radiographs and bile acid testing to rule out concurrent hepatic disease.

There are several treatment options for cloacal papillomas. Because they can spontaneously regress and recur, the author does not treat papillomas unless there is bleeding or discomfort. Larger papillomas result in tenesmus and constipation and should be removed. Electrocautery, radiosurgery, cryosurgery, and chemical cautery have all been used with varying degrees of success. A simple technique for chemical cautery involves the application of silver nitrate to the abnormal tissue. Using silver nitrate–tipped sticks, carefully apply the chemical only to the affected tissue. Immediately flush the area with saline or water to remove any excess silver nitrate to prevent damage to the adjacent normal tissue.

ABDOMINAL DISTENSION

Abdominal enlargement or distension is not always obvious in birds because of the extensive feather covering and the typical avian posture. A client may observe the onset of weakness, a reluctance or inability to fly, and labored breathing. Any space-occupying mass or fluid in the avian coelomic cavity can result in partial compression of the air sacs and respiratory distress. These birds may initially appear to have a primary respiratory disorder. During physical examination, a discrete mass may be palpated, or the abdomen may feel "full." Subtle masses or organomegaly may not be palpable because of the large sternal covering in most species. In budgerigars with abdominal tumors, the presence of a "sternal lift" may indicate a mass deeper in the abdomen. If the abdomen is enlarged, a wet cotton ball can be used to part the feathers and wet the skin for closer examination. An enlarged liver is sometimes seen protruding from under the sternum (Fig. 26–14). Transillumination with a bright light source across the abdominal wall may reveal a mass or the presence of ascites.

It is important to differentiate nonpathologic causes of abdominal enlargement. Active egg-laying hens can have an enlarged abdomen from oviductal activity. Most neonate birds and some adult passer-

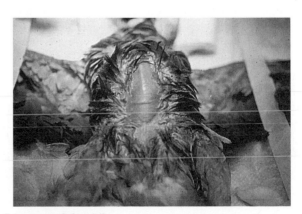

Figure 26–14

The liver is seen extending caudal to the sternum in this African grey parrot with hepatomegaly.

ine species normally have a "full" abdomen on palpation. The workup of abdominal enlargement includes complete clinical pathology data to determine general metabolic state and organ involvement. Contrast radiographs are usually needed to delineate the gastrointestinal tract and determine organomegaly. Ultrasound is possible in many cases. In the author's practice, detailed imaging has been possible in cockatiels and budgerigars using a 7.5-MHz finger probe. Fine needle aspiration (25- or 27-gauge) of a visible mass can provide valuable cytologic information in some birds. Be careful performing blind needle aspirates in small birds with hepatomegaly; some of these birds have coagulopathies and can hemorrhage excessively. Aspirate a small amount of ascitic fluid for analysis as well as to alleviate intra-abdominal pressure and tachypnea. Exploratory laparotomy can be done when the bird's condition is stable.

MALDIGESTION/MALABSORPTION

The development of a maldigestion syndrome in birds is characterized by the presence of whole seeds or undigested material in the droppings (see Color Fig. 26–11A). This may not initially be noted by the owner and can be an incidental finding during routine checkups. Weight loss and lethargy may accompany maldigestion, or the bird may appear normal. Birds with PDS can have concurrent regurgitation and limb weakness or ataxia. Melena may also be present, indicating gastrointestinal bleeding or ulceration.

Visually examine the droppings. Smear the feces out on white paper to evaluate fecal contents. Large, bulky stools may actually contain bits of foreign matter that can be identified. In small birds (e.g., budgerigars, cockatiels, and lovebirds) pieces of millet or grit may be found in the droppings. Birds that overeat grit supplements can have digestion problems; in other cases, the addition of a small amount of grit may be beneficial. Pancreatic disease can result in bulky droppings (see later). Food allergy is thought to affect birds but is poorly documented. Gastric neoplasia may result in maldigestion and malabsorption. Mycotic infections in the koilin lining of the ventriculus can affect the grinding function of the gizzard. Viral or bacterial gastroenteritis can also disrupt digestive processes.

PDS is a common cause of whole seeds in the droppings.

The etiology of gastroenteric disorders is not always identified ante mortem (Table 26–8). Take survey radiographs to rule out gastrointestinal foreign bodies, grit impaction, or proventricular dilatation. Add contrast material to evaluate mural lesions and to assess transit time. Birds with gastric dilatation often have striking radiographic changes. (See Figs. 13–25, 13–26, Chapter 13, Radiology.) Perform hematology, plasma biochemistry, and fecal Gram's stain as a minimum data base. Fecal flotation, direct wet mount, and tests for *Giardia* species should also be considered. Treatment is symptomatic and based on initial diagnosis. Grit supplements should be removed if they are excessively consumed, or added in small amounts if not previously available to the bird.

DISORDERS OF THE EXOCRINE PANCREAS

The avian exocrine pancreas functions in a similar manner to that in mammals. Avian pancreatic enzymes are important to the chemical phase of digestion in the small intestine, and disruption in the normal production of these enzymes results in maldigestion and the passage of abnormal feces (see Color Fig. 26–11E). It is difficult to diagnose pancreatic disease ante mortem in birds. Blood tests are not always diagnostic, and radiographic changes involving the pancreas are rare.[106] Endoscopy or

T a b l e 2 6 – 8
CAUSES OF UNDIGESTED FOOD IN DROPPINGS

- Gastroenteritis
  Bacterial (especially gram-negatives)
  Mycobacteriosis
- Gastrointestinal parasitism
  Giardia
  Helminths
  Coccidia
- Candidiasis *(C. albicans)*
- Foreign body obstruction
- Grit impaction
- Lack of grit
- Proventricular dilatation syndrome
- Pancreatic disease
- Liver disease
- Food allergy
- Gastric neoplasia
- Koilin abnormalities

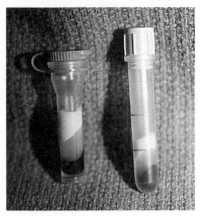

Figure 26–15

Severe lipemia. This blood sample was collected from an obese Amazon parrot.

laparotomy is possible in some larger species. Certain clinical signs may suggest pancreatic involvement—polyuria; polydipsia; polyphagia; weight loss; bulky, pale droppings; and undigested food in the feces. Lipemia may be present (Fig. 26–15).

The avian pancreas can be affected by several inflammatory and degenerative diseases. Reported pancreatic lesions in companion birds include pancreatic necrosis and atrophy, pancreatitis, neoplasia, lipidosis, hemochromatosis, and fibrosis.[107–113]

Etiology of pancreatic disease in birds is not always identified. Obesity and diets high in fat are speculated to be predisposing factors in the development of acute pancreatic necrosis and pancreatitis. Quaker parrots may be predisposed to pancreatic necrosis.[108] Chlamydiosis has also been implicated in cases of pancreatitis and necrosis.[107, 114] Viral infections involving the pancreas can occur; herpes virus (Pacheco's disease), adenovirus (lovebirds; cockatoos), polyoma virus, and paramyxovirus (type 3) may play a role in the development of pancreatic lesions.[107, 110] Pancreatic atrophy is a feature of the stunting and runting syndrome of poultry; it is speculated that there may be a viral etiology associated with this condition.[115] Large amounts of ingested zinc can accumulate in the pancreas and cause degenerative changes.[77, 80] Selenium deficiency in juvenile chickens results in pancreatic atrophy and fibrosis.[116] Pancreatic adenocarcinoma is also reported.[104, 107, 117] There is no specific therapy for the treatment of acute pancreatitis in the bird. Follow therapeutic protocols recommended in small animals—aggressive parenteral fluid therapy, broad-spectrum antibiotics, and dietary management. Supplement with vitamin E and selenium. Consider the addition of plant-based enzymes to assist in the digestion of the high-cellulose diets typical of grain-eating birds (Hi-Vegi-Lip, Freeda Vit, $\frac{1}{4}$ of a 2400 g tablet for each small parrot in every feeding).[19] Prognosis is guarded.

HEPATOBILIARY DISORDERS

Many avian diseases involve the hepatobiliary system. Clinical signs of liver disease in birds are variable, ranging from mild inappetence and inactivity to acute hemorrhage and sudden death. Signs are often silent or inapparent until disease is advanced. This may in part reflect the large functional reserve capacity and regenerative ability of the liver. As much as 80% of liver tissue must be lost before signs of impairment are perceptible. The diagnosis of liver disease is therefore difficult even under ideal conditions.

Some clinical signs are highly suggestive of liver involvement (Table 26–9) but none of these are pathognomonic. Dyspnea is commonly associated with ascites or space-occupying organomegaly. A green or yellow discoloration to the urates may result from biliverdinuria and is a common finding with liver disease in birds (see Color Fig. 26–11D). Physical findings associated with liver disease are nonspecific but may include weight loss, poor

Table 26–9

CLINICAL SIGNS OF LIVER DISEASE

- Nonspecific signs
  - Anorexia
  - Lethargy
  - Weight loss
  - Weakness
  - Diarrhea
  - Poor feathering
  - Polyuria/polydipsia
- More specific signs
  - Green urates
  - Abdominal swelling
  - Ascites
  - Coagulopathy
  - Melena
  - Bloody droppings
  - Bruised nails and beak
  - Overgrown beak (budgerigars)

feathering, overgrowth and bruising of the beak and nails, and pallor. Jaundice is rare in birds. Hepatomegaly is sometimes palpable, and an enlarged liver may be seen extending ventrally from beneath the sternum (see Fig. 26–14). In some birds, the only indication of an underlying hepatopathy might be an abnormal screening blood test on a postpurchase examination.

Diagnosis of Liver Disease

Clinical Pathology

Key differences exist between the hepatobiliary physiology of birds and mammals. It is generally considered that birds do not develop jaundice because bilirubin elevations are not observed with avian hepatobiliary dysfunction. In most mammalian species, the major pathway for bilirubin formation is through the oxidation of heme to biliverdin with subsequent reduction to bilirubin. Birds lack biliverdin reductase and, instead, excrete unconjugated biliverdin into bile as the endproduct of heme catabolism.[118, 119] Unlike unconjugated bilirubin in mammals, biliverdin is readily excreted into the urine and does not accumulate in the tissues. Biliverdin is the major avian bile pigment and is responsible for the green discoloration seen in the urates of birds with liver disease. The measurement of total bilirubin levels in plasma is not helpful in the diagnosis of liver disease in birds. The yellow appearance sometimes observed in avian plasma should not be mistaken for jaundice; carotene pigments from the diet may be responsible for this color.

Enzymes

Plasma enzyme activity is often used clinically to assess liver disease. The tissue distribution of "liver enzymes" varies between mammals and birds and may also vary between individual avian species. Evaluation of liver disease in birds can be difficult because of the nonspecific nature of avian plasma enzymes. Alanine aminotransferase (ALT or SGPT) is a liver-specific enzyme in dogs and cats but has variable activity in avian hepatocytes. Lactate dehydrogenase (LDH) is highly concentrated in the avian liver but is found in other tissues, and the relatively short plasma half-life makes measured values inconclusive. Aspartate aminotransferase (AST or SGOT) has high activity in avian hepatocytes but is also found in other tissues, particularly skeletal muscle. Alkaline phosphatase (AP) has a high tissue distribution in small intestine, kidney, and bone and is rarely elevated with hepatocyte damage.

Although most avian clinicians look at AST values in the assessment of liver disease, any muscular injury, including injections, can also elevate AST values. Creatine kinase (CK) is a muscle-specific enzyme and should be a part of a "liver panel." CK levels can determine if muscle damage has occurred in cases of AST elevation, but cannot rule out if both liver *and* muscle injury have taken place. Following an intramuscular injection, for example, both the CK and the AST levels are elevated. Because the plasma half-life of CK is very short, CK levels may return to normal before AST and can lead to an erroneous diagnosis of liver disease. To help avoid some interpretation difficulties, pretreatment blood testing should be done whenever possible. It is important to ask the bird owner detailed questions regarding possible muscle injury (e.g., recent injections at another clinic, muscle injury during capture, or in the case of racing pigeons, recent flight or training). Other diagnostic tests are necessary, such as plasma bile acids and radiographs.

Bile Acids

Plasma bile acid concentrations can be useful in detecting liver disease and in differentiating liver from muscle damage in cases of AST elevations. Bile acids are synthesized by the liver from cholesterol and are the main constituents of bile. Following a meal, bile is secreted into the small intestine, where it facilitates the digestion of dietary fats. Bile acids are then actively reabsorbed from the small intestine and travel through the portal circulation back to the liver for recycling. This pathway is known as the "enterohepatic cycle." In the healthy state, fasting bile acid concentrations circulate at a basal level. Not all species have a gall bladder (psittacines, pigeons), but the physiology of bile acid release should be the same regardless of the anatomic presence of a gall bladder. It has been demonstrated that postprandial bile acid levels do not significantly differ between nonpsittacine species with and without gall bladders.[120, 121] Individual pre- and postprandial levels can be variable in psittacine species.[122]

The plasma levels of bile acids rely on the integrity of the enterohepatic circulation and hepatobiliary system. A disruption in hepatic uptake, storage, or perfusion interferes with the uptake of bile acids from the circulation and results in elevated values. The bile acids test is specific for liver function. Several studies have shown the test to be useful in detecting liver disease in birds.[123–125] A single plasma sample is recommended for testing plasma bile acids in birds. Lipemic or hemolyzed samples interfere with the assay and can falsely elevate values. The recommended assay is an enzymatic procedure that requires a very small sample (Sigma Diagnostic Procedure 450, St. Louis).[126] Because there may be a degree of variability in bile acid values between laboratories, normal reference values should be determined by each laboratory that performs the assay. The test should be validated for use in avian species and calibrated before being offered commercially to the practitioner. In the author's laboratory testing, normal fasting plasma bile acid values in Amazon and African grey parrots are less than 100 μmol/L. Values in the 90 to 120 μmol/L range are considered suspicious and should be repeated. Similar bile acid values have been obtained in pigeons[120]; other values have been published for psittacine species.[122] Although bile acid concentrations in the "suspicious" range are occasionally observed, values in the 150 μmol/L to 400 μmol/L are more typical of fulminant liver disease.

Imaging Techniques

Radiographs

Radiographs are an essential component of the diagnostic workup of liver disease in birds. Used in conjunction with results of both clinical and laboratory findings, radiographs provide a more thorough evaluation of the liver. Radiographs supply information about the size of the liver, the displacement of other organs, and the presence of concurrent disease processes. Radiographs are always indicated before surgical or endoscopic biopsy of the liver. Sedation or isoflurane anesthesia is usually necessary to obtain diagnostic films. Poor positioning

can create "pseudolesions" on the radiographs and result in interpretation difficulties.

Assess patient condition prior to taking films; severely compromised birds should be in stable condition prior to having radiographic examination. Take advantage of the anesthesia to complete the diagnostic workup (e.g., draw blood, perform a fine-needle aspirate of an enlarged liver lobe, check the cloaca for papillomas, or place a probe on the abdomen for an ultrasonographic image). All birds should be fasted prior to radiographs; anesthesia and recumbency can induce regurgitation and possible aspiration.

Radiology is useful in identifying hepatomegaly and ascites in birds. Contrast radiographs are usually necessary for added detail, especially in birds with ascites or gastrointestinal dilatation. A dilated, fluid-filled proventriculus can mimic a large liver radiographically, and oral contrast (barium or iohexol) must be administered to delineate the gastrointestinal tract. Hepatomegaly can be readily identified radiographically. (See Fig. 13–27, Chapter 13, Radiology.)

Liver disease does not always result in a grossly enlarged liver. Hepatic fibrosis or cirrhosis, for example, may result in a smaller hepatic silhouette. There is a degree of variability of normal liver size between some species of birds (e.g., large macaws often appear to have a subjectively smaller liver radiographically than other psittacines). Base a diagnosis of liver disease on the results of clinical findings and blood testing in conjunction with radiographic findings. Ultrasound is useful in some cases (see later).

Ultrasonography

Ultrasonography can provide detailed imaging under certain conditions. The liver is difficult to image in a small (cockatiel) or medium-sized bird (mynah) unless there is abdominal effusion or pronounced organomegaly. With the bird held in an upright position, it is a relatively simple procedure that can often be done without sedation. Using a 6.5- or 7.5-MHz finger probe, place the transducer caudal to the sternum and direct the beam cranially. The air sacs interfere with ultrasound imaging, but if the probe is kept centrally along the caudal rim of the sternum, the air sacs are avoided. Ultrasound is best used to identify and characterize hepatic lesions. Neoplasms or granulomas may appear as discrete hyperechoic areas throughout the liver. It is also useful to rule out other abdominal diseases that may be difficult to interpret radiographically. Ultrasound-guided fine needle biopsy of the liver can be performed to obtain samples for cytology.

Liver Biopsy

In many birds, a specific etiology or morphologic diagnosis can be obtained only through tissue biopsy. Because liver biopsy is not without potential complications, both risks and benefits need to be considered prior to the biopsy. Indications for liver biopsy include persistently elevated AST (>330 IU/L), elevated bile acids (>150 μm/L), radiographic changes, and lack of response to therapy. Biopsy findings can provide prognostic information and aid in guiding the management of the disease (Figs. 26–16, 26–17).

Etiology of Liver Disease

There are many possible causes of liver disease in birds (Table 26–10). Because the liver is involved with so many metabolic functions, any disruption in normal physiologic activities can result in hepatic damage. Liver impairment may result from toxins, metabolic disorders, infectious disease, malnutrition, neoplasia, and degenerative disorders. Liver disease can be primary, such as with chlamydiosis, or it can be secondary to other diseases such as

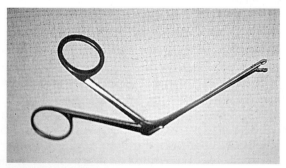

Figure 26–16

Alligator-type biopsy forceps with a 3-mm cup. (Hartmann-Citelli forceps, Baxter Healthcare Corporation, McGraw Park, IL.)

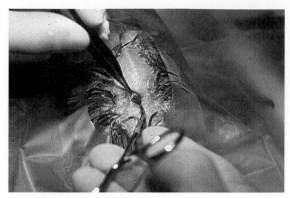

Figure 26–17

Nonendoscopic liver biopsy in an African grey parrot with hepatomegaly. A keyhole incision is made just caudal to the sternum to visualize the liver.

hypothyroidism or obesity. Unfortunately with avian species, the etiology of hepatic damage is not always identified. Much of what is known about avian liver diseases is based on liver biopsy, response to therapy, and postmortem examination. Although it is ideal to biopsy every suspected case of hepatic disease in birds, this is often not possible because of the size and the compromised state of most sick birds at the time of presentation.

There is still much to learn about the pathophysiology and etiology of hepatobiliary disease in birds. In this section, a review of some of the more common causes of liver disease is presented. More detailed information on specific etiologies can be found in other chapters of this book.

Infectious Diseases

Bacterial Hepatitis

Bacterial hepatitis is common in birds and may result from infection with a large number of different bacterial species. Bacterial hepatitis may be a sequela to septicemia or may result from an ascending cholangiohepatitis, especially in association with concurrent enteritis. Although infection by many different bacteria is possible, the gram-negative bacteria of the family Enterobacteriaceae are a particular problem in most avian species. The Enterobacteriaceae can be primary pathogens or can function as secondary invaders in association with immune-suppression and gastrointestinal flora

T a b l e   2 6 – 1 0

COMMON CAUSES OF HEPATIC DISEASE IN BIRDS

Infectious
- Bacteria
    Gram-negative (Enterobacteriaceae)
- Chlamydiosis
- Mycobacteriosis
- Viruses
    Adenovirus
    Herpes virus (Pacheco's disease)
    Polyoma virus
    Reovirus
- Trematodes (especially cockatoos)

- Protozoa
    Atoxoplasma
    Histomonas meleagridis
    Leukocytozoon simondi
    Microsporidia
    Trichomonas gallinae
    Toxoplasma

Noninfectious
- Aflatoxicosis
- Fatty liver (lipidosis)
- Hemochromatosis (iron storage disease)
- Neoplasia
    Cholangiocarcinoma
    Lymphoma
    Adenoma
- Amyloidosis
- Cirrhosis

disruptions. *E. coli, Salmonella, Klebsiella, Pasteurella, Serratia, Yersinia, Campylobacter,* and *Pseudomonas* are common isolates. *M. avium* can cause a granulomatous hepatitis usually in association with multiorgan involvement and a chronic wasting disease. Chlamydial hepatitis should always be considered in birds with signs of liver disease (see later).

Diagnosis of bacterial hepatitis can be made from histologic examination and bacterial culture of a liver biopsy specimen. Some organisms may be fastidious and difficult to grow on standard media (e.g., *Mycobacterium, Chlamydia,* and *Campylobacter*). Special cytologic stains, such as acid-fast stains for mycobacteria, are necessary on some biopsy samples and should be requested when submitting the sample. (See Chapter 18, Bacteriology.) Therapeutic success depends on the pathogenicity of the organism, the degree of damage to the liver parenchyma, and the duration of infection prior to treatment. Chronic cases are often associated with fibrosis, cirrhosis, and other irreversible parenchymal damage.

Chlamydiosis

Chlamydiosis is one of the more common causes of bacterial hepatitis in psittacines and should always be considered in pet birds with signs of liver disease. Other avian species are also at risk including Columbiformes and passerines. *Chlamydia psittaci* is an intracellular bacteria that causes multiorgan infection. Differences in host susceptibility and strain virulence affect the clinical progression of disease. Clinical signs vary between species and can range from chronic unthriftiness to acute anorexia, diarrhea, and dyspnea. "Lime green" urates are a common clinical sign in acutely affected birds (see Color Fig. 26–11D). However, this is not pathognomonic for chlamydiosis. The yellow-green color seen in the urates of birds indicates a hepatopathy that has many potential causes, one of which may be chlamydial infection.

A singular laboratory test to obtain a definitive diagnosis of chlamydial infection is not available at present. Clinical diagnosis can be challenging and usually requires interpretation of several different laboratory tests (see Chapter 23, Chlamydia). Liver biopsy can confirm infection; identification of chlamydial organisms is aided by the use of special stains (PVK, Gimenez, or Macchiavello's). Treatment is always recommended; affected birds rarely recover spontaneously. Antibody production during active disease is not protective, and recovered birds are susceptible to reinfection. Bird owners need to be warned of the zoonotic potential of chlamydiosis.

Viral Infections

Viruses can affect the liver exclusively or in conjunction with multisystemic disease. In companion birds, herpes virus, polyoma virus, adenovirus, and reovirus have been associated with hepatitis.

Inclusion body hepatitis refers to an inflammatory disease of the liver that results from intracellular viral inclusion bodies. In both companion and wild birds, at least three different viruses may be associated with inclusion body hepatitis: herpes virus, polyoma virus, and adenovirus.[127–129] These viruses produce characteristic intranuclear inclusion bodies in hepatocytes of avian species. Tentative viral differentiation is based on the histologic lesion produced in the liver, the appearance of the inclusion bodies, and the size of the viral particle as identified by electron microscopy (see Chapter 19, Virology).

Pacheco's disease virus is a herpes virus that affects psittacine species and has long been associated with flock outbreaks and aviary mortality.[130–133] The clinical picture may vary somewhat between species, but most often the disease results in sudden death in susceptible birds. Herpes virus infections typically produce focal hepatic necrosis with intranuclear eosinophilic inclusions. Herpes virus inclusion body hepatitis occurs in nonpsittacine species as well.[18, 134–137] Polyoma virus infection is also associated with an acute hepatic necrosis; acute death is not uncommon in juvenile psittacines.[138–142] The appearance of extensive subcutaneous hemorrhages is typical in affected birds. Amphophilic or basophilic intranuclear inclusions are suggestive of polyomavirus disease. Adenovirus infection has been associated with a fatal intranuclear inclusion body hepatitis.[129, 143–146] Affected birds die with few premonitory signs. Extensive hepatic necrosis with large basophilic intranuclear inclusion bodies has been observed in affected birds. Reovirus-like particles have been associated with necrotizing hepatitis, especially in African grey parrots.[147, 148] Inclusion bodies are not typically observed.

Protozoa

Protozoal hepatopathy is not uncommon and may be caused by any one of several different protozoal types. Flagellate protozoans from the gastrointestinal tract can spread and invade multiple sites, including the hepatobiliary system. *Trichomonas gallinae* is most commonly found in pigeons and raptors but can also be seen in passerine and psittacine species. *Histomonas meleagridis* is a flagellate that results in enterohepatitis ("blackhead" in turkeys) in gallinaceous birds. Coccidian parasites can also produce varying degrees of liver disease in

birds. *Atoxoplasma* species infection is common in canaries and other passerine species. *Toxoplasma gondii* liver infection has been reported in mynahs, finches, and lories, and can potentially affect many different avian species.[149–152] *Sarcocystis falcatula* is a coccidian parasite that is known for devastating outbreaks in psittacine flocks. Characteristic necropsy findings in one zoo outbreak included pulmonary hemorrhage, hepatomegaly, and splenomegaly.[153] Microsporidian (*Encephalitozoon* species) infections have been identified in the liver and kidneys of lovebirds.[154, 155] The protozoan hemoparasites *Leukocytozoon* and *Plasmodium* may be associated with hepatomegaly.

Trematode Infection

Trematodiasis can result in liver and bile duct disease. Imported birds (Old World species) represent the majority of reported cases of fluke infection. Hepatic trematodiasis is a problem in some imported cockatoos.[100, 101, 156] Chronic infection can result in bile duct obstruction and hepatomegaly. Histologic lesions are characterized by hepatic fibrosis and bile duct hyperplasia. Diagnosis is based on identification of trematode eggs on direct fecal smears and on necropsy findings. Treatment may not result in clinical improvement.

Noninfectious Disorders

Hemochromatosis

Iron storage disease or hemochromatosis results from the pathologic accumulation of iron in various tissues. This differs from hemosiderosis, which is defined as the excessive accumulation of iron in hepatocytes without the alteration of normal tissue morphology. Iron storage disease can occur in many tissues, but the liver is most frequently involved. Ramphastids (toucans, toucanettes, aracaris), mynah birds, starlings, birds of paradise, and the currassow are most commonly affected, although other species are at risk. Although the complete pathogenesis is unknown, it is thought to be related to abnormal iron metabolism that may be aggravated by a high amount of dietary iron.[157] Sudden death without premonitory signs is common in affected toucans. In mynah birds, dyspnea, hepatomegaly, and ascites are common clinical findings.[158] Cardiomyopathy may result from the accumulation of iron in the myocardium. Initial diagnosis is based on clinical signs, history, and the presence of hepatomegaly and abnormal liver function tests. Definitive diagnosis must be made through hepatic biopsy and iron staining techniques. Blood iron testing results may not be conclusive in all species.[159] Immediate therapy includes stabilization of the acutely dyspneic bird and supportive care. Long-term therapy is based on weekly phlebotomy of 1% of body weight and maintenance on a low iron diet (>100 ppm) (see Chapter 51, Toucans and Mynahs).

Deferoxamine (Desferal, CIBA), a chelating agent, has sometimes been used in birds with variable results. Recently, successful therapy of hemochromatosis with deferoxamine was reported in a channel-billed toucan.[160]

Hepatic Lipidosis

Hepatic lipidosis, or fatty liver infiltration, is relatively common in some species of birds. Psittacine birds most commonly affected with fatty liver disease include budgerigars, Amazon parrots, cockatiels, lovebirds, and Quaker parrots.[161] Fatty liver hemorrhagic syndrome occurs in some egg-laying chickens. Fatty liver disease can have multiple causes and may actually be a culmination of several factors, including a genetic predisposition. Excessive consumption of high energy, high fat (all-seed) diets with restricted exercise may lead to fatty degeneration. Deficiency of lipotrophic factors such as choline, biotin, and methionine may play a role in the development of hepatic lipid accumulation. Thyroid dysfunction may promote obesity and the development of lipomas. Toxins such as aflatoxin can result in fatty changes in the liver (see later). Diabetes mellitus is an important cause of hepatic lipidosis in dogs and cats, and may play a similar role in diabetic birds. Steroid administration, such as methylprogesterone treatment in egg-laying hens, can result in hepatic lipidosis.

Clinically, psittacines suffering from hepatic lipidosis are slightly overweight or obese. Typical history includes an acute onset of anorexia, varying degrees of lethargy, and abnormal droppings (biliverdinuria). The liver is enlarged radiographically and sometimes palpably in the smaller species.

Budgerigars may have overgrown nails and beak with hemorrhages. On biochemical profiles, the liver function tests are often abnormal (AST and bile acids) and the cholesterol is high. Some birds have grossly lipemic plasma that can interfere with biochemical testing (see Fig. 26–15).

Take care when performing jugular venipuncture in the smaller species (budgerigars); underlying hepatopathy can lead to excessive hematoma formation and collapse. Definitive diagnosis is made on liver biopsy. Affected birds require immediate and aggressive supportive care to include fluid therapy, oral lactulose (0.3 ml/kg every 8 hours) to prevent ammonia formation and absorption, and nutritional support. Eliminate fat in the diet and replace with long-chain complex carbohydrates, fructose, and lipotrophic vitamins.

Toxins

Toxic liver disease results from certain agents that are hepatotoxic. (See Chapter 35, Toxic Diseases.) Known hepatotoxins in small animals and birds include mycotoxins (see later), heavy metals (lead, copper, arsenic), certain drugs (methoxyflurane, halothane, anticonvulsants, dimetronidazole, quinacrine), insecticides, and some plants (gossypol, castor bean, oleander, hemlock). Multiple factors are thought to predispose an individual to toxic liver injury, including individual susceptibility and nutritional status. Diets containing adequate high-quality protein, specifically the lipotrophic factors methionine and choline, can protect against some forms of hepatic insult. The duration of exposure is important in cases in which toxins have a cumulative effect. Hepatotoxins result in necrosis of parenchymal cells. When hepatocellular necrosis begins, it is replaced with fibrosis or lipidosis. The process may be self-perpetuating even if the agent is no longer present.[162] Cirrhosis can result from widespread hepatic fibrosis and scarring.

Aflatoxicosis

Aflatoxicosis occurs when a bird is exposed to the toxic chemical metabolites (aflatoxins) produced by certain species of *Aspergillus* fungi (*A. fumigatus* and *A. parasiticus*). The toxin-producing strains are widely distributed and can grow on a variety of food or feed types. Peanuts, nuts, cereals, and corn are at a particular risk for production of aflatoxins. In the author's practice, most cases of suspected aflatoxicosis were in seed-eating Amazon parrots with a particular preference for peanuts. Aflatoxin production is optimal in warm, dark, and humid environmental conditions. Refrigeration and proper storage of seeds can prevent the production of the toxin.

Aflatoxin B_1 is the most toxic of the aflatoxins. It is a known hepatotoxin that results in depression, poor weight gain, anorexia, and hepatomegaly. Histologic changes in the liver include fatty infiltration, bile duct hyperplasia, and fibrosis. Aflatoxins can also be carcinogenic.[163] Definitive diagnosis of aflatoxicosis in birds is difficult. Liver biopsy results can be suggestive of mycotoxic disease; however, identification of the toxin in a particular batch of seeds is difficult and seed testing is usually inconclusive. There is no specific treatment for aflatoxicosis.

Amyloidosis

Amyloidosis refers to the deposition of abnormal hyaline-like substance primarily within the liver, kidney, and spleen. Primary amyloidosis is considered very uncommon in veterinary medicine.[162] Secondary or reactive systemic amyloidosis is associated with chronic infectious or inflammatory conditions. Amyloid A deposition is stimulated by chronic diseases that involve antibody-antigen production. As this material accumulates in the liver, anoxia and necrosis develop, and the liver becomes enlarged with rounded edges. Diagnosis is based on liver biopsy and special stains of histologic specimens to confirm the presence of amyloid. In birds, amyloidosis is most common in waterfowl and may be secondary to chronic infection with aspergillosis, bumblefoot, or tuberculosis. There are rare reports of amyloidosis in psittacines.[164] In the author's practice, an African grey parrot with a chronic intraocular infection was diagnosed with hepatic amyloidosis. Progressive amyloidosis can be ultimately fatal.

Therapy is directed at correcting the underlying infection but is not always successful. The use of colchicine may be beneficial in blocking the formation of amyloid in dogs and may be considered for use in avian species as well.[165] Ascorbic acid therapy may also be useful.

Neoplasia

Hepatic neoplasia can be primary or metastatic. The most common hepatic tumor reported in birds is cholangiocarcinoma, with a high rate of occurrence in Amazon parrots.[102–104, 166–168] Hepatoma, hemangioma, fibrosarcoma, adenocarcinoma, hepatocellular carcinoma, biliary adenoma, hepatic lymphosarcoma, and lymphoid leukosis are all known to occur in birds.[169] There may be a relationship between the presence of hepatic neoplasia and cloacal papillomas and prolapse in Amazon parrots. (See earlier, Cloacal Prolapse.)[102–104] Aflatoxins are potentially carcinogenic and may play a role in the development of hepatobiliary neoplasia.

Therapeutic Considerations

The clinical objectives of treatment for liver disease involve support of the patient until a diagnosis can be made, symptomatic therapy, and a specific attempt to eliminate the causative agent. Specific therapy is directed at the causative agent, and symptomatic and supportive care is provided regardless of the etiology. Unfortunately in avian medicine, the specific etiologic agent of liver disease is often undetermined. If determined, the agents may not be responsive to treatment, such as viruses, or the primary agent is no longer present at the time of diagnosis, such as toxins. Some types of hepatopathies, when diagnosed, respond very poorly to therapy (e.g., amyloidosis, cirrhosis, and neoplasia). Regardless, every attempt should be made to determine the cause of hepatic disease.

Supportive Care

Supportive care must begin immediately in the acutely sick bird. The presence of anemia, ascites, and hepatomegaly can result in respiratory distress. Handle these birds minimally initially and provide an oxygenated incubator in a low-stress, isolated area. Ascitic fluid can be aspirated in the dyspneic bird as a temporary measure to provide immediate relief. Be careful with paracentesis; fluid removal can result in protein (albumin) depletion and hypovolemia and is meant only for abrupt relief and diagnostic purposes. Diuretics such as furosemide can be used initially in an attempt to control ascites.

Both replacement and maintenance fluids are needed; intravenous or intraosseous administration is ideal. Be careful in handling anemic or dyspneic birds; the protracted restraint necessary for the placement of an indwelling catheter may induce fatalities in the severely compromised avian patient. Subcutaneous administration of fluids may prove safer initially, and a catheter can be placed later if needed. Consider one initial intravenous bolus of fluids, dextrose, and corticosteroids in the hypoglycemic, dehydrated patient. Some birds with liver disease are hypoalbuminemic, and the administration of fluids may result in edema. The use of synthetic plasma colloid agents has been preliminarily investigated in avian species.[170] The intravenous or intraosseous administration of colloid hetastarch (Hespan, DuPont Pharmaceuticals, Wilmington, DE) at 10 to 15 ml/kg every 8 hours for one to four treatments may be effective in severe, nonresponsive hypoalbuminemic states.

Diet Therapy

Dietary therapy must be considered in both acute and chronic liver disease. Acutely sick birds are inappetent or anorexic and require gavage feedings three to four times daily. An easily digestible, protein-restricted, low-residue diet is optimal for the management of hepatic failure. Hypovitaminosis is common in liver disease both as a sequela to the actual disease process as well as from a primary dietary deficiency. Hypovitaminosis occurs in 70% of people with hepatic disease; important vitamin deficiencies include those of the B-complex vitamins and deficiencies of vitamins A, E, D, and K.[152] Supplement avian patients with injectable multivitamins. The fat-soluble vitamins A and D_3 should be used sparingly (e.g., once or twice initially at weekly intervals); vitamin K and B-complex vitamins are given daily.

Lactulose

Lactulose is often used in the treatment of hepatic disease. It is a synthetic, nonabsorbable dissacharide that is administered per os. Lactulose is fermented in the gut by bacteria into acetic and lactic acid. This results in the reduction of pH and the

subsequent ionization of ammonia to prevent its absorption in the colon. Lactulose is useful in helping to reduce hepatic encephalopathy and can be administered with minimal side effects in most birds (0.3 ml/kg orally every 8–12 hours).

Glucocorticoids

Glucocorticoids are often used in the treatment of chronic active hepatitis in mammals, but their use is controversial in avian medicine. Infectious agents are often an underlying component of liver disease in birds and they are not always identified. The use of corticosteriods can exacerbate an infectious hepatitis and is contraindicated in suspect cases.

Colchicine

Colchicine is an antimitotic agent that also has some anti-inflammatory properties. Although specifically labeled for use in gout in people, it may be valuable as an antifibrotic agent in the control of hepatic fibrosis.[171, 172] The author has used colchicine (0.04 mg/kg orally every 6–12 hours) in psittacines for prolonged periods without adverse reactions. The use of colchicine for hepatic fibrosis is considered controversial. It is difficult to document histologically whether the drug actually blocks the progression of fibrosis in the liver but clinical improvement may be seen.

Specific therapy must be directed at the suspected agent. Viral hepatitis is generally not treatable, but acyclovir has been used with some success in controlling outbreaks of Pacheco's disease.[173, 174] Bacterial infections require appropriate antimicrobial therapy based on culture and sensitivity testing. Doxycycline is the drug of choice in treating chlamydiosis. Begin doxycycline therapy immediately while awaiting laboratory results if chlamydial hepatitis is suspected. Successful treatment of hepatic mycobacteriosis is possible in some cases,[85, 86] but carefully consider the zoonotic potential before recommending or beginning therapy.

References

1. Gill FB: Ornithology, ed 2. New York, WH Freeman, 1994.
2. Duke GE: Alimentary canal: Anatomy, regulation of feed-

ing, and motility. In Sturkie PD (ed): Avian Physiology, ed 4. New York, Springer-Verlag, 1986, pp 269–288.

3. Hegde SN: Composition of pigeon milk and its effect on growth in chicks. Indian J Exp Biol 11:238–239, 1973.

4. Lumeij JT: Gastroenterology, hepatology, nephrology. In Ritchie BW, Harrison GJ, Harrison LR (eds): Avian Medicine: Principles and Application. Lake Worth, FL, Winger Publishers, 1994, pp 484–521, 522–537, 538–555.

5. Nott HMR, Taylor EJ: Nutrition of Pet Birds. In Burger IH (ed): The Waltham Book of Companion Animal Nutrition. Oxford, Pergamon Press, 1993, pp 69–84.

6. Brue RN: Nutrition. In Ritchie BW, Harrison GJ, Harrison LR (eds): Avian Medicine: Principles and Application. Lake Worth, FL, Winger Publishers, 1994, pp 63–95.

7. Ruckebush L, Phaneuf L-P, Dunlop R: Physiology of Small and Large Animals. Philadelphia, BC Decker, 1991.

8. King JR, Murphy ME: Periods of nutritional stress in annual cycles of endotherms: Fact or fiction? Am Zool 25:955–964, 1985.

9. Murphy ME, King JR: Sparrows discriminate between diets differing in valine or lysine concentrations. Physiol Behav 45:423–430, 1989.

10. King AS, McLelland J: Digestive System, ed 2. London, Bailliere Tindall, 1984, pp 84–109.

11. King AS, McLelland J: Integument, ed 2. London, Bailliere Tindall, 1984, pp 23–42.

12. Campbell TW: Cytology of the Upper Alimentary Tract: Oral Cavity, Esophagus, and Ingluvies. Ames, Iowa State University Press, 1988, pp 45–49.

13. Clubb SL: Avian pox in cage and aviary birds. In Fowler M (ed): Zoo and Wild Animal Medicine. Philadelphia, WB Saunders, 1986, pp 213–220.

14. McDonald SE, Lowenstine LJ, Ardans AA: Avian pox in blue-fronted Amazon parrots. J Am Vet Med Assoc 179:1218–1222, 1981.

15. Gerlach H: Avipoxvirus. In Ritchie BW, Harrison GJ, Harrison LR (eds): Avian Medicine: Principles and Application. Lake Worth, FL, Wingers Publishing, 1994, pp 865–874.

16. Winterfield RW, Clubb SL, Schrader D: Immunization against psittacine pox. Avian Dis 29:886–890, 1985.

17. Fudge AM: Psittacine vaccines. Vet Clin North Am Small Anim Pract 21:1273–1279, 1991.

18. Gerlach H: Herpesviridae. In Ritchie BW, Harrison GJ, Harrison LR (eds): Avian Medicine: Principles and Application. Lake Worth, FL, Wingers Publishing, 1994, pp 874–885.

19. Ritchie BW, Harrison GJ: Formulary. In Ritchie BW, Harrison GJ, Harrison LR (eds): Avian Medicine: Principles and Application. Lake Worth, FL, Wingers Publishing, 1994, pp 457–478.

20. Parrott T: Clinical treatment regimes with fluconazole (abstract). Proc Assoc Avian Vet, 1991, pp 15–16.

21. Panigrahy B, Clark FD, Hall CF: Mycobacteriosis in psittacine birds. Avian Dis 27:1166–1168, 1983.

22. Henderson GM, Gulland FM, Hawkey CM: Haematological findings in budgerigars with megabacterium and Trichomonas infections associated with 'going light.' Vet Rec 123:492–494, 1988.

23. Murtaugh RJ, Jacobs RM: Trichomoniasis of the crop in a cockatiel. J Am Vet Med Assoc 185:441–442, 1984.

24. Garner MM: Trichomoniasis in a blue-fronted Amazon parrot. J Assoc Avian Vet 6:17–20, 1992.

25. Baker JR: Trichomoniasis, a major cause of vomiting in budgerigars. Vet Rec 118:447–449, 1986.

26. Murphy J: Psittacine trichomoniasis (abstract). Proc Assoc Avian Vet, 1992, pp 21–24.

27. Petrak ML, Gilmore CE: Neoplasms. In Petrak ML (ed): Diseases of Cage and Aviary Birds. Philadelphia, Lea & Febiger, 1982, pp 606–637.

28. Chin RP, Barr BC: Squamous-cell carcinoma of the pharyngeal cavity in a Jersey black giant rooster. Avian Dis 34:775–778, 1990.

29. Anderson WI, Steinberg H: Primary glossal squamous-cell carcinoma in a Spanish cochin hen. Avian Dis 33:827–828, 1989.

30. Cooper JE, Lawton MP, Greenwood AG: Papillomas in psittacine birds (letter). Vet Rec 119:535, 1986.

31. Graham DL: Wasting/proventricular dilation disease, a pathologists view (abstract). Proc Assoc Avian Vet, 1991, pp 43–44.

32. Ramsay EC, Drew ML, Johnson B: Trichomoniasis in a flock of budgerigars (abstract). Proc Assoc Avian Vet, 1990, pp 309–311.

33. Sasipreeyajan J, Newman JA: Goiter in a cockatiel (Nymphicus hollandicus). Avian Dis 32:169–172, 1988.

34. Murase T, Ikeda T, Goto I, et al: Treatment of lead poisoning in wild geese. J Am Vet Med Assoc 200:1726–1729, 1992.

35. Morgan RV, Moore FM, Pearce LK, Rossi T: Clinical and laboratory findings in small companion animals with lead poisoning: 347 cases (1977–1986). J Am Vet Med Assoc 199:93–97, 1991.

36. Redig PT, Stowe CM, Barnes DM, Arent TD: Lead toxicosis in raptors. J Am Vet Med Assoc 177:941–943, 1980.

37. Mautino M: Avian lead intoxication (abstract). Proc Assoc Avian Vet, 1990, pp 245–247.

38. McDonald SE: Lead poisoning in psittacine birds. In Kirk RW (ed): Current Veterinary Therapy IX. Philadelphia, WB Saunders, 1986, pp 713–718.

39. Arnall L: The digestive system. In Arnall L, Keymer IF (eds): Bird Diseases. Neptune City, TFH Publications, 1975, p 223.

40. Pare JA, Hunter B: Ingluviolith in a cockatiel (Nymphicus hollandicus). J Assoc Avian Vet 7:139–140, 1993.

41. Murtaugh RJ, Ringler DJ, Petrak ML: Squamous cell carcinoma of the esophagus in an Amazon parrot. J Am Vet Med Assoc 188:872–873, 1986.

42. Turrel JM, McMillan MC, Paul-Murphy J: Diagnosis and treatment of tumors of companion birds II. AAV Today 1:159–165, 1987.

43. McMillan MC: Avian gastrointestinal radiography. Comp Contin Ed Pract Vet 5:273–278, 1983.

44. Goring RL, Goldman A, Kaufman KJ, et al: Needle catheter duodenostomy: A technique for duodenal alimentation of birds. J Am Vet Med Assoc 189:1017–1019, 1986.

45. Degernes LA, Davidson GS, Kolmstetter C, et al: Preliminary report on the use of total parenteral nutrition in birds (abstract). Proc Assoc Avian Vet, 1992, pp 19–20.

46. Quesenberry KE, Hillyer EV: Supportive care and emergency therapy. In Ritchie BW, Harrison GJ, Harrison LR (eds): Avian Medicine: Principles and Application. Lake Worth, FL, Wingers Publishing, 1994, pp 382–416.

47. Bauck L: Vomiting in the young macaw (abstract). Proc Assoc Avian Vet, 1992, pp 126–128.

48. Flammer K: Avian antibacterial therapeutics: Selecting an antibiotic (abstract). Proc Assoc Avian Vet, 1988, pp 109–118.

49. Van Sant F: Resolution of an esophageal stricture in a hyacinth macaw (abstract). Proc Assoc Avian Vet, 1992, pp 177–179.

50. Lutz ME, Wilson RB: Psittacine proventricular dilatation syndrome in an umbrella cockatoo. J Am Vet Med Assoc 198:1962–1964, 1991.

51. Joyner KL, Kock N, Styles D: Encephalitis, proventricular and ventricular myositis, and myenteric ganglioneuritis in an umbrella cockatoo. Avian Dis 33:379–381, 1989.

52. Mannl A, Gerlach H, Leipold R: Neuropathic gastric dilatation in psittaciformes. Avian Dis 31:214–221, 1987.

53. Clark FD: Proventricular dilatation syndrome in large psittacine birds. Avian Dis 28:813–815, 1984.

54. Vice CA: Myocarditis as a component of psittacine proventricular dilatation syndrome in a Patagonian conure. Avian Dis 36:1117–1119, 1992.

55. Suedmeyer WK: Diagnosis and clinical progression of three cases of proventricular dilatation syndrome. J Assoc Avian Vet 6:159–163, 1991.

56. Gaskin JM, Homer BL, Eskelund KH: Preliminary findings in avian viral serositis: A newly recognized syndrome of psittacine birds. J Assoc Avian Vet 5:27–34, 1991.

57. Phalen DN: An outbreak of psittacine proventricular dilatation syndrome (PPDS) in a private collection of birds and an atypical form of PPDS in a Nanday conure (abstract). Proc Assoc Avian Vet, 1986, pp 27–34.

58. Walsh MT: Radiology. In Harrison GJ, Harrison LR (eds): Clinical Avian Medicine and Surgery. Philadelphia, WB Saunders, 1986, pp 201–233.

59. McCluggage D: Proventriculotomy: A study of select cases (abstract). Proc Assoc Avian Vet, 1992, pp 195–200.

60. Doolen M: Crop biopsy—a low risk diagnosis for neuropathic gastric dilatation (abstract). Proc Assoc Avian Vet, 1994, pp 193–196.

61. Rae MA, Merryman M, Lintner M: Gastric neoplasia in caged birds (abstract). Proc Assoc Avian Vet, 1992, pp 180–189.

62. Leach MW, Paul-Murphy J, Lowenstine LJ: Three cases of gastric neoplasia in psittacines. Avian Dis 33:204–210, 1989.

63. Levine BS: What is your diagnosis? Intramural mass in the proventriculus. J Am Vet Med Assoc 185:911–912, 1984.

64. Baker JR: A survey of causes of mortality in budgerigars (Melopsittacus undulatus). Vet Rec 106:10–12, 1980.

65. Schmidt RE, Dustin LR, Slevin RW: Proventricular adenocarcinoma in a budgerigar and a grey-cheeked parakeet. AAV Today 2:140–142, 1988.

66. Gerlach H: Gram-positive bacteria of clinical importance. In Ritchie BW, Harrison GJ, Harrison LR, (eds): Avian Medicine: Principles and Application. Lake Worth, FL, Wingers Publishing, 1994, pp 965–983.

67. Bangert RL, Cho BR, Widders PR, et al: A survey of aerobic bacteria and fungi in the feces of healthy psittacine birds. Avian Dis 32:46–52, 1988.

68. Joyner KL: Microbiologic techniques for the avian practitioner. In Kirk RW (ed): Current Veterinary Therapy X. Philadelphia, WB Saunders, 1989, pp 780–786.

69. Fudge AM, Reavill DR, Rosskopf WJ: Clinical aspects of avian pseudomonas infections: A retrospective study (abstract). Proc Assoc Avian Vet, 1992, pp 141–155.

70. Dorrestein GM, Buitelaar MN, van der Hage MH, Zwart P: Evaluation of a bacteriological and mycological examination of psittacine birds. Avian Dis 29:951–962, 1985.

71. Kaneene JB, Taylor RF, Sikarskie JG, et al: Disease patterns in the Detroit Zoo: A study of the avian population from 1973 through 1983. J Am Vet Med Assoc 187:1129–1131, 1985.

72. Orosz SE, Chengappa MM, Oyster RA, et al: Salmonella enteritidis infection in two species of psittaciformes. Avian Dis 36:766–769, 1992.

73. Flammer K, Drewes LA: Species-related differences in the incidence of gram-negative bacteria isolated from the cloaca of clinically normal psittacine birds. Avian Dis 32:79–83, 1988.

74. Baker JR: Megabacteriosis in exhibition budgerigars [see comments]. Vet Rec 131:12–14, 1992.

75. Rae MA, Rosskopf WJ: Mycobacteriosis in passerines (abstract). Proc Assoc Avian Vet, 1992, pp 234–242.

76. Graham DL: Endoventricular mycosis: An avian pathologist's perspective (abstract). Proc Assoc Avian Vet, 1994, pp 279–282.

77. Droual R, Meteyer CU, Galey FD: Zinc toxicoses due to ingestion of a penny in a gray-headed chachalaca (Ortalis cinereiceps). Avian Dis 35:1007–1011, 1991.

78. Henderson BM, Winterfield RW: Acute copper toxicosis in the Canada goose. Avian Dis 19:385–387, 1975.

79. Van Sant F: Zinc toxicosis in a hyacinth macaw (abstract). Proc Assoc Avian Vet, 1991, pp 255–259.

80. Howard BR: Health risks of housing small psittacines in galvanized wire mesh cages. J Am Vet Med Assoc 200:1667–1674, 1992.

81. Reece RL, Dickson DB, Burrowes PJ: Zinc toxicity (new wire disease) in aviary birds. Aust Vet J 63:199, 1986.

82. Dhillon AS: An outbreak of enteritis in a psittacine flock (abstract). Proc Assoc Avian Vet, 1988, pp 185–188.

83. Shima AL, Osborn KG: An epornitic of Salmonella typhimurium in a collection of lories and lorikeets. J Zoo Wildl Med 20:373–376, 1989.

84. Gerlach H: Gram-negative bacteria of clinical importance. In Ritchie BW, Harrison GJ, Harrison LR (eds): Avian Medicine: Principles and Application. Lake Worth, FL, Wingers Publishing, 1994, pp 950–965.

85. Rosskopf WJ, Woerpel RW: Successful treatment of avian tuberculosis in pet psittacines (abstract). Proc Assoc Avian Vet, 1991, pp 238–251.

86. VanDerHeyden N: Update on avian mycobacteriosis (abstract). Proc Assoc Avian Vet, 1994, pp 53–62.

87. Erlandsen SL, Bemrick WJ: SEM evidence for a new species, Giardia psittaci. J Parasitol 73:623–629, 1987.

88. Panigrahy B, Craig TM, Glass SE: Intestinal parasitism in budgerigars. J Am Vet Med Assoc 179:573–574, 1981.

89. Giddings RF: Treatment of flukes in a toucan. J Am Vet Med Assoc 193:1555–1556, 1988.

90. Scholtens RG, New JC, Johnson S: The nature and treatment of giardiasis in parakeets. J Am Vet Med Assoc 180:170–173, 1982.

91. Panigrahy B, Mathewson JJ, Hall CF, Grumbles LC: Unusual disease conditions in pet and aviary birds. J Am Vet Med Assoc 178:394–395, 1981.

92. Blagburn BL, Lindsay DS, Hoerr FJ, et al: Cryptosporidium sp. in the proventriculus of an Australian diamond firetail finch (Staganoplura bella: Passeriformes, Estrildidae). Avian Dis 34:1027–1030, 1990.

93. Goodwin MA: Cryptosporidiosis in birds—a review. Avian Pathol 18:365–384, 1989.

94. Latimer KS, Steffens WL, Rakich PM, et al: Cryptosporidiosis in four cockatoos with psittacine beak and feather disease. J Am Vet Med Assoc 200:707–710, 1992.

95. Lindsay DS, Blagburn BL, Hoerr FJ: Small intestinal cryptosporidiosis in cockatiels associated with Cryptosporidium baileyi-like oocysts. Avian Dis 34:791–793, 1990.

96. Goodwin MA, Krabill VA: Diarrhea associated with small-intestinal cryptosporidiosis in a budgerigar and in a cockatiel. Avian Dis 33:829–833, 1989.

97. Bronsdon MA: Rapid dimethyl sulfoxide-modified acid-fast stain of Cryptosporidium oocysts in stool specimens. J Clin Microbiol 19:952–953, 1984.

98. Greiner EC, Ritchie BW: Parasites. In Ritchie BW, Harrison GJ, Harrison LR (eds): Avian Medicine: Principles and Application. Lake Worth, FL, Wingers Publishing, 1994, pp 1007–1029.

99. Rosskopf W Jr, Woerpel RW: Pet avian conditions and syndromes of the most frequently presented species seen in practice. Vet Clin North Am Small Anim Pract 21:1189–1211, 1991.

100. Kazacos KR, Dhillon AS, Winterfield RW, Thacker HL: Fatal hepatic trematodiasis in cockatoos due to Platynosomum proxillicens. Avian Dis 24:788–793, 1980.

101. Quesenberry KE, Tappe JP, Greiner EC, et al: Hepatic trematodiasis in five cockatoos. J Am Vet Med Assoc 189:1103–1105, 1986.

102. Potter K, Connor T, Gallina AM: Cholangiocarcinoma in a yellow-faced Amazon parrot (Amazona xanthops). Avian Dis 27:556–568, 1983.

103. Coleman CW: Bile duct carcinoma and cloacal prolapse. J Assoc Avian Vet 5:87–89, 1991.

104. Hillyer EE, Moroff S, Hoefer H, Quesenberry KE: Bile duct carcinoma in two out of ten Amazon parrots with cloacal papillomas. J Assoc Avian Vet 5:91–95, 1991.

105. Graham DL: Internal papillomatous disease (abstract). Proc Assoc Avian Vet, 1988, p 31.

106. McMillan MC: Imaging techniques. In Ritchie BW, Harrison GJ, Harrison LR (ed): Avian Medicine: Principles and Application. Lake Worth, FL, Wingers Publishing, 1994, p 255.

107. Graham DL, Heyer GW: Diseases of the exocrine pancreas in pet, exotic, and wild birds: A pathologists perspective (abstract). Proc Assoc Avian Vet, 1992, pp 190–193.

108. Graham DL: Acute pancreatic necrosis in quaker parrots (*Myiopsitta monachus*) (abstract). Proc Assoc Avian Vet, 1994, pp 87–88.

109. Candeletta SC, Homer BI, Garner MM, Isaza R: Diabetes mellitus associated with chronic lymphocytic pancreatitis in an African Grey parrot (Psittacus erithacus erithacus). J Assoc Avian Vet 7:39–43, 1993.

110. Simpson VR: Suspected paramyxovirus 3 infection associated with pancreatitis and nervous signs in Neophema parakeets. Vet Rec 132:554–555, 1993.

111. Quesenberry KE, Liu SK: Pancreatic atrophy in a blue and gold macaw. J Am Vet Med Assoc 189:1107–1108, 1986.

112. Pass DA, Wylie SL, Forshaw D: Acute pancreatic necrosis of galahs (Cacatua roseicapilla). Aust Vet J 63:340–341, 1986.

113. Phalen DN: Acute pancreatic necrosis in an umbrella cockatoo (abstract). Proc Assoc Avian Vet, 1988, pp 203–205.

114. Gerlach H: Chlamydia. In Ritchie BW, Harrison GJ, Harrison LR (eds): Avian Medicine: Principles and Application. Lake Worth, FL, Wingers Publishing, 1994, pp 984–996.

115. Rosenberger JK, Olson NO: Reovirus infection. In Calnek BW (ed): Diseases of Poultry. Ames, Iowa State University Press, 1991, pp 639–647.

116. Thompson JN: Impaired lipid and vitamin E absorption related to atrophy of the pancreas in selenium deficient chicks. J Nutr 100:797–809, 1970.

117. Swartout MS, Wyman M: Pancreatic carcinoma in a cockatiel. J Am Vet Med Assoc 191:451–452, 1987.

118. Tenhunen R: The green color of avian bile: A biochemical explanation. Scand J Clin Lab Invest 27:9, 1971.

119. Lin GL, Himes JA, Cornelius CE: Bilirubin and biliverdin excretion by the chicken. Am J Physiol 226:881–885, 1974.

120. Lumeij JT: Fasting and postprandial bile acid concentrations in racing pigeons (*Columbia livia domestica*) and mallards (*Anas platyrhynchus*). J Assoc Avian Vet 5:197–200, 1991.

121. Lumeij JT, Remple JD: Plasma bile acid concentrations in response to feeding in peregrine falcons (*Falco peregrinus*). Avian Dis 36:1060–1062, 1992.

122. Flammer K: Serum bile acids in psittacine birds (abstract). Proc Assoc Avian Vet, 1994, pp 9–12.

123. Lumeij JT, Meidam M, Wolfswinkel J, et al: Changes in plasma chemistry after drug induced liver disease or muscle necrosis in racing pigeons (*Columbia livia domestica*). Avian Pathol 17:865–874, 1988.

124. Bromidge ES, Wells JW, Wight PAL: Elevated bile acids in the plasma of laying hens fed rapeseed meal. Res Vet Sci 39:378–382, 1985.

125. Hoefer HL, Moroff S: The use of bile acids in the diagnosis of hepatobiliary disease in the parrot (abstract). Proc Assoc Avian Vet, 1991, pp 118–119.

126. Mashige F, Tanaka N, Maki A: Direct spectrophotometry of total bile acids in serum. Clin Chem 27:1352–1356, 1981.

127. Gaskin JM: Psittacine viral diseases: A perspective. J Zoo Wildl Med 20:249–264, 1989.

128. Pass DA: Inclusion bodies and hepatopathies in psittacines. Avian Pathol 16:581–597, 1987.

129. Goodwin MA, Davis JF: Adenovirus particles and inclusion body hepatitis in pigeons. J Assoc Avian Vet 6:37–39, 1992.

130. Panigrahy B, Grumbles LC: Pacheco's disease in psittacine birds. Avian Dis 28:808–812, 1984.

131. Gough RE, Alexander DJ: Pacheco's disease in psittacine birds in Great Britain 1987 to 1991. Vet Rec 132:113–115, 1993.

132. O'Toole D, Haven T, Driscoll M, Nunamaker C: An outbreak of Pacheco's disease in an aviary of psittacines. J Vet Diagn Invest 4:203–205, 1992.

133. Cartwright M, Spraker TR, McCluggage D: Psittacine inclusion body hepatitis in an aviary. J Am Vet Med Assoc 187:1045–1046, 1985.

134. Schuh JC, Sileo L, Siegfried LM, Yuill TM: Inclusion body disease of cranes: Comparison of pathologic findings in cranes with acquired versus experimentally induced disease. J Am Vet Med Assoc 189:993–936, 1986.

135. Aini I, Shih LM, Castro AE, Zee YC: Comparison of herpesvirus isolates from falcons, pigeons and psittacines by restriction endonuclease analysis. J Wildl Dis 29:196–202, 1993.

136. Charlton BR, Barr BD, Castro AE, et al: Herpes viral hepatitis in a toucan. Avian Dis 34:787–790, 1990.

137. Saik JE, Weintraub ER, Diters RW, Egy MAE: Pigeon herpesvirus: Inclusion body hepatitis in a free ranging pigeon. Avian Dis 30:426–428, 1986.

138. Graham DL, Calnek BW: Papovavirus infection in hand-fed parrots: Virus isolation and pathology. Avian Dis 31:398–410, 1987.

139. Bernier G, Morin M, Marsolais G: A generalized inclusion body disease in the budgerigar (Melopsittacus undulatus) caused by a papovavirus-like agent. Avian Dis 25:1083–1092, 1981.

140. Kingston RS: Budgerigar fledgling disease (papovavirus) in pet birds. J Vet Diagn Invest 4:455–458, 1992.

141. Jacobson ER, Hines SA, Quesenberry K, et al: Epornitic of papova-like virus-associated disease in a psittacine nursery. J Am Vet Med Assoc 185:1337–1341, 1984.

142. Ritchie BW, Niagro FD, Latimer KS, et al: Polyomavirus infections in adult psittacine birds. J Assoc Avian Vet 5:202–206, 1991.

143. Gomez-Villamandos JC, Mozos E, Sierra MA, et al: Inclusion bodies containing adenovirus-like particles in the intestine of a psittacine bird affected by inclusion body hepatitis. J Wildl Dis 28:319–322, 1992.

144. Scott PC, Condron RJ, Reece RL: Inclusion body hepatitis associated with adenovirus-like particles in a cockatiel (Psittaciformes; Nymphicus hollandicus). Aust Vet J 63:337–378, 1986.

145. Jack SW, Reed WM: Further characterization of an avian adenovirus associated with inclusion body hepatitis in bobwhite quail. Avian Dis 34:526–530, 1990.

146. Bryant WM, Montali RJ: An outbreak of fatal inclusion body hepatitis in zoo psittacines (abstract). Proc First Int Conf Zool Avian Med, 1987, p 473.

147. Graham DL: Characterization of a reo-like virus and its

isolation from and pathogenicity for parrots. Avian Dis 31:411–419, 1987.

148. Wilson RB, Holscher M, Hodges JR, Thomas S: Necrotizing hepatitis associated with a reo-like virus infection in a parrot. Avian Dis 29:568–571, 1985.

149. Hartley WJ, Dubey JP: Fatal toxoplasmosis in some native Australian birds. J Vet Diagn Invest 3:167–169, 1991.

150. Helman RG, Jensen JM, Russell RG: Systemic protozoal disease in zebra finches. J Am Vet Med Assoc 185:1400–1401, 1984.

151. Howerth EW, Rich G, Dubey JP, Yogasundram K: Fatal toxoplasmosis in a red lory (Eos bornea). Avian Dis 35:642–646, 1991.

152. Dhillon AS, Thacker HL, Winterfield RW: Toxoplasmosis in mynahs. Avian Dis 26:445–459, 1982.

153. Hillyer EV: An outbreak of *Sarcocystis* in a collection of psittacines. J Zoo Wildl Med 22:434–445, 1991.

154. Lowenstine LJ, Petrak MI: Microsporidiosis in two peach-faced lovebirds. In Montali RJ, Migaki G (eds): Comparative Pathology of Zoo Animals. Washington DC, Smithsonian Institution Press, 1980, pp 365–368.

155. Randall CJ, Lees S, Higgins RJ, Harcourt-Brown NH: Microsporidian infection in lovebirds (*Agapornis* spp.). Avian Pathol 15:223–231, 1986.

156. Kock MD, Duhamel GE: Hepatic distomiasis in a sulphur-crested cockatoo. J Am Vet Med Assoc 181:1388–1389, 1982.

157. Gosselin SJ, Kramer LW: Pathophysiology of excessive iron storage in mynah birds. J Am Vet Med Assoc 183:1238–1240, 1983.

158. Randell MG, Patnaik AK, Gould WJ: Hepatopathy associated with excessive iron storage in mynah birds. J Am Vet Med Assoc 179:1214–1217, 1981.

159. Worell AB: Further investigations in ramphastids concerning hemochromatosis (abstract). Proc Assoc Avian Vet, 1993, pp 98–107.

160. Cornelissen H, Ducatelle R, Roels S: Successful treatment of a channel-billed toucan (*Ramphastos vitellinus*) with iron storage disease by chelation therapy: Sequential monitoring of the iron content of the liver during the treatment period by quantitative chemical and image analyses. J Avian Med Surg 9:131–137, 1995.

161. Murphy J: Psittacine fatty liver syndrome (abstract). Proc Assoc Avian Vet, 1992, pp 78–82.

162. Hardy RM: Diseases of the liver and their treatment. In Ettinger SJ (ed): Textbook of Veterinary Internal Medicine, vol. II. Philadelphia, WB Saunders, 1989, pp 1479–1527.

163. Campbell TW: Mycotic diseases. In Harrison GJ, Harrison LR (eds): Clinical Avian Medicine and Surgery. Philadelphia, WB Saunders, 1986, pp 464–471.

164. Swanson JR, Veatch J, Trieb DK: CNS symptoms in a tucuman Amazon (*Amazona tucumana*) due to amyloidosis in the brain (abstract). Proc Assoc Avian Vet, 1994, pp 275–277.

165. Loeven KO: Hepatic amyloidosis in two Chinese Shar Pei dogs. J Am Vet Med Assoc 204:1212–1216, 1994.

166. Anderson WI, Dougherty EP, Steinberg H: Cholangiocarcinoma in a 4-month-old double yellow-cheeked Amazon parrot (Amazona autumnalis). Avian Dis 33:594–599, 1989.

167. Elangbam CS, Panciera RJ: Cholangiocarcinoma in a blue-fronted Amazon parrot (Amazona estiva). Avian Dis 32:594–596, 1988.

168. Allen JL, Martin HD, Crowley AM: Metastatic cholangiocarcinoma in a Florida sandhill crane. J Am Vet Med Assoc 187:1215, 1985.

169. Leach MW: A survey of neoplasia in pet birds. Semin Avian Exotic Pet Med 1:52–64, 1992.

170. Stone EG, Redig PT: Preliminary evaluation of hetastarch for the management of hypoproteinemia and hypovolemia (abstract). Proc Assoc Avian Vet, 1994, pp 197–199.

171. Boer HH: Colchicine therapy for hepatic fibrosis in a dog. J Am Vet Med Assoc 185:303, 1984.

172. Hoefer HL: Hepatic fibrosis and colchicine therapy. J Assoc Avian Vet 5:193, 1991.

173. Norton TM, Gaskin J, Kollias GV, et al: Efficacy of acyclovir against herpesvirus infection in Quaker parakeets. Am J Vet Res 52:2007–2009, 1991.

174. Norton TM, Kollias GV, Clark CH, et al: Acyclovir (Zovirax) pharmacokinetics in Quaker parakeets, Myiopsitta monachus. J Vet Pharmacol Ther 15:252–258, 1992.

Karen Rosenthal
Susan Orosz
Gerry M. Dorrestein

27

Nervous System

Susan Orosz

Anatomy of the Central Nervous System

SPINAL CORD

The spinal cord is approximately the same length as the vertebral column in birds. For this reason, birds do not have a cauda equina that would be useful for cerebral spinal fluid (CSF) taps. Instead, the nerves travel laterally through their respective intervertebral foramina. Like mammals, birds have two enlargements of the spinal cord—the cervical and lumbosacral. Their relative size is dependent on function. Birds that fly have a larger cervical enlargement, whereas ratites have a larger lumbosacral enlargement. Within the dorsal midline of the lumbosacral enlargement is a cleft or rhomboidal sinus that is filled with a gelatinous material, which is called the "glycogen body." It consists of glycogen cells that are innervated by unmyelinated nerves. This structure is unique to birds and its function remains unknown. The meninges of the spinal cord are the same as in mammals, except that there is an epidural space in the cervical and thoracic regions that is filled with a gelatinous material. It is thought that this material acts as a cushion for the cord in this region because of the great mobility and length of the neck in birds.

Most birds have more spinospinal pathways than mammals, and their lateral and ventral white columns of tracts are much larger than the dorsal column (Fig. 27–1). The ascending tracts have been explored mostly in pigeons. The dorsal column is similar to the fasciculus gracilis and fasciculus cuneatus of mammals. It remains uniform in size throughout the length of the cord, suggesting that axons ascend for only several segments. The dorso-lateral ascending bundle is similar to the dorsal spinocerebellar tract of mammals, which is stimulated by muscle receptors. Nerve fibers originate in the gray matter in a similar location to Clarke's column, and ascend ipsilaterally to enter the cerebellum via the caudal cerebellar peduncle. Unlike mammals, this tract serves only the brachial plexus and hence the wing musculature. The ventrolateral ascending bundle is activated by muscle afferents from the hind limb only and arises from the gray matter in that region. Fibers decussate and ascend through the cord and brainstem to enter the cerebellum by the rostral cerebellar peduncle, where they decussate a second time in the commissure. There is a dorsolateral fasciculus similar to the tract of Lissauer, the ventral spinothalamic tract of mammals, which transmits information about pain to the thalamus. In addition, there is a lateral column that is suggestive of the dorsal spinothalamic tract, which transmits tactile information and may also transmit pinprick pain, temperature, and light touch. The spinoreticular tract ascends bilaterally to the reticular formation of the brainstem and probably provides somatosensory information for pain localization. Birds also have a propriospinal system which is homologous to the fasciculus proprius of mammals. It is a multisynaptic pathway for the transmission of pain fibers that are nonlocalizing and is part of the reticular activating system.

Little is known about the descending pathways in the spinal cord. The majority of these tracts are fairly long spinospinal axons. There are two tracts in the lateral column that are known in birds. The rubrospinal tract originates in the red nucleus of the

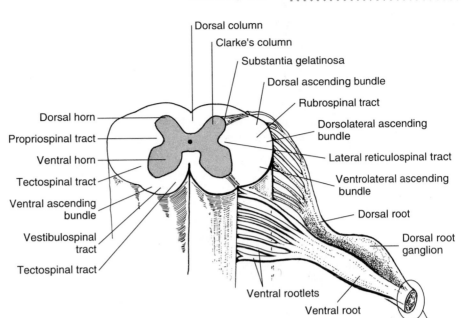

Figure 27-1

Diagram of the location of fiber tracts and anatomic components of the spinal cord. The dorsal column sends information on conscious proprioception, whereas the dorso- and ventrolateral ascending bundles convey unconscious proprioception. The propriospinal tract surrounds the gray matter to form a multisynaptic pathway carrying pain fibers. Vestibulospinal and tectospinal tracts stimulate extensor motor tone, and the rubrospinal tract stimulates flexor motor tone.

midbrain or mesencephalon. Fibers decussate as they leave the red nucleus and descend on the contralateral side of the cord to end near motoneurons that enhance flexor tone. The lateral spinoreticular tract ends near the nucleus intermedius of the gray matter, which in mammals represents the preganglionic fibers that affect visceral motor function. The ventral column contains a number of tracts. One is similar to the pyramidal tract in that it is thought to arise from the archistriatum of the forebrain, decussate in the pyramids, and then descend in both the dorsal and ventral columns to synapse on motoneurons of the cervical region only. The vestibulospinal tract originates from the medial longitudinal bundle, divides into a medial and lateral tract, and ends near motoneurons that stimulate extensor tone. The tectospinal tract arises from the optic tectum and oculomotor nuclei to descend to the upper cord segments. This tract is involved in the coordination of eye and trunk movements for tracking.

BRAIN AND BRAINSTEM

The brainstem of birds has evolved from the reptilian brain, and its appearance and architecture are similar to that of mammals (Fig. 27–2). However,

the forebrain, consisting of the diencephalon and the telencephalon, has undergone divergent lines of evolution, making it extremely difficult to recognize homologous structures. For example, the neocortex developed on the surface of the cerebral hemispheres in mammals, but in birds the cortical cells are found deep within the cortex. Another interesting and important finding is that birds have a unique ability to repopulate collections of neurons and re-establish tracts within the central nervous system (CNS). This occurs during the breeding season, particularly for the development of song. It is unknown at this time if birds can regenerate nuclei and tracts after trauma.

Birds have a subarachnoid cistern between the cerebellum and the dorsal medulla; however, it is extremely difficult to collect CSF from a live bird. There are no grossly visible medial and lateral foramina of the fourth ventricle for release of CSF into the subarachnoid space. It is thought that the fluid moves out by diffusion or possibly by microscopic pores. Birds have arachnoid granulations in their dural venous sinuses for drainage of CSF out of the ventricular system.

CRANIAL NERVES

The olfactory nerve arises from cell bodies within the mucosa that converge to form a trunk in the

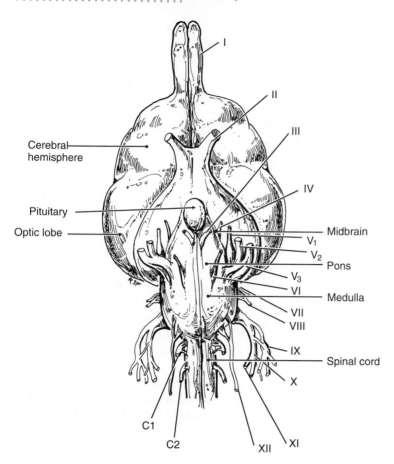

Cerebral
hemisphere

Pituitary

Optic lobe

I

II

III

IV

V₁

Midbrain

V₂

Pons

V₃

VI

Medulla

VII

VIII

IX

Spinal cord

X

C1

C2

XII

XI

F i g u r e 2 7 – 2

Schematic representation of the ventral view of the brain and brainstem, indicating the origin of the cranial nerves. The cortex does not have sulci and gyri.

caudal nasal cavity. This trunk enters the skull through an olfactory foramen, in contrast to entry through the cribriform plate of mammals.

The optic nerve represents fibers from the ganglion cells of the retina. They become myelinated as they penetrate the sclera. Almost all of the fibers decussate at the optic chiasm to continue as the optic tract. These fibers project to the principal optic nucleus of the thalamus, which is similar to the lateral geniculate body of mammals. The cross-sectional diameter of the optic nerve of birds is at least as large as their cervical spinal cord, which suggests that birds are highly visual animals. In addition, fibers enter the mesencephalic colliculus or optic tectum, which in birds is so large that it is commonly called the "optic lobe." Cranial nerves III, IV, and VI supply the muscles to the eye and orbit in birds. These extraocular muscles are very small in birds. Birds move their heads for tracking, instead of using extraocular muscles.

The oculomotor nerve originates from its nucleus, which is similarly located in mammals, ventral to the mesencephalic aqueduct in the rostral midbrain. The nerve leaves the skull through its own separate foramen or the optic foramen and then divides into dorsal and ventral branches. The dorsal branch supplies the dorsal rectus and the levator palpebrae superioris, whereas the ventral branch innervates the ventral rectus, medial rectus, and ventral oblique muscles and the ciliary ganglion. The trochlear nerve arises from its nucleus just caudal to the oculomotor nerve. As in mammals, the axons swing dorsally to decussate over the cerebral aqueduct. The nerve travels through the trochlear foramen to supply the dorsal oblique muscle. The abducent nerve arises from the ventral medulla and runs in the dural venous sinus to escape through the abducent foramen. This nerve supplies the lateral rectus and the two muscles that move the third eyelid—the pyramidalis and quadratus muscles.

The trigeminal nerve originates ventral to the mesencephalic colliculus or optic tectum. This large nerve swells to form the trigeminal ganglion and then divides into an ophthalmic nerve and a combined maxillary/mandibular nerve that separates as it leaves the skull. The ophthalmic nerve or V_1 branches as the iridociliary nerve, which is sensory to the eyeball. The ophthalmic nerve continues through the orbit dorsally to divide rostrally into medial and lateral branches. The lateral branch receives sensory information from the upper eyelid; skin of the forehead; comb, if present; and the rostral portion of the nasal cavity. The medial branch is sensory to the nasal septum, nasal mucosa, the hard palate, and the Herbst corpuscles along the upper edge of the maxillary rhamphotheca or beak.

The maxillary nerve or V_2 divides into three branches after it emerges from the skull. The supraorbital nerve is one branch. It provides sensory information from the conjunctiva and skin of the upper lid and dorsolateral surface of the head. The infraorbital nerve is small compared with that of mammals. It is sensory to the lower eyelid, conjunctiva, and skin of the rictus that surrounds the angle of the mouth. The nasopalatine nerve is the third branch of the maxillary nerve. It arises from the sphenopalatine ganglion and thus receives post-ganglionic parasympathetic fibers from the facial nerve. It receives fibers (sensory from V_2) from the lacrimal gland and from the receptor endings on the tomium of the maxillary rhamphotheca. The mandibular nerve, V_3, emerges from either the maxillomandibular foramen or the mandibular foramen. It supplies motor fibers to the muscles of mastication and sensory fibers to the skin and mucosa of the rictus, the mandibular rhamphotheca, and the floor of the rostral portion of the oropharynx.

The facial nerve emerges from the ventrolateral medulla to enter the internal acoustic meatus with cranial nerve (CN) VIII. It traverses the facial canal and enlarges slightly to demarcate the geniculate ganglion (special visceral afferent cell bodies for taste) before dividing into the palatine and the hyomandibular nerves. The palatine nerve is comparable to the greater superficial petrosal nerve of mammals. It divides into a dorsal branch that provides post-ganglionic fibers from the ethmoidal ganglion to the gland of the nictitans, to the nasal gland, as well as to glands of the nasal and rostral palatine mucosa. The ventral branch arises from the sphenopalatine ganglion and gives off post-ganglionic parasympathetic fibers to the glands of the nasal mucosa and caudal part of the hard palate. The hyomandibular nerve innervates the mandibular depressor muscle, which is similar to the caudal belly of the digastricus muscle and the stylohyoid muscle. The chordi tympani nerve innervates the rostral mandibular salivary gland. Axons sending information concerning taste from the maxillary and mandibular rhamphotheca most likely travel with V_2 and V_3, not the chordi tympani nerve, to the nucleus solitarius in the medulla.

The vestibulocochlear nerve has a vestibular component that innervates the ampullary cristae and the maculae of the utricle and saccule. It also has a cochlear component that has processes that arise along the basilar membrane of the cochlea, which discriminates sounds.

The glossopharyngeal nerve arises in the ventral caudal medulla in close association with cranial nerves X and XI. The proximal ganglion of IX fuses with X, and fibers from its distal ganglion anastomose with the vagus nerve. Therefore, it is impossible to distinguish pure IX from X dysfunction clinically. After these anastomoses, the glossopharyngeal nerve divides into three nerves. The lingual nerve provides sensory fibers and taste to the tongue and parasympathetic supply to the lingual salivary glands. The laryngopharyngeal nerve innervates the muscles of the larynx and provides sensory fibers to the larynx and oropharynx. The third branch is the descending esophageal nerve, which supplies the esophagus and trachea. This nerve anastomoses with the recurrent laryngeal nerve to supply the crop. The ninth cranial nerve does not supply the carotid body in birds like it does in mammals.

After the vagus combines with the glossopharyngeal nerve to form a common ganglion, it descends out of the skull though a separate foramen. It receives fibers from the cranial cervical ganglion and then reanastomoses with cranial nerve IX. The vagus nerve continues down the cervical region with the jugular vein and at the thoracic inlet expands into the distal vagal ganglion. It is thought that these fibers are visceral afferents. The vagus nerve provides innervation to the carotid body; fibers to the thymus, parathyroids, and ultimobranchial glands; baroreceptors in the aorta and/or pulmonary trunk; afferents from the heart and lung; musculature and mucosa of the esophagus, crop, trachea, and syrinx; parasympathetic supply to the heart and lungs and by the abdominal vagus; and parasympathetic supply to the proventriculus, ventriculus, duodenum, liver, and possibly the spleen.

The accessory nerve has a spinal component consisting of the first two cervical cord segments that ascend through the foramen magnum to join with the brainstem component. This nerve becomes enclosed in a common sheath with the vagus while it is still in the skull cavity. It then continues out of the foramen in this manner. Some of the fibers branch out of this sheath to innervate the dorsal cervical muscles, whereas the remainder are thought to travel with the vagus. This dispersion makes it difficult to distinguish cranial nerve dysfunction on neurologic examination.

The same problem occurs with the hypoglossal nerve. Rootlets emerge from the medulla to form two trunks that combine with the first cervical nerve as the hypoglossocervical nerve. This nerve then anastomoses with cranial nerves IX and X. This combined nerve then branches as the descending cervical nerve, which supplies the tracheal muscles; the laryngolingual ramus, which innervates the intrinsic tongue musculature of psittacines; and the tracheal nerve, which supplies the intrinsic muscles of the syrinx.

SPINAL NERVES

The spinal nerves are numbered consecutively from the first to the last. The first pair of nerves move out of the vertebral canal laterally between the occipital condyle and the atlas. The last pair of spinal nerves traverse the intervertebral foramen between the last free caudal vertebra and the pygostyle. Each of the remaining nerves emerges through an intervertebral foramen. However, in the synsacrum, they split into a dorsal and ventral branch before leaving by their respective foramina. The anatomy of the spinal nerves is similar to that of mammals. Dissections in domestic fowl demonstrate that the sympathetic chain in the thoracic and synsacral regions fuses with their respective dorsal root ganglia, which most likely occurs in other species of birds as well. The thickness of the spinal nerves varies with the function of the musculoskeletal system in each re-

gion. Nerves that are relatively large can be found in the cervical region and in the brachial and lumbosacral plexuses. The musculature of the cervical region provides tremendous flexibility of the head and neck.

The brachial plexus contributes innervation to the thoracic limb or the wing. It is often formed from the ventral rami of four or five spinal nerves, which combine and then emerge as two to three trunks. After various divisions of the trunk, a ventral fascicle, which innervates the flexors of the wing, and a dorsal fascicle, for the extensors, are formed. The nerves associated with flexion include the pectoral nerves to the pectoralis musculature that provide the downstroke for the wing; the medianoulnar nerve, which further divides into the median (brachialis muscle and flexors of the carpus and digits) and ulnar (some of the flexors of the carpus and digits) nerves; the bicipital nerve, which innervates the biceps brachii muscle for flexion of the forelimb; and the ventral propatagial nerve, which is sensory to the ventral propatagial area of the leading edge of the wing. The dorsal fascicle divides into the axillary nerve, which innervates the deltoid muscles, which elevate the shoulder; nerves to the triceps muscles, which extend the elbow; and the radial nerve, which supplies the extensors of the carpus and digits and sensory supply to the dorsal propatagial area.

The lumbosacral plexus innervates the musculature of the pelvic limb of the bird. It is formed from the ventral rami of approximately eight spinal nerves of which the first three become the lumbar plexus and the last five to six form the sacral plexus. The lumbar plexus is adjacent to the cranial division of the kidney, whereas the sacral plexus actually runs through the parenchyma of the middle division.

The two major nerves derived from the lumbar plexus are the femoral and the obturator nerves. The former supplies the dorsolateral surface of the ilium, the extensors of the knee (femorotibialis and iliotibialis) and the ambiens muscle medially. The obturator nerve supplies the puboischiofemoralis muscles, or adductors of the leg.

The sacral plexus innervates the flexor cruris medialis and lateralis, muscular rami to the proximal muscles of the leg, and ends as the ischiatic nerve. This nerve travels through the parenchyma of the middle division of the kidney. Nerve dysfunction resulting from renal masses in budgies results in non–weight-bearing lameness. The ischiatic nerve divides into the fibular or peroneal nerve and usually two tibial nerves. The fibular nerve supplies the flexors of the intertarsal joint or the hock and the extensors of the digits. The tibial nerve supplies the extensors of the intertarsal joint (gastrocnemius) and flexors of the digits.

Physiology of the Brain and Special Senses

Gerry M. Dorrestein

Birds exhibit greater intelligence than is implied by the popular slur "birdbrain." They outperform mammals in many laboratory problem-solving experiments. Two-way verbal communication experiments with an African grey parrot have revealed advanced abstracting and conceptual abilities.

The evolution of the avian brain has taken a different course from that of mammals. The basis for avian intelligence lies in the hyperstriatum layer of the forebrain, primarily in tissue called the Wülst. Particularly exciting have been the identification of the brain centers for control of song in passerine birds and the definition of the neural pathways that control this complex motor skill. Another example of the relationship between brain development and behavior in birds is the control of spatial memory by the enlarged hippocampus of the forebrain in seed-caching birds. For instance, the Clark's nutcracker hides an average of two pine seeds in each of 1400 to 2000 caches to survive the winter and early spring.[1] The ability to recall the precise locations of about 2000 caches for spans of as long as 8 or 9 months reflects a phenomenal spatial memory.

Birds have a full repertoire of well-developed senses. Large eyes and well-developed optic lobes of the brain provide excellent vision, including an ability to follow small moving objects. Some birds may also have the most highly developed color vision of any vertebrate. The hearing of birds generally is good but not extraordinary, except perhaps for the ability of homing pigeons to hear extremely low frequencies (infrasound) and the ability of barn owls to pinpoint sounds made by potential prey. Birds are sensitive to slight differences in barometric pressure and to magnetism. The senses of smell, taste, and touch are also better developed in birds than once was thought.[2]

PHYSIOLOGY OF COMMUNICATION

Birds typically use two modes of communication, visual and acoustic (vocal) signals. Avian displays serve primarily as a means of identification and of communicating locomotory intentions (attack, escape, move, or stay still) or other intentions such as a desire to mate, play, or claim ownership. Visual displays function in concert with plumage color and plumage elaborations.

Complementing the use of visual displays to mediate social interactions are rich vocabularies of sounds. These vocalizations are used to mediate social interactions over long distances. Avian vocalization may be inherited, learned, or invented. The calls of chickens and doves are inherited. Learning guides vocalization development in songbirds, parrots, and hummingbirds. Although birds such as African grey parrots and Northern mockingbirds add new vocalizations to their repertoires throughout their lives, vocal learning is most intensive in early age. Observations of and experiments on the development of singing behavior of hand-reared baby birds have revealed four key periods that influence adult vocalization. These periods of song learning are an early critical learning period, a long silent period, and two practice periods, which involve subsong production and song crystallization.

The critical learning period is the early period during which information is stored for use in later stages of learning. In most species, the critical learning stage lasts less than a year, sometimes much less. The silent period is a long period (up to 8 months) in which syllables learned during the early critical learning period are stored without practice or rehearsal. The subsong period (up to a few months) is analogous to infant babbling. It is a period of practice without communication. Long, soft, unstructured series of syllables and ill-formed sounds are produced (plastic song). In the next practice period (song crystallization), the young bird transforms plastic song into real song by selecting a few syllables from its unstructured repertoire, perfecting them, and then organizing them into "correct patterns and timings." Auditory feedback is essential for song development.[2]

Transferring this knowledge to the "speaking ability" of hand-raised companion parrots could mean that it takes at least 2 years before "communication" can be expected. This is true assuming that in the first year much time is spent in "training" the bird.

MIGRATION AND NAVIGATION

Migration allows year-round activity, unlike dormancy and hibernation, and is the means by which many animals live through severe seasons. The advantage of migration is that birds can exploit seasonal feeding opportunities while living in favorable climates throughout the year. The costs of migration are potentially great. It takes radical physiologic adjustments and sustained fine-tuning to survive such extended travel. In general, among land birds migrants achieve moderate levels of reproductive success and adult survivorship, whereas residents sacrifice productivity for high survivorship (tropical residents) or survivorship for high productivity (temperate residents).

In captivity, migratory species can, when stimulated by changes in day length, show migratory behavior, including early moult, premigratory fattening, and migratory restlessness (Zugunruhe).

In their daily routine and on annual migrations, birds navigate great distances, sometimes across unfamiliar terrain. Homing pigeons return to their lofts by flying as much as 800 Km per day from unfamiliar places.

Birds rely on acute visual memories for short-distance travel and local orientation. Homing pigeons often ignore obvious landmarks until they come within their home area, where they use large buildings to make a final correction toward home. Well-trained homing pigeons can fly "blind" back to their lofts. When they reach the vicinity of their lofts, they hover and land much like helicopters.

Migratory birds and pigeons also use the position of the sun to guide them by day. Birds maintain their direction when they migrate at night by using the stars. The solar compass compensates for the ever-changing position of the sun in the course of the day. The stellar compass probably does not, but instead focuses on the constellations close to the North Star, the fixed axis of rotation of the night sky.

Pigeons can smell their way home. It appears that olfactory cues may supplement other navigation systems. Recent studies confirm that birds use the earth's magnetic fields to define their initial compass directions and then add celestial compass information onto this foundation.[3] A pigeon's ability to use magnetic compass information develops before solar compass abilities are manifest. On their first flight, juvenile homing pigeons record the general direction of their outbound journey, which is based on magnetic field information. Young pigeons do not establish a home direction if they are transported in a distorted magnetic field from their nest on the first trip or they are made to carry magnets on their maiden flight. Pigeons do not inherit a knowledge of solar compass positions but calibrate their solar compass in reference to their initial magnetic compass.[4] Orientation by magnetic field information alone is practiced when clouds obscure celestial cues. Specialized photoreceptors in the visual system appear to be sensitive to a bird's orientation relative to these fields.

Some, perhaps most, migratory songbirds inherit genetic programs that route them to traditional wintering grounds by controlling their orientations and flight distance.[2]

Disorders of the Avian Nervous System

Karen Rosenthal

Neurologic disease is a common problem in pet birds. A 3-year retrospective study identified more than 80 cases of avian neurologic disease.[5] The clinician's objectives for the diagnosis and management of a possible neurologic disorder include: (1) determining if a neurologic lesion is causing disease; (2) localizing the lesion in the nervous system; (3) estimating the extent of the lesion in the nervous system; (4) determining the pathologic process; and (5) determining the prognosis and treatment protocol.[6]

Many of the neurologic examination methods used to evaluate mammalian responses are not useful or appropriate in birds. Clinical tests frequently used in mammals, such as CSF aspiration, are difficult or impossible to do in birds.

HISTORY

Establishing a diagnosis of neurologic disease depends on the clinical history and the results of a systematic neurologic examination. Because an avian neurologic examination protocol has yet to be established, the signalment and a detailed history are essential in the diagnosis of neurologic disease. The signalment may provide important clues for a diagnostic plan, although very few diagnoses can be positively ruled in or out based on signalment.[6] Age ranges often have certain disease syndromes associated with them.[7] Epilepsy and congenital malformations are more likely to occur in younger birds. Neoplasia and degenerative changes are seen more often in the older patient.

Neurologic disease signs can be either acute and blatant or chronic and insidious. A thorough history is necessary to establish the duration of signs and the present disease status. A history of past or present illnesses could support a diagnosis of a multisystemic or metabolic disorder. General information regarding the health history and drug therapy of the bird is essential.[7] Questions regarding the environment include the type of cage housing the bird, whether it chews on objects in the house, what types of toys are in the cage, and if there is exposure to toxic products. A complete diet history should include what is offered and what is actually eaten, what vitamin and mineral supplements are given, and whether the diet has been changed recently. The possibility of recent trauma is discussed. This is very important in flighted birds because head trauma from flying into windows or fans is common.

A description of the onset, course, duration, and symmetry of the neurologic problem gives important insight into the possible disease mechanism.[7] Congenital disease usually produces clinical signs near hatching. Inflammation, nutritional disorders, and metabolic disease can be acute or chronic but are usually progressive unless therapy is instituted. Traumatic and vascular accidents have an acute onset, but signs remain static or may improve. Toxic effects can be acute or chronic and may progress if the toxin is not removed.

EXAMINATION

The neurologic evaluation of the avian patient begins with a complete physical examination. The avian neurologic examination ideally should adhere to the same systematic evaluation as has been developed for mammals.[6, 7] In practice, this may not be possible. Neurologic examination techniques such as wheelbarrowing and hemiwalking cannot be adequately assessed in birds. In addition, because of anatomic differences, it is much more difficult to obtain an uncontaminated CSF aspiration from a bird than from a mammal.[8]

One objective of the neurologic examination is to locate a lesion and determine if the disease is focal, multifocal, or diffuse.[7] Serial neurologic examinations performed over days or weeks allow determination of disease progression and allow one to view signs that are intermittent.

The veterinarian can obtain a general impression of the bird's behavior by observing its response to the environment.[6] This is best done in an area of the hospital that is quiet. The mental status of the patient reflects brain function, specifically that of the cerebrum, limbic system, hypothalamus, or midbrain.[7] The mental status can be described as alert, dull, stuporous, or comatose. The patient is also described as oriented and appropriate or disoriented and inappropriate.

As with other animals, birds have 12 cranial nerves. These can have sensory, motor, or mixed function. The function of some nerves is unknown.[8] Cranial nerve tests are used to evaluate the function of cranial peripheral nerves and specific anatomic regions of the brainstem, from the prefrontal anatomic regions of the brainstem, from the prefrontal cortex and hypothalamus caudally to the medulla.[7] Each cranial nerve should be evaluated separately, but this may not be possible in birds because the more caudal nerves are characterized by numerous anastomoses.[8] Some cranial nerves cannot be fully assessed. For example, because the sphincter and dilator muscles of the avian pupil are striated, the assessment of the function of cranial nerve III (pupillary light reflex) is equivocal.[8] However, isolated cranial nerve dysfunction occurs rarely in avian species.[9]

Olfactory Nerve

This nerve (cranial nerve I) is sensory in birds, as it is in mammals.[8] It is difficult to assess the function of this nerve in pet birds. A behavioral response to a noxious odor is the test used in mammals.[6]

Optic Nerve

This nerve (cranial nerve II) is entirely sensory and is the largest cranial nerve.[8] Vision is assessed by observation of the animal's movements in unfamiliar surroundings.[6] A menace response, used to evaluate vision in mammals, may be elicited in birds by bringing a finger or hand to the eye causing a blink or a pulling away of the head.[6, 10]

Oculomotor Nerve

This nerve (cranial nerve III) is somatic and also has parasympathetic fibers that are efferent to the ciliary body and iris.[8] In mammals, this nerve is tested with the pupillary light response and presence of pupil symmetry. This test is hampered in birds because of striated muscle in the avian iris. Damage to the motor aspect of this nerve could lead to a strabismus.[10]

Trochlear Nerve

This nerve (cranial nerve IV) is motor to the dorsal oblique muscle of the eye.[8] Lesions in this nerve are difficult to evaluate but may be seen as a lateral rotation of the eye.[6]

Trigeminal Nerve

The ophthalmic nerve branch of cranial nerve V is the main sensory nerve of the nasal cavity and the wall of the eyeball.[8] It is sensory to the upper eyelid, skin of the forehead, nasal mucosa, the palate, the upper beak, and bill tip organ.[8] The maxillary nerve branch is sensory to the skin of the lower eyelid and rictus. The mandibular nerve branch is motor to the muscles of mastication.[8] A lesion in the motor branch of this nerve causes a weakness in the jaw or a dropped jaw if the lesion is bilateral. A lesion in the sensory branch of the nerve causes a lack of response when the appropriate skin areas are stimulated.[6]

Abducent Nerve

This nerve (cranial nerve VI) is motor to the lateral rectus muscle of the eyeball and the striated muscles of third eyelid.[8] Lesions of this nerve may cause a medial strabismus and/or change in the position of the third eyelid.[6]

Facial Nerve

The hyomandibular branch of cranial nerve VII innervates muscles of the mandible. The parasympathetic portion of the nerve innervates the gland of the nictating membrane, the nasal mucosa, salivary glands, and taste buds.[8] A lesion in this nerve may cause weakness of the jaw. A lesion in the parasympathetic branch may affect the glandular response.

Vestibulocochlear Nerve

This nerve (cranial nerve VIII) innervates the ear and provides information about hearing and equilibrium or balance.[8] Head tilt, nystagmus, and vestibular ataxia are characteristic signs seen in mammals having dysfunction of this nerve. Results of simple tests for hearing such as hand clapping are difficult to evaluate in birds.

Glossopharyngeal Nerve

The lingual branch of this nerve (cranial nerve IX) replaces the lingual branch of cranial nerve V in mammals and innervates the epithelium of the tongue.[8] It also has branches that descend into the neck.

Vagus Nerve

In some species the vagus (cranial nerve X) gives off branches to the larynx and pharynx.[8] It also gives off branches to the carotid body, thyroid, parathyroid, heart, esophagus, and crop.[8]

Accessory Nerve

The main branch of this nerve (cranial nerve XI) innervates the cucullaris muscle, which may be homologous to the trapezius muscle in mammals.[8] It may be difficult to assess a lesion in this nerve except if atrophy of the affected muscle is apparent.[6]

Hypoglossal Nerve

This nerve (cranial nerve XII) supplies the tracheal muscles and parts of the syrinx.[8]

Postural Reactions

Proprioceptive position evaluation tests such as wheelbarrowing, hopping, hemiwalking, and placing are difficult or impossible to do in birds because of their bipedal stance. Evaluation of these reactions can be misinterpreted because of the general uncooperativeness of the avian patient.

Motor System

A consistent examination protocol to test the avian upper and lower motor neuron system is yet to be established. In mammals, upper motor neuron deficits cause paralysis, hyperreflexia, and late and mild muscle atrophy.[6] Decreased proprioception and decreased pain perception may accompany upper motor neuron disease. Lower motor neuron disease in mammals causes paralysis, hyporeflexia, and early and severe muscle atrophy.[6] Anesthesia of the innervated area may accompany lower motor neuron disease. In avian species it is difficult to evaluate these motor tracts. Evaluation of the reflexes in mammals is done with the mammal in lateral recumbency, a very unnatural position for birds. Therefore, determining if a disorder such as paralysis is the result of a lesion in the upper or lower motor system and determining its location are challenges for the avian clinician.

NEUROLOGIC DISEASE SIGNS

Seizures

Clinical Signs

A seizure is a paroxysmal, uncontrolled, transient electrical discharge from the neurons of the brain.[7] Seizures in birds can be mild to severe, generalized or partial, and frequent or infrequent.[11] Seizures can be spontaneous or can be induced by external stimuli.[12] Avian seizures can begin with short periods of disorientation with head and body ataxia followed by loss of grip on the perch. The bird then may remain rigid or have major motor activity for varying lengths of time.[10] Signs of a seizure also include falling off the perch with subsequent tremoring and extension of the wings and legs.[13] Unconsciousness can accompany the seizures. Birds can also develop status epilepticus. Postictal activity in birds is variable.[10]

Lesion Localization

A seizure is the result of a disturbance in the CNS; specifically, a seizure indicates a lesion rostral to the midbrain (Fig. 27–3).[7] Systemic disease such as hypoglycemia may induce seizures. Both extracranial and intracranial disease cause seizures by altering the electrical activity of the brain.

Diagnosis

The clinician must first determine whether a seizure has occurred. A seizure must be differentiated from episodes of syncope or weakness. The diagnosis of seizure is based on history, observation of the seizure activity, and ancillary tests, such as hematologic profiles and diagnostic imaging (Fig. 27–4).

Differential Diagnosis

Generalized seizures are most often associated with epilepsy, metabolic disorders, or nutritional disease. Partial seizures are most often associated with infection, trauma, or neoplasia.[7]

Degenerative. Hydrocephalus has been reported as a cause of seizures.[13, 14] In birds, this is typically diagnosed postmortem. However, in mammals it can be found ante mortem by computed tomography (CT) and magnetic resonance imaging (MRI).[7]

Idiopathic. Epilepsy is the most common idiopathic cause of seizures. Intermittent seizures with no other abnormalities can indicate epilepsy, especially if there is a long history of seizures.[12] In chickens, epilepsy has been found to have a genetic basis.[12] Epilepsy is usually a diagnosis of exclusion.[9, 15] Epilepsy may be acquired as a result of a cerebral insult and residual brain damage.

Infectious. Acute septicemia resulting from an infectious agent can cause seizures.[15] Mycotoxicoses can lead to seizures.[16] Velogenic viscerotropic Newcastle disease infections are reported to cause seizures.[15] Aberrant parasite migration in the brain causes seizures.[15]

Metabolic. Hypoglycemia and hypocalcemia are common metabolic imbalances that induce seizures.[15] Seizures associated with hypocalemia have long been recognized in African grey parrots.[17, 18] Vitamin D_3 deficiency may play a role in the pathogenesis of this syndrome because most affected birds are fed a vitamin D_3–deficient diet. Seizures may be associated with hepatic encephalopathy in pet birds.[15] In mammals, it is theorized that toxic substances produced in the gastrointestinal tract, normally cleared by the liver, are responsible for hepatic encephalopathy.[7]

Neoplastic. Brain neoplasms are an important cause of seizures.[15] Typically, neoplasia is a necropsy diagnosis, but it may be found ante mortem with a CT or MRI scan. Pituitary tumors are a well-documented cause of seizures, especially in budgerigars.[19]

Nutritional. Thiamine deficiency is reported as a nutritional cause of seizures in fish-eating birds.[20]

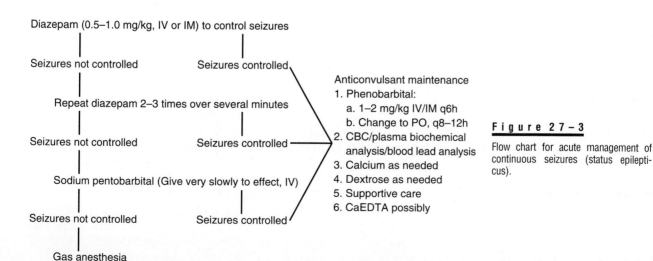

Figure 27–3

Flow chart for acute management of continuous seizures (status epilepticus).

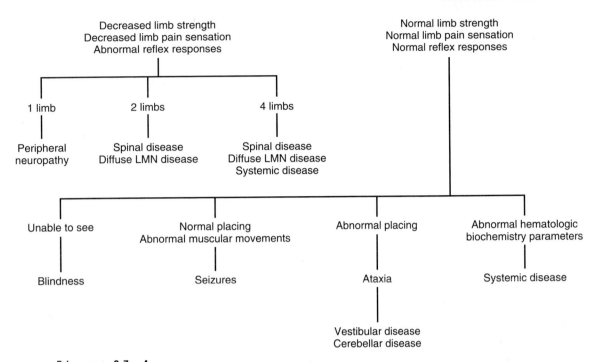

F i g u r e 2 7 – 4

Flow chart for lesion localization in a bird with an abnormal gait or abnormal flight. LMN = lower motor neuron.

This commonly results from ingesting fish that contain thiaminase.

Toxic. Toxins suspected of causing seizures include lead, zinc, aflatoxins, insecticides, and polytetrafluoroethylene.[9, 15] Lead poisoning is a well-known cause of seizures and other neurologic signs in pet birds.[14, 21] Lead poisoning is diagnosed with a blood lead assay. In the author's hospital, 10 to 15 μg/dl is considered the upper limit of the normal range for blood lead concentration. Radiographs aid in the diagnosis. Diagnosis of other toxic causes of seizures is usually based on history of exposure.

Traumatic. A common cause of seizures in psittacine birds is head trauma.[15]

Vascular. An acute, ischemic infarction in the brain can cause seizures.[15] A systemic cause of the infarction should be investigated, but physical evidence of a vascular incident may be difficult to identify on postmortem examination.

Blindness and Abnormal Eye Movements

Clinical Signs

Blindness may be difficult to assess in a bird, especially if it is unilateral. Blindness is recognized by an inability to avoid obstacles in the cage or environment; however, cage-bound birds that are familiar with their environment may not appear blind.[10] Blindness is suspected when pupils are fixed and dilated or birds are startled when caught. Blindness may be associated with exophthalmia.

Lesion Localization

Visual deficits are the result of lesions within the eyeball or are associated with lesions of innervation to the eye.[7] A thorough ophthalmologic examination rules out blindness associated with structural disease within the eye itself. Neurologic disease affects the retina, optic nerve, optic chiasm, optic tract, or optic areas of the brain.[7] Pituitary tumors can put pressure on or invade the optic chiasma and should be considered when blindness is bilateral.[22] If nystagmus or abnormal eye deviation is present, cranial nerves III, IV, and VI may be involved.[10] To locate the lesion in mammals, techniques such as menace response, pupillary light response, CT scan, MRI, electroretinography, and electroencephalography are used.[7] Many of these techniques are not practical or applicable to birds, and lesion location is sometimes difficult to achieve. In birds, the optic nerve fibers decussate almost completely at the optic chiasma, and pupillary responses and accommodation can be asymmetrical.[23] Some abnormalities such as anisocoria that aid in lesion localization in mammals are not as useful in birds because of voluntary motor control of pupil size.[8]

Diagnosis

Diagnosis of blindness is based on the ability of a bird to react to objects brought within its normal line of vision.

Differential Diagnosis

The most common cause of blindness in birds is not neurologic disease, but rather is a structural disorder, such as cataracts.[24]

Infectious. An infection that affects the visual centers of the brain can lead to blindness. Toxoplasmosis is an infectious cause of blindness that affects the retina, the optic nerve, or the brain.[25] Either unilateral or bilateral blindness can be expected.[25] *Toxoplasma* infection is suspected in birds with a positive blood antibody titer.[26]

Metabolic. Severe metabolic disease (e.g., hypoglycemia), hepatic encephalopathy, and osmotic disturbances are reported to cause blindness.[7]

Neoplastic. Neoplasia at any site along the visual pathway produces visual deficits.[7] A space-occupying lesion in the brain is considered when bilateral blindness is present. Pituitary tumors in budgerigars cause bilateral blindness, mydriasis, and exophthalmos.[22, 27, 28] Polyuria, polydipsia, and color pattern changes of the feathers can accompany the neurologic signs of a pituitary tumor.[29] In one report, blindness, exophthalmos, and seizures were associated with a mass around the optic nerve that extended into the optic chiasma.[14] The mass was determined to be a carcinoma of unknown origin.[14] Neoplasia is difficult to diagnosis ante mortem even when imaging diagnostics such as CT and MRI are used.

Nutritional. Thiamine deficiency has been associated with blindness in dogs.[7]

Toxic. Toxic causes of blindness include lead and hexachlorophene ingestion.[15]

Traumatic. Trauma can produce blindness by destroying the eye, the nerves that innervate the eye, or the visual area of the brain. Blunt trauma to the head or eye can cause retinal detachment followed by blindness.[24] Retinal detachment is diagnosed with an ultrasonic eye examination.

Paresis of One Limb

Clinical Signs

Paresis of a wing or leg is common. Asymmetrical wing droop without a fracture is usually a sign of neurologic dysfunction.[10] Little or no movement is elicited from the affected wing. Denervation causes rapid atrophy of the associated muscle group.[7] Birds with a paretic leg develop a weak gait, have a weak or absent withdrawal response, are unable to grasp, and have muscle atrophy of the proximal limb. Severe neurologic disease of the leg is evident when knuckling of the digits or contraction of the leg is apparent.[10] Partial limb paresis is possible and is seen in such diseases as the "curled toe" syndrome.[20, 27]

Lesion Localization

Total paresis of one limb, especially if acute, suggests an injury to either the brachial or sacral plexus, including the avulsion of the roots of the spinal nerves from the plexus. Paresis or paralysis of a wing with no other neurologic abnormalities is caused by an ipsilateral disease process of the brachial plexus or individual nerves of the wing. Paresis or paralysis of the leg is caused by an ipsilateral disease process of the lumbosacral plexus or the individual nerves to the legs.[7] A unilateral thoracolumbar spinal cord lesion could cause paresis of one leg. Toxins, such as lead, have been associated with edema, fragmentation, and inflammation of the myelin sheaths of nerves.[30]

Diagnosis

The diagnosis of a paretic wing or leg is based on history, clinical signs, and physical examination.

Radiographs are used to rule out fractures. The closer the nerve injury is to the muscle it must re-innervate, the better the prognosis for anatomic contact and re-innervation of the muscle before fibrosis occurs.[7]

Differential Diagnosis

Fractures and dislocations are common non-neurologic causes of unilateral limb paresis. Paralysis of one limb is usually caused by trauma or neoplasia.[7]

Infectious. Velogenic viscerotropic Newcastle disease has been reported to cause unilateral paralysis.[31] Unilateral leg paralysis resulting from ascarids has been described.[32] Chlamydial infection and aspergillosis are two infectious causes of unilateral limb paresis.[15]

Inflammatory. Inflammatory diseases such as neuritis and encephalitis are reported to cause unilateral limb paresis.[15]

Metabolic. Metabolic disorders such as hypocalcemia and hypoglycemia must be considered when unilateral paresis is present.[33]

Neoplastic. Tumors involving part of the brachial plexus can account for unilateral wing paralysis.[10] Renal and gonadal tumors cause unilateral leg paresis by compromising the sciatic nerve.[27, 32, 34] The most common clinical sign associated with renal and gonadal tumors is unilateral leg paresis progressing to paralysis, which results from direct pressure of the mass on the sciatic nerve trunk.[34] This occurs commonly in the budgerigar. Tumors can be palpated, found with diagnostic imaging, or diagnosed at necropsy.

Nutritional. Riboflavin deficiency in poultry leads to myelin degeneration of the sciatic nerve, a disease called "curled toe."[35] Other vitamin and mineral deficiencies such as calcium deficiency can cause unilateral limb paresis.[15]

Toxic. Lead poisoning is considered even when there is paresis of only one limb.[30]

Traumatic. Fractures and dislocations are frequently accompanied by peripheral nerve dysfunction and unilateral paralysis. Function normally returns after swelling has resolved and the abnormality is corrected. Paresis of a wing or leg can result from a traumatic brachial or sacral plexus avulsion, respectively.[34, 36] Trauma to the obturator nerve can cause unilateral leg paresis.[15]

Bilateral Limb Paresis, Paralysis, and Ataxia

Clinical Signs

Paresis of the limbs is weakness with retention of some voluntary movement and pain perception. Paraplegia is the loss of voluntary movement, usually accompanied by the loss of motor function and deep pain. Presence of paraplegia carries a very poor prognosis. It usually results from a severe, bilateral spinal cord lesion.[7]

Lesion Localization

Bilateral limb paresis must be differentiated from weakness of non-neurologic origin.[10] Gait deficits with no cranial nerve abnormalities are most commonly caused by either thoracolumbar spinal cord lesions or bilateral peripheral nerve disease.[7] Gait deficits resulting from peripheral lesions may mimic ataxia of either cerebellar or vestibular origin. Bilateral leg paresis indicates that the lesion is most likely in the thoracolumbar spinal cord and is the result of focal, multifocal, or diffuse disease.[7] Ante mortem diagnosis of a spinal lesion in birds is challenging because of the inability to do a myelogram. A diagnosis may be reached using imaging techniques such as CT and MRI. Spinal cord lesions are usually a postmortem diagnosis.

Diagnosis

The diagnosis of bilateral paresis is based on history, clinical signs, physical examination, and results of clinical tests. Ataxia from lesions rostral to the spinal cord and muscular weakness should be ruled out.

Differential Diagnosis

Young animals with bilateral paraparesis, paraplegia, and ataxia may have nutritional disease or congenital abnormalities of the spinal cord or vertebrae. Older animals may have degenerative or neoplastic disease.[7] Nonprogressive bilateral disease is associated with trauma, disc herniation, infarction, or thrombosis. Progressive disease is seen with neoplasia, degenerative disease, and infections.[7]

Congenital. Congenital spinal cord or vertebral malformations are most evident in young animals.[7]

Degenerative. Ruptured intervertebral discs and cervical spondylosis have been reported to cause compression of the spinal cord leading to bilateral pelvic limb paresis and recumbency in birds.[37, 38] In mammals, cervical spinal lesions are more likely to cause tetraparesis than bilateral paresis. Bilateral limb paresis in birds has been attributed to arteriosclerosis.[19]

Infectious. Eastern equine encephalitis virus has been reported to cause leg paresis in finches and pheasants.[39] Velogenic viscerotropic Newcastle disease can cause bilateral paralysis.[31] Chronic *Yersinia pseudotuberculosis* infection in Piciformes leads to leg paralysis.[40] Paralysis of the legs is reported in cockatiels with psittacosis.[41] Fungal infections are known to cause bilateral limb paresis.[15] This is reportedly the result of aspergillosis in the peripheral nerves or spinal cord.[42, 43]

Metabolic. Hypocalcemia is seen with bilateral limb paresis.[33]

Miscellaneous. Dystocia (egg binding) can lead to bilateral leg paresis.[15] This results in part from pressure of the egg on the nervous innervation of the limbs.

Neoplasia. Renal tumors can account for bilateral leg paresis.[27] Spinal cord neoplasia can cause bilateral limb paraplegia.[7]

Nutritional. Vitamin E and selenium deficiency can lead to bilateral limb paresis.[15]

Toxic. Lead poisoning is a very important differential diagnosis when paresis of both limbs is present.[30]

Traumatic. Trauma to the spinal cord and vertebrae can lead to bilateral limb dysfunction.[7]

Vascular. An infarction or thrombosis can lead to bilateral paresis, although the degree of paresis may be asymmetrical.[7]

Tetraparesis

Clinical Signs

Paresis of all four limbs can be acute, chronic, static, or progressive. Birds with motor dysfunction of all four limbs are unable to fly or walk and appear ataxic.

Lesion Localization

Lesions causing tetraparesis are usually central rather than peripheral. Disease origin is above the foramen magnum or is a focal cervical spinal cord disorder, multifocal or diffuse spinal cord disease, or diffuse neuromuscular disease.[7]

Diagnosis

Tetraparesis must be differentiated from diffuse muscle disease, skeletal disease, or severe depression from metabolic disease.[6] The history, physical examination, and ancillary tests are essential factors in the diagnosis.

Differential Diagnosis

The differential diagnosis for tetraparesis includes any disease process that affects multiple areas of the CNS. In mammals, acute tetraparesis is most commonly associated with toxins, spinal cord injury, or intravertebral disc herniation. Chronic progressive tetraparesis is associated with metabolic disease, neoplasia, or infection.[7] In mammals, young animals are more likely candidates for congenital disorders and trauma whereas older animals are more commonly affected by neoplasia.[7]

Degenerative. Degenerative diseases have not been described in birds but are a well-known cause of four-limb motor dysfunction in dogs (cervical disc disease, cervical spondylopathy).[6]

Idiopathic. A progressive tetraparetic syndrome in lorikeets has been described. It begins with bilaterally clenched feet and an inability to extend the phalanges, and progresses to paralysis of the legs and eventually the wings.[44] Although lesions were seen in the spinal cord and brainstem, a definitive diagnosis has not been made. A virus or protozoa is suspected.[34, 44]

Infectious. There is a report of disseminated cryptococcosis causing tetraparesis in a macaw.[45] The cerebral meninges were affected but brain parenchyma was not.

Metabolic. Extracranial causes such as hypocal-

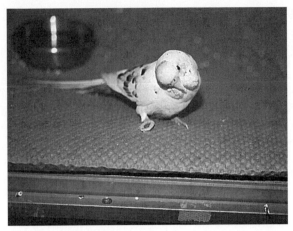

Figure 27–5

Neurologic disease in a budgerigar with signs of ataxia, head tilt, and unilateral knuckling while standing.

cemia and hypoglycemia should be considered in the differential diagnosis of tetraparesis.[33]

Neoplastic. Diffuse, multifocal, or cervical neoplasia of the spinal cord causes tetraparesis.

Toxic. Toxicities from agents such as lead can cause tetraparesis.[30]

Traumatic. A severe cervical spinal cord injury leads to tetraparesis.

Vascular. In dogs, fibrocartilaginous embolization is a well-documented cause of lateralizing paresis, including tetraparesis.[6]

Ataxia of Head and Limbs

Clinical Signs

Ataxia is characterized by a broad-based stance and uncoordinated movements of the head or limbs.[6] Cerebellar gait incoordination (dysmetria) is manifested by excessive, exaggerated, jerky movements of the limbs. Clinical signs are described as whole body tremors and intention tremors with weakness, dysmetria, or hypermetria.[46] Birds may show an inability to fly and walk or they may do so with an unsteady gait.[47] Frequently the first sign of incoordination is falling off the perch.[48] Lesions of the cerebellum in birds produce variable effects, but disorders of posture and movement are the main feature.[8] Cerebellar disease produces an increase in muscle tone leading to strong extension of the

wings, legs, tail, and neck with severe swaying. Torticollis and opisthotonos (muscle spasms resulting in lateral recumbency and dorsiflexion of the neck and extensor rigidity) may also be present.[49] The patient is alert and responsive if only the cerebellum is affected.[7] Walking in circles has been reported.[50]

Lesion Localization

In mammals, ataxia and head incoordination are produced by lesions in the cerebellum, vestibular system, or proprioceptive areas (Figs. 27–5 to 27–7).[7] Lesions reported in the avian literature are rarely localized to the vestibular or proprioceptive tracts. In mammals, ataxia and circling due to a cerebellar lesion are differentiated from signs resulting from vestibular and proprioceptive lesions. Vestibular lesions are characterized by a head tilt, circling, rolling, and nystagmus, which can lead to ataxia.[7] Peripheral vestibular lesions involve disease of the inner ear and the vestibular nerve. Central vestibular lesions disturb the brainstem, vestibular nuclei, and the flocculonodular lobe of the cerebellum.[7] Head tilt and torticollis may be the result of a primary ear infection and not a CNS disease. However, brain inflammation can result from extension of otitis externa.[14] A proprioceptive lesion causes loss of balance and proprioceptive deficits leading

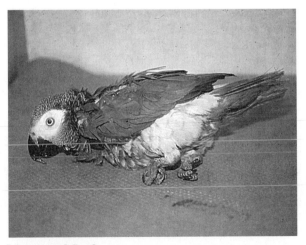

Figure 27–6

Neurologic disease in an African grey parrot exhibiting signs of knuckling and ataxia.

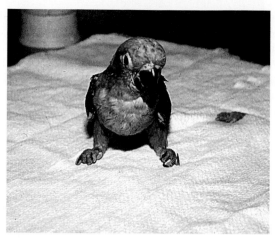

Figure 27-7

Neurologic disease in a conure exhibiting signs of knuckling and ataxia.

to ataxia without the presence of tremors, nystagmus, or head tilt.

In the avian literature, the differentiation between head tilt and head incoordination is seldom appreciated. This differentiation is important for lesion localization. Head ataxia and head tremors are the result of cerebellar disease, whereas head tilt is not characteristic of cerebral or cerebellar disease.[7] It may be that vestibular disease is frequently grouped with cerebral and cerebellar diseases in birds. This is likely because vestibular disease is difficult to differentiate in avian patients; methods used to assess vestibular disease in mammals (tympanic membrane examination, swimming, hopping, and placing) are not practical in birds.[3] Confusingly, reports also describe lesions causing ataxia, intention tremors, incoordination, and even head tilt to be located in the cerebrum in birds.[14] In avian patients with cerebellar disease, it is not uncommon on histopathologic examination to find areas other than the cerebellum affected, such as the cerebrum and medulla.[51, 52] Meningitis can also accompany cerebellar disease.[53] These discrepancies between signs and histologic lesions may, in part, result from functional differences between birds and mammals, misinterpretation of signs, or lesion misinterpretation.

A thorough neurologic examination is very important. A blind bird can be disoriented and appear uncoordinated or ataxic. Ataxia of the head and limbs characterizes some avian seizures.[10]

Diagnosis

To assess movement, the patient is placed on a surface and locomotion is observed. An unsteady gait, inability to fly, inability to right when fallen over, and whole body tremors are characteristic of cerebellar defects.[47] The bird is placed on a perch and observed for the ability to hold onto the perch.[46] Food is placed near the bird and the presence of intention tremors is determined.[46] Because the cerebellum controls the rate, range, and force of movement, any change in these characteristics may indicate cerebellar disease. Histopathology of the CNS offers the definitive diagnosis. CSF from a bird with cerebrospinal nematodiasis yielded only reactive lymphocytes and macrophages.[51] If trauma is suspected, there may be external signs of inflammation around the head and a history of trauma. Erythematous areas on the skull may represent hemorrhage into the skull bones and meninges.[19]

Differential Diagnosis

Most diseases that affect the cerebellum are diagnosed at necropsy. Advanced imaging diagnostics such as CT and MRI may indicate a lesion ante mortem, but a complete diagnosis may not be discerned until postmortem examination.

Congenital. Hereditary ataxia is a recessively inherited disease that affects pigeons, especially young pigeons.[54]

Degenerative. Cerebellar degeneration has been associated with toxins including lead.[30] Encephalomalacia in the cerebellum of conures has been shown to cause weakness and ataxia.[14]

Developmental. Cerebellar degeneration (e.g., from ceroid lipofuscinosis), hypoplasia, atrophy, or failure to develop all cause signs of cerebellar disease in young birds.[14, 47, 55, 56]

Idiopathic. There are numerous reports of cockatiels, especially the lutino variety, having "night frights" or episodes of incoordination with no apparent cause or cure.[32]

Infectious. A nonpurulent encephalitis may be seen with viral diseases.[57] Velogenic viscerotropic Newcastle disease virus causes ataxia and torticollis in budgies.[58] Paramyxovirus groups 1 and 3 cause opisthotonos, torticollis, tremors, clonic-tonic paralysis of the limbs, and ataxia.[31, 57-61] Ataxia of the head and limbs has been associated with Eastern equine encephalitis virus.[62] *Salmonella* produces neuromotor signs such as ataxia in affected pigeons.[40, 54] *Mycoplasma* infections are a cause of cerebellar disease.[53] Other infections that can cause cerebellar disease include *Sarcocystis,* cerebrospinal nematodiasis (*Baylisascaris* species), and toxoplasmosis.[19, 46, 49–52]

Inflammatory. Torticollis resulting from a lymphoplasmacytic meningoencephalitis and associated with moderate mortality has been observed in *Pionus* species and *Neophema* species.[34] Encephalomyelitis, encephalopathies, and meningitis are all possible causes of cerebellar disease.[15, 30]

Neoplastic. Various cerebellar and cerebral tumors and space-occupying lesions are reported to produce ataxia.[14] Carcinoma, chondroma, and lymphosarcoma are a few of the neoplasms that have been reported.[14]

Nutritional. Folic acid deficiency causes head ataxia due to neck muscle paralysis.[34] Encephalomalacia from vitamin E deficiency is known to cause ataxia, head tilt, circling, and torticollis in chicks and budgerigars.[19, 20, 34] Pantothenic acid deficiency has been shown to cause ataxia.[35] Opisthotonos and ataxia are associated with thiamine deficiency.[19, 34, 62] Dietary deficiencies are diagnosed by history, examination of the food, and response to treatment.

Toxic. Numerous toxins are reported to cause signs of cerebellar disease. Two of the many manifestations of lead poisoning are ataxia and tremors.[21] Toxins such as strychnine produce ataxia, tremors, and even seizures.[63] An organophosphate pesticide, chlorpyrifos (Dursban), has been reported to cause incoordination.[64] Dimetridazole toxicity in budgies causes tremors, ataxia, and incoordination.[34, 56, 65, 66] A similar effect is seen with metronidazole and fenbendazole.[56, 65]

Traumatic. Head trauma is an important differential diagnosis of cerebellar disease.[19, 27, 34]

Vascular. Acute ischemic infarction can result in head ataxia.[9]

Disorders of the Face, Tongue, and Larynx

Clinical Signs

The neurologic basis of disorders of the face, tongue, and larynx is cranial nerve dysfunction. However, isolated cranial nerve dysfunction rarely occurs in birds.[9]

Lesion Localization

A loss of beak strength for climbing or eating may be localized to cranial nerve V.[10] Dysphagia or atrophy of the tongue may be associated with abnormalities of cranial nerves IX, X, and XII.[10] Cranial nerve dysfunction resulting from brainstem lesions is characterized by multiple cranial nerve involvement.[6]

Diagnosis

Diagnosis is confirmed by a thorough neurologic examination of the cranial nerves followed by electromyography.[9]

Differential Diagnosis

There are very few reported differential diagnoses for disorders of the face, tongue, and larynx. Differential diagnoses of third eyelid dysfunction include cranial nerve neuritis, encephalitis, and postpox lesions.[15] Paralysis of the mouth occurs with temporomandibular dislocations.[15] Paralysis of the jaw or mouth in cockatiels has been labeled the "cockatiel paralysis syndrome" and is reportedly responsive to vitamin E and selenium.[33]

Signs of Systemic or Multifocal Disease

Clinical Signs

The first step in management of a neurologic problem is the localization of the disease process. When localization is not possible, a multifocal, systemic, or diffuse disease is suspected.[6] A multifocal lesion is suspected when the signs and neurologic examination indicate that two or more components of the nervous system are involved.[6] For example, a space-occupying lesion can affect both the cerebrum (polyphagia, polydipsia) and cerebellum (ataxia).[67] Birds with generalized encephalitis exhibit diverse signs such as tremors, ataxia, inability to fly, torticollis, depression, and paresis. Birds with blindness, ataxia, incoordination, polyuria, and polydipsia have been shown to have extensive pituitary tumors that affect multiple areas of the brain. Birds with multifocal neurologic disease can exhibit generalized whole body tremors and loss of strength.[68]

Lesion Localization

To be considered a multifocal disease, the lesion should be found in at least two areas of the nervous system.

Diagnosis

Many causes of diffuse disease in birds are found only at necropsy and are confirmed by histopathologic examination. Nonprimary neurologic disease must be ruled out. For example, generalized muscle weakness or damage can result in signs resembling generalized neurologic disease. Cranes affected with fusariomycotoxicosis presented with progressive weakness, but histopathologic lesions revealed skeletal muscle damage and degeneration.[69]

Differential Diagnosis

Infectious. Infectious diseases that affect multiple areas of the body cause diffuse neurologic and systemic signs. Paramyxovirus type 1 in pigeons and Newcastle disease both cause generalized neurologic symptoms.[70, 71] Paramyxovirus causes lesions in the brain, spinal cord, and meninges, which lead to generalized neurologic disease.[70] Other infectious agents that have been reported to cause multifocal neurologic disease in birds include *Amoeba* species, *Mycobacterium* species, and *Sarcocystis* species.[14] Generalized encephalitis and neurologic signs are reported with bacterial diseases such as salmonellosis, streptococcosis, and staphylococcosis.[19] *Listeria monocytogenes* infection causes torticollis, whole body tremors, paresis, and stupor.[40, 72] Toxoplasmosis is reported to cause systemic neurologic signs such as torticollis, circling, paralysis, and blindness.[32, 34] Chronic psittacosis can cause diverse neurologic signs such as tremors, convulsions, opisthotonos, and torticollis, especially in African grey parrots, cockatoos, and Amazon parrots.[41] Aspergillosis involving the CNS can cause signs of ataxia and paralysis.[34, 73] Whole body weakness, depression, and ataxia are some of the vague neurologic signs reported with proventricular dilatation syndrome.[9, 74]

Inflammatory. A report on *Pionus* species parrots indicates that a lymphoplasmacytic inflammation is responsible for encephalitis, myelitis, and meningitis (spinal and cerebral). Affected birds exhibited multifocal signs of tremors, circling, ataxia, torticollis, weakness, paresis, and depression. The diagnosis was made at necropsy.[75] Any cause of encephalitis or meningitis can show clinical signs of a diffuse lesion.

Metabolic. Extracranial disease can cause diffuse neurologic signs. This is true of metabolic disease caused by hypoxia, renal dysfunction, and hepatic encephalopathy.[11, 76, 77]

Miscellaneous. Lafora body neuropathy has been reported to cause systemic disease signs.[68]

Neoplastic. If both cerebellar and cerebral signs are present, a space-occupying lesion should be considered. For example, a tumor of the pineal gland can impinge on both the cerebrum and the cerebellum.[67] Other tumors reported in the brain include gliomas, choroid plexus tumors, hemangiomas, and metastatic tumors.[19]

Toxic. A toxic reaction to the antiparasiticide levamisole can lead to multifocal nervous system signs such as ataxia, mydriasis, and leg and wing paralysis.[65] Flaccid paralysis of the skeletal musculature and tongue, bulbar paralysis of the skeletal musculature and tongue, bulbar paralysis, and diarrhea are all seen in botulism.[40] Classically, a limp neck is described from paralysis of the neck muscles.[34]

Traumatic. Diffuse trauma can lead to multisystemic neurologic signs.

Vascular. Ischemic infarctions have been reported in the brains of birds. Multifocal neurologic signs such as blindness, ataxia, paresis, and seizures are seen with an ischemic infarction of the CNS.[19, 34] Ischemic infarctions can be associated with an abundance of lipemic serum.

References

1. Balda RP, Kamil AC: A comparative study of cache recovery by three corvid species. Anim Behav 38:486–495, 1989.

2. Gill FB: Ornithology, ed 2. New York, WH Freeman and Company, 1994.
3. Wiltschko W, Wiltschko R: Magnetic orientation in birds. Curr Ornithol 5:67–121, 1988.
4. Wiltschko W, Wiltschko R, Keeton WT, et al: Growing up in an altered magnetic field affects the initial orientation of young homing pigeons. Behav Ecol Sociobiol 12:135–142, 1983.
5. Quesenberry KE, Hillyer EV, Putter L: Neurologic disorders in caged birds: A retrospective review of cases. Proc Assoc Avian Vet, 1988, 175–176.
6. Oliver JE, Lorenz MD: Handbook of Veterinary Neurologic Diagnosis. Philadelphia, WB Saunders, 1983.
7. Chrisman CL: Problems in Small Animal Neurology. Philadelphia, Lea & Febiger, 1991.
8. King AS, McLelland J: Birds: Their Structure and Function. Philadelphia, Baillière Tindall, 1984.
9. Lyman R: Neurologic disorders. In Harrison G, Harrison L (eds): Clinical Avian Medicine and Surgery. Philadelphia, WB Saunders, 1986, pp 486–490.
10. Lyman R: Neurologic examination. In Harrison G, Harrison L (eds): Clinical Avian Medicine and Surgery. Philadelphia, WB Saunders, 1986, pp 282–285.
11. Walsh MT: Seizuring in pet birds. Proc Assoc Avian Vet, 1985, pp 121–128.
12. George DH, Munoz DG, McConnell M, Crawford RD: Megalencephaly in the epileptic chicken: A morphometric study of the adult brain. Neuroscience 39(2):471–477, 1990.
13. Wack RF, Lindstrom JG, Graham DL: Internal hydrocephalus in an African grey parrot (Psittacus erithacus timneh). J Assoc Avian Vet 3(2):94–96, 1989.
14. Shivaprasad HL: Diseases of the nervous system in pet birds: A review and report of diseases rarely documented. Proc Assoc Avian Vet, Nashville, 1993, pp 213–222.
15. Harrison GJ, Rosskopf WJ, Woerpel RW, et al: Differential diagnosis based on clinical signs. In Harrison G, Harrison L (eds): Clinical Avian Medicine and Surgery. Philadelphia, WB Saunders, 1986, pp 115–150.
16. Wyatt RD, Colwell WM, Hamilton PB, Burmeister HR: Neural disturbances in chickens caused by dietary T-2 toxin. Appl Microbiol 26(5):757–761, 1973.
17. Hochleithner M: Convulsions in African grey parrots. Proc Assoc Avian Vet, Seattle, 1989, pp 78–81.
18. McDonald LJ: Hypocalcemic seizures in an African grey parrot. Can Vet J 29(11):928–930, 1988.
19. Hasholt J, Petrak ML: Diseases of the nervous system. In Petrak M (ed): Diseases of Cage and Aviary Birds. Philadelphia, Lea & Febiger, 1982, pp 468–477.
20. Lowenstine LJ: Avian nutrition. In Fowler M (ed): Zoo and Wild Animal Medicine. Philadelphia, WB Saunders, 1986, pp 201–212.
21. Morris PJ, Jensen J, Applehans F: Lead and zinc toxicosis in a blue and gold macaw (Ara ararauna). Proc Am Assoc Zoo Vet, Scottsdale, 1985, pp 13–17.
22. Bauck L: Pituitary neoplastic disease in 9 budgies. Zoo Avian Med Proc, Hawaii, 1987, pp 87–89.
23. Schaeffel F, Wagner H: Barn owls have symmetrical accommodation in both eyes, but independent pupillary responses to light. Vision Res 32(6):1149–1155, 1992.
24. Small E, Burke TJ: Diseases of the organs of special senses. In Petrak M (ed): Diseases of Cage and Aviary Birds. Philadelphia, Lea & Febiger, 1982, pp 491–496.
25. Vickers MC, Hartley WJ, Mason RW, et al: Blindness associated with toxoplasmosis in canaries. J Am Vet Med Assoc 200(11):1723–1725, 1992.
26. Orosz SE, Mullins JD, Patton S: Evidence of toxoplasmosis in two ratites. J Assoc Avian Vet 6(4):219–222, 1992.
27. Beach JE: Diseases of budgerigars and other cage birds. Vet Rec 74(2):63–68, 1962.
28. Petrak ML, Gilmore CE: Neoplasms. In Petrak M (ed): Diseases of Cage and Aviary Birds. Philadelphia, Lea & Febiger, 1982, pp 606–637.
29. Curtis-Velasco M: Pituitary adenoma in a cockatiel (Nymphicus hollandicus). J Assoc Avian Vet 6(1):21–22, 1992.
30. Hunter B, Wobeser G: Encephalopathy and peripheral neuropathy in lead-poisoned mallard ducks. Avian Dis 24(1):169–178, 1980.
31. Clubb SL: Velogenic viscerotropic Newcastle disease. In Fowler ME (ed): Zoo and Wild Animal Medicine. Philadelphia, WB Saunders, 1986, pp 221–226.
32. Ryan TP: Nervous disorders in pet birds. Mod Vet Prac Sept/Oct:481–483, 1987.
33. Harrison GJ, Woerpel RW, Rosskopf WJ, Karpinski LG: Symptomatic therapy and emergency medicine. In Harrison G, Harrison L (eds): Clinical Avian Medicine and Surgery. Philadelphia, WB Saunders, 1986, pp 362–375.
34. Paul-Murphy J: Avian neurology. Proc Assoc Avian Vet, New Orleans, 1992, pp 420–432.
35. Gries CL, Scott, ML: The pathology of thiamine, riboflavin, pantothenic acid and niacin deficiencies in the chick. J Nutrit 102:1269–1286, 1972.
36. De Lahunta A, Smiley LE, Bonda M, et al: Avulsion of the roots of the brachial plexus in five birds. Comp Anim Pract 2(2):38–40, 1988.
37. Hultgren BD, Wallner-Pendleton E, Watrous BJ, Blythe LL: Cervical dorsal spondylosis with spinal cord compression in a black swan (Cygnus atratus). J Wildl Dis 23(4):705–708, 1987.
38. Emerson CL, Eurell JC, Brown MD, et al: Ruptured intervertebral disc in a juvenile king penguin (Aptenodytes patagonica). J Zoo Wildl Med 21(3):345–350, 1990.
39. Curtis-Velasco M: Eastern equine encephalomyelitis virus in a lady gouldian finch. J Assoc Avian Vet 6(4):227–228, 1992.
40. Gerlach H: Bacterial diseases. In Harrison G, Harrison L (eds): Clinical Avian Medicine and Surgery. Philadelphia, WB Saunders, 1986, pp 434–453.
41. Gerlach H: Chlamydia. In Harrison G, Harrison L (eds): Clinical Avian Medicine and Surgery. Philadelphia, WB Saunders, 1986, pp 457–463.
42. Bygrave AC: Leg paralysis in pheasant poults (Phasianus colchicus) due to spinal aspergillosis. Vet Rec 109:516, 1981.
43. Greenacre CB, Latimer KS, Ritchie BW: Leg paresis in a black palm cockatoo (Probosciger aterrimus) caused by aspergillosis. J Zoo Wildl Med 23(1):122–126, 1992.
44. McOrist S, Perry RA: Encephalomyelitis in free-living rainbow lorikeets (Trichoglossus haematodus). Avian Pathol 15:783–789, 1986.
45. Clipsham RC, Britt JO: Disseminated cryptococcosis in a macaw. J Am Vet Med Assoc 183(11):1303–1305, 1983.
46. Jacobson ER, Gardiner CH, Nicholson A, Page CD: Sarcocystis encephalitis in a cockatiel. J Am Vet Med Assoc 185(8):904–906, 1984.
47. Reece RL, Butler R, Hooper PT: Cerebellar defects in parrots. Aust Vet J 63(6):197–198, 1986.
48. Raphael BL, Clemmoms RM, Nguyen HT: Glioblastoma multiforme in a budgerigar. J Am Vet Med Assoc 177(9):923–925, 1980.
49. Myers RK, Monroe WE, Greve JH: Cerebrospinal nematodiasis in a cockatiel. J Am Vet Med Assoc 183(10):1089–1090, 1983.
50. Kazacos KR, Reed WM, Thacker HL: Cerebrospinal nematodiasis in pheasants. J Am Vet Med Assoc 189(10):1353–1354, 1986.

51. Armstrong DL, Montali RJ, Doster AR, Kazacos KR: Cerebrospinal nematodiasis in macaws due to *Baylisascaris procyonis*. J Zoo Wildl Med 20(3):354–359, 1989.

52. Kazacos KR, Wirtz WL: Experimental cerebrospinal nematodiasis due to *Baylisascaris procyonis* in chickens. Avian Dis 27(1):55–65, 1983.

53. Chin RP, Daft BM, Meteyer CU, Yamamoto R: Meningoencephalitis in commercial meat turkeys associated with *Mycoplasma gallisepticum*. Avian Dis 35:986–993, 1991.

54. Zwart P: Pigeons and doves (Columbiformes). In Fowler ME (ed): Zoo and Wild Animals Medicine. Philadelphia, WB Saunders, 1986, pp 439–446.

55. Reece RL, MacWhirter P: Neuronal ceroid lipofuscinosis in a lovebird. Vet Rec 122:187, 1988.

56. Reece RL, Scott PC, Barr DA: Some unusual diseases in the birds of Victoria, Australia. Vet Rec 130:178–185, 1992.

57. Gerlach H: Viral diseases. In Harrison G, Harrison L (eds): Clinical Avian Medicine and Surgery. Philadelphia, WB Saunders, 1986, pp 408–433.

58. Proctor SJ, Erickson GA, Gustafson GA: Neurologic lesions in velogenic viscerotropic Newcastle disease virus in parrots, budgerigars, and canaries. Ann Meet Am Assoc Vet Lab Diagnostics, 1974, pp 115–122.

59. Leach MW, Higgins RJ, Lowenstine LJ, Shor B: Paramyxovirus infection in a Moluccan cockatoo (*Cacatua moluccensis*) with neurologic signs. Assoc Avian Vet Today 2(2):87–90, 1988.

60. Simpson VR: Suspected paramyxovirus 3 infection associated with pancreatitis and nervous signs in *Neophema* parakeets. Vet Rec 132:554–555, 1993.

61. VanDerHeyden N, Reed WM: Paramyxovirus group 3 infection in cockatiels. Assoc Avian Vet Today 1(2):53–54, 1987.

62. Ward FP: Thiamine deficiency in a peregrine falcon. J Am Vet Med Assoc 159(5):599–601, 1971.

63. Cheney CD, Vander Wall SB, Poehlmann RJ: Effects of strychnine on the behavior of great horned owls and red-tailed hawks. J Raptor Res 21(3):103–110, 1987.

64. Mohan R: Dursban toxicosis in a pet bird breeding operation. Proc Assoc Avian Vet, Phoenix, 1990, pp 112–114.

65. Harrison GJ: Toxicology. In Harrison G, Harrison L (ed): Clinical Avian Medicine and Surgery. Philadelphia, WB Saunders, 1986, pp 491–499.

66. Lancaster MJ, Hooper LN: Neuronal necrosis in budgerigars treated with dimetridazole. Aust Vet J 68(8):280–281, 1991.

67. Wilson RB, Holscher MA, Fullerton JR, Johnson MD: Pineoblastoma in a cockatiel. Avian Dis 32:591–593, 1988.

68. Britt JO, Pater MB: Lafora body neuropathy in a cockatiel. Comp Anim Pract March:31–33, 1989.

69. Roffe TJ, Stroud RK, Windingstad RM: Suspected fusariomycotoxicosis in sandhill cranes (*Grus canadensis*): Clinical and pathologic findings. Avian Dis 33:451–457, 1989.

70. Barton JT, Bickford AA, Cooper GL, et al: Avian paramyxovirus Type 1 infections in racing pigeons in California. 1. Clinical signs, pathology, and serology. Avian Dis 36:463–468, 1992.

71. Clubb SL, Graham DL: An outbreak of viscerotropic velogenic Newcastle disease in pet birds. Proc Am Assoc Zoo Vet, 1980, pp 105–109.

72. Sinn LC: Listeriosis in birds. Proc Assoc Avian Vet, Houston, 1988, pp 189–198.

73. Campbell TW: Mycotic diseases. In Harrison G, Harrison L (eds): Clinical Avian Medicine and Surgery. Philadelphia, WB Saunders, 1986, pp 464–471.

74. Woerpel R: Proventricular dilatation and wasting syndrome: Myenteric ganglioneuritis and encephalomyelitis of psittacines; an update. Proc Assoc Avian Vet, Toronto, 1984, pp 925–928.

75. Lowenstine LJ, Joyner K, Fowler M: Lymphoplasmacytic encephalitis, myelitis, and meningitis in a group of *Pionus* spp. parrots. Proc 34th West Poult Dis Conf, 1985, pp 25–28.

76. Randell MG: Nutritionally induced hypocalcemic tetany in an Amazon parrot. J Am Vet Med Assoc 179(11):1277–1278, 1981.

77. Spaulding MG, Kollias GV, Calderwood-Mays MB, et al: Hepatic encephalopathy associated with hemochromatosis in a toco toucan. J Am Vet Med Assoc 189(9):1122–1123, 1986.

Barbara L. Oglesbee
Susan Orosz
Gerry M. Dorrestein

28

The Endocrine System

Anatomy of the Endocrine System

Susan Orosz

The endocrine glands and their hormones in birds are similar in some respects to those described in mammals. Endocrine glands release hormones into the peripheral circulation to act on at least one target organ distal to the parent gland. Target organs include the various cells and tissues that are affected by the hormone. The hormone binds to their specific receptors, which may be on the cell surface (usually proteins or polypeptide hormones) or within the cytoplasm or the nucleus (steroid hormones). In this classic interpretation, the endocrine glands include the hypothalamo-hypophyseal complex, the thyroid glands, the parathyroid glands, ultimobranchial bodies, adrenal glands, pancreatic islets, gonads, and the endocrine cells of the gastrointestinal (GI) tract (Fig. 28–1). Additionally, there are compounds with properties similar to hormones that are not understood as well. These include, for example, melatonin from the pineal gland, somatostatin from the liver and pancreatic islets, and substances from the carotid bodies.

HYPOTHALAMOHYPOPHYSEAL COMPLEX

The hypothalamohypophyseal complex is composed of the hypothalamus, a connective stalk, or tuber cinereum, and a ventral hypophysis or pituitary gland (Fig. 28–2). The pituitary gland has two embryologic origins that help to segregate the two different ways that it functions. The more rostral portion is the adenohypophysis that is formed by an evagination from the roof of the mouth (Rathke's pouch) and is of ectodermal origin. The neurohypophysis arises from the ventral outgrowth of the diencephalon of the developing brain. The adenohypophysis of mammals consists of the pars distalis, pars tuberalis, and the pars intermedia. There is no pars intermedia in birds; its function is included in that of the pars distalis. The pars tuberalis is a stalk of tissue that connects the hypophysis to the pars distalis and covers the median eminence dorsally. The neurohypophysis consists of the pars nervosa, the infundibulum, and the median eminence. The median eminence and infundibulum are a direct continuation of the hypothalamus and are difficult to distinguish grossly. The pars nervosa or neural lobe can be distinguished from the hypothalamus by its ventral-caudal projection from the infundibular stalk.

The blood supply to the hypophysis is derived from the internal carotid arteries. They form a capillary plexus within the hypothalamus and the median eminence of the neurohypophysis. This primary capillary plexus continues as the portal vein of the hypophysis. The portal vein travels through the pars tuberalis before dividing into a second plexus in the pars distalis. This portal system in some birds can be divided into two zones—a rostral and a caudal zone—that are distinct in their drainage pattern. The capillary plexus in the rostral median eminence drains via portal veins to the rostral portion of the pars distalis. It is through this blood vascular hookup that releasing factors of the hypothalamus and median eminence control the release of hormones of the pars distalis. The pars distalis is

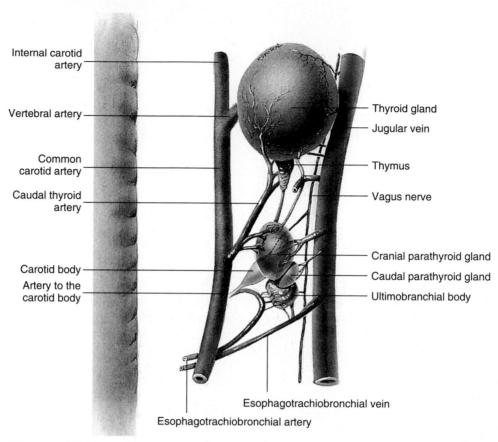

Internal carotid
artery

Vertebral artery

Common
carotid artery

Caudal thyroid
artery

Carotid body

Artery to the
carotid body

Thyroid gland

Jugular vein

Thymus

Vagus nerve

Cranial parathyroid gland

Caudal parathyroid gland

Ultimobranchial body

Esophagotrachiobronchial vein

Esophagotrachiobronchial artery

F i g u r e 2 8 – 1

Diagram of the endocrine system.

not innervated by hypothalamic axons. This is in
direct contrast to the neurohypophysis, which is
controlled by the release of neurotransmitters from
axonal terminals that extend into the pars nervosa.
These two different ways that cells of the hypophysis are controlled reflect their two different embryologic origins. In the pars distalis, there is a blood
vascular transmission of releasing factors to the adenohypophysis. In the neurohypophysis, there is axonal transmission of releasing factors.

The majority of the tissue that comprises the adenohypophysis is the pars distalis. It is composed of
secretory follicles with a central lumen of a basophilic substance or colloid. It is similar to the arrangement of the thyroid gland. Seven cell types
are recognized because of their different staining
affinities. However, staining affinity does not correlate completely with the type of hormone released
from the cell.

The two gonadotropins of the adenohypophysis
are follicle-stimulating hormone (FSH) and luteinizing hormone (LH). Both are glycoproteins that are
made up of two subunits. Each hormone has differences in chemical composition when compared
among species. This makes it difficult to measure
the concentration of each hormone in serum. FSH
in the male bird acts to increase testicular size by
increasing the diameter of seminiferous tubules,
causing differentiation of Sertoli cells and stimulating spermatogenesis. LH acts to stimulate and differentiate Leydig cells to produce testosterone.

Gonadotropins are also important in ovarian activity; however, their exact roles are unknown. LH
is known to be involved in ovulation in birds. Both
LH and FSH are important for steroidogenesis in
the ovary. However, LH may be the principal player
in, at least, the larger follicles. It acts to increase
progesterone and testosterone production in granu-

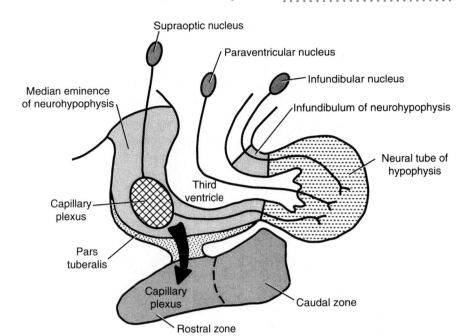

Figure 28–2

Diagrammatic representation of the hypothalamohypophyseal system. Three nuclei are depicted that transmit hormones to the neural lobe of the hypophysis. Additionally, the two capillary plexuses of the hypothalamohypophyseal portal system are shown. The second plexus goes to both the rostral and caudal zones.

losa cells. Progesterone may induce the preovulatory surge of LH in the hen.

These gonadotropins are controlled by releasing hormones (RH) from the hypothalamus. Luteinizing hormone releasing hormone (LHRH) is found within cells in the preoptic nucleus and tuberoinfundibular neurons that extend into the median eminence. This releasing hormone is secreted into the portal veins where it is transported to the adenohypophysis. Norepinephrine is thought to play the major role for the release of LHRH.

Thyrotropin or thyroid stimulating hormone (TSH) is a glycoprotein with two subunits (α and β). Its α subunit is the same as that of LH. TSH is under the control of thyrotropin releasing hormone (TRH), which is released from the median eminence into the portal system. TRH stimulates the thyrotropic cells of the adenohypophysis to secrete TSH. TSH causes circulating levels of T_4 and T_3 to increase, and it increases the concentration of colloid droplets and the uptake of phosphate and iodide for the manufacture of T_3 and T_4. Increasing TRH results in an increase in T_3 and T_4 via TSH, but the magnitude of the increase of each varies among species.

Prolactin is secreted from cells in the rostral area of the adenohypophysis. Although the hypothalamus exerts an inhibition of prolactin release in mammals, the feedback controls of prolactin are not well understood in birds. Dopamine may be important for inhibiting the release of prolactin. Additionally, its stimulatory release by a releasing factor is not established. It is thought that TRH may be prolactin releasing hormone in birds. Prolactin increases with injections of norepinephrine, serotonin, or histamine and is influenced by the breeding season and prostaglandins. Prolactin is involved in the reproductive system and carbohydrate metabolism. It stimulates the production of crop milk by increasing the mucosal cells of the crop epithelium in columbiformes. Additionally, prolactin increases broodiness or incubation and nesting behavior in both males and females. It decreases gonadal activity by suppressing gonadotropin secretion in both sexes. Prolactin also produces hyperglycemia in birds and stimulates hepatic lipogenesis. It does not affect the other fat stores of the body. Prolactin is thought to assist in changes of metabolism associated with premigratory behavior and nesting.

Growth hormone (GH) or somatotropin is produced and secreted from somatotropic cells in the caudal zone of the pars distalis. The release of GH is under hypothalamic control and is influenced by three factors, which include: (1) the stimulatory effect of TRH; (2) the stimulatory effect of GH releasing factor (GRF); and (3) the inhibitory effect of somatostatin. Various neurotransmitters may affect GH either directly or indirectly. Norepinephrine, epinephrine, and serotonin reduce the plasma levels of GH. Plasma levels of GH are also reduced by prostaglandins E_1, E_2, and $F_{2\alpha}$, insulin, and glucagon. However, plasma levels increase with nutritional deprivation and by chronic feed restriction in chickens. Low thyroxin levels are associated with higher than normal levels of GH, and the concentration of GH drops with the administration of androgens.

Adrenocorticotropic hormone or ACTH is produced from a much larger protein that is broken down to form β-endorphin, α- and β-melanophore stimulating hormone (MSH), and ACTH. ACTH and its associated polypeptides are produced in corticotropic cells in the rostral zone of the pars distalis. ACTH stimulates adrenal cortical cells to produce and release corticosterone and other glucocorticoids. ACTH is increased in the circulation with a variety of stresses including handling, immobilization and anesthesia, fasting, extremes of temperature, and endotoxemia. Although its control is poorly understood, ACTH is presumably released when corticotropin releasing factor (CRF) is increased in the portal circulation. The control and physiologic mechanisms of action of β-endorphin and MSH is unknown.

There are two major hormones of the neurohypophysis—arginine vasotocin (AVT) and mesotocin (MT). These are produced by cells that are distinct from each other, but that lie in both separate and overlapping areas of the hypothalamus. The hormones are transported down the axonal terminals by carrier proteins or neurophysins where they are stored in the pars nervosa for release. AVT differs from the mammalian antidiuretic hormone (ADH) by one amino acid residue. Two major actions of AVT are the control of water reabsorption and oviductal contraction during oviposition. AVT also has an antidiuretic effect by decreasing glomerular filtration in the kidneys. It is released when the osmolarity of the blood increases or when the sodium chloride (NaCl) concentration rises. AVT in the hen results in contraction of the distal oviduct, primarily the uterus or shell gland, causing a rapid rise in intrauterine pressure. Oxytocin is not considered to cause uterine contraction. The role of mesotocin is unknown.

THYROID GLANDS

The thyroid glands are dark red, oval, paired glands that are situated just cranial to the thoracic inlet, medial to the jugular veins and lateral to the trachea. The thyroid glands are further placed in the notch formed from the branching of the brachiocephalic trunk into the common carotid and subclavian arteries. The glands are well vascularized by the cranial and caudal thyroid arteries that branch from the common carotid artery. The veins of the thyroid glands drain into the jugular vein (see Fig. 28–1). There are both parasympathetic and sympathetic nerves to the glands. The glands are composed of follicles consisting of a simple columnar epithelium with a central cavity of colloid. The majority of this eosinophilic colloid material is presumed to be thyroglobulin, a storage form of T_3 and T_4. Between the follicles are spaces filled with connective tissue, a capillary plexus, and nerves. The thyroid gland in birds does not have the C cells that secrete calcitonin, as in mammals. This cell type is found in the ultimobranchial bodies. However, in pigeons the C cells are located in the thyroid gland. Iodine is concentrated in the thyroid glands as in mammals; however, avian thyroglobulin has a greater percentage of iodine than that of mammals. Therefore, the effects of dietary deficiencies are more exaggerated in birds and may include goiter. Enlarged thyroid glands resulting from iodine deficiencies may get so large that they block the movement of foodstuffs down the esophagus.

It is thought that thyroglobulin can be converted to both T_3 and T_4. It has been found that T_4 can be converted to T_3 in the peripheral circulation. More T_4 is released than T_3 from the thyroid glands. In the bloodstream, either form is bound to albumin, which has a similar affinity for each. It is thought that the biologic effect is the same when T_3 is compared with T_4. Both hormones have a much shorter half-life in birds when compared with mammals. This fact results in measurable fluctuations in T_3 and T_4, making it difficult to interpret a single value for hypo- or hyperthyroidism.

PARATHYROID GLANDS

The parathyroid glands usually consist of two pairs of small, yellow-colored organs just caudal to the thyroids. They are often fused to each other, and the more cranial one is usually larger. During embryonic development they are associated with the thymus. Histologically, each gland is composed of groups and cords of columnar or chief cells that synthesize, package into vesicles, and secrete parathyroid hormone or PTH. This hormone is involved in calcium and phosphorus metabolism. Birds that are administered PTH exogenously exhibit a rapid but transient rise in plasma calcium. This rise is more rapid than that shown in mammals. The initial part of the rise is probably the result of increased tubular reabsorption of calcium. The second portion is more sustained and may result from increased osteoclastic activity and release of calcium from medullary bone.

Birds are very different than mammals in their calcium metabolism. Birds produce significant quantities of medullary bone, which acts as a calcium repository for eggshell formation. This process, osteomyelosclerosis, begins approximately 10 days prior to laying and is induced by increased levels of circulating estrogens and/or androgens. Birds are capable of laying an egg daily, which requires a large amount of calcium. For this reason, they must have a highly effective and efficient system for calcium metabolism. In addition to producing a rise in plasma calcium, PTH also causes a reduction in plasma phosphorus. This serum decrease in phosphorus is the result of a reduction in tubular reabsorption and an increase in tubular secretion. PTH also is involved in the renal synthesis of 1,25-dihydroxyvitamin D_3.

ULTIMOBRANCHIAL BODIES

The ultimobranchial bodies are small, pink, flattened glands located caudal to the parathyroid glands. They are found just craniolateral to the origins of the common carotid arteries. The left body may be attached to the caudal parathyroid gland. These bodies are not encapsulated. Histologically, they consist of C cells arranged in small groups or cords. Parathyroid cells are intermingled with interconnected vesicles. Vesicles that have a lumen are filled with a carbohydrate-protein complex and an accumulation of lymphoid tissue. The C cells of the ultimobranchial bodies secrete calcitonin. However, the role of calcitonin in calcium metabolism

in birds is unknown. It does not appear to lower serum levels of calcium, but may play a role in limiting extensive bone resorption by PTH.

ADRENAL GLANDS

The adrenal glands are small, yellowish, ovoid glands tucked into the dorsal body wall on either side of the caudal vena cava and abdominal aorta. They are just cranial to the kidney and the gonads. These glands may be fused in rheas. In many species, the male bird may have an appendix epididymis that may extend into the adrenal gland, or adrenal tissue may be found within the epididymis. There may also be an adrenal portal system between each gland, and the abdominal wall musculature. The arterial supply to the adrenal glands is from the cranial renal artery and the venous return is into the caudal vena cava.

Cranial and caudal sympathetic ganglia are found within the fibrous capsule of the glands. Unmyelinated post-ganglionic fibers synapse with a number of chromaffin cells that are found in the medulla. Unlike the distinct histologic region of the adrenals of mammals, the outer cortex of avian adrenals is not well differentiated from the inner medulla. The cortical tissue accounts for approximately 70 to 80% of the gland and is intermixed with medullary tissue. There are two different chromaffin cell types that can be distinguished cytochemically and ultrastructurally. One type secretes norepinephrine, and the other secretes epinephrine. The cortical cells are arranged in anastomosing and branching cords that appear to have two zones—an outer subcapsular zone and an inner zone. It is the outer zone that secretes aldosterone, whereas the inner zone secretes corticosterone.

The adrenal glands of birds secrete considerably more corticosterone than aldosterone; the proportions of each are somewhat species-dependent. In the biosynthesis of corticosterone from cholesterol, other hormones are produced, including progesterone, pregnenolone, androstenedione, testosterone, and estradiol. The level of circulating corticosterone is dependent in part on its affinity and binding capacity of its two principal transport proteins—transcortin or corticosteroid-binding protein (CBG) and albumin. When adrenal hormones are bound to these proteins they are less able to pass through cell membranes where they would normally bind to cytosolic receptors. The concentration of these transport proteins is influenced by a variety of factors such as thyroxine, testosterone, and hypophysectomy. All three decrease CBG. The level of corticosterone in the blood is regulated by the hypothalamohypophyseal complex. Corticosterone releasing factor (CRF) causes the release of ACTH, which causes the release of corticosterone within minutes. However, this response is partially dependent on the specificity of the ACTH in individual species. Corticosterone levels provide a negative feedback to the hypothalamus. Glucocorticoids, including dexamethasone, block the release of corticosterone at either basal or stress levels. Various types of stress normally cause an increase in corticosterone release.

Birds differ from mammals in that corticosterone has both glucocorticoid and mineralocorticoid activity. In terms of its mineralocorticoid activity, it increases the glomerular filtration rate but decreases the secretion of potassium. Corticosterone has been shown to increase food intake and increase glycogenolysis, lipolysis, gluconeogenesis, protein metabolism, and plasma glucose. Increased levels above the basal rate adversely affect the immune system by causing an involution of the cloacal bursa, lymphoid tissue of the spleen and the thymus, and suppressing both humoral and cell-mediated immunity. In chickens, increased concentrations of corticosterone result in an increased susceptibility to viral infections. The granulocyte cell line is increased with elevated levels of corticosterone, but their phagocytic capability is impaired, making birds less resistant to bacterial infections as well. Corticosterone levels are high at oviposition and have diurnal rhythm with the higher level at dawn.

Aldosterone secretion is based on the blood volume of the glomerulus and the concentration of sodium in the blood vascular space. When the blood volume is reduced or the sodium concentration increases, the cells of the juxtaglomerular apparatus release renin into the bloodstream. Renin converts circulating angiotensinogen to angiotensin I. Angiotensin I is then presumably converted to angiotensin II, which stimulates aldosterone release. ACTH may also cause release of aldosterone.

Norepinephrine and epinephrine are released from separate cell types as the result of neural stimulation or blood-borne factors, including ACTH. The physiologic actions of norepinephrine and epinephrine include glycogenolysis by epinephrine and gluconeogenesis by norepinephrine. Lipogenesis is inhibited by both; both are important in the regulation of blood pressure. However, it is unknown if these actions are the result of catecholamine release from the adrenal chromaffin cells or from other locations.

PANCREAS

The majority of the pancreas lies in the two limbs of the duodenum within the dorsal mesentery. The pancreas is often divided into three lobes, as described in domestic fowl. These include the dorsal, ventral, and splenic lobes. The dorsal and ventral lobes are often united so that they appear as a continuous mass. However, they may be separated, as in the case of the pigeon and domestic duck. The splenic lobe may arise either from the dorsal or ventral lobe as it continues cranially. The exocrine portion of the pancreas is drained by one to three ducts that open into the distal portion of the ascending duodenum in close apposition to the openings of the bile or the hepatoenteric ducts. The exocrine cells secrete amylase, lipases, trypsin, and other proteases and bicarbonate.

The endocrine portion of the pancreas contains three types of islets, which vary according to the lobe and the species. The dark islets are composed primarily of alpha cells, with some delta cells. The light islets contain a mixture of both beta and delta cells. The mixed islets have all three cell types—alpha, beta, and delta cells. The dark islets of birds are large, irregularly shaped and not distinctly separated from the exocrine pancreas. The light islets by contrast are compact, rounded to elliptical in shape, and distinct from the exocrine tissue.

The alpha cells secrete glucagon, which is thought to be the major regulator of carbohydrate metabolism. The levels of glucagon in the blood are much higher than they are in mammals. Glucagon stimulates glycolysis in the liver, thereby elevating blood glucose levels. In addition, glucagon is also lipolytic and increases circulating levels of free fatty acids. The beta cells secrete insulin. Although insulin in birds affects carbohydrate metabolism, it is basically an anabolic hormone. It stimulates glycogenesis, lipogenesis, and protein synthesis. Circulating levels are much lower than those in mammals.

The delta cells secrete somatostatin. Somatostatin is thought to act as a regulator of glucagon and insulin and "fine-tunes" their release. In addition, the pancreas contains cells that secrete avian pancreatic polypeptide or APP. The exact function of this hormone is not entirely known. At higher than physiologic levels, it causes glycogenolysis and hyperglycerolemia, but at lower levels it stimulates the release of gastrin.

Physiology of the Endocrine System

Gerry M. Dorrestein

THE ROLE OF THE PANCREAS IN INTESTINAL MOTILITY

The hormonal regulation of the motility of the intestine and the exact pancreatic involvement in birds is still confusing. In mammals the arrival of the acid chyme into the duodenal lumen starts the principal secretin-mediated phase of pancreatic secretion. Only during this limited pH window is a large amount of secretin released from a zone of the duodenal mucosa containing the inactive form of the hormone (prosecretin). Like mammals, in birds the gut enzymes cholecystokinin (CCK) and APP are involved. CCK stimulates mostly exocytosis of acinar enzymes of the pancreas like the other gut hormone gastrin, but it also increases secretion of bicarbonate. CCK greatly potentiates secretin and vasoactive intestinal polypeptide (VIP) effects on bicarbonate secretion in mammals. VIP seems to be much more active in birds than secretin. Bicarbonate neutralizes the acid chyme in the lumen of the small intestine. Both CCK and APP cause depression of gastric and duodenal motility and slow gastric emptying, and both may be involved in satiety. APP also increases gastric secretion of pepsin and hydrogen. In sheep the half-life of secretin is 3 minutes, and it is metabolized in the kidney.[1, 2] The increased pH in the duodenum allows the gastric emptying again.

In a macaw, the author has seen a clinical case with maldigestion and passing of feces with excessive amylum and fat. This indicated the absence of pancreatic enzymes. The affected birds had voluminous, pale, and greasy feces. Treatment with trypsin turned the food intake as well as the consistency of the feces back to normal. However, when the treatment was stopped after 6 weeks, the feces stayed normal. This case was suggestive of a nonstimulated exocrine pancreas resulting from no acid production in the proventriculus.

The exocrine pancreatic enzymes are secreted in the duodenum and include amylase, lipase, trypsin, and chymotrypsin, which facilitate degradation of carbohydrates, fats, and proteins, respectively. Trypsin and chymotrypsin are secreted as inactive precursors, and they become active only when they enter the duodenum. The activator is the locally produced enzyme enterokinase, which changes trypsinogen to trypsin. This prevents the pancreas from being digested by its own enzymes.[1]

Barbara Oglesbee

Diseases of the Endocrine System

DIABETES MELLITUS

Diabetes mellitus, an abnormality of glucose homeostasis characterized by polyuria, polydipsia, glycosuria, polyphagia, and weight loss, has been reported in several species of birds. Most reports of diabetes mellitus in granivorous birds are of disease experimentally induced by partial or complete pancreatectomy. Spontaneously occurring diabetes mellitus has been reported in several species of birds, including the budgerigar, toucan, pigeon, Amazon parrot, African grey parrot, cockatiel, and red-tailed hawk.[3, 8, 10, 15, 23, 30, 36] It is anecdotally reported to be especially common in budgerigars and cockatiels.

The pathophysiology of diabetes mellitus in birds, including the relative roles of insulin and glucagon, is much debated. In both mammals and birds, the net effect of glucagon secretion is to increase serum glucose concentration by stimulating gluconeogenesis, lipolysis, and glycogenolysis. The action of insulin is diametrically opposed to that of glucagon, in that its secretion serves to decrease serum glucose concentrations by stimulating tissue uptake and storage and use of glucose.

Some significant differences are known to exist between granivorous birds and mammals. The pancreatic islets in the species of granivorous birds studied (chickens, ducks, and geese) have a substantially higher percentage of glucagon-secreting alpha cells as compared with the mammalian pancreas. The pancreatic islets of these birds consist of 50% α and 37% insulin-secreting beta cells, versus human pancreatic islets, which consist of 20% α cells and 70% beta cells.[13, 28] Correspondingly, the plasma glucagon-to-insulin ratio (G/I) in granivorous birds studied is 5 to 10 times higher than that of mammals.[3, 30, 33] Because of these differences, it is widely believed that birds in general (including pet birds) are far more dependent on glucagon for carbohydrate metabolism, and that insulin plays little or no role.[4, 7, 15, 30, 32, 34] The latter assumption was further supported by early studies of pancreatectomized ducks and chickens in which only a transient

hyperglycemia was observed, with blood glucose levels returning to normal.[3, 12] It is now generally accepted that these were flawed studies in that the small splenic lobe of the pancreas, containing most of the glucagon-secreting alpha cells, was not removed.[12, 22, 32, 33] In later studies in which complete pancreatectomies were performed, profound hypoglycemia leading to death was observed if these birds were not supplied with exogenous glucagon and glucose.[32, 33] The apparent resistance to insulin seen in some species of birds was used to further support the theory that insulin plays little to no role in glucose homeostasis in birds.[13, 15] This insulin resistance was demonstrated in experiments showing that domestic fowl were up to 250 times more resistant to exogenous insulin than mammals.[13] Accordingly, data from a combination of these early studies have been used to support the hypothesis that neither an insulin deficiency nor peripheral insulin resistance played a significant role in the development of diabetes in birds (including pet birds).

Substantial evidence exists, however, illustrating that insulin does, in fact, play an important role in carbohydrate homeostasis in several different species of birds. For example, pancreatectomized domestic fowl, in addition to becoming hypoglycemic, were shown to be glucose intolerant during glucose tolerance testing.[30, 32] These studies of pancreatectomized fowl demonstrate that a lack of insulin does result in impaired glucose tolerance (as in mammalian diabetes), and a lack of glucagon leads to hypoglycemia. It also appears that domestic fowl are not as resistant to the effects of insulin as once believed. In early studies demonstrating insulin resistance in these species, the types of insulin used were always of mammalian source. Substantial insulin resistance does not occur, however, when insulin of an avian source is used.[13] Furthermore, resistance to mammalian insulin has not been reported in clinical cases of spontaneously occurring diabetes mellitus in psittacines. Additional support for the role of insulin in avian glucose homeostasis comes from a study in which diabetes mellitus was produced in ducks by insulin antibodies. In this study, an injection of anti-insulin serum produced immediate hyperglycemia in both normal and pancreatectomized ducks, demonstrating the essential role of insulin in the regulation of blood glucose in this species.[22] Although the relative importance of glucagon in carbohydrate metabolism may be greater in some birds than in mammals, insulin still appears to play a significant role.

Although it is generally accepted that glucagon is the dominant hormone in glucose regulation in chickens and ducks, one must take care when extrapolating this information to all species of birds, including pet birds. There are many examples illustrating that generalizations applicable to glucose metabolism in chickens are not applicable to other species. For instance, pancreatectomized geese demonstrated pronounced *hyper*glycemia, leading to death (as opposed to the hypoglycemia seen in other domestic fowl).[33] Carnivorous birds are similar to mammals in both their pancreatic islet cell composition and G/I ratio.[15, 33, 36] A limited study of captive toucans suggests that glucose regulation in this species is significantly different, in that glucose loading did not suppress glucagon levels in diabetic or normal toucans, as it does in granivorous birds.[23] In another report of three diabetic pet birds, two had elevated serum glucagon concentrations with normal insulin concentrations. The third diabetic bird, however, had a two- to three-fold decrease in serum glucagon concentrations, as compared with normal birds of that species.[15]

In a recent report of diabetes mellitus in an African grey parrot, insulin-dependent diabetes (similar to type I diabetes in man) was diagnosed. In this report, the parrot had significantly decreased serum insulin concentration in the face of fasting hyperglycemia, ketonuria, and pancreatic atrophy on postmortem examination.[8] The author has seen a similar case in which a diabetic scarlet macaw was diagnosed as insulin-dependent based on a fasting serum glucose concentration of 1600 mg/dl, with a serum insulin concentration of only 0.56 μU/ml (compared with 5.8–9.1 μU/ml in other Psittaciformes).[15, 39] These differences among various avian species suggest that the pathophysiologic mechanisms behind diabetes mellitus may be significantly disparate, depending on the species of birds affected.

Clinical Signs

Clinical signs of diabetes mellitus in pet birds are similar to those observed in affected mammals. Polyuria and polydipsia may be severe, such that the bird empties its water dish several times daily and the cage bottom becomes soaked with urine. Most affected birds have a voracious appetite. Despite this, weight loss is marked and usually rapid. In some cases, especially those with concurrent disease, nonspecific signs such as depression, lethargy, vomiting, or anorexia may be seen.

Diagnosis

The diagnosis of diabetes mellitus is based upon clinical signs, together with presence of persistent glycosuria and elevated fasting serum glucose. The normal range for serum glucose in pet birds is significantly higher than that observed in mammals, with ranges from 250 to 500 mg/dl, depending on the species. One should be cautious, however, not to base the diagnosis of diabetes mellitus on fasting serum glucose alone, because many birds may develop a significant transient hyperglycemia when stressed.

The urine may be tested for glucose with urine reagent test strips (Keto-Diastix). The bird must be polyuric so that a sample can be obtained. The liquid portion of the dropping should be aspirated with a syringe, avoiding fecal contamination, which may falsely elevate glucose readings. Normal avian urine is reported to be "negative" or "trace" on the urine reagent strip.[29] Glycosuria in the presence of hyperglycemia differentiates diabetes mellitus from primary renal glycosuria. The presence of ketones in the urine of birds is considered to be abnormal. Although this may be suggestive of ketoacidosis, ketone body metabolism in birds appears to be very different than in mammals, making the value of testing for ketones questionable.

If possible, serum insulin and glucagon concentrations should be determined at the same time in which fasting hyperglycemia is documented. Significantly decreased serum insulin concentrations in the face of hyperglycemia and glycosuria suggest a diagnosis of insulin-dependent diabetes.

It is the author's experience that some birds presenting with clinical manifestations of diabetes mellitus have other concurrent disease. Therefore, a complete blood count, serum chemistry profile, and radiographs are recommended.

Treatment

Birds that are depressed, dehydrated, anorectic, and/or vomiting should be maintained on intraosseous fluids. Acid-base and electrolyte disorders noted from the serum chemistry profile should be corrected. (See Chapter 48 for details on fluid therapy.) Treatment of an underlying disorder is essential for the successful management of diabetes mellitus.

The bird should be hospitalized when insulin therapy is begun to initially regulate the serum glucose. A serial blood glucose curve should be performed, measuring blood glucose concentrations initially, then every 2 to 3 hours for 12 to 24 hours. This is especially important in birds, because many species of birds tend to be erratic in their response to insulin therapy. Furthermore, the peak and duration of effect of insulin preparations currently available are unknown in avian species. The glucose blood curve aids in determining a proper dosage of insulin individually titrated to the patient.

If the bird is ill and requires intraosseous fluid therapy, the author begins therapy with Regular Insulin at 0.1 to 0.2 U/kg. Serum glucose concentrations are monitored every 1 to 2 hours, and the dosage is adjusted until blood glucose concentration is maintained within normal range. When the bird is stable, eating, no longer vomiting, and all electrolyte and acid-base disorders have been corrected, therapy with longer-acting NPH or Ultralente insulin is begun. Birds with uncomplicated diabetes that are not ill are immediately begun on NPH or Ultralente insulin, but should likewise be hospitalized for a serial blood glucose curve, adjusting the insulin dosage until blood glucose concentration is maintained within the normal range. Dosages vary significantly between birds, and should be individually titrated. Reported dosages range from 0.067 to 3.3 U/kg intramuscularly (IM) q 12 to 24 hours.[13, 21] Insulin may be diluted with sterile water and remains stable under refrigeration for 30 days.

When an initial dosage of insulin has been determined, the bird is released from the hospital on insulin injections to be administered by the owner. In most cases, twice-daily injections are necessary.

The goals of long-term home management are to eliminate weight loss and reduce the clinical signs of polyphagia, polyuria, and polydipsia. The value of strict control of hyperglycemia must be weighed against the possibility of inducing hypoglycemia, which could be immediately life-threatening. If the urine is to be used to monitor insulin therapy at home, it is necessary to maintain a slight hyperglycemia and subsequent polyuria to obtain a urine sample for testing. The urine is monitored with test reagent strips two to three times daily, at the time of each insulin injection and once in the middle of the day. Urine glucose should be maintained at a slightly positive or "trace" level, and the insulin dosage adjusted accordingly.

It is important to advise the owner of the signs of hypoglycemia such as ataxia, disorientation, shivering, lethargy, or seizures. If such episodes occur, oral glucose supplementation may be given if the bird is capable of swallowing. Oral supplementation should not be attempted in birds that are convulsing. Severe episodes of hypoglycemia may require treatment with parenteral dextrose. The insulin dosage must be decreased following hypoglycemic episodes.

As with diabetic mammals, a high fiber diet should be offered. High fiber diets combat obesity, decrease postprandial fluctuations in blood glucose, and slow glucose absorption from the intestinal tract. It has been suggested that a change in diet from dog kibble to a commercial softbill diet may have decreased the need for insulin in one diabetic toucan.[23]

Ideally, the bird should return to the hospital for serial blood glucose monitoring several days after the initiation of insulin therapy, because it is likely that several days are required for glucose homeostasis to equilibrate (as is the case in mammals). The serial blood glucose curve should also be reevaluated whenever clinical signs of diabetes and glycosuria become persistent, or every 2 to 3 months in the bird with well-controlled diabetes. The lack of knowledge of the pathophysiologic mechanism behind diabetes mellitus in avian species commonly kept as pets requires strict monitoring of the diabetic bird and flexibility on the part of the veterinarian.

Transient Diabetes Mellitus

The author has treated psittacine birds with two cases of diabetes that appeared to be transient or induced, similar to a condition encountered in cats. A yellow-naped Amazon parrot and a scarlet macaw were diagnosed with diabetes mellitus based on clinical signs of polyuria and polydipsia, polyphagia, severe weight loss, and persistent hyperglycemia with glycosuria. After several weeks of insulin therapy, the need for insulin slowly declined and was ultimately discontinued when all clinical signs, hyperglycemia, and glycosuria resolved. In the case of the Amazon parrot, this occurred twice over a period of several years, the second episode occurring following an injection of Depo-Provera given by another veterinarian. The scarlet macaw became profoundly hyperglycemic (serum glucose 1000–1600 mg/dl) and symptomatic for diabetes as often as once or twice yearly. These episodes were correlated with acute exacerbations of chronic air sacculitis and bronchopneumonia. Two of these episodes required temporary insulin therapy in addition to treatment of the primary disorder. However, in the remainder of these episodes, the manifestations of diabetes mellitus resolved with treatment of the underlying air sacculitis and bronchopneumonia alone, without the use of insulin.

The condition may be similar to one encountered in some cats, which appear to be able to compensate for their diabetes without developing clinical signs for prolonged periods. Clinical signs of diabetes may begin during episodes of severe stress or underlying disease, and insulin therapy is required. Upon resolution of the underlying disorder, many of these cats spontaneously recover from their insulin dependence.[11] Cats with transient or induced diabetes mellitus are generally non–insulin-dependent, unlike the macaw mentioned above, which had significantly decreased serum insulin concentrations.

DISEASES OF THE THYROID GLAND

Hypothyroidism

Primary hypothyroidism has been documented in chickens, pigeons, and in a scarlet macaw. Hypothyroidism is widely believed to be the cause of several skin and feathering disorders in pet birds.[15, 18, 25–27] These descriptions, however, have been based upon the results of resting serum T_4 concentrations, the favorable response to L-thyroxine ad-

ministration, or on extrapolation from experimental models in poultry. As in mammals, a low resting serum T_4 concentration alone is unreliable in the diagnosis of primary hypothyroidism. Euthyroid mammals may have falsely lowered basal serum T_4 concentration attributable to stress, drug treatment, or a number of acute or chronic systemic diseases. Likewise in birds, serum T_4 concentrations may be influenced by stress, infections, environmental temperature, food intake, drugs, and handling.[12, 20] The lack of provocative thyrotropin-stimulation testing makes the diagnosis of hypothyroidism in most cases reported in pet birds questionable.

Clinical Signs

Only one case of hypothyroidism in a psittacine bird confirmed by TSH-stimulation testing has been reported. In this case, the clinical manifestations of hypothyroidism were similar to those seen in mammals. Obesity and nonpruritic feather loss with loss of feather regrowth were evident. Hematologic and serum biochemical abnormalities included a mild leukocytosis, nonregenerative anemia, hypoalbuminemia, and hypercholesterolemia. Feather loss in areas inaccessible to automutilation or plucking is compatible with a diagnosis of hypothyroidism, warranting further investigation. In nonpsittacine species, experimental thyroidectomy has been shown to delay molt; retard regrowth of new feathers; and alter the size, color, and structure of new feathers.[35] Other clinical signs that have been reported to be associated with low resting serum T_4 concentrations include lipomas, dry skin, feather picking, and pododermatitis. In these reports, however, the diagnosis of hypothyroidism was not confirmed.

Diagnosis

The diagnosis of hypothyroidism is based on characteristic clinical signs coupled with the failure to respond to provocative TSH-stimulation testing. Clinical signs and low basal serum T_4 concentrations alone may be suggestive of hypothyroidism, but are not diagnostic. Response to L-thyroxine therapy is not itself confirmatory of a diagnosis. Many conditions seen in pet birds may resemble the clinical signs seen in hypothyroidism, and these signs may improve with L-thyroxine supplementation, even in birds with normal thyroid function. Furthermore, basal serum T_4 concentrations in pet birds are significantly lower than those reported in mammals. Protocols for TSH testing have been developed for pigeons and psittacines.[10, 14, 18] Reported protocols vary significantly, including TSH doses ranging from 0.1 to 2.6 IU/kg, to 0.1 to 2.0 IU per bird, and post-TSH sampling times varying from 0.5 to 16 hours. The most recent protocol developed for psittacine birds recommends a TSH dosage of 1 IU/kg IM, followed by a post-TSH sampling time of 6 hours.[12] Reference values for basal serum T_4 concentrations are available for some species of commonly kept birds and may vary substantially.[16, 18, 25, 27] In all TSH stimulation protocols reported, however, there was at least a doubling of serum T_4 concentration over baseline after TSH administration. Therefore, a basal serum T_4 concentration that fails to double following TSH testing supports a diagnosis of hypothyroidism.

Treatment

Suggested regimens for thyroid replacement treatment in birds generally involve drinking water–based treatment, ranging from ¼ tablet to 2 tablets of 0.1 mg L-thyroxine/4 oz of drinking water.[9, 26] In one report, a psittacine bird with confirmed hypothyroidism responded favorably to an L-thyroxine dosage of 0.02 mg/kg orally q 12 hours.[24] This dosage was extrapolated from mammalian treatment protocols of 0.01 to 0.02 mg/kg po q 12 hours. No pharmacologic data are currently available to confirm the proper administration of thyroid hormone replacement therapy in pet birds. If treatment is attempted, the bird should be monitored and the dosage adjusted on the basis of clinical response, signs of toxicity, and postmedication serum T_4 concentrations.

GOITER

Iodine deficiency resulting in diffuse thyroid hyperplasia has been reported in budgerigars, cockatiels, canaries, and pigeons.[6, 7, 31] The disease appears to be especially common in budgerigars. In one re-

port, 85% of budgerigars examined at necropsy had some degree of thyroid abnormality, and 23.8% had died as a direct result of thyroid hyperplasia.[6] The disease is associated with a deficiency of iodine in seed mixtures commonly fed to these birds. Iodine is necessary for the production of thyroid hormone. If deficient, insufficient serum concentrations of thyroxine are available to inhibit the production of TSH by the anterior pituitary. As a result, excessive quantities of TSH cause proliferation of thyroid follicular epithelium and accumulation of follicular colloid, resulting in severe thyroid gland enlargement.

Clinical Signs

Clinical signs of goiter appear to be directly related to the space-occupying effects of thyroid gland enlargement, and not to decreases in serum T_4 concentration. In affected birds, the thyroid glands may be 100 to 200 times normal size. Dyspnea, often severe, may be seen as a result of tracheal compression by the thyroid glands. This is usually accompanied by a characteristic squeak with each inspiration. Regurgitation, repeated attempts at swallowing, and crop emptying disorders have been reported as a result of esophageal compression.[5]

Diagnosis

The diagnosis of goiter is based on a history of a dietary iodine deficiency and characteristic clinical signs. The enlarged thyroid glands are generally not palpable because of their location within the anterior thoracic cavity.

Treatment

Birds that are severely dyspneic should be handled minimally and placed in an oxygen-rich environment. Daily injections of 0.01 to 0.03 ml of 20% sodium iodide have been recommended, but are indicated only under life-threatening conditions.[7, 15] In most cases, oral supplementation in the form of iodized seed or administration of a dilute Lugol iodine solution to the drinking water is sufficient for treatment. Goiter may be prevented by dietary supplementation of approximately 20 μg of iodine per week.[7] Most commercially available formulated diets should contain sufficient quantities of iodine to prevent goiter.

ADRENAL DISORDERS

There are currently no documented cases of spontaneously occurring cases of either hypo- or hyperadrenocorticism in birds. A high percentage of adrenal pathology has been reported to occur in psittacine birds during routine necropsy, but ante mortem confirmation of adrenal disease in these birds is lacking.[28] Adrenal tumors have also been reported in birds, especially budgerigars; however, ante mortem information is unavailable on these cases.[5, 7] Previous clinical case reports that suggested a diagnosis of hypoadrenocorticism were based on the failure of basal cortisol concentrations to rise following ACTH-stimulation testing. In all species of birds investigated, however, corticosterone and not cortisol was shown to be the major glucocorticoid hormone secreted by the adrenal gland, and should be the hormone measured if ACTH-stimulation testing is performed.[17, 37, 40] Protocols for ACTH stimulation testing have been developed for psittacines, raptors, and pigeons.[17, 19, 37, 40] If adrenal disease is suspected, diagnostic confirmation is achievable using one of these protocols.

References

1. Duke GE: Alimentary canal: Anatomy, regulation of feeding, and motility. In Sturkie PD (ed): Avian Physiology, ed 4. New York, Springer-Verlag, 1986, pp 269–288.
2. Ruckebush L, Phaneuf L-P, Dunlop R: Physiology of Small and Large Animals. Philadelphia, BC Decker, 1991.
3. Altman RA, Kirmayer AH: Diabetes mellitus in the avian species. J Am Anim Hosp Assoc 12:531–537, 1976.
4. Barrington EJ: Trends in comparative endocrinology. Am Zool 15:255–270, 1975.
5. Beach JE: Diseases of budgerigars and other cagebirds. A summary of post mortem findings. Vet Rec 74:10–15, 1962.
6. Blackmore DK: The pathology and incidence of thyroid dysplasia in budgerigars (Melopsittacus undulatus). Vet Rec 75:1068–1072, 1965.
7. Blackmore DK, Cooper JE: Diseases of the endocrine system. In Petrak ML (ed): Diseases of Cage and Aviary Birds, ed 2. Philadelphia, Lea & Febiger, 1982, pp 478–490.
8. Candeletta SC, Homer BL, Garner MM, et al: Diabetes mellitus associated with chronic lymphocytic pancreatitis in an African grey parrot (Psittacus erithacus erithacus). J Assoc Avian Vet 7(1):39–43, 1993.
9. Clubb SL: Therapeutics individual and flock treatment regimens. In Harrison GJ, Harrison LR (eds): Clinical Avian Medicine and Surgery. Philadelphia, WB Saunders, 1986, pp 237–355.
10. Douglass M: Diabetes mellitus in a Toco Toucan. Mod Vet Pract 62:293–295, 1981.
11. Feldman ED, Nelson RW: Feline diabetes mellitus. In Kirk RW (ed): Current Veterinary Therapy IX. Philadelphia, WB Saunders, 1986, pp 1000–1005.
12. Harms CA, Hoskinson JJ, Bruyette DS, et al: An experimental model of hypothyroidism in psittacine birds. Proc Assoc Avian Vet, 1993, pp 250–253.
13. Hazelwood RL, Kimmel JR, Pollock GH: Biological characterization of chicken insulin activity in rats and domestic fowl. Endocrinology 83:1331–1340, 1968.
14. Lothrop CD: Diseases of the thyroid gland in caged birds. Proc Assoc Avian Vet, 1984, pp 85–94.
15. Lothrop C, Harrison GJ, Schultz D, et al: Miscellaneous diseases. In Harrison GJ, Harrison LR (eds): Clinical Avian Medicine and Surgery. Philadelphia, WB Saunders, 1986, pp 531–534.
16. Lothrop CD, Loomis MR, Olsen JH: Thyrotropin stimulation test for evaluation of thyroid function in psittacine birds. J Am Vet Med Assoc 186(1):47–48, 1985.
17. Lothrop CD, Olsen JH, Loomis MR, et al: Evaluation of adrenal function in psittacine birds, using the ACTH stimulation test. J Am Vet Med Assoc 187(11):1113–1115, 1985.
18. Lothrop CD, Olsen JH, Loomis MR: Endocrine diagnosis of feathering problems in psittacine birds. Proc Am Assoc Zoo Vet, 1983, pp 144–147.
19. Lumeij JT, et al: Action of ACTH upon plasma corticosterone concentrations in racing pigeons (Columba livia domestica). Avian Pathol 16:199–204, 1987.
20. Lumeij JT, Westerhof I: Clinical evaluation of thyroid function in racing pigeons (Columbia livia domestica). Avian Pathol 17:63–70, 1988.
21. Mirsky IA, Nelson N, Grayman I, et al: Studies on normal and depancreatized domestic ducks. Am J Physiol 135:223–229, 1941.
22. Mirsky AI, Jinks R, Perisutti G: Production of diabetes mellitus in the duck by insulin antibodies. Am J Physiol 206:133–135, 1964.
23. Murphy J: Diabetes in toucans. Proc Assoc Avian Vet, 1992, pp 165–170.
24. Oglesbee BL: Hypothyroidism in a scarlet macaw. J Am Vet Med Assoc 201(10):1599–1601, 1992.
25. Parrot T: Pododermatitis in three amazon parrots, and treatment with L-thyroxine. Proc Assoc Avian Vet, 1991, pp 263–264.
26. Rosskopf WJ, Woerpel RW: Remission of lipomatous growths in a hypothyroid budgerigar in response to L-thyroxine therapy. Vet Med/Sm Animal Clinician 78:1415–1418, 1983.
27. Rosskopf WJ, Woerpel RW: Normal thyroid values for common pet birds. VM/SAC 77:409–412, 1982.
28. Rosskopf WJ, Woerpel RW, Richkind M, Woerpel RW, Lane RA: Pathogenesis, diagnosis and treatment of adrenal insufficiency in psittacine birds. Cal Vet 5:26–29, 1982.
29. Rosskopf WJ, et al: The practical uses and limitations of the urinalysis in diagnostic pet avian medicine: with emphasis on the differential diagnosis of polyuria, the importance of cast formation in the avian urinalysis, and case reports. Proc Assoc Avian Vet, 1986, pp 61–73.
30. Ryan CP, Walder EJ, Howard EB: Diabetes mellitus and islet cell carcinoma in a parakeet. J Am Anim Hosp Assoc 18:139–142, 1982.
31. Sasipreeyajan J, Newman JA: Goiter in a cockatiel (Nymphicus hollandicus). Avian Dis 32:169–172, 1988.

32. Sitbon G, Strosser MT, Gross R, et al: Endocrine factors in intermediary metabolism, with special reference to pancreatic hormones. In Avian Endocrinology. New York, Academic Press, 1980, pp 251–270.

33. Sitbon G, Laurent F, Mialhe A, et al: Diabetes in birds. Horm Metab Res 12:1–9, 1980.

34. Smith HA, Jones TC, Hunt RD, et al: Veterinary Pathology, ed 4. Philadelphia, Lea & Febiger, 1972.

35. Voikevic AA: The Feathers and Plumage of Birds. New York, October House, 1966, pp 91–215.

36. Waller-Pendleton E, Rogers D, Epple A: Diabetes mellitus in a red-tailed hawk (Buteo jamaicensis). Avian Pathol 22:631–635, 1993.

37. Walsh MT, Beldegreen RA, Clubb SL, et al: Effect of exogenous ACTH on serum corticosterone and cortisol concentrations in the Moluccan cockatoo (Cacatua moluccensis). Am J Vet Res 46(7)1584–1587, 1985.

38. Zenoble RD, Kemppainen RJ, Young DW, et al: Endocrine response of healthy parrots to ACTH and thyroid stimulating hormone. J Am Vet Med Assoc 187(11)1116–1118, 1985.

39. Zenoble RD, Kemppainen RJ: Endocrinology of birds. In Kirk RW (ed): Current Veterinary Therapy IX. Philadelphia, WB Saunders, 1986, pp 702–705.

40. Zenoble RD, Kemppainen RJ, Young DW, et al: Effect of ACTH on plasma corticosterone and cortisol in eagles and condors. J Am Vet Med Assoc 187:1119–1120, 1985.

Karen Rosenthal
Michael Miller
Susan Orosz
Gerry M. Dorrestein

29

Cardiovascular System

Anatomy of the Cardiovascular System

Susan Orosz

Birds have a larger heart compared with body mass than do mammals. The heart itself is located in the middle and slightly cranial in the thoracic portion of the thoracoabdominal cavity. Unlike that of mammals, the heart is surrounded below its base by the lobes of liver and not the lungs. This relationship can be seen easily radiographically.

The heart, as in mammals, has four chambers, and although its anatomy (Fig. 29–1) is similar in general, there are several differences. In some bird species, the sinus venosus and the right and left pulmonary veins are partially separated from the atria. For example, the right cranial and the caudal vena cava form a sinus venosus that is partially

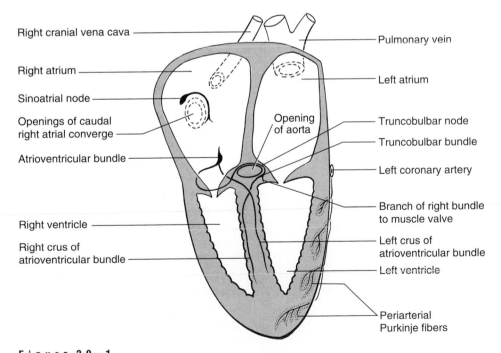

Right cranial vena cava

Right atrium

Sinoatrial node

Openings of caudal right atrial converge

Atrioventricular bundle

Right ventricle

Right crus of atrioventricular bundle

Pulmonary vein

Left atrium

Opening of aorta

Truncobulbar node

Truncobulbar bundle

Left coronary artery

Branch of right bundle to muscle valve

Left crus of atrioventricular bundle

Left ventricle

Periarterial Purkinje fibers

F i g u r e   2 9 – 1

Anatomy of the heart.

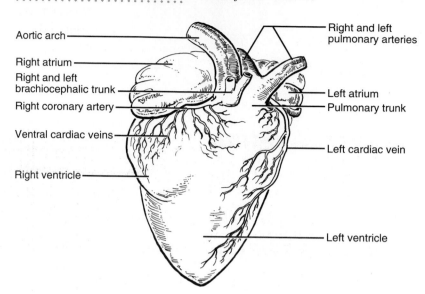

Aortic arch

Right atrium

Right and left
brachiocephalic trunk

Right coronary artery

Ventral cardiac veins

Right ventricle

Right and left
pulmonary arteries

Left atrium

Pulmonary trunk

Left cardiac vein

Left ventricle

F i g u r e 2 9 – 2

Ventral surface of the heart.

separated from the right atrium. Another difference is that the right atrioventricular (AV) valve does not have chordae tendineae associated with its flap.

The myocytes of cardiac muscle are much smaller in diameter but have a larger surface area than those of mammals. These characteristics allow for more rapid depolarization of cardiac muscle, a factor that is extremely important with a rapid heart rate. In addition, birds have fibrous rings around the base of each of the chambers that act as an internal skeleton. This skeleton prevents a general spread of excitation, thereby requiring the impulse to move from the atria into the ventricles via the AV node. The pacemaker of the heart of birds is the sinoatrial (SA) node. The cells of the node have an increased frequency of depolarization compared with the rest of the cardiac muscle. The wave of depolarization moves through the atrial myocardial cells to the AV node. Depolarization continues through the conducting system via the AV bundle. Birds have an additional pathway, the right AV ring, which surrounds the area of the right AV opening (see Fig. 29–1). This ring joins with the truncobulbar node found at the base of the aorta. From here, the impulses travel back to the AV bundle at its crura into right and left branches. This arrangement may enhance rapid depolarization of the ventricles. The relatively large size of the Purkinje cells that form

the conduction system also improves rapid depolarization.

The aorta of birds is derived from the right aortic arch instead of the left. For this reason, the aortic arch curves to the right in birds. After the coronary arteries branch off, the aorta subdivides into right and left brachiocephalic trunks and a descending aorta (Fig. 29–2). These trunks divide into a common carotid artery, which ascends up the neck, and a subclavian artery, which continues out the wing. The common carotid artery divides shortly after its origin into a vertebral artery and an internal carotid artery. The internal carotid arteries may be paired or may fuse as they ascend up the neck in a ventral groove of the vertebral column.

There are several portal systems in birds. The hepatoportal system is made up of two veins that drain the stomach (proventriculus and ventriculus), spleen, and intestines. This system forms an anastomosis with the coccygeomesenteric vein or the caudal mesenteric vein. This vein also drains into another portal system, the renal portal system. The renal portal system and its clinical significance are described in the chapter on the urinary system (see Chapter 36). The hepatoportal system has a number of connections with the systemic circulation, primarily through the proventriculus and its connections with the cranial vena cava on the left.

Physiology of the Avian Cardiac System

Gerry M. Dorrestein

The circulatory system of birds is matched to the demands of their metabolism.[1] Avian hearts are 50 to 100% larger and are more powerful than those of mammals of the corresponding body size.

The cardiac output averages 100 to 200 ml of blood per kilogram of mass per minute in birds. A large proportion of the oxygenated cardiac output from the left ventricle goes directly to the legs for the purpose of heat loss.[2] The legs in some species get three times as much blood per heartbeat as the pectoral muscles and twice as much as the head, the next most important target. Together, the legs and brain receive 10 to 20% of the total cardiac output.

Birds and mammals achieve high cardiac outputs in different ways. Normal resting heart rates in birds (up to 500 g body weight) range from 150 to 350 beats per minute and average about 220. Although avian hearts beat more slowly at rest than mammalian hearts, their cardiac outputs are similar because of large stroke volumes. Not only is the avian heart large, but the ventricles empty more completely than those of mammals on each contraction. In addition, at high heart rates, the ventricle fills more completely between contractions.[2] The avian ventricle is made up of more muscle fibers than the mammalian ventricle. Each fiber is thinner and its cells contain more mitochondria. The thinness of avian fibers speeds up the transfer of oxygen.

The high-performance features of the avian heart lead to high arterial blood pressures, up to 300 to 400 mm Hg in some species. (A blood pressure of 150 mm Hg is high for a human.) Not surprisingly, heart failure, aortic rupture, and hemorrhage are common causes of death in birds that are frightened or otherwise stressed. Also contributing to morbidity is the stiff structure of the avian arteries, which improves smooth, peripheral blood flow but increases susceptibility to atherosclerosis.[2]

Specialized diving birds have a mechanism through selective vasoconstriction and bradycardia that rations the available oxygen sparingly to the central nervous system, sensory organs, and endocrine glands by stopping the blood flow to most other organs and skeletal muscles during a dive.

Cardiac Disease

Karen Rosenthal
Michael Miller

Heart disease in avian patients is an underrecognized problem. There are few reports of heart disease in birds.[3, 7, 14, 19, 23] Numerous reasons can be cited. Heart disease in mammals is often detected by the presence of heart murmurs. Many veterinarians do not routinely perform auscultation on the heart of avian patients and, even for those who do, hearing a murmur is extremely challenging because of the rapid heart rate. Some cardiac diagnostic tests are intrinsically more difficult to do in birds than in mammals. Air interface from the air sacs makes it troublesome to produce ultrasonographic imaging of the heart in birds. It is cumbersome and time-consuming to perform electrocardiography on birds routinely. Finally, the lack of normal values for all heart assessment tests in birds makes interpretation of diagnostic test results difficult at best.

SIGNS OF HEART DISEASE

The paucity of case reports impedes the ability to summarize the most common signs seen with heart disease in birds. The number of signs occurring in an individual is variable, but heart disease signs become more numerous and obvious with increased severity of cardiac disease.[12]

Ascites

Ascites is a consistent sign of right-sided and generalized heart failure.[10, 12, 18] There are many causes of ascites. Right-sided heart failure leading to increased preload and compromise of the vascular system eventually causes fluid leakage into the coelom. Right-sided heart failure also leads to hepatic congestion, which is another cause for ascites. Right-sided heart failure in poultry is associated with cardiac enlargement, causing passive congestion of the liver and resulting in ascites.[24] Renal disease can occur as a result of heart disease and is also a cause of ascites.

Asymptomatic Disease

Birds, like mammals, can die from heart disease without ante mortem signs.

Cough

Cough is a common presentation in mammals but may be rare in birds with cardiac disease. Even though birds do not possess a diaphragm, they are able to cough because other areas of the respiratory system such as the pharynx, trachea, bronchi, pleura, and pericardium initiate coughing.[8] In mammals, it is the compression of the left bronchus between the enlarged left side of the heart and the left aorta that elicits a cough in heart disease.[12] This does not happen in birds with left-sided heart enlargement because the aorta curves to the right and not to the left.

Dyspnea

Dyspnea is a common sign of heart disease in birds. Open-mouth breathing and an extremely exaggerated effort of the abdominal musculature are manifestations of dyspnea in birds. A thorough physical examination of the dyspneic bird is often impossible; handling is kept to a minimum until the bird is less dyspneic. Dyspnea is partially caused by the collapse and loss of air capillaries in the lungs because of the chronic edema associated with heart failure.[24] Dyspnea is also a result of ascites that limits the expansion of the air sacs. Similarly, an enlarged liver from passive congestion due to heart failure acts as a space-occupying mass, limiting the ability of the air sacs to expand and producing

dyspnea. Dyspnea is not pathognomonic of heart disease; any disorder that negatively affects the respiratory system of birds can lead to dyspnea.

Exercise Intolerance

Exercise intolerance is a hallmark of cardiac disease in mammals. This is also true in birds, although exercise intolerance is less obvious in birds that live in cages. It is more evident in free-flying birds.

Muffled Heart Sounds

Fluid accumulation around the heart muffles heart sounds. In birds, as in mammals, fluid buildup in the pericardial sac suppresses heart sounds. Ascites also muffles heart sounds in birds because there is no diaphragm to separate ascitic fluid from the thoracic cavity. A condition unique in birds, enlargement of the liver by passive congestion, can cause a muffling of heart sounds because the liver partly envelops the heart.

Murmurs

A heart murmur is one of the most common signs of heart disease in mammals. A murmur may or may not be associated with clinical heart disease. The investigation of heart disease is imperative when a murmur is auscultated. A murmur is characterized as systolic or diastolic, graded on its intensity, and located by the area of loudest intensity. These designations are almost impossible in birds because of the rapid heart rate.

Palpable Coelomic Masses

Liver enlargement due to chronic passive congestion is a common sequela to heart disease.[12] An enlarged liver not only is palpable but frequently is seen through the thin coelomic skin as a red mass. If tense ascites is present, it may not be possible to palpate the liver.

Pulse Deficits

Pulse deficits in mammals are detected when the heart is auscultated and the pulse is palpated simultaneously. In birds, this aspect of heart disease is difficult to assess because of the rapid heart rate.

DIAGNOSIS OF HEART DISEASE

The complete cardiac data base includes signalment, history, physical examination, auscultation, whole body radiographs, electrocardiogram (ECG), echocardiograms, complete blood count, serum metabolic assessment, cytologic evaluation of fluid aspirations, and blood cultures.

Signalment

Because there are few case reports regarding heart disease in pet birds, it is almost impossible to characterize the type of bird (i.e., by age, sex, species) that is more likely to have heart disease. Mynah birds are prone to heart disease owing to the effects of iron storage disease on the heart tissue.[17] Descriptions of congenital heart lesions are lacking in birds, as are descriptions of acquired heart lesions in older pet birds. The latter may be so because of the relatively young age of most large parrots currently kept as pets; most birds are less than 20 years of age, whereas their potential lifespan is 60 to 80 years.

History

A thorough history of a bird with heart disease should emphasize diet, clinical signs, and previous disease history.

Physical Examination

The physical examination is routine. Particular attention is paid to heart auscultation, presence of ascites, and assessment of breathing quality and exercise intolerance.

Auscultation

Auscultation of a bird's heart is hindered by the rapid heart rate and the listener's inability to discern individual heart sounds. Restraint, stress, and disease all may cause the heart rate to rise, making it even more difficult for the veterinarian to auscultate the heart. The best approach is to listen to the bird free from stress or placed under anesthesia because the heart rate usually declines during anesthesia. The heart is auscultated over the left and right thoracic regions and over the dorsum. Murmurs, even if heard, are difficult to characterize (i.e., systolic versus diastolic) because of the rapid heart rate. In mammals, the area where the murmur is heard the loudest helps identify the area of the heart where the murmur originates from.[8] The small avian heart makes identification of the murmur location difficult. Muffled heart sounds may be the result of ascites or pericardial effusion. Auscultation over the dorsum is muffled if there is pulmonary edema or pleural effusion. Although the unique anatomy and physiology of avian patients preclude auscultation as a rich source of information, it allows detection of murmurs and arrhythmias and should be a part of every physical examination, especially when heart disease is suspected.

Radiographs

Radiographs allow determination of the size and shape of the heart. Liver size is assessed, as is presence of ascites. The great vessels, lungs, and air sacs are visualized and evaluated. In all reports of heart disease in birds, the most common radiographic characteristics are changes in the cardiac-hepatic silhouette.[3, 7, 14, 19, 23]

Both lateral and ventral-dorsal views are recommended. The normal heart size varies with species and is either normal or increased with heart disease. The normal heart on the ventral-dorsal view forms a cardiac-hepatic waist where the heart tapers toward its apex and silhouettes with the tapered dorsal aspect of the liver. This gives an hourglass appearance on radiographs (Fig. 29–3).[20] A ventral-dorsal radiograph affords a view of the right-sided aortic arch and the pulmonary arteries (Fig. 29–4).[20] The lateral view of the heart offers views of the ascending aorta, the pulmonic arteries, and the cau-

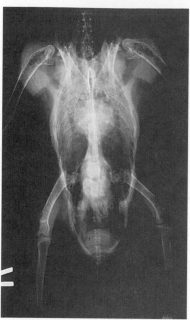

F i g u r e   2 9 – 3

Normal ventral-dorsal radiographic appearance of the cardiac-hepatic silhouette in a blue and gold macaw.

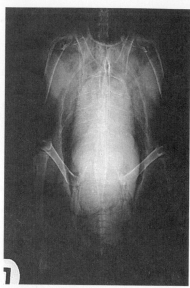

F i g u r e   2 9 – 5

Ventral-dorsal radiographic appearance of an African grey parrot with pericardial effusion. The engorged pericardial sac produces an enlargement of the heart shadow. Radiographically, this is indistinguishable from cardiomegaly.

dal vena cava.[20] Microcardia, usually associated with hypovolemia caused by dehydration, is rarely the result of heart disease, whereas cardiomegaly is usually correlated with heart disease. The heart shadow increases with both cardiomegaly and pericardial effusion (Figs. 29–5 and 29–6). Radiographically, the difference is indiscernible.

In mammals, distortion of the normal heart shape can indicate the type of heart disease present. Although this may be possible to do in birds, the lack of normal values and species variation makes this type of assessment infeasible. Positioning is extremely important in the determination of heart size in birds. Poor positioning can lead to false conclusions regarding the shape of the heart.

Great vessels are easily visualized on radio-

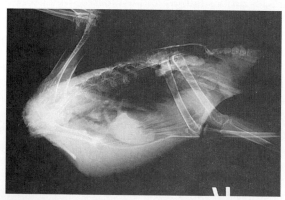

F i g u r e   2 9 – 4

Normal lateral radiographic appearance of the great vessels and their association with the heart.

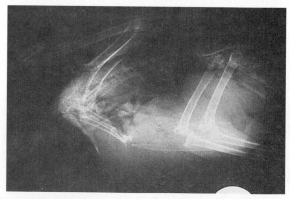

F i g u r e   2 9 – 6

Lateral radiographic appearance of an African grey parrot with pericardial effusion. The engorged pericardial sac produces an enlargement of the heart shadow. Radiographically, this is indistinguishable from cardiomegaly.

graphs. These include the aorta and pulmonary vessels (see Fig. 29–4). When viewed end on, great vessels appear round and are radiopaque. The enlargement of these vessels can signify heart disease. In the lateral view, vessels are seen emanating from the heart.

Ascites is easily recognized radiographically. A decrease in radiographic detail is the hallmark of fluid accumulation in the coelom and can be confirmed by fluid aspiration. Because of the lack of a diaphragm, ascitic fluid bathes not only the abdomen but also the thoracic region.

Liver congestion is common in heart disease, especially right-sided heart failure. This is identified radiographically as an enlarged hepatic silhouette. An enlarged liver obscures the hourglass-shaped cardiac-hepatic waist on the ventral-dorsal view. The lateral view shows caudal displacement of the ventriculus and intestines, whereas the proventriculus is displaced dorsally.

Electrocardiography

The ECG is an important element in the diagnosis of heart disease. Electrocardiography is a modality best used to detect cardiac arrhythmias and conduction disorders but is also useful to characterize chamber size and even metabolic disorders (i.e., potassium increases). The indications for an ECG recording are cardiac arrhythmias, suspected heart disease (i.e., signs such as coughing, lethargy), murmurs, radiographic heart changes, metabolic disease, syncopal episodes, seizures, presurgical screen, intraoperative monitoring, and evaluation of cardiotoxic drugs. It is used less frequently in birds because of lack of patient compliance, lack of normal values, and difficulty in easily attaching the leads to birds.

A number of methods have been published describing how to perform an ECG in the avian patient.[14, 16] Some recommend recording an ECG in the awake patient and some in the anesthetized patient. In our hospital, ECG recordings are done exclusively on anesthetized patients because the slightest movement disrupts the ECG recording. We prefer birds in dorsal recumbency for ECG monitoring, and most awake birds do not lie still in this position. We attach ECG leads to 25-gauge needles that pierce the skin; this is not well tolerated in

conscious birds. Finally, restraint of an unanesthetized bird could significantly alter the heart rate and character of the rhythm.[16] Anesthesia predictably lowers the heart rate. According to Lumeij and Ritchie, the only differences between the ECG recording in awake versus anesthetized birds are the heart rate and the QT interval.[14]

We place the bird in dorsal recumbency with wings and legs fully extended. Four electrodes are attached in the following manner: one in each prepatagial area and one each in the medial thigh region. Needles (25-gauge) are placed through the skin in these areas, carefully avoiding blood vessels in the wing (Fig. 29–7). Acoustic gel on the skin, in our experience, improves conduction better than alcohol on the electrodes. Accordingly, if the ECG is monitored during a surgical procedure in which electrocautery is used, gel is preferred over alcohol. Very accurate and repeatable ECG results are obtained from this method. With the widespread use and availability of isoflurane gas anesthesia, it is safe to anesthetize even seriously ill patients. Typically, we obtain a six-lead ECG recording with a long lead II.

Normal cardiac values were first established in poultry but are reported in a limited number of pet bird species.[14, 16, 25] The normal heart rate, as recorded by ECG, varies greatly between species and even among individuals of the same species. This is because of differences in the type and length of restraint, positioning, and anesthesia. Effects on the avian heart rate are induced by exercise, age, cli-

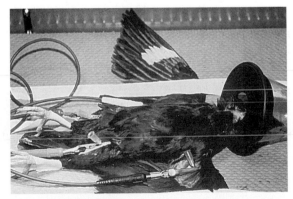

F i g u r e   2 9 – 7

Mynah bird with ECG electrodes attached by needles placed subcutaneously through the skin.

mate conditions, stress, drugs, toxins, diet, and blood pressure.[14]

Avian heart rates vary between 150 and 1000 beats per minute.[14, 16, 22, 25] Recommendations include a recording chart speed of 100 mm/sec and 1 cm equal to 1 mV. The P wave (atrial depolarization), the QRS complex (ventricular depolarization), and the T wave (ventricular repolarization) are all recognizable deflections of the avian ECG. A slow chart speed may hide the T wave in the P wave because of the rapid avian heart rate. Another explanation for the fusion of the P and T waves is that the atrium depolarizes before the ventricle completely repolarizes from the last heart cycle.[22] The most unique aspect of the avian ECG is the negative deflection of QRS in leads II, III, and aVF. The mean electrical axis of the ventricles is normally negative in leads II, III, and aVF and measures between −83° and −162°.[14, 16] The difference in the QRS complex configuration and the mean electrical axis between birds and mammals is explained by the complete penetration of Purkinje fibers throughout the ventricular free walls in birds. In addition, ventricular depolarization begins subepicardially and spreads through the myocardium to the endocardium.[14] In mammals there is subendocardial termination of those fibers.[16]

Normal values for ECG intervals and amplitudes vary among species (Table 29–1). Values for very few species have been recorded and published. Because the R wave is small or absent in leads II and III, the P-S interval is described in birds rather than the P-R interval.[22] In general, the amplitude of all waves of the avian ECG recording is relatively low.[22]

There is a lack of information correlating abnormal ECG recordings with cardiac pathology in birds. It may well be that changes in the avian ECG reflect the same pathophysiologic changes seen in mammals. Detection of arrhythmias is by auscultation or a combination of auscultation and pulse palpation. Complete characterization of the arrhythmia is best done with ECG. Arrhythmias are evaluated in the context of the clinical history. An occasional arrhythmia in an asymptomatic bird requires nothing more than observation. Arrhythmias associated with anesthesia, hypothermia, hypoxia, sepsis, and drugs may occur without significant underlying heart disease.[16] Frequent or consistently appearing arrhythmias demand more investigation and possibly treatment.

It is important to identify clinically significant arrhythmias, because these can degenerate into malignant beats and may lead to cardiac arrest and death. Mechanisms of cardiac arrhythmias include individual or concurrent abnormalities in impulse initiation (automaticity), conduction (including reentry), triggered activity (early and delayed after depolarization), and anisotropy (differential conduction speeds, longitudinally versus horizontally).

Numerous arrhythmias are reported in birds. These include atrial premature complexes, junctional complexes, ventricular premature complexes, atrial tachycardia, atrial flutter, atrial fibrillation, ventricular tachycardia, AV block, AV dissociation, and toxicity-associated (e.g., digoxin) and intraventricular conduction disturbances.[15, 16] Pathologic lesions in the AV node or bundle may cause the AV block.[22] Because of the rapid heart rate of avian patients, many of these arrhythmias are not appar-

Table 29–1

REPORTED RANGES FOR ECG VALUES IN BIRDS

Parameter	Budgie	Amazon Parrot	Racing Pigeon	African Grey Parrot
P-S (sec)	0.01–0.04	0.04–0.08	0.045–0.070	0.040–0.055
QRS (sec)	0.01–0.03	0.01–0.03	0.013–0.016	0.010–0.016
MEA	−83 to −108	−90 to −162	−83 to −99	−79 to −103
P (sec)	0.01–0.02	0.01–0.02	0.015–0.02	0.012–0.018
HR (bpm)	600–750	275–780	160–300	340–600
P (mV)	NA	NA	0.4–0.6	0.25–0.55
QS (mV)	NA	NA	1.5–2.8	0.9–2.2

Data from Lumeij J, Ritchie B: Cardiology. In Ritchie B, Harrison G, Harrison L (eds): Avian Medicine. Lake Worth, FL, Wingers Publishing, pp 695–722; Miller M: Avian cardiology. Proc Assoc Avian Vet, 1986, pp 87–102; Zenoble R: Electrocardiology in the parakeet and parrot. Comp Cont Ed 3:711–714, 1981.

NA = not available; MEA = mean electrical axis; HR = heart rate.

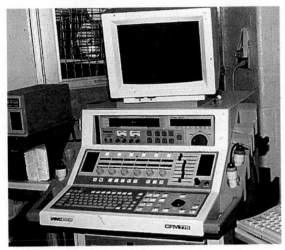

Figure 29-8

Color flow Doppler echocardiograph machine.

ent upon auscultation. These arrhythmias are found only when ECG is performed.

Dilated cardiomyopathy changes the ventricular mean electrical axis from negative to positive (i.e., +170°).[16] Hypokalemia causes SA block and AV block.[16] Thiamine deficiency results in sinus bradycardia, S-T segment depression, and ventricular premature complexes.[16] Vitamin E deficiency causes ventricular premature complexes, sinus bradycardia, sinus arrest, and S-T segment elevation.[14, 16] Sinus bradycardia is induced by vagal stimulation and various anesthetic agents. This is reversed with atropine.[14]

Known causes of ventricular premature complexes in birds include hypokalemia, thiamine deficiency, vitamin E deficiency, and digoxin toxicity.[14] AV block is seen in birds. First degree block is seen with anesthetic agents and is reversed with atropine. Second degree block has been noted in asymptomatic parrots and those with heart disease.[14] Third degree heart block is described with hypokalemia and severe cardiomegaly.[14]

Echocardiography

Echocardiography is the definitive method in the diagnosis of heart disease ante mortem, especially cardiomyopathy and valvular disease. No other imaging modality gives a real-time view of heart func-

tion. Echocardiography measures the long and short axes of the heart and allows the examiner to identify global and regional changes in cardiac structure and function.[21] Chamber size, wall thickness, and contractility are all measured. Echocardiography has severe limitations in birds because of the difficulty in obtaining a clear acoustic window of the heart owing to interference by air in the air sacs. Ascites and liver congestion from heart disease improve visualization of the heart.

A problem with echocardiography is the lack of published normal values, especially because what is normal for one species may not be normal for another. Echocardiography describes heart function, heart shape, valvular function, and pericardial status. The best view is obtained by placing a 7.5- or 10-MHz transducer under the caudal edge of the keel, directing the beam toward the heart. This gives a four-chambered view (Figs. 29–8 and 29–9).

Aspiration

Aspiration of fluid and tissue can aid in the diagnosis of heart disease. Aspiration of coelomic fluid and pericardial fluid helps clinicians characterize the type of heart disease. For example, ascites or pericardial effusion described as a modified transudate is consistent with cardiomyopathy. Mesothelial hyperplasia is present in pericardial effusion due to cardiomyopathy. Cultures (aerobic, anaerobic, and fungal), cytology results, and special stains

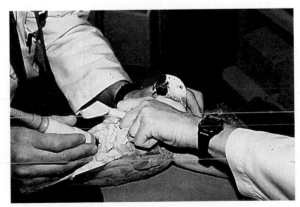

Figure 29-9

African grey parrot being restrained for echocardiographic imaging. The patient is awake and in dorsal recumbency. The probe is being held at the caudal edge of the keel.

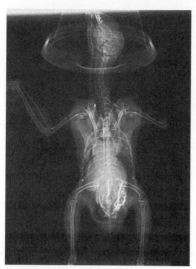

Ventral-dorsal radiograph of a mynah bird with congestive heart failure. Note the loss of the cardiac-hepatic hourglass silhouette owing to both cardiomegaly and hepatomegaly.

of the aspirated fluid help determine if infectious disease is causing heart failure. Fine needle aspiration of a large liver may reveal congestion, a diagnosis consistent with cardiac disease.

Differential Diagnosis

The differential diagnosis of cardiac disease depends on the clinical signs of the patient. The most common differential diagnoses include diseases of the respiratory system and the liver.

HEART DISEASE PATHOPHYSIOLOGY

Cardiac disease involves the myocardium, pericardium, endocardium, AV valves, outflow tract valves, impulse-forming and conduction systems, and major blood vessels. Although lesions of these anatomic areas of the heart are well described in mammals, descriptions are lacking in avian medicine.

Myocardium

Myocardial disease is either inflammatory or noninflammatory and can be the result of multiple causes.[16] Edema of the myocardium is noted in poultry with right-sided heart failure.[24] Round heart disease is a spontaneously occurring cardiomyopathy of the myocardium in fowl.[5, 6, 14] This is characterized by cardiomegaly caused by ventricular dilatation leading to congestive heart failure and eventually death.[5, 6] In chickens, right heart hypertrophy and dilatation with ascites leading to right heart failure are associated with developmental disease, inflammatory disease, and phosphorus-deficient diets.[10, 11] Vitamin E and selenium deficiency can cause myopathy leading to death.[13, 14] A thin left free wall and associated ascites were noted in a number of mynahs. The predominant sign was dyspnea, and the ultimate cause was most likely iron storage disease.[14] Myocardial tumors are included in a differential diagnosis of myocardial disease.

Congestive heart failure is described sparingly in birds.[17, 19, 23] It is accompanied by one or more of the following abnormalities: cardiomegaly, ascites, distention of the right jugular vein, liver enlargement, abdominal distention, and dyspnea[14, 17, 19] (Figs. 29–10 to 29–13; see Color Fig. 29–12). Furazolidone toxicity has been implicated as a cause of cardiomegaly.[23] Myocardial disease was a lesion frequently reported in one study of birds of prey.[4]

Pericardium

Pericardial effusion is found in association with right-sided heart failure, pericarditis, hypoproteinemia, and ascites (Fig. 29–14; see Figs. 29–3 and 29–4). One author states that pericardial effusion is

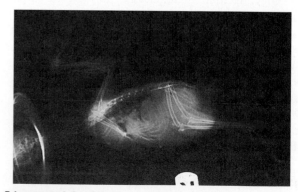

Lateral radiograph of a mynah bird with congestive heart failure. Both cardiomegaly and hepatomegaly are present.

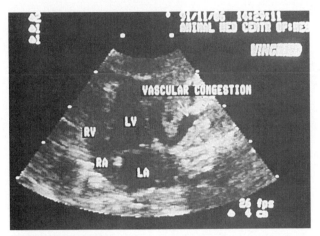

Figure 29-13

Four-chamber color flow Doppler echocardiographic image of a mynah bird with congestive heart failure. Both the left atrium and ventricular chambers are enlarged. There is also vascular congestion in the liver. (RV = right ventriculus, RA = right atrium.)

common in birds, but clinically this disease state is rarely recognized.[14] Pericardial effusions can be transudates, modified transudates, exudates, and hemorrhages. Aspiration of the pericardial fluid is essential to differentiate the type of fluid that is present. Various infectious agents (*Mycobacterium, Chlamydia, Salmonella*, various gram-negative and gram-positive bacteria) have been implicated in infectious pericarditis.[14]

Valvular Disease

Valvular diseases are congenital, inflammatory, degenerative, or the result of myocardial disease. Valvular insufficiency in one report occurred from the histopathologic lesions of mitral endocardiosis with resulting left atrial distention and left ventricular hypertrophy.[3] Bacterial endocarditis of the left and right AV valves was noted in a swan.[9] Valvular endocarditis is reported in a variety of avian species. Bacteria such as streptococci, staphylococci, and coliforms have been implicated.[14] Signs are consistent with valvular insufficiency and resulting heart failure.

HEART DISEASE TREATMENT

The first priority in the treatment of heart disease is to correct life-threatening problems.[12] Treatment

protocols for heart disease in birds are largely empiric and are usually based on mammalian pharmacokinetics.

Inotropic Medications

Positive inotropes, such as digoxin, improve the contractility of the failing heart, thereby enhancing cardiac output and function.[19] Digoxin is indicated in birds with poor contractility and myocardial failure. Digoxin therapy starting at 0.02 mg/kg every 24 hours is recommended.[19] The therapeutic range in mammals is 0.8 to 2.4 ng/ml and is used as a guideline for therapy in birds.[21] Digoxin therapy can have serious, life-threatening side effects and is used with caution. Treatment is monitored by ECG recordings and serial serum digoxin concentrations. Digoxin can lower heart rate and cause arrhythmias. Cardiac arrhythmias including bradycardia, AV block, supraventricular arrhythmias, and atrial fibrillation are common signs of toxicity.[21]

Diuretics

Diuretics are the mainstay of cardiac treatment, and most have a wide therapeutic range. The most commonly used diuretic, furosemide, is a loop diuretic, and this decreases both preload and afterload on the heart. It also diminishes ascites, which allows birds to breathe with less effort. Our initial dosage is 2.2 mg/kg every 12 hours, given intravenously, intramuscularly, or orally. Side effects of furosemide

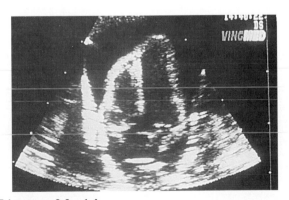

Figure 29-14

Four-chamber color flow Doppler echocardiographic image of an African grey parrot with pericardial effusion.

administration include hypovolemia and hypokalemia.[14] Diuretic treatment can be monitored with daily body weight measurements, especially in animals with significant effusions.[12]

Vasodilators

Angiotensin-converting enzyme inhibitors, balanced vasodilators, decrease both preload and afterload and are an effective treatment for mammals. Their use in birds has not been reported.

Diet Changes

There is speculation that heart disease in poultry is related to deficiencies in certain amino acids, selenium, and vitamin E.[24] It is not known if this is true in pet birds or if treatment with these dietary supplements would be beneficial by the time disease is recognized.

References

1. Jones DR, Johansen K: The blood vascular system. Avian Biol 2:157–285, 1972.
2. Gill FB: Ornithology, ed 2. New York, WH Freeman and Company, 1994.
3. Beehler B, Montali R, Bush M: Mitral valve insufficiency with congestive heart failure in a Pukeko. J Am Vet Med Assoc 177:934–937, 1980.
4. Cooper J, Pomerance A: Cardiac lesions in birds of prey. J Comp Pathol 92:161–168, 1982.
5. Czarnecki C: Review: Cardiomyopathy in turkeys. Comp Biochem Physiol 77A:561–598, 1984.
6. Einzig S, Staley N, Mettler E, et al: Regional myocardial blood flow and cardiac function in naturally occurring congestive cardiomyopathy of turkeys. Cardiovasc Res 14:396–407, 1980.
7. Ensley P, Hatkin J, Silverman S: Congestive heart failure in a greater hill mynah. J Am Vet Med Assoc 175:1010–1013, 1979.
8. Gompf R: History taking and physical examination of the cardiovascular system. In Tilley L, Owens J (eds): Manual of Small Animal Cardiology. New York, Churchill Livingstone, 1985, pp 3–24.
9. Harari J, Miller D: Ventricular septal defect and bacterial endocarditis in a whistling swan. J Am Vet Med Assoc 183:1296–1297, 1983.
10. Julian R, Friars G, French H, Quinton M: The relationship of right ventricular hypertrophy, right ventricular failure, and ascites to weight gain in brooder and roaster chickens. Avian Dis 31:130–135, 1986.
11. Julian R, Summers J, Wilson J: Right ventricular failure and ascites in broiler chickens caused by phosphorus-deficient diets. Avian Dis 30:453–459, 1985.
12. Knight D: Pathophysiology of heart failure. In Ettinger S (ed): Textbook of Veterinary Internal Medicine. Philadelphia, WB Saunders, 1989, pp 899–922.
13. Liu S, Dolensek E, Tappe J: Cardiomyopathy and vitamin E deficiency in zoo animals and birds. Heart Vessels Suppl 1:288–293, 1985.
14. Lumeij J, Ritchie B: Cardiology. In Ritchie B, Harrison G, Harrison L (eds): Avian Medicine: Principles and Applications. Lake Worth, FL, Wingers Publishing, 1994, pp 695–722.
15. Matthews N, Burba D, Cornick J: Premature ventricular contractions and apparent hypertension during anesthesia in an ostrich. J Am Vet Med Assoc 198:1959–1961, 1991.
16. Miller M: Avian cardiology. Proc Assoc Avian Vet, 1986, pp 87–102.
17. Panigrahy B, Senne D: Diseases of mynahs. J Am Vet Med Assoc 199:378–381, 1991.
18. Peacock A, Pickett C, Morris K, Reeves J: Spontaneous hypoxaemia and right ventricular hypertrophy in fast growing broiler chickens reared at sea level. Comp Biochem Physiol 97A:537–541, 1990.
19. Rosenthal K, Stamoulis M: Diagnosis of congestive heart failure in an Indian Hill Mynah Bird (Gracula religiosa). J Assoc Avian Vet 7:27–30, 1993.
20. Rubel G: Birds. In Rubel G, Isenbugel E, Wolvekamp P (eds): Atlas of Diagnostic Radiology of Exotic Pets. Philadelphia, WB Saunders, 1991, pp 76–175.
21. Sisson D: The clinical evaluation of cardiac function. In Ettinger S (ed): Textbook of Veterinary Internal Medicine. Philadelphia, WB Saunders, 1989, pp 923–938.
22. Sturkie P: Heart: Contraction, conduction and electrocardiography. In Sturkie P (ed): Avian Physiology. New York, Springer-Verlag, 1986, pp 167–190.
23. Wack R, Kramer L, Anderson N: Cardiomegaly and endocardial fibrosis in a secretary bird (Sagittarius serpentarius). J Assoc Avian Vet 8:76–80, 1994.
24. Wilson J, Julian R, Barker I: Lesions of right heart failure and ascites in broiler chickens. Avian Dis 32:246–261, 1988.
25. Zenoble R: Electrocardiography in the parakeet and the parrot. Comp Cont Ed 3:711–714, 1981.

J. M. Smith
T. E. Roudybush

30

Nutritional Disorders

REPRODUCTIVE NUTRITIONAL DISORDERS

Breeding birds require a higher plane of nutrition than birds at maintenance. This is primarily true of the female, because of the increased demands of egg production. Nutritional deficiency is almost never seen in the male if the nutrition is adequate for the female. Nutritional requirements of the hen rise in direct proportion to the number of eggs she lays in succession. Even a single pet that is laying infertile eggs has increased nutritional requirements resulting from the draw from her body's stores.

Clinical Signs

Clinical signs of malnutrition in breeding birds include cessation or decrease in egg production, abnormal eggshells, bone fractures in the female, egg binding, uterine or cloacal prolapse, infertility, decreased hatchability of fertile eggs, and decreased livability of hatchlings.

In a breeding flock, the typical manifestation of chronic malnutrition is initial good production, fertility, hatchability, and chick size and livability early in the season followed by gradual decreases in reproductive success with each successive clutch. Late in the season the owner may also see chronic infections, egg binding, uterine prolapses, and bone fractures. Examination of unhatched late-season eggs shows a high percentage of eggs with cracks, holes, desiccation, and mid- to late-incubation embryo deaths.

Etiologies

Deficiencies of total protein or essential amino acids, most likely lysine, methionine, or tryptophan,

cause reduced egg production. The hen will not produce an egg deficient in protein, so she stops production instead. Protein may become deficient on an all-seed diet during mid or late breeding season, depending on the number of eggs laid. Birds that lay only two or four eggs per year are unlikely to become protein deficient even on a diet averaging 9% protein. The level appropriate for breeders varies with egg production, but even in poultry the requirement is 14.5% or less.

Calcium deficiency is manifested initially as eggshell thinning and increased eggshell conductance. Hatchability decreases because of cracked or broken eggs and desiccation of the embryo resulting from excessive moisture loss. As calcium deficiency progresses and the hen's calcium stores are depleted, one may see egg binding, prolapsed cloaca and/or uterus, bone fractures in the hen, and eventually cessation of egg-laying. In studies conducted at University of California, Davis, researchers found that cockatiel hens fed 0.05% calcium produced thin-shelled eggs with higher-than-normal water conductance, which results in embryo mortality due to desiccation unless incubation humidity is raised to compensate. Cockatiel hens fed 0.3% calcium produced as many as 15 eggs with normal shell thickness, normal water conductance, and no evidence of bone thinning.[1] Commercial seed mixes have calcium levels of about 0.05%.

Calcium deficiency is implicated as one of several causes of egg binding and prolapse because of the responsiveness of these conditions to calcium administration. It is theorized that calcium deficiency causes smooth and skeletal muscle weakness resulting in unproductive straining to lay the egg. In addition, abdominal muscle tone and contractility of the oviduct may be lost, allowing prolapse to occur more easily.

The earlier-described signs may also be caused by vitamin D_3 deficiency. Vitamin D_3 is required for regulating absorption of calcium from the intestine. A diet may be adequate in calcium but the calcium is not absorbed because of a vitamin D_3 deficiency.

Decreased fertility caused by nutritional deficiency in the male is usually associated with decreased sperm count, decreased sperm motility, or abnormal sperm. Most of the information available is derived from poultry. Vitamin E deficiency was shown to cause sterility in male chickens, even causing degenerative changes in the testes leading to permanent sterility with prolonged deficiency.[2, 3] Harrison reported a case in which semen samples collected from Amazon parrots showed few sperm present. The birds had been maintained on a diet of frozen vegetables, fresh fruit, and a parrot treat. Upon administration of fat-soluble vitamins, sperm quantity and quality increased.[4] Harrison also reported a "vitamin E and selenium responsive syndrome" in cockatiels and other psittacines. Decreased flock fertility was one of the signs of this syndrome. A positive response was seen when the birds were fed supplements of vitamin E and selenium. Giardiasis was diagnosed and proposed as the underlying cause of the deficiency resulting from a malabsorption syndrome.[5]

Vitamin A deficiency has also been shown to cause decreased sperm count, decreased sperm motility, and abnormal sperm morphology in poultry. In one report, egg production in hens ceased with vitamin A deficiency prior to a decrease in hatchability.[6] Another report described decreased hatchability with embryo death occurring primarily in early incubation.[7]

Other indirect causes of infertility may be obesity or malnutrition leading to increased susceptibility to diseases such as gram-negative bacterial infections or chlamydiosis.

Decreased hatchability of fertile eggs may be caused by several nutritional deficiencies. Other non-nutritional causes of reduced hatchability should also be ruled out. Effects of specific nutrient deficiencies on hatchability are taken from research in poultry. Researchers have begun comparing vitamin and mineral analyses of unhatched ratite eggs with those of chicken eggs, assuming that the levels should be comparable.[8] This may become a useful tool for determining nutritional causes of impaired hatchability.

To date, there are no published reports of controlled studies on nutrient deficiencies affecting psittacine hatchability. Table 30–1 lists the effects of specific nutrient deficiencies on poultry embryos. In general, if increased embryo mortality is seen, the parents' diet should be investigated.

Diagnosis and Treatment

Take a careful history of flock, or pair, reproductive performance including egg production, hatchability, developmental stages of embryo death, hatchling performance, and number of infertile eggs. In cases of embryo mortality, evaluate egg storage and incubation conditions, paying particular attention to possibilities of power outages, fluctuating or inadequate temperatures, poor ventilation, and improper humidity.

Decreasing performance over the course of a breeding season is a common occurrence in marginal nutritional deficiencies. Advise breeders to do break-outs on all clear incubated eggs to distinguish fertile from infertile eggs. Examine embryos to determine approximate stage of development at death, for lesions or deformities, and to culture or perform histopathologic examinations to rule out infectious causes. Examine the eggshells for small cracks, holes, or thinning. Determining whether a production problem is due to infertility, eggshell abnormalities, or embryo mortality is important for proper diagnosis, treatment, and prevention.

Evaluate the parents' diet, making determinations based on what is consumed, not just offered. Certain hens in a flock fed cafeteria-style or offered free-choice mineral supplements may not choose appropriate foods in adequate amounts. Plain seed diets are deficient in some vitamins and minerals required for breeding. Table 30–2 shows the nutrient composition of some seeds commonly included in psittacine diets. Nutrient levels deficient for breeding poultry have been highlighted. This comparison is made because only poultry breeding requirements are known. When extrapolating psittacine breeding requirements, remember that breeding poultry may each lay 200 to 360 eggs per year. A parrot laying 10 eggs per year has considerably lower nutrient requirements. However, com-

Table 30–1

EFFECTS OF SPECIFIC VITAMIN AND MINERAL DEFICIENCIES ON DEVELOPING POULTRY (CHICKEN AND TURKEY) EMBRYOS

Nutrient	Effect of Deficiency
Vitamin A	Early incubation mortality
Vitamin D₃	Stunting, soft bones
Vitamin E	Mortality at 2–4 days (severe deficiency), mortality late in incubation (moderate deficiency), hemorrhages
Vitamin K	Late incubation mortality, hatching mortality, hemorrhages
Riboflavin	Mid-incubation mortality, dwarfing, edema, club down
Pantothenic acid	Late incubation mortality, subcutaneous edema and hemorrhage
Pyridoxine	Mortality
Biotin	Mortality in first or last week of incubation, chondrodystrophy, webbed feet, dwarfing
Folic acid	Mortality at internal pip Deformed beak and bent tibiotarsus
B₁₂	Mid-incubation mortality, hemorrhages, perosis, edema, fatty liver
Manganese	Late incubation mortality, chondrodystrophy
Iodine	Late incubation mortality, delayed hatch time, delayed yolk resorption, dwarfing
Iron	Pale, poorly visible extraembryonic blood vessels in candled eggs
Zinc	Skeletal abnormalities of head, limbs, spine

Data from Austic RE, Scott ML: Nutritional deficiency diseases. In Hofstad MS (ed): Diseases of Poultry, ed 8. Ames, Iowa State University Press, 1984, pp 38–64; and Subcommittee on Poultry Nutrition: Symptoms of nutritional deficiencies in chickens and turkeys. In Subcommittee on Poultry Nutrition (ed): Nutrient Requirements of Poultry, ed 6 and ed 8. Washington, DC, National Academy of Sciences, ed 6, 1971, pp 5–11; ed 8, 1984, pp 12, 17.

Table 30–2

NUTRIENT COMPOSITION OF SEEDS COMMONLY INCLUDED IN PSITTACINE DIETS

	Leghorn Breeder	Corn	Proso Millet	Oat Groats (Dehusked)	Rape	Sunflower 95% DM	Rye
Ca (%)*	3.4	**0.03**	**0.03**	**0.08**	1.33	**0.12**	**0.07**
Cu (mg/kg)	8.0	**4.0**		7.0	8.0	**3.5**	8.0
Fe (mg/kg)	60.0	300.0	79.0	82.0	182.0	70.0	69.0
Mg (%)	0.05	0.14	0.18	0.13	0.07	**0.038**	0.14
Mn (mg/kg)	60.0	**5.0**		**31.0**	46.0	23.9	66.0
P (total %)	0.32	**0.29**	0.34	0.48	0.39	0.84	0.37
K (%)	0.15	0.37	0.48	0.39	2.98	0.92	0.52
Se (mg/kg)	0.10	**0.08**					0.44
Na (%)	0.15	**0.03**		**0.06**	0.05		**0.03**
Zn (mg/kg)	65.0	**14.0**		**0.0**			**36.0**
Biotin (mg/kg)	0.15	**0.08**					**0.06**
Choline (mg/kg)		567.0	489.0	1264.0		3000.0	479.0
Folic acid (mg/kg)	0.35	0.3		0.6			0.7
Niacin (mg/kg)	10.0	28.0	26.0	11.0		54.0	21.0
Pantothenic acid (mg/kg)	10.0	**6.6**	12.2	15.4		43.0	**9.1**
Vitamin A (IU/kg)	4000.0					**500.0**	
Vitamin B₆ (mg/kg)	4.5	5.3		**1.2**			**2.9**
Riboflavin (mg/kg)	3.8	**1.4**	4.2	**1.3**		**2.0**	**1.9**
Thiamine (mg/kg)	0.8	3.8	8.1	7.2		20.0	4.2
Vitamin B₁₂ (μg/kg)	4.0						
Vitamin E (mg/kg)	10.0	25.0		16.0			17.0
Vitamin K (mg/kg)	0.5	**0.2**					
Vitamin D₃ (ICU/kg)	500.0	0.0	0.0	0.0	0.0	0.0	0.0

Data from Subcommittee on Poultry Nutrition: Symptoms of nutritional deficiencies in chickens and turkeys. In Subcommittee on Poultry Nutrition (ed): Nutrient Requirements of Poultry, ed 8. Washington DC, National Academy of Sciences, 1984, pp 12, 17; and Subcommittee on Feed Composition: United States-Canadian Tables of Feed Compositions, ed 3. Washington DC, National Academy Press, 1982; and Grau CR: Sunflower seeds for psittacines. Exotic Bird Rep 1:6, 1983.

*Calcium levels are compared with 0.3%, which has been determined to support egg-laying in cockatiels.

†Highlighted figures do not meet the nutrient requirements of breeding poultry.

§100% dry matter, unless otherwise noted.

monly fed seeds are likely to be low in calcium, copper, manganese, phosphorus, selenium, sodium, zinc, biotin, choline, vitamin A, vitamin D, vitamin K, and riboflavin for sustained production in psittacines. It is commonly believed that seeds are high in phosphorus, because seeds have a low calcium/phosphorus ratio, but both nutrients are deficient for sustained egg-laying. The deficiency of calcium is more severe than the deficiency of phosphorus, however.

Homogeneous foods containing vitamin and mineral supplementation offer the advantage of eliminating the hazards of individual food choices.

If infertility is determined to be the problem, rule out the many non-nutritional causes of infertility, and investigate possible nutritional causes. The hen should be examined for excessive abdominal fat. If obesity is a problem, follow the treatment guidelines outlined in the section on Adult Nutritional Disorders.

Infertile birds on an all-seed diet with little or no vitamin supplementation, or given vitamin-rich foods cafeteria-style, may be deficient in vitamins A and E. Injectable forms of these vitamins may be given. Injacom 100 (Roche), an injectable form of vitamins A and D_3, is administered at a dosage of 0.0007 ml/g body weight. Seletoc (Schering), vitamin E and selenium, is given at 0.01 ml/100 g body weight. Prevention requires increasing vitamin A in the consumed diet to approximately 4000 IU/kg feed and vitamin E to approximately 10 IU/kg feed. Examine infertile birds for evidence of *Giardia* species or other parasites that may be affecting absorption of ingested nutrients.

In cases of decreased hatchability of fertile eggs or poor chick livability, advise the owner to supplement the diet with a multiple vitamin and mineral product. Supplementation is best accomplished by providing a nonchoice food item such as a mash or pellet. Supplementation via drinking water is quite variable and may be insufficient for bird species that drink very little water.

Egg binding is usually first seen as a hen hunched over, tail pointed straight down, fluffed up either on a perch or on the floor. Physical examination shows a large, hard mass cranial to the pelvic bones. After egg binding the owner should be advised to increase levels of calcium and vitamin D_3 in the diet, calcium to 0.5 to 0.9% and vitamin D_3 to 200 international chick units (ICU)/kg diet. If the hen is obese, a weight-loss program should also be initiated. Some hens may be prone to egg binding

because of hereditary factors affecting egg size and pelvic conformation.

Hens with unusual bone fractures caused by simple maneuvers such as flying, landing, or routine handling should be treated with calcium and vitamin D_3 injections and dietary improvement. They should be discouraged from egg production while their depleted bone stores are replenished. This may be accomplished by removing the hen from her mate or flock if colony-bred, and denying her access to a nest box. If she continues to lay infertile eggs, administer medroxyprogesterone (Depoprovera, Upjohn), 3 mg/100 g body weight, to inhibit ovulation. Monitor progress by radiography after 2 to 3 months of reproductive rest.

Other manifestations of calcium or vitamin D_3 deficiency may be treated initially with injectables. Treatment and prevention may continue by provision of adequate dietary supplementation.

GROWTH AND DEVELOPMENTAL NUTRITIONAL DISORDERS

Rapidly growing chicks require the highest concentration of essential nutrients per *calorie* of energy intake. Growing birds fed diets just adequate for maintenance of their parents will die. Adult birds can be maintained on diets with as little as 4% protein with a good balance of essential amino acids, but cockatiel chicks, for example, fed 5% protein all died by 4 weeks of age.[13] Chicks fed 10% protein experienced 50% mortality by the same age.

In birds, except the Columbiformes, there is no evidence that parents use their body stores to enrich the diet fed to the chicks.[14] It is important to ensure that the diet offered to the parents during chick feeding is adequate for the chicks and not just adequate for the parents. Achieving this is complicated by the lack of information on the nutrient requirements for growth for most birds.

Poor-Growth Syndrome

Clinical Signs

Nutrient deficiencies, including underfeeding, during growth can result in a variety of clinical manifestations. Stunting, poor growth, weakness, and slow development are all part of the same continuum. In cockatiels, stunting is characterized by a large head relative to the body, failure of the normal transition of small pink feet to larger black feet at 10 to 13 days of age, and low body weights at weaning. Frequently, nutritionally deficient chicks with full crops continue to beg as long as the feeder is present without respect to the timing or frequency of feeding. Some nutritionally deficient chicks at the age of maximum body weight (about 3½ weeks in cockatiels) exhibit mild to extreme resistance to feeding with violent regurgitation, biting, and screaming. Crop stasis is a frequent result of a nutrient deficiency and can vary from slow crop emptying to complete cessation.

Abnormal feathering in growing chicks is usually manifested as reduced or absent feathering. This is usually associated with a generally poor condition and extremely reduced growth—perhaps 50 to 70% of normal. Severely compromised chicks can experience even poorer growth with virtually no feathering. Late weaning is also the result of failure of the bird to grow at its potential.

Etiology

Most nutritional deficiencies manifest these clinical signs. The regurgitation seen in this syndrome must be differentiated from that which occurs spontaneously in chicks that have been fed in excess of their capacity. These chicks assume a characteristic posture in which the chick usually holds its head still and back farther than chicks that have not been overfilled. This occurs commonly during hand-feeding with chicks at the age of maximal body weight when their crops shrink at the end of growth.

Failure to wean can have a number of nutritional causes. It is important to differentiate between those cases in which the chick fails to take any food on its own and those in which the chick takes inadequate amounts to maintain its body weight. If no food is eaten, management conditions should be checked. Chicks that do not have access to water often fail to eat dry foods. The amount of water available from hand-feeding may be inadequate to stimulate intake of seeds or other dry foods.

Weaning appears to be a developmental and not a learned process.[15] When normal chicks reach the age of weaning, their previous experience with food and water appears to make no difference in their weight or age of weaning. The single most important factor in weaning is that the bird grow at its potential. This means that chicks should grow rapidly to a peak body weight (about 100 g in cockatiels) by the time they normally reach peak weight (3–3½ weeks in cockatiels) and decline to weaning weight (80–85 g in cockatiels) before the age of weaning (by about 4–4½ weeks in cockatiels). Weaning should take place at this weight at the normal age of weaning (6–7 weeks in cockatiels), after which weight is maintained or slow growth occurs. Chicks that achieve weaning weight without reaching normal peak weights may experience impaired weaning. Reduced growth rates have been shown to delay weaning and in extreme cases to cause a failure to balance food and water intake in chicks. In some cases the abilities to wean and to balance food and water intake may be permanently affected.

A discussion of some of the nutrient deficiencies that have been investigated and that can result in this syndrome follows.

Protein can be fed in excess to growing birds. Roudybush and Grau have shown that a diet of 35% protein results in growth inhibition and behavioral abnormalities in cockatiels.[13] Twenty-five percent protein resulted in normal growth, but behavioral abnormalities still occurred. Twenty percent protein was shown to be adequate for maximal growth and normal behavior. Chicks fed 18% protein or less experienced reduced growth. Stunting and 50% mortality by 4 weeks occurred in chicks maintained at 10% protein.

Balancing food and water in hand-fed birds is essential. The consistency of a diet, however, is not a good measure of the amount of water it contains. The proper dilution of the diet during hand-feeding is about 20 to 25% dry weight and 75 to 80% water.[13] In younger birds a more dilute diet may be needed, and in older birds a drier diet may be adequate. When a diet that is too dilute is fed, chicks experience, in order of onset, increased or excessive begging, emaciation, crop stasis, increasingly dark-colored droppings, crop infection, lethargy, and death. Birds affected by excess water in the diet have low hematocrits and suffer from emaciation and overhydration.

Birds that are dehydrated immediately cease growing and exhibit dry wrinkled skin and slow food passage. Cockatiel chicks fed 50% solids all died within 7 days.[13]

Other causes of this syndrome that have been investigated in a preliminary way are riboflavin, lysine, and pantothenic acid deficiencies. It is safe to assume that many trace nutrient and amino acid deficiencies result in this syndrome as well.

Diagnosis

Diagnosis of nutritional diseases is often difficult, and many times a specific diagnosis is not needed. Many nutritional deficiencies produce the syndrome under discussion. Fortunately, diet evaluation can be easier in some cases than diagnosis of the bird from signs. If commercial diets are involved, the manufacturer can be contacted to see if there have been other problems with that lot. If not, the diet is unlikely to be the cause of disease. If the diet has been formulated by the client, a few specific nutrients, such as total protein (20% of dry weight), calcium (0.9%), phosphorus (0.6% available), water (70–80%), and sources of trace nutrients can be evaluated from the recipe. If these nutrients are within the acceptable range, other nutrients can be checked.

Evaluation of the efficiency of feed conversion or the amount of feed (dry weight) consumed per unit of body weight gain (live postprandial weight) is useful. The more efficiently feed is converted to body weight, the more nearly adequate the diet composition and food intake are under most conditions. As a diagnostic tool in rapidly growing birds, feed efficiency can be measured before and after diet changes and the results compared.

$$\text{Feed efficiency} = \frac{\text{Dry weight of feed eaten during trial}}{\text{Final weight of chick} - \text{Beginning weight of chick}}$$

$$\text{Dry weight of feed eaten} = \frac{\text{Wet weight eaten} \times 100\%}{\% \text{ of solids in food}}$$

Relatively small increases in feed intake as a proportion of body weight can result in a marked increase in feed efficiency, because all of the added food is available for weight gain when the needs for maintenance have been met. Birds should always be weighed at the same time each day, usually before the first feeding of the day, to be consistent

in treatment and to avoid the added and variable weight of a full gut and crop.

Treatment and Prevention

Any deficiency, excess, or imbalance found in the diet should be corrected or, if the diet is found to be grossly inadequate, it should be replaced with a diet that has been shown to be adequate. If the needed diet changes are extreme, time must be allowed for the chick to adapt to the new levels and types of substrate. Liver enzyme levels including those involved in gluconeogenesis, glycolysis, lipogenesis, and so forth may need to adjust to handle these changes. This process takes about 3 days in animals that have been tested. New diets should be mixed with old diets in decreasing proportions for 2 to 3 days if the changes are extreme. Most developmental disorders can be reversed if treated soon enough, but severely stunted birds may never reach their potential adult condition. Failure to wean, like stunting, appears to be permanent. In severe cases the ability to balance food and water intake as adults is not regained. The prognosis for these birds is poor.

Metabolic Bone Disease

Clinical Signs

Metabolic bone disease may be seen as bone malformations including spraddle-legged chicks, fractures, folding fractures, rickets, beak malformations, and crooked toes. Reduced growth and poor condition are usually also seen.

Etiology

Metabolic bone disease is related to deficiencies of calcium, phosphorus, vitamin D_3, or to an improper ratio of calcium to phosphorus in the diet.

An excess of either calcium or phosphorus results in the sequestering of the other in the form of an insoluble calcium phosphate. In the gut this results in reduced absorption and availability of the element found in low concentrations. The ratio of calcium to phosphorus in most diets for growth needs to be in the range of 1:1 to 2:1, with 3:2 being common.

There are ample data from poultry work to conclude that levels of calcium in excess of 1.2% of the diet involve risking toxic effects,[16] including decreased body weight gain,[17] reduced growth rate and poorer feed conversion,[18] depressed feed intake and increased mortality,[19] and, in pullets 8 to 20 weeks of age, nephrosis, visceral gout, calcium urate deposits, high mortality, and reduced feed consumption and weight gains.[20]

Diagnosis

If clinical and/or radiographic examination reveals folding fractures, decreased bone density, or other bone formation abnormalities, the diet should be evaluated.

Treatment and Prevention

Calcium levels should be about 0.9% and available phosphorus about 0.6% of the dry matter. There should also be a source of vitamin D$_3$, which makes about 500 to 2000 ICU available per kilogram of diet. Correct the underlying dietary deficiency or imbalance.

Feather Achromatosis

Clinical Signs

Feather achromatosis shows up as lack of normal pigmentation in feathers.

Etiology

Achromatosis can occur because of specific deficiencies but is not a consistent response among species. In dark breeds of chickens, turkeys, and quail, a lysine deficiency in growing birds results in achromatosis of the wing feathers over a broad range of levels of lysine.[21] This has been considered pathognomonic for a lysine deficiency. Achromatosis has not been observed with a lysine deficiency in either cockatiels or squab. In some spe-

cies, multiple deficiencies may result in achromatosis, even though lysine deficiency is not one of them. In preliminary work with cockatiels, chicks fed diets marginal in riboflavin showed achromatosis of the wing feathers, and a choline deficiency produced achromatosis of varying intensity in 30 to 40% of the chicks. Although the quantitative requirement for choline in cockatiels is not known, the level is lower than in poultry, and deficiency produces achromatosis.

Diagnosis

Achromatosis is usually seen on the long feathers of the wing and occasionally on the tail. Often the affected feathers are normal in color at the base and the tip.

Treatment and Prevention

If there are no other clinical signs, the bird need not be treated. Achromatosis disappears at the chick's first molt. Prevention consists of feeding an adequate diet to growing chicks. The level of lysine needed by growing cockatiels is 0.8% of the diet.

Lactose Intolerance

Clinical Signs

Diarrhea, abdominal distention, anorexia, and poor growth rate may be seen.

Etiology

Milk products can be either a concentrated source of essential nutrients or a source of dietary problems, or both. The significance of milk products in the diet depends on which products are used and what proportion of the diet they compose. The main problem with milk products in the feeding of birds is inability to digest lactose. Birds that have been tested cannot digest lactose and suffer from diarrhea when the diet reaches a level of 10 to 30% on a dry-weight basis.[22, 23] Thus, lactose in milk products should be avoided when possible. When a milk product is used, the total amount of lactose in the diet should be limited. Some of the milk products that contain significant amounts of lactose include dried skim milk, which is 50% lactose and dried whey, which can reach 70% lactose. Some milk products such as cheeses and yogurts contain little or no lactose and can be used safely in the diets of birds. The use of lactase to digest lactose should be avoided in birds. Galactose, one product of lactose digestion, is toxic to birds.

Diagnosis

Rule out other causes of diarrhea and determine amount of lactose in the diet.

Treatment and Prevention

Limit the amount of lactose in the diet.

Vitamin D Toxicity

Clinical Signs

Crop stasis, weight loss, depression, polyuria, hematuria, accumulation of white material in the subcutis have been reported.[24]

Etiology

The level of vitamin D required in the diet to produce hypervitaminosis D is not well defined. The requirement for vitamin D in poultry diets is about 200 ICU per kilogram of diet. It is likely that most birds can tolerate 100 times this amount or 20,000 ICU per kilogram of diet.[10] The high incidence of toxicity in macaws[25] implies that there may be a greater sensitivity to vitamin D in some species than there is in poultry. In most cases these birds were fed commercially prepared diets to which a vitamin supplement had been added.[25] It is likely that commercial hand-feeding formulas are, in general, not excessive in levels of vitamin D and that without supplementation they will not produce toxicity.

Diagnosis

Radiographs may show abnormal calcification in kidneys and various other soft tissues and increased intramedullary bone production. Necropsy and histopathologic examination reveal abnormal calcification of soft tissues.[24]

Treatment and Prevention

Low protein diets, sodium bicarbonate, allopurinol, aspirin, and other supportive treatments may be attempted. Reduce the level of vitamin D in the diet.

Gout

Gout in chicks is not likely to be associated with nutrition. The primary nutritional cause of gout in birds is a vitamin A deficiency. Young birds are likely to suffer other signs of vitamin A deficiency before the onset of gout.

ADULT NUTRITIONAL DISORDERS

Nonbreeding adult birds have lower nutritional requirements than do growing or breeding birds. Unfortunately, there is little published information on the nutritional requirements for maintenance of any species of bird. In chickens, maintenance requirements of protein (3.5%), calcium (0.05%), phosphorus (0.1%), and potassium (0.06%) have been estimated, but other nutrients have not been determined.[12] Because maintenance requirements are likely to be quite low, deficiencies often take years to become clinically apparent. Secondary disorders caused by an underlying, subclinical nutritional deficiency are more likely to be seen.

Nutritional excesses may also cause disease in adult birds. These disorders may be readily apparent, as with obesity, or they may remain subclinical for varying amounts of time, as with fatty liver disease.

Chronic Malnutrition Syndrome

Clinical Signs

Adult birds suffering from chronic malnutrition may show skin and feather disorders. The feathers may appear dull and tattered, with barb defects visible. They may have color abnormalities such as pale yellows instead of bright yellow or orange, or black replacing greens. The skin may appear dry and flaky. The owner may complain that the bird scratches itself too much and has excessive dander.

Another common sign of chronic malnutrition is increased susceptibility to infections, manifesting as frequent upper respiratory infections. Any number of gram-negative bacteria species may be cultured from these birds.

Etiology

Often the condition is a multifactorial nutritional deficiency, caused by years of inadequate or marginal nutrition, such as an unsupplemented all-seed diet or a non-nutritional, imbalanced human-food diet. Considering the nutrient composition of seed diets, the most common deficiencies seen are vitamin A, calcium, vitamin K, sodium, and vitamin B_{12}.

Diagnosis is derived from clinical signs and dietary history.

Treatment and Prevention

Supplement the diet with a multivitamin and mineral mix, preferably in the food, or switch to a more balanced diet, such as a maintenance pellet.

Vitamin A Deficiency

Clinical Signs

Chronic sinusitis, recurring bacterial infections, hyperkeratosis of sinuses or skin of legs and feet, and white nodular oral plaques are seen.

Etiology is all-seed diets, which are very low in vitamin A.

Diagnosis

Clinical signs, dietary history, and response to administration of vitamin A are diagnostic. Biopsy of lesions showing hyperkeratinization may also be useful for definitive diagnosis.

Treatment and Prevention

Severe cases of vitamin A deficiency should be treated initially with intramuscular injection of vitamin A (Injacom 100, 0.7 ml/kg body weight). Blocked sinuses may need to be further treated by removal of excess keratinized material. The diet should be adjusted to contain 4000 IU/kg feed.

Calcium or Vitamin D₃ Deficiency

Clinical Signs

Seizures and convulsions are most commonly seen in African grey parrots.[26] Pathologic fractures, egg binding, scoliosis, and folding fractures are more commonly seen in other species.

Etiology

It is unclear why African grey parrots appear to be predisposed to hypocalcemia.[27, 28] Relatively few adult grey parrots on all-seed, low calcium diets actually exhibit signs of hypocalcemia. It has been suggested that African greys may have poorly functional, or fewer, osteoclasts, making them less efficient at mobilizing calcium from bone stores in times of need.[29] To date, data to substantiate this theory have not been published or presented.

Diagnosis

Serum calcium levels less than 8.0 mg/dl may be associated with hypocalcemic seizures. Low serum calcium levels are often seen in asymptomatic African greys. Response to calcium injection is also diagnostic and is the diagnostic test of choice in the case of a convulsing bird.

Treatment and Prevention

Give injectable calcium initially, and adjust dietary calcium and vitamin D_3 to 0.3% and 200 ICU/kg of feed, respectively. Injectable calcium (Calphosan, Carleton Corp.) is given at a dosage of 0.5 to 1.0 ml/kg body weight intramuscularly.

Obesity

Clinical signs

Excessive abdominal fat (distended abdomen) and subcutaneous fat may be found on physical examination, especially prominent in the submandibular and clavicular areas, and along the sides of the breast, groin, and abdomen. The bird often has a wider stance than normal. Feathering may appear to have bald spots where feather tracts have separated because of underlying fat accumulation. Lipomas may be seen.

Etiology

Obesity is caused when energy intake exceeds energy expenditure for a long period of time.

Treatment

Increase energy expenditure or decrease energy intake, or both. The most effective way to overcome obesity is a combination of the two. Increasing exercise is effective in reducing appetite; and so both measures increase energy expenditure and decrease energy intake. Food and water may be placed at opposite ends of the cage; cage or flight area may be increased; or the bird may be given more exercise out of the cage. The next steps are to regulate energy intake. These include (1) regulation of food intake by offering a measured amount of food; (2) changes in food composition to reduce caloric density; and (3) decrease of fat in the diet.

The bird must be closely monitored to assess the rate of weight loss and whether any newly substituted diet is being consumed. Weight loss should not be more than a sustained 3% of the bird's body weight per week.

Lipomas may be reduced or eliminated by weight reduction alone or with treatment with L-thyroxine (Synthroid, 0.1 mg), 1 tablet per 4 oz of drinking water for 1 to 4 months.

Hepatic Lipidosis—Fatty Liver

Clinical Signs

Anorexia, regurgitation, and depression may be seen. Often, signs remain subclinical prior to death.

Etiology

Fatty liver can result from a variety of problems, the most common of which are toxic insult and malnutrition. Fatty liver from malnutrition results from the inability of the liver to mobilize fat, which is present either from deposition directly in the liver from the diet or, more importantly, fat that is synthesized from carbohydrate or protein in the liver. Mobilization of this fat requires the formation of lipoproteins as the form of fat carried out of the liver. Three specific types of deficiencies that can inhibit formation of lipoprotein inhibit the mobilization of hepatic fat and cause fatty liver: protein-calorie malnutrition with nearly adequate calories but inadequate protein, methionine deficiency, and choline deficiency.

Diagnosis

Radiographs showing enlarged liver, enlarged and pale liver seen on laparoscopy, liver biopsy, and serum chemistries showing greatly elevated liver enzymes are diagnostic.

Treatment and Prevention

Birds that have fatty livers should be fed about 800 mg choline, 0.2% methionine, and 12% protein per kilogram feed, until they recover. The primary cause of the fatty liver should be investigated to ensure that toxic insult and disease are not continuing causes of the disease.

Iron Storage Disease—Hepatic Hemochromatosis

Clinical Signs

Dyspnea, abdominal distension (hydrops ascites), and weakness are seen with hepatic hemochromatosis. The syndrome is commonly seen in toucans, birds of paradise, and mynahs, but it is also reported in many other species.

Etiology

Iron storage is an often observed but poorly understood syndrome. Iron excess has been observed in a number of species[30-33] and remains a problem in many pet and zoo birds. In general, fructivorous, insectivorous, and omivorous birds accumulate more iron in their livers than carnivorous, piscivorous, and granivorous birds, even within the same order.[65] Diets with 100 ppm of iron or less have been recommended to reduce dietary sources of iron, because most birds shown to have the disease had been consuming diets in excess of 100 ppm of iron. Because in a practical situation diets with less than 100 ppm of iron are difficult to formulate, this observation may prove to be more in line with what is available to feed birds than what is needed to prevent excessive iron storage. Even diets with 100 ppm of iron are in excess of the requirements for growth of poultry, which generally require 60 to 80 ppm.[10] Higher iron levels in the diet are no problem in birds who have a high duodenal mucosal blockage, such as chickens. No problems were seen in chicken flocks maintained on diets containing 250 to 300 ppm iron for 10 years. In birds that are prone to develop an iron storage syndrome in the liver, diets with 50 to 60 ppm of iron can induce an iron liver concentration of over 50 μg/g wet tissue.[66] Even in birds that normally have a low iron content in the liver, such as pigeons and doves, high daily doses can induce the iron storage syndrome.[67]

Some other possible causes influencing iron storage in the liver are stresses related to disease exposure (immunologic stress),[34-36] crowding, and nutritional stress related to periodic starvation associated with diet changes,[37] because disease occurs with high frequency in recently imported birds.[38] Another stress that has been shown to be associated with increased iron stores is intoxication with heavy metals.[39]

Diagnosis

Radiographs reveal enlarged liver and ascites. Liver biopsy reveals hemochromatosis.

Treatment and Prevention

One effective treatment, phlebotomy, is usually performed in conjunction with low iron diets.[68] A less invasive treatment has been documented using deferoxamine (100 mg/kg q24h, SC) combined with a low iron diet (65 ppm) for periods as long as 4 months until the iron content in the liver of a toucan was normalized.[66]

Vitamin K Deficiency

Clinical Signs

Vitamin K deficiency is manifested as excessive bleeding or bruising associated with trauma or delayed clotting time.

Etiology

A long-term, unsupplemented all-seed diet may lead to vitamin K deficiency.

Diagnosis

History, clinical signs, and dietary history may lead to a presumptive diagnosis of vitamin K deficiency.

Treatment and Prevention

Give injectable vitamin K, initially at a dosage of 1.0 to 2.0 mg/kg body weight intramuscularly (IM) every 12 to 24 hours, and adjust diet to 0.5 ppm vitamin K.

Goiter

Clinical Signs

Swelling in the clavicular area with associated respiratory noises, dyspnea, voice changes or loss of voice, and regurgitation are characteristic of goiter caused by iodine deficiency, which is prevalent in budgerigars.

The sole etiology is iodine deficiency.

Diagnosis, Treatment, and Prevention

Iodine deficiency is diagnosed by physical examination, characteristic clinical signs, and/or response to oral or injectable iodine treatment. Minor cases may be treated with oral iodine supplementation in the drinking water. Mix a stock solution from Lugol solution or potassium iodide (1 g/10 ml deionized water) by mixing 2 ml iodine solution into 30 ml water. Mix 1 drop of the stock solution per ounce of drinking water. Give as the sole source of drinking water for 1 week or until signs disappear. Give twice weekly thereafter as a preventative. For critical cases, when birds are severely dyspneic, administer oxygen, dexamethasone, and 0.01 to 0.03 ml of 20% sodium iodide in breast muscle once daily for 3 to 5 days.[40]

Vitamin E/Selenium Deficiency

Clinical Signs

Paralysis or paresis, tremors, incoordination, and torticollis may be seen with vitamin E/selenium deficiency. Harrison reports a vitamin E/selenium–responsive syndrome in cockatiels characterized by eyelid paralysis, weak bite, weak perching grip, partial tongue paralysis, hyperactivity or inactivity, and voice abnormalities.[5]

Etiology

Etiologies may be long-term unsupplemented all-seed diets, maldigestion or malabsorption syndromes, or ingestion of rancid fat or oil.

Diagnosis

The diagnosis is determined by clinical response to vitamin E/selenium injections, dietary history, and fresh fecal or fecal trichrome examination.

Treatment and Prevention

Administer injectable vitamin E/selenium (Seletoc), 0.01 ml/100 g body weight IM. Adjust dietary level to 10 IU per kilogram of feed.

INTERACTIONS BETWEEN DISEASE STATES AND NUTRITION

Immunologic Stress

Birds exhibit a physiologic stress response to a wide variety of environmental changes, making them more susceptible to diseases or allowing recurrence of latent diseases being carried asymptomatically.

It is well known that many nutrient deficiencies can affect the immune system adversely, and providing minimum requirements results in reestablishing normal immune function. Recent medical research has provided more and more evidence that certain nutrients actually act as immunostimulants when given in pharmacologic amounts. Although many of these studies have been conducted in mammals, several have used turkeys and chickens with similar results.

In poultry, feeding pharmacologic doses of vitamin A (1000–60,000 IU/kg feed) results in enhanced immune function because of a variety of mechanisms. These enhanced immune functions translated into increased resistance to infection and decreased mortality upon disease challenge.[41–43]

Carotenoids, such as beta carotene, have also been shown to have immunostimulatory properties distinct from their pro-vitamin A activity. Beta carotene has many of the same effects on the immune system as vitamin A. In addition, beta carotene is a better antioxidant than vitamin A, and it enhances antitumor immune functions, whereas vitamin A does not.[41, 42] Vitamin E is known as an antioxidant and has been used to stabilize fats in products for many years. Pharmacologic doses of vitamin E (60–300 mg/kg feed) protect phagocytic cells from self-damage caused by the presence of free radicals and reactive oxygen molecules produced to combat bacterial infections. Vitamin E also enhances immune responses in a variety of ways.[43–45] In studies with poultry, pharmacologic doses of vitamin E reduced morbidity and mortality associated with _Escherichia coli_ challenge or cold and light stress.[43, 45]

There are interactions between vitamin E and other nutrients that affect immune function and are worthy of note. Selenium enhances vitamin E immunostimulation but does not replace it when supplemented alone without vitamin E.[45] Vitamin A, when given at pharmacologic doses with vitamin E, does not potentiate its effects and seems to actually have an antagonistic effect.[43, 45] Vitamin C acts synergistically with vitamin E as an antioxidant. Vitamin C spares vitamin E consumption during oxidation reactions of phagocytic cells.[46–48] Increased dietary vitamin C also increases immune system function and responsiveness.[49] Almost all the bird species kept as cage or aviary birds are capable of synthesizing vitamin C. This process occurs predominantly in the kidneys of primitive orders and in the livers of more advanced orders of birds. Ability to synthesize vitamin C does not prevent birds from being able to efficiently absorb dietary vitamin C from the gastrointestinal tract. Certain conditions of stress, vitamin deficiencies, and infection can interfere with the biosynthesis and metabolism of vitamin C in vitamin C–synthesizing species.[49, 50]

The clinical conclusion suggested by results of research conducted to date is that pharmacologic doses of vitamin A, beta carotene, vitamin E, or vitamin E and vitamin C may be used to prevent disease, prevent immunosuppression due to stress or disease, and reduce the morbidity and mortality in the face of a disease outbreak. Given the potential toxicity of vitamin A and its possible antagonistic effects on vitamin E, the other choices would probably be safer to use. Although pet birds synthesize vitamin C, supplementation may be advisable under conditions of stress, infectious disease, or when significant liver damage is diagnosed.

Poultry research has been providing evidence that diets high in n-3 fatty acids (found in fish oils and fish meal) cause decreased responsiveness of macrophages to interferon and cause decreased production of factors that modulate white blood cell (WBC) activity. Birds fed diets high in the n-6 fatty acids (found in corn, vegetable oils, and poultry fat) show full responsiveness of macrophages and increased production of WBC modulators.[51]

Meal frequency has been found to greatly affect immune response. Short periods of feed deprivation increase cellular and humoral immunity in chicks. Overconsumption of feed causes decreased immunoglobulin production and decreased delayed-type hypersensitivity.[51] More research in adult birds is needed to determine if meal feeding would be more desirable than the typical ad libitum feeding generally practiced in aviculture today.

When a bird becomes ill owing to infection, often one of its first responses is to stop eating. The current dogma in veterinary medicine is usually to immediately begin parenteral or enteral supplementation. Current research suggests that this may be ill-advised. In chicks undergoing immunologic stress, growth decreases both from reduced feed consumption and inefficiencies of feed conversion to lean tissue. After the stress is resolved, compensatory growth occurs and trace mineral and amino acid requirements increase above normal. Immunologic response is enhanced by brief periods of starvation. In adults, nitrogen excretion increases during immune response, and it is not prevented by increasing the levels of amino acids in the diet. Certain trace minerals (iron, copper, zinc) are consumed by the immune response, and serum levels drop. Supplementation with these trace minerals during the immune response increases morbidity and mortality. The requirements for these trace minerals increases after the immune response as the bird replenishes its depleted stores.[51–53] Anorexia due to stress or infection may be a defense, and the fact that it has been a highly conserved response throughout evolution suggests that it provides survival advantage.[53] Therefore, force-feeding and parenteral mineral supplementation should probably be avoided early in an infection process in birds with adequate body weight. If the bird loses a significant amount of weight (5–10% body weight in a lean bird), force-feeding should be resorted to.

Drug Therapy and Nutrition Interactions

Some drug therapies exert direct effects on the patient's nutritional status; others may exert indirect effects. The indirect effects are the most commonly encountered.

Medication via drinking water is often chosen because of the ease of administration, especially in groups of birds, and because it eliminates handling stresses on the birds. Many medications are unpalatable to most birds and may result in refusal to drink. When a bird stops drinking water, it very shortly thereafter refuses to eat dry foods. Soon the patient is dehydrated and anorectic in addition to the original malady. Medications with a bitter taste are the most likely to cause this, but even fruit-flavored syrups may be refused by some birds simply because the water tastes or smells different. Effects of bitter medications may be eliminated by mixing sweeteners or fruit juices into the medicated water.

Advise owners to watch their birds' drinking behavior and observe the birds' droppings daily when medicating the drinking water. If droppings become scant and dark green, the bird has probably stopped drinking and eating because of unpalatable water.

Medication via feed is another route chosen for ease of administration on both owner and birds. This route is most reliable and useful when the bird has been previously prepared. Trying to have a sick bird accept a mash, pellet, or treat for the first time is not likely to be successful. Advise your clients to accustom their healthy birds to treats (such as grapes, yogurt, applesauce) that may someday hide oral medications; to mashes that may someday be medicated with any number of oral medications; or pellets that may someday be replaced by medicated pellets.

Some drugs may cause adverse side effects of nausea and anorexia. Trimethoprim-sulfamethoxazole has this effect in individuals of a variety of species, but side effects are especially prevalent in macaws and pigeons. Vomiting or regurgitation is also occasionally seen in these birds. LA-200, a long-acting injectable form of oxytetracycline, and chloramphenicol have been reported to cause anorexia in some individuals of several psittacine species.

Sulfa drugs, such as sulfamethazine, sulfaquinoxaline, and sulfamerazine, may cause a hemorrhagic syndrome consisting of subcutaneous hemorrhages, splenic enlargement and infarction, anemia, and increased clotting times. It is thought that the sulfas eradicate cecal flora responsible for producing vitamin K, leaving the bird deficient. Research in poultry shows that clinical signs can be reduced or partially prevented by supplementation with vitamin K, but the syndrome does appear to have other components involved.[54] Administer vitamin K when treating birds with a significant ceca with sulfa drugs.

Tetracyclines have an affinity for binding with divalent cations present in the intestinal tract, forming nonabsorbable complexes. Calcium, magnesium, and iron may all be bound, but calcium is the mineral of concern because of its prevalence compared with the others. When treating birds with oral forms of tetracycline, oxytetracycline, or chlortetracycline, mineral supplements containing calcium should be removed from the diet. Pellets medicated with chlortetracycline are required to have no more than 0.7% calcium. When treating flocks with chlortetracycline for 45 days, advise the owner to discontinue breeding to prevent calcium deficiency in egg-laying hens and growing chicks. Doxycycline has a much lower affinity for forming complexes with calcium, and thus oral forms of doxycycline may be administered without reducing the calcium level in the diet.[55]

Prolonged treatment with testosterone or medroxyprogesterone may predispose birds to obesity. The owner should be advised to monitor the bird's weight once or twice monthly, instituting diet restrictions or increased exercise if weight gain occurs.

Anticonvulsant therapy (phenobarbital, primidone, phenytoin) may result in a megaloblastic anemia because of decreased absorption of folic acid. Another possible nutritional side effect is osteomalacia from decreased calcium absorption and altered vitamin D metabolism.[56, 57]

Neomycin has been reported to cause malabsorption of fats, carotene, iron, glucose, vitamin B_{12}, sodium, potassium, and calcium.[58, 59]

Kidney Disease and Gout

In birds, gout is a common sequela of kidney disease and may not prove to be a nutritional disease except under unusual circumstances, such as in a calcium toxicity resulting in renal calcification and urolithiasis or a deficiency of vitamin A resulting in keratinization of the kidneys.[60, 61] Gouty chickens selected for their propensity to develop gout required 70% protein to produce the disease.[62]

Kidney stress can be reduced by lowering dietary levels of minerals, fat-soluble vitamins, and protein. The protein source should have as near as possible a balanced profile of amino acids to reduce the need for excess protein to include all the essential amino acids and thereby transamination reactions.

Liver Disease

As part of the treatment of liver disease, diets that reduce stress and the need for liver function may facilitate recovery. Many functions of the liver can be reduced by either eliminating or lowering the substrates upon which the liver must work. This can be accomplished, in part, by replacing these substrates with substrates that are metabolized in other organs. An example of this is the branched-chain amino acids (BCAA) (isoleucine, leucine, and valine), which are transaminated in peripheral tissues. Use of high levels of BCAA reduces the need for transamination reactions in the liver to produce dispersible amino acids by allowing this production to take place in peripheral tissues. Aromatic amino acids (phenylalanine, tyrosine) are poorly metabolized in liver disease and need to be reduced in the diet. Total protein should be reduced to about 8% of the diet, with a molar ratio of branched-chain amino acids to aromatic amino acids of 2:1. Energy should be available from high levels of fat and carbohydrate. Vitamin A should be reduced to a minimum to avoid accumulation in the liver (less than 1500 IU/kg feed).

Maldigestion/Malabsorption

Nutritional deficiency signs may be seen in birds eating normal amounts of a nutritionally adequate diet if they are suffering from some degree of maldigestion or malabsorption. Feed birds a low-fat diet with elevated levels of vitamins and minerals and medium-chain triglycerides.[63] If pancreatic insufficiency is diagnosed, add pancreatic enzymes to the diet (Viokase powder, ⅛ tsp/kg, mixed into moist food 15 minutes prior to feeding).

Yeast Infection

Yeast infections with *Candida albicans* can be caused, in part, by improper diet. Candidiasis caused by other management problems can be exacerbated by certain nutrients. Diets should be free of simple carbohydrates and sugars such as sucrose, glucose, dextrose, honey, corn syrup, molasses, and maltose. Complex carbohydrates are less likely to support growth of *Candida*. Deficiencies of vitamin A, thiamin, riboflavin, and pyridoxine, vitamin C, and selenium increase susceptibility to candidiasis.[64] Because stress and immunosuppression often predispose hand-fed birds to candidiasis, nutritional treatment and prevention of immunologic stress are also applicable.

References

1. Roudybush TE, Grau CR, Limberg LA: Unpublished data, 1986.
2. Austic RE, Scott ML: Nutritional deficiency diseases. In Hofstad MS (ed): Diseases of Poultry, ed 8. Ames, Iowa State University Press, 1984, p 46.
3. Subcommittee on Poultry Nutrition: Symptoms of nutritional deficiencies in chickens and turkeys. In Subcommittee on Poultry Nutrition: Nutrient Requirements of Poultry, ed 6. Washington, DC, National Academy of Sciences, 1971, p 7.
4. Harrison GJ: Reproductive medicine. In Harrison GJ, Harrison LR (eds): Clinical Avian Medicine and Surgery. Philadelphia, WB Saunders, 1986, p 627.
5. Harrison GJ: Preliminary work with selenium/vitamin E responsive conditions in cockatiels and other psittacines. Proc Assoc Avian Vet 1986, Miami, pp 257–262.
6. Paredes JR, Garcia TP: Vitamin A as a factor affecting fertility in cockerels. Poult Sci 38:3–7, 1959.
7. Austic RE, Scott ML: Nutritional deficiency diseases. In Hofstad MS (ed): Diseases of Poultry, ed 8. Ames, Iowa State University Press, 1984, pp 38–64.
8. Angel CR: Research update: Age changes in digestibility of nutrients in ostriches and nutrient profiles of status of the hen and chick. Proc Assoc Avian Vet 1993, Nashville, pp 275–281.
9. Subcommittee on Poultry Nutrition: Symptoms of nutritional deficiencies in chickens and turkeys. In Subcommittee on Poultry Nutrition (ed): Nutrient Requirements of Poultry, ed 6. Washington DC, National Academy of Sciences, 1971, pp 5–11.
10. Subcommittee on Poultry Nutrition: Symptoms of nutritional deficiencies in chickens and turkeys. In Subcommittee on Poultry Nutrition (ed): Nutrient Requirements of Poultry, ed 8. Washington DC, National Academy of Sciences, 1984, pp 12, 17.
11. Subcommittee on Feed Composition: United States-Canadian Tables of Feed Composition, ed 3. Washington DC, National Academy Press, 1982.
12. Grau CR: Sunflower seeds for psittacines. Exotic Bird Rep 1:6, 1983.
13. Roudybush TE, Grau CR: Food and water interrelations and the protein requirement for growth of an altricial bird, the cockatiel (*Nymphicus hollandicus*). J Nutr 116:552, 1986.
14. Roudybush TE, Grau CR: Unpublished data, 1986.
15. Roudybush TE: Weaning of cockatiels. Proc West Poult Disease Conf 35:162–165, 1986.
16. National Research Council: Calcium. In Mineral Tolerance of Domestic Animals. Washington DC, National Academy of Sciences, 1980, pp 131–141.
17. Urban L: Chicken feeding trials with diets containing sufficient phosphorus and increasing calcium carbonate. Nutr Abstr 30:691, 1960.
18. Smith H, Taylor JH: Effect of feeding two levels of dietary calcium on the growth of broiler chickens. Nature 190:1200, 1961.
19. Fangauf R, Vogt H, Penner W: Studies of calcium tolerance in chickens. Arch Geflugelk 25:82, 1961.
20. Shane SM, Young RJ, Krook L: Renal and parathyroid changes produced by high calcium intake in growing pullets. Avian Dis 13:558, 1969.
21. Rutter WJ, Krickevsky PE, Scott HM, Hansen, RG: The metabolism of lactose and galactose. Poult Sci 32:706–715, 1953.
22. Spivey Fox MR, Briggs GM: Effect of dietary lactose upon chicks fed purified diet. Poult Sci 964–968, 1959.
23. Grau CR, Roudybush TE, Vohra P, et al: Obscure relations

of feather melanization and avian nutrition. World Poult Sci 45:241, 1989.

24. Takeshita D, Graham DL, Silverman S: Hypervitaminosis in baby macaws. Proc Assoc Avian Vet 1986, p 341.

25. Graham, D: Personal communication, 1987.

26. Hochleithner M: Convulsions in African grey parrots. Proc Assoc Avian Vet 1989, pp 78–81.

27. Lewandowski AH, Campbell TW, Harrison GJ: Clinical Chemistries. In Harrison GJ, Harrison LR (eds): Clinical Avian Medicine and Surgery. Philadelphia, WB Saunders, 1986, p 198.

28. Rosskopf WJ, Woerpel RW: Psittacine conditions and syndromes. Proc Assoc Avian Vet, 1990, pp 432–433.

29. Murphy J: Personal communication, 1986.

30. Griner LA: Pathology of Zoo Animals. San Diego, Zoological Society of San Diego, 1983.

31. Lowenstine LF, Petrak ML: Iron pigment in the livers of birds. In Montali RJ, Migaki G (eds): The Comparative Pathology of Zoo Animals. Washington DC, Smithsonian Institution Press, 1980, pp 127–135.

32. Taylor JJ: Iron accumulation in avian species in captivity. Dodo, J Jersey Wildl Preserv Trust 21:126–131, 1984.

33. Kincaid AL, Stoskopf MK: Passerine dietary overload syndrome. Zoo Biol 6:79–88, 1987.

34. Bafundo KW, Baker DH, Fitzgerald PR: The iron-zinc interrelationship in the chick as influenced by *Eimeria acervulina* infection. Poult Sci 63:59, 1984.

35. Bafundo KW, Baker DH, Fitzgerald PR: *Eimeria acervulina* infection and the zinc-cadmium interrelationship in the chick. Poult Sci 63:1828–1832, 1984.

36. Bafundo KW, Baker DH, Fitzgerald PR: Zinc utilization in the chick as influenced by dietary concentrations of cadmium and phytate and by *Eimeria acervulina* infection. Poult Sci 63:2430–2437, 1984.

37. Borch-Johnsen B, Nilssen KJ: Seasonal iron overload in Svalbard reindeer liver. J Nutr 117:2072–2078, 1987.

38. Clubb, S: Personal communication, 1986.

39. McDonald SE, Lowenstine LJ: Lead toxicosis in psittacine birds. In Proc 25th Int Symposium Diseases of Zoo Animals, Vienna, 1983, pp 183–196.

40. Lathrop, Jr CD, Harrison GJ: Miscellaneous diagnostic tests. In Harrison GJ, Harrison LR (eds): Clinical Avian Medicine and Surgery. Philadelphia, WB Saunders, 1986, p 293.

41. Bendich A: Carotenoids and the immune response. J Nutr 119:112–115, 1989.

42. Chew BP: Symposium: Immune function: Relationship of nutrition and disease control. J Dairy Sci 70:2732–2743, 1987.

43. Tengerdy RP, Brown JC: Effect of vitamin E and vitamin A on humoral immunity and phagocytosis in *E. coli* infected chickens. Poult Sci 56:957–963, 1977.

44. Tengerdy RP, Heinzerling RH, Nockels CF: Effect of vitamin E on the immune response of hypoxic and normal chickens. Infect Immun 5(6):987–989, 1972.

45. Tengerdy RP: Effect of vitamin E on immune responses. In Machlin LJ (ed): Vitamin E: A Comprehensive Treatise, vol. 1. New York, Marcel Dekker, 1980, pp 429–444.

46. Ginter E: Interactions between vitamins C and E and cytochrome P450. In Miguel J, Quintanilha AT, Weber H (eds): Handbook of Free Radicals and Antioxidants in Biomedicine, vol. 2. Boca Raton, CRC Press, 1989, pp 95–104.

47. Niki E: Synergistic inhibition of oxidation by vitamin E and vitamin C. In Ching Kuang Chow (ed): Cellular Antioxidant Defense Mechanisms, vol 2. Boca Raton, CRC Press, 1988, pp 112–122.

48. Bendich A: Interaction between vitamins C and E and their effect on immune responses. In Miguel J, Quintanilha AT, Weber H (eds): Handbook of Free Radicals and Antioxidants in Biomedicine, vol. 2. Boca Raton, CRC Press, 1989, pp 153–160.

49. Combs GF Jr: Vitamin C. In Combs GF: The Vitamins. San Diego, Academic Press, 1992, pp 223–249.

50. McDowell LR: Vitamin C. In McDowell LR: Vitamins in Animal Nutrition. San Diego, Academic Press, 1989, pp 365–387.

51. Klasing K: Physiological immunomodulation in poultry. 43rd North Central Avian Disease Conf Proc, 1992, pp 38–43.

52. Klasing K: Nutrition and metabolism of trace minerals during stress. Proc Animal Nutr Conf, 1994, pp 27–36.

53. Klasing K, Johnstone BJ, Benson BN: Implications of an immune response on growth and nutrient requirements of chicks. In Haresign W, Cole DJA (eds): Recent Advances in Animal Nutrition. Oxford, Butterworth and Heinemann, 1991, pp 135–146.

54. Klasing K: Personal communication, 1993.

55. Peckham MC: Poisons and Toxins. In Hofstad MS (ed): Diseases of Poultry, ed 8. Ames, Iowa State University Press, 1984, p 784.

56. Pfizer Laboratories: Drug insert technical information for Vibramycin, January, 1988.

57. Hahn TJ: Anticonvulsant drug induced mineral disorders. In Roe DA, Campbell TC (eds): Drugs and Nutrients: The Interactive Effects, vol. 21. New York, Marcel Dekker, 1984, pp 409–427.

58. Basu TK: Drug-nutrient Interactions. London, Croom Helm, 1988, p 42.

59. Holtzapple PG, Schwartz SE: Drug-induced maldigestion and malabsorption. In Roe DA, Campbell TC (eds): Drugs and Nutrients: The Interactive Effects, vol. 21. New York, Marcel Dekker, 1984, pp 475–477.

60. Altman RB: Noninfectious diseases. In Fowler ME (ed): Zoo and Wild Animal Medicine. Philadelphia, WB Saunders, 1986, p 506.

61. Halliwell WH: Toxic and metabolic conditions in birds of prey. In Fowler ME (ed): Zoo and Wild Animal Medicine. Philadelphia, WB Saunders, 1986, p 432.

62. Petersen DW: Personal communication, 1974.

63. Zeman FJ: Clinical Nutrition and Dietetics, ed 2. New York, Macmillan Publishing Co, 1991, pp 218–279.

64. Odds FC: Candida and Candidiosis, ed 2. London, Bailliere-Tindall, 1988, p 102.

65. Dierenfield E, Sheppard CD: Investigations of hepatic iron levels in zoo birds. Proc 8th Dr. Scholl Conference on Nutrition in Captive Wild Animals, 1989, pp 101–104.

66. Cornelissen H, Ducatelle R, Roels S: Successful treatment of a channel-billed toucan (*Ramphastos vitellinus*) with iron storage disease by chelation therapy: Sequential monitoring of the iron content of the liver during the treatment period by quantitative chemical and image analyses. J Avian Med Surg 9:131–137, 1995.

67. Dorrestein GM, Grinwis GM, Dominguez L, Jagt E van der, Beynen AC: An induced iron storage syndrome in doves and pigeons: A model for hemochromatosis in mynah birds? Proc Assoc of Avian Vet, 1992, pp 108–112.

68. Worell A: Phlebotomy for the treatment of hemochromatosis in two sulphur-breasted toucans. Proc Assoc Avian Vet, 1991, pp 9–14.

Katherine Quesenberry
Susan Orosz
Gerry M. Dorrestein

31

Musculoskeletal System

Anatomy of the Musculoskeletal System

Susan Orosz

SKULL

The avian skull is characterized by large orbits, a relatively large brain case, and pneumatized spaces between the laminae of bone. Birds have retained some reptilian anatomy such as a single occipital condyle, the formation of the mandible or lower jaw from approximately six small bones, the articulation of the mandible to the cranium through the quadrate bone, and the movable nature of the quadrate and pterygoid bones.

The upper or maxillary jaw is primarily made up of the premaxillary and nasal bones, with the maxillary bone contributing to only a small extent (Fig. 31–1). The lower jaw or mandible is the result of the fusion of five small membrane bones with the articular bone; these bones were derived embryologically from the cartilages of the pharyngeal or gill arches. This is in contrast to mammals, in which the mandible consists of a single bone. Each mandibular ramus is fused by a symphysis in both mammals and birds. In mammals, however, two of these bones—the articular and quadrate bones—have been relegated to an auditory function and are termed the incus and malleus. The quadrate bone of birds is crucial as the link between the mandible and the cranium.

Birds are also distinct from mammals by the movements of their jaws. Cranial kinesis is one of the distinctive features possessed by most birds and allows movement of the maxillary jaw while the brain case stays motionless. Birds possess elastic areas or zones in the rostral portion of the skull that allow bending of the bones. These areas consist of multiple thin laminae of bone stacked on top of each other and separated by connective tissue. Pneumatization is absent in these elastic zones.

Prokinesis is one type of cranial kinesis. Birds with maxillas capable of cranial kinesis move them as a unit in relation to the cranial vault. Anatomically, these birds have a short elastic zone between the brain case and the nasal and premaxillary bones of the maxillary jaw and have small, oval, bony nasal openings. Gallinaceous birds and psittacines are included in the movement of this group. Psittacines have more flexibility in the maxillary jaw because this elastic zone is replaced by an articular joint.

Another type of cranial kinesis is rhynchokinesis, in which only the more rostral end of the maxillary jaw moves as opposed to the entire maxilla. Birds with this type of jaw have large nasal openings (schizorhinal) as a consequence of a dorsal bar, a pair of ventral bars, and a pair of nasal bars that connect the tip of the bill to the caudal maxillary jaw. Muscle forces act on the tip and move it in relation to the rest of the maxilla. Birds in this group include most of the shore birds, pigeons, and hummingbirds.

The sutures between the bones of the skull are not retained in most birds and are no longer present soon after hatching, except in ratites. Another feature of birds that fly is the presence of pneumatic areas between the tables of bone in the tympanic and nasal cavities. Although most diagrams show the diverticuli of the infraorbital sinus as balloons

517

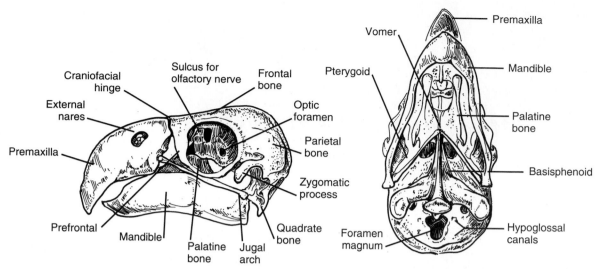

F i g u r e   3 1 – 1

The skull of the parrot—lateral and ventral views. The parrot has a prokinetic jaw that is unique because of its craniofacial synovial joint or hinge, whereas most birds have an elastic zone. This allows the premaxilla greater flexibility of movement.

of air that invade the skull, in actuality they are not. Instead, the spaces consist of a honeycomb of bony spicules that bridge the outer and inner laminae and are lined by the respiratory epithelium of the infraorbital sinus. An understanding of this anatomy helps the clinician to appreciate the difficulty in resolving upper respiratory tract disease.

VERTEBRAL COLUMN

Most avian vertebrae are fused to each other to provide a rigid framework for the muscles. The exception is in the cervical region where there is an increased number of vertebrae that are more mobile compared with those in mammals. Because of the fusion of the avian vertebral column, it is often difficult to distinguish the number of vertebrae.

The vertebral column can be subdivided into cervical, thoracic, and free caudal vertebrae, as well as a synsacrum and a pygostyle (Fig. 31–2). The synsacrum represents a fusion of the caudal thoracic, lumbar, sacral, and caudal vertebrae. Distal fusion of caudal vertebrae forms the pygostyle, where the rectrices or tail feathers insert. It is often difficult to distinguish the cervical from the thoracic vertebrae. However, by convention, a thoracic vertebra has a complete rib that articulates with the

sternum or ends near it. The number of cervical vertebrae range from 11 or 12 in psittacines and up to 25 in swans. The articular surfaces of the bodies of the cervical vertebrae are highly mobile and their range of motion differs from proximal to caudal. This results in the S-shaped appearance of the neck. The great mobility of the neck of birds is important for carrying out additional functions. This is the result of the thoracic limbs being confined to flight and the bill taking on the function of grooming and manipulating objects. The cervical vertebrae (except the atlas) have small rib-like components and a transverse foramen for the vertebral artery. This artery supplies the spinal cord and brain. The atlas articulates with a single occipital condyle.

The first thoracic vertebra has its rib attached to the sternum. In most birds, the first of the thoracic vertebrae fuse to form a single bone, the notarium. This bone probably functions to provide a rigid supportive beam for flight. There are from three to ten thoracic vertebrae, with psittacines having approximately eight. Uncinate processes project caudodorsally from the ribs. Because the last rib of psittacines does not usually have an uncinate process, it is used as a surgical landmark. Uncinate processes, although associated with ribs, form from an independent center of ossification and may not fuse with the rib or may not develop. In addition to vertebral ribs, there are sternal ribs. They repre-

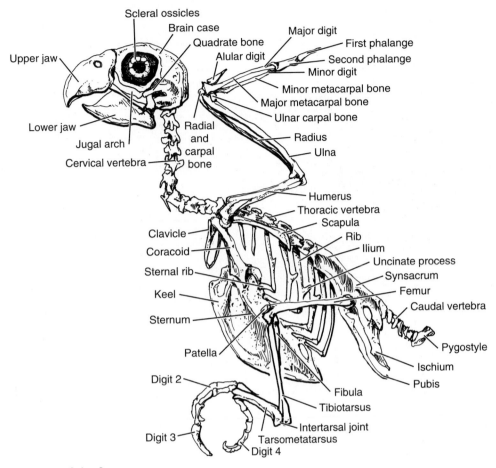

Figure 31–2

Skeleton of a psittacine—lateral view.

sent the ossified costal cartilages of mammals. The increased strength afforded by their ossification may be important to withstand the forces exerted by the contraction of the pectoral muscles.

In psittacines, approximately eight lumbar and sacral vertebrae and several caudal thoracic and caudal vertebrae fuse to form the synsacrum. The synsacrum is also important for providing a centrally rigid structure for flight. Its fusion to the ilium is important for transferring support of the body to the pelvic limbs. Caudal vertebrae are of variable numbers in birds. Psittacines commonly have eight caudal vertebrae. The pygostyle and caudal vertebrae are well developed in species that use their tails in support and climbing.

The sternum is a ventral plate of bone that is much more extensive in birds than in mammals. It

provides protection for the thoracoabdominal cavity and, with its ventrally directed keel, provides an important surface area for attachment of the flight muscles. The flight muscles include the large and powerful pectoral muscle that provides the downstroke and the smaller supracoracoideus muscles that provide the upstroke. Palpation of the flight muscles in relation to the ventrally directed keel or carina is an important part of the physical examination. The anatomy of this area is also important for administering intramuscular injections. Most birds that possess a carina or keel are called "carinates." The length and strength of the keel is related to the power of flight. In ratites, there is no keel because these birds are ground-dwellers and have a reduction in function or size of the wings. They have a reduced or absent pectoral muscle mass. The name

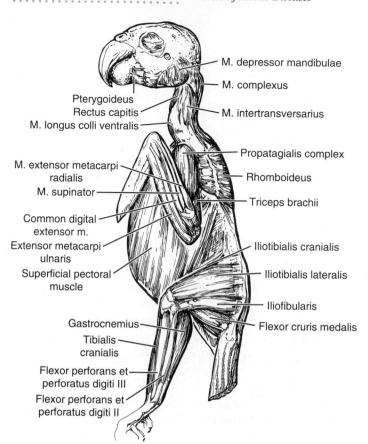

M. depressor mandibulae

M. complexus

M. intertransversarius

Pterygoideus
Rectus capitis
M. longus colli ventralis

Propatagialis complex

M. extensor metacarpi
radialis

Rhomboideus

M. supinator

Triceps brachii

Common digital
extensor m.

Extensor metacarpi
ulnaris

Iliotibialis cranialis

Superficial pectoral
muscle

Iliotibialis lateralis

Iliofibularis

Gastrocnemius

Tibialis
cranialis

Flexor cruris medalis

Flexor perforans et
perforatus digiti III

Flexor perforans et
perforatus digiti II

Figure 31–3

The muscles of a psittacine—lateral view.

"ratite" comes from the Latin word for raft, a boat without a keel.

Like mammals, birds have both epaxial and hypaxial muscles associated with movement of the vertebral column (Fig. 31–3). These muscles are more completely developed in the neck region, where fine control of the head and neck is essential for the everyday activities of a bird. The large dorsal-most proximal cervical muscle is the complexus muscle. It is often described as the pipping muscle and possibly serves to help in the break-out from the egg. The remainder of the vertebral muscles are reduced in development as a consequence of vertebral fusion to form a rigid framework for flight. The exception is the muscles that act on the tail. These muscles are well developed to help in the control of pitch during flight.

The muscles associated with breathing are similar to those of mammals. The muscles of inspiration are the external intercostal muscles and the costo-sternalis muscle. Expiration is an active process in birds, requiring muscular exertion. The muscles of expiration are the internal intercostal muscles and the abdominal musculature. The abdominal musculature includes the external and internal m. obliquus abdominis, the m. transversus abdominis, and the m. rectus abdominis. In a number of species, however, there is a variable amount of reduction of these muscles.

THORACIC GIRDLE AND WING

The thoracic girdle is formed from the coracoid, clavicle, and scapula and these in turn articulate with the humerus. The coracoid bone is short and thick to act as a strut to support the wing and attach it to the sternum. It acts to hold the wing away from the sternum, which keeps the thoracic cage from collapsing in on itself during the powerful downstroke. The coracoid, in combination with the clavicle and scapula and the ribs, helps to suspend the sternum and hence the viscera during gliding flight.

The clavicles may fuse to form a furcula or may be attached by cartilage or fibrous connective tissue, as in the parrot. In some parrots and ratites, the clavicles may be absent or much reduced. The furcula and clavicles function as a transverse spacer bar to keep the wings apart. In addition, the clavicles provide the proximal attachment for the pectoralis muscles.

The scapula is attached to the ribs by ligaments. The length is proportional to the strength of the flight of a particular species. Together with the coracoid and clavicle, the bones articulate proximally to form a triosseal canal or foramen. The foramen triosseum transmits the supracoracoideus muscle and tendon. This change in direction produced by the foramen is important for the mechanical advantage required for the upstroke.

The skeleton of the thoracic limb or wing is made up of the humerus, radius, ulna, alula, carpometacarpus, the major digit with two phalanges, and the minor digit with one phalanx. When the wing is folded, the humerus lies against the body wall. It is a short broad bone with a slight curve to it. The pectoral muscles attach onto the pectoral crest medially, and the supracoracoideus muscle inserts onto the dorsal tubercle dorsally. On the medial surface of the dorsal tubercle is a foramen that allows for the extrathoracic portion of the clavicular air sac to enter. Because the humerus is pneumatized, when fractured it may transmit bacterial and/or other foreign material to the remainder of the respiratory system.

The radius and ulna work together as a unit with their ligamentous attachments. They act like a reciprocal apparatus so that the wing flexes or extends in concert. The ulna is more caudal in location to the radius and is a larger bone. The secondary remiges or flight feathers insert directly onto this bone on its caudal margin. The ulna is often used for the placement of an intraosseous catheter.

The manus or hand has undergone a reduction of its skeletal elements, in part to produce a flat strong base for the attachment of the primary flight feathers or primary remiges. These primary remiges attach to the carpometacarpus dorsally. The carpus has only radial and ulnar carpal bones. Its function is restricted to flexion and extension of the joint. The carpometacarpus represents a partial fusion of the major and minor metacarpal bones both proximally and distally, leaving an intraosseous space between them. The major metacarpal bone articulates with the major digit, which has two phalanges. The minor metacarpal bone articulates with its minor digit.

The supracoracoideus muscle provides for the upstroke of the wing or elevation of the humerus. This muscle lies deep to the pectoral muscles on the ventral surface of the sternum and keel. It ascends through the foramen triosseum to insert on the dorsal tubercle of the humerus. The direction change is important for lifting the wing. The supracoracoideus muscle is most pronounced in birds that gain altitude rapidly after takeoff. The pectoralis muscles may be subdivided into superficial and deep. The superficial pectoral muscle is responsible for the downstroke, while the deep pectoral muscle is thought to provide for rapid adjustment to wind changes during soaring flight. Other muscles that are important surgical landmarks of the humerus include the tensor propatagialis complex proximally and dorsally; the biceps brachii along its cranial margin; and the triceps brachii along its caudal margin. The tensor acts to tense the propatagial tendons—the longus, which runs along the leading edge of the wing, and the brevis, which inserts along the proximal antebrachium. By tensing the propatagium, the bird achieves a smooth air flow over the wing's surface. The biceps brachii is the main flexor of the antebrachium, whereas the triceps is the main extensor.

Flexion and extension are the primary movements at the carpus. However, these movements at the carpus act as a unit with those of the elbow. It can be likened to the reciprocal apparatus of a horse. The main extensor of the carpus is the extensor metacarpi radialis on the craniodorsal surface, whereas the major flexor is the flexor carpi ulnaris on its ventral surface.

The carpometacarpus has undergone considerable fusion so that it provides a flattened surface for the insertion of the primary remiges dorsally. The phalanges are relatively immovable except for the alular digit. There are small intrinsic muscles that act to flex (flexor alulae), extend (extensor brevis alulae), abduct (abductor alulae), and adduct the alula (adductor alulae).

PELVIC GIRDLE AND HIND LIMB

The pelvic girdle is made up of three bones that are partially fused to each other. These are the ilium, ischium, and pubis. The pelvic girdle is fused to the synsacrum. The pubic bones are not fused ventrally, except in the ostrich. There is an antitrochanter on the dorsal ilium, which articulates with a facet on the dorsal trochanter of the femur. This additional articulation helps to reinforce the femoral attachment to the pelvis. The acetabulum is deep and has a foramen centrally. Subluxation of the femur is infrequent because of these anatomic characteristics. However, if subluxations do occur, they are usually directed craniodorsally. Ventrally, on the pelvis, bilaterally directed renal fossae are present for each of the caudal divisions of the kidneys.

The pelvic limb is composed of a femur, tibiotarsus, fibula, tarsometatarsus, a metatarsal bone, and usually four digits. Ostriches have two digits with four phalanges each, whereas rheas and emus have three digits with four phalanges. Birds with four digits usually have the following: digit I with two phalanges; digit II with three phalanges; digit III with four phalanges; and digit IV with five phalanges.

The femur is a short and stout bone. It slopes forward cranioventrally and is tucked against the body wall. The femur articulates with the tibiotarsus and the patella. The patella is a sesamoid bone of the femorotibialis muscle, which is similar to the quadriceps muscle of mammals. The tibiotarsus represents a fusion of the proximal tarsal bones to the tibia. Lateral to the tibiotarsus is a fibula. The hock represents an intertarsal joint. This is because the proximal row of tarsal bones is fused to the tibia and the distal row is fused to the metatarsus, forming the tarsometatarsus. Its shape is partially dependent on the locomotor skills of the particular species; it is wider in birds that walk and run and longer and narrower in divers.

The pelvic limb functions mainly to enable locomotion and perching. The actions of the hip joint of birds are mainly flexion and extension, with some medial and lateral rotation of the femur. There is no abduction and adduction of the leg at the hip. The main flexor of the hip is the iliotibialis cranialis. The extensors include the iliofemoralis lateralis and the pubo-ischio-femoralis. Flexion and extension are the primary actions of the knee joint. The flexors of the knee include the flexor cruris medialis and lateralis and the iliotibialis lateralis muscles. The femorotibialis complex of muscles is like the quadriceps group in mammals and acts to extend the knee joint. Its tendon of insertion also has a sesamoid portion, the patella.

The hock joint undergoes flexion and extension. The primary flexor is the tibialis cranialis muscle that lies along the cranial region of the tibiotarsus. The main extensor is the gastrocnemius muscle, which provides the power stroke of the foot. Power stroke is particularly important in water birds. Medial rotation can also occur in some species to reduce drag. This action is provided by the fibularis or peroneus brevis muscle that is closely associated with the tibialis cranialis muscle on the cranial surface of the tibiotarsus.

The main actions of the digits are flexion and extension. The main extensor muscle is the extensor digitorum longus; passerines further extend their first digit with the extensor hallucis longus. Flexion is provided by three groups of muscles—superficial, intermediate, and deep. The superficial flexors are the flexor perforati digit II, III, and IV muscles. The intermediate flexors are the flexores perforantes et perforati digiti II and III muscles. The deep flexors are the flexor hallucis longus and the flexor digitorum longus muscles.

When birds perch, the tendons of the digital flexors are tensed and the small sprocket-like projections from these tendons interdigitate to hold the tendons in place. This reduces the amount of energy required to perch.

Physiology of the Musculoskeletal System

Gerry M. Dorrestein

FLIGHT

Structural adaptations for flight dominate avian anatomy. Fusions and reinforcements of light-weight, air-filled bones are among the adaptations of the avian skeleton for flight. Of particular importance are the keeled sternum, which supports the powerful pectoralis and supracoracoideus flight muscles, and the strut-like arrangement of the pectoral girdle. A bird's flying ability is correlated with the size of its keel; some flightless birds lack the keel completely (e.g., the ostrich). The tendons of the ventrally located supracoracoideus muscles pass through the triosseal canal to dorsal insertions on the humerus.

The power for flight derives from the metabolic activity in the cellular fibers of flight muscles, some of which have an extraordinary capacity for aerobic metabolism. The extremes of the variation are the red and the white fibers, but intermediate fiber types exist.

The sustained contraction power of red muscle fibers results from oxidative metabolism of fat and glucose. These narrow fibers have high surface-to-volume ratios and short diffusion distances, which aid the uptake of oxygen. They also contain abundant myoglobin, mitochondria, fat, and enzymes that catalyze the chain of metabolic reactions, which is known as the Krebs cycle.

Sustained flight power derives from a high concentration of red muscle fibers in the flight muscles. The dark red breast muscle of pigeons consists mostly, but not exclusively, of red fibers. Conversely, the white breast muscles of fowl have a low proportion of red fibers. White muscle fibers are powered by products of anaerobic metabolism; they are capable of a few rapid and powerful contractions, but they fatigue quickly as lactic acid (a product of anaerobic metabolism) accumulates.[1]

The form of the wing and of the individual flight feathers is that of an airfoil, which generates a force called lift as air passes over and is deflected downward by the asymmetrical surfaces. Control of flight is achieved through changes in wing and wing feather positions and through the use of slots between feathers. Gliding birds exploit rising air currents, both heated thermals and slope-deflected air, to gain altitude without the exertion of flapping.

Flight power requirements are least at intermediate flight speeds, but birds often fly faster or slower than this speed to maximize distances traveled or to feed. Birds are the only vertebrates that can land with precision on elevated or arboreal perches.

Some birds have become flightless, particularly those that live on remote islands and lack mammalian predators. Specialized diving birds rely either on hindlimb locomotion or wing-propelled underwater locomotion. Some diving birds have traded aerial flight for underwater flight using highly modified flipper-like wings (e.g., penguins).

Disorders of the Musculoskeletal System

Katherine Quesenberry

Disorders of the musculoskeletal system occur frequently in pet birds. Many diseases that primarily involve other organ systems also involve the musculoskeletal system. Although traumatic injuries are seen most frequently, other causes of musculoskeletal disorders include malnutrition, parasitism, metabolic abnormalities, neoplasia, and disorders of unknown etiology. Many clinical syndromes that initially appear musculoskeletal in origin are actually associated with the neurologic or integumentary system.

MUSCULAR DISORDERS

Soft Tissue Trauma

Soft tissue trauma can result from accidental injury or self-inflicted mutilation. Common causes of accidental injury are bite wounds from mammals or other birds; flight injuries; falls; constriction injuries from leg bands; and entrapment in chains, string, wire, or toys. Self-inflicted injury includes mutilation of the pectoral muscles, axilla, flank, legs, feet, or toes. Self-mutilation is seen most frequently in Moluccan and umbrella cockatoos, Quaker parakeets, lovebirds, some conures, and Amazon parrots. The type and severity of the injury vary with the etiology.

Bite Wounds

Birds with bite wound injuries from a mammal are usually presented with a known history of trauma. Bite wounds most commonly result from attack by a dog, cat, or larger bird. Puncture wounds and lacerations from mammals are inflicted most often along the back and tail base. Wing or tail feathers may be ripped from the follicles, leaving the skin torn or severely bruised. Bite wounds from larger birds are frequently crushing injuries of the beak or head (Fig. 31–4). Birds housed in outdoor aviaries are occasionally attacked by wild predators such as raccoons.

Birds with bite wounds should first have their

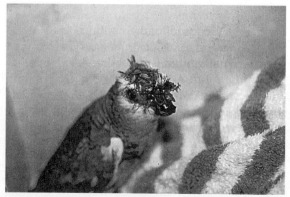

Figure 31–4

Severe head trauma in an Amazon parrot caused by a bite from a macaw.

condition stabilized. Administer supportive care including oxygen, intravenous or subcutaneous fluids, and heat as needed. Flush wounds copiously with sterile saline, and excise necrotic or devitalized tissue. Administer a parenteral, broad-spectrum bactericidal antibiotic. Long-term management consisting of antibiotic therapy, wound debridement, and bandage changes may be necessary, depending on the severity of the wound.

Cat bite wounds are commonly associated with infections with *Pasteurella multocida*. Accordingly, antibiotics such as penicillin derivatives effective against *P. multocida* should be used. Cat bite wounds that initially appear superficial and uncomplicated often become severely infected, with necrotizing myositis and dermatitis. The prognosis should always be guarded even with the most superficial cat bite wounds, and the wounds must be treated aggressively and closely monitored.

Traumatic Injuries

Injuries associated with flight or falls are seen frequently in young birds and birds that have had extensive wing clips. Birds with extensive wing clips and young, heavy-bodied birds that are learning to fly are frequently presented for treatment of sternal wounds (Fig. 31–5). This type of injury occurs when the bird tries to fly but falls to the ground, landing on its sternum. The skin may split, and an oval, open wound results along the cranial keel bone. Successful treatment involves use of a hydroactive wound dressing such as Biodres (DVM Pharmaceuticals, Inc., Miami, FL) and changing the dressing every 2 to 3 days until the wound is healed. Surgical closure is sometimes necessary in chronic cases. Reopening of the wound frequently occurs if the bird again falls on its sternum. If the flight feathers are extensively cut or shattered, removing these affected feathers to force regrowth may be indicated.

Similar to sternal wounds are tail wounds. Many birds fall on the tail area, causing a horizontal tearing of the skin and muscles caudal to the cloaca on the ventral pygostyle. The resulting wound can be superficial or more extensive with torn muscles. Complications occur from contamination with urates and feces, and this area is difficult to bandage. Clean and debride the area as needed before

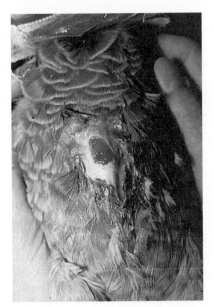

Figure 31-5

Sternal wound in an African grey parrot, 1 week after original injury. The bird's wings were clipped extensively, and the bird fell on its sternum while attempting to fly. The wound was bandaged with a hydroactive wound dressing.

applying a semiocculsive wound dressing such as Tegaderm (3M Animal Care Products, St. Paul, MN), changing to a hydroactive dressing when infection is controlled. If the wound is fresh and contamination is minimal, a hydroactive dressing can be directly applied. Secure the dressing by wrapping it around the tail and apply bandage tape as needed. A collar is usually necessary, because most birds pick at the wound. Administer broad-spectrum systemic antibiotics. With chronic or extensive wounds, surgical debridement and closure is often successful.

Traumatic wing or leg injuries, without fractures, may occur from a fall, catching a leg or wing in cage wire, or wedging the leg in the chain of a hanging toy. A common history is that the owner was absent for several hours or overnight, and returned to find the pet bird with the leg caught or wrapped in a chain. Birds may show lameness or have a wing droop, and the area may be grossly swollen. Palpate the area carefully to detect fractures. Wet the feathers around the area with alcohol or water to improve detection of injuries. Bruises are usually apparent as a dark purple or, in older injuries, green discoloration of the soft tissues.

Injuries to the back or head such as bruises are also usually apparent. Radiographs may be needed to determine if a fracture is present when limbs are grossly swollen. Treatment is variable, depending on the type of injury. Cage rest or supportive bandages can be used. Severe injuries to the leg with interruption of the blood supply may lead to eventual necrosis of the digits. In these birds, closely monitor the affected leg over several days to weeks to decide which tissues or digits are nonviable. Amputate or debride nonviable tissue when this determination is made.

Self-mutilation

Self-mutilation is a poorly understood problem that occurs in several species. Self-inflicted wounds are most common along the sternum (cockatoos), flank, or axilla (lovebirds, conures, and Quaker parakeets). In Amazon parrots, a different syndrome occurs. Areas of skin on the feet become hyperemic, followed 1 to 2 days later by the formation of vesicles that appear to be subdermal. These vesicles rupture, and the involved skin then becomes blackened. The lesions are apparently irritative, because the bird chews at these areas of the feet. Although many veterinarians consider self-mutilation a behavioral problem, the etiology is unknown. Viral disease and a hypersensitivity syndrome to bacteria or environmental agents are possible causes.[2, 3] Hypothyroidism has also been suspected as a cause.[4] (See Chapter 32, Avian Dermatology, for a more comprehensive discussion.)

Soft Tissue Swelling

Soft tissue swelling or masses can be soft or firm, diffuse or discrete, and infiltrative or nodular and pedunculated. Diffuse swelling most commonly occurs along the long bones of the metacarpus, radius and ulna, elbow, or tibiotarsus. Diffuse swelling may be indurated or soft and may vary in color depending on the cause. Nodular soft tissue masses can occur anywhere on the wing, leg, body, or head.

Noninfectious causes of diffuse soft tissue swelling include soft tissue trauma, as previously described, fractures, iatrogenic trauma, and neoplasia.

Bone fractures produce swelling and bruising that initially appears erythematous but changes to a greenish-blue color after 1 to 2 days. A fracture is often detectable by gentle palpation and can be confirmed with radiographs. Iatrogenic causes of swelling include bandages applied too tightly, restricting blood flow and resulting in edema of the distal limb. This can occur from overflexion of the wing when a figure-eight bandage is applied. Pronounced inflammation and edema can occur after surgery that requires extensive resection or wound closure with tension across the suture line, but the inflammation and edema usually resolve within several days. Inflammation with resultant swelling and edema of the feather follicle can occur if silver nitrate is used for hemostasis following removal of a mature or blood feather.

Nodular soft tissue swelling can result from a variety of causes. Feather cysts are seen in many species, but are most common in canaries. (See Chapter 32, Avian Dermatology.) These can vary from solitary nodules to irregular, large, multilobulated masses occurring along a feather tract on the body or at the base of the flight feathers. Feather cysts can be debrided or, more successfully, excised surgically.

Nodular granulomas can be infectious or noninfectious in origin. Bacterial granulomas are uncommon but can occur. Large nodular abscesses resulting from *Serratia marcescens* were reported in a blue and gold macaw.[5] Infection with *Mycobacterium* species can produce swelling of variable size and shape. Firm swelling of the left periocular area, right submandibular area, and an area proximal to the right metatarsal joint caused by *M. tuberculosis* was reported in a red-lored Amazon parrot.[6] Irregular lobular swellings of the legs have been reported in various Amazon parrots and confirmed positive for acid-fast organisms by biopsy or fine-needle aspirate testing.[7, 8] Treatment of mycobacteriosis is controversial.[9]

Subcutaneous and muscular nodules caused by hypopal acariasis are common in wild bird species, and have been reported in many species including pigeons, cranes, cattle egrets, owls, pelicans, toucans, and woodpeckers.[10–17] This parasitic nymphal stage of free-living adult mites can cause small, white, cyst-like structures in subcutaneous tissues and muscles of the limbs and breast muscles, and are found in numerous visceral organs.[13] The hy-

popi are usually found at necropsy and have little if any effect on the host. However, if treatment is elected, ivermectin may be effective.[18]

Neoplasia arising from connective tissue or muscle can cause either diffuse or nodular swelling (see Chapter 34, Neoplasia). Fibrosarcomas and fibromas are usually firm, white to gray, and circumscribed; the margins of fibrosarcomas are usually irregular.[19] Fibrosarcomas may occur on the wing, leg, head, beak, cere, and trunk. Fibromas may involve the skin or subcutaneous tissues of the leg, wing, beak, neck, face, or sternum.[20] Rhabdomyosarcomas are tumors of striated muscle origin that occur uncommonly as firm, gray to red-brown masses, usually of the wing, shoulder, or dorsal lumbar muscles (Fig. 31–6).[18] Rhabdomyomas are benign tumors of striated muscle origin and are rare in birds. Leiomyosarcomas are the most common tumors of muscles reported in birds.[20] They may arise from smooth muscle of any location.

Liposarcomas can occur in the subcutaneous tissues of pet birds and have been reported as firm, palpable, white nodules in the muscles of the breast, neck, legs, abdomen, wings, and back of a Canada goose *(Branta canadensis)*.[21] Myelolipomas are rare, but they may occur as slowly enlarging, broad-based semisoft subcutaneous masses.[22] Xanthomas commonly occur as diffuse, yellow, indurated swellings along the wings but also can appear as discrete nodular masses (Fig. 31–7).[20] Periarticular xanthomatosis involving the carpal and metacarpal joints with secondary bony proliferation has been reported in a kestral.[23] A cystadenoma was described anterior to the left eye in an African

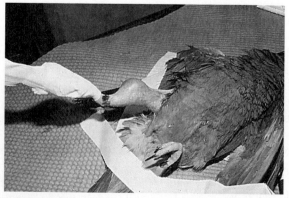

Figure 31–6

Rhabdomyosarcoma on the tibiotarsus of an Amazon parrot.

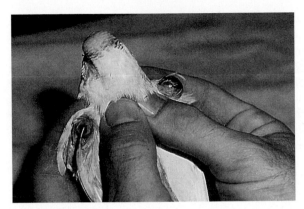

Figure 31-7

Xanthomas occurring as discrete nodular masses on the dorsal wing surfaces of a parakeet.

grey parrot.[24] The growth was large, multilobulated, and cystic. A neuroma involving the right ramus of the mandible was reported in an ostrich.[25] The mass was large, firm, and rounded, and may have occurred as a result of previous laceration of the mandible. Neuromas also occur following beak amputation in chickens.[26]

Diagnosis of a swelling or mass is based on clinical appearance, history, and diagnostic tests. Radiographs are needed to detect bony involvement of diffuse swelling or an extensive mass. A cytologic examination of a fine-needle aspirate may give a presumptive diagnosis. A wedge or excisional biopsy is preferred but is not always possible because of the nature or location of the swelling or size limitations of the bird. If an iatrogenic cause is suspected, a careful review of the history and treatment techniques is suggested.

Treatment varies with the etiology. Fractures are repaired surgically or with coaptation splinting. A discrete mass can usually be removed surgically, whereas a diffuse mass such as a fibroma or a sarcoma is often difficult to excise. Radiation therapy or chemotherapy are treatment options for nonresectable neoplasia.

Weakness and Myopathies

Generalized weakness in a bird can be a diagnostic dilemma. Differentiating muscle weakness from weakness associated with neurologic, toxic, or metabolic disease is often very difficult. Myopathies

that cause weakness can be inherited, traumatic, nutritional, infectious, toxic, or metabolic in origin. Birds that show generalized weakness are usually paretic, unable to walk, and may sometimes sit on their metatarsi with their weight resting on the keel bone. Paretic birds kept in wire cages often balance themselves by holding on to the cage wire with their beaks.

Inherited Myopathies

Inherited myopathies have not yet been described in pet birds. However, three well-described, inherited myopathies occur in poultry. These include inherited muscular dystrophy of chickens, deep pectoral myopathy of turkeys and broilers, and focal myopathy of turkeys.[27] These myopathies are in part related to selection for rapid growth and inbreeding of certain lines.

Capture and Nutritional Myopathies

Capture myopathy has been infrequently described in birds, including waterfowl, cranes, wild turkeys, and finches.[28-32] Skeletal muscle lesions of capture myopathy are characterized by rhabdomyolysis; serum concentrations of creatine kinase (CK) and aspartate aminotransferase (AST) are elevated. It is speculated that selection for rapid growth rates in domestic turkeys, in which growth of muscle fibers outpaces that of connective tissue, coupled with limited exercise may predispose birds to focal muscle necrosis when they are subjected to capture or sudden physical exertion.[27] This syndrome could occur in other captive birds that have little exercise and are pushed to rapid growth rates.

Nutritional myopathy caused by vitamin E and selenium deficiency is very similar to capture myopathy. Vitamin E deficiency may be a factor in capture myopathy.[33] Hypovitaminosis E and selenium deficiency have been postulated as possible causes of cockatiel paralysis syndrome.[34] This syndrome is most common in lutino cockatiels infected with *Giardia* or *Hexamita* species. Infestation is characterized by a variety of clinical signs including weakness, clumsiness, spraddle leg, paresis of the lower eyelid, death of young in the nest, and weak nestlings. Vitamin E and selenium–responsive syndromes have also been seen in blue and gold macaws, severe macaws, eclectus parrots, and African grey parrots.[34] Vitamin E deficiency can occur in fish-eating birds that eat an unsupplemented diet of frozen fish.[35]

Toxic Myopathies

Toxic myopathy resulting from suspected fusariomycotoxicosis has been described in sandhill cranes.[36] The most prominent clinical sign was a flaccid paralysis of the neck, progressing to loss of ability to fly and ataxia. Histologic lesions of skeletal muscle included hemorrhages, granulomatous myositis, thrombosis, and vascular degeneration. A trichothecene mycotoxin produced by *Fusarium* species from moldy peanuts was implicated as the cause. Pathology was caused by vascular damage that resulted in widespread hemorrhage in skeletal muscle. Myopathies associated with therapeutic levels of monensin added to the feed has been described in turkeys.[37] Monensin and other anticoccidials added to commercial poultry feeds at higher than recommended levels can also cause skeletal myopathy.

Parasitic Myopathies

Sarcocystosis has been described as a cause of muscular disease in psittacine and Columbiforme Old World species.[38-40] Although the acute pneumonitis form of sarcocystosis is more common, it is theorized that birds infected with a sublethal dose develop clinical muscular disease instead.[41] The causative agent, *Sarcocystis falcatula*, is a heteroxenous coccidian parasite that alternates between a sexual, intestinal phase in the definitive host and an asexual, multiorgan and muscular cyst phase in the intermediate host. Opossums are the only definitive hosts, shedding sporulated oocysts in the stool, but cockroaches and flies can act as transport hosts of fecal oocysts. *S. falcatula* can infect psittacine, Columbiforme, and passerine birds; Anseriformes and Galliformes appear to be resistant.[41] Birds present with weakness in the wings, legs, or both and may not be able to fly or walk. Mild to moderate muscle wasting may be present. Budgerigars experimentally infected with *S. falcatula* developed inter-

stitial myocarditis, myositis, nephritis, splenitis, and encephalitis.[42] Cysts were first noted in skeletal muscle 8 days after infection and matured 2 to 7 weeks after infection. Most cysts in the pectoral and heart muscle degenerated 28 to 42 days after infection. Inflammation in the striated muscle was strongly related to myocyte degeneration and weakly to meront burden, suggesting that inflammatory cell response was primarily related to muscle cell necrosis and not to the parasites themselves. The recommended treatment of the muscular form of sarcocystosis is at least a 6-week course of pyrimethamine (0.5 mg/kg PO every 12 hours) and trimethoprim/sulfadiazine (30 mg/kg PO every 8 hours).[41] Birds are sometimes unresponsive to treatment, and relapses are common.

Degenerative Myopathies

Degenerative myopathy is common in young ratites. In one report, clinical signs included depression, reluctance to move or rise, and rapid death. Histologic lesions included cardiac and skeletal muscle degeneration.[43] Selenium and vitamin E deficiency was speculated as a possible cause. In another report, 20 ostrich chicks died at or within 1 week of hatching.[44] Fifteen of the chicks had acute degenerative changes in the complexus and pelvic limb muscles. Selenium and vitamin A and E deficiencies were ruled out by biochemical examination. High humidity during incubation and malpositioning were cited as probable causes.

Metabolic Muscular Atrophy

Metabolic causes of muscular atrophy and weakness are common. Any debilitating or generalized disease can cause inanition, as does any lesion or injury of the beak, oral cavity, esophagus, and crop that interferes with normal digestion and absorption of nutrients.[45] Weight loss and muscle weakness are the result. In a clinical condition of muscle weakness, a full diagnostic workup including hematology and biochemical analysis, radiographs, and often muscle biopsy is necessary to learn the cause.

Table 31-1
DIFFERENTIAL DIAGNOSIS FOR LAMENESS

Usually Unilateral	Usually Bilateral	Bilateral or Unilateral
Renal neoplasia	Spinal trauma	Dyschondroplasia
Leg trauma	Myopathies	Osteochondrosis
Coxofemoral luxation	Nutritional imbalances	Osteomyelitis
Stifle luxation	Gout	Degenerative joint disease
Leg or foot fractures		Arthritis
		Tenosynovitis
		Pododermatitis
		Hereditary factors
		Bony neoplasia

SKELETAL DISORDERS

Lameness

Lameness in birds can occur from a variety of causes. Besides the soft tissue injuries previously discussed, causes of lameness include developmental problems and degenerative disorders, genetic factors, infectious disease, nutritional imbalances or deficiencies, environmental factors, and primary musculoskeletal disorders (Table 31–1).

Developmental and Degenerative Causes

Lameness resulting from dyschondroplasia and osteochondrosis is most common in fast-growing poultry but does occur in other species. Dyschondroplasia is characterized by a proliferation of unmineralized and avascular cartilage arising below the epiphyseal plate and extending into the metaphysis. Osteochondrosis is described as degeneration or necrosis of the growth or ossification centers, followed by abnormal endochondral ossification. Osteochondrosis can occur as subchondral bone cysts, physitis or epiphysitis, or osteochondrosis dessicans. In poultry, tibial dyschondroplasia is associated with genetic factors, growth rates of long bones, dietary composition, flock management, and intoxication with fungicides and mycotoxins.[46] Osteomyelitis as an acute complication of dyschondroplasia was reported in turkeys.[47] Pain associated with osteomyelitis was thought to be the main cause of lameness in these birds. Atraumatic avulsion of the trochanteric muscles associated with osteochondrosis occurs in poultry, affecting the nonarticular,

lateral aspect of the avian femoral trochanter.[48] Birds exhibit severe lameness, and on pathology examination, trochanteric muscle insertions are found to have avulsed, and the lateral metaphyseal defect is usually lined with granulation tissue. Osteochondrosis and tendon avulsion are suspected to occur in cranes,[49] and a subchondral bone cyst has been reported in an ostrich.[50]

One study in turkeys assessed pain associated with degenerative hip disorders.[51] Affected birds given daily injections of betamethasone exhibited more spontaneous activity and sexual activity than affected birds given a placebo. This study supports the use of pain medication and anti-inflammatory agents in management of degenerative skeletal disorders in birds. Radiographically, degenerative joint disease may be apparent as periarticular lipping, sclerosis of subchondral bone, and osteophytes.[52]

Vertebral abnormalities can be associated with lameness or ataxia. Scoliosis is a common condition of genetic etiology in chickens, and a cause-and-effect association with this condition and slipped tendons has been suggested.[53] This correlation may occur from torsional stresses at the trochlea of the tibiotarsus or possibly an interaction between the pull of tendons and growing bones. Cervical dorsal spondylosis with spinal cord compression has been reported in a black swan with clinical signs of ataxia.[54] Noninflammatory, degenerative changes of the synovial joint cartilage were associated with the spondylosis.

Hereditary factors are implicated in lameness and limb disorders in psittacines,[54] ratites, and other long-legged birds.[49, 56, 57] Lameness associated with genetic factors is first noted during the early growth and developmental stages in young birds. (See Chapter 6, Pediatrics, for further discussion.)

Infectious Causes

Infectious causes of lameness can result from teno-synovitis, arthritis, osteomyelitis, and pododermat-itis or cellulitis. Many bacteria have been associated with synovitis and arthritis in birds, including *Staphylococcus* species, *Actinobacillus* species, *Escherichia coli*, *E. rhusopathiae* (ducks and geese), *M. avium*, *Mycoplasma* species, *P. multocida*, and *Salmonella* species.[3] Infection can result after a traumatic wound or from hematogenous spread. Birds usually develop unilateral or bilateral swollen joints; the tibiotarsal-tarsometatarsal joints are most commonly affected in psittacines (Fig. 31–8). The humeral-radial/ulnar joint is a frequent site of arthritis associated with *Salmonella* species in pigeons and doves. Experimentally, healthy chickens with no known stress factors have developed bacteremia, osteomyelitis, and septic arthritis after inoculation with *Staphylococcus aureus*.[58]

Tenosynovitis in chickens is associated with *Staphylococcus* infection, and is characterized by fibrinopurulent exudate, edema, synovial cell hyperplasia, fibrosis of tendon sheaths, and tendon rupture.[59] Reovirus is also implicated in this condition and produces similar gross lesions. Histologically, reovirus is characterized by diffuse lymphocytic inflammation of the tendon, peritendineum, and synovium, whereas *Staphylococcus* infection causes focal purulent synovitis. Fibrosis occurred 10 weeks after infection in experimental birds, after which lesions could not be differentiated histologically. Tenosynovitis associated with reovirus and *Staphylococcus* has also been reported in pheasants.[60] In these birds, it was postulated that reovirus infection predisposed birds to tendon strain, with the damaged tendons becoming a focus for bacterial infection.

Diagnosis of septic arthritis is based on radiographic appearance of the affected joints, cytologic examination of a joint aspirate, biopsy of the synovial membrane, and bacterial culture and sensitivity testing. Radiographs of the affected joint are needed to detect whether osteolysis or joint effusion is present[52] (Fig. 31–9). Joint effusion may be the only radiographic change with acute septic arthritis. As the infection progresses and becomes chronic, loss of joint space occurs from destruction of articular cartilage, and osteolysis and periosteal changes may occur.

Various treatment protocols are used in treatment of septic arthritis. Joint lavage, performed by through-and-through or surgical technique, is useful to remove purulent debris containing bacteria, bacterial products, cartilage-destroying enzymes, and fibrin deposits.[61, 62] Appropriate antibiotic therapy is indicated based on bacterial culture and sensitivity test results. Antibiotics can be administered systemically or through intra-articular injection. Topical steroids and dimethyl sulfoxide (DMSO) are sometimes used, but birds should be closely monitored for signs of immunosuppression or opportunistic fungal infection.

Severe joint infections with pronounced bone involvement are sometimes unresponsive to therapy. Fusion of the affected joint in a functional position has been successful in treatment of some psittacines. The purpose of fusion is to stop progression of the infection and remove pain. An autogenous bone graft using cancellous bone harvested from the keel bone is used to pack the joint after surgical debridement. The joint is stabilized by a modified Kirschner-Ehmer–type apparatus, with pins and connecting bars placed above and below the affected joint. Healing and fusion occurs after 6 to 8 weeks.

Nutritional Causes

Nutritional imbalances are important factors in bone problems that may cause lameness. Imbalances of calcium, phosphorus, vitamin D_3, and other nutrients are factors in development of angular limb

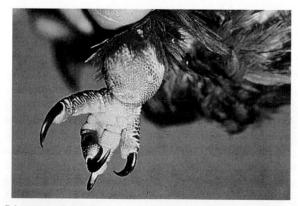

Figure 31–8

Swollen tarsometatarsal joint in a macaw with septic arthritis.

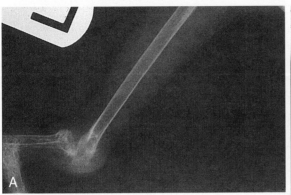

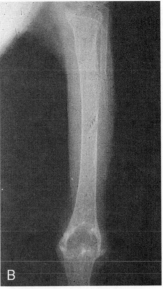

Figure 31–9

Mixed proliferative and osteolytic lesion with soft tissue swelling resulting from septic arthritis of the tibiotarsal-tarsometatarsal joint in a macaw. Lateral *(A)* and dorsoventral *(B)* views.

deformities and dyschondroplasia. However, these conditions are probably caused by an interplay of many factors, including trauma, use of poor footing substrate, genetic factors, and incubation problems. Angular limb deformities are common in young psittacines, ratites, and poultry. Leg deformities in young psittacines usually occur as either bowing of

the tibiotarsus with lateral rotation of the femur or tibiotarsus, or splay leg (Fig. 31–10).[63] (See Chapter 6, Pediatrics.) Initially leg problems in ratites may not involve angular limb deformities, but deformities may result if the problems are not corrected early.[56] Besides nutritional factors, factors contributing to leg problems in ratites include genetics, incubation, inadequate exercise, trauma, and muscular adductor weakness. Angular limb deformities occur primarily in ratites younger than 3 months of age during the period of rapid growth.

The interplay of calcium, phosphorus, vitamin D_3, and bone abnormalities has been studied extensively in poultry. Experimental results show that the problem is complex and multifactorial. Excessive dietary vitamin D_3 together with high-density housing stress factors lead to an increased incidence of angular leg deformities in chickens.[64] Stress appears to increase the severity of the deformities; the level of excess vitamin D_3 does not. In another study, chickens with valgus-varus deformity had decreased plasma levels of vitamin D metabolites.[65] Vitamin D_3 deficiency is classically associated with rickets in poultry.[66, 67] Controversy exists concerning the potency of different vitamin D metabolites. Injection of a specific vitamin D_3 metabolite, 24,25-dihydroxycholecalciferol $(24,25(OH)_2D_3)$, has been found to have a direct local effect on healing of rachitic lesions, whereas $1,25(OH)_2D_3$ did not.[68] However, it has also been found that $1,25(OH)_2D_3$

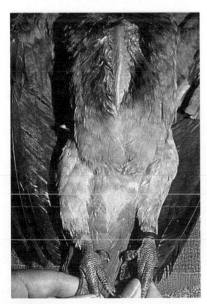

Figure 31–10

A young African grey parrot with bowing deformities of the tibiotarsal bones and the sternum resulting from nutritional bone disease.

prevents rickets, whereas high doses impair skeletal development. Similarly, 24,25(OH)$_2$D$_3$ corrects plasma calcium homeostasis but can exacerbate cartilage lesions, probably because of stimulation of chondrocyte proliferation and failure of mineralization.[66] Vitamin D metabolites have been fed at different levels to poultry on calcium-deficient diets to study effects on prevention of tibial dyschondroplasia.[69–71] Results show that 1,25(OH)$_2$D$_3$ exerts powerful effects on the incidence of dyschondroplasia, but the exact mechanism is unknown. These studies exemplify the importance of vitamin metabolism in bone growth and maturation, but illustrate the need for more studies in this important area.

Other nutritional factors may also play a role in bone growth. High dietary protein levels, excess vitamin A, excess vitamin E, manganese deficiency, and copper deficiency have all been suggested as factors in leg deformities.[66, 72] Intestinal diseases that cause malabsorption in very young birds can result in a malabsorption syndrome, leading to skeletal abnormalities.[73, 74]

Management of angular limb deformities is based on the age of the bird, degree of normal bone calcification, size and weight of the bird, and economic factors. Conservative management techniques include the use of bandages, hobbles, casts, splints, and support devices. Severe angular deformities often require surgical correction. (See Chapter 42, Orthopedic Surgery, and Chapter 6, Pediatrics.) Dietary imbalances must be addressed.

Environmental and Traumatic Causes

Environmental factors such as population density, surface footing, and lack of exercise are among factors that influence bone density, growth, and maturation. These factors are subtle, but in a population of birds experiencing bone abnormalities, their influence must be considered.

Traumatic injury is a common cause of lameness in adult birds. Fractures of the leg and feet are common injuries in pet birds. Traumatic injury is a common problem in captive long-legged birds, including cranes, herons, storks, and ratites.[49] These birds have little supportive soft tissue distal from the mid-tibiotarsus, and injuries involving the tendons, ligaments, and bones often occur. Diagnosis of fractures is based on history, physical examination, and radiographic appearance. Bandaging techniques and surgical repair are described in other chapters.

Coxofemoral luxations occasionally occur in psittacines. Birds develop nonweight-bearing lameness of acute onset. Luxations usually occur craniodorsally, but cranioventral luxation can occur.[75] On palpation, a dorsal-cranial displacement of the femoral head may be palpated, and radiographs can confirm the diagnosis. The luxation can be repaired by closed reduction and a spica splint in some birds. An open reduction or a femoral head ostectomy may be necessary for luxations that cannot be reduced by closed manipulation or that are chronic. (See Chapter 42, Orthopedic Surgery.)

Stifle luxation is rare in birds and usually results from trauma.[76] Affected birds show nonweight-bearing lameness. Repair of stifle luxation requires that the luxated joint be first reduced and immobilized. The joint is permanently stabilized by fibrous ankylosis using internal or external fixation methods, or joint fusion (ankylosis). (See Chapter 42, Orthopedic Surgery.)

Gout

Articular gout is a common cause of lameness in parakeets and small psittacines. The cause of gout in birds is not known, but is thought to result from kidney disease or possibly high dietary levels of protein; in humans, this disease is genetically determined. Urate crystals are deposited in the synovial tissues of the joints and subcutaneously. Affected birds are usually middle-aged to older with clinical signs of weakness, inability to perch, shifting leg lameness, and a shuffling gait that results from difficulty in walking. White tophi are often visible subcutaneously around the joints and along the long bones and digits (Fig. 31–11). Diagnosis is based on physical examination, history, and increased uric acid levels on plasma biochemical analysis.

Drugs that may be effective in the treatment of gout in psittacines include oral allopurinol (Zyloprim, Burroughs Wellcome), colchicine, colchicine/probenecid, or combination therapy. Allopurinol reduces the synthesis of uric acid by inhibiting xanthine oxidase, which is needed to convert hypoxanthine to xanthine to uric acid.[77] The concentration

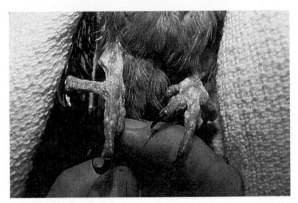

Figure 31–11

Severe gout with visible subcutaneous tophi in a cherry-headed conure.

of the insoluble urates and uric acid in tissues and plasma decreases, and the concentrations of the more soluble xanthines and hypoxanthines increase. Uricosuric drugs (probenecid and sulfinpyrazone) increase uric acid excretion by a direct action on the renal tubules. However, both of these drugs may inhibit excretion of uric acid if given in subtherapeutic doses.[77] Therefore, these drugs should be used very cautiously in birds because their pharmacokinetics are unknown in these species. Colchicine acts by preventing migration of neutrophils into the joints through interference with neutrophil motility. This may prevent production of inflammatory glycoprotein by neutrophils after phagocytosis of urate crystals.[77] Experience with psittacines using combination therapy of allopurinol and colchicine has shown that treated birds have a positive clinical response, which is associated with a regression of tophi deposits and a decrease in plasma uric acid level. Conversely, a study in red-tailed hawks showed that oral administration of allopurinol caused severe hyperuricemia and induced gout in three of six birds.[78] It was theorized that renal damage in these birds may have resulted from deposition of xanthine crystals, the precursor of uric acid. Renal damage may also have resulted from the formation of oxypurinol, an endproduct of allopurinol that is insoluble and nephrotoxic. From this study it may be concluded that allopurinol is contraindicated in treatment of gout in red-tailed hawks. However, raptors and psittacines differ in their normal dietary protein intake (carnivorous vs. granivorous species), and this may be a factor in drug metabolism and clinical response.

Neoplasia

Renal neoplasia is a common cause of lameness in budgerigars and is rare in other species. (See also Chapter 34, Neoplasia, and Chapter 36, Urogenital Disorders). Lameness is most commonly unilateral, but bilateral lameness can be seen.* Typically, affected budgerigars are 4 to 5 years of age or older, and are presented with lameness of a slowly progressive onset. On physical examination, palpable muscle atrophy of varying severity is usually present in the affected leg. The lameness may be only slight, with the leg held out from the body, or severe, with the leg held down and usually behind the perch (Fig. 31–12). The toes are usually positioned straight or curled. Polyuria, weight loss, and abdominal distention may be present. An abdominal mass is sometimes palpable caudally and laterally on the affected side. Plain films or contrast radiographs or ultrasound are useful to confirm the diagnosis.

Other neoplasias that may cause lameness are as described under soft tissue swellings and include fibrosarcomas, fibromas, rhabdomyosarcomas, and rhabdomyomas. Subcutaneous neoplasms such as lipomas, liposarcomas, and myelolipomas may cause lameness if they interfere with normal perching or movement.[22] Osteosarcomas are rare tumors

---

*Altman R, personal communication.

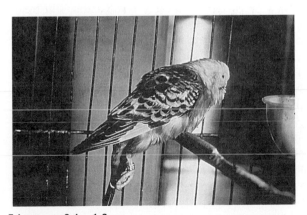

Figure 31–12

Parakeet with non–weight-bearing lameness resulting from renal neoplasia.

in captive and wild birds, and they can cause lameness depending on the area of involvement.[79] Diagnosis of neoplasia is based on radiographic appearance and biopsy and histopathology results. (See Chapter 34, Neoplasia, for further discussion.)

Wing Droop

Wing droop usually indicates a fracture, luxation, or traumatic soft tissue or nerve injury of the proximal wing or shoulder joint. Fractures of the humerus are usually palpable with or without visible soft tissue injury. Fractures of the coracoid occur frequently and may not be obvious on physical examination. Coracoid fractures should be suspected if there is an obvious wing droop and a humeral fracture is not palpable. By carefully tracing both coracoid bones with digital palpation, a coracoid fracture can often be detected. Radiographs are needed to confirm the diagnosis. (Coracoid fractures are discussed in Chapter 42, Orthopedic Surgery.)

Luxations of the shoulder joint are uncommon in birds, but do occur in raptors.[80] Shoulder luxations may be accompanied by an avulsion fracture of the ventral tubercle of the proximal humerus. Luxation can usually be managed by a figure-eight bandage to the body; surgical repair of the avulsion fracture may be necessary. Elbow luxations occur occasionally in free-ranging raptors because of trauma to the distal wing while the bird is in flight.[80] Repair requires reduction and stabilization of the joint.

A wing droop commonly results from soft tissue injury to the muscles of the shoulder joint. Bruising or soft tissue injury may be apparent on physical examination. Radiographs are negative for fractures. Treatment usually involves cage rest for a few days, with or without a supportive bandage immobilizing the wing to the body.

Nerve damage or brachial plexus avulsion resulting in wing droop can occur as a result of several causes including trauma, viral disease, or toxicity. Viral neuropathy resulting from paramyxovirus may result in wing droop.[34] Wing droop is occasionally seen with lead toxicity. (See Chapter 27, Nervous System, for more detailed discussion.)

Neoplasia involving the shoulder joint, humerus, or other bones of the wing is an uncommon cause of wing droop. The types of neoplasia that may affect the wing are as described under lameness.

Feet and Digits

Constriction Injuries

Constriction injuries to the leg or digits occur commonly. Constriction wounds of the metatarsus are usually a result of trauma involving the leg band. The bird may injure its foot or catch the leg band on a toy or wire and struggle to free itself. This causes soft tissue trauma and edema of the metatarsus. The swelling causes the leg band to become too tight, and further swelling proximal and distal to the leg band results, with accompanying pressure necrosis of the soft tissues under the band (Fig. 31–13). Small plastic or light metal bands on small birds are easily removed with band-cutting and spreading scissors. If the leg is severely swollen or the metal cannot be cut easily, a dental drill works very well in removing the band atraumatically (Fig. 31–14). Even with extensive soft tissue trauma, most lesions heal well after the band is removed and the wound is treated.

Bandage the leg with a supportive wrap, using a hydroactive or semiocclusive wound dressing over the constriction injury to promote healing. Administer systemic antibiotics if the injury is severe and secondary bacterial infection is suspected. Occasionally, fractures occur under the band, requiring

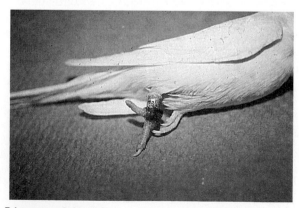

F i g u r e 3 1 – 1 3

Leg band constriction injury in a parakeet, with swelling and pressure necrosis of the leg.

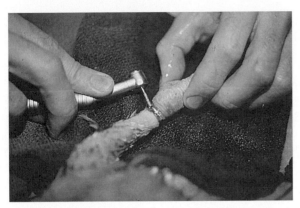

Figure 31–14

Use of a dental drill to remove the leg band from an Amazon parrot with a constriction injury.

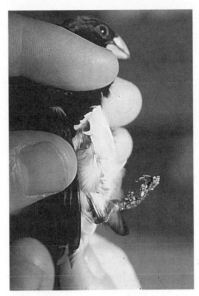

Figure 31–16

Constriction injury causing avascular necrosis of the foot of a finch.

orthopedic management or, in severe injuries, amputation of the foot.

Entanglement of strings or nesting material around the feet and digits is common in small psittacines and passerines. Fine nesting material wrapped around the leg digits may be difficult to see with the naked eye, but can usually be teased up from the constricted tissue. Wounds usually heal well after the strings are removed and circulation is restored. Some constricting wounds are so severe that the digit may be almost completely self-amputated (Fig. 31–15). If the foot or digits are blackened and the nails do not bleed when cut, the foot or affected digit should be amputated (Fig. 31–16). If viability is questionable, wait several days to a week before deciding to amputate; often, healing occurs when

swelling resolves. As with leg band injuries, apply a wound dressing and bandage the foot until it is healed.

Constricted toe syndrome is seen frequently in psittacine birds. This syndrome is characterized by an annular band of tissue around one or more digits that causes swelling and possibly eventual necrosis of the digit distal to the band. The appearance is similar to that of constrictive injury produced by entanglement of strings or fibers, discussed previously. The etiology is unknown; low brooder humidity or fractures of the digits have been proposed as causes.[63] Conservative therapy consisting of debridement of the band and necrotic tissue, followed by warm water soaks, massage, and hydroactive dressings may be successful with mild lesions. Correction of the problem is possible with surgical removal of the annular band and anastomosis of the skin, leaving a release incision to allow for swelling without constriction.[81] Hydroactive dressings should be applied over the wound to keep the wound moist and prevent formation of a scab with recurrence of the constriction.

Pododermatitis

Pododermatitis is common in captive birds and can occur from a variety of causes. In severe forms,

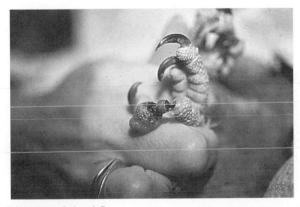

Figure 31–15

Severe constriction injury of the digit of an Amazon parrot. The digit is almost completely self-amputated.

this condition is termed "bumblefoot," and is a debilitative condition in birds of prey. (See Chapter 52, Raptors, and Chapter 32, Avian Dermatology.) In caged birds, pododermatitis is most often associated with obesity, lack of exercise, and poor perching surfaces. Caged birds commonly are kept on smooth wooden dowel perches. This type of perch is unnatural in that the perching surface and diameter are unvariable. Pressure is constantly applied to the same areas of the feet, leading to callus formation, erythema, and occasionally open lesions secondarily infected with bacteria. Treatment of pododermatitis in caged birds usually involves bandaging the feet with a wound dressing and a soft padded bandage. Birds that are only mildly affected may not need bandaging; instead they can be provided with clean, soft perching surfaces. Perches can be wrapped with cast padding and Vetrap (3M Animal Care Products, St. Paul, MN) until the lesions are healed. Systemic and topical antibiotics may be indicated with open lesions, and long-term therapy and management may be necessary. Attention also must be given to the diet; high fat diets or diets deficient in vitamin A must be corrected. Management of this condition includes providing perches of variable sizes and surfaces and encouraging exercise.

Traumatic Injuries

Traumatic toe injuries are among the most common injuries seen in clinical practice. Injuries can occur from entrapment in toys, strings, clips, or cage doors; bite injuries from other birds; or crushing injuries from doors or furniture. Often shear-type injuries are present, with the skin sheared from one or more surfaces of the toe. The nail may be avulsed or traumatized. Initially, the wound is treated as any open wound, with attention to hemostasis and cleansing. With severe toe injuries in which viability is questionable, bandaging the injured toe with a hydroactive or semiocclusive dressing for several days is often prudent until viability can be determined. Wounds that initially appear very severe often heal well with proper wound management. Systemic antibiotics are usually indicated until healing is progressing well and the wound shows no evidence of infection or nonviable tissue. If damage

to the toe or nail does progress to avascular necrosis, amputation is necessary.

Subcutaneous Filariasis

Localized swelling of one or more digits or subcutaneous nodules on other areas of the foot caused by infestation with filarid nematodes is occasionally seen in psittacines.[82, 83] One or more adult nematodes of *Pelecitus* species is found in these swellings. The involved digits are usually diffusely swollen and often discolored, with no evidence of constriction injury (Fig. 31–17). The nematodes must be surgically removed.

BONY INFILTRATES

Although not necessarily indicative of skeletal disease, bony infiltrates are often noted radiographically in birds. The cause is variable, ranging from normal physiologic processes to neoplastic and infectious diseases.

The most common cause of radiographic bony infiltrates is normal medullary bone formation in association with egg-laying. Hens normally begin accumulating calcium in medullary bone for the formation of eggshells during the 10 days before oviposition. This process, termed "polyostotic hyperostosis" or osteomyelosclerosis, is under the influence of estrogen and testosterone and is independent of calcium intake.[84] Radiographically this

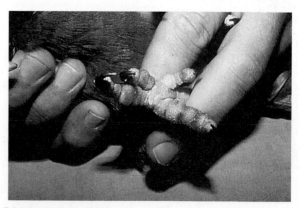

Figure 31–17

Swelling and discoloration of the fourth digit of a conure. Nematodes of *Pelecitus* species were found in the digit.

is observed as medullary opacity in nonpneumatic long bones, which is most noticeable in the femur, tibiotarsus, radius, and ulna. Bones may have a mottled appearance if deposition is patchy, and occasionally discrete nodular bone densities are found on the ribs, vertebrae, or pubic bones.[52] Osteomyelosclerosis also can be seen in hens with reproductive abnormalities, including ovarian and oviductal tumors,[85] ovarian cysts, and egg yolk peritonitis, and in males with gonadal tumors.

Primary bone neoplasia is rare and usually is seen radiographically as areas of osteolysis. However, osteoblastic tumors with periosteal reactions do occur.[52, 79]

Bony infiltrates may be apparent radiographically with mycobacteriosis. Bone marrow infiltrates occur most frequently in *Brotegeris* species; clinically, lameness is a common physical finding. Pathologic lesions are most common in the long bones of the leg.

Diagnosis of problems associated with bony infiltrates requires a good history and physical examination, interpreted in association with results of clinical laboratory tests. In hens with a history of reproductive activity, further workup of the bony infiltrates is not necessary in normal birds. In birds with suspected pathologic abnormalities, examination of a bone marrow aspirate may be indicated.

References

1. Gill FB: Ornithology, ed 2. New York, WH Freeman and Company, 1994.
2. Rosskopf WJ: The psittacine mutilation syndrome: Management, incidence, possible etiology and therapy. Proc Assoc Avian Vet, Seattle, 1990, pp 301–304.
3. Gerlach H: Bacteria. In Ritchie BW, Harrison GJ, Harrison LR (eds) Avian Medicine: Principles and Application. Lake Worth, FL, Wingers Publishing, 1994, pp 949–983.
4. Parrott T: Pododermatitis in three Amazon parrots, and treatment with L-thyroxine. Proc Assoc Avian Vet, Chicago, 1991, pp 263–264.
5. Quesenberry KE, Liu SK: Pancreatic atrophy in a blue and gold macaw. J Am Vet Med Assoc 189:1107–1108, 1986.
6. Brown R: Sinus, articular and subcutaneous *Mycobacterium tuberculosis* infection in a juvenile red-lored Amazon parrot. Proc Assoc Avian Vet, Seattle, 1990, pp 305–308.
7. Loudis BG. Soft tissue involvement of avian tuberculosis and attempted treatment—a case study. Proc Am Assoc Zoo Vet, Calgary, 1991, pp 246–247.
8. Rosskopf WJ, Woerpel RW, Asterino R: Successful treatment of avian tuberculosis in pet psittacines. Proc Assoc Avian Vet, Chicago, 1991, pp 238–251.
9. VanDerHeyden N: Update on avian mycobacteriosis. Proc Assoc Avian Vet, Reno, 1994, pp 53–61.
10. Boyd EM: Deutonymphs as endoparasites of the Eastern belted kingfisher and the Eastern green heron in North America. Proc Entomol Soc Washington, 1967, 69:73–81.
11. Fain A: Les hypopes parasites des tissus cellulaires des oiseaux (Hypodectidae: Sarcoptiformes). Bull l'Institut Royal Sci Naturelles Belg 43:1–139, 1967.
12. Fain A: A new heteromorphic deutonymph (hypopus) of a sarcoptiform mite parasitic under the skin of a toucan. J Nat Hist 2:459–461, 1968.
13. Hendrix C, Kwapien RP, Porch JR: Visceral and subcutaneous acariasis caused by hypopi of *Hypodectes propus bulbuci* in the cattle egret. J Wild Dis 23(4):693–697, 1987.
14. O'Connor BM: A new genus and species of Hypoderidae (Acari:Astigmata) from the nest of an owl (Aves: Strigiformes). Acarologia 22:299–304, 1981.
15. Pence DB, Courtney CH: The hypopi (Acarina: Hypoderidae) from the subcutaneous tissues of the brown pelican, *Pelecanus occidentalis carolinensis* Gmelin. J Parasitol 59:711–718, 1973.
16. Pence DB: *Toucanectes dryocopi* sp. n. (Acarina: Hypoderidae) from the pileated woodpecker, *Dryocopus pileatus* L. J Parasitol 57:1318–1320, 1971a.
17. Spurlock GM, Emlen JT: *Hypodectes chapini* n. sp. (Acarina) from the red-shafted flicker. J Parasitol 28:341–344, 1942.
18. Clubb SL: Therapeutics: Individual and flock treatment regimens. In Harrison GJ, Harrison LR (eds): Clinical Avian Medicine and Surgery. Philadelphia, WB Saunders, 1986, pp 327–355.
19. Schmidt RE: Morphologic diagnosis of avian neoplasms. Semin Avian Exotic Pet Med 1(2):73–79, 1992.
20. Latimer KS: Oncology. In Ritchie BW, Harrison GJ, Harrison LH, (eds): Avian Medicine: Principles and Application. Lake Worth, FL, Wingers Publishing, 1994, pp 640–672.
21. Doster A, Johnson JL, Duhamel GE, et al: Liposarcoma in a Canada goose *(Branta canadensis).* Avian Dis 31:918–920, 1987.
22. Latimer KS, Rakich PM: Subcutaneous and hepatic myelolipomas in four exotic birds. Vet Pathol 32:84–87, 1995.
23. Haley PJ, Norrdin RW: Periarticular xanthomatosis in an American kestrel. J Am Vet Med Assoc 181(11):1394–1396, 1982.
24. Hochleithner M: Cystadenoma in an African grey parrot (*Psittacus erithacus*). J Assoc Avian Vet, 4(3):163–165, 1990.
25. Tully TN, McClure JR, Morris JM, Cho D-Y: Post-transectional submandibular neuroma in an ostrich (*Struthio camelus*). J Assoc Avian Vet, 7(2):75–76, 1993.
26. Gentle MJ: Neuroma formation following partial beak amputation (beak trimming) in the chicken. Res Vet Sci 41:383–388, 1986.
27. Wilson B: Developmental and maturational aspects of inherited avian myopathies. Proc Soc Exp Biol Med 194(2):87–96, 1990.
28. Carpenter JW, Thomas NJ, Reeves S: Capture myopathy in an endangered sandhill crane *(Grus canadensis pulla).* J Zoo Wild Med 22:488–493, 1991.
29. Dabbert CB, Powell KC: Serum enzymes as indicators of capture myopathy in mallards *(Anas platyrhynchos).* J Wild Dis 29(2):304–309, 1993.
30. Spraker TR, Adrian WJ, Lance WR: Capture myopathy in wild turkeys (*Meleagris gallopavo*) following trapping, handling and transportation in Colorado. J Wild Dis 23(3):447–453, 1987.
31. Windingstad R, Hurley SS, Sileo L: Captive myopathy in a free-flying greater sandhill crane (*Grus canadensis tabida*) from Wisconsin. J Wild Dis 19:289–290, 1983.
32. Young E: Leg paralysis in the greater flamingo and lesser flamingo. Intl Zoo Yearbook 7:226–227, 1967.

33. Hulland TJ: Muscles and tendons. In Jubb KVF, Kennedy PC, Palmer N (eds): Pathology of domestic animals, ed 3. New York, Academic Press, 1985, pp 139–199.

34. Bennett RA: Neurology. In Ritchie BW, Harrison GJ, Harrison LR (eds): Avian Medicine and Surgery: Principles and Application. Lake Worth, FL, Wingers Publishing, 1994, pp 721–747.

35. Nichols DK, Montali RJ. Vitamin E deficiency in captive and wild piscivorous birds. First Intl Conf Zoo Avian Med, Oahu, 1987, pp 419–421.

36. Roffe TJ, Stroud RK, Windingstad RM: Suspected fusariomycotoxicosis in sandhill cranes *(Grus canadensis)*: Clinical and pathologic findings. Avian Dis 33:451–457, 1989.

37. Cardona CJ, Bickford AA, Galey FD, et al: A syndrome in commercial turkeys in California and Oregon characterized by a rear-limb necrotizing skeletal myopathy. Avian Dis 36:1092–1101, 1992.

38. Bicknese EJ, Murnane RD, Rideout RA, et al: A pathologic muscular form of *Sarcocystis* in two species of exotic Columbiformes. Proc Joint Meeting Am Assoc Zoo Vet/Am Assoc Vet, Oakland, 1992, pp 186–190.

39. Bolon B, Greiner EC, Mays MBC: Microscopic features of *Sarcocystis falcatula* in skeletal muscle from a Patagonian conure. Vet Pathol 26:282–284, 1989.

40. Todd KS, Gallina AM, Nelson WB: Sarcocystis species in psittaciforme birds. J Zoo Anim Med 6:21–24, 1975.

41. Bicknese EJ: Review of avian sarcocystosis. Proc Assoc Avian Vet, Nashville, 1993, pp 52–58.

42. Smith JH, Neill PJG, Box EC: Pathogenesis of *Sarcocystis falcatula* (Apicocomplexa: Sarcocystidae) in the budgerigar *(Melopsittacus undulatus)* III. Pathologic and quantitative parasitologic analysis of extrapulmonary disease. J Parasitol 75(2):270–287, 1989.

43. Rae M: Degenerative myopathy in ratites. Proc Assoc Avian Vet, New Orleans, 1992, pp 328–335.

44. Philbey AW, Button C, Gestier AW, et al: Anasarc and myopathy in ostrich chicks. Aust Vet J 68(7):237–240, 1991.

45. Graham D: Generalized muscle atrophy and fat depletion: An avian pathologist's perspective. Assoc Avian Vet, Nashville, 1993, pp 87–91.

46. Wu W, Cook ME, Chu Q, Smalley EB: Tibial dyschondroplasia of chickens induced by fusarochromanone, a mycotoxin. Avian Dis 37:302–309, 1993.

47. Wyers M, Cherel Y, Plassiart G: Late clinical expression of lameness related to associated osteomyelitis and tibial dyschondroplasia in male breeding turkeys. Avian Dis 35:408–414, 1991.

48. Duff SRI: Avulsion of muscles from the femoral trochanter in the fowl. J Comp Pathol 95(3):383–392, 1985.

49. Curro TG, Langenberg J, Paul-Murphy J: A review of lameness in long-legged birds. Proc Assoc Avian Vet, New Orleans, 1992, pp 265–270.

50. Tully TN, Pechman RD, Cornick J, Morris JM: A subchondral cyst in the distal tibiotarsal bone of an ostrich *(Struthio camelus)*. J Avian Med Surg 9(1):41–44, 1995.

51. Duncan IJH, Geatty ER, Hocking PM, Duff SRI: Assessment of pain associated with degenerative hip disorders in adult male turkeys. Res Vet Sci 50:200–203, 1991.

52. McMillan MC: Imaging techniques. In Ritchie BW, Harrison GJ, Harrison LR, (eds): Avian Medicine: Principles and Application. Lake Worth, FL, Wingers Publishing, 1994, pp 246–326.

53. Droual R, Bickford AA, Farver TB: Scoliosis and tibiotarsal deformities in broiler chickens. Avian Dis 35:23–30, 1991.

54. Hultgren BD, Wallner-Pendleton E, Watrous BJ, Blythe LL: Cervical dorsal spondylosis with spinal cord compression in a black swan *(Cygnus atratus)*. J Wild Dis 23(4):705–708, 1987.

55. Clipsham RC: Correction of pediatric leg disorders. Proc Assoc Avian Vet, Chicago, 1991, pp 200–204.

56. LaBonde J, Miller R, Michel C: Conservative orthotic management of angular limb deformities in ratites. Proc Assoc Avian Vet, Reno, 1994, pp 143–145.

57. Tully TN: Examination and joint isolation for lameness in ratites. Proc Assoc Avian Vet, Reno, 1994, pp 141–142.

58. Daum RS, Davis WH, Farris KB, et al: A model of *Staphylococcus aureus* bacteremia, septic arthritis, and osteomyelitis in chickens. J Orthop Res 8(6):804–813, 1990.

59. Hill JE, Rowland GN, Glisson JR, Villegas P: Comparative microscopic lesions in reoviral and staphyloccal tenosynovitis. Avian Dis 33:401–410, 1989.

60. Curtis PE, Al-Mufarrej SI, Jones RC, et al: Tenosynovitis in young pheasants associated with reovirus, staphylococci and environmental factors. Vet Rec 131(13):293, 1992.

61. Tully TN, Morris M: A treatment protocol for non-responsive arthritis in companion birds. Proc Assoc Avian Vet, Reno, 1994, pp 45–49.

62. Lindstrom JG: A surgical approach to chronic septic arthritis in a blue and gold macaw: A case report. Proc Assoc Avian Vet, Seattle, 1990, pp 210–214.

63. Flammer K, Clubb SL: Neonatology. In Ritchie BW, Harrison GJ, Harrison LR (eds): Avian Medicine: Principles and Application. Lake Worth, FL, Wingers Publishing, 1994, pp 805–838.

64. Cruickshank JJ, Sim JS: Effects of excess vitamin D_3 and cage density on the incidence of leg abnormalities in broiler chickens. Avian Dis 31(2):332–338, 1987.

65. Newbrey JW, Baksi SN, Dhillon AS, et al: Histomorphometry and vitamin D metabolism of valgus-varus deformity in broiler chickens. Avian Dis 32:704–712, 1988.

66. Leeson S, Summers JD: Some nutritional implication of leg problems with poultry. Br Vet J 144(1):81–92, 1988.

67. Hedstrom OR, Cheville NF, Horst RL: Pathology of vitamin D deficiency in growing turkeys. Vet Pathol 23:485–498, 1986.

68. Lidor C, Atkin I, Ornoy A, et al: Healing of rachitic lesions in chicks by 24R,25-dihydroxycholecalciferol administered locally into bone. J Bone Min Res 2(2):91–98, 1987.

69. Rennie JS, Whitehead CC, Thorp BH: The effect of dietary 1,25-dihydroxycholecalciferol in preventing tibial dyschondroplasia in broilers fed on diets imbalanced in calcium and phosphorus. Br J Nutr 69:809–816, 1993.

70. Edwards HM: Efficacy of several vitamin D compounds in the prevention of tibial dyschondroplasia in broiler chickens. J Nutr 120(9):1054–1061, 1990.

71. Edwards HM, Elliot MA, Sooncharernying S: Effect of dietary calcium on tibial dyschondroplasia. Interaction with light, cholecalciferol, 1,25-dihydroxycholecalciferol, protein, and synthetic zeolite. Poult Sci 71(12):2041–2055, 1992.

72. Tang K-N, Rowland GN, Veltmann J Jr: Vitamin A toxicity: Comparative changes in bone of the broiler and leghorn chicks. Avian Dis 29(2):416–429, 1985.

73. Perry RW, Rowland GN, Glisson JR: Poult malabsorption syndrome. II. Pathogenesis of skeletal lesions. Avian Dis 35:694–706, 1991.

74. Perry RW, Rowland GN, Foutz TL, Glisson JR: Poult malabsorption syndrome. III. Skeletal lesions in market-age turkeys. Avian Dis 35:707–713, 1991.

75. Martin HD, Kabler R, Sealing L: The avian coxofemoral joint. J Assoc Avian Vet, 1(1):22–30, 1989.

76. Rosenthal K, Hillyer E, Mathiessen D: Stifle luxation repair in a Moluccan cockatoo and a barn owl. J Assoc Avian Vet, 6(4):235–238, 1992.

77. Rang HP, Dale MM, Ritter JM, Gardner P: Pharmacology. New York, Churchill Livingstone, 1995, pp 258–259.
78. Lumeij JT, Redig PT: Hyperuricaemia and visceral gout induced by allopurinol in red-tailed hawks *(Buteo jamaicensis)*. Proc Deutsche Vet Gesellschaft, 1992, pp 265–269.
79. Liu S-K, Dolensek EP: Osteosarcoma with multiple metastases in a Panama boat-billed heron. J Am Vet Med Assoc 181(11):1396–1398, 1982.
80. Martin H, Ritchie BW: Orthopedic surgical techniques. In Ritchie BW, Harrison GJ, Harrison LR (eds): Avian Medicine: Principles and Application. Lake Worth, FL, Wingers Publishing, 1994, pp 1137–1169.
81. Bennett RA, Harrison GJ: Soft tissue surgery. In Ritchie BW, Harrison GJ, Harrison LR (eds): Avian Medicine: Principles

and Application. Lake Worth, FL, Wingers Publishing, 1994, pp 1097–1136.
82. Greve JH, Graham DL, Nye RR: Tenosynovitis caused by *Pelecitus calamiformis* (Nematoda: Filarioidea) in the legs of a parrot. Avian Dis 26:431–436, 1982.
83. Allen JL, Kollias GV, Greiner EC, Boyce W: Subcutaneous filariasis (*Pelecitus* sp.) in a yellow-collared macaw *(Ara auricollis)*. Avian Dis 29:891–894, 1985.
84. Johnson AL: Reproduction in the female. In Sturkie PD (ed): Avian Physiology, ed 4. New York, Springer-Verlag, 1986, pp 403–431.
85. Stauber E, Papageorges M, Sande R, Ward L: Polyostotic hyperostosis associated with oviductal tumor in a cockatiel. J Am Vet Med Assoc 196(6):939–940, 1990.

Louise Bauck
Susan Orosz
Gerry M. Dorrestein

32

Avian Dermatology

Susan Orosz

Anatomy of the Integument

The avian skin is much thinner and more delicate than that of mammals. It is infrequently attached to a few muscles. It has bony attachments, primarily in the manus or distal wing and the feet or pes. The skin consists of an epidermis, dermis, and a subcutaneous layer with its neurovascular supply. The epidermis in birds is roughly equally divided between living and dead cells, with an approximate thickness of only 10 cells in the domestic fowl. The basal layer, stratum basale or germanitivum, has cells that divide and push cells toward the surface. The most superficial layer is the stratum corneum, which is composed of horny dead cells. The dermis is also relatively thin compared with that of mammals and is the site for feather development from a dermal papilla. The dermis includes a superficial layer in which thickness varies according to the age of the bird and location on the body. The superficial layer contains an outer layer of compact connective tissue that is predominantly collagen. There is an inner layer with small smooth muscles that attach to the feather and the skin to change the elevation of the feather. There is a deeper subcutaneous layer, which is composed of loose connective tissue and fat and some striated muscle for the regulation of skin tension.

The horny bill is called the rhamphotheca, which consists of a hard keratinized epidermis with an underlying dermis that becomes continuous with the periosteum of the premaxilla or mandible. The outer layer of the rhamphotheca is like the stratum corneum and may be very thick and hard. This is particularly true at the tip of the beak. The epider-mis often is thrown into folds on its basal surface, thereby allowing dermal projections or papillary pegs to be found closer to the surface. Within these dermal or papillary pegs are mechanoreceptors (Herbst corpuscles for food discrimination) and sensory receptors similar to Merkel cells. The sensory supply to the maxillary rhamphotheca is the ophthalmic and maxillary divisions of cranial nerve V; the mandibular rhamphotheca is supplied by the mandibular division of cranial nerve V. There can be a variety of anomalies of the beak that may be associated with hereditary problems; interruption of growth from improper nutrition, causing a twisting of the beak; as well as traumatic insults that damage the stratum basale or germanitivum and the dermis from which the beak grows.

The claws or nails surround the distal phalanx of each of the digits. The epidermis is highly keratinized, particularly on its dorsal ridge and two lateral walls. This dorsal ridge grows faster than the ventral plate, which helps produce the curvature. Claws may be associated with the alular digit (rheas and ostriches), major digit (ostriches, emus, kiwis, and cassowaries), or minor digit (ostriches). The nonfeathered area of the legs is the podotheca, which is composed of scales. Scales are raised epidermal plates that are highly keratinized. They may become lifted with trauma or as the result of infestation with *Knemidocoptes* mites, which burrow under the scales.

The uropygial gland is also called the preen gland or oil gland and is particularly prominent in waterfowl. This holocrine gland is found dorsally at the base of the tail. It is raised and somewhat heart-shaped and is drained by a papilla dorsocaudally. The papilla is covered by a tuft of feathers. The papilla may drain by a single or by multiple ducts. The secretion, composed of extruded cells with their lipid content, is spread by the bill over feathers during preening. However, the uropygial gland is not essential for waterproofing. A number of birds, including emus, ostriches, and Amazon parrots, do not have this gland. It is inconstant in many pigeons, and in other parrots and macaws. The gland is present in African grey parrots and budgerigars.

Footpads in birds are formed by a thickening in the skin over the ventral interphalangeal region. These thickenings are derived from both epidermis and dermis. The footpad can be likened to the frog area of the horse, which is designed to withstand compression on the impact of landing. Bumblefoot is the condition whereby the footpad becomes infected and abscessed.

There are a number of different feather types. They include contour, semiplume, filoplume, bristle, down, and powder down feathers. Feathers are arranged in tracts or pterylae. Spaces without contour feathers are called apteryia and may be filled with down.

Contour feathers are those that cover the body and provide feathers for flight (remiges) and for the tail (rectrices) (Fig. 32–1 *A* and *B*). Remiges are divided into the "primaries" and "secondaries." The primary remiges insert dorsally from the carpus distally along the carpometacarpus and phalanges. There are often 10 primaries. They are numbered from one to 10 from the carpus outward. The secondary remiges insert dorsally along the ulna. Remiges are "covered over" by feathers called coverts. Coverts can also be found over the external ear canal and over the base of the tail.

Each of the contour feathers is attached to a feather follicle where the new feather emerges during a molt. The anatomy of the contour feather can also be used when describing other feather types. The main shaft of the feather is called the scapus (Fig. 32–2). The scapus is subdivided into the portion with the vane or vexilla and base or calamus that is unvaned. The vaned portion of the feather may have barbs or plumes. Barbs are slender but stiff filaments that contain hooks or barbules that also project at roughly 45° angles from the barbs. They act to zipper the barbs together to give the

feather a tight smooth appearance, which is important for waterproofing and for flight. The plumes appear as downy-like barbs because they do not contain the barbules.

Semiplume feathers are fluffy in appearance. The rachis is longer than the length of their longest barb. Barbules are not present. These feathers often lie along the margin of feather tracts or pterylae.

Filoplumes are found in close association with the follicle of each contour feather (Fig. 32–3). They have a long calamus with a short tuft of barbs at their free end. Unmyelinated nerve endings are found at their follicles. Herbst corpuscles, with their encapsulated nerve endings, are found adjacent to them. These feathers may be involved in providing sensory information about the orientation of the adjacent contour feathers.

Bristles have a stiff scapus (Fig. 32–4). They may have a few barbs at their proximal ends but often do not. Bristles are found at the base of the eyelids, nares, and mouth. Like filoplumes, they are thought to have a sensory function because they have encapsulated nerve endings at their base.

Down feathers (Fig. 32–5) are opposite in definition from semiplume feathers. The rachis of down feathers is shorter than the longest barbs or may be absent altogether. Down feathers in various species may be absent entirely, as in ratites, passerines, and pigeons; may be restricted to certain sites; or may cover the entire body surface, as in ducks and penguins.

Powder down feathers may be of any feather type and are often found in specified areas of the body. These feathers shed a "powdery" keratin from their outer sheaths.

Feathers are molted by extrusion of the old feather from its base. This results from growth of epidermal cells that form a cap over an epidermal collar covering a dermal papilla (Fig. 32–6). This structural arrangement of the feather follicle can be thought of as an invagination of the skin so that its lining consists of an outer epidermal layer with an inner dermal sone. At its base is a point that is lined by an epidermal layer of cornified cells. The dermal papilla is at the bottom of the feather follicle where it receives blood supply from the dermis below. Beneath this layer is the dermis, which is continuous with the dermal papilla. As the feather grows from its papilla, the central pulp cavity consists of a dermis with an axial artery and vein. This stage

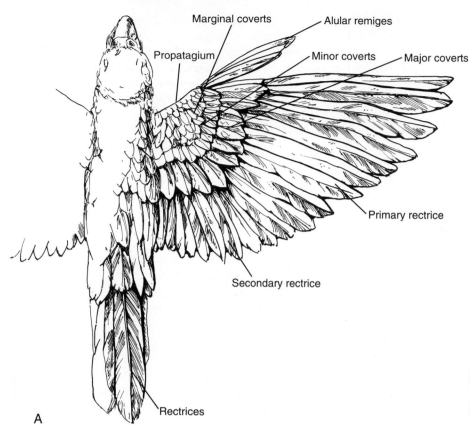

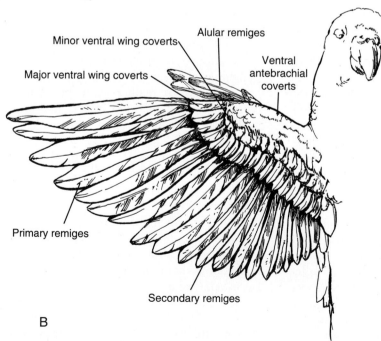

F i g u r e 3 2 – 1

Feather tracts of the wing of a psittacine. *(A)* Dorsal view of the wing. *(B)* Ventral view of the wing.

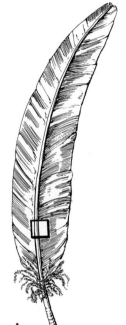

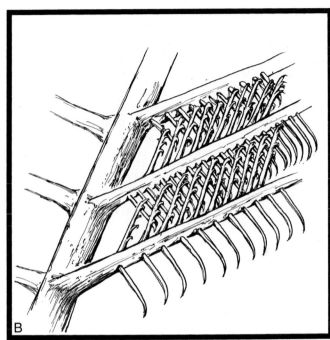

Figure 32–2

(A) Anatomy of a contour feather. *(B)* Detail of this feather type showing the relationship of barbs and barbules.

A

B

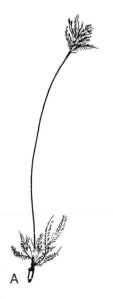

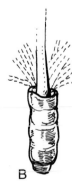

A

B

Figure 32–3

Anatomy of the filoplume feather. *(A)* Filoplumes often have a long shaft with a tuft of barbs or barbules at the end. Some filoplumes do not have a short tuft at the end. *(B)* Proximal end of the filoplume. These feathers are thought to provide sensory information.

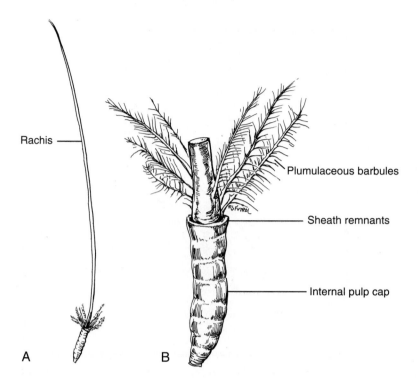

Rachis

Plumulaceous barbules

Sheath remnants

Internal pulp cap

A

B

F i g u r e   3 2 – 4

Anatomy of a bristle feather. *(A)* Bristle feathers have a stiff rachis. *(B)* Close-up showing the barbs and plumulaceous barbules. These feathers may have a mechanoreceptor function.

F i g u r e   3 2 – 5

Anatomy of the down feather. *(A)* Down feathers have a rachis that is shorter than the longest barb or it may be absent altogether. *(B)* Detail of a down feather. There are numerous barbs with noninterlocking barbules.

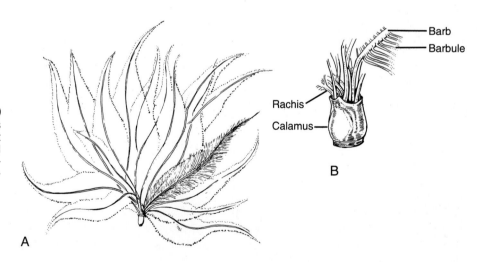

Barb

Barbule

Rachis

Calamus

A

B

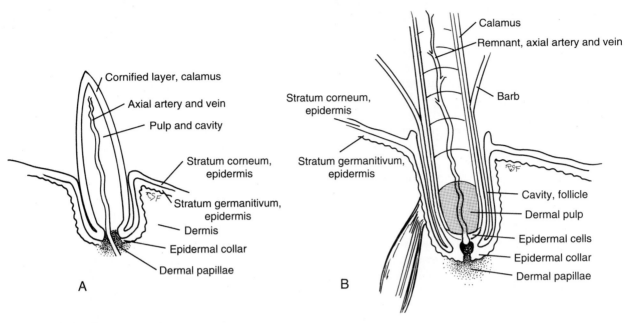

Figure 32-6

Feather development. *(A)* Longitudinal section of a developing feather. *(B)* Longitudinal section of a mature feather.

in development is also called the "blood feather." The outer keratin sheath is of epidermal origin and protects the developing feather that is found within it. The pulp cavity including its vessels will become the scapus. The vessels retreat normally when the feather is at its normal length and the keratin sheath is ready to be removed to become a mature feather.

Physiology of Avian Dermatology

Gerry M. Dorrestein

FEATHERS

Feathers are the most distinctive feature of avian anatomy. Collectively referred to as plumage, feathers are unique structures of the skin that provide insulation for controlling body temperature, aerodynamic power for flight, and colors for communication and camouflage. Feathers also perform secondary roles. Modified feathers are important in swimming, sound production, hearing, protection, cleanliness, water repellency, water transport, tactile sensation, and support.[1]

Function of Feathers

The most conspicuous feathers are the vaned contour feathers that include the smaller contour feathers covering the body surface and the larger flight feathers of the wings and tail. The smooth overlapping arrangement of vaned feathers reduces air turbulence in flight. The tiny, flat contour feathers that cover a penguin's body create a smooth, almost scaly, surface that reduces friction during swimming.

The flight feathers of the tail attach to the pygostyle and function primarily in steering and braking during flight.

Down feathers have loosely entangled barbules and, by trapping air in a layer next to the skin, provide an excellent natural, lightweight thermal insulation. Powder down assists in cleaning of the plumage.

Semiplumes enhance thermal insulation, fill out the aerodynamic contours of body plumage, and serve as courtship ornaments.

Hairlike filoplumes monitor the movement and position of adjacent vaned feathers. Disturbance of a filoplume's enlarged tip is transmitted by the long, thin shaft to sensory corpuscles at its base, which then signal the muscles at the base to adjust the feather's position. Filoplumes associated with the flight feathers aid aerodynamic adjustments. Those in association with contour feathers may also help to monitor airspeed; filoplumes are absent in penguins and in ostriches and other flightless ratites.

Bristles are specialized feathers with both sensory and protective functions (e.g., eyelashes of ostriches, facial feathers of raptors). Corresponding to their sensory functions, bristles, like filoplumes, have sensory corpuscles at their bases.

The Feather Coat

The feather coat of most birds consists of thousands of feathers. In general, the feather coats of birds weigh two to three times as much as their bones. In most birds the feathers are not attached to the skin evenly or uniformly. There are feather tracts (pterylae) and featherless skin regions (apteria). The functional significance of pterylae and apteria has not yet been established. The bases of adjacent feathers are linked by an elaborate network of tiny muscles, which elevate and depress feathers for courtship displays or heat regulation. The apteria probably facilitate wing and leg movements and provide spaces for tucking these appendages beneath the feather coat. Apteria themselves may also facilitate heat loss; penguins lack them.

Feather Care

Daily care of the feathers is essential. In most birds the uropygial gland or preen gland secretes a rich oil of waxes, fatty acids, fat, and water, which, when applied externally with the bill, cleans feathers and preserves feather moistness and flexibility. The waxy secretion of the preen gland also helps to regulate the bacterial and fungal flora of feathers. Birds may preen their feathers as often as once an hour while resting. They draw the long flight feathers individually and firmly through the bill to restore the vane's integrity and to remove parasites. Feather-chewing parasites damage the structural integrity of feathers, reducing both winter survival and attractiveness of male pigeons to females.[2] Feather damage reduces the insulation quality of feathers and thereby causes metabolic heat production to increase by 8.5%.[3]

Birds groom and delouse head and neck feathers by vigorous scratching. Crippled and one-legged birds cannot scratch their heads properly and may accumulate large, uncontrolled populations of lice on their heads.

A dust-like substance resembling talcum powder is present on the contour feathers of many birds (e.g., parrots, cockatoos, pigeons). Special feathers called powder downs, which are dispersed throughout the feather coat, continuously slough this waterproofing powder of keratin particles 1 μm in diameter from the surface of their barbs.

Feather Growth

Except for cases of accidental loss of feathers and their immediate regrowth, feather replacement takes place regularly with age and with season, and is termed "moult." New feathers grow from specialized pockets of epidermal and dermal cells called follicles, which periodically produce new feathers. The new feather grows rapidly, and toward the end of its growth the basal cells form a simple cylindrical callus that anchors the mature feather in the follicle. The emerging new feather then pushes its predecessor out of the follicle.

The follicle grips the feather at the calamus by a combination of muscular tightening and friction. Substantial force is required to pull a feather from its grip. The tight grip of follicular muscle, which is controlled by the autonomic nervous system, may relax when a bird becomes frightened. The resultant loss of feathers is known as fright loss.

Moult and Plumage

Every bird goes through a series of plumages in its lifetime. The first natal down plumage may consist of a few scattered down feathers (psilopaedic, e.g., parrots, pigeons) or it may be a dense, fuzzy covering like that in ducklings and chicks (ptilopaedic). They are soon replaced by a more substantial set of downy or vaned feathers. When the juvenile bird approaches independence, its immature plumage is completed with tail and wing feathers.

In most species, an adult bird typically moults after breeding, replacing its entire plumage (basic plumage). It may keep its new set of feathers for 12 months, or it may replace some plumage before nesting the following year, converting sober camouflage plumage to a brightly colored plumage (alternate plumage) for territorial display.[1]

Moulting in most birds follows a regular sequence within each feather tract. The usual sequence for the primary flight feathers is from the innermost primary outward to the last feather of the wingtip. The staggered replacement of the primaries and secondaries of the wings in most birds produces only small, temporary gaps in the wing surface and only a small reduction of flight power. The tail feathers in most species typically moult centrifugally from the innermost pair to the outermost pair.

Physiology of Moult

Moult and preparations for migration are triggered by changes in day length and can be experimentally manipulated. The endocrine pathways that tie moult to photoperiod are not well defined, but the endocrine hormones clearly affect the timing and course of moult. Historically, thyroid hormone was thought to regulate moult in birds, but the relationship is not a simple or direct one; rather, indirect interactions between thyroid activity and gonadal cycle probably are involved.[1]

Moult typically follows breeding and often precedes migration. Few species breed and moult at the same time. Some female hornbills moult while imprisoned in sealed nest cavities, incubating eggs and brooding young. Tropical birds moult more predictably than they breed, because reproduction may be tied to irregular periods of rain. Desert birds, such as the zebra finch of Australia, moult on a regular schedule but nest whenever the predictable rains begin, stopping the moult temporarily to do so. Moult resumes after nesting is completed.

The gonadal hormones, androgens and estrogens, appear to inhibit moult, because moult begins as the level of the hormones in the bird's breeding cycle decreases.[4] Experimental injections of gonadal hormones into moulting birds slow or even stop moult. Moult cycles, however, are not directly coupled to gonadal cycles because castrated birds continue to moult on schedule.

Moult is a period of intense physiologic change.[5] Accompanying the replacement of worn feathers is the synthesis of keratin by the skin, increased amino acid metabolism, increased cardiovascular activity to supply blood to the growing feathers, shunting of water to the developing feathers, changes in bone metabolism and calcium distribution, and a daily cycling of the body protein content, plus increased need for iron for red blood cell production and for calcium for bone formation. Together these metabolic changes impose substantial hidden energy costs beyond those required simply to convert amino acids into feather proteins. Only 7% of the energy used by moulting birds is actually incorporated into feathers themselves.

Birds that lose feathers as a result either of disease or plucking have higher nutritional demands to compensate for this loss. In addition to the amino acid requirements (cystine [methionine], lysine, and arginine) for new feather growth, partially feathered birds experience increased heat loss. This results in an increase in metabolic rate of up to 60% with a concomitant increase in energy demands for heat production and feather regrowth. Energy intake by defeathered birds is about 85% higher than for those with normal feathering (at 22°C).[6]

Louise Bauck

● ● ● ● ● ● ● ● ● ● ● ● ● ● ●

Avian Dermatology

Avian dermatology is an important and complex subject. Because owners often seem to evaluate a pet bird by viewing it, abnormalities of the skin and feathers are noticed much more quickly than changes in weight or other nonvisual signs. Presenting complaints involving feather loss are one of the most frequent problems seen in avian practice. Much of avian dermatology is still poorly understood, particularly dermatologic expressions of hypersensitivities or allergies. Viral skin disorders are also just now coming under increasing scrutiny.

Establishing an etiologic diagnosis can be extremely difficult in birds with dermatologic disease. A complete and detailed history contained within the medical record is essential and can be expedited by having the owner fill out a programmed form. Encourage owners to allow biopsy procedures and other diagnostic tests by introducing all of the options and prioritizing each test.

FEATHER ABNORMALITIES

Feather Mutilations

Feather picking, plucking, and chewing may represent one or more manifestations of compulsive behavior or (between individuals) actual aggression (Fig. 32–7). It may also be a natural expression of

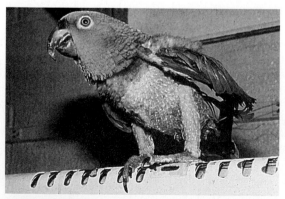

F i g u r e 3 2 – 7

Yellow-nape Amazon parrot with severe feather plucking.

genuine pruritis or pain from a physical pathology, or these factors may trigger or influence initial episodes of feather mutilation. Some affected birds start by demonstrating *excessive grooming* behavior, perhaps because of boredom, frustration ("displacement" activities), or poor feather and skin quality.[7] Feather mutilators demonstrate behavior patterns with habitual or repeated acts that are very resistant to occupational or drug therapies.[8] Primates held in zoologic establishments exhibit overgrooming and self-mutilation behaviors, as do dogs and cats. In humans, similar behaviors are grouped as self-injurious behavior (SIB)[9] or obsessive-compulsive disorders (OCD).[10]

Passerine Plucking

Some passerine species are more likely to engage in plucking behavior than others. Of the commonly kept small passerines, feather plucking is a common component of *aggression* and is typified by loss of feathers on the back, head, and (less commonly) trunk. Males generally pluck females and subordinate males, although dominant females can also engage in feather plucking.[11] Most plucking incidents occur in closely confined, stressed populations. Aggressive plucking is particularly common in the zebra finches, red-eared waxbills, golden-breasted waxbills, and orange-cheeked waxbills. It is uncommon between cutthroats, nuns, java finches, or silverbills. Society finches (Bengalese) sometimes show evidence of picking only on the tail. It is unclear if self-mutilation is also involved in some of these cases. Feather picking is uncommon in canaries and most softbills.

Differential diagnoses for passerine birds should include mite infestations and fungal skin infections. Lice infestations are seen in canaries and other passerines, but are rarely associated with self-mutilation. Diagnosis of feather picking in a passerine bird should include a thorough evaluation and examination of the environment, as well as skin scrapings and cultures.

Treatment of intraspecific aggression in a large

group is difficult because instigators are hard to identify, often having normal feathers themselves. Increasing the number of perches and water and feed containers and providing "baffles" or visual barriers may help.[11]

Psittacine Feather Mutilations

Psittacines are well known for self-mutilation of feathers and skin, but intraspecific aggression or even overgrooming by a contact bird may also play a role. Breeding hen cockatoos may have feather loss on the head resulting from the attentions of the male.[12] Many macaws pick a second bird once the habit has been established on themselves. Eclectus males are often dominated and *stressed* by the hens, and self-mutilation of the feathers is a common problem in males of this species. *Parent birds* of some species may pluck the feathers of their offspring. This is particularly true of male cockatiels, which may pluck the back and neck feathers of the chick, and may also kill chicks in some instances.

Self-mutilation of the feathers is well known in the African grey parrot (especially in wild-captured individuals).[13] This species has been known to denude the entire body from the neck down. However, as with most feather mutilators, a more typical (and less severe) pattern includes removal of the external portion of the contour feathers of the chest. A moth-eaten "downy" appearance results. This behavior may then progress to actual plucking or to more widespread chewing of the wing, leg, or tail feathers. Macaws and cockatiels often demonstrate patterns of feather removal that begin with the wings or legs. Amazons and Moluccan cockatoos seem to mutilate feathers less commonly than other species, but are well-known skin mutilators.[14] Chewing of the wing and tail primaries is another common type of feather mutilation. Often no other feathers are touched. This is a less serious form of mutilation, but resolution is difficult to judge because the shortened and damaged quills are frequently retained for more than 1 year.

Differential Diagnoses of Feather Mutilations and Plucking

Wing-clipped birds have little protection for emerging pin feathers. A bumped feather may trigger a pain response resulting in progressive mutilation of the damaged feather and other feathers around it. Other common *painful* or *pruritic* etiologies may include trauma, neoplastic or xanthomatous lesions, viral eruptions, fungal or bacterial skin or follicular infections, and (rarely) parasitic infestations. Moult-associated pruritus and/or poor skin condition (possibly associated with low humidity or inadequate diet) may be contributing factors to feather destruction.

Bacterial pulpitis is an unusual but possible triggering factor. *Pulpitis* is described as a primary pulp infection or the localization of an infectious or septicemic process in the vascular pulp.[15] A related condition has been seen in waterfowl when wings are trimmed short, exposing the hollow quill to water.[16] Water and algae collect on the quill (calamus) and cause irritation to the follicle. Excessive preening may be a clinical sign.[16]

Allergic reactions are suspected in birds but are difficult to diagnose or confirm. Suggested hypersensitivities include fungal infections (*Pityrosporum* species)[17], pollen, *Staphylococcus* species, peanuts and other food items,[18] and *Giardia* species.[19] In a retrospective study of skin biopsies of 213 psittacine birds with feather loss or feather picking, hypersensitivity reactions were tentatively diagnosed in 78 birds, primarily in cockatiels, conures, and macaws.[15] Hypersensitivity is difficult to diagnose in birds because of the differences between mammals and birds in inflammatory response. Histologic appearance associated with suspected hypersensitivity-induced dermatitis in birds has been described as multiple angiocentric cellular infiltrations.[17]

The *Myialges* mange mite, found primarily in grey-cheeked parakeets, is uncommon but has been reported in association with pruritus.[13] However, behavioral feather plucking is common in grey-cheeks. *Myialges* has also been reported as a cause of pruritus and scaling of the skin on a lilac-crowned Amazon.[20] An unidentified sarcoptic mange mite was also reported in association with pruritus on the wings and legs of a green-wing macaw.[15] *Knemidocoptes* has been reported in the macaw[21]; the author has seen this on the hocks and feet of imported green-wing macaws. Like many other parasites, prevalence is usually lower in hand-raised (vs. imported) birds, particularly when birds are bred in indoor facilities. Lice are rare in all psittacines and are unlikely to cause pruritus except in extremely heavy infestations. Lice are usually very host-specific; this may have facilitated their control in captive propagation.

Pruritus is probably not involved in some feather mutilation syndromes. In the wild, psittacines expend considerable time and energy searching for food, water, and roosting and nesting sites. [7,8] Normal social interactions also demand a portion of their time. The powerful beaks of most psittacines are needed for husking, shelling, and peeling food sources, as well as for processing the nesting site. The time needed for these activities and the physical outlet for which the bird evolved are modified in captivity. Pet birds may also suffer separation anxiety or frustration when confined alone in a cage when their owners depart for varying lengths of time. [7,8] Many psittacine species live in groups in nature and may be stressed when separated from other birds or substitute social companions.

Diagnosis of these conditions depends on a careful evaluation of the history, and routine diagnostic tests including a CBC, blood chemistries, and bacterial and or fungal cultures. Skin biopsies, cytology, and skin scrapings are useful if inflammation or skin lesions are visible. Deoxyribonucleic acid (DNA) probe tests for psittacine beak and feather disease (PBFD) are often indicated.

Treatment of Feather Mutilations in Psittacines

The treatment of self-mutilation behavior in most species focuses on a *multidisciplinary* approach. When a pathologic etiology has been ruled out or corrected, the owners should be provided with educational material explaining feather mutilation and detailing the complex nature of habitual behavior. [22] Occupational therapy designed to displace destructive behavior away from feathers is often helpful (see later), as are measures designed to lower emotional and physical stress. A change of environment, alteration of the nutritional content of the diet and the provision of a mate may or may not be helpful. Increasing exercise and ensuring adequate sleep may decrease self-mutilation. [8]

Drug therapy usually involves anxiolytics, tranquilizers, or opioid antagonists (Table 32–1). The safety, efficacy, and pharmacologic effects of these drugs are poorly documented in birds. None of

these drugs are specifically labeled for use in birds. Clomipramine, doxepin, naltrexone, and haloperidol have been used to treat feather mutilation in pet birds [9,10,23–25] with some reported success. Fluoxetine has been used clinically in some birds with mixed results.* However, any type of drug therapy should be combined with altered management techniques for best results.

Steroids are rarely used in the management of feather mutilation. Hypersensitivity may be uncommon in birds. Steroids can cause immunosuppression in birds, and their use has been linked to aspergillosis. [26] Bitter sprays are ineffective as a management tactic. Psittacines rarely seem influenced by the application of bitter substances, possibly because of differences from mammals in taste sensations.

The use of restraint or Elizabethan collars is controversial. Restraint collars are generally effective only as long as they are worn. Exceptions include early cases of feather mutilation and birds in which skin or feather pathology is still present. Quality of life should be considered before long-term use of an Elizabethan collar is contemplated. For anxious birds, a lightweight, clear plastic small-diameter collar can be placed for a 24-hour trial prior to fitting a more effective collar. Extension-type collars (tube collars) have also been recommended, but they frequently interfere with the normal resting posture of the bird and may be inappropriate. Combinations of extension and flange collars are much preferred to extension collars, but they are generally heavier than a film collar and are commercially available for only a few species.† Some species (such as the Moluccan cockatoo) are particularly difficult to humanely collar because of their extremely long neck.

Feather mutilators may be helped by decreasing the time available for inappropriate behavior or by providing an alternate means of expression to displace chewing behavior. For example, the time spent in certain types of feeding behavior can be increased by feeding whole food items, using "feeder puzzles," or feeding small amounts at multi-

---

*Heidi Hoefer, DVM, personal communication, 1994.

†Editor's note: A number of clinicians report moderate to good results with restraint collars, particularly during the acute or pruritic phase. One type of collar made of high-impact plastic is almost indestructible and comes in two sizes to fit parrots to macaws (Veterinary Specialty Products, Boca Raton, Fl).

T a b l e   3 2 – 1

PHARMACEUTICAL AGENTS USED IN TREATING FEATHER AND SKIN MUTILATION

Drug	Dose	How Supplied/Administered
Clomipramine[4] (Anafranil) Basel Pharmaceuticals, Summit, NJ 07901	0.5–1.0 mg/kg PO BID	10 mg tablet: make 1 mg/ml solution in sterile water; refrigerate up to 7 days
Doxepin[18] (Sinequan) Roerig, New York, NY 10017	0.5–2.5 mg/kg PO BID	
Haloperidol[19] (Haldol) McNeil Pharmaceuticals, Raritan, NJ 08869	0.02–0.05 mg/kg PO SID	2 mg/ml oral liquid
Naltrexone[3] (Trexan) DuPont Multi-Source Products, Garden City, NY 11530	1.5 mg/kg PO SID	50 mg tab: make a 5 mg/ml solution in sterile water; refrigerate up to 3 months
Medroxyprogesterone[13] (Depo-Provera) Upjohn Co, Kalamazoo, MI 49001	25–50 mg/kg IM SQ once every 6–12 wk	Injectable

ple locations outside of the cage. Commercially available seed in a pressed "berry" or nugget form may be useful because this food is relatively *labor-intensive*. Spray millet is relished by most large parrots and also takes time to consume. The total nutritional plan should be carefully reviewed in conjunction with such a program.

Chew toys constructed from such materials as rawhide, leather, wood, rope, or other chewable products also provide a good chewing outlet for many parrots. Toy safety should be discussed with the owner. Many parrots enjoy chewing on twigs, bark, branches and even 2″ × 4″ wood boards. Standard dowel-type perches can be replaced with fresh, clean branches. This adds interest to the environment as well as providing for chewing behavior, and is undoubtedly a more natural substrate for the feet. Commercial aviaries frequently use natural perches, replacing remnants every 4 to 6 weeks. Citrus, willow, alder, maple, eucalyptus, and apple prunings have all been used successfully.[8]

Feather Loss

Feather loss or absence *without* plucking also occurs commonly in pet birds. Some conditions have a suspected genetic component, such as feather absence on the posterior aspect of the head in some lutino cockatiels. Some types of feather loss may be metabolic in nature. Hypothyroidism has recently been reported in the scarlet macaw,[27] and has been diagnosed in Amazon parrots as well.[28] Some types of feather loss are poorly understood, such as canary baldness.

Hypothyroidism and hyperadrenalism have been discussed in the literature in association with feather loss,[19] but little definitive evidence for diagnosis was given. *Hypothyroidism* in pet psittacines has been associated with excess fat deposition over the legs and abdomen and a delayed moult, as well as a diffuse loss of contour feathers.[27,28]

Diagnosis of suspected hypothyroidism includes screening for hematologic and biochemical abnormalities of nonregenerative anemia, mild heterophilia, hypercholesterolemia, and hypoalbuminemia. Biopsy results in a scarlet macaw with reported hypothyroidism included hyperkeratosis and vacuolar degeneration of the follicular epithelium.[27] Suspected hypothyroidism in pet budgerigars has also been described[29]; reported signs include poor feather quality, loss of feather pigmentation, and down feather protrusion in obese inactive budgerigars. Thyrotropin stimulation testing is not always possible in budgerigars because of their small blood volume. The nutritional status of budgerigars with suspected hypothyroidism should be evaluated, with particular attention to iodine. Thyroid hyperplasia and hypothyroidism are not generally linked, but it may be possible for chronically iodine-deficient birds to show some thyroid insufficiency.

Viral infections are an important cause of actual feather loss. Some viral skin infections may cause pruritic or nonpruritic skin eruptions, but viruses such as polyoma virus and PBFD virus may cause a primary feather loss.

The PBFD virus is known to infect a wide range of Old World Psittaciformes,[30] and may occasionally affect New World species. Clinically, it is seen most frequently in cockatoo species. Affected chicks may exhibit an acute form,[31] which is often manifested by hemorrhage into the shafts of developing feathers (particularly wing primaries) followed by their loss a few days later. Classic forms of PBFD (in weaned juveniles or young adults) often show diffuse feather loss, with reduced, atrophied, or malformed feathers (Fig. 32–8).[31] In cockatoos, down feathers on the hips and flanks may appear shortened, with very little powder and fluff formation.

Diagnosis of PBFD is covered in detail in Chapter 19. The most sensitive and specific test is the DNA probe test.[32] Biopsies are also highly specific, but viral inclusions may not always be present in the sections submitted or in subclinical or preclinical cases. Treatment of affected cockatoos is mainly palliative.

Polyoma virus infection has also been associated with feather loss or atrophy. In young budgerigars, infection may cause early nestling mortality or may result in feather loss in a variety of patterns. In fledglings, the feather loss has been described as a

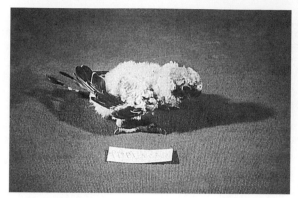

Figure 32–9

One of a variety of feather abnormalities in parakeets surviving a polyoma virus infection.

loss or lack of down feathers and filoplumes on the trunk, head, and neck.[33] North American *"French" moult* has been described as a lack of wing and tail primaries in weaned budgerigars[12] and may or may not be associated with polyoma virus (Fig. 32–9). In Australia, young budgerigars with a bilateral symmetrical loss of wing and tail primaries have been diagnosed with PBFD virus.[34] However, as is often true with affected budgerigars in North America, some of these birds apparently recover[34] (scarlet macaws affected with PBFD virus have also been reported to recover[32]). Polyoma virus infection is considered a significant cause of mortality in domestically raised large psittacines,[33] but feather lesions in surviving birds are rare. Polyoma virus infection has also been reported as a cause of feather abnormalities in young finches (Fig. 32–10).[35]

Diagnosis may be accomplished through the use of biopsies and a DNA probe test.[17,32] Histologic lesions have been described as inflammation of the perifollicular dermis and pulp, with enlargement of the cells of the epidermal collar. Karyomegaly and pale or granular intranuclear inclusions are present. (See Chapter 19, Virology.)

Changes in the Feather Color and Structure

In addition to feather changes that result from self-mutilation (transection, stripping, fraying, and wearing), feather changes can be caused by many other factors.

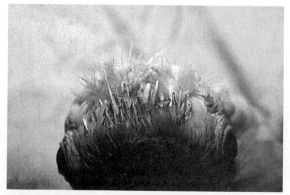

Figure 32–8

Retained and hemorrhagic pin feathers in the crest of an umbrella cockatoo with PBFD.

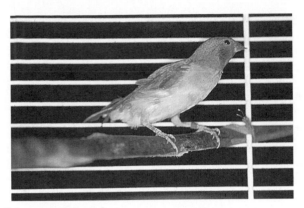

F i g u r e   3 2 – 1 0

Missing wing primaries and tail feathers, with overgrown underbeak in a young Gouldian finch infected with polyoma virus.

Overgrooming, or the cumulative effects of aging in a feather (as it is groomed repeatedly), may possibly contribute to a color change. A physical loss of the metallic green pigment in many Amazons and conures results in a darkening or blackening of the feather. This blackening has also been associated with stress and poor nutrition.[36] General darkening with an oily appearance (possible lack of powder down) has been reported in young cockatiels and may be associated with stress.[37] Lack of powder down in cockatoos affected with PBFD virus often results in darkening (soiling) of the feathers, particularly on the head.[38] The PBFD virus has also been suspected to cause a loss of pigment in certain affected vasa parrots, resulting in a color change from gray to white; this has also been reported in some transiently affected scarlet macaws.[32]

Feather color may also be influenced by certain nutritional deficiencies, particularly amino acid deficiencies.[39] A change in color after moulting in some species may be associated with the provision or removal of certain coloring agents, such as beta-carotene or canthaxanthin (a synthetic reddening agent). Many color changes are associated with maturation and sexual dimorphism. A link between pigment loss and hypothyroidism has been speculated in the budgerigar.[29] Pituitary neoplasia has also been reported as a cause of feather pigment changes.[40]

Bars or bands of pigment loss and textural changes have been noted in several species, particularly in the macaw. These bars are usually seen on the tail and have been associated with stress during feather eruption.[39] Areas of constriction are also seen frequently in the feathers of birds affected by PBFD virus, but these are usually near the base of the feather shaft. PBFD also causes hemorrhage into the shaft of the feather[41] and stunted, clubbed, or persistent pin feathers.

Clubbed feathers are also seen in canaries, and are thought to be a genetic problem associated with *encysted feathers*. Psittacines occasionally have encysted feathers, which usually occur as a single smooth mass on the wing or tail. An important differential diagnosis is fibrosarcoma, which may also present as a mass on the wing.[42] Xanthomas also occasionally present as a nodular mass in this location. Chronic feather pluckers may sometimes have small multiple follicular cysts. Multiple and recurring feather cysts are most common in canaries, particularly in "soft-feathered" or "type" breeds, such as the border, Gloucester, and Norwich canaries.[43]

Diagnosis of a feather cyst is sometimes accomplished by the use of a needle aspirate or exploratory incision (for smooth cysts). Caution is advised because hemorrhage from a mass such as a fibrosarcoma can be significant. In canaries, diagnosis is aided by the often characteristic appearance of the encysted feathers. Cysts generally appear in mature birds as a dry or crusted "lump" or mass, principally on the pectoral and scapular (back) feather tracts (Fig. 32–11). Physical examination usually reveals the presence of several developing cysts. The encysted feather rarely shows the black crusts that are more characteristic of advanced fibrosarcoma.[42] Most feather cysts in canaries are fenestrated or

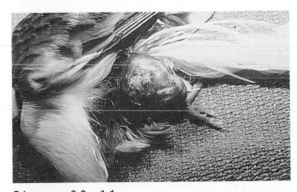

F i g u r e   3 2 – 1 1

Large feather cyst on the back of a canary.

only partially covered with skin. Cyst contents often appear papery or filamentous.

Treatment of feather cysts is usually simple, although repeated treatments may be required. A common treatment technique is to carefully remove the contents of the cyst through a small skin incision or through the various openings in the skin. The base of the follicle is cauterized with silver nitrate. Anesthesia may or may not be necessary. Hemorrhage is rare. A more permanent treatment technique is excision of the follicle and sometimes the adjacent areas of feather tract.[43,44] Coagulation of the cyst lining by radiosurgery is also effective. However, recurrence at another site is common in canaries. Regular (twice yearly) visits to remove the most bothersome feather cysts are often necessary for long-term management.

"Straw feathering" is a lethal disorder that appears to be hereditary in canaries. Feathers fail to emerge from the feather sheath, leaving a straw-like appearance.[45] "Feather duster" is a term that describes another lethal genetic disorder in budgerigars (Fig. 32–12). Gigantism along with long filamentous feathers occurs; affected birds usually die shortly after weaning.[46a] Filamentous feathers in cockatoos have been associated with enlarged adrenal glands.[46b]

SKIN ABNORMALITIES

Many other skin conditions that do not involve feather loss, removal, or change are important in pet birds. These conditions have been divided ac-

cording to etiologic agent to facilitate discussion. Table 32–2 lists some common nodular transformations for easy reference.

Bacterial Conditions

Primary bacterial skin infections are relatively uncommon in pet birds. Skin biopsies of birds with feather and skin mutilation have shown that a small portion of these birds may have either a primary or secondary bacterial infection of the skin or follicle.[15] (See also preceding discussion under Differential Diagnosis of Feather Abnormalities.) *Staphylococcus* species are suspected as the most common pathogen.[15] A primary bacterial dermatitis known as gangrenous dermatitis occurs in which staphylococcal or clostridial infections are found. (See following discussion under Skin Abnormalities of Uncertain Etiology.) Bacterial pyodermas in pet birds have been described as areas of inflammation with infiltrating heterophils; bacteria may or may not be present.[17] Focal granulomatous dermatitis resulting from mycobacteriosis is also seen. Heterophils, macrophages, and plasma cells are seen with acid-fast bacteria present within macrophages.[17]

Diagnosis of bacterial dermatitis is based on results of bacterial culture, skin biopsy, and cytology.

Treatment of most bacterial pyodermas involves appropriate antibiotic therapy based on culture and sensitivity testing. Topical creams are often helpful if used judiciously. The treatment of mycobacteriosis is controversial.

Bumblefoot

Bumblefoot (pododermatitis) is a common and important disease of captive raptors, zoo species, and certain pet species. In pet birds, it is most common in heavy-bodied, inactive psittacines, particularly cockatiels, budgerigars, and Amazon parrots. *Staphylococcus* species are frequently isolated, along with a variety of less common bacteria. *Mycoplasma* species infection has also been diagnosed in a raptor.[47] Bumblefoot is marked by an abnormal appearance of the plantar surface of the foot or feet, and in raptors there is usually a distinct and obvious swelling. In pet species, the lesion appears to be somewhat flattened with a central area of necrosis (Fig.

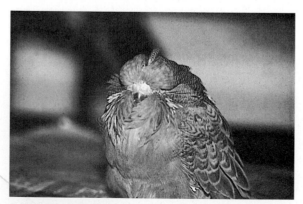

F i g u r e 3 2 – 1 2

Feather duster anomaly in a young parakeet.

Table 32-2

DIFFERENTIAL DIAGNOSES FOR MASSES OF THE SKIN, SUBCUTIS, AND ADJACENT TISSUES

Common Location(s)	Typical Appearance	Species Usually Affected	Differential Diagnoses
Face, extremities	Firm, fixed, +/− ulcerated	Budgerigar, other psittacines	Fibrosarcoma
Head, trunk	Smooth, yellowish	Canary, cockatoo	Lymphosarcoma
Abdomen, wing	Quilted, +/− nodular yellowish	Budgerigar, cockatoo, cockatiel	Xanthoma
Chest, abdomen	Smooth, soft, yellowish gray	Budgerigar, cockatoo	Lipoma
Feet, face, mouth	Proliferative	Budgerigar, finch, cockatiel	Papilloma (noncloacal)
Face, nostril	Firm, encapsulated	Any	Granuloma (fungal, bacterial)
Trunk, wing, tail	Firm, smooth or rough (dry and crusted in canary)	Canary, macaw, Amazon, cockatiel	Feather cyst
Rump (uropygial)	Firm, crusted	Budgerigar	Keratoacanthoma
Toes	Gray, finger-like projections	Cockatoo, macaw	Foot herpes
Toes, wingtips	Hard, smooth, off-white	Cockatiel, other psittacines	Tophi (gout)
Toes (plantar surface)	Yellowish, finger-like projections	Canary, goldfinch	Tasselfoot (*Knemidocoptes*)
Trunk, neck, leg	Firm subcutaneous mass or masses	Larger psittacines	Mycobacterial granuloma

32–13).[48] Differential diagnoses should include articular gout and fibrosarcoma or other neoplastic conditions.

Treatment must address the sometimes multifactorial etiology because this condition appears to be an artifact of a captive life style. Under feral conditions, relatively pristine perches are found for roosting, and they are usually resilient and of varying diameters. A hard wooden dowel that has been the principal perch for years at a time represents a departure from natural conditions. Nutritional deficiencies such as hypovitaminosis A have also been suggested as contributing disease factors in pet species.[49] A review of husbandry procedures is recommended.

Currently, "wet" or moist bandaging techniques are popular. After surgical debridement (removal of crusts and debris, and culture and sensitivity of the lesion recess if possible) an ointment is placed under a gauze pad, which may then be wrapped in cellophane and covered with Vetrap (3M Animal Care Products, St. Paul, MN). Alternatively, a thick plantar pad may be developed into a ball-type bandage.[50] Acrylic "shoes" designed to elevate the central portion of the foot and relieve all pressure from the lesion have also been suggested for therapy.[51]

Bandages (except for a shoe technique) are usually changed every 3 to 4 days.[47] Preparation H (Whitehall Laboratories, NY) and topical combination antibiotic ointments have both been used in treating bumblefoot lesions. Concurrent systemic antibiotic therapy is often recommended at the beginning of therapy.[48] Choose antibiotics that target gram-positive organisms. Avoid the use of aminoglycosides or other antibiotics that are not suitable for relatively long or repeated treatment periods and that do not work well in the presence of organic debris.

Perches should be wrapped in a safe, soft, inexpensive (replaceable) covering such as foam wraps, cotton cast padding covered with Vetrap, or paper toweling. Artificial turf coverings on perches have been used in treatment of lesions in raptors, but

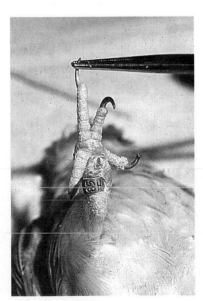

Figure 32-13

Parakeet with bumblefoot lesions and nail deformities. This obese bird was maintained on incorrect perches and an improper diet.

they must be attached securely and still be easy to remove for frequent washings.

Abscesses and Granulomas

Abscesses and granulomas are most common when they involve the sinuses of the head. However, they have been reported in other locations (particularly fungal granulomas).[52] Collections of infectious debris in subcutaneous pockets often involve the infraorbital sinus, with nasal and other granulomas also being found. (See Chapter 25, Respiratory Disease.) Cutaneous masses suspected to be granulomas are usually differentiated from neoplasia by cytologic examination of a needle aspirate and/or biopsy. Macaws may suffer from miliary facial granulomas, although this condition has not been well described in the literature. *Mycobacterium tuberculosis* was confirmed as the cause of miliary facial granulomas in a green wing macaw.*

Viral Conditions

Viral agents are also capable of causing cutaneous changes. In addition to PBFD virus, pox viruses are well known for their effects on the skin and mucous membranes. Pox lesions have been reported in a wide variety of pet birds. Usually each virus is limited to a species or class of bird; however, lesions are often similar, and some cross-species infections can occur. Most pox lesions are found on the head, with the eyes and mouth of the bird frequently affected. Occasionally, lesions occur on the feet. Large crusts or plaques, sometimes flattened and sometimes massive, transform the tissues. Oral lesions are often white in appearance. Differential diagnoses may include trichomoniasis, vitamin A deficiency lesions, candidiasis, papillomas, and bacterial infections.

Diagnosis is difficult to confirm in the live bird because safe biopsy of a tissue section large enough for histopathologic examination in these sensitive locations may be difficult. Cytologic examination of impression smears may be helpful. In group outbreaks, mortalities often occur in associated birds. Histologic examination of tissues usually reveals the characteristic intracytoplasmic inclusions.

---

*Heidi Hoefer, DVM, personal communication, 1995.

Commonly affected species include canaries (imported), lovebirds, and imported blue-fronted Amazons. Vaccinations are available for some species and should be administered well *before* shipping if there is any likelihood of infection.

Treatment of pox infection is nonspecific. Good nursing care is essential. Extra vitamin supplementation and a high plane of nutrition are recommended.[53] Anorexic birds should receive supplemental gavage feedings. Crusted eyes usually benefit from gentle cleaning and the sparing application of a broad-spectrum antibiotic ophthalmic ointment. Systemic antibiotics given prophylactically to prevent secondary bacterial infections are probably not helpful, except possibly in canaries.

Herpes virus lesions have been reported on the skin of pet birds, particularly the feet of cockatoos.[49] The typical appearance is a gray to white, pale or crusted area (Fig. 32–14). Mutilation of lesions is uncommon. Diagnosis may be difficult because the feet are easily damaged by biopsy procedures. Differential diagnoses should include thermal burns, trauma, self-trauma, papillomas, and bacterial infections.

Classic *papilloma* lesions have been reported to affect the feet and mouth of finches, budgerigars, and cockatiels.[54] The lesions appear grayish, dry, and proliferative. Oral and cloacal papillomas occur commonly in New World Psittaciformes. Lesions range from small blister-like areas on the rim of the larynx (often progressing into cauliflower-like lesions) to large, red proliferative masses on the mucosa of the cloaca. These are primarily diseases

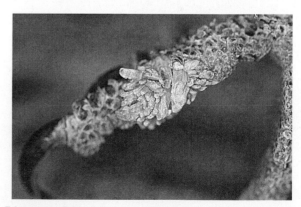

F i g u r e 3 2 – 1 4

Papilloma-like lesions on the toe of a Moluccan cockatoo. The biopsy was negative for viral inclusions.

of the mucous membranes and not skin. Although a papilloma virus has not been isolated from these lesions, the epidemiology suggests an infectious disease.[37] Herpes virus has been isolated in association with this condition, but its role in the disease process is not known.[55]

Metaplastic Skin Changes

Many neoplasms affect the skin surface of birds. (See Chapter 34, Neoplasia.) Fibrosarcomas are primarily subcutaneous masses but may distort or ulcerate the skin surface (Fig. 32–15). These masses are found primarily on the head and extremities[41] and are one of the most common tumors in these locations. A fibrosarcoma is generally firm, protrusive, and well vascularized. Traumatic or primary ulceration is often present in advanced lesions. Prognosis is generally good if complete excision or amputation is possible.

Lymphosarcomas are also common on the head and neck,[36,50] but may have a more yellow and softer character. Lymphosarcoma, including a cutaneous expression, was treated with some success in a young Moluccan cockatoo with combination chemotherapy (prednisone, vincristine, cyclophos-

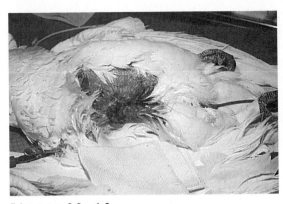

Figure 32–16

Squamous cell carcinoma of the skin in a cockatoo.

phamide, doxorubicin, L-asparaginase, gamma interferon, and astragalus).[57] Cutaneous pseudolymphoma has been reported in a macaw[58] and responded well to treatment with chlorambucil. Squamous cell carcinomas affecting the skin are occasionally seen (Fig. 32–16). Differential diagnoses for these and other skin masses should include granulomas (mycobacterial, fungal, others), lipomas, and xanthomas. A biopsy is highly recommended to rule out a neoplasm in a bird with mutilation and ulceration.

Diagnosis of neoplasia usually depends on histologic examination of the excised mass or tissue. Treatment decisions are based on the type of neoplasm involved and its location and size.

Xanthomatosis is a condition of uncertain etiology. Xanthomas are defined as yellowish nodules or plaques, caused by lipid or cholesterol ester accumulations in the cytoplasm of affected cells.[59] Diagnosis is based on microscopic examination, that shows the characteristic foamy appearance of the cytoplasm. "Cholesterol clefts" are also evident.[42] Xanthomas occur regularly in budgerigars and occasionally in other species as yellowish to orange thickened (sometimes "quilted" looking) skin patches.[41,42] The thigh, wingtip, and abdomen are usually affected (see Color Fig. 32–17). The abdominal wall is often the site of xanthomatous skin change if there is abdominal distension, such as that caused by a lipoma or "hernia" (see Color Fig. 32–18). These lesions do not appear as pruritic as lesions on the extremities. Differential diagnoses include inflammatory or neoplastic processes.

Treatment is usually based on the complete surgi-

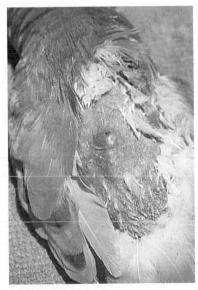

Figure 32–15

Fibrosarcoma causing a raised lesion on the skin of the back of a parakeet.

cal excision of lesions, particularly pruritic lesions. The open wound should be closed as completely as possible; if open areas are present, a bandage and dressing should be used until second-intention healing has progressed. An Elizabethan collar is often necessary until the wound is healed.

Parasitic Conditions

Skin changes can be seen (without pruritis) in birds affected by the knemidocoptic mange mite. *Knemidocoptic mange* is seen frequently in the budgerigar, in which it typically causes a white crusting eruption on the beak and around unfeathered skin surfaces such as the beak commissures, palpebral areas ("scaley face"), hocks, and vent. In canaries and goldfinches, the plantar surface of the foot is commonly affected ("tasselfoot").[48] Knemidocoptic mange has occasionally been reported on the legs of wild-caught green-wing macaws (see earlier) and (more rarely) on the beaks and faces of other species.

Diagnosis can be aided by the close inspection of the lesions (magnification is useful). A characteristic "pinhole" appearance can often be seen. The holes represent the tunnels or burrowing sites of the mites. A skin scraping usually reveals the mites without difficulty.

Systemic treatment with ivermectin at 200 μg/kg subcutaneously is effective, and may be combined with topical treatment (i.e., the sparing application of mineral oil on the lesions). Topical "spot-on" and oral administration are also successful. Topical application consists of up to 1 drop of the bovine formulation of ivermectin (10 mg/ml) applied topically to the skin directly over the neck. Treatment is repeated at 7- to 10-day intervals for two to three total applications.

The red mite (*Dermanyssus* species) does not usually have a significant effect on the skin surface, being primarily a blood-sucking mite that remains on the host only at night.[41] It is normally considered to be a parasite of passerine and gallinaceous birds. However, it has been suggested that it may cause local irritations, particularly on the feet of canaries.[60] Differential diagnoses for foot lesions include foreign body (thread) necrosis, hyperkeratosis, nutritional deficiencies, idiopathic gangrenous necrosis,[12] and pox.

The red mite is not normally recovered with scrapings, but diagnosis is based on seeing the mite on the host or on cage bars, toys, nests, and other objects in heavy infestations. The mites may vary in appearance but are sometimes grayish in color. If mites are suspected but cannot be detected on the host or cage, a white sheet can be placed over the cage at night. The cover is checked in the morning for the small dark bodies of the mites.

Treatment with ivermectin has been used, as have pyrethrin dusts or sprays and even dichlorvos strips. The northern fowl mite (*Ornithonyssus* species) is not as frequently reported in caged birds, but the same treatment methods can be used.

Local inflammation from *nematode* parasites has been reported in pet birds. Microfilarial concentrations in the feet and toes have been suggested to cause local inflammation in some imported neotropical species.[12,48] Ivermectin is the treatment of choice[48] but little information is available on its efficacy.

Fungal Infections

Cutaneous yeast infections have been reported in pet avian species[52] but are best known in turkeys and waterfowl, which may suffer from cutaneous candidiasis in the vent region.[26] Pet birds (including a cockatiel, mynah, and an eclectus parrot) have been reported with cutaneous yeast infections, with most of lesions on the head.[15,52] Eliminating predisposing factors and using ketoconazole have been suggested for treatment.[15]

Dermatophyte infections are uncommon in the pet bird but have been reported in domestic fowl. In the chicken, the wattles are a frequent target site.[26]

SKIN AND FEATHER CONDITIONS OF UNCERTAIN ETIOLOGY

A variety of dermatologic conditions have yet to be well defined in terms of etiology. Some of these conditions appear to be readily recognized between affected individuals and may appear in the literature as "syndromes."

One such problem has been described as "Amazon foot necrosis," "psittacine mutilation syn-

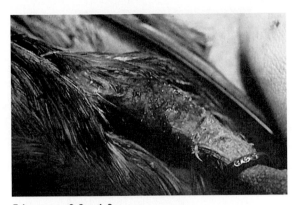

Figure 32-19

Amazon foot necrosis affecting the leg.

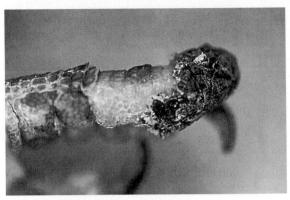

Figure 32-21

Amazon foot necrosis. This bird had necrotic lesions on the toes only, with no injury or foreign bodies involved. This bird was in the adjacent cage to the bird shown in Figure 32-19.

drome,"[13] and "Pacific Northwest mutilation syndrome."[7] Amazon parrots are most frequently affected, and their appearance is of variable amounts of skin necrosis on the wings and legs or feet (Figs. 32-19 to 32-21). Single or multiple lesions may be present. Mutilation is often present, but the original areas of necrosis may arise independently of the self-mutilation. A red-black blister-like appearance (feet or metatarsus) and blackened areas of gangrenous necrosis or crusting (wing, leg, or toe) have been described, sometimes in association with mutilation wounds.[13] The etiology of this condition is unknown. The lesions tend to recur. Speculation on etiology has included viral agents, bacterial disease or hypersensitivity and allergic conditions including food allergy.[13, 61] Gram-positive

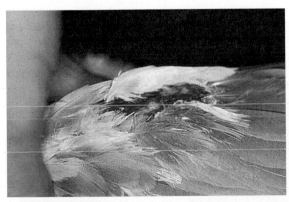

Figure 32-20

Amazon foot necrosis. This bird (same bird as in Fig. 32-19) had wingtips and legs involved in addition to black, blistering lesions on the foot. Biopsy showed inflammation only.

cocci have been noted in Gram's stains of tissue lesions from affected parrots. This condition is somewhat suggestive of gangrenous dermatitis in the chicken, which has been ascribed to either primary or secondary infection with *Staphylococcus* species or *Clostridium* species.[62] Black or brown necrosis of the skin can occur in a variety of locations including the legs, toes, and wings. Affected poultry may develop toxemia and die within 24 hours.[62]

Diagnostic procedures should include cytology and histology studies. Small biopsies may be removed from lesion margins, including some normal skin if possible. Aerobic and anaerobic cultures may be taken from deep portions of the lesion (if possible).

Topical treatment with a broad-spectrum antibiotic or antibiotic/antifungal/steroid combination may be tried. Systemic steroids may have serious side effects, and there is no evidence at present to warrant their use. Systemic antibiotics such as piperacillin, cefotaxime, or chloramphenicol should be used until culture and sensitivity results are known. A dressing and bandage (particularly over leg and foot lesions) are usually helpful in controlling pain and pruritis, and they also increase the contact time of topical medications. Many Amazons tolerate a bandage, or at least are unable to completely remove the bandage before it is due to be changed. A restraining collar may be needed. In mildly affected birds or those with chronic recurrences, topical astringents such as Domeboro solu-

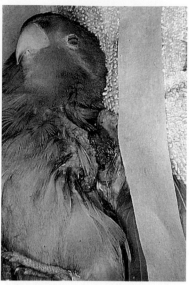

Figure 32-22

Dermal ulcer in a peach-faced lovebird. Biopsy showed inflammation only. The wingweb is a characteristic location for this syndrome.

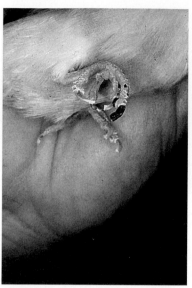

Figure 32-24

Hemorrhagic necrosis of nails in a parakeet. The condition is of unknown etiology.

tion (Miles Laboratories, Elkhart, IN) sprayed on the legs and feet may decrease pruritis. Dilute antibacterial solutions (chlorhexidine) sprayed topically on the feet and legs may reduce the surface population of bacteria and decrease the severity or frequency of recurrences. Drug therapy with anxiolytics or other agents may also be helpful in preventing self-mutilation. Many veterinarians consider the classic Amazon parrot cases to be cyclic or even seasonal (recurrence is common).[13]

Lovebirds also suffer from a well-described but poorly understood localized dermatitis. A shallow *ulcer* appears on the wingweb, axilla, rump, or thigh (Fig. 32–22). The lesion is apparently intensely pruritic. Healing or partial healing may occur if the lesion is protected, but the lesion quickly recurs when the lovebird resumes mutilation. This appears to be different from the more spontaneous skin mutilations of the chest and neck in cockatoos. Pox virus has been implicated in the lovebird but not

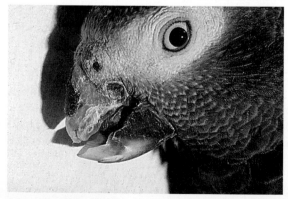

Figure 32-23

Timneh parrot with a traumatic impact slough of the upper beak (collision with a wall).

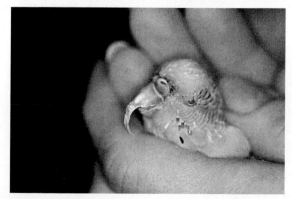

Figure 32-25

Overgrown beak with hemorrhagic streaks in a parakeet with concurrent hepatic adenocarcinoma.

proved. A biopsy or biopsies from lesion margins is suggested. Prognosis is guarded for resolution.

Canary "baldness" has been described in the lay literature. Previously well-feathered canaries develop a feather loss incorporating all or most of the head.[12, 36] In affected birds usually there is no evidence of skin pathology consistent with infectious disease, including fungal, bacterial, and parasitic pathogens.

In Australia, a syndrome reported as "budgerigar short tail disease" is a significant problem in budgerigar aviaries. A progressive and symmetrical thickening, shortening, and clubbing of tail feathers occurs. A virus is suspected.[46]

BEAK AND NAIL CONDITIONS

Some beak and nail conditions have already been discussed under other headings. PBFD may cause an overgrowth of beak and/or nails, and is well known for producing a palatine crust (necrosis) inside the beak, often before other abnormalities can be detected. Splitting, cracking, and sloughing of the beak may eventually occur.

Parasitic conditions such as knemidocoptic mange often result in beak overgrowth in budgerigars. Malformation may result in a "crow-like" beak. The pinhole tunnel entrances can often be spotted on affected beaks. Nails are rarely affected. "Tasselfoot" is the equivalent mange condition in passerines. The face and beak are usually not affected. The nails sometimes develop a corkscrew appearance, with excess scaliness of the foot (see the discussion in the previous section).

Fungal and bacterial diseases also occasionally cause beak problems in pet birds. However, published reports of primary fungal or bacterial problems are rare. Primary beak necrosis caused by *Aspergillus* species in an African grey parrot has been seen by the author, although cere and nasal deformations are more common.[52] Candidiasis has been reported in the lower beak of cockatiels, ostriches, and other birds.[26, 45] Bacterial disease is a common sequela of *trauma,* particularly with penetrating injuries to the beak created in cockatoo mate aggression. Alexandrine and greatbill parrots may also create penetrating beak injuries during disagreements. Aggression is also a frequent cause of toe and nail loss. Impact trauma and hematoma

formation may occasionally cause sloughing of the beak (Fig. 32–23).

Cere problems are seen, independent of fungal infections. "Brown hypertrophy of the cere" is common in budgerigar hens. Although this is not usually considered harmful, careful debridement results in an improved appearance. The etiology is not known, but hormonal and nutritional causes have both been implicated.[45] Cere color changes in the budgerigar are often the result of gonadal neoplasms; Sertoli cell tumors in the budgerigar male are especially associated with a change from blue to brown.[42, 45]

Nail blackening is sometimes seen along with gangrenous toe necrosis (independent from foreign body or thread necrosis) (Fig. 32–24). Although the problem has not been investigated in great detail, it is usually associated with stress. Septicemia has been suggested as a possible cause.[12, 45] Streaks of hemorrhage along with overgrowth have also been noted in both beaks and nails of various psittacine birds, especially budgerigars (Fig. 32–25). Liver dysfunction has been implicated.[36, 45]

Neoplastic conditions are an important cause of beak malformations in pet birds. Fractures, sloughs, and growths can result. Fibrosarcoma is the most frequently identified tumor.[42] Biopsy of accessible soft or germinal tissue is necessary for diagnosis.

References

1. Gill FB: Ornithology, ed 2. New York, WH Freeman and Company, 1994.
2. Clayton DH: Mate choice in experimentally parasitized Rock Doves: Lousy males lose. Am Zool 30:251–262, 1991.
3. Booth DT, Clayton DH, Block BA: Experimental demonstration of the energetic cost of parasitism in wild hosts. Proc R Soc London [Ser B] 253:125–129, 1994.
4. Hahn TP, Swingle J, Wingfield JD, Ramenofsky M: Adjustments of the prebasic moult schedule in birds. Ornis Scand 23:314–321, 1992.
5. Murphy ME, King JR: Energy and nutrient use during moult by white-crowned sparrows, *Zonotrichia leucophrys gambelii*. Ornis Scand 23:304–313, 1992.
6. O'Neill SJB, Blanave D, Jackson N: The influence of feathering and environmental temperature on heat production and efficiency of utilizing of metabolizable energy by the mature cockerel. J Agric Sci 77:293–305, 1971.
7. Rosenthal K: Differential diagnosis of feather picking in pet birds. Proc Assoc Avian Vet Nashville, 1993, pp 108–112.
8. Bauck L: Avian dermatology. Proc Am Anim Hosp Assoc (Seattle), 1993, pp 39–40.
9. Turner R: Trexan (naltrexone hydrochloride) use in feather picking in avian species. Proc Assoc Avian Vet, Nashville, 1993, pp 116–117.

hydrophthalmos) simulates exophthalmos (see Abnormal Palpebral Fissure Size). Anterior globe displacement results from orbital trauma, inflammation, infection, or neoplasia. Traumatic skull fractures may involve the bony orbit; major neurologic dysfunction may be present. Post-traumatic orbital hemorrhage causes exophthalmos uncommonly in birds compared with mammals. Idiopathic harderian gland inflammation causing proptosis has been noted in several psittacines.* Orbital abscesses extending from paranasal sinuses have been noted in Amazon and African gray parrots.* Orbital neoplasia is relatively rare. Lymphoreticular neoplasms[38, 39]; adenocarcinoma and osteosarcoma in budgerigars[40]; sarcomas, optic nerve glioma in caged birds[41, 42]; pituitary chromophobe adenoma[43]; and medulloepithelioma in two cockatiels[44] have been reported.

Clinical Signs

The globe is deviated anteriorly within the orbit. Eyelid closure may be incomplete or inconsistent, which may result in exposure keratitis manifest as corneal ulceration and/or neovascularization with scarring and conjunctivitis. Nictitans movement may be restricted or absent. Serous, mucoid, or mucopurulent discharge may be evident. Birds may exhibit facial rubbing. Periocular cutaneous changes may include eyelid swelling, feather loss, depigmentation, and/or excoriation. If optic nerve function is compromised, direct pupillary light reflex may be diminished or absent and vision may be reduced. Anorexia and altered behavior may be noted.

Diagnosis

Perform a complete physical examination with careful attention to evaluation of the respiratory and nervous systems. Perform a complete bilateral ocular examination, noting asymmetry if exophthalmos is unilateral; rule out buphthalmos by comparison with or measurement of the fellow eye. Perform tonometry if feasible. Consider skull radiography to identify sinus or osseous pathologic changes.[45] If available, ultrasonography, computerized tomography, or magnetic resonance imaging may be useful.

Consider an orbital biopsy or a fine needle aspirate if exophthalmos is pronounced and the bird is relatively large.

Treatment

Following traumatic injury, treat life-threatening conditions first. When the bird's condition is stable, treat for exposure keratopathy and potential infection with topical bacitracin-neomycin-polymyxin B ointment (Neosporin, Burroughs Wellcome, Research Triangle Park, NC) three to four times daily until the condition resolves and eyelid (especially nictitans) functions return. Consider the use of systemic corticosteroids at an anti-inflammatory dose (e.g., 0.2 mg/30 g body weight prednisolone twice daily [bid] per os) if traumatic optic neuropathy is suspected. Reduce the dosage if polyuria and polydipsia become excessive. Corticosteroids are immunosuppressive and must be used cautiously in birds with systemic infections or infected wounds. Broad spectrum systemic antibiotic therapy is usually indicated. Prognosis for vision is determined by the extent of intraocular and optic nerve injuries and their sequelae.

Suspected orbital inflammation should be considered infectious in origin unless otherwise indicated. Begin systemic antibiotic administration and continue treatment through resolution of the problem. If the condition fails to improve in 10 to 14 days, consider an alternate antibiotic or reassess the etiology of the exophthalmos. Consider orbital exploratory surgery for nonresponsive cases. Removal of inspissated pus via superior and/or inferior approaches has been successful.*

If neoplasia is suspected or proved by biopsy or aspirate tests, recommend exenteration of the orbit, which consists of enucleation and removal of all orbital soft tissues. Before surgery, assess likelihood of metastasis or association with primary systemic disease or neoplasia elsewhere with abdominal and thoracic radiography, hematology, and serum chemistry testing.

Enucleation may be indicated for eyes with catastrophic traumatic injury, ocular perforation resulting from exposure keratopathy, intractable uveitis, or intraocular neoplasia. It may be done by the conventional transpalpebral or lateral approaches.

---

*Murphy CJ, personal communication.

*Murphy CJ, personal communication.

Two modifications of these approaches are potentially useful in some birds. One modification involves incision and collapse of the globe prior to enucleation.[46] This procedure may be useful because the equatorial diameter of the globe may exceed that of the anterior orbit but is contraindicated if infectious endophthalmitis is present or suspected. This method alters tissue architecture and may adversely influence ocular histopathologic evaluation. Second, a transaural approach to enucleation has been devised in owls, which have very large tubular globes. The anterior auricular margin is transected, which facilitates globe removal through the lateral aspect of the orbit.[46]

With all surgical approaches to enucleation, remove the third eyelid, conjunctiva, and eyelid margins. The orbital septum is poorly defined in birds; thus, reconstruction of an anterior orbital tissue plane to prevent postoperative sinkage is not usually possible. Appose skin margins and anterior auricular margin, if transected, with the surgeon's choice of suture (Fig. 33–6).

Evisceration with intrascleral prosthesis implantation has been reported in an African grey parrot.[47] In the author's experience the technique has proved unsatisfactory.

Prevention

If bird is a pet or other captive, assess the reasons for traumatic injury and eliminate or correct them, as feasible.

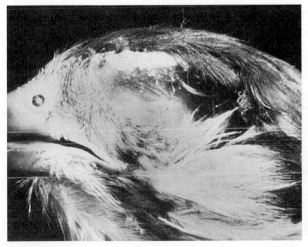

F i g u r e 3 3 – 6

Kestrel following enucleation of the eye. (Courtesy of C. J. Murphy.)

Periocular Swelling

Etiology

Focal or diffuse periocular swelling may result from disorders involving the eyelids (less commonly, the conjunctiva), infraorbital sinus (where present), or nasal gland (where present). Causes of eyelid disorders include trauma, infections, nutritional deficiency, and neoplasia. In addition to swelling, trauma may cause eyelid laceration, hemorrhage, or excoriation. Bacterial, viral, and parasitic infections may involve the eyelids. Staphylococcal blepharoconjunctivitis has been reported in imported Amazon parrots in Japan.[48] Severe fibrinopurulent blepharoconjunctivitis in chickens and turkeys has been described associated with infection with *Staphylococcus hyicus, Escherichia coli,* and *Streptococcus* species; systemic disease was not identified clinically or at necropsy.[49] *Pasteurella multocida* causes blepharoconjunctivitis in turkeys.[50] Hemolytic *Actinobacillus* infection has been associated with blepharitis in waterfowl.[51] Eyelid swelling has been reported with malaria infection (*Plasmodium* species) in canaries and domestic poultry.[30] Bilateral supraorbital abscesses from *Pseudomonas aeruginosa* infection were reported in an Amazon parrot.[52]

Poxvirus infection affects the eyelids and periocular skin in many susceptible species, including quail,[53, 54] peafowl,[55] pigeons,[56] waterfowl,[57] Amazon parrots,[58] canaries,[59–61] mynahs,[62] conures,[63] raptors,[3, 64] and other passerine and gallinaceous birds.[65, 66] Infection with a papilloma-like virus was associated with proliferative eyelid lesions in an African grey parrot.[67] Goose parvovirus causes blepharitis and enteritis.[68] Papovavirus inclusions were reported from the eyelids of budgerigars.[69]

In budgerigars and other aviary and companion birds, *Knemidokoptes pilae* may cause proliferative, scaly, protuberant lesions of the cere and eyelids. Other *Knemidokoptes* species may cause similar lesions in poultry and wild passerines.[70] Periocular myiasis occasionally occurs in wild and aviary birds.

Vitamin A deficiency may cause conjunctival hyperkeratosis and swollen eyelids that may mimic poxvirus and other infections.[71–74]

Eyelid and conjunctival neoplasms are rare. Reports include a benign basiloid cell tumor in a budgerigar,[75] histiocytic sarcoma of the lower eyelid

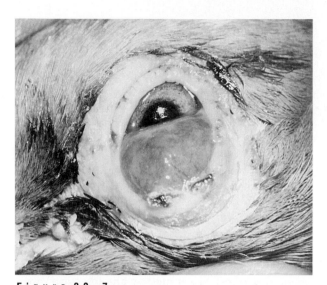

Figure 33-7

Pigeon with eyelid abscess.

in a great horned owl,[76] a mastocytoma of the lower lid in a chicken,[77] and cystadenoma in an African grey parrot.[78] A subconjunctival hibernoma and a benign neoplasm of brown fat was successfully removed from a domestic goose.[79] The mass was ventrolateral to the eye and involved the pyramidalis muscle tendon.

Infraorbital sinusitis, especially common in psittacines, may cause swelling medial and ventromedial to the globe.[5] It is usually associated with generalized respiratory system diseases. Idiopathic nasal or salt gland inflammation in turkeys has caused swelling above the globe. Hyperplasia of this gland may occur in waterfowl given drinking water high in sodium.[80]

Clinical Signs

Eyelids and/or periocular areas appear generally or focally swollen, erythematous, and/or scaly (Figs. 33-7, 33-8). The palpebral fissure width may be reduced and the nictitans may be partially prolapsed (Fig. 33-9). Eyelid and periocular feather loss may be prominent. Serous, mucoid, or mucopurulent discharge may be present, even to the degree of matting the eyelids together. Conjunctival hyperemia or swelling and/or facial swelling may be evident. Facial rubbing may be evident. With eyelid lacerations the palpebral margin is focally interrupted or absent.

Poxvirus infection may occur as a mild form causing proliferative periocular and facial lesions or a severe generalized form involving the skin generally as well as fibrinonecrotic lesions of the oral cavity and respiratory tract (Fig. 33-10).[65] In psittacines, unilateral or bilateral blepharitis develops 10 to 14 days after infection, followed by conjunctivitis with ocular discharge. Ulcerative keratitis and uveitis may follow. After 2 to 3 weeks, scabs form along

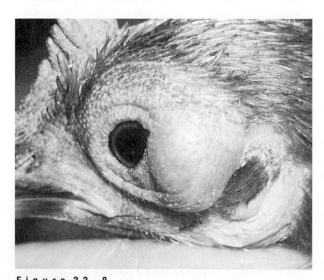

Figure 33-8

Chicken with periocular masses associated with Marek's disease.

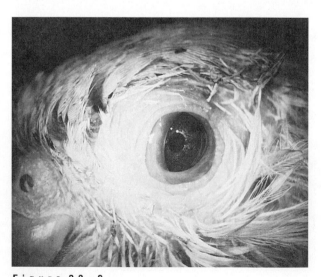

Figure 33-9

Red-rumped parakeet with periorbital sinusitis.

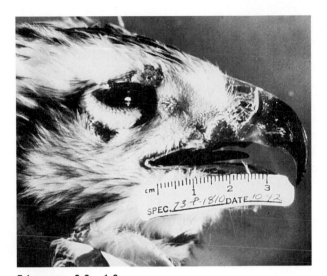

Figure 33-10

Red-tailed hawk with avian pox.

the eyelid margins, sealing them. Eventually, the scabs fall off. The ocular form often precedes the generalized infection. In psittacines, residual ocular problems are common, including eyelid deformities, loss of periocular pigmentation and filoplumes, corneal neovascularization and degeneration, chronic corneal erosion, symblepharon formation, epiphora due to nasolacrimal puncta and duct occlusions, uveitis, cataract, and phthisis.[81]

Diagnosis

Perform a careful and complete ocular examination with the aid of magnification. Consider skin scrapings to rule out *Knemidokoptes,* or a skin biopsy or cytologic examination to confirm poxvirus infection, suspected neoplasia, or nasal gland enlargement. With poxvirus infection, epidermal hyperplasia with ballooning degeneration, intraepithelial vesicles, and eosinophilic intracytoplasmic inclusions are seen on histopathologic examination of a skin biopsy section. Brick-shaped pox virions may be demonstrable by electron microscopy. Consider bacterial culture and sensitivity submission from lesions. Review the history and diet to rule out trauma and hypovitaminosis A. If conjunctival or corneal lesions are prominent, pursue the diagnostic evaluation for conjunctivitis or keratoconjunctivitis (see Conjunctivitis/Keratoconjunctivitis). Perform a physical examination and/or radiography

to rule out respiratory disease or signs of vitamin A deficiency (e.g., oral lesions or periorbital swellings). Following trauma, rule out retained ocular and periocular foreign bodies (e.g, gunshot) by examination and radiography. Assess the integrity of the globe by inspection and *gentle* digital palpation. Marked hypotony may suggest corneal or scleral perforation.

Treatment

If lagophthalmos is present and associated with eyelid swelling (especially of the lower lid) or facial nerve paralysis, lubricate the cornea with sterile petrolatum ointment (Lacri-Lube, Allergan Pharmaceuticals, Irvine, CA, or equivalent) three to four times daily. Consider temporary tarsorrhaphy if adequate lubrication is not feasible. Remove crusts and discharge as needed with warm wet soaks and eyewash. Instill topical corticosteroid/antibiotic ointment or a solution to relieve post-traumatic inflammation *only if corneal ulceration is absent.*

Therapy for poxvirus infection is aimed at prevention of secondary bacterial and fungal infections with topical and systemic antibiotics. Parenteral vitamin A (10,000 to 25,000 IU/300 g body weight) may limit severity of the disease if given early in its course. The eyelids should be cleansed gently with dilute baby shampoo and opened daily. The eyes should be irrigated daily with a merbromin eyewash (add 1 oz. of 2% merbromin [Mercurochrome, Hynson, Wescott, and Dunning, Cockeysville, MD] to 4 oz. eyewash solution). Scabs should be allowed to fall off naturally to avoid excessive scarring.[81, 82] To prevent spread of infection, isolate affected birds, implement vector control, and practice meticulous sanitation and hygiene procedures.

Provide parenteral and dietary vitamin A supplementation to effectively control the deficiency.[71-74]

Surgically excise neoplasms if they are small and circumscribed. Obtain surgical biopsy specimens from large neoplasms prior to definitive therapy. Consider cryotherapy if neoplasms are large or diffuse.

Repair eyelid lacerations with appropriately small (e.g., 5–0 to 9–0) absorbable suture material (e.g., polyglactin 910) and magnification. Single-layer closure is recommended for all but large birds, in which a subcutaneous layer may be placed. Anatomic apposition of the eyelid margins, avoiding a marginal knot that may traumatize the cornea, is optimal. A cruciate suture pattern with the knot tied away from the eyelid margin is satisfactory.

Prevention

For infectious diseases, quarantine new additions to an aviary or flock and isolate affected birds early. For hypovitaminosis A, ensure adequate dietary sources or provide a vitamin supplement. Commercial vaccines are available for chickens, turkeys, pigeons, canaries, and psittacines.

Conjunctivitis and Keratoconjunctivitis

Etiology

Conjunctivitis may be caused by trauma, vitamin A deficiency, infectious organisms, and toxic reactions. Trauma may be associated with handling, shipping, self-induced cage injury, and fights with other birds. Possible infectious causes include bacteria, mollicutes (*Mycoplasma, Ureaplasma, Acholeplasma*), viruses, fungi, nematodes, and trematodes.

A survey of the conjunctival flora of normal psittacines has been reported.[83] No bacterial growth was reported from the conjunctival sacs of 41% of 151 birds. Isolates from the remaining birds were primarily gram-positive organisms, including *Staphylococcus epidermidis*, α-hemolytic streptococci, *Corynebacterium* species, and *Staphylococcus aureus.* Gram-negative organisms were isolated from only 1% of the specimens. Bacterial isolation was more frequent from birds at an import station than from privately owned pets. In another survey of conjunctival flora from both psittacine and other captive exotic birds, 83% of 117 samples yielded bacterial isolates and 48% yielded fungal isolates. Seventy percent of the bacterial isolates were gram-positive, most frequently *Staphylococcus* and *Corynebacterium,* and 30% were gram-negative. Identity of fungal organisms was not reported.[84]

Conjunctivitis in passerine birds has been associated with numerous infectious agents: Newcastle disease, paramyxovirus (PMV-2), poxvirus, cytomegalovirus, *Streptococcus* species, *Erysipelothrix rhusiopathiae, Clostridium botulinum, Mycobacterium avium* serotype 2, *Escherichia coli, Pseudomonas aeruginosa, Bordetella avium, Chlamydia psittaci, Mycoplasma* species, and *Candida albicans.*[85] An epidemic of conjunctivitis and fatal respiratory disease was reported in Gouldian and other Australian finches; a cytomegalovirus was found in electron micrographs of conjunctiva. Light microscopy showed intranuclear inclusions in karyomegalic epithelial cells of the conjunctiva, esophagus, and respiratory tract.[86] Previously, conjunctivitis in Gouldian finches had been reported from Austria and Switzerland.[86] Conjunctivitis associated with endophthalmitis due to toxoplasmosis was reported in canaries.[87]

Keratoconjunctivitis alone and combined with systemic disease has been associated with chlamydiosis in psittacines,[88] waterfowl,[89] and other species. The role of *Mycoplasma* in conjunctivitis is uncertain in birds other than domestic poultry, in which it causes primarily sinusitis with secondary conjunctivitis.[90] Infectious coryza, caused by *Hemophilus paragallinarum,* causes conjunctivitis in poultry.[91]

A conjunctivitis syndrome has been reported in cockatiels.[82] The cause remains unknown. *Mycoplasma* and adenovirus infections have been suspected but not proved. Conjunctivitis may accompany any upper or lower respiratory infections in domestic and wild birds. In domestic poultry, infectious laryngotracheitis, duck plague, Newcastle disease, influenza A, infectious bronchitis, quail bronchitis viruses, turkey and pigeon herpesviruses, adenovirus, and pneumovirus cause conjunctivitis.[92] *Aspergillus* species conjunctivitis has been reported in young chickens.[30]

Unusual causes of conjunctivitis in birds have been reported occasionally. Cryptosporidial infection has been associated with conjunctivitis in pheasants,[93] a duck,[94] and a peacock,[95] and conjunctivitis and sinusitis in turkeys.[96] *Mycobacterium avium* was cultured from conjunctival granulomas on the nictitans of an ostrich.[97] *Actinobacillus suis* was isolated from a Canada goose with severe blepharoconjunctivitis.[98]

Parasites are sometimes found behind the nictitans. These include the spirurids *Ceratospira* and *Oxyspirura* species in psittacines, mynahs, and domestic and wild birds[30, 82, 99]; the trematode *Philophthalmus gralli* in ostriches, waterfowl, and other species[100–102]; and the nematodes *Thelazia* species in a Senegal parrot[103] and *Setaria* in passerines.[85]

Among other problems, photosensitization from

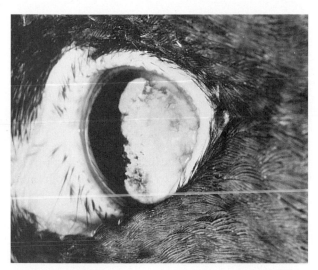

Figure 33–11

Idiopathic lipoidal degeneration of the cornea in a falcon.

ingestion of certain plants (*Ammi* [Bishop's weed] and *Cymopterus* species) and ammonia burn from unsanitary housing conditions cause toxic conjunctivitis, blepharitis, and keratitis in ducks and geese.[104, 105]

Ulcerative and nonulcerative keratitides in birds have been associated with handling and cage trauma,[82] injuries and burns in raptors,[20, 31, 106] possibly infectious agents,[82] and general anesthesia. In mynahs, chronic keratoconjunctivitis with proliferation of inferior palpebral conjunctiva may develop in association with self-induced cage trauma.[82]

Crystalline corneal deposits of unknown cause in the corneal epithelium and stroma were found at necropsy in 8.7% of birds at a quarantine station, most commonly in cockatiels, budgerigars, ring-necked parakeets (*Psittacula krameri*), Amazon parrots, and Gouldian finches.[69] Similar deposits have been noted following poxvirus infection in Amazon parrots.*

Punctate keratitis has been reported in imported Amazon parrots, rarely associated with sinusitis.[82] Bilateral keratopathy of unknown cause was reported in a young barred owl. Dense white corneal opacities were correlated histologically with deep neovascularization and extensive fibroblast proliferation.[107] Idiopathic lipoidal corneal degeneration has been seen bilaterally in four falcons (three pere-

---

*Clubb SL, personal communication.

grines, one prairie falcon) (Fig. 33–11). Neutral lipid and cholesterol deposits were noted in the stroma with subepithelial fibrosis.[108]

Clinical Signs

Hyperemia, blepharospasm, variable photophobia, chemosis, and serous to mucopurulent discharge characterize conjunctivitis. Extensive chemosis may cause or simulate eyelid swelling. Nictitans motility may be impaired; the third eyelid may remain partially prolapsed. If ocular discharge is copious, the eyelid margins may become sealed together. With chronicity, periocular feather loss and self-trauma may occur (Fig. 33–12).

Signs of keratitis include photophobia; blepharospasm; and corneal opacity, erosion or ulceration; or neovascularization. Hypopyon may develop with bacterial corneal ulceration. Progressive ulceration may result in ocular perforation with uveal prolapse and endophthalmitis. Mild conjunctivitis usually accompanies all but the most minor keratitis.

Diagnosis

Before instillation of any collyria or topical anesthetic solution, collect swab specimens from the cornea and/or conjunctiva for potential submission for viral, bacterial, or fungal culture. Perform an ocular examination under magnification as completely as the clinical signs and the size of the eye allow.

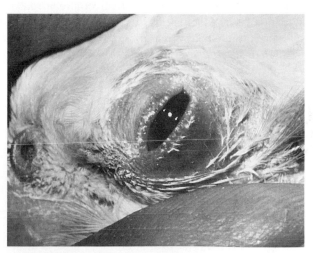

Figure 33–12

Cockatiel with idiopathic keratoconjunctivitis.

Stain the cornea with fluorescein to identify corneal erosion and ulceration. After instillation of topical anesthesia, collect specimens for conjunctival and/ or corneal cytology and Gram's stain. Carefully examine *under magnification* the conjunctival sacs and nictitans for parasites, using a traumatic forceps to manipulate the nictitans to inspect the bulbar and palpebral surfaces completely.

Exfoliative conjunctival cytologic specimens should be evaluated for type of cellular response (inflammatory vs. noninflammatory; suppurative vs. nonsuppurative) and presence of inclusions typical of infectious agents. Routinely prepare extra slides for Gram's and other special stains (e.g., acid-fast, Gimenez, periodic acid-Schiff [PAS]), which may be indicated by initial cytologic test results. The presence of even small numbers of bacteria, especially if located intracellularly in neutrophils or epithelial cells, may be significant. Birds affected with chlamydiosis may show conjunctival epithelial cell hyperplasia and infiltration with heterophils, lymphocytes, macrophages, and plasma cells. Intracytoplasmic chlamydial elementary bodies may be seen on Giemsa- or Gimenez-stained conjunctival epithelial smears, and antigen may be demonstrated by immunofluorescent antibody (IFA) testing; negative cytologic and IFA results do not rule out infection. *Chlamydia* may be cultured from conjunctival sacs. Isolation in embryonated chicken eggs[88] or mouse brain inoculation may be more sensitive than identification on conjunctival smears. *Mycoplasma* inclusions are small basophilic dots peppering the surface of conjunctival epithelial cells. Pursuit of viral inclusions on conjunctival smears is usually futile. Submission of surgically obtained conjunctival biopsy specimens for histopathologic testing may be indicated if other diagnostic efforts are nonproductive.

The cost and historically nonspecific yield of viral, fungal, and bacterial cultures (including *Chlamydia* and *Mycoplasma*) discourage routine submission of samples from most avian patients. Consider selective cultures for recurrent problems in individual birds and in flock outbreaks. Chlamydial serology may indicate active infection if the titer is high or a rise in titer is documented in paired blood samples (see Chapter 23).

Complete physical examination is always indicated, even when the presenting complaint appears to be confined to the eye; many causes of external eye disease are in fact systemic diseases. Diagnostic pursuit of nonocular signs may be more useful than combination of ocular signs alone. The role of hypovitaminosis A in the promotion or maintenance of respiratory and ocular disease is unclear; despite this, if signs of deficiency are evident, consider that lack of vitamin A may be associated with the ocular clinical signs.[65]

If corneal infiltrates or deposits become extensive, proliferative, or vision-threatening, consider biopsy under general anesthesia. This is rarely indicated. Conjunctival masses should be evaluated histologically following surgical biopsy.

Treatment

The objectives of treatment for conjunctivitis and nonulcerative keratoconjunctivitis are: (1) elimination or prevention of infection, and (2) reduction of inflammation. Treat suppurative (kerato) conjunctivitis of undocumented cause with broad-spectrum topical antibiotic (e.g., bacitracin–polymyxin B–neomycin, tetracycline, chloramphenicol) ointment four times daily (qid) or solution every 3 to 4 hours for 7 to 14 days, then reassess for improvement. If clinical signs suggest infectious respiratory illness, prescribe an appropriate oral or parenteral broad-spectrum antibiotic (see Chapter 25). Treat conjunctival nematodes and trematodes by removal with forceps under topical anesthesia; if this is impossible owing to size or numbers, consider topical instillation of 0.125% demecarium bromide (Humorsol, MSD, West Point, PA),[103] topical ivermectin (0.005–0.05 mg),[109] or 5% carbamate powder.[101] Single doses are recommended to minimize toxicity. The conjunctival sac should be flushed thoroughly after treatment to remove the parasites. Elimination of bacterial or parasitic infection will resolve the inflammation. If chemosis is excessive, treat with 5% sodium chloride ointment (AKNaCl 5%, Akorn, Abita Springs, LA) three times daily (tid) for a few days.

Treat nonsuppurative conjunctivitis judiciously with topical corticosteroid ointment four times daily (qid) or solution every 3 to 4 hours *if corneal ulceration is absent*. The cause of at least some nonsuppurative conjunctivitis is probably viral; thus, the possibility exists that corticosteroids could exacerbate clinical signs. Schedule frequent followup examinations to monitor for local and systemic side effects (e.g., polyuria, polydipsia, systemic infections).

The objectives of treatment of ulcerative keratitis are: (1) prevention or elimination of infection, and (2) support or reconstruction of the cornea as needed. Note that anterior uveitis resulting from ulceration is not controllable in birds with topical 1% atropine as in mammals because of the predominance of striated muscle in the iris. Treat noninfected ulcers and erosions (typified by superficial nature, sharp border, lack of miosis and surrounding corneal infiltrate, and clear anterior chamber) with broad-spectrum topical antibiotic ointment qid or solution every 3 to 4 hours until resolved. Schedule frequent followup visits initially to confirm the benign nature and course of the lesion. Treat infected ulcers (typified by severe blepharospasm, progressive deepening, gray or yellow corneal infiltrate, miosis, and variable aqueous flare or hypopyon) aggressively. Choose an antibiotic based on corneal scraping cytologic and Gram's stain results; gentamicin or tobramycin for gram-negative organisms, ciprofloxacin (Ciloxan, Alcon Laboratories, Fort Worth, TX) or chloramphenicol for gram-positive organisms. Consider administration of a subconjunctival antibiotic once daily (e.g., gentamicin) for the first few days; this may be impractical in small species. (*Note: Calculate the maximal safe systemic dose of the antibiotic selected and do not exceed this dose by subconjunctival and/or topical administration,* that is, no greater than 10 mg/kg/day dose of gentamicin in most avian species.[110]) Administer topical antibiotic frequently (ointments q 4 h, solutions q 2 h) until ulcer progression is static, then reduce frequency to maintain this status until healed. Consider confining a fractious or highly stressed bird to a small cage and spraying solutions into the eyes through a 25-gauge needle attached to a tuberculin syringe. (*Note: Topical drugs are absorbed systemically and toxicity is possible!*) Thus, reduce intensive antibiotic treatment as soon as prudent.

If corneal ulceration threatens perforation, consider applying cyanoacrylate adhesive (Vetbond, 3M Animal Care Products, St. Paul, MN) to the defect under general anesthesia. Hold the eyelids apart; dry the cornea with a sterile cotton swab and apply *one small drop* of adhesive delivered through a 27- or 30-gauge needle to the ulcer bed and allow to dry (a few seconds to more than 1 minute).

Continue antibiotic therapy topically until the adhesive plug spontaneously extrudes in a few days to a few weeks. Note that conjunctival flaps are technically difficult or impossible to perform in birds because of the small size of most avian eyes and the relative immobility of the bulbar conjunctiva. Note also that the nictitans is too mobile to hold sutures and serve as a protective flap. Partial temporary tarsorrhaphy may be considered for protection of moderately deep ulcers. However, observation and treatment of the lesion is compromised. For tarsorrhaphy, place partial thickness horizontal mattress or simple interrupted sutures through the eyelid margins with small (5–0 or 6–0) absorbable or nonabsorbable suture material without stents. Suture corneal lacerations and perforations with 7–0 to 11–0 absorbable simple interrupted sutures (e.g., polyglactin 910, Vicryl, Ethicon, Somerville, NJ). Consider temporary tarsorrhaphy placement for protection. Treat with a topical and systemic broad-spectrum antibiotic for 14 to 21 days. Consider using an Elizabethan collar to discourage self-trauma. Provide nursing and supportive care for birds with external eye disease associated with systemic viral infections.

Prevention

Isolate birds with (kerato)conjunctivitis to minimize spread of infectious diseases. Minimize trauma associated with handling and cage design. For domestic poultry, consider vaccination prophylaxis for infectious coryza and viral infections (infectious bronchitis and laryngotracheitis, duck plague, Newcastle disease, Marek's disease, avian encephalomyelitis).

Uveitis

Etiology

The causes of uveitis in birds include trauma, infections, immune-mediated inflammation, and neoplasia. Both blunt and perforating trauma may cause anterior and/or posterior uveitis, often associated with hemorrhage. Hyphema was the most frequent ocular finding in a retrospective survey of ocular examinations of 931 raptors.[106] Iridocyclodialysis, iris tears, lens rupture, and/or fracture of scleral ossicles may occur.[106, 111, 112] Reflex anterior uveitis

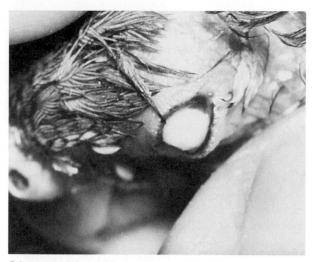

Figure 33–13

Bourke's parrot with endophthalmitis.

resulting from corneal ulceration appears to occur in birds as well as in mammals.

Viral, bacterial, mycotic, and protozoal infections cause uveitis. Avian encephalomyelitis virus causes iridocyclitis and cataract in chickens.[113, 114] Marek's disease, a herpesvirus infection of chickens, causes moderate to severe anterior uveitis and uveal lymphoma.[115] Fowl cholera in turkeys (*Pasteurella multocida* infection) may cause panophthalmitis.[50] Septicemia due to any bacterial infection (e.g., salmonellosis,[69, 116] *Mycoplasma gallisepticum* infection)[117] may cause uveitis. Mycotic endophthalmitis has been associated with disseminated aspergillosis in turkeys[30, 118] and ocular candidiasis in ducks,[119] a budgerigar,[69] and chickens.[30] Toxoplasmosis has caused chorioretinitis and blindness in canaries.[87] Immune-mediated uveitis may develop as mature cataracts undergo resorption.[120, 121] Granulomatous uveitis was reported in a great horned owl.[122] In the delayed amelanotic strain of chickens, spontaneous immune-mediated uveitis occurs in association with acquired intolerance to melanin. These chickens develop secondary cataract and retinal degeneration and white plumage.[123] In addition to herpesvirus–induced ocular lymphomatosis in chickens, primary uveal neoplasia has been reported: medulloepithelioma in two cockatiels[44]; iris melanoma, iris hemangioendothelioma, and anterior uveal rhabdomyosarcoma in chickens[40]; and iris melanoma in a great horned owl.[124]

Clinical Signs

Signs of active anterior uveitis include photophobia, blepharospasm, corneal edema, aqueous flare, hypopyon, vitreous opacity, hypotony or secondary glaucoma, miosis, dyscoria, iris thickening or discoloration, rubeosis irides, and/or anterior or posterior synechiae (Fig. 33–13). Signs of active posterior uveitis include focal to diffuse retinal edema, hemorrhage, and/or detachment and/or vitreal opacity. Vision may be decreased or absent with either iridocyclitis or choroiditis.

Sequelae of chronic uveitis include diffuse corneal edema, posterior synechiae causing pupillary seclusion and iris bombé, anterior synechiae, secondary glaucoma (buphthalmos in birds is uncommon), cataract, retinal atrophy or chronic detachment, and blindness (Figs. 33–14 and 33–15).

Diagnosis

Diagnosis of uveitis is based on identification of a combination of typical ocular clinical signs. Perform a complete physical examination to identify concurrent systemic disease. Perform necropsy on birds that die and submit appropriate tissue samples for pathologic assessment. Submit blood samples for a hemogram and serum or plasma biochemical panel. Perform aqueous or vitreous paracentesis

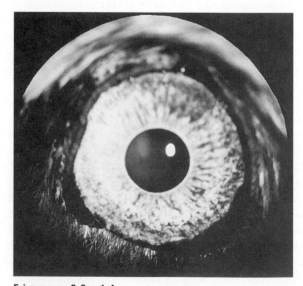

Figure 33–14

Great horned owl with iris atrophy.

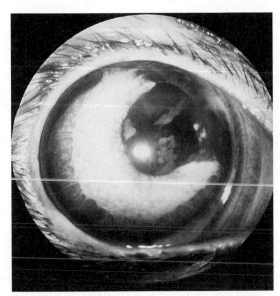

Figure 33-15

Bald eagle with post-traumatic dyscoria and cataract.

judiciously if hypopyon or vitreal cloudiness is marked and other diagnostic tests are inconclusive. Identification of glaucoma in birds is problematic; Schiotz tonometry has not been validated for birds and the instrument's size is too large for many species of interest. In large birds with unilateral ocular disorders, tonometry may be feasible, with the normal fellow eye providing the reference value for intraocular pressure (see Clinical Examination).

Treatment

Objectives of therapy for uveitis include (1) elimination of the cause, (2) control of inflammation, (3) preservation of the pupil, and (4) prevention and treatment of secondary glaucoma. Prescribe specific systemic antibiotic therapy for bacteremia. Consider lensectomy for chronic lens-associated uveitis (this is expensive and may be impractical for small birds). Prescribe topical antibiotic and corticosteroid therapy for symptomatic treatment of inflammation; observe for systemic side effects (polyuria, polydipsia, etc.). Mydriasis cannot be achieved by topical therapy (e.g., atropine) in birds, and pupil preservation is best accomplished by adequate control of inflammation. The safety and efficacy of the topical and oral medications routinely prescribed for mammals for glaucoma are unproven for birds. Enucle-

ate eyes suspected to harbor neoplasia after ruling out metastasis or a distant primary site by physical examination and radiography.

Prevention

Identify viral causes of uveitis in poultry early and isolate or eliminate infected birds. Consider vaccination of poultry for Marek's disease and avian encephalomyelitis. Identify and treat minor corneal ulceration early to prevent progression.

Cataract

Etiology

Cataract, opacity of any portion of the lens or its capsules, may be associated in birds with malformations, genetic disorders, nutritional deficiency, trauma, senescence, toxic effects, and other ocular disorders (e.g., uveitis, retinal degeneration).[125] Developmental ocular malformations have been described in raptors. Malformations include microphakia, cataract, and formation of abnormal lens material (lentoid), along with uveal and retinal dysplasia and retinal detachment.[31] Hereditary autosomal recessive cataract has been reported in Norwich and Yorkshire canaries.[126] Cataract and optic nerve hypoplasia were noted in turkeys.[127] Spontaneous cataract associated with crooked toes has been reported in Brahma chickens.[128] Maternal vitamin E deficiency in turkeys produce cataract in offspring.[30] Blunt or perforating trauma may cause focal or diffuse lens opacity. Cataract in aged birds is commonly noted,[129] especially in long-lived psittacines.[130] Dinitrophenol fed to chicks caused cataract.[30] Avian encephalomyelitis has been associated with iridocyclitis and cataract in chickens.[113, 114] Chronic uveitis and generalized retinal degeneration of any cause promote secondary cataract formation. The cause of cataract may be inapparent (e.g., as in a large proportion of captive-reared bobwhite quail[131] and chicken flocks.[132] Lens opacities in a quail flock[131] and in turkeys[133] were first noted in the axial anterior cortex and posterior cortex after 3 months of age. Progression to maturity occurred by 10 months of age, continuing to hypermaturity in many older birds. Among eye lesions noted in birds that died in quarantine, cataract unassociated with inflammation was the most frequent lesion found at necropsy (15.4% of 24 birds). It occurred most commonly in cockatiels, Amazon parrots, and budgerigars.[69]

Clinical Signs

Lens opacities identified by direct or retroillumination may be small and focal to diffuse and may involve the capsules, cortices, and/or nucleus (Fig. 33–16). Hypermature cataracts are distinguished from incipient cases by their flat, shrunken appearance and the presence of a deep anterior chamber. Dyscoria and posterior synechiae suggest prior or current uveitis but do not distinguish whether uveitis was the cause or result of inflammation (Fig. 33–17). Lens luxation or subluxation may accompany longstanding cataract or precede it.[106, 121, 122, 134] Vision loss is proportionate to the extent of cataract if other serious intraocular disease is absent. If globe size is reduced, the potential causes may be congenital microphthalmos or acquired phthisis.

Treatment

Treat lens-associated uveitis to the desired effect with topical corticosteroid preparations. Consider cataract surgery in blind birds if evidence of other intraocular disease is absent: synechiae, unresponsive mydriasis, extensive corneal opacity, retinal at-

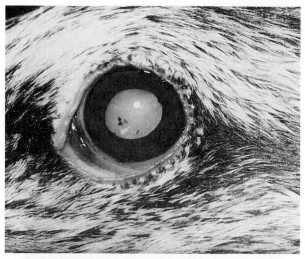

F i g u r e   3 3 – 1 7

Mallard duck with a hypermature cataract. Note the focal posterior synechiae and uveal pigment on the anterior lens capsule.

rophy or detachment. Lensectomy by needle discission and aspiration, and conventional extracapsular extraction or ultrasonic phacoemulsification can be successful in birds. Satisfactory results have been reported in an Andean condor,[129] a screech owl and peregrine falcon[135]; mallard duck[136]; a cockatiel, Amazon parrots, cockatoos, eagles, and several owl and hawk species.* Guarded results were reported in a barred owl with a luxated lens[134] and an African kite.[137]

Prevention

Treat traumatic ocular injury and other uveitides aggressively and early with topical corticosteroids to minimize chronic uveitis sequelae.

Retinopathy and Optic Neuropathy

Etiology

Disorders of the retina include malformation, degeneration, inflammation, and detachment or separation. Retinal dysplasia has been described in raptors, including a prairie falcon[138] and red-shouldered hawks, a kestrel, a great horned owl, and a screech owl,[139] in a kestrel/peregrine hybrid,[140] and

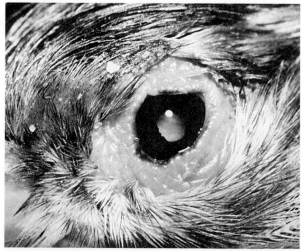

F i g u r e   3 3 – 1 6

Canary with a mature cataract.

---

*Murphy CJ, personal communication.

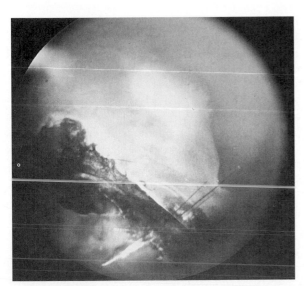

F i g u r e 3 3 – 1 8

Great horned owl fundus; hemorrhage is associated with feather displaced into the vitreous.

in chickens.[141, 142] Several developmental retinal degenerations have been described in chickens.[143–146] Idiopathic retinal degeneration has been recorded in a budgerigar.[147] Retinal and uveal calcification of unknown cause was noted at necropsy in ring-necked parakeets.[69] Traumatic injury is the most commonly implicated cause of posterior segment lesions, especially in raptors.[3, 139] Choroiditis associated with bacteremia or viremia may develop.[69] Toxoplasmosis causing chorioretinitis was noted in chickens.[30] Idiopathic retinal detachment was reported in young captive-reared pheasants (*Phasianus colchicus*) from several areas of the United Kingdom.[148]

Optic neuropathy may be associated with malformation, trauma, inflammation, neoplasia, or chronic glaucoma. Optic nerve hypoplasia and cataract of unknown cause were noted in turkey poults.[127] Trauma is probably the most common cause, resulting in direct injury and/or neuritis. Chromophobe adenomas of the pituitary have been reported in budgerigars[43] and a cockatiel,[149] causing optic nerve compression, atrophy, and blindness. The prevalence of spontaneous chronic glaucoma in birds is unknown.

Clinical Signs

Focal or multifocal retinopathy or optic neuropathy may not interfere with vision, resting pupil size, or direct pupillary light responses. Extensive retinal and optic nerve lesions cause vision loss, variable tonic mydriasis, and impairment of direct pupillary responses. Unilateral lesions cause anisocoria. Progressive cataract may follow extensive retinal degeneration or detachment. Funduscopic signs of retinal degeneration include focal to diffuse depigmentation, hyperpigmentation, and loss of distinct choroidal vascular pattern. Following acute traumatic injury, pre- and intraretinal hemorrhages and vitreal hemorrhage around the pecten are common. Retinal edema and detachment appear as focal to diffuse indistinct gray areas that may appear elevated. Retinal tears usually appear as linear defects in normal attached retina or in edematous detached retina. The optic nerve head is not normally visible, being obscured by the pecten (Figs. 33–18, 33–19, and 33–20).

Diagnosis

Assess vision-directed behavior in a cage, natural surroundings, or loose under handler supervision. Perform indirect (preferably) or direct ophthalmoscopy. Pathologic mydriasis, if present, facilitates examination; if funduscopy seems unusually easy to perform, consider that to be suggestive of retinal or optic nerve dysfunction. If the deficit is unilateral,

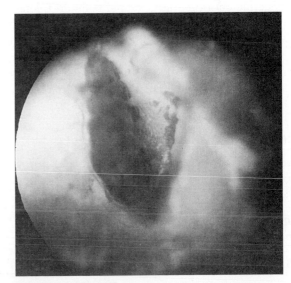

F i g u r e 3 3 – 1 9

Screech owl with hemorrhage around the pecten.

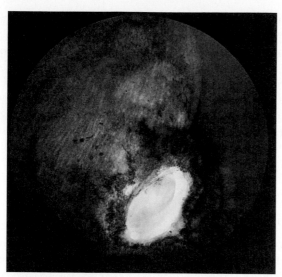

Figure 33–20

Great horned owl fundus with a healed pellet hole in the posterior sclera.

compare the fundus appearance with that of the normal fellow eye.

Treatment

Treat acute traumatic retinopathy and/or optic neuropathy systemically with broad-spectrum antibiotics and anti-inflammatory doses of corticosteroids. Prescribe specific systemic antibiotic therapy for septicemic chorioretinitis. Retinal tears and detachments are not operable. If retinal detachment is the result of inflammatory choroidal effusion, reattachment may occur after systemic corticosteroid therapy. Glaucomatous optic atrophy is usually present and is irreversible when avian glaucoma is suspected or confirmed.

Prevention

Promptly diagnose and treat septicemia and posterior uveitis. Prevent or minimize traumatic incidents.

Blindness With Normal Pupil Sizes and Responses

Etiology

Central nervous system lesions above the lateral geniculate body may be the result of malformations,

trauma, infections (bacterial, viral, parasitic, fungal), toxic effects, and neoplasia. Reversible blindness has been reported in budgerigars as a result of lead and hexachlorophene toxicoses.[21]

Clinical Signs

Variable unilateral or bilateral blindness with normal resting pupil sizes and pupillary light responses characterize central lesions. Additional major or minor neurologic signs may be evident, including disorientation, seizures, abnormal behavior, coma, and others.

Diagnosis

Perform complete neurologic, physical, and ocular examinations. Pursue systemic disease evaluation if indicated.

Treatment

Treat specific systemic disease, if possible. Consider systemic anti-inflammatory corticosteroid therapy, especially immediately after trauma. Implement attentive nursing and supportive care. Prognosis for functional improvement and survival is usually guarded but may not necessarily be hopeless, especially after trauma.

Prevention

Minimize handling and environmentally associated trauma. Base other recommendations upon associated systemic disease, if present.

THE EAR

Anatomy

As in mammals, the ear in birds is the organ of hearing and balance and is composed of external, middle, and inner parts. The external ear lacks a pinna, the middle ear has only one bony ossicle instead of three as in mammals, and the auditory portion of the inner ear lacks a coiled cochlea duct, represented instead by a short lagena.[4]

The external ear opening is hidden by feathers. The surrounding skin is loose and can be drawn forward by a dermo-osseous muscle dorsal to the meatus. When the skin is drawn forward, the oval meatus narrows to a vertical slit. The auditory canal extends obliquely downward and backward; the external orifice lies rostral and dorsal to the tympanum. A bony shelf projects from the dorsal wall of the canal and appears to block easy access to the tympanum.[4]

The middle ear cavity with its columella bone and extracolumella cartilage transmits sound vibrations from the tympanum to the vestibular window of the inner ear. Auditory tubes connect the middle ears with the pharynx, opening into a common median ostium rather than by an orifice on either side of the nasopharynx as in mammals.[4]

The inner ear consists of three semicircular ducts within bony canals with associated ampullae, connected to the sacculus, utriculus, cochlear duct, and lagena (Fig. 33–21). The eighth cranial nerve receives both vestibular and auditory sensory fibers.[4]

Auditory abilities of the canary and budgerigar have been investigated.[150, 151]

Hearing

Most birds approach the levels of discrimination of simple sounds found for humans and other mammals. However, pitch discrimination is restricted to a narrower range in birds, with less sensitivity to higher and lower tones.[152] Temporal resolution is approximately 10 times faster than in man; individual notes of songbirds are not discernible to man unless the song is slowed.[152] With the exception of nocturnal birds, birds are capable of locating sound sources roughly equivalent to this ability in humans. In contrast, the acuity of sound localization of the barn owl surpasses that of any terrestrial mammal tested thus far.[152] In addition, the ear position in owls is asymmetrical, allowing one ear to be more sensitive to sounds below the horizontal plane, and the other sensitive to sounds above the horizontal plane. Most birds cannot hear ultrasonic vibrations, but some nocturnal species use echo location, producing short pulses of 4 to 8 kHz. These sounds, audible to man, are used for obstacle location during flight. Penguins also appear to hunt by echo location while underwater.[152] Vocal learning and the development of specific vocalizations (songs) are prominent among many species. Psychoacoustic tests have determined some sex differences in perception of vocal signals.[153]

Clinical Problems

Clinical problems with the ear in birds are uncommon.

Otitis Externa

Etiology

Inflammation of the ear canal is occasionally seen in birds. Bacterial infection is most often implicated, although fungal infections are possible. Squamous cell carcinoma originating from the external ear canal has been seen in a Quaker parrot.*

Clinical Signs

Pruritus is usually present, with the bird scratching at the ear canal with its claws or rubbing its head against the perch. A serous to purulent discharge may be noted, and the soft tissue around the ear canal is inflamed and swollen. Feathers may be missing or matted with discharge around the opening of the ear canal.

Diagnosis

Swab the ear canal for cytology and Gram's staining of the exudate. Submit a sample of exudate for bacterial and/or fungal culture and sensitivity testing. If a mass is present, submit a biopsy sample for histopathologic examination.

Treatment

Use topical antibiotic or antifungal solutions applied two to three times daily into the ear canal. Avoid products containing corticosteroids; ophthalmic antimicrobial preparations without steroids are convenient to use. Excise soft tissue masses under anesthesia using sharp dissection or, preferably, electrosurgery.

---

*Quesenberry K, personal communication.

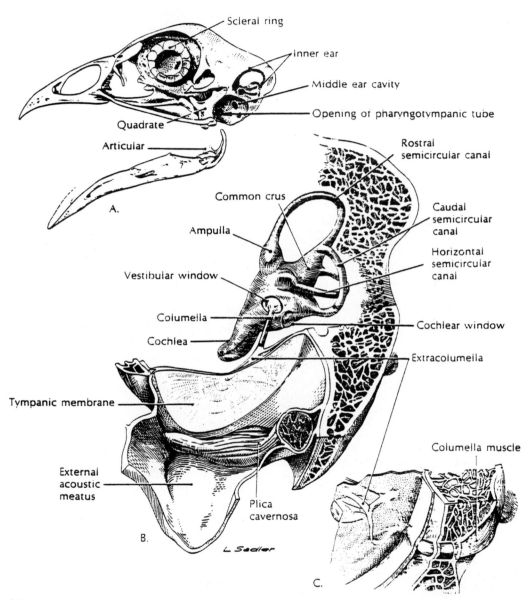

Figure 33–21

Ear schematic. (From Evans HE: Anatomy of the budgerigar. In Petrak ML [ed]: Diseases of Cage and Aviary Birds, ed 2. Philadelphia, Lea & Febiger, 1969.)

Otitis Media and Interna

Etiology

Septicemia may cause otitis media and interna.[154] *Pseudomonas aeruginosa* infection was reported in an African grey parrot.[155] Chronic *Pasteurella multocida* infection is a frequent cause in poultry.[156] Other causes of otitis media and interna are poorly characterized. Vascular or cardiac disease with associated anemia, drug overdosage, and possible dietary deficiencies have been incriminated.[21] Harvest mites of the family Trombiculidae may enter the auditory canal and cause vertigo.[21] Cranial trauma may cause hemorrhage or inflammation.[45]

Clinical Signs

Torticollis, loss of balance, and inability to fly may be evident. If the condition is bilateral, deafness may be noted.

Diagnosis

Examine the external ear and canal as completely as possible. Perform a complete physical examination. Consider a hemogram and skull radiography to evaluate tympanic bullae.

Treatment

Consider broad-spectrum systemic antibiotic therapy for suspected bacterial otitis media and interna. Provide supportive care.

Prevention

Identify and treat septicemia early. Minimize opportunities for self- and environmentally-induced head trauma.

Hemorrhage from the Ear

Etiology

Benign neoplasia of unspecified type was reported to be the cause of hemorrhage in one Amazon parrot.[157] Head trauma may damage the external canal or tympanum and result in hemorrhage.

Clinical Signs

Acute or chronic bleeding from the external meatus is present, with or without signs of vestibular dysfunction.

Diagnosis

Diagnostic measures are the same as for otitis media and interna.

Treatment

The benign neoplasm reported was successfully removed by fulguration.[157] Consider broad-spectrum antibiotic therapy.

Prevention

Minimize opportunities for head trauma.

TASTE AND SMELL

Birds have relatively few taste buds but are capable of some taste discrimination.[21] Taste buds are primarily confined to regions of epithelium that are glandular and noncornified. The taste buds lie on the base of the tongue and the roof and floor of the oropharynx. Presumably, disorders involving the oral cavity may affect taste.

The sense of smell is generally poorly developed in birds. The olfactory bulbs of seedeating birds are quite small.[21]

Problems with taste and smell cannot be directly assessed clinically. Oropharyngeal disorders probably do cause dysfunction, and this may contribute to anorexia associated with some systemic diseases.

References

1. Duke-Elder SS: The eyes of birds. In The Eye in Evolution, vol. 1. London, Henry Kimpton, 1958, pp 401–428.
2. Murphy CJ, Dubielzig RR: The gross and microscopic structure of the golden eagle (*Aquila chrysaetos*) eye. Prog Vet Comp Ophthal 3(2):74–79, 1993.
3. Murphy CJ: Raptor ophthalmology. Compendium on Continuing Education for the Practicing Veterinarian 9(3):241–259, 1987.
4. Evans HE: Anatomy of the budgerigar. In Petrak ML (ed): Diseases of Cage and Aviary Birds. Philadelphia, Lea & Febiger, 1969, pp 45–112.

5. Walsh MT: Clinical manifestations of cervicocephalic air sacs of psittacines. Compendium on Continuing Education for the Practicing Veterinarian 6(9):783–792, 1984.

6. Phillips AF, Clubb SL: Psittacine neonatal development. In Schubot MM, Clubb KJ, Clubb SL (eds): Psittacine Aviculture. Loxahatchee, Fl, Aviculture and Breeding Center, 1992, pp 12–1 to 12–26.

7. Fix AS, Arp LH: Conjunctiva-associated lymphoid tissue (CALT) in normal and *Bordetella avium*-infected turkeys. Vet Pathol 26:222–230, 1989.

8. Fix AS, Lawrence HA: Morphologic characterization of conjunctiva-associated lymphoid tissue in chickens. Am J Vet Res 52(11):1852–1859, 1991.

9. Oliphant LW, Johnson MR, Murphy CJ, Howland H: The musculature and pupillary response of the great horned owl iris. Exp Eye Res 37:583–595, 1983.

10. Oliphant LW: Pteridines and purines as major pigments of the avian iris. Pigment Cell Res 1(2):129–131, 1987.

11. Murphy CJ: Ocular lesions in birds of prey. In Fowler ME (ed): Zoo and Wild Animal Medicine. Current Therapy, ed 3. Philadelphia, WB Saunders, 1993, pp 211–220.

12. Levine J: Consensual pupillary responses in birds. Science 122:690, 1955.

13. Murphy CJ, Howland HC: Owl eyes: Accommodation, corneal curvature, and refractive state. J Comp Physiol 151:277–284, 1983.

14. Waldvogel JA: The bird's eye view. Am Sci 78:342–353, 1990.

15. Wood CA: The Fundus Oculi of Birds Especially as Viewed by the Ophthalmoscope. Chicago, Lakeside Press, 1917, p 181.

16. Brach V: The functional significance of the avian pecten: A review. Condor 79:321–327, 1977.

17. Braekevelt CR: Fine structure of the pecten of the pigeon (*Columba livia*). Ophthalmology (Basel) 196:151–159, 1988.

18. Bellhorn RW: Ophthalmologic disorders of exotic and laboratory animals. Vet Clin North Am 3:345–356, 1973.

19. Davidson MG: Ophthalmology of exotic pets. Compendium on Continuing Education for the Practicing Veterinarian 7(9):724–736, 1985.

20. Greenwood AG, Barnett KC: The investigation of visual defects in raptors. In Recent Advances in the Study of Raptor Diseases. West Yorkshire, Chiron Publications, 1981, p 131.

21. Small E, Burke TJ: Diseases of the organs of special sense. In Petrak ML (ed): Diseases of Cage and Aviary Birds, ed 2. Philadelphia, Lea & Febiger, 1982, pp 491–496.

22. Verschueren CP, Lumey JT: Mydriasis in pigeons (*Columba livia domestica*) with d-tubocurarine: Topical instillation versus intracameral injection. J Vet Pharmacol Ther 14:206–208, 1991.

23. Mikaelian I, Paillet I, Williams D: Comparative use of various mydriatic drugs in kestrels (*Falco tinnunculus*). Am J Vet Res 55(2):270–272, 1994.

24. Davis GS, Siopes TD, Peiffer RL, Cook C: Morphologic changes induced by photoperiod in eyes of turkey poults. Am J Vet Res 47(4):953–955, 1986.

25. Korbel R: Tonometry in avian ophthalmology. Proc VIII Symp Avian Dis, University of Munich, March, 1992, pp 281–291.

26. Schmidt V, Seidel B: Augenkrankheiten der Vogel. In Augenkrankheiten der Haustiere. VEB Gustav Fischer Verlag Jena Publishers, 1988, pp 237–261.

27. Kern TJ, Murphy CJ, Heck WR: Partial upper eyelid agenesis in a peregrine falcon. J Am Vet Med Assoc 187:1207, 1985.

28. Buyukmihci NC, Murphy CJ, Paul-Murphy J, Hacker DV: Eyelid malformation in four cockatiels. J Am Vet Med Assoc 196(9):1490–1492, 1990.

29. Flach M, Dausch D, Wegner W: Augenanomalien bei Zebrafinken. Kleiner-Prax 25:505–509, 1980.

30. Mustaffa-Babjee A: Specific and nonspecific conditions affecting avian eyes. Vet Bull 10:681, 1969.

31. Buyukmihci NC, Murphy CJ, Schulz T: Developmental ocular disease of raptors. J Wildl Dis 24:207–213, 1988.

32. Takatsuji K, Sato Y, Lizuka S, et al: Animal model of closed angle glaucoma in albino mutant quails. Invest Ophthalmol Vis Sci 27(3):396–400, 1986.

33. Takatsuji K, Tohyama M, Sato Y, Nakamura A: Selective loss of retinal ganglion cells in albino avian glaucoma. Invest Ophthalmol Vis Sci 29(6):901–909, 1988.

34. de Kater AW, Smyth JR, Rosenquist RC, Epstein DL: The slate turkey: A model for secondary angle closure glaucoma. Invest Ophthalmol Vis Sci 27(12):1751–1754, 1986.

35. Smith ME, Becker B, Podos S: Light-induced angle-closure in the domestic fowl. Invest Ophthalmol 8:213–221, 1969.

36. Ashton WL, Pattison M, Barnett KC: Light-induced eye abnormalities in turkeys and the turkey blindness syndrome. Res Vet Sci 14(1):42–46, 1973.

37. Kinnear A, Lauber JK, Boyd TA: Genesis of light-induced avian glaucoma. Invest Ophthalmol 13(11):872–875, 1974.

38. Paul-Murphy JR, Lowenstine L, Turrel JM, Murphy CJ: Malignant lymphoreticular neoplasm in an African gray parrot. J Am Vet Med Assoc 187:1216–1217, 1985.

39. Rambow VJ, Murphy JC, Fox JG: Malignant lymphoma in a pigeon. J Am Vet Med Assoc 179:1266–1268, 1981.

40. Dukes TW, Pettit JR: Avian ocular neoplasia—a description of spontaneously occurring cases. Can J Comp Med 47:33–36, 1983.

41. Arnall L: Anesthesia and surgery in cage and aviary birds. II. A regional outline of surgical conditions. Vet Rec 73:173–178, 1961.

42. Arnall L: Anesthesia and surgery in cage and aviary birds. III. A systematic outline of surgical conditions. Vet Rec 73:188–192, 1961.

43. Blackmore DK, Cooper JE: Diseases of the endocrine system. In Petrak ML (ed): Diseases of Cage and Aviary Birds, ed 2. Philadelphia, Lea & Febiger, 1982, p 479.

44. Schmidt RE, Becker LL, McElroy JM: Malignant intraocular medulloepithelioma in two cockatiels. J Am Vet Med Assoc 189(2):1105–1106, 1986.

45. Paul-Murphy JR, Kobleh PD, Stern B, Penninck DG: Psittacine skull radiography: Anatomy, radiographic technique, and patient application. Vet Radiol 21(4):218–224, 1990.

46. Murphy CJ, Brooks DE, Kern TJ, et al: Enucleation in birds of prey. J Am Vet Med Assoc 183(11):1234–1237, 1983.

47. Neumann U, Kummerfield N: Implantation of an ocular prosthesis in a gray parrot. Tierarztl Prax 11(2):195–199, 1983.

48. Shimakura S, Sawa H, Yamashita T, Hirai K: An outbreak of ocular disease caused by staphylococcal infection in Amazon parrots (*Amazona aestiva*) imported into Japan. Jpn J Vet Sci 43:273–275, 1981.

49. Cheville NF, Tappe J, Ackermann M, Jensen A: Acute fibrinopurulent blepharitis and conjunctivitis associated with *Staphylococcus hyicus*, *Escherichia coli*, and *Streptococcus* sp. in chickens and turkeys. Vet Pathol 25:369–375, 1988.

50. Olson LD: Ophthalmia in turkeys infected with *Pasteurella multocida*. Avian Dis 25(2):423–430, 1980.

51. Hacking MA, Sileo L: Isolation of a hemolytic *Actinobacillus* from waterfowl. J Wildl Dis 13:69–73, 1977.

52. Tully TN, Carter TD: Bilateral supraorbital abscesses associ-

ated with sinusitis in an orange-winged Amazon parrot (*Amazona amazonica*). J Assoc Avian Vet 7(3):157–158, 1993.

53. Davidson WR, Kellogg FE, Doster GL: An epornitic of avian pox in wild bobwhite quail. J Wildl Dis 16(2):283–297, 1980.

54. Poonacha KB, Wilson M: Avian pox in pen-raised bobwhite quail. J Am Vet Med Assoc 179:1264, 1981.

55. Al Falluji MM, Tantawi HH, Al-bana A, Sheikhly S: Pox infection among captive peacocks. J Wildl Dis 15(4):597–600, 1979.

56. Dodd K: Pox in racing pigeons. Vet Rec 95:41–43, 1974.

57. Montgomery RD, Chowdhury KA: Avian pox in a whistling swan. J Am Vet Med Assoc 177:930–931, 1980.

58. MacDonald SE, Lowenstine LJ, Ardans AA: Avian pox in blue-fronted Amazon parrots. J Am Vet Med Assoc 179:1218, 1981.

59. Johnson BJ, Castro AE: Canary pox causing high mortality in an aviary. J Am Vet Med Assoc 189:1345–1347, 1986.

60. Bigland CH, Whenham GR, Graesser FE: A pox-like infection in canaries—report of an outbreak. Can Vet J 3:347, 1962.

61. Cavill JP: Canary pox—report of an outbreak in roller canaries. Vet Rec 76:463, 1964.

62. Panigrahy B, Senne DA: Diseases of mynahs. J Am Vet Med Assoc 199(3):378–381, 1991.

63. Emanuelson S, Carney J, Saito J: Avian pox in two black-masked conures. J Am Vet Med Assoc 173(9):1249–1250, 1978.

64. Graham DD, Halliwell WH: Viral diseases of birds of prey. In Fowler ME (ed): Zoo and Wild Animal Medicine. Philadelphia, WB Saunders, 1981, p 260.

65. Millichamp NJ: Exotic animal ophthalmology. In Gelatt KN (ed): Veterinary Ophthalmology, ed 2. Philadelphia, Lea & Febiger, 1991, pp 680–705.

66. Ensley PK, Anderson MP, Costello ML, et al: Epornitic of avian pox in a zoo. J Am Vet Med Assoc 173:1111, 1978.

67. Jacobson ER, Mladinich CR, Clubb S, et al: Papilloma-like virus infection in an African gray parrot. J Am Vet Med Assoc 183(11):1307–1308, 1983.

68. Gough RE: Goose parvovirus infection. In Calnek BW (ed): Diseases of Poultry, ed 9. Ames, Iowa State University Press, 1991, pp 684–690.

69. Tsai SS, Park JH, Hirai K, Hakura C: Eye lesions in pet birds. Pathology 22:95–112, 1993.

70. Arnall L, Keymer IF: Bird Diseases. Neptune City, TFH Publications, 1975, pp 164–168.

71. Koschmann JR: Vitamin A deficiency in caged birds. Texas Vet Med J 48:25, 1986.

72. Zwart B: Vitamin A deficiency in parrots. XXI Intl. Symp. Uber die Erkrankungen der Zootiere. Berlin, Academie-Verlag, 1979.

73. Dorrestein GM, Zwart P: Practical aspects of vitamin A-deficiency in parrots and cockatoos. Proc Voorjaarsdagen Netherlands Sm Anim Vet Assoc, Amsterdam, 1980, pp 142–146.

74. Konstantinov A: A contribution to the pathomorphology of vitamin A deficiency in chickens. Zentralbl Veterinarmed [A] 19:407–416, 1972.

75. Brightman AH, Burke TJ: Eyelid tumor in a parakeet. Mod Vet Pract 59:683, 1978.

76. Sacré BJ, Oppenheim YV, Steinberg H, Gould WJ: Presumptive histiocytic sarcoma in a great horned owl. J Zoo Wildl Med 23(1):113–121, 1992.

77. Patnaik GM, Mohanty D: A case of avian mastocytoma. Indian Vet J 47(4):298–303, 1970.

78. Hochleitner M: Cystadenoma in an African grey parrot (*Psittacus erythacus*). J Assoc Avian Vet 4(3):163–166, 1990.

79. Murphy CJ, Bellhorn RW, Buyukmihci NC: Subconjunctival hibernoma in a goose. J Am Vet Med Assoc 189(9):1109–1110, 1986.

80. Riddell C, Roepke D: Inflammation of the nasal gland in domestic turkeys. Avian Dis 35:982–985, 1991.

81. Karpinski LG, Clubb SL: Post pox ocular problems in blue-fronted Amazon and blue-headed pionus parrots. Proc Assoc Avian Vet, Boulder, CO, 1985, p 91.

82. Karpinski LG, Clubb SL: Clinical aspects of ophthalmology in caged birds. In Current Veterinary Therapy IX. Philadelphia, WB Saunders, 1986, pp 616–621.

83. Zenoble RD, Griffith RW, Clubb SL: Survey of bacteriologic flora of conjunctiva and cornea in healthy psittacine birds. Am J Vet Res 44:1966–1967, 1983.

84. Wolf ED, Amass K, Olsen J: Survey of conjunctival flora in the eye of clinically normal, captive exotic birds. J Am Vet Med Assoc 183(11):1232–1234, 1983.

85. Gylstorff I, Grimm F: Vogel-krankheiten. Stuttgart, Verlag Engen Ulmer, 1987, pp 267–275.

86. Desmidt M, Ducatelle R, Uyttebroeck E, et al: Cytomegalovirus-like conjunctivitis in Australian Finches. J Am Avian Vet 5(3):130–136, 1991.

87. Vickers MC, Hartley WJ, Mason RW, et al: Blindness associated with toxoplasmosis in canaries. J Am Vet Med Assoc 200(11):1723–1725, 1992.

88. Surman PG, Schultz DJ, Tham VL: Keratoconjunctivitis and chlamydiosis in cage birds. Aust Vet J 50:356–362, 1974.

89. Farmer H, Chalmers WSK, Coolcock PR: *Chlamydia psittaci* isolated from the eyes of domestic ducks (*Anas platyrhynchos*) with conjunctivitis and rhinitis. Vet Rec 110(59):346–347, 1982.

90. Yoder HW, Yamamoto R, Kleven SH, Rowland GN: Mycoplasmosis. In Calnek BW (ed): Diseases of Poultry, ed 9. Ames, Iowa State University Press, 1991, pp 196–235.

91. Yamamoto R: Infectious coryza. In Calnek BW (ed): Diseases of Poultry, ed 9. Ames, Iowa State University Press, 1991, pp 186–195.

92. Calnek BW: Diseases of Poultry, ed 9. Ames, Iowa State University Press, 1991.

93. Randall CJ: Conjunctivitis in pheasants associated with cryptosporidial infection. Vet Rec 118:211, 1986.

94. Mason RW: Conjunctival cryptosporidiosis in a duck. Avian Dis 30:598–600, 1986.

95. Mason RW, Hartley JW: Respiratory cryptosporidiosis in a peacock chick. Avian Dis 24:771–776, 1980.

96. Current WL: Cryptosporidiosis in turkeys. In Calnek BW (ed): Diseases of Poultry, ed 9. Ames, Iowa State University Press, 1991, pp 801–802.

97. Hood HB: Eye pathology in an adult male ostrich (*Struthio camelus*). Proc Am Assoc Zoo Vet, 1978.

98. Maddux RL, Cgengappa MM, McLaughlin BG: Isolation of *Actinobacillus suis* from a Canada goose (*Branta canadensis*). J Wildl Dis 23:483, 1987.

99. Greve JH: Parasitic diseases. In Fowler ME (ed): Zoo and Wild Animal Medicine. Philadelphia, WB Saunders, 1981, p 233.

100. Schmidt RE, Toft JD: Ophthalmic lesions in animals from a zoologic collection. J Wildl Dis 17(2):267–275 1981.

101. Greve JH, Harrison CJ: Conjunctivitis caused by eye flukes in captive-raised ostriches. J Am Vet Med Assoc 177:909, 1980.

102. Nollen PM, Murray HD: *Philophthalmus gralli:* Identification, growth characteristics and treatment of an oriental eye fluke of birds introduced into the continental United States. J Parasitol 64:178, 1978.

103. Brooks DE, Greiner EC, Walsh MT: Conjunctivitis caused by *Thelazia* sp. in a Senegal parrot. J Am Vet Med Assoc 183:1305, 1983.

104. Egyed MN, Shlosberg A, Eilat A, Malkinson M: Chronic lesions in geese photosensitized by *Ammi majus*. Avian Dis 19(4):822–827, 1975.

105. Riddell C: Vesicular dermatitis and photosensitization. In Calnek BW (ed): Diseases of Poultry, ed 9. Ames, Iowa State University Press, 1991, p 854.

106. Murphy CJ, Kern TJ, McKeever K, et al: Ocular lesions in free-ranging raptors. J Am Vet Med Assoc 181:1302, 1982.

107. Murphy CJ, Kern TJ, MacCoy DM: Bilateral keratopathy in a barred owl. J Am Vet Med Assoc 179:1271, 1981.

108. Dubielzig RR, Murphy CJ, Kern TJ, et al: Corneal lipoidal degeneration in aged falcons. Vet Pathol 29(5):468, 1992.

109. Thomas-Baker B: Ivermectin as a treatment for ocular nematodiasis in birds. Proc Am Assoc Zoo Vet, Chicago, 1986, p 99.

110. Clark CH: Pharmacology of antibiotics. In Harrison GJ, Harrison LR (eds): Clinical Avian Medicine and Surgery. Philadelphia, WB Saunders, 1986, p 323.

111. Murphy CJ, Kern TJ, Riis RC: Intraocular trauma in a red-tailed hawk. J Am Vet Med Assoc 181(11):1390–1391, 1982.

112. Lindley DM, Hatchcock JT, Miller WM, DiPinto MN: Fractured scleral ossicles in a red-tailed hawk. Vet Radiol 29:209, 1988.

113. Barber CW, Blow WL: A genetic influence on cataract formation among white leghorn incrosses following an outbreak of avian encephalomyelitis. Avian Dis 7:495–500, 1963.

114. Bridges CH, Flowers AI: Iridocyclitis and cataracts associated with an encephalomyelitis in chickens. J Am Vet Med Assoc Jan. 132:79–84, 1958.

115. Rigdon RH: Cataracts in chickens with lymphomatosis. Am J Vet Res 20:647–654, 1959.

116. Silva EN, Hipolito D, Grecchi R: Natural and experimental *Salmonella arizonae* 18:74, 732 (Ar. Til, 7,8) infection in broilers. Bacteriological and histopathological survey of eye and brain lesions. Avian Dis 24:631–636, 1980.

117. Power J, Jordan FT: Unilateral enlargement of the eye in chicks infected with a strain of *M. gallisepticum*. Vet Rec 99(6):102–103, 1976.

118. More EN: *Aspergillus fumigatus* as a cause of ophthalmitis in turkeys. Poult Sci 32:796–799, 1953.

119. Crispin SM, Barnett KC: Ocular candidiasis in ornamental ducks. Avian Pathol 7:49–59, 1978.

120. Schmidt RE: Hypermature cataract in a crested mynah, *Leucospar rothschildi*. J Wildl Dis 19:158–159, 1983.

121. Anderson GA, Buyukmihci N: Phacoanaphylactic endophthalmitis in an owl. Vet Pathol 20:776–778, 1983.

122. Miller WH, Boosinger TR, Maslin WR: Granulomatous uveitis in an owl. J Am Vet Med Assoc 193:365, 1988.

123. Fite KV, Montgomery N, Whitney T, et al: Inherited retinal degeneration and ocular amelanosis in the domestic chicken *(Gallus domesticus)*. Curr Eye Res 2(2):109–115, 1982.

124. Fournier GA, Albert DM, Bachrach A, Lamping KA: Symbol of Boston's Museum of Science: An eye tumor. N Engl J Med 308:782–783, 1983.

125. Keymer IF: Cataracts in birds. Avian Pathol 6:335–341, 1977.

126. Slatter DH, Bradley JS, Vales B, et al: Hereditary cataracts in canaries. J Am Vet Med Assoc 183:872–874, 1983.

127. Barr BC, Murphy CJ, Yan Ghazihaneen G, Bellhorn RW: Cataracts and optic nerve hypoplasia in turkey poults. Avian Dis 32:469–477, 1988.

128. Chmielewski N, Render JA, Schwartz L, et al: Spontaneous cataract and crooked toes in Brahma chickens. Avian Dis 37(4):1151–1157, 1993.

129. Moore CP, Pickett JP, Beehler B: Extracapsular extraction of senile cataract in an Andean condor. J Am Vet Med Assoc 187:1211–1214, 1985.

130. Clubb SL, Karpinski L: Aging in macaws. J Assoc Avian Vet 7(1):31–33, 1993.

131. Krehbiel JD: Cataracts in bobwhite quail. J Am Vet Med Assoc 161:634–637, 1972.

132. Critchley KL, Tham VL: Cataracts in a chicken flock. Aust Vet J 60:223–224, 1983.

133. Rigdon RH, Ferguson TM, Couch JR: Spontaneous cataracts in turkeys. Am J Vet Res 20:961–965, 1959.

134. Brooks DE, Murphy CJ, Quesenberry KE, Walsh HT: Surgical correction of a luxated cataractous lens in a barred owl. J Am Vet Med Assoc 183:1298–1299, 1983.

135. Kern TJ, Murphy CJ, Riis RC: Lens extraction by phacoemulsification in two raptors. J Am Vet Med Assoc 185:1403–1406, 1984.

136. Hacker DV, Shifrin M: Cataract extraction in a mandarin duck. J Am Anim Hosp Assoc 24:679–682, 1988.

137. Van Niekerk WH, Petrick SW: Unilateral lentectomy in a black-shouldered kite. J S Afr Vet Assoc 61(3):124–125, 1990.

138. Dukes TW, Fox GA: Blindness associated with retinal dysplasia in a prairie falcon, *Falco mexicanus*. J Wildl Dis 19:66–69, 1983.

139. Buyukmihci NC: Lesions of the ocular posterior segment of raptors. J Am Vet Med Assoc 187:1121–1124, 1985.

140. Murphy CJ, Buyukmihci NC, Bellhorn RW, et al: Retinal dysplasia in a hybrid falcon. J Am Vet Med Assoc 187:1208, 1985.

141. Randall CJ, Wilson MA, Pollock BJ, et al: Partial retinal dysplasia and subsequent degeneration in a mutant strain of domestic fowl (rdd). Exp Eye Res 37:337–347, 1983.

142. Ulshafer RJ, Allen CB: Ultrastructural changes in the retinal pigment epithelium of congenitally blind chickens. Curr Eye Res 4(10):1009–1021, 1985.

143. Ulshafer RJ, Allen C, Dawson WW, Wolf ED: Hereditary retinal degeneration in the Rhode Island red chicken. Exp Eye Res 39:125–135, 1984.

144. Randall CJ, McLachlan I: Retinopathy in commercial layers. Vet Rec 105:41–42, 1979.

145. Curtis PE, Baker JR, Curtis R, Johnston A: Impaired vision in chickens associated with retinal defects. Vet Rec 120:113–114, 1987.

146. Cheng KM, Schoffner RN, Gelatt KN, et al: An autosomal recessive blind mutant in the chicken. Poult Sci 59:2179–2182, 1980.

147. Tudor DC, Yard C: Retinal atrophy in a parakeet. Vet Med Small Anim Clin 73:85, 1978.

148. Randall CJ, Bygrave AC, McLachlan I, Bickwell SR: Retinal detachment in the pheasant *(Phasianus colchicus)*. Avian Pathol 15:687–695, 1986.

149. Curtis-Velasco M: Pituitary adenoma in a cockatiel *(Nymphicus hollandicus)*. J Assoc Avian Vet 6(1):21–22, 1992.

150. Dooling RJ, Mulligan JA, Miller JD: Auditory sensitivity and song spectrum of the common canary *(Serinus canarius)*. J Acoust Soc Am 50(2):700–709, 1971.

151. Dooling RJ, Saunders JC: Hearing in the parakeet *(Melopsittacus undulatus)*:absolute thresholds, critical ratios, frequency difference limens, and vocalizations. J Comp Physiol Psychol 88(1):1–20, 1975.

152. King AS, McLelland J: Special sense organs. In King AS, McLelland J (eds): Birds, Their Structure and Function. Philadelphia, Ballière-Tindall, 1984, pp 284–314.

153. Dooling RJ: Hearing in birds. In Webster DB, Fay RR,

Popper A (eds): The Evolutionary Biology of Hearing. New York, Springer-Verlag, 1992, pp 545–560.

154. Arnall L, Keymer IF: Anatomy and physiology. In Bird Disease. London, TFH Publications, 1976, pp 19–77.

155. Munger LL, Pledger T: *Pseudomonas* infection of the middle ear. Proc Assoc Avian Vet, Nashville, 1993, pp 254–255.

156. Olsen LD: Gross and histopathological description of the cranial form of chronic fowl cholera in turkeys. Avian Dis 10:518–529, 1966.

157. Harrison GJ: Selected surgical procedures. In Harrison GJ, Harrison LR (eds): Clinical Avian Medicine and Surgery. Philadelphia, WB Saunders, 1986, p 381.

Robert E. Schmidt
Katherine Quesenberry

34

Neoplasia

Robert E. Schmidt

Neoplastic Diseases

A wide variety of neoplastic diseases is seen in pet avian species. Often presenting as masses or space-occupying lesions, their gross appearance is varied and must be differentiated from non-neoplastic proliferative conditions. For a systemic differential approach to the diagnosis of these conditions, a variety of techniques, including physical examination, clinical laboratory tests, radiographs, and cytologic and biopsy examinations, should be used. This section reviews the differential diagnosis of neoplastic diseases by organ system of occurrence. For an extensive reference list on neoplasia in pet birds, published articles[1] should be consulted.

TUMORS OF THE SKIN AND SUBCUTIS

Epithelial

With the exception of viral-induced papillomas,[2] the specific etiology of epithelial tumors is not known. Although several tumor types may occur anywhere in the skin, others are localized by virtue of their cell of origin, which can be a diagnostic consideration. Aspiration or impression cytologic examination can be used to differentiate epithelial neoplasia from non-neoplastic diseases, but biopsy provides the most reliable diagnostic tool. Treatment for external tumors includes surgery, cryosurgery, radiation, and possibly chemotherapy.[3]

Papillomas may occur anywhere in the skin and usually present with a narrow base. Trauma can lead to superficial necrosis and crust formation. Be-

nign tumors of basal cell origin (epitheliomas) are also occasionally seen. These neoplasms must usually be differentiated from follicular cysts by biopsy. Adenomas and carcinomas of the uropygial gland are localized to the pygostyle region, and present as variably sized masses that may be superficially ulcerated. Gross appearance of carcinomas shows more infiltration and less well-differentiated margins. The primary differential diagnoses are squamous cell carcinoma, adenitis of the uropygial gland, or vitamin A deficiency leading to glandular metaplasia and hyperkeratosis. Primary diagnostic methods are cytologic examination and biopsy of the lesion.

Otic gland carcinomas are unusual; their appearance is of a proliferative lesion in the ear canal. Depending on the age of the lesion, there is a variable degree of necrosis and destruction of normal tissue (see Chapter 33, Special Senses). These tumors may be invasive, and radiographic evidence of bone destruction may be present. Granulomatous otitis is a primary differential diagnosis, with biopsy of the lesion usually needed for conclusive differentiation.

Basal and squamous cell carcinomas can occur anywhere in the skin. They are usually broad-based masses, often with central areas of ulceration (Fig. 34–1). Tumor margins may not be distinct. Highly anaplastic squamous tumors can contain large amounts of scirrhous connective tissue stroma, which can cause cytologic confusion with mesenchymal tumors. Biopsy is the diagnostic method of choice.

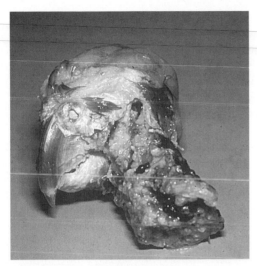

Figure 34–1

Squamous cell carcinoma involving the face with formation of a large necrotic mass.

A common non-neoplastic problem of the skin of birds is follicular cyst formation (Fig. 34–2). Cysts are circumscribed lesions that must be differentiated from benign epithelial tumors and bacterially induced abscesses. Follicular cysts usually contain keratin, which grossly is yellow-white and can appear caseous, resembling the material seen in avian abscesses. Negative culture results may indicate that the lesion is not a primary infection, but positive culture results may not be meaningful because fol-

licular cysts can become secondarily infected. Granulomatous lesions may be the result of bacteria, fungi, foreign body penetration, or idiosyncratic reactions to vaccination. Primary methods for differential diagnoses include culture and biopsy.

Mesenchymal

Various mesenchymal tumors have been reported in pet birds. With some exceptions, exact diagnosis is difficult without histologic examination. These tumors appear as firm or soft swelling; cytologic examination often can only characterize the lesion as being of mesenchymal origin.

Lipomas are characterized grossly as lumps of fat. They are seen in all species, but are more common in budgerigars (Fig. 34–3).[4] Differential diagnoses include liposarcomas, but the latter are usually firmer and more infiltrative. Liposarcomas are rarely reported.[5]

Fibrosarcomas are commonly reported tumors[6]; however, in the author's experience, fibromas are less often seen. Both tumors present as firm masses that are usually gray-white on cut-section (Fig. 34–4). The borders of sarcomas are irregular. Fibrosarcomas have a moderate to high potential for recur-

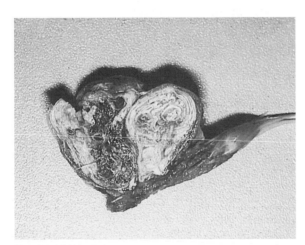

Figure 34–2

Benign feather cyst in a canary. The central caseous-appearing material has a laminated appearance that suggests keratin.

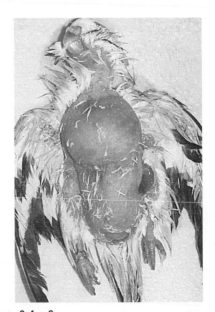

Figure 34–3

Common presentation of subcutaneous lipoma in a budgerigar.

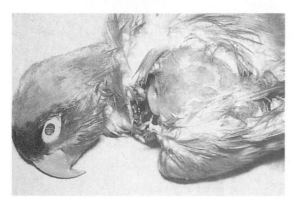

F i g u r e 3 4 – 4

Large fibrosarcoma of the shoulder of a lovebird. Overlying feather loss is present. (From Schmidt RE: Morphologic diagnosis of avian neoplasms. Semin Avian Exotic Pet Med 1(2):74, 1992.)

rence, and occasionally metastasis is seen. They can occur in any location on the body.

Hemangiomas are more common than hemangiosarcomas. Benign vascular tumors are usually circumscribed, dark red-black masses found in the skin and subcutis (Fig. 34–5). Grossly, a primary differential diagnosis is melanoma. Hemangiosarcomas are not often grossly distinctive, particularly more anaplastic tumors. These neoplasms are found in the skin and subcutis, and may also be present in bone, with a variable amount of bone lysis seen radiographically. Their gross appearance varies from firm and gray-red to softer dark red masses somewhat similar to hemangiomas.

Neoplasia of the lymphatic vessels is not reported in pet birds. The author has seen only one case that morphologically appeared to be a lymphangioma. At gross examination, the tumor was not specific, and the diagnosis was made based on numerous endothelial-lined channels seen histologically, with no erythrocytes present.

Lymphosarcomas can be found in the skin and subcutis as well as other organs. They usually present as gray-yellow thickenings that can be multifocal or diffuse. Primary differential diagnoses include inflammatory lesions and xanthomas. A "pseudolymphoma" of the skin has been reported.[7] The exact classification of the lesion was not determined. Morphologically, it was difficult to rule out a cutaneous lymphosarcoma.

Mast cell tumors are infrequently reported in birds[8] and apparently have not been seen in common pet species. They present no specific gross features, and must be differentiated by cytologic or histologic examination.

Non-neoplastic lesions that must be differentiated from others include xanthomas and granulomas. Xanthomas are yellow, thickened areas that occur commonly in pet birds. Diagnosis is by cytologic examination or biopsy. Granulomas have been previously described.

Melanocytic tumors are infrequently described[9, 10] but are occasionally seen in psittacine birds. Malignant melanoma appears to be more frequent, based on the limited literature and cases observed. These tumors are brown-black with infiltration into the surrounding tissues and irregular borders. The beak and face appear to be common sites of tumor formation among the few cases seen (Fig. 34–6).

TUMORS OF THE RESPIRATORY SYSTEM

Upper Respiratory System

Small squamous papillomas are often seen on the mucosa adjacent to the choana. These are often multiple gray-white structures that can be inflamed in some birds. Although a viral etiology has been suggested, the cause is not known. Squamous cell carcinomas may also arise in this area and can infiltrate into the nasal sinuses. Carcinomas have poorly defined margins and associated hemorrhage and necrosis of surrounding tissue. A primary differential diagnosis is carcinoma of the nasal or sinus

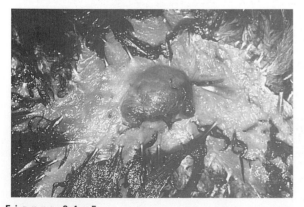

F i g u r e 3 4 – 5

Hemangioma in a macaw. Typical presentation as a circumscribed red-black mass.

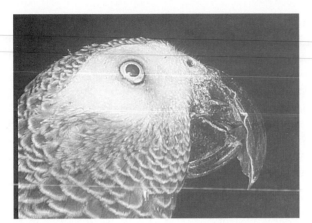

Figure 34–6

Malignant melanoma presenting as an irregular black lesion associated with beak necrosis in an African grey parrot. (Courtesy of Dr. Irv Ingram, All Creatures Animal Hospital, Phoenix, AZ.)

mucosa. Both squamous carcinoma and nasal carcinoma may appear as gray to red infiltrative masses that distort bone and soft tissue in the nasal and facial portions of the skull (Fig. 34–7).

Radiographically, bone lysis and possibly reactive proliferation are seen. Cytologic examination of the nasal cavity may be difficult to interpret, particularly if there is a secondary infection. Biopsy is the most reliable method for diagnosis. Non-neoplastic conditions that may mimic neoplasia include granulomas, severe vitamin A deficiency leading to metaplasia and severe hyperkeratosis, and non-neoplastic cysts.

Lower Respiratory System

Primary carcinomas of the lung and/or air sac are infrequently seen and are not well documented. They usually appear as large masses in which exact origin is difficult to determine (Fig. 34–8). If respiratory disease is suspected clinically, radiographic appearance indicates a space-occupying lesion. Initially, clinical presentation may be as a mass that becomes visible externally, or perhaps as signs referable to involvement of the spinal cord because of invasion of the spinal column by the tumor. There is no specific gross identifying feature, and the diagnosis is made histologically.

Both metastatic carcinomas and sarcomas have been seen in birds. They can appear as single or multiple lesions in the lungs, and there is usually a history of previous primary tumor diagnosis. As with primary tumors, gross features are not diagnostic.

Granulomas that form as a result of infectious disease and inhalation of foreign material constitute the primary non-neoplastic differential diagnosis. These may be somewhat characteristic grossly (i.e.,

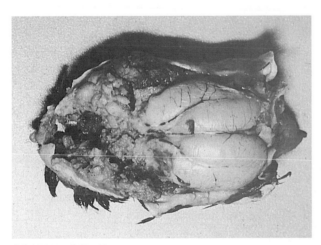

Figure 34–7

Nasal/sinus carcinoma that has severely distorted the anterior portion of the head and face in a conure. The tumor is extending caudally into the brain.

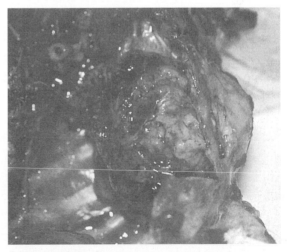

Figure 34–8

Replacement of lung by primary pulmonary carcinoma in a Moluccan cockatoo. (From Schmidt RE: Morphologic diagnosis of avian neoplasms. Semin Avian Exotic Pet Med 1(2):176, 1992.)

aspergillosis). However, culture, cytologic, and/or histopathologic examination are necessary for an exact diagnosis.

TUMORS OF THE GASTROINTESTINAL SYSTEM

Oral Cavity

As mentioned with the upper respiratory system, squamous papillomas can form within the oral mucous membrane. These are usually small, gray-white lesions that can become necrotic and secondarily inflamed.

Malignant tumors of the oral cavity include squamous cell carcinoma and carcinoma of the submucosal salivary glands. At gross examination tumors may be indistinguishable, presenting as variably sized infiltrative lesions that are gray, yellow, or white. Hemorrhage and foci of necrosis and inflammation can be present. Tumors are infiltrative and may distort soft tissue and bone. If bone is invaded, radiographs show lysis and possibly new bone production. Cytologic examinations can be used to diagnose carcinoma, but histologic examination of biopsies is the most reliable method of differential diagnosis.

Non-neoplastic differential diagnoses include granulomas of all types, and histologic examination is often necessary to differentiate these lesions. Vitamin A deficiency can lead to metaplasia and hyperkeratosis of submucosal salivary glands. The gross appearance is of large masses of yellow-white material, and cytologic examination may indicate the presence of keratin and possibly secondary infection and inflammation. Because keratin can also be seen in squamous cell carcinoma, biopsy may be needed for diagnosis.

Esophagus

Papilloma and squamous cell carcinoma can occur in the esophagus. They are grossly and histologically similar to those seen in the oral cavity. They may be suspected when there is a problem with swallowing of food, or when regurgitation is a primary clinical sign. Radiography may indicate a space-occupying lesion that can be seen by endos-

copy. Positive diagnosis may require biopsy, particularly with large papillomas that occasionally are reported.

Proventriculus and Ventriculus

Infiltrative carcinoma, primarily located at the proventricular/ventricular junction, is reported in a variety of psittacine birds. The greatest incidence is in *Brotogeris* species.[11, 12] Clinical signs include regurgitation and chronic wasting. Contrast radiography may indicate an area of ulceration or a space-occupying lesion, but grossly these tumors can be difficult to detect because they tend to infiltrate laterally in the wall of the ventriculus and proventriculus (Fig. 34–9). Histologic examination is necessary to confirm the diagnosis. Extension of the tumor into the mesentery and liver is seen, and metastasis occurs occasionally.

Differential diagnosis includes granulomas due to various causes. Because there is a high incidence of this tumor in *Brotogeris* species, avian mycobacteriosis is a primary differential diagnosis. Mycobacteriosis is common in gray-cheeked parakeets and can cause similar clinical signs as well as gross lesions if stomachs are affected.

Intestines

Papillomas can be seen throughout the intestinal tract and are similar to those previously reported.

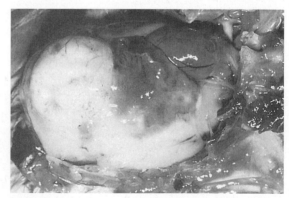

F i g u r e   3 4 – 9

Proventricular carcinoma with thickening of the proventricular wall and extension to the liver, which is adhered to the proventriculus. (From Schmidt RE: Morphologic diagnosis of avian neoplasms. Semin Avian Exotic Pet Med 1(2):75, 1992.)

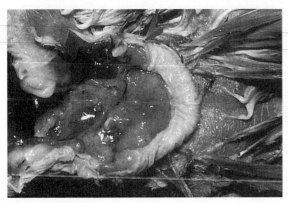

Figure 34–10

Cloacal papilloma in a macaw. Foci of hemorrhage are seen. (From Bauck L: Clinical approach to pet bird neoplasms. Semin Avian Exotic Pet Med 1(2):70, 1992.)

Adenoma of the large intestine has also been reported.[13] Intestinal carcinoma is an infrequent occurrence in the author's experience. Carcinomas can be space-occupying and infiltrative into the intestinal wall, with ulceration and secondary infection sometimes seen. Histologic examination is necessary to differentiate tumors from areas of focal infection and inflammation.

Tumors of smooth muscle are infrequently seen. Both benign and malignant varieties occur and are grossly similar, presenting as red-gray masses in the wall of the intestinal tract. Because metastasis is rare, histologic examination is needed to differentiate leiomyoma from leiomyosarcoma.

The primary non-neoplastic differential diagnosis is chronic inflammation with the formation of a space-occupying lesion. Impression smears, microbiology, and histopathology may be used to determine the etiology.

Cloaca

Papillomas are common in the cloaca, particularly in some species of Amazon parrots and macaws (Fig. 34–10). These are single or multiple proliferative lesions and can be diagnosed by biopsy. Cloacal carcinomas are less common and are infiltrative, leading to thickening of the cloacal wall, necrosis, hemorrhage, and possibly adhesions of the cloaca to the other abdominal organs.[14]

Non-neoplastic lesions can mimic both papillo-

mas and carcinomas. Inflammatory thickening or polyp formation at the mucocutaneous junction and cloacal prolapse must be distinguished from papilloma formation, and chronic inflammation with the formation of granulomas or abscesses must be differentiated from carcinoma. Cytology and culture results may be of benefit, but histologic examination is usually the method of choice for definitive diagnosis.

TUMORS OF THE LIVER AND PANCREAS

Primary hepatic tumors can arise from bile ducts, hepatocytes or hepatic stromal connective tissue, and smooth muscle. Primary vascular or lymphoid tumors can also occur, and are discussed in other sections of this chapter. Hepatocellular adenomas and carcinomas may vary in color from tan to purple and are often friable.[15, 16] Adenomas may appear circumscribed, but carcinomas have irregular, difficult-to-define borders. These tumors can be solitary in one liver lobe (Fig. 34–11), or occasionally multiple in several lobes.

Bile duct carcinomas may present as solitary or multiple gray-white lesions that usually are firm and have irregular borders (Fig. 34–12). Metastasis of primary hepatocellular or biliary carcinomas is infrequently reported, but a possible association with intestinal tract papillomas has been suggested.[17] If there is a relationship, the causal factors have not yet been identified. Differential diagnosis of primary hepatic adenomas and carcinomas is done by histopathologic examination.

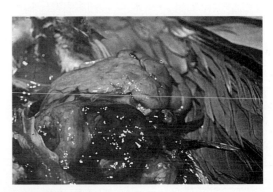

Figure 34–11

Hepatocellular carcinoma. Severely enlarged and distended liver lobes are seen.

Primary hepatic tumors of smooth muscle or fibrous connective tissue origin appear as firm masses. Their size and degree of infiltration of surrounding parenchyma vary, with malignant tumors having less well-defined margins. These tumors are usually yellow, gray, or red grossly, and may have foci of hemorrhage and necrosis.

Various potential metastatic tumors can involve the liver. These may appear as multiple foci in liver lobes, but there are no distinguishing features to suggest origin, unless a lesion is found at another site that can be presumed to be a primary tumor. Definitive diagnosis is made by histologic examination. Because the primary tumor site may sometimes be small and less prominent than metastases, careful search for the primary tumor should be done.

Tumors of pancreatic parenchyma vary in size and gross presentation. They are usually gray-white and may appear as discrete masses in the area of the pancreas and duodenal loop of the intestine (Fig. 34–13). With progression, there is often infiltration of the intestine, and there can be loss of normal architecture with adhesions involving much of the upper and portions of the lower intestinal tract. Normal pancreas may not be apparent in advanced cases.

Tumors of the islets of Langerhans may be difficult to see grossly, but the tumors can be functional, leading to hypoglycemia.[18] In gross appearance, small nodular foci are present within pancreatic parenchyma. Metastasis to the liver or spleen is possible.

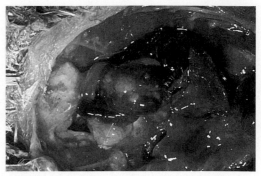

Figure 34–13

Pancreatic carcinoma in a cockatiel. Nodular masses are replacing the pancreas and infiltrating into the duodenal loop of the intestine.

Non-neoplastic lesions of the liver and pancreas that must be differentiated include various chronic infections that can cause abscesses and granulomas. Idiopathic pancreatitis with secondary fat necrosis can also lead to the formation of nodular masses.

TUMORS OF THE CARDIOVASCULAR SYSTEM

Hemangiosarcoma can occur in the myocardium. This tumor is similar to hemangiosarcomas found in other organs, and has been previously described. Lymphosarcoma can also involve the myocardium and is described in another section. Primary rhabdomyosarcoma of the avian heart has not been reported, and the author has not seen any example of this tumor.

TUMORS OF THE URINARY SYSTEM

Renal tumors are most frequently seen in budgerigars.[19] Adenomas may be confined to the renal fossa, but carcinomas are often infiltrative, leading to pressure on nerve roots and paralysis. These tumors are irregular, nodular, and red-brown or gray (Fig. 34–14). Radiographically, there may be some bone lysis. Histologic examination may be needed to properly classify the tumor as benign or malignant, particularly if there is no obvious infiltration of surrounding tissues.

Differential diagnoses include adrenal and gonadal tumors involving the cranial pole of the kid-

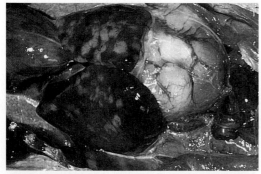

Figure 34–12

Bile duct carcinoma that is present in both right and left liver lobes. (Courtesy of Dr. Mike Murray, Avian and Exotic Animal Clinic of Monterey, CA.)

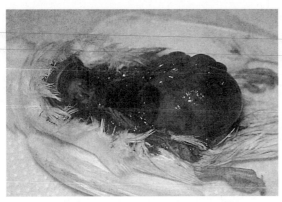

Figure 34-14

Large renal carcinoma in a budgerigar. The tumor is displacing other organs. (From Schmidt RE: Morphologic diagnosis of avian neoplasms. Semin Avian Exotic Pet Med 1(2):76, 1992.)

ney and infections leading to granuloma formation. The latter can be associated with hematogenous infection or extension of air sac granulomas. Birds with severe urate deposition in ureters or medullary cones can present with enlarged swollen kidneys. Histologic examination is often necessary for a definitive diagnosis.

TUMORS OF THE REPRODUCTIVE SYSTEM

Female Reproductive System

Ovarian tumors have been reported most frequently in budgerigars and cockatiels. These tumors appear as masses that may fill a large portion of the abdominal cavity. Ovarian tumors may also be implanted throughout the peritoneal cavity. Ovarian granulosa cell tumors have been described as yellow, lobulated, and irregular.[20] Ovarian adenoma and adenocarcinoma are rarely reported in pet birds and have not been well described.

Tumors arising in the oviduct or uterus can become quite large before the bird is presented for examination, and grossly it may be difficult to distinguish them from ovarian tumors. Histologic differentiation can be difficult, particularly if tissue from several portions of the reproductive tract is not examined.

Abscesses and granulomas must be differentiated from tumors. Birds that are egg-bound may also present with abdominal swelling, which is another non-neoplastic differential diagnosis.

Male Reproductive System

Testicular tumors are uncommon, but both Sertoli's cell tumors and seminoma have been reported.[20, 21] The affected testicle is grossly enlarged and the tumors may be gray to yellow (Fig. 34–15). Seminomas may be somewhat more friable than Sertoli's cell tumors. Differential diagnosis is by histologic examination. Primary diagnostic considerations are tumors of the adrenal gland or cranial portion of the kidney.

TUMORS OF THE ENDOCRINE SYSTEM

Pituitary Gland

Histologically, pituitary tumors have been regarded as common in budgerigars.[22, 23] A pituitary adenoma has been reported in a cockatiel.[24] A 1992 report places pituitary tumors as the most common neoplasm involving the brain.[24] The clinical presentation includes neurologic signs referable to a space-occupying lesion, as well as various signs referable to endocrine abnormalities including polyuria, cere-

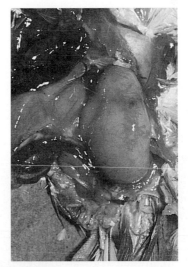

Figure 34-15

Seminoma that has greatly enlarged and displaced abdominal organs.

bral abnormalities, and changes in the cere. Exophthalmos and blindness have also been reported. Radiographically, there may be lysis of bones of the skull. The tumors are red-brown and grow by expansion (adenomas) and infiltration (carcinomas). Differential diagnosis includes tumors of central nervous system origin and abscesses or granulomas involving the inner ears, base of the brain, or retropharyngeal area.

Thyroid Gland

Thyroid tumors are seen in a variety of birds, but are most commonly reported in cockatiels and budgerigars.[25] Tumors are located just above the thoracic inlet, vary from gray to red-brown, and are sometimes palpable. Adenomas grow by expansion; carcinomas, which occur less frequently, are differentiated by irregular borders and invasion of surrounding tissue. Functional changes resulting from hormonal alterations are not well documented.

The primary differential diagnosis is thyroid gland hyperplasia. Hyperplasia usually occurs bilaterally, which distinguishes it from adenoma formation. If unilateral, the morphologic difference is difficult to determine. Other differential diagnosis includes a thymic tissue tumor in the same area as the thyroid gland, and the possibility of ultimobranchial cyst formation.

Parathyroid Gland

Tumors of the parathyroid gland are not documented in birds. However, if there is clinical evidence of possible parathyroid gland hyperfunction, neoplasia must be ruled out. Primary and secondary hyperplasia are other differential considerations.

Adrenal Gland

Primary tumors of the adrenal gland have not been documented in pet avian species, but the condition probably exists, based on undocumented disease descriptions by avian practitioners. Tumors originating in both interrenal (cortical analogue) and chromaffin (medullary analogue) cells are possible, and clinical signs referable to hormonal imbalances, as seen in mammals, may be expected. At laparoscopy or necropsy, primary differential diagnosis includes tumors and granulomas involving the gonads or the cranial pole of the kidney.

TUMORS OF HEMATOPOIETIC AND LYMPHOID TISSUE

Thymus

Lymphosarcoma is seen in the thymus, as well as in other organs.[26] Thymic tissue occurs in the neck region from the upper cervical area to the thoracic inlet and neoplastic masses can occur throughout this area. These tumors are usually circumscribed and gray-white. They may present as solitary masses but can be associated with generalized lymphosarcoma. Primary epithelial thymomas are rarely seen, but have been reported in a budgerigar[27] and should be considered in the differential diagnosis of thymic neoplasia. Depending on the exact location of the tumor, other diagnoses include thyroid neoplasia and hyperplasia as well as non-neoplastic thymic cysts. At gross examination, the latter may be fluid-filled rather than solid. Cytologic or histologic examination is necessary for confirmation of the diagnosis.

Spleen

Neoplastic enlargement of the spleen is usually the result of lymphosarcoma or myeloid neoplasia (Fig. 34–16). Histologic examination is needed for a definitive diagnosis. Affected spleens are often markedly enlarged and may be mottled red, purple, and gray-white. In large lesions, foci of necrosis and hemorrhage may be seen. The enlargement is usually uniform with smooth borders, although irregular nodules are seen in some tumors.

Metastatic tumors are occasionally seen in the spleen. They usually occur as an irregular enlargement or as multiple foci that are firm and tan, gray, or white. A variety of non-neoplastic differential diagnoses are possible, including chlamydiosis, bacterial infections, and severe amyloidosis.

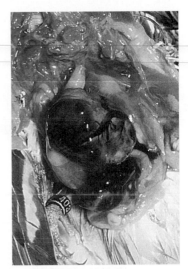

Enlarged spleen in a budgerigar with a myeloproliferative disorder.

SYSTEMIC LYMPHOSARCOMA AND MYELOPROLIFERATIVE DISORDERS

Infiltration of any organ or tissue by malignant lymphoid or myeloid cells is possible. Tumors often present as areas of yellow-gray thickening that are variable in size and shape. Diffuse involvement of parenchymal organs can occur (Fig. 34–17) and grossly must be differentiated from various inflammatory conditions or degenerative diseases such as amyloidosis. Impression smears and/or histologic examination are needed for diagnosis. In some birds only a single organ is grossly involved, whereas in others, multiple organs may be affected. Unfortunately many birds with lymphosarcoma are not leukemic, and peripheral blood smear examination may not be helpful in diagnosis. There does not appear to be any particular species or age predilection for lymphoid or myeloid neoplasia.

Bone Marrow

Lymphosarcoma and myeloid neoplasms are seen in bone marrow. These diagnoses are usually made by a combination of clinical signs involving anemia and results of bone marrow smears or biopsy. Gross distortion of bones is rare.

TUMORS OF THE MUSCULOSKELETAL SYSTEM

Bone

The author has seen at least two neoplastic masses that histologically were considered osteomas. Tu-

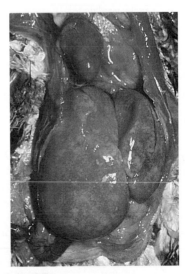

F i g u r e   3 4 – 1 7

Lymphosarcoma in a cockatiel. The liver is markedly enlarged and mottled.

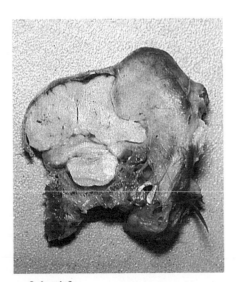

F i g u r e   3 4 – 1 8

Osteoma of the skull of a conure. Bone enlargement is impinging on the brain.

mors were grossly hard and gray-white and grew by expansion (Fig. 34–18). They could not be cut by a sharp scalpel, which is a gross feature leading to a differential diagnosis. Based on the hardness of the lesion, osteosarcoma also has to be considered. Osteosarcomas are usually seen in the long bones[28] and occur as firm swellings (Fig. 34–19). Their borders are not as well differentiated as those of osteomas. With sarcomas there is often abundant proliferative new bone formation and bone lysis that can be seen on radiographs.

Chondroma and chondrosarcoma may occur in the same areas as tumors of osteoblasts.[29] Few reports are found in the literature and they are infrequent in the author's experience. Granulomatous disease of bone, particularly mycotic infections and mycobacteriosis, must also be considered in the differential diagnosis, based on gross characteristics. Histologic examination is usually necessary to differentiate neoplasia from inflammation and other tumors.

Striated Muscle

Rhabdomyosarcoma has been reported in pet birds[30] but is infrequently seen. These tumors arise in striated muscle and may appear gray to red-brown. Tumor margins are indistinct. Histologic examination is needed to differentiate rhabdomyosarcoma from other soft tissue sarcomas. A rhabdomyoma reported in the eyelid of a pigeon was described as nodular masses of abnormal muscle fibers.[31]

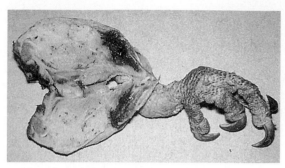

Figure 34–19

Destruction of the femur of an African grey parrot by an osteosarcoma. (From Schmidt RE: Morphologic diagnosis of avian neoplasms. Semin Avian Exotic Pet Med 1(2):77, 1992.)

TUMORS OF THE SPECIAL SENSES

Ear

Tumors of the external ear have been discussed with skin tumors.

Eye

Primary ocular neoplasia is infrequently reported in pet birds[32] (see Chapter 33). Clinical presentation is often of buphthalmos or exophthalmos. In advanced cases there may be an orbital mass that is not grossly recognizable as a globe. Histologic examination is needed to determine tumor type and to differentiate primary from possibly metastatic tumors, retrobulbar tumors, or inflammatory lesions and abscesses.

Treatment of Neoplasia | Katherine Quesenberry

The use of chemotherapy and radiation therapy in the treatment of neoplasia in birds is new and unexplored in avian medicine. Very few clinical reports have been published concerning these treatment methods in birds. Cancer is most commonly treated in birds by surgical excision of neoplastic masses where possible, or surgical amputation of limbs with nonresectable masses. However, surgical resection or amputation cannot be used in birds with diffuse neoplasia or nonresectable masses. As the population of pet birds has increased and many pet birds are aging, neoplasia will be seen more commonly in geriatric birds. Therefore, we must learn more about treatment methods for cancer in birds to provide high-quality veterinary care for these birds.

Therapy of neoplasia in any animal often requires combined treatment methods to achieve a degree of success. Surgical resection and debulking procedures are commonly used with chemotherapy or radiation treatments. Some neoplastic processes are treated with only one treatment modality. The course of therapy chosen must be based on the type and location of the tumor, the degree of infiltration, and knowledge of how the tumor behaves in other animals. Consultation and collaboration with a veterinary oncologist is very important in the treatment of neoplasia in birds.

CHEMOTHERAPY

Prednisone is used in birds as a palliative therapy in several neoplastic disorders.[3, 33–35] It is sometimes used in budgerigars with renal neoplasia in an attempt to slow clinical progression. Beneficial effects if any are unknown.

Doxorubicin is a naturally occurring antineoplastic agent that is often used in mammals. It is commonly used as part of a combined treatment protocol in the treatment of solid sarcomas. Doxorubicin has been used in treating osteosarcoma in a blue-front Amazon parrot after the tumor mass was debulked with radiosurgery.[36] A dosage of 60 mg/m^2 was injected intravenously once a month for 4 months. The parrot was premedicated with diphenhydramine (1 mg) 30 minutes before treatment, and treatment was given while the bird was anesthetized with isoflurane. The bird was in remission at the time of the report, although it was unknown if the positive response was the result of chemotherapy, radiosurgery, or the combination of both.

Cisplatin, a platinum-containing compound with antineoplastic activity, is commonly used to treat osteosarcomas, squamous cell sarcomas, and other sarcomas. Its use is associated with a high incidence of toxicosis in mammals, resulting in gastrointestinal signs, bone marrow depression, and nephrotoxicosis; therefore, it is usually used in a combined treatment protocol. Intratumoral injection of cisplatin given in a repositol matrix was used in the treatment of facial fibrosarcoma in a blue and gold macaw.[37] The bird was treated with orthovoltage radiation using 4 Grey

(Gy) three times a week for 11 treatments, following initial surgical debulking of the tumor. The tumor had increased in size after the sixth radiation treatment, and cisplatin was added to the therapeutic protocol. Injections of cisplatin were given before the eighth and eleventh radiation therapy sessions. Following completion of therapy, the tumor was in remission for 29 months before recurrence.

Chlorambucil was used successfully in the treatment of cutaneous pseudolymphoma (lymphocytoma) in a juvenile blue and gold macaw.[7] Chlorambucil, an alkylating agent related to nitrogen mustard, is relatively nontoxic and is used commonly in the treatment of lymphomas in mammals. Initially, chlorambucil (20 mg/m^2) was given at 14-day intervals for three treatments. All cutaneous lesions had regressed at the end of the 6-week treatment period. New lesions developed 12 weeks later, and treatment was repeated for an additional 6 weeks at the same dosage. No evidence of recurrence was present 2.5 years after cessation of therapy.

Combination chemotherapy has been used in the treatment of lymphosarcoma in a Moluccan cockatoo[38] and lymphocytic leukemia and malignant lymphoma in a Pekin duck.[39] The cockatoo was treated with a cyclic protocol of prednisone (25 mg/m^2 orally daily), cyclophosphamide (200 mg/m^2 intraosseously weekly), vincristine sulfate (0.75 mg/m^2 intraosseously weekly), doxorubicin (30 mg/m^2 intraosseously every 3 weeks), asparaginase (400 IU/kg intramuscularly weekly), and alpha interferon (15,000 U/m^2 subcutaneously every 48 hours for three treatments). Treatment was continued over a period of 13 weeks. A partial response was achieved for solid tumors during the treatment period, and the cockatoo tolerated chemotherapy well. The duck was treated with vincristine sulfate (0.5 mg/m^2 on week 1; 0.75 mg/m^2 on weeks 2–4), prednisone (2.2 mg/kg every 12 hours), and chlorambucil (1 mg twice weekly). The duck clinically improved for 4 weeks, before it was euthanized. Necropsy results showed diffuse pneumonia, airsacculitis, peritonitis, and diffuse lymphoma involving the liver, spleen, intestines, bone marrow, lungs, air sacs, and kidneys.

RADIATION THERAPY

Orthovoltage (low energy) x-ray teletherapy was used in the treatment of a periorbital mass in an

chronic exposure to a fine metal powder. This also may not be visible on radiographs.

Blood lead levels above 20 μg/dl (0.2 ppm) are suggestive of lead poisoning, especially if clinical signs consistent with lead toxicosis are present. Clinical signs have been correlated with blood levels as low as 15 μg/dl (0.15 ppm),* whereas other species (chickens) may appear clinically normal with blood lead levels as high as 800 μg/dl (8 ppm).[2] Tissue lead levels of above 3 to 6 ppm are considered significant.

Serum or plasma zinc concentrations can be useful to diagnose zinc toxicosis. However, samples must be collected in tubes specifically designed for trace mineral determination, or in plastic containers. Conventional tubes may add extraneous zinc to the sample. Serum zinc levels above 200 μg/dl (2 ppm) are diagnostic for zinc toxicosis. In the authors' experience, birds suffering from zinc toxicosis usually have serum levels above 1000 μg/dl (10 ppm). Tissue zinc levels are best recovered from the pancreas, kidney, and liver.

Treatment

Three goals should be met when treating heavy metal poisoning[2]: (1) the patient's condition must be stabilized, (2) the source of the metal must be removed, dislodged, or flushed, and (3) the heavy metal must be removed from the tissues of the bird with chelating agents.

Supportive therapy often includes correcting fluid and electrolyte imbalances because GI disturbances may be the dominant clinical signs in birds with acute toxicity. Oral electrolyte solutions may be used when vomiting is not present. Subcutaneous fluid administration is often combined with intravenous bolus therapy. Severely ill birds may benefit from the installation of a jugular catheter with a port for intermittent fluid administration; intraosseous catheters are another possible route for fluid administration. Anticonvulsants, primarily diazepam (0.5–1.0 mg/kg intramuscularly [IM], one to three times daily), are sometimes indicated if seizures are severe.[8, 9] Dexamethasone (1–2 mg/kg IM or subcutaneously [SC] once) may also be indicated to decrease cerebral edema.[10]

Anemia may be severe. Iron replacement therapy and rarely homologous blood transfusion may be warranted. Heat and humidity from an intensive care unit should be provided. Gavage feeding may be necessary after vomiting or convulsions have been controlled. Perches and open water bowls should be removed from cages of birds that have seizures to prevent accidental trauma or drowning.

Radiography is useful in monitoring the success of a removal and dislodgement program. If possible, radiographs should be taken at the beginning of treatment to detect the number and size of metal particles or fragments, if present. However, in a critically ill bird, radiography may have to be postponed until several days after the treatment has begun and the bird is clinically stable. If a number of small fragments are present in the ventriculus, treatment with lubricating agents (such as feline laxatives, hairball remedies, and mineral oil) and bulk or combination agents (such as oral cellulose products and peanut butter) are usually helpful in moving them out into the distal GI tract. Such agents should be given two to three times daily (mineral oil should be administered carefully by gavage tube). Oral magnesium sulfate (Epsom salts) acts as a mild cathartic and also precipitates lead as lead sulfate ($PbSO_4$), preventing further absorption.[10] A few granules can be mixed with honey or 50% dextrose and given orally twice daily. Small fragments may be removed by these methods over a period of 1 to 3 weeks. Progress may be followed by weekly radiography. Positioning is not essential to count the fragments, and followup radiographs may be done by simply placing the patient on the radiographic cassette without restraint.

Large metal foreign bodies may not pass readily through the GI tract. These larger pieces may sometimes be retrieved or flushed by endoscopy (usually aided by an ingluvotomy procedure).[11, 12] Blind flushing techniques also have been described in detail.[11] If these techniques are unsuccessful in removing large metal fragments, a ventriculotomy may be considered. Altman's technique[13] is recommended, although some foreign bodies also can be removed with a caudal, ventral incision near the exit of the ventriculus. Pellets and other metal pieces exterior to the digestive tract are usually removed by conventional surgery.

Chelating agents are available in both oral and injectable forms. However, the majority of informa-

---

*Quesenberry K, personal communication, 1995.

tion on efficacy in avian species has involved injectable calcium ethylenediaminetetraacetate (CaEDTA) (Calcium Disodium Versonate, Riker Laboratories, Northridge, CA). A short course of CaEDTA is not harmful when used at appropriate dose ranges and may be used in unconfirmed cases to monitor response to therapy.[8] With chronic heavy metal toxicosis, dramatic response to therapy is not always evident, as it often is in acute lead poisoning. CaEDTA is generally given at a dose of 30 to 35 mg/kg twice daily for 5 days. The undiluted 20% solution (200 mg/ml) of CaEDTA may cause a painful reaction at the injection site but can be given intramuscularly if necessary. The solution is best diluted with isotonic saline to a final concentration of no greater than 1% (10 mg/ml) and is given subcutaneously. The effective concentration of plasma CaEDTA is prolonged by subcutaneous administration, as compared with intravenous injection, and enhances elimination of lead from the bone.[10] CaEDTA chelates lead directly from the bone but not from the soft tissues. Lead is removed from the soft tissues by equilibration with the bone over time, thus sometimes requiring multiple treatments.[10]

In mammals, CaEDTA can cause acute necrotizing nephrosis, but this has not been documented in birds. To avoid this complication, chelation therapy should be limited to 5 days with a rest period of 5 to 7 days between additional treatment courses. Treatment should be continued until blood lead levels are normal. If metal densities remain in the GI tract after blood levels are normal, radiographs and blood lead levels should be repeated at routine intervals until the metal densities have been passed.

Oral chelating agents are sometimes used as followup therapy for birds discharged from the hospital still requiring chelation therapy. Oral agents are not generally used in acute situations because affected birds tend to vomit and because of insufficient data on efficacy. The best known oral agent is D-penicillamine (Cuprimine, Merck, Rahway, NJ). It is usually made into a suspension for avian use and must then be refrigerated according to the manufacturer. Stability in suspension is unknown, but suspensions should probably be remade every 5 days. A dose of 55 mg/kg orally twice daily has been suggested, although ranges from 30 to 90 mg/kg q12h also have been reported.[14]

PHARMACOLOGIC AGENTS

Many therapeutic agents have the potential for toxicity if given at a dose that is not tolerated by an individual bird or species. Individual variation accounts for some drug reactions, but few pharmacologic agents have been extensively studied in birds, and the potential for adverse effects must always be considered. Written notations in the medical record should aways show that an owner has been informed of the off-label status of a drug regimen.

Certain groups of birds are well known for their sensitivities. Lories and many finches have been reported for various drug sensitivities,[1] although this may be the result of medication placed in drinking water. A bird with the very small body weight of a finch (often less than 10 g) has a relatively small margin of error for certain drugs, and the uncertainties of water consumption may cause an error to be made. This is particularly true when young are being raised or if climactic conditions are hot or dry. Lories are often maintained on a powdered diet, and water consumption may be higher than for some other psittacine species. Parakeets originate from areas with arid climates, and are likely to be underdosed.

Macaws have been reported to be sensitive to a variety of therapeutic agents that may cause GI disturbances.[15] Some of these agents include doxycycline oral suspensions, sulfa/trimethoprim suspensions, and antifungal imidazoles such as ketoconazole (Table 35–1). As more data become available on new drug usage in large psittacines, other sensitivities throughout the group will undoubtedly be found. Until then, caution is warranted when dealing with these large and valuable birds.

INHALANT TOXINS

The efficiency of the avian respiratory system makes birds more susceptible to gases or fumes in the household or aviary and can often result in acute death. The majority of exposures occurring in the home are a result of inappropriate use in proximity to pet birds. Smoke from cooking or burning material and fumes from aerosols or cleaning agents are frequent causes of inhalant toxicosis (Table 35–2). Any strong odor from a household product can be

T a b l e   3 5 – 1

REPORTED DRUG REACTIONS AND TOXICOSES

	Drug	Species	Reactions/Toxicoses
Antibiotics	Aminoglycosides (gentocin, amikacin)	All	At higher than recommended doses or in dehydrated birds, these drugs can cause nephrotoxicity and neuromuscular blockade.
	Cephalosporins	All	At higher than normal doses or in debilitated young birds, these drugs may cause hepatotoxicity and renal toxicity.
	Macrolides (clindamycin, erythromycin, tylosin)	All	Gastrointestinal upset and diarrhea can occur. At doses greater than 40 mg/kg IM of tylosin, anaphylactic-like reactions have been observed in cockatiels.
	Nitrofurazone powder 9.2%	Softbills, lories, grass parakeets	At a dose of 1 tsp/gal, ataxia, convulsions, and death have been observed. The recommended dose for these birds is ½ tsp/gal.
	Sulfas (vetasulid)	All	Hypersensitivities and hemorrhagic syndrome have been observed.
	Tetracyclines (oxytetracycline, doxycycline)	All	With IM parenteral administration, tissue necrosis and inflammation at injection sites can occur.
	Trimethoprim-sulfas	Macaws	Regurgitation, facial flushing, and depression have occurred.
	Quinolones (enrofloxacin, ciprofloxacin)	All	Dyspnea and muscle tremors have been observed with injectable doses greater than 70 mg/kg; articular cartilage erosions and lameness have been reported in young animals (but apparently not in young psittacines).
	Doxycycline oral suspension	Macaws	Vomiting has been seen in the young macaw when maintained at 50 mg/kg q24h.
Parasiticides	Diazinon	All	Problems occur when food or water sources are contaminated. Weakness, muscle tremors, and death in young birds may occur.
	Dimetridazole	Pigeons, budgerigars, cockatiels	When used in drinking water, ataxia, neurologic disorders, and death have been observed.
	Fenbendazole	Finches, canaries, quail, pigeons, and young birds	When used at 10 ml/l, neurologic signs and death may occur.
	Ivermectin	Finches, budgerigars	Most toxic reactions involve intramuscular use in smaller birds. Lethargy, depression, and death can occur.
	Levamisole 13.56%	All	When used parenterally or at 10 ml/gal, most species show emesis. Tissue necrosis at injection sites and hepatotoxicity have been reported.
	Praziquantel 56.8 mg/mL	Finches	Depression and death have been reported from parenteral administration.
Miscellaneous Drugs	Aventyl HCl	All	Hyperactivity and agitation have occurred.
	Flunixin	All	Regurgitation may be observed when used frequently or in high doses.
	Calcium	Primarily young birds	Nephrosis, visceral urates, parathyroid dysfunction, and retarded growth have been observed.
	Gamma globulin (human)	All	Vomiting, weakness, and conjunctival edema have been observed after repeated injections.
	Levothyroxine	Amazons, budgerigars	Reactions are individual, but owners should be warned for hyperactivity, aggression, or lethargy.
	Medroxyprogesterone	All; cockatiels are most often reported	A transitory diabetes as well as lethargy, obesity, and fatty liver have been observed. Reactions are more common with repeated injections.
	Acetylcystine	All	Hypersensitivity reactions have been observed with neubulization therapy. Clinical signs include dyspnea, prolapsed nictitans, and anaphylaxis.
	Phenobarbital	All	Excitement or depression may be observed when elixir is used in the drinking water.
	Vitamin A	All	Reactions are due to excessive use. Young birds suffer from osteodystrophy and parathyroid hypertrophy. Adults show a burnt-orange color in the skin, which is prone to drying and cracking.
	Vitamin D_3	Juvenile macaws are most sensitive	Increased soft tissue calcification is the primary underlying problem for most reactions in baby birds. Dietary levels should be monitored closely for both breeding adults and chicks.
	Itraconazole	African grey parrots	Vomiting, anorexia, and death have been reported even at low doses.
	Ketoconazole, fluconazole	All	Gastrointestinal disturbances including anorexia and vomiting are possible with many imidazoles.
	Flucytosine	Young psittacines	Feather abnormalities have been seen in prefledgling birds maintained on flucytosine.

Amended from LaBonde, Vet Clin North Am, 1991[18].

potentially toxic (see Household Toxins). Standard ventilators or stove-top filters do not sufficiently clear the air of toxic particles. When gases or fumes are present in the home or aviary, the birds should be removed from the house and the windows opened for ventilation. After a toxic inhalant exposure occurs, the veterinarian needs to treat the clinical signs presented. Remedies may include adminis-

T a b l e 3 5 – 2

INHALANT HOUSEHOLD TOXINS

Ammonia and strong bleach
Automobile exhaust, carbon monoxide
Bug bombs, pesticide strips and sprays
Burning foods and cooking oils
Chemical sprays (i.e., disinfectants, deodorizers, furniture polish)
Fluoropolymers from spray starch
Glues, paints, and nail polish and remover
Hair permanent solutions and hair sprays
Hair dryer fumes (primarily from new hair dryers)
Leaded gasoline fumes
Most non-stick cookware surfaces
Mothballs (naphthalene, paradichlorobenzene)
Self-cleaning ovens
Smoke (tobacco or any other source)

Data from Wells, J Am Vet Med Assoc, 1983[17]; Beasly, Vet Clin North Am, 1990[19]; Dumonceau et al, in Ritchie et al (eds): Avian Medicine, 1994[20]; and Humphreys, Veterinary Toxicology, 1988[28].

tration of oxygen, anti-inflammatory drugs, diuretics for pulmonary edema, broad-spectrum antibiotics, and supportive fluid and heat therapy.

Polytetrafluoroethylene (PTFE) poisoning, or polymer fume fever, is one of the more common airborne toxic events reported in birds.[16, 17] Sources of PTFE are non-stick surfaces on products such as cookware, drip pans, heat lamp covers, irons, and ironing board covers. The gas is emitted when the surface undergoes pyrolysis at 280°C (536°F) and the PTFE is degraded. Sudden death is the most common history, but mild exposures may result in moist rales, dyspnea, ataxia, depression, or anxious behavior. At necropsy, hemorrhagic and edematous lungs are the most common findings, which are consistent with any irritant gas exposure.[18]

The primary cause of death in most cases of smoke inhalation toxicosis is carbon monoxide (CO). There are, however, other irritant (aldehydes, hydrogen chloride [HCl], sulfur dioxide) and nonirritant (CO, carbon dioxide [CO_2], hydrogen cyanide) gases as well as particulate matter that can cause severe respiratory trauma. Carbon monoxide from incomplete combustion of fires, combustible engines (such as poorly ventilated vehicles), and some poorly maintained furnaces can result in sudden death. Carbon monoxide does not injure the lungs, but it decreases the oxygen-carrying capacity of hemoglobin in the blood, resulting in dyspnea, depression, ataxia, nausea, and death. Carbon dioxide buildup lowers available oxygen and acts as a respiratory stimulant, resulting in increased inhalation of other toxic constituents of smoke. Hydrogen cyanide causes cellular inability to use oxygen, further complicating smoke inhalation.[19]

The primary concern with irritant gases (aldehydes, HCl, sulfur dioxide) is delayed, complicated pulmonary failure.[19] Clinical problems may not surface for days. Therefore, persistent monitoring and treatment should continue for days to 3 weeks after smoke exposure.

Treatment of smoke inhalation includes access to fresh air immediately followed by emergency therapy as needed. Oxygen given in a dark, stress-free environment is used to stabilize the bird's conition. If available, humidified oxygen or nebulized saline in oxygen minimizes drying of secretions and seeding of bacteria. Bronchodilator therapy can be used to alleviate reflex bronchospasms. Fluid therapy aids in cardiac output and enhances oxygen delivery to tissues. Corticosteroids should be used only if life-threatening circulatory shock is suspected.

Tobacco smoke from passive inhalation can produce chronic respiratory problems, increased susceptibility to bacterial invasion, ocular irritation, and some dermatologic problems most commonly on the feet or face.[5] Coughing, sneezing, and conjunctivitis are the most common clinical signs. The ingestion of nicotine can also cause problems such as vomiting, diarrhea, hyperexcitability, seizures, and death. Therapy for secondary illnesses resulting from tobacco exposure helps only if the bird is removed from chronic exposure.

MISCELLANEOUS HOUSEHOLD TOXINS

Many common household products are potentially toxic to birds. Many products can be used safely around birds if used correctly with proper ventilation, but are toxic if inappropriate use occurs. Pet bird owners should always be questioned about exposure to household products, aerosols, or cleaning agents when any bird presents with an unexplained illness. Many owners are unaware of the sensitivity of birds to commonplace products. This author (LaBonde) has seen an Amazon parrot that exhibited severe respiratory distress after an owner applied a spray-on antistain protectant to a nearby sofa.

Birds should be treated according to their clinical signs and condition. Clinical signs of exposure to some common household products and appropriate therapy are outlined in Table 35–3.[18, 20–23]

PESTICIDES

The inappropriate use of pesticides can result in exposure of birds through inhalation, ingestion of contaminated food or water sources, and skin absorption from surfaces with pesticide residues. Insecticides and rodenticides are the most commonly reported agents causing toxicoses of indoor or aviary birds. Indoor environments with poor ventilation increase the potential of pesticide exposure even at times when the product is used properly. Some insecticides, such as carbamates (5% carbaryl, carbofuran, methyl carbamates) and pyrethrins, can be used safely around birds with proper ventilation and application. However, ingestion or inhalation from excessive preening or ingestion from contaminated feed sources can result in a dose-related toxicosis. Detrimental effects from chronic exposure to low doses of pesticides have yet to be determined but could contribute to increased susceptibility to

disease from immunosuppression, and poor fertility or hatchability.

Organophosphates (OP) and carbamates such as chlorpyrifos, diazinon, 5% carbaryl, malathion, dichlorvos, and dieldrin are found in insecticides and fertilizers. Clinical signs of toxicosis vary depending on the age and species of the bird and the degree of exposure. The inhibition of acetylcholinesterase (AChE) is the cause for most clinical signs including anorexia, diarrhea, crop stasis, ataxia, tremors, seizures, and paralysis. Less commonly observed signs include dyspnea, moist rales, and bradycardia. In raptors, clinical signs reported have been spastic nictitans, muscle tremors, inability to fly, rapid respiration, and rigid paralysis.[24–26] In breeding facilities, a decrease in hatchability and hatchling size, and a decrease in egg production can occur from chronic low-grade exposure.[27] Teratogenic effects such as scoliosis, lordosis, stunting, and cerebellar defects have been reported.[20]

An infrequent organophosphorus ester–induced delayed neuropathy has been described in mammals and in Amazon parrots.[25] The onset occurs 7 to 21 days after exposure and is not associated with

Table 35–3
MISCELLANEOUS TOXINS

Agent	Clinical Effects	Therapy
Alcohol (distilled)	Lethargy, anorexia, regurgitation, death	Fluids; quiet, dark area
Aluminum chloride (deodorants)	Oral irritant, hemorrhagic gastroenteritis, ataxia, and nephrosis	Lavage crop and proventiculus carefully; GI protectants
Ammonia	Respiratory irritation, immunosupression	Supportive care; fresh air
Chlorine	Photophobia, conjunctivitis, dyspnea, chemical burns, and ulcerations	Irrigation with cool water; oral dilution with water or milk; GI protectants
Chocolate	Caffeine and theobromine are the toxins producing depression, regurgitation, and diarrhea	Supportive therapy and fluids; GI adsorbents
Detergents		
Anionic	Alkaline products that cause dermal irritation, vomiting, and diarrhea	Lavage with water or milk; supportive therapy
Cationic	Fabric softeners, germicides, and sanitizers (quaternary compounds) that cause GI corrosion vomiting, and depression	Milk, water, or egg whites orally followed with activated charcoal
Pine oils (phenols)	Gastroenteritis, vomiting, ulcers, CNS depression, seizures, nephrosis	Milk or egg whites orally; aggressive supportive therapy
Furniture polish	Petroleum-based products cause CNS depression, mucosal irritation, and hepatorenal damage	Lavage but avoid aspiration and monitor for pneumonia; aggressive support
Matches	Potassium chloride can cause GI irritation, vomiting, methemoglobinemia	Supportive treatment; monitor for methemoglobinemia
Nicotine	Ingestion can cause depression, cyanosis, and dyspnea; coma and death can occur	Adsorbents and cathartics; supportive therapy
Hexachlorophene	Found in soaps and deodorants; blindness may occur	GI adsorbents and support
Sodium chloride (salt)	Polydypsia, depression, excitement, hemoglobinemia, ataxia, death	Cerebral edema should be treated with diuretics and fluids (D₅W, 2.5% dextrose)

AChE inhibition. The neuropathy target esterase is inhibited by prolonged exposure to the OP molecule. Clinical signs include weakness, ataxia, and decreased proprioception that progresses to paralysis. The paralysis observed in Amazon parrots progresses in an ascending direction.

The diagnosis of OP or carbamate toxicosis is often based on a history of recent exposure or use in the household. Most warning labels apply to the safety of humans or other mammals and do not take into account the high sensitivity of birds to these chemicals. Cholinesterase analysis of whole blood or brain tissue may establish exposure, but paired samples from nonexposed birds may be required. Most toxicology laboratories do not have reference ranges for avian cholinesterase, and local or state veterinary laboratories should be consulted before submitting samples. Insecticide residues can be identified from suspected food or food containers, GI contents, liver, body fat, and skin.[28]

Antidotes for OP or carbamate toxicity should be instituted within the first 24 hours of exposure to be effective because OP irreversibly binds to AChE. Atropine (0.2 to 0.5 mg/kg IM) every 3 to 4 hours until cessation of clinical signs is the treatment of choice for OP or carbamate toxicity. One-fourth of the initial dose can be given intravenously (IV). Pralidoxime chloride (2-PAM, Ayerst) can be given at 10 to 20 mg/kg every 8 to 12 hours in conjunction with atropine. If no response to 2-PAM is observed after the first dose, caution should be used with repeated doses. The use of 2-PAM in carbamate exposures is controversial because of reports indicating a reduction in the protective effects of atropine when 2-PAM is used. The AChE-OP bond can require several days to achieve spontaneous decay; therefore, close monitoring of the bird is important. Atropine has little or no effect on nicotinic receptor sites, and when used alone does not counteract OP neuromuscular paralysis.[25, 26, 28]

Supportive therapy includes washing exposed skin or feathers with mild detergent. If ingestion has occurred, activated charcoal and cathartic treatment is indicated. Concurrent administration of medications such as phenothiazines, theophylline, diazepam, fluids, and heat are beneficial as needed.

Anticoagulant rodenticides include products such as warfarin, brodifacoum, and indanedione derivatives. The mechanism of action is interference with vitamin K recycling. Warfarin is a first-generation anticoagulant and requires multiple- or large-dose ingestions to reach toxic levels. It has a shorter half-life than brodifacoum and does not require the length of therapy necessitated by brodifacoum exposure (5–7 days for warfarin and 2 weeks or more for brodifacoum).[29, 30] Brodifacoum has a prolonged half-life and can be lethal with a single ingestion. Clinical signs range from depression and anorexia to subcutaneous hemorrhage, bleeding from the nares, and oral petechiation.[18]

The treatment of choice is vitamin K_1 (0.2–2.2 mg/kg IM) every 4 to 8 hours until stable, then daily. The duration of treatment depends on the type of anticoagulant ingested, the dose, and clinical signs. Birds should be rechecked up to 2 weeks after treatment to detect recurrence of clinical signs.

Other pesticides causing avian toxicoses are crimidine (Castrix), zinc phosphide, alphachloralose, and chlorophenols.[28] Treatment for crimidine ingestion is pyridoxine and diazepam. Zinc phosphide ingestion is treated with supportive therapy and 5% sodium bicarbonate gavaging solution. Alphachloralose is an avicide used for pigeon overpopulation; toxicosis is treated with anticonvulsants. Other avicides include 4-aminopyridine or 4-AP (Avitrol), which causes disorientation and vocalization, and 2-chloro-4-acetotoludine (CAT) and 3-chloro-p-toludine (CPT), which cause liver and kidney necrosis. Chlorophenols are used for termite control and as herbicides or fungicides. Mortalities have been reported from contaminated bedding.

TOXIC PLANTS

The most common questions from bird owners related to toxins involve the ingestion of houseplants and certain foods. Plant toxicoses are rare, and many sources reporting toxic plants have been extrapolated from lists of plants toxic to mammals. Significant evolutionary adaptations, physiologic variations, and variable digestive transit times between birds and mammals may explain why ingestion of many plants is tolerated by birds but not by mammals. Many birds eat only parts of a plant, avoiding the toxin, whereas mammals tend to eat larger portions. Clinical studies and case reports have shown a wide variation in avian species tolerance to reportedly toxic plants. Many clinical reports have not addressed the potential of herbicide or pesticide residues contributing to toxic reactions. Plants reported to cause toxic reactions in birds are listed in Table 35–4.

Many birds are curious chewers or browsers, and determining the amount of plant ingested or just shredded is difficult. The majority of plant-related reactions result in oral irritation or mild GI upsets. Some plants considered toxic to mammals have been force-fed to birds with no deleterious effects. For example, budgerigars appear to be much more resistant to the effects of cardiac glycosides compared with mammals. Similarly, *Prunus* species containing cyanogenic glycosides, such as choke cherry, peach, almond, and laurels, have been listed as potential toxins in pet birds and fowl, but documentation is rare or nonexistent. Philodendrons have been considered safe by some practitioners because of their use in aviaries with no problems.[20] However, lethargy and vomiting from ingestion have been observed and documented. This discrep-

Table 35–4

PLANTS CLINICALLY REPORTED TO CAUSE TOXIC REACTIONS IN PET BIRDS, WATERFOWL, GAMEFOWL, AND RATITES

Avocado (*Persea americana*)
Bishops weed (*Acgopodium podograria*)
Black locust (*Robina pseudoacacia*)
Blue-green algae (*Microcystis aeruginosa*)
Burdock (*Arctium minus*)
Camel bush (*Trichodesma incanum*)
Castor bean (*Ricinus communis*)
Clematis (*Montana rubens*)
Coffee bean (*Sesbania drumundii*)
Diffenbachia (*Diffenbachia* spp)
Elephants ear (*Colocasia* or *Alocasia* spp)
Ergot (*Claviceps purpurea*)
Lily of the valley (*Convallaria majalis*)
Locoweed (*Astragalus emoryanus*)
Maternity plant (*Kalanchoe* spp)
Milkweed (*Asclepias* spp)
Nightshade (*Solanum* spp)
Oak (*Quercus* spp)
Oleander (*Nerium oleander*)
Parsley (*Petroselinum sativum*)
Philodendron (*Philodendron scandens*)
Poinsettia (*Euphorbia pulcherrima*)
Pokeweed (*Phytolacca americana*)
Precatory bean (*Arbus precatoius*)
Rhododendron (*Rhododendron simsii*)
Tobacco (*Nicotiana* spp)
Virginia creeper (*Parthenocissus* spp)
Yew (*Taxus media*)

Adapted from LaBonde, Vet Clin North Am 1991[18].

Table 35–5

PLANT TOXICOSES IN BUDGERIGARS (B) AND CANARIES (C)

Plant	Bird
Avocado (*Persea americana*)	B
Black locust (*Robina pseudoacacia*)	B
Clematis (*Montana rubens*)	B
Diffenbachia (*Diffenbachia* spp)	C
Foxglove (*Digitalis pupurea*)	C
Lilly of the valley (*Convallaria majalis*)	B
Lupinus spp	C
Oleander (*Nerium oleander*)	B, C
Philodendron (*Philodendron scandens*)	B
Poinsettia (*Euphorbia pulcherrima*)	B
Rhododendron (*Rhododendron simsii*)	B
Virginia creeper (*Parthenocissus quinquefolio*)	B
Yew (*Taxus media*)	B, C

Data from LaBonde, Vet Clin North Am, 1991[18]; Kenny et al, Proc Am Assoc Zoological Parks and Aquariums, 1987[29]; Lawerence et al, J Wildl Dis, 1985[30]; Arai et al, J Am Vet Med Assoc, 1992[31]; Hargis et al, J Am Vet Med Assoc, 1989[32].

ancy may be the result of species variation and dose.

Clinical studies in budgerigars and canaries have provided useful information on the effects of plants known to be toxic to birds (Table 35–5). The most common clinical signs observed are lethargy and regurgitation. With avocado toxicosis, weakness, depression, anorexia, tachypnea, and death can be observed. Small birds such as canaries and budgies seem to be more susceptible.[31, 32] However, one author (LaBonde) has observed death in cockatiels and depression with regurgitation in an Amazon parrot. In two separate cases, one cockatiel suffered sudden death, and another was depressed for 36 hours before death. Pulmonary congestion is the primary concern. The toxin responsible for avocado poisoning has not been identified.

Treat birds with suspected plant toxicoses according to their clinical signs, with treatment directed toward the principal toxin of the plant. Activated charcoal, cathartics, bulk diets, or mineral oil can be helpful in preventing further absorption. Birds with stomatitis may need gavage feeding. Supplemental fluids and supportive care may be needed.

PREVENTION

Prevention of toxicosis includes counseling the owner of a new bird on the dangers of common toxic substances (lead, zinc, PTFE, chocolate, avocados, etc.). The purchase of domestically produced national or international brandname cages and feed bowls is recommended to avoid exposure to toxins from cages. Examination and treatment of new galvanized wire (if necessary) is recommended. Removal of dangerous items from the household such as leaded weights and pellets is the best course of preventive action. Careful use of household pesticides is warranted.

References

1. Marshall R: Avian anthelmintics and antiprotozoals. Semin Avian Exotic Pet Med 2(1):37, 1993.
2. LaBonde J: Avian toxicities. Proc Assoc Avian Vet, Houston, 1988, pp 159–174.
3. VanSant F: Zinc toxicosis in a hyacinth macaw. Proc Assoc Avian Vet, Chicago, 1991, pp 255–259.
4. Mazliah I, Barron S, Bental E, et al: The effects of long-term lead intoxication on the nervous system of the chicken. Neurosci Lett 101:253–257, 1989.
5. Lloyd M: Heavy metal ingestion: Medical management and gastroscopic removal. J Assoc Avian Vet 6:25–29, 1992.
6. Howard BR: Health risks of housing small psittacines in galvanized wire mesh cages. J Am Vet Med Assoc 200(11):1667–1674, 1992.
7. Buck WB, Osweiler GD, VanGelder GA: Clinical and Diagnostic Toxicology, 2nd ed. Dubuque, IA, Kendall Hunt Publishers, 1976, p 321.
8. Worell A: Therapy of noninfectious avian disorders. Semin Avian Exotic Pet Med 2(1):42–47, 1993.
9. Bond M: Intravenous catheter therapy. Proc Assoc Avian Vet, Nashville, 1993, pp 8–14.
10. Kowalczyk DF: Clinical management of lead poisoning. J Am Vet Med Assoc 184(7):858–860, 1984.
11. VanSant F: Avian gastrointestinal tract surgery. Semin Avian Exotic Pet Med 2(2):91–96, 1993.
12. Clipsham R: Introduction to psittacine pediatrics. Vet Clin North Am Small Anim Pract 21(6):1361–1392, 1991.
13. Altman RB: Avian neonatal and pediatric surgery. Semin Avian Exotic Pet Med 1(1):34–39, 1992.
14. Mautino M: Avian lead intoxication. Proc Assoc Avian Vet, Phoenix, 1990, pp 245–247.
15. LaBonde J: Avian toxicology. Vet Clin North Am Small Anim Pract 21(6):1329–1342, 1991.
16. Lyman R: Polytetrafluoroethylene toxicity. In Harrison GJ, Harrison LR (eds): Clinical Avian Medicine and Surgery. Philadelphia, WB Saunders, 1986, p 87.
17. Wells R: Fatal toxicosis in pet birds caused by overheated cooking pan lined with polytetrafluoroethylene. J Am Vet Med Assoc 182(11):1248–1250, 1983.
18. LaBonde J: Avian toxicology. Vet Clin North Am 21(6):1329–1342, 1991.
19. Beasly V: Smoke inhalation. Vet Clin North Am 20(2):545, 1990.
20. Dumonceaux G, Harrison G: Toxins. In Ritchie B, Harrison G, Harrison L (eds): Avian Medicine: Principles and Application. Lake Worth, FL, Wingers Publishing, 1994, pp 1030–1052.
21. Fowler M: Disinfectant and insecticide usage around birds and reptiles. In Kirk RW (ed): Current Vet Therapy VIII. Philadelphia, WB Saunders, 1983, pp 606–611.
22. Kore AM, Kiesche-Nesselrodt A: Toxicology of household products and disinfectants. Vet Clin North Am 20(2):525–538, 1990.
23. Julian R, Hoerr F: Poisons and toxins and mycotoxicoses. In Calneck B (ed): Diseases of Poultry, ed 9. Ames, Iowa State University Press, 1991, pp 863–916.
24. Alexander J: Probable diazinon poisoning in peafowl, a clinical description. Vet Rec 113(20):470, 1983.
25. LaBonde J: Two clinical cases of exposure to household use of organophosphate and carbamate insecticides. Proc Assoc Avian Vet, New Orleans, 1992, pp 113–118.
26. Ritchie B: Organophosphate poisoning in *Columba livia*. Am Avian Vet Today 1(1):23, 1987.
27. Mohan R: Dursban toxicosis in a pet bird breeding operation. Proc Assoc Avian Vet, Phoenix, 1990, pp 112–114.
28. Humphreys DJ: Veterinary Toxicology, ed 3. London, Balliere Tindal, 1988.
29. Kenny D, Kinsey M: Brodifacoum toxicity in avian species at the Denver Zoological Gardens. Regional Proc Am Assoc Zoological Parks and Aquariums, 1987, pp 447–455.
30. Lawrence J, Henny C, Grove R, et al: Effects of pelletized anticoagulant rodenticides on California Quail. J Wildl Dis 21(4):392–394, 1985.
31. Arai M, Stauber E, Shropshire CM: Evaluation of selected plants for their toxic effects in canaries. J Am Vet Med Assoc 200(9):1329–1331, 1992.
32. Hargis AM, Stauber E, Casteel S, et al: Avocado (Persea americana) intoxication in caged birds. J Am Vet Med Assoc 194(1):64, 1989.

Susan Orosz
Gerry M. Dorrestein
Brian L. Speer
· · · · · · · · · · · · · · ·

36

Urogenital Disorders

Susan Orosz
· · · · · · · · · · · · · ·

Anatomy of the Urogenital System

THE URINARY SYSTEM

The kidneys of birds are fixed to the ventral depressions of the synsacrum or the ventral fossa. The kidneys are paired and each one is divided into a cranial, middle, and caudal division in most species (Fig. 36–1*A*). The divisions of the kidneys of birds may be distinct externally as in psittacines and Galliformes, indistinct as in passerines, or the caudal divisions may be fused to each other as in herons, puffins, and penguins. These lobules are not homologous to the lobes of the kidneys of mammals. The spinal nerves of the lumbar and sacral plexuses run through the parenchyma of the kidneys. This is an important clinical consideration in birds with lameness resulting from renal tumors.

The renal lobule may be seen on the surface of the kidney as a small rounded projection. In cross-section, it represents a pear-shaped wedge of both cortical and medullary tissue between interlobular veins of the renal-portal system and interlobular collecting tubules. Each lobule is supplied by an intralobular artery and an intralobular vein, which is the reverse of that present in mammals (Fig. 36–1*B*). The cortical region is the widest, proximal end of this pear-shaped wedge. It consists of both cortical and medullary type nephrons. The cortical portion of the lobule drains into more than one medullary region and drainage occurs toward the medulla. The medullary region or cone is the smaller portion of the pear and is the area where the medullary loops or loops of Henle and the collecting tubules are found. Each lobe is composed of a cone-shaped bundle of medullary collecting tubules that drain into a single collecting duct.

There are two types of nephrons in birds. The cortical type is reptilian in form, and the medullary type is mammalian in form. The cortical type is urecotelic, producing urates, whereas the medullary type produces urine. The renal corpuscles of birds are composed of a glomerular or Bowman capsule, which is indented by a glomerular tuft of capillaries. Both nephron types have this anatomic arrangement. The corpuscles are arranged radially around the centrally located intralobular or efferent vein. The renal corpuscles of birds are considered to be less complex anatomically than those found in mammals.

Cortical nephrons have their proximal and distal convoluted tubules confined to the cortical region of the kidney. The proximal convoluted tubule is found in the periphery of the lobule and occupies approximately one-half of the total length of the nephron. The intermediate segment is short and convoluted and its distal convoluted tubule is closely associated with the intralobular vein. The cortical type nephrons excrete uric acid by filtering it through their glomeruli and by secreting it mainly from the peritubular capillary plexus into the proximal convoluted tubules.

The proximal and distal convoluted tubules of the medullary type nephron are also in the cortical region. However, the intermediate segment of the tubule is the loop of Henle, and it is found in the medulla as medullary cones. There can be both short and long loop mammalian type nephrons.

Collecting tubules may be found superficially between lobules in the cortical region or in the medullary cone where they combine to form a collecting duct. A counter-current multiplier is present in the medullary cone, which is capable of producing concentrated urine. However, the degree of concentration is much less in birds than it is in mammals.

The arterial supply to the kidneys is from the cranial, middle, and caudal renal arteries from the abdominal aorta. These arteries subdivide to form the intralobular arteries, which further divide to form the afferent glomerular arteries, and they in turn form the glomeruli. The glomerulus of birds is less complex than that found in mammals, forming two to three capillaries that continue as the efferent glomerular arteriole. The peritubular capillary plexus arises, in part, from the efferent arterioles. The plexus then drains into the centrally located intralobular veins. In the medullary region are vasa recta that arise from the afferent glomerular arterioles. They in turn drain into the venulae recta, which again drain into the intralobular veins. In addition, there are interlobular veins at the periphery of the lobule that arise from the renal portal system. These veins are continuous with the peritubular capillary plexus as well.

The renal portal system is a venous vascular ring that allows blood to be shunted in several directions—the caudal vena cava; caudal mesenteric vein and hence to the liver; the internal verte-

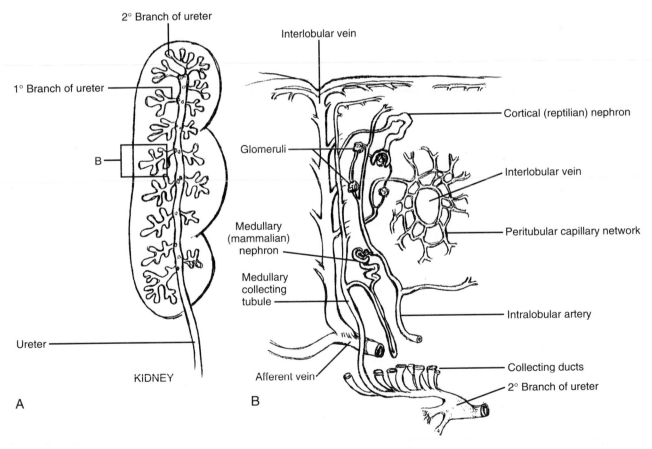

Figure 36-1

Diagram of the kidney of the bird. *(A)* Ventral view of the kidney and its collecting system. The kidney is composed of three divisions—cranial, middle, and caudal. The ureter collects urine and urates from the collecting tubules. Its lining consists of a pseudostratified columnar epithelium that secretes mucus to help move the urates down the tract. Inset *(B)* Diagram of the nephron types in a renal lobule. Birds have both cortical (reptilian) nephrons and medullary (mammalian) nephrons.

bral venous plexus of the vertebral column; and the peritubular capillary plexus. This anatomic arrangement has important implications with drug metabolism, particularly when drugs are given in the muscle of the leg or thigh.

The vascular ring includes the cranial and caudal renal portal veins and their anastomoses (Fig. 36–2). The right and left cranial renal portal veins are connected with the cranial renal veins and are a continuation of the common iliac veins. The cranial renal portal veins anastomose with the internal vertebral venous plexus, allowing blood to go from the pelvic limb through the kidneys and then into the venous system of the spinal cord. The right and left caudal renal portal veins anastomose with each other and the coccygyomesenteric veins. The internal iliac and ischiatic veins feed into the caudal portion of the ring formed by the right and left caudal renal portal veins. There is a renal portal valve in the common iliac vein where the cranial renal portal vein arises. When the valve is open,

blood is shunted away from the kidney into the caudal vena cava and hence the systemic circulation. This valve is opened by action of adrenergic fibers. It is closed by action of histamine or acetylcholine released from cholinergic fibers. When closed, blood from the pelvic limb is shunted into the portal system and then into the parenchyma of the kidney. Approximately two-thirds of the renal blood volume is derived from portal flow. This suggests that the renal portal system provides the majority of the uric acid for elimination in the peritubular capillary plexus and the cortical nephrons.

The ureter begins along the medial edge of the cranial division of the kidney and continues in a groove ventrally and usually medially. The ureter opens into the dorsal wall of the urodeum, a compartment of the cloaca. The ureter should be identified and avoided when a kidney biopsy is performed. The lining of the ureter is a mucus-secreting pseudostratified columnar epithelium. The mucus produced is important in moving uric acid and

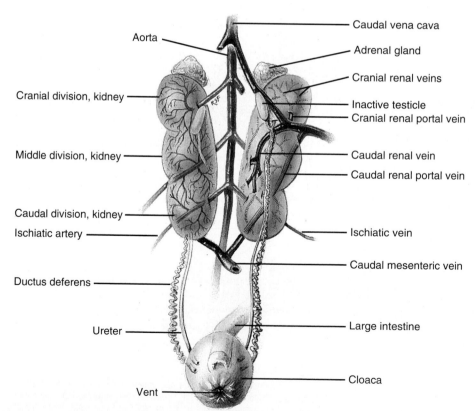

Aorta
Cranial division, kidney
Middle division, kidney
Caudal division, kidney
Ischiatic artery
Ductus deferens
Ureter
Vent

Caudal vena cava
Adrenal gland
Cranial renal veins
Inactive testicle
Cranial renal portal vein
Caudal renal vein
Caudal renal portal vein
Ischiatic vein
Caudal mesenteric vein
Large intestine
Cloaca

F i g u r e 3 6 – 2

Diagram of the urogenital tract of a male bird *(ventral view)*. The blood supply to the kidneys is also shown. The renal portal system of the bird is important in the metabolism of drugs and as an avenue for movement of infectious agents or metastatic cells.

urates down the ureter into the urodeal portion of the cloaca. Urate precipitation could result in the obstruction of the ducts.

FEMALE REPRODUCTIVE SYSTEM

Although the female avian embryo has two gonads and oviducts, usually only the left side develops. The right ovary and oviduct usually regress and disappear by adulthood. However, both ovaries are often retained in a number of raptor species and within individuals of other orders. The right oviduct is less frequently retained in various species but is more commonly found in birds of prey. These are important anatomic considerations when surgically sexing birds.

Mesodermal germ cells migrate into the ovaries to become part of the germinal epithelium. As the embryo develops, its germ cells undergo three phases of oogenesis. In the first phase, the oogonia, or germ cells, actively divide for a defined period of time and then stop at the prophase of the first maturation division. In the second phase, the germ cells grow in size to become primary oocytes. In domestic fowl, this phase occurs at approximately the time of hatch. During the third phase oocytes complete the first maturation division to become secondary oocytes. The completion of the second maturation period results in an ovum.

The ovarian medulla consists of blood vessels that are arranged as irregular vascular zones, interstitial cells, autonomic nerve fibers, and smooth muscle. These ova are located peripherally in the cortex of the ovary. The surface of the ovary is covered by parietal peritoneum with an underlying layer of dense connective tissue, the tunica albuginea. The ovary is suspended by a dorsal mesentery, the mesovarium. It receives its vascular supply from the cranial renal artery, which often has numerous short branches. Often there are two ovarian veins that drain blood flow directly into the caudal vena cava. Because the stalk of the cranial renal artery is short, ovariectomy is technically extremely difficult. The ovary is located just caudal to the adrenal gland and near the cranial tip of the cranial division of the kidney along the body wall. It lies deep to the abdominal air sac, which forms an ovulation pocket in domestic fowl near the time of the lay. This pocket is thought to help retrieve the ovulated ovum with its yolk into the oviduct opening.

The oviduct enlarges around the time of sexual activity to occupy the dorsal portion of the left intestinal-peritoneal portion of the coelomic cavity. Seasonal growth and differentiation is under hormonal control. The oviduct is divided into five parts: the infundibulum, magnum, isthmus, shell gland or uterus, and vagina (Fig. 36–3).

The wall of the oviduct is lined by a mucosa composed primarily of ciliated epithelial cells with unicellular mucous glands or goblet cells. The submucosa has mucosal folds that spiral slightly and vary in height and thickness. Submucosal tubular glands (except in the vagina) have glandular grooves in the infundibulum. The muscularis mucosa has an inner layer of circular smooth muscle and an outer layer of longitudinal smooth muscle.

The infundibulum is subdivided into the more proximal funnel that narrows down into the tubular portion or the chalaziferous region. The funnel portion consists of a very thin wall with low mucosal folds. It is this funnel that surrounds and engulfs the ovulated ovum with its yolk to draw it into the

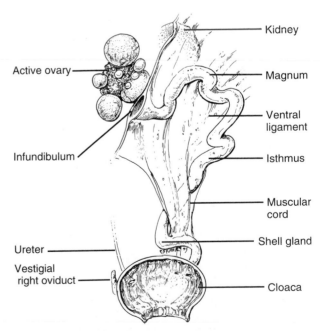

Figure 36–3

Diagram of the female reproductive tract of the bird *(ventral view)*. The ovary sits just distal to the adrenal and proximal to the cranial division of the kidney against the dorsal body wall. Most birds have only a left ovary and oviduct.

oviduct. At the beginning and at the end of the lay cycle, the oviduct and the ovary may not be synchronous, resulting in ovulation without infundibular capture. This is called internal laying. The yolk may be resorbed or it may lead to peritonitis. The mechanism by which peritonitis occurs after internal laying is not well understood. It is in the funnel portion of the oviduct where fertilization occurs.

The tubular portion of the infundibulum is thicker-walled with taller branching folds than in the funnel portion. Beneath these folds are branched convoluted tubular glands that produce the chalaza, the fibrous bands that suspend the yolk within the egg. In this region, a thin but dense layer of albumin is added to surround the yolk (Fig. 36–4). In some species, there are sperm host glands in this region that maintain sperm for fertilization for a variable period of time.

The magnum is distinguished histologically by the large mucosal folds that result from the numerous branched tubular glands. The majority of albumen is added in this region by these glands, along with sodium, magnesium, and calcium. This release of albumen as the yolk passes along the magnum may be controlled by mechanical, neural, and endocrine factors.

In domestic poultry, a narrow translucent band separates the next portion of the oviduct, the isthmus, from the magnum. However, this band is not present in psittacines. The isthmus is short and the

mucosal folds are less prominent. The tubular glands in this region are unique in that they produce sulfur-containing proteins. These proteins are incorporated into the shell membranes, which are also produced in the isthmus. A small amount of albumin is added to the developing egg as it passes through this region. Calcification may be initiated while the egg is still in the isthmus.

As the egg travels down the oviduct, the majority of its time is spent in the uterus, or shell gland. There are two portions—a short, relatively narrow region where the egg traverses relatively rapidly and a pouch-like region where it spends a longer period of time. It is in the pouch-like portion that the calcification proceeds to completion. "Plumping" of the egg most likely occurs in the more proximal, short narrow region. Plumping is a process whereby a large amount of water and solutes are added relatively quickly. The mucosal lining is characterized by a large number of leaf-like lamellar folds that press against the surface of the egg. These folds increase the surface area to improve completion of calcification and plumping.

The vagina is separated from the uterus by a vaginal sphincter. In most species, it is a passageway for the rapid exit of the egg out of the oviduct into the urodeum. However, the egg may remain for a longer period to allow for hardening of the shell in some species. At the uterovaginal junction are sperm host glands for storage of sperm. Sperm viability is maintained for extended periods. In the

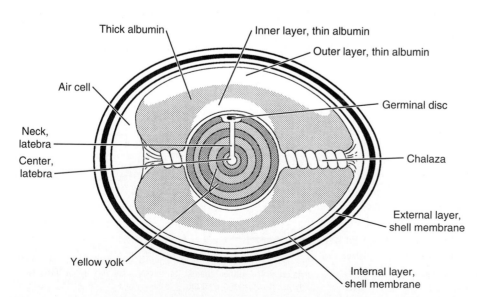

Figure 36–4

Diagram of an egg, longitudinal section. The light area is the thin albumin, whereas the stippled area is the thick albumin. The central area of yellow yolk can be layered as yellow and white strata. There is a central latebra that is part of the yellow yolk. The germinal disc, when fertilized, will become the embryo.

turkey, viability may be maintained for up to several months.

MALE REPRODUCTIVE SYSTEM AND CLOACA

The testes are paired, ovoid organs that lie near the cranial pole of the kidney (Fig. 36–5). They are slightly caudal to the adrenal glands. Each testicle is suspended by a short mesentery or mesorchium that protrudes into each intestinal peritoneal cavity and is partially surrounded medially by the abdominal air sac. The testes change in size and color based on hormonal fluctuations that alter sexual activity. This increased size is the result of the increased length and diameter of the seminiferous tubules and the numbers of Leydig or interstitial

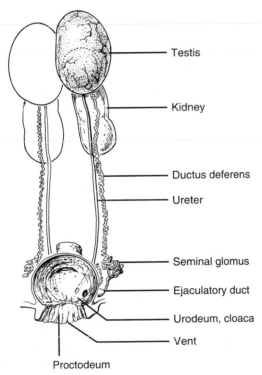

Figure 36–5

Diagram of the male reproductive system of a passerine during breeding season *(ventral view)*. The epididymis is attached to the testis dorsally and is not well demarcated into segments in the bird. During breeding season, each testicle enlarges and the ductus deferens elongates at its distal end, the seminal glomus. The glomus often protrudes on either side of the vent, allowing for the determination of sex.

cells. In general, increased size is the result of increasing serum concentrations of follicle stimulating hormone (FSH) and luteinizing hormone (LH). These physiologic processes occur during the nuptial or culmination phase of the reproductive cycle. Often the inactive testicle is white to yellow in color because of the accumulation of lipid in the interstitial cells. In some species, the immature or inactive testicle is black because of a large number of melanocytes. When these birds become sexually active, their testicles turn gray and possibly even white from the increased volume of the seminiferous tubules.

Birds do not have septa that divide the testicles into lobules as occurs in mammals. In addition, there are no mediastinum testes. Unlike mammals, the seminiferous tubules of birds anastomose with each other. Each seminiferous tubule is composed of a lining of spermatogonia and sustentacular or Sertoli cells. The spermatogonia divide to form primary spermatocytes. They then divide to form secondary spermatocytes. As the spermatocytes progress toward the lumen, they undergo a maturation process to become spermatids. The spermatids mature into spermatozoa or sperm. Maturation proceeds with the head end of each of the spermatozoa embedded in the sustentacular cells. These nurturing cells extend the width of the epithelium to provide support for the developing spermatozoa. The Sertoli cells may also produce steroid hormones, or at least bind testosterone, and are phagocytic.

The sperm, when mature, detach from the Sertoli cells and travel down the lumen of the seminiferous tubules. In most species, these tubules converge into a smaller number of short straight tubules that continue as the rete testes. The rete is a meshwork of tubules embedded in connective tissue. Both the rete testes and the straight tubules are lined by a low cuboid epithelium of sustentacular cells. The rete testes are located dorsomedially to each testicle, adjacent to the epididymis.

The Leydig, or interstitial cells, are found between seminiferous tubules. They are light-colored and eosinophilic with hematoxylin-eosin stain because of the large concentration of smooth endoplasmic reticulum and droplets of cholesterol. The smooth endoplasmic reticulum is involved in the conversion of the cholesterol to steroid hormones, with testosterone and androstenedione being the major androgens. These hormones stimulate the development of secondary sex characteristics; courtship behavior such as coloration and song; and the development and maturation of the tubules of the male system, particularly the ductus deferens.

The epididymis of the bird is hidden, because of its dorsomedial location on the testicle and its small size compared to that of mammals. It is not divided into a head, body, and tail, but is composed of many efferent ductules that drain the rete testes or straight tubules. A number of these efferent ductules drain into the main epididymal duct along its length, again a difference from mammals. The epididymal duct is relatively short and straight and is lined by nonciliated pseudostratified columnar epithelium. This epithelium is secretory and provides some of the seminal fluid. Sperm may be stored in the epididymis or in the seminal glomus of more seasonal birds. Some birds have an appendix epididymis that extends cranially into the adrenal glands. The efferent ductules of this tissue may secrete androgens following castration.

The epididymis continues as the ductus deferens. The ductus deferens is closely associated with the ureter dorsomedially in the coelom. It can be distinguished from the latter by its zigzag appearance. It was originally thought that the seminal glomus was similar to the seminal vesicles, but further anatomic studies showed otherwise. In passerines, each ductus elongates distally during the culmination phase of the reproductive cycle to form a ball of tissue, the cloacal promontory, that can project into the cloaca. This protrusion can be used to sex these birds during the breeding season. Birds with a seminal glomus use it as the main storage site for sperm. The ductus is composed of pseudostratified squamous epithelium that is nonciliated and has less secretory function when compared with the epididymis. There are no accessory sex glands in birds.

The semen of birds is derived in part from the sustentacular cells and epithelial cells that line the male reproductive tract. A lymph-like fluid is produced from the lymphatic folds in the floor of the proctodeum. This fluid is thought to be harmful to spermatozoa because of the presence of clotting factors and the high concentrations of chlorine and calcium.

The spermatozoa of birds are either simple or complex (Fig. 36–6). The complex type is found in passerines, whereas the simple type is found in the other species. Like mammals, each spermatozoon is composed of an acrosome, head, and tail. In the simple type of spermatozoon, the acrosome is attached to the head only at its rostral-most point. The head is long and slender and the tail is long and moves in an undulating manner. In the complex type, the entire sperm is spiral in appearance. This type moves by rotating along its longitudinal axis.

The Cloaca

The cloaca is the terminal receptacle for the fecal material from the digestive system (Fig. 36–7); the urine and urates from the urinary system; and egg(s) or semen from the reproductive system. In its dorsal wall is the cloacal bursa, or bursa of Fabricius, which is involved in B lymphocyte development and maturation. The cloaca is divided into the coprodeum, the urodeum, and the proctodeum.

The coprodeum is the cranial-most compartment, and is a direct continuation of the rectum or large intestine. In most birds, it is marked only by expansion of the rectal lumen. In ratites, there is a rectocoprodeal fold that partially separates the two regions. The urodeum is partially separated by the coprodeum and proctodeum by two mucosal folds. The coprourodeal fold is circumferential and acts as a diaphragm that holds fecal material behind it. When the coprodeum is filled with feces, it can protrude into the urodeum and even through the vent. Feces are then deposited directly out of the vent without mixing of urates. The uroproctodeal fold hangs from the roof the cloaca. The urinary and genital ducts empty into the dorsal wall of the urodeum. The ureters are often dorsomedial and the genital ducts open laterally to the ureters. The ureters open directly into the urodeum and are often difficult to visualize. In ratites, they open onto papillae. The left oviduct opens ventrolateral to the ureter onto a small mound. In ducks, geese, and swans, it is closed by a membrane until the bird reaches sexual maturity.

The proctodeum is a small compartment between the uroproctodeal fold and the external cloacal orifice or vent. In the dorsal wall of the proctodeum is the cloacal bursa or the bursa of Fabricius. The cloacal bursa is the site of B lymphocyte production and maturation in the bird. B lymphocytes are an

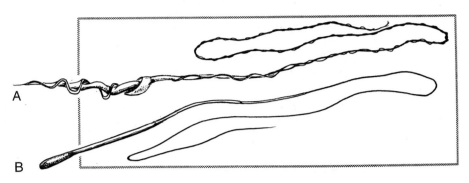

Figure 36-6

Diagram of avian sperm types. *(A)* Complex sperm of passerines. *(B)* Simple sperm type found in most birds.

integral part of humoral immunity. Early in the bird's development, this gland has a duct that opens into the proctodeum so that cells within the bursa can be exposed to fecal antigens for stimulation. Galliformes, in addition to having a cloacal bursa, have a dorsal proctodeal gland that is found just caudal to the cloacal bursa. This gland has lymphocytes that are admixed with mucosal glands. In quail, there is a frothy secretion that is extruded from multiple ducts during coitus. In addition, birds can have lateral proctodeal glands. The function of the dorsal and lateral proctodeal glands is unknown.

The vent is a transverse slit in domestic fowl and other Galliformes and a circular opening in psittacines. The sphincter muscle that surrounds the opening has both an outer circular and an inner transverse striated muscle layer. In addition, birds have a transverse muscle that originates on the pelvic bone and/or caudal vertebrae. It interdigitates with the sphincter muscle that surrounds the vent. When the transverse muscle contracts, it pulls the vent ventrocranially, which is important during breeding. In the male, this muscular action allows for the cloaca to be directed over the female's cloaca. The levator muscle originates ventrally on the tail head and inserts ventrally onto the vent and/or the phallus. It pulls the vent caudally after copulation and defecation.

The phallus (Fig. 36–8) may be present as a nonprotrusible structure (in Galliformes), a protrusible one (in ratites, Anseriformes), or be absent (in Psittaciformes). The non-intromittent phallus is found on the floor of the lip of the vent. Domestic chickens and turkeys have this type of phallus. It consists of a median and two lateral phallic bodies. Lateral to the phallic bodies are lymphatic folds on the ventrolateral floor of the proctodeum. These folds and phallic bodies are connected by a lymphatic meshwork. It is the lymphatic flow through

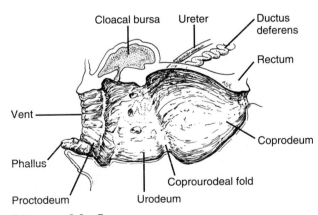

Cloacal bursa   Ureter   Ductus deferens

Rectum

Vent

Coprodeum

Phallus

Proctodeum   Urodeum   Coprourodeal fold

Figure 36-7

Diagram of the right side of the cloaca of a male fowl *(longitudinal section)*. The cloaca is subdivided into compartments—the coprodeum stores the fecal material and the urodeum stores the urinary products. The ductus deferens or oviduct empties into the urodeum. Any of these products moves through the third portion of the cloaca, the proctodeum.

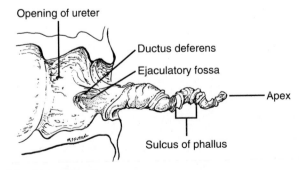

Opening of ureter

Ductus deferens

Ejaculatory fossa

Apex

Sulcus of phallus

Figure 36-8

Diagram of the cloaca of a duck *(longitudinal section)* demonstrating an everted, erect phallus. There are two types of phalluses—non-intromittent and intromittent. Psittacine and passerine birds, for example, do not have a phallus.

these structures that results in tumescence. The lymphatic folds and lateral phallic bodies have a greater accumulation of fluid than that of the median phallic body, thereby producing eversion and a groove for semen to travel. The phallus contacts the everted oviduct opening where semen is deposited.

An intromittent phallus can be of two types—one without a ventral cavity (in ostriches, kiwis, and tinamous), and one with a cavity (in emus, rheas, cassowaries, and Anseriformes) where the phallus lies at rest. The former type of phallus consists of paired fibrolymphatic bodies with a dorsal sulcus for semen to travel. This phallus lies on the floor of the cloaca and partially everts during micturition and defecation. Tumescence occurs by increased lymphatic flow and stasis into an elastic vascular body within the distal end of phallus. The latter type of phallus is also found in the floor of the cloaca but is enclosed in a sac or cavity. The proximal end usually stays within the cavity and does not engorge. Only the distal end everts on engorgement by lymphatic fluid.

Gerry M. Dorrestein

Physiology of the Urogenital System

KIDNEYS AND OTHER EXCRETORY SYSTEMS

Excretion of water and nitrogenous wastes by birds combines processing by the kidneys and the intestines and, in some species, the action of salt-secreting glands. Avian kidneys differ in structure and function from those of reptiles or mammals. Urine produced by the kidneys mixes with fecal components in the lower intestine, where additional water can be resorbed as needed.

The most conspicuous physiologic adaptation for promoting water economy in birds is the excretion of nitrogenous wastes in the form of uric acid, white crystals that are synthesized in the liver and that give bird droppings their usual color. Ninety percent of its secretion is by tubular secretion from reptilian type nephrons and therefore largely independent of urine flow. Excretion of nitrogen as urea (in mammals) in aqueous solution requires flushing by large quantities of water, but uric acid can be excreted as a semisolid suspension (colloid solution) in which each molecule of uric acid contains twice as much nitrogen as a molecule of urea. Therefore, birds require only 0.5 to 1.0 ml of water to excrete 370 ml of nitrogen as uric acid, whereas mammals require 20 ml of water to excrete the same amount of nitrogen as urea. Birds concentrate uric acid in the cloaca, just prior to defecation, to amazing levels—up to 3000 times the acid level in their blood.

Gout, a precipitation of uric acid on serosa or in joints (visceral or articular gout), should be regarded as a clinical sign of any severe renal dysfunction that causes a chronic, moderate hyperuricemia.[1]

Water typically constitutes 75 to 90% of the excrement of birds with access to plenty of water, but can drop to 55% in desert-dwelling birds.

Although avian kidneys can concentrate nitrogenous wastes, they usually cannot concentrate salt or electrolytes much above normal blood levels. This is the result of the short loops of Henle in the avian kidney, presumably associated with the excretion of uric acid instead of urea. Birds with a high salt intake, like sea birds, rely on extrarenal structures called "nasal salt glands."

ANNUAL CYCLES OF BIRDS

The typical year of most birds has only three main, sequential tasks: breed, moult, and survive until the following breeding season. Migration can complicate this annual pattern.

In areas where the climate is very stable and day length is unchanged, birds normally start to nest when the rains begin. Adults begin to moult shortly after the young have left the nest and continue moulting until the beginning of the "dry" season, when food starts to become scarce. When heavy rains resume and food supplies increase, gonads increase in size and the cycle repeats itself. Similar sequences of reproduction and moult occur in residents of northern temperate locations. The trigger in this situation is the increasing length of daylight in the spring.

This annual cycle involves an orderly sequence of complex integrated behavioral and physiologic conditions. A network of physiologic controls regulates the schedules of reproduction, moult, sleep, feeding, and migration.

In the cells of all plants and animals, biologic clocks control the release of hormones and other chemicals that regulate metabolism, reproduction, and behavior.

Birds possess an elaborate system of biologic clocks. Neuroendocrine systems synchronize cellular rhythms so that the entire bird is organized internally and appropriately synchronized with its periodically altering environment.

Biologic clocks, called circannual cycles, are synchronized to the annual cycle of the earth's revolution around the sun. In constant environments, circannual cycles tend to drift. Seasonal changes in day length probably entrain the endogenous circannual rhythms.[2]

Other biologic clocks, called circadian rhythms, match the daily 24-hour cycle of the earth's rotation on its axis. Twilight triggers a switch in animal physiology from diurnal to nocturnal systems. This rhythm is not exactly 24 hours in length, but external light-dark cycles adjust the endogenous rhythm, keeping it synchronized with the 24-hour cycle.

The Role of Photoperiod

Seasonal reproduction by birds has favored the evolution of a control system that synchronizes the physiologies of individuals with the environment. Day length, or photoperiod, plays a key role in this control system. Specifically, the avian photoperiodic control system uses two kinds of information: environmental light, which stimulates neural receptors, and clock information from an internal circadian cycle, which enables the bird to measure day length. This system allows birds to respond at the mean optimal time for reproduction, to synchronize

reproductive function in mating pairs, and to terminate reproductive function—three fundamental requirements for control of the annual reproductive cycle.

In temperate zone bird species, the gonadal cycles are predominantly controlled by the photoperiod. The longer days in early spring stimulate gonad development and, in some species, the pre-alternate moult and spring migration. Supplemental information such as warmer temperature, rainfall, and the springtime display behavior of other individuals provide fine-tuning of physiologic events of breeding and, as a result, the increased secretion of sexual hormones.

The pineal gland (hypophysis cerebri) has been regarded as the probable location of the biologic clock and the mechanisms of photosensitivity in birds, but unlike the glands in reptiles, avian pineal glands do not house the primary light receptors. In addition, birds do not monitor day length visually, as do mammals, but do so by means of special receptors in the hypothalamus. After stimulation of the photoreceptors directly, neurosecretory cells in the hypothalamus induce the release of neurohormones in the neural portion (median eminence) of the pituitary (epiphysis), which links this organ to the midbrain. The released neurohormones are then carried in the blood to the anterior pituitary gland, where they induce the synthesis and release of luteinizing hormone (LH) and follicle-stimulating hormone (FSH). LH stimulates gonad activity, and the combination with FSH, with release lagging behind that of LH, stimulates the ovaries and testes to make gametes.

Circadian rhythms include a limited photosensitivity period each day, during which external light can stimulate receptors in the brain, which in turn triggers a series of physiologic reactions. As day length increases, so does the chance that there will be daylight during that short photosensitive period. Not only does the chance of overlap, or coincidence, rise with increasing day length, but the duration of the period of overlap also rises. The amount of overlap enables birds to measure day length (Fig. 36–9).

After birds have bred, the shortening days of late summer stimulate the main moult. The gonadal cycle normally concludes with a rapid collapse and reabsorption of gonad tissue. Then there follows a photorefractory period, during which long days do

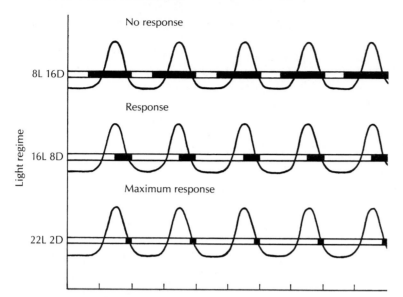

Figure 36–9

The external coincidence model suggests that day length is measured by the increased amount of time that daylight periods *(open bars)* coincide with the photosensitive phase of the circadian rhythm (oscillation peaks). (L = number of hours of light; D = number of hours of dark.) Response was measured in terms of gonadal enlargement, which was greatest for a 22-hour light and 2-hour dark cycle. (From Gill FB: Ornithology. New York, Freeman and Co, 1995, p 271.)

not induce gonad regrowth. The mechanisms of photorefractory physiology are still a mystery, but the phase relationships of two different circadian rhythms may be responsible.

The photorefractory period is best developed in migratory temperate zone species. It is weak or absent in most tropical zone species examined to date, where rainfall usually defines breeding seasons. The photorefractory period in adults seems to be an adaptation for scheduling moult and migratory preparations during the favorable conditions of late summer by discontinuing reproductive activity while days are still long.

Finally, the very short days of early winter, which inhibit gonadal growth, terminate the refractory period, and thereby restore sensitivity to the stimulus of long photoperiods, and the cycle begins anew.

Short winter days are essential to the control of the annual cycle; the gonads do not grow in response to the long days in spring unless the bird has experienced a prior period of short day lengths.

It is easy to change a bird's hormonal physiology by changing day length or photoperiod. This is common practice in canary breeding. Simulating the seasons by increasing or decreasing day lengths can bring captive birds into breeding condition, can cause them to moult more often than normal, and can cause them to accumulate premigratory fat.

Breeding Seasons

Guiding the evolution of the timing of seasonal physiologic controls have been such factors as the timing of adequate food supplies for both parents and their young, availability of nest sites, locations of favorable climates, and areas or times of low predation risk, all of which ornithologists call "ultimate factors."[2] Over many generations, the control systems are tuned to the best average time for reproduction.

Proximate factors are the external conditions that actually induce reproduction. The correct habitat, new vegetation or abundant food, the ritualized displays and aggression among neighbors, and social stimulation in general are all proximate factors that help to bring on the final stages of gonadal enlargement and ovarian development. For desert-dwelling birds and species from the tropical lowlands, rainfall usually defines the breeding activity. Temperature is probably the most important modifier of annual gonadal cycles. In American robins the combination of temperature and humidity were the best predictors of the nesting period. Robins typically had nests with young in late April and early May when the relative humidity was about 50% and the temperatures were between 7° and

18°C. Certain localities where robins do not breed fall outside the species-defined climate space.[3]

Tropical nesting seasons last longer than those in the temperate zone and sometimes permit nesting for 6 to 10 months, or even, in some cases, throughout the year.

Many of the ultimate and proximate factors influence breeding results in captivity.

Diseases of the Urogenital System

Brian L. Speer

Diseases of the avian urogenital system are comparatively less commonly diagnosed in clinical practice than are those of other organ systems. In addition, the volume of literature documenting end-stage organ disease accounts for a large percentage of these diagnoses. These observations suggest that the profession has considerable room for improvement in areas of earlier detection of urogenital system disease, therapy, and preventative management. A key complicating issue clinically is that most early signs are very mild and nonspecific until a fairly advanced stage of urogenital disease has been reached.

Although this chapter predominantly describes the more commonly recognized signs of urogenital system diseases and their diagnostic approaches, it also emphasizes early consideration of these diseases in our differential diagnosis and more aggressive approaches in diagnosis as well as therapy and preventative management.

THE URINARY SYSTEM

Clinical Signs Associated with Renal Disease

Abnormal Urinary Output (Polyuria, Anuria, Oliguria)

"Normal" urine output and water intake vary immensely among birds of different species, age, and physiologic state. When presented with a client complaint of excessive or inadequate urinary output, the initial step required of the practitioner is to use experience and observation to assess if there is a true abnormality present (Table 36–1). Frequently, the urine output described is within normal limits for the species and age of the bird. A common presenting complaint of "diarrhea" often proves to be polyuria on further inquiry and physical examination. Urinary output should be evaluated by volume and color criteria for both its urine and urate component. Other clinical signs in addition to polyuria may be noted during initial physical examination, and they may help to further characterize a differential diagnosis (Fig. 36–10).

Polyuria has been traditionally accepted as one of the classic signs of renal disease in birds, although oliguria and anuria are also noted. Characterized by a true and persistent increase in urinary output and water intake, polyuria is a fairly nonspecific sign that requires diagnostic and interpretive effort on the part of the veterinary practitioner. Polyuria is usually not accompanied by an increase in uric acid or urate excretion concurrently. Oliguria and anuria can also be caused by multiple nonurogenital system sources, severe dehydration being perhaps the most common general cause noted. Cloacal diseases including cloacaliths, neoplasia, and cloacitis may at times be characterized by anuria, oliguria, or stranguria. To further complicate the clinical picture, many cases of renal disease in birds have not been associated with appreciable changes in urinary output.

Polydipsia

Polydipsia, when it occurs with polyuria, is similarly linked to renal disease in birds. Polydipsia may be either the cause of polyuria (e.g., behavioral etiologies) or the result of polyuria (e.g., renal disease, endocrine disease). The diagnostic approach

Table 36-1

ASSESSMENT FLOW CHART FOR ABNORMAL URINARY OUTPUT

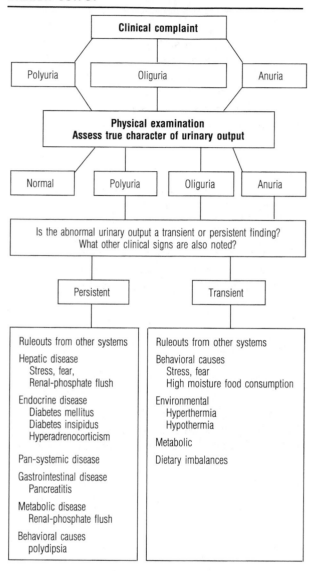

Clinical complaint

Polyuria — Oliguria — Anuria

Physical examination
Assess true character of urinary output

Normal — Polyuria — Oliguria — Anuria

Is the abnormal urinary output a transient or persistent finding?
What other clinical signs are also noted?

Persistent — Transient

Ruleouts from other systems
Hepatic disease
Stress, fear,
Renal-phosphate flush
Endocrine disease
Diabetes mellitus
Diabetes insipidus
Hyperadrenocorticism
Pan-systemic disease
Gastrointestinal disease
Pancreatitis
Metabolic disease
Renal-phosphate flush
Behavioral causes
polydipsia

Ruleouts from other systems
Behavioral causes
Stress, fear
High moisture food consumption
Environmental
Hyperthermia
Hypothermia
Metabolic
Dietary imbalances

Abnormal Urine or Urate Color

Yellow to green urates or urine is suggestive of hemolysis or liver disease. Green-colored urine can be seen in birds with gastrointestinal stasis. Idiopathic, reddish brown urine has been described in some hand-fed psittacine babies that seem to be otherwise healthy with normal growth patterns. This observation is reportedly more common in birds that are receiving an animal protein–based diet and usually resolves when the diet is switched to a plant protein–based formula.[1] Red-colored urine may be attributed to hematuria, and the presence of hematuria in any form is abnormal. Blood that is in the urine may originate from the gastrointestinal (GI) tract, oviduct, kidneys, testicles, or cloaca. Renal diseases associated with visible or occult hematuria include renal neoplasia, bacterial and viral nephritis, and some forms of toxic nephropathies. Occult hematuria tends to correlate well with suspected renal neoplasia in budgerigars, but septicemia should also be included in the differential diagnosis. Red, pink, or tan urates caused by hemoglobinuria are seen commonly in birds with lead poisoning, particularly in Amazon parrots.

General Signs of Renal Disease

Many clinical signs associated with renal disease in birds are similar to those seen in mammals (Table 36–2). Birds are usually lethargic, weak, and anorexic. Birds may regurgitate or vomit, which are signs related to GI stasis and may result from uremia or general ill health. Both signs are common in psittacine pediatrics, wherein dehydration or vita-

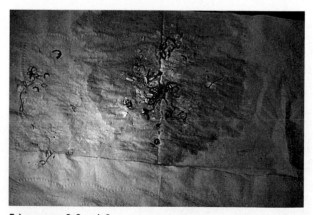

Figure 36-10

True polyuria is a fairly nonspecific sign, requiring diagnostic and interpretive effort on the part of the clinician. This cockatiel was diagnosed with diabetes mellitus based on polyuria, persistent hyperglycemia, and glucosuria. Note the increased urinary volume with normal fecal and uric acid components to the droppings.

to this clinical observation is similar to that described with polyuria.

Table 36-2

GENERAL CLINICAL SIGNS ASSOCIATED WITH RENAL DISEASE

Clinical Signs Similar to Those in Mammals	Clinical Signs Different from Those in Mammals
Lethargy	Articular and visceral gout
Anorexia	Constipation
Regurgitation and vomiting	Lameness
Weakness	Inability to fly
Dehydration	Delayed development in hand-fed
Abdominal mass	chicks
Abdominal distention	

min D_3 toxicosis are frequent causes of renal disease.[4] GI signs are also seen in adult birds in more severe or advanced forms of renal disease. Dehydration may be either the cause or effect of renal disease in avian species (Fig. 36–11).

Abdominal distention is a general sign related to nephromegaly or ascites. Nephromegaly should be included in differential diagnoses involving an abdominal mass. Ventral displacement of the ventriculus, detected by contrast radiography, palpation, ultrasonography, or abdominal transillumination, may support a clinical diagnosis of nephromegaly.

Many other clinical signs of renal disease in birds are not seen in mammals. Birds may develop articular or visceral gout from any severe renal dysfunction that results in chronic, moderate, or severe hyperuricemia. Subcutaneous urate tophi may be

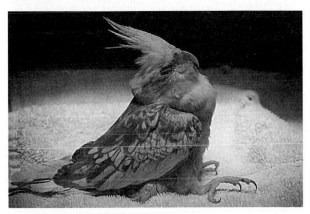

Figure 36-11

This cockatiel was in an advanced stage of renal failure. No forewarning signs were noted by the owners. Even in this stage of disease, the profound dehydration and cachexia are fairly nonspecific signs.

visible with articular gout, particularly on the feet, metatarsal joints, and joints of the wing. Birds may be unable to fly as a general sign related to uremia, physical weakness, or articular gout. Lameness is often the first sign noted in psittacine birds with neurologic deficits resulting from renal neoplasia, particularly in budgerigars. Neurologic deficits and lameness are attributable to direct compression, invasion, or impingement of the branches of the lumbosacral plexus that passes through the kidneys. Lameness may also result from articular gout and uric acid–induced arthritis.

Early recognition and diagnosis of renal disease is frequently difficult because many signs are nonspecific. As a result, visible signs of renal disease are often not detected until the disease process is well advanced. Subclinical disease is probably much more common than is now recognized clinically. Through a complete clinical differential diagnosis and the use of urinalysis, endoscopy, and renal biopsy, early recognition, diagnosis, and treatment of renal disease may be possible.

Diagnostic Tools

Plasma Uric Acid

Elevations of plasma uric acid values above available reference values for the age and species of the bird in question may support a tentative diagnosis of renal dysfunction.[5] Hyperuricemia, however, is neither uniquely specific nor sensitive for renal disease. In general, nonprotein nitrogen substances in plasma, such as uric acid, are elevated only when renal function is below 30% of its original capacity. Uric acid synthesis occurs in both the liver and renal tubules.[6] Uric acid excretion occurs independently of the rate of tubular water reabsorption in birds. Although serum uric acid level is believed to be the best means available to test for renal function, it is not sensitive enough to rely on as a sole means of patient evaluation.

Urea

In most avian species, urea concentration (blood urea nitrogen [BUN]) is considered to have little value in the detection of renal disease. Urea has been shown to be a sensitive indicator of the general state of hydration in birds, however, and has been shown to be of value in detecting early renal disease in pigeons.[7] Although some avian reference laboratories report this value as part of their biochemical profiles, its clinical value in the diagnosis of renal disease remains questionable.

Creatinine

Serum creatinine is viewed to be a poor diagnostic test in birds, perhaps because of their excretion of creatine before its conversion to creatinine.[8] Elevations in creatinine have been described in association with some avian diseases in the past.[9] As for BUN, the clinical value of serum creatinine in the diagnosis of avian renal disease remains unproved.

Urinalysis

The kidneys normally excrete a pasty white to yellow urate and a sparse, clear and colorless watery urine. It is this watery component that can be separated from the urates for analysis, if indicated. Urine for detailed analysis should be collected from an impervious surface as soon as possible after it is excreted. The avian urinalysis should include cytologic testing and determination of the pH, glucose, sediment, color, and specific gravity. The presence of casts or blood is suggestive of possible renal disease.

A urinalysis is indicated if renal disease is suspected, and is a valuable diagnostic tool in general veterinary medicine.[1, 5] Unfortunately, despite its high diagnostic value, urinalysis is not routinely done in avian practice. The presence of an abnormal specific gravity, casts, proteinuria, glucosuria, ketonuria, or hematuria can have significant value in the clinical evaluation of a polyuric avian patient. Urinalysis, if performed and interpreted appropriately, can become a significant tool that aids in early detection of renal disease, and should be a routine portion of the medical workup of the avian patient with suspected renal disease.

Radiology

Radiographic evaluation of the kidneys offers significant potential diagnostic benefit. Increases in renal size or density may support a tentative diagnosis of renal disease. Renal mineralization and nephromegaly are frequently encountered radiographic abnormalities suggestive of renal disease. The identification of renomegaly or other radiographic abnormalities is an indication for endoscopy or biopsy for definitive diagnosis in the stable patient.

Endoscopy and Renal Biopsy

Endoscopy provides direct visual assessment of kidney appearance, as well as that of adjacent organs, and is an invaluable source of information in the evaluation of renal disease in birds. With the new developments in endoscopic equipment, the diagnostic advantage and lower risk of renal biopsy should prove to be of immense benefit in the earlier detection of renal disease in birds. Polyuria, polydipsia, and infertility are all specific urogenital signs of disease that may warrant endoscopy as a portion of the diagnostic workup. This potential should be discussed with the client at the onset of a medical workup, and client acceptance will be greater if the procedure is indicated later on. The recommended sites for renal biopsy are either the middle or caudal divisions, because the cranial renal artery may be easily lacerated or torn if the cranial renal division is biopsied (Fig. 36–12).

Histologically, nephrosis characterizes noninflammatory degenerative lesions of the kidney that may be either acute or chronic. The nephrosis that results from gentamicin toxicosis is in this category. Nephritis or glomerulonephritis is usually a multifocal condition with suppurative lesions. These cases may also show degenerative lesions of the tubules or interstitial nephritis. Nephritis is common in bacterial or other infectious renal diseases.

General Supportive Therapy of Renal Disease

Fluids

Dehydration, if not treated properly, can rapidly result in an augmentation of renal disease in most bird species. This is primarily because uric acid is eliminated by tubular secretion and its rate is

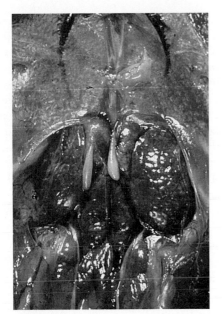

Figure 36–12

The recommended site for renal biopsy is either the middle or caudal renal divisions, because the cranial renal artery may be easily torn.

independent of hydration status of the bird. Uric acid that is actively secreted into renal tubules without regular removal by diuresis can result in sludging or accumulation of urates within the kidneys. Fluids may be administered by gavage or by subcutaneous, intravenous, or interosseous routes, depending on the clinical circumstance. Mannitol, furosemide, and sodium bicarbonate may help increase urinary output in oliguric or anuric patients.

Antibiotics

Depending on the etiologic agent suspected, broad-spectrum antibiotics of a non-nephrotoxic nature are an important consideration in patients with suspected renal disease with poor clinical stability. Because an estimated 50% of nephritis patients have bacterial disease, antibiotic therapy should be a key component of supportive care for renal disease of birds.[1, 10]

Control of Hyperuricemia

If hyperuricemia is suspected or known, allopurinol may be used in conjunction with fluid therapy to attempt to inhibit uric acid synthesis (allopurinol) and increase uric acid secretion.

Low Protein Diet

Initially, gavage feeding of very low protein baby foods may help stabilize birds with clinically confirmed or suspected renal disease. Once stabilized, maintaining a lower dietary protein intake may help improve prognosis for renal disease outcome, particularly in those birds with chronic disease.

RENAL DISEASES

Infectious Diseases

Viruses

Several viral infections are capable of producing polyuria as a clinical sign, although none is characterized by polyuria or renal disease alone. The renal disease and polyuria encountered with most viral diseases represent components of a systemic infection.

Polyoma virus is the best known virus affecting the kidneys of caged birds[11, 12] (Fig. 36–13). Adenovirus[13, 14] and pox[15] have been described in association with renal lesions in caged birds. Proventricular dilatation syndrome (PDS), infectious bronchitis virus (chickens), Newcastle virus, paramyxovirus (pigeons), and other unidentified viral inclusions have also been mentioned in association with renal disease in caged birds.[4]

Polyomavirus infection may be diagnosed ante mortem by polyomavirus probe of a cloacal swab sample. However, a negative polyoma virus probe does not eliminate polyoma virus from the differential diagnoses. Persistent hematuria noted on urinalysis in young hand-fed psittacines with suspicious clinical signs may suggest renal disease, including polyomavirus infection.[16] Renal biopsy should be regarded as the best diagnostic tool to yield positive identification of a viral or other etiologic agent associated with renal disease.

With the exception of herpesvirus, there are no specific treatments available for viral diseases. Treatment protocols for avian species with viral nephritis generally include basic supportive care

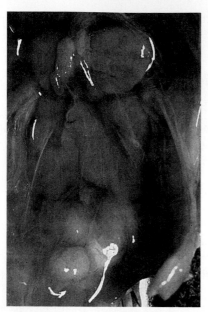

Figure 36-13

This young macaw died of systemic polyoma virus infection. Note the pale color to the organs, nephritis, and bursitis present in this case.

and clinical management of the multisystemic disease processes that are generally present. Herpes infections may respond favorably to acyclovir, although the potential nephrotoxic nature of this drug needs to be considered when treating birds with nephropathies.[17]

Bacteria

The majority of bacterial renal disease is associated with multisystemic disease processes.[10] Less frequently, ascending infections are encountered. Renal lesions that may be present with bacterial infections include granulomas, interstitial nephritis, nephrosis, and glomerulopathy.

Etiologic agents of bacterial renal disease that have been described include *Staphylococcus* species,[18] *Streptococcus* species,[18] *Listeria* species,[19–21] *Escherichia coli*[1, 10, 18] *Klebsiella* species,[22] *Salmonella* species,[21] *Yersinia* species,[20] *Proteus* species,[10, 18] *Pseudomonas* species,[10] *Mycobacterium* species,[1] and *Chlamydia psittaci*.[23]

Diagnosis of bacterial renal disease may be supported by urinalysis, urine culture and sensitivity testing, blood culture testing, renal aspirate, or renal biopsy. Remember that interpretation of results of urinalysis and urine cultures must be done with care, because it is difficult to obtain a pure and clean sample of urine.

Treatment depends on the specific agent identified and severity of disease at the time of diagnosis. Because of the relatively high incidence of bacterial renal disease in caged birds, antibiotic therapy with a non-nephrotoxic broad-spectrum antibiotic is indicated when renal disease is suspected or confirmed. Antibiotics such as the penicillins, which are predominantly cleared by renal tubular secretion or filtration, may demonstrate a shorter half-life in a polyuric avian patient, and this factor should be considered in the therapeutic regimen.

Fungi

Fungal renal disease is comparatively uncommon. Renal disease may result from involvement from adjacent lesions or from renal infarction resulting from arterial and venous thrombi containing fungal hyphae.

Parasites

Parasitic renal diseases of caged birds are comparatively uncommon. *Isospora* species,[24] *Eimeria* species,[1] *Cryptosporidium* species,[25] Encephalitozoon species,[1] and *Microsporidium* species infections[26–28] are reported.

Toxic Diseases

Hypervitaminosis D_3 and aminoglycoside nephrotoxicosis are the two best known causes of renal disease in caged birds. Both have been associated with polyuria and with diffuse nephrosis identified on histologic examination of tissue obtained by renal biopsy or at necropsy (Figs. 36–14, 36–15). Heavy metal toxicosis, mycotoxic disease, salt toxicosis, and severe muscle damage (myoglobinuria) have been associated with renal disease.[1] Allopurinol may be nephrotoxic to red-tailed hawks.[29] Polyuria has been mentioned in association with glucocorticoid and medroxyprogesterone therapy in

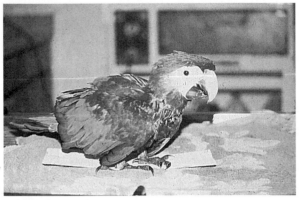

Figure 36-14

This 8-week-old macaw exhibited crop stasis and delayed development. Serum uric acid at the time of presentation was 72 mg/dl, and ultimately a diagnosis of hypervitaminosis D was made. This bird survived after aggressive supportive care.

caged birds.[1] Oak toxicosis has been confirmed in a cassowary, and renal lesions were noted.[30]

A history of exposure to heavy metals, nephrotoxic drugs, or supplementation with excessive levels of vitamin D_3 may support a tentative diagnosis of toxic nephropathy. Confirmation of the severity and specific nature of suspected renal disease is made by renal biopsy, if indicated.

Treatment depends on the specific nature of the toxin that is suspected or confirmed. Supportive care, removal of the source of the toxin, and anti-

dotal or chelation therapy are important considerations.

Neoplastic Diseases

Polyuria is least commonly noted as an initial sign of renal neoplasia, as compared with unilateral or bilateral leg paresis and abdominal distention. Budgerigars have a particularly high incidence of primary renal tumors, although renal neoplasms have been observed in both free-range and caged birds of numerous species. Specific tumors reported include renal carcinoma, renal adenoma, embryonal nephroma, and metastatic tumors from other primary sites, lymphoma being the most common in one report[31] and adenocarcinoma in another.[32]

Renal tumors of the budgerigar are extremely common, and most are challenging to diagnose early (Fig. 36–16). Early signs may include painful behavior, twitching, or subtle changes in the use of a leg. During the annual physical examination, a ventral or caudoventral displacement of the ventriculus on abdominal palpation may be the first sign of a problem. This displacement is most frequently seen as a result of organomegaly, including nephromegaly in this case. As these tumors progress, progressive cachexia and weight loss may be seen or more frequently *felt* by the examining veterinarian, many times even prior to the owner's awareness of the existence of a problem. Polyuria is uncommonly noted. As the size of the mass progresses, abdominal distention may be noted. When the neoplasm invades or presses on the nerve supply to one or

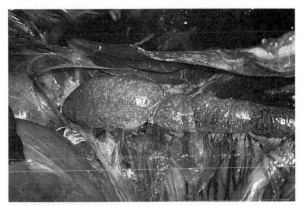

Figure 36-15

This emu died of renal failure attributed to gentamicin nephrotoxicosis. Serum uric acid climbed from 32 mg/dl at presentation to 76 mg/dl at the time of death. Articular gout and early visceral gout were noted at necropsy in addition to the nephromegaly and tophi seen here. Oddly, this bird never showed polyuria, as might have been anticipated.

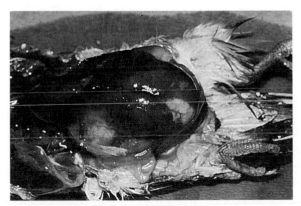

Figure 36-16

Renal adenocarcinoma in a budgerigar.

both legs, lameness, weakness, or inability to stand may be observed. Diagnosis may be supported by urinalysis, with hematuria noted in many cases. Hematuria should not be viewed as diagnostic for renal neoplasia, however, because toxicoses or infectious nephritis may also yield a similar observation. Radiography often supports the clinical suspicion of nephromegaly or organomegaly, but contrast GI studies may be required to determine the organ that is enlarged. The cranial division of the kidney is the most common location for the budgerigar renal adenocarcinoma or adenoma.[33] Ultrasonographic examination of these birds also aids in determining where an abdominal mass may be located. Because of the comparatively small size of the budgerigar, renal biopsy is a more challenging procedure than in most larger species. Renal neoplasms are also quite vascular and pose significant risk of hemorrhage, particularly when renal tumors are well advanced and associated with abdominal distention and significant organ displacement.

Early diagnosis of renal neoplasia is difficult, at best. As a result, supportive care and palliative treatments are most commonly described. Clinical history, careful physical examination, urinalysis, aspiration cytology, and renal biopsy may all play a beneficial role in obtaining a specific diagnosis of renal neoplastic disease. Analgesia may be a viable recommendation in the short term.[33]

Care should be taken by the attending avian clinician to avoid overdiagnosing or underdiagnosing renal neoplasms in companion birds. Euthanasia should be recommended at the first visit only if the patient is unequivocally diagnosed and is deteriorating rapidly.[33] A healthy respect for the nature of the human-animal bond is extremely important in these types of advanced cases, because often the owners do not expect a diagnosis of terminal illness when presenting their lame budgerigar for examination.

Nutritional Deficiency

Vitamin A deficiency is incriminated in renal disease. Metaplastic changes of the ureters and collecting ducts and decreased secretions of mucus in these structures can contribute to ureteral obstruction and post-renal failure. Vitamin A deficiency is also reported to increase precipitation of urates within the urinary system by causing a drop in production of the mucus that would normally dilute the urate suspension in the tubules.[34]

Hypovitaminosis A should be considered in oliguric and anuric renal patients with hyperuricemia, and parenteral vitamin A should be included in their supportive care treatment protocols.

Miscellaneous Diseases

Amyloidosis

Renal amyloidosis is fairly common in waterfowl, shorebirds, and gulls but is less commonly diagnosed in caged bird species.[10] A clinical diagnosis of renal disease is supported by history and urinalysis, and amyloidosis is confirmed by renal biopsy. "Amyloidosis" is a general term applied to several diseases characterized by the deposition of one or several forms of amyloid. Specific lesions may involve the renal artery, arterioles, and basement membranes of the glomerulus and tubules. The gross appearance of amyloid-infiltrated kidneys may be enlarged, firm, pale, or waxy organs. Amyloid-infiltrated tissues stain brown with iodine, and the brown color changes to blue with the addition of sulfuric acid.[10] The causes of amyloidosis remain multifactorial and unclear, and treatment other than supportive care is not documented.

Gout

Articular and visceral gout is a common diagnosis in bird species, and can often be attributed to renal disease. Gout is believed to be the result of hyperuricemia, and renal disease processes leading to transient or persistent hyperuricemia should be considered in the clinical differential diagnosis of most avian gout.

Birds with articular gout initially may show ill-defined signs, including lameness, joint swelling, reluctance to walk, decreased activity, or pain (Fig. 36–17).[35] Shifting from leg to leg or a reluctance to fly may be seen during examination or noted on careful history-taking. Visceral gout is rarely diagnosed ante mortem. The most common clinical sign of visceral gout is sudden death. Earlier signs that may be observed include anorexia and polyuria.

A diagnosis of gout is made through a combina-

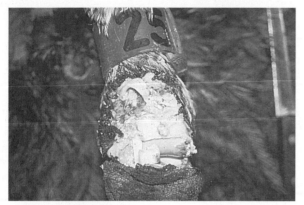

Figure 36-17

Articular gout can be extremely painful and severe, as is evident in the tibiotarsal-metatarsal joint of an emu.

tion of diagnostic tools and their careful interpretation. Cytologic examination of aspirates of swollen joints and the identification of sharp, needle-shaped crystals with inflammatory cells is an excellent supportive or confirmatory test.[36] Chemically, the murexide test can be used to confirm the presence of urates and to differentiate urates from calcium deposits.[37] A drop of nitric acid is mixed with the crystals on a slide, the slide is slowly flamed dry, and one drop of ammonia is added. If a red to purple color appears, urates are present. An elevated serum or plasma uric acid concentration may be present on biochemical analysis, although an elevated uric acid concentration alone does not definitively characterize renal disease or gout. Patients may have a normal serum uric acid concentration. Many gout patients have elevations in creatine kinase (CK) and aspartate aminotransferase (AST) concentrations, and some demonstrate leukocytosis with relative heterophilia. Urinalysis may be helpful in the diagnosis of renal disease, and the presence of blood, glucose, protein, or casts may be noted in some cases. Radiography may reveal urate tophi or mineralization in kidneys, joints, or other soft tissues.[38] Laparoscopy may be helpful in the identification of urate deposits.[39] Gross postmortem examination may reveal the accumulation of white uric acid tophi on the serosal surfaces of internal organs (visceral gout) or in the joints (articular gout). On some occasions, urate deposits may be noted only in the kidneys, pericardium, or liver.[40]

The causes of gout are numerous and may be multifactorial. Any disease process resulting in hyperuricemia can result in the development of articular or visceral gout.[34] Renal causes include obstructive ureteral disease, dehydration, renal tubular disease, and infectious renal disease of viral or bacterial origin. Nonrenal causes include hereditary causes[34, 41] and dietary causes including intake of excessive protein.[42] Many nutritional causes have been mentioned, including excessive calcium supplementation,[34, 41] dietary sodium and potassium imbalances,[34] hypervitaminosis A,[43] hypervitaminosis D_3,[44] hypervitaminosis B,[35] and magnesium and phosphorus deficiency.[35]

Treatment of gout in avian species is similar to that of humans, and may include allopurinol, colchicine, low protein diets, and other treatments based on the nature of renal disease if diagnosed as a primary cause. Response to therapy seems to be quite variable, possibly because of the multifactorial nature of this disease. General guidelines for the treatment of gout are to (1) seek a careful primary diagnosis or cause of gout if possible; (2) identify and correct metabolic imbalances that may be present; (3) avoid use of nephrotoxic drugs when possible; (4) provide nutrition appropriate for the patient at the current stage of disease; (5) provide an environment as free of stress as possible; (6) reduce serum uric acid concentration with drug and fluid therapy if possible; (7) keep the constantly changing metabolic status of the patient in mind and adjust the supportive care frequently.[35]

THE REPRODUCTIVE SYSTEM

Unlike many other avian systems, the reproductive system directly incorporates production-oriented medicine in many ways. The discussion presented here addresses specific diseases of the genital system as well as some production concerns, such as infertility, that veterinarians are frequently asked to address.

Reproductive Disorders of the Female

Egg Binding and Dystocia

Egg binding is defined as the failure of an egg to pass through the oviduct at a normal rate. This may or may not be associated with dystocia, which involves the mechanical obstruction of oviposition or cloacal function because of the egg's presence in the distal oviduct.[45] Dystocia should be expected to be a more advanced clinical sign than egg binding alone.

Egg binding is characterized by multifactorial and species-variant causes. These causes may include, but are not limited to, smooth muscle functional deficits of the oviduct, mechanical tears or damage to the oviduct, oviduct infections, excessive egg-laying and subsequent fatigue of the oviduct, systemic disease processes, nutritional deficiencies or excesses (vitamin E_1, selenium, calcium), obesity, inadequate exercise, genetic predisposition, and concurrent stressors such as hypo- or hyperthermia. Many of the predisposing factors to egg binding are diagnostic challenges in an individual bird.

The clinical signs of egg binding and dystocia vary according to severity, degree of secondary complications present, and size and species of the bird affected. Small species such as finches, canaries, and cockatiels are frequently the most severely affected. Common general signs include an acute onset of depression, abdominal straining, and occasionally sudden death. Other signs may include lameness (usually the left leg in larger birds) and bilateral leg paralysis or pariesis. Waterfowl may show abdominal distention, lameness, or respiratory difficulty (Fig. 36–18). Ratites rarely show signs other than persistent reproductive behavior and a

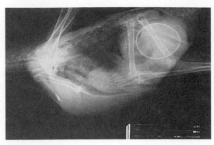

F i g u r e   3 6 – 1 9

This blue and gold macaw was egg bound. The oviduct was ruptured, and the egg was free in the abdominal cavity. Cause of the initial binding was attributed to a *Proteus* salpingitis diagnosed at the time of surgery.

cessation of egg-laying. Egg-bound ostrich hens have been known occasionally to pass one egg around a bound egg.

The diagnosis of egg binding is based on clinical signs, physical examination, and supportive diagnostic tests, including ultrasonography and radiography (Fig. 36–19). Care should be taken during the physical examination of caged birds or others that are clinically unstable to expedite time to diagnose and minimize stress. Ultrasonography is invaluable as a diagnostic tool in ratites, because the contractile nature of the oviduct is particularly important as a diagnostic aid. Bound hens lack the normal "rocking" motion of the egg in the oviduct when scanned. This rocking motion, or lack thereof, can also be appreciated in waterfowl, but is not detectable in psittacine species.

Therapy is dictated by the severity of the clinical signs and the patient's condition. General guidelines include stabilizing the patient's condition and correcting the likely cause of egg binding.[45] Fluid therapy, parenteral calcium, and heat are adequate for minimally depressed patients. The passive delivery of steam in a nonstressful manner has traditionally been recognized as a conservative home or hospital therapy.

Manual "delivery" of the egg can be done with careful digital pressure, taking care to not induce oviduct or cloaca prolapse in the process. If prolapsed tissues are present, cleaning and repair of significant lacerations or tears and replacement are required following removal of the egg. In critical cases, in addition to basic supportive care, ovocentesis and implosion of the egg may be a less stressful and safer approach.

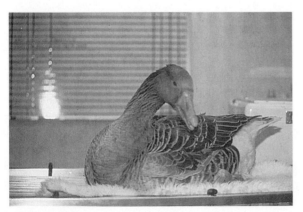

F i g u r e   3 6 – 1 8

Clinical signs of egg binding vary immensely among species. This egg-bound goose was presented by her owners for a perceived respiratory problem, and her most obvious sign was respiratory difficulty.

Ovocentesis can be accomplished through cloacal access or, most commonly, through transabdominal aspiration. Oxytocin has traditionally been used in dystocia cases when no physical obstruction to oviposition is suspected. Sometimes multiple injections have been used and recommended. More recently, prostaglandins have been shown to induce powerful oviductal contractions and help expel the retained egg. Arginine vasotocin has been shown to induce oviposition in domestic avian species through its likely effect of increasing prostaglandin release from the oviduct tissues. Surgical removal of retained eggs is most commonly performed in large bird species such as ratites. At the time of surgery, both biopsy and culture of the oviduct are indicated to detect infectious agents, and the oviduct should be flushed in a normograde manner prior to closure.

Prolapse of the Oviduct

Oviductal prolapses are seen most frequently subsequent to dystocia. Predisposing factors may include malnutrition, salpingitis, cloacitis, and soft shelled or abnormal eggs. Treatment includes removal of the egg (which may or may not be still present), cleaning the exposed tissues, application of topical anti-inflammatory preparations, repairing lacerations or traumatic lesions, and gently replacing the tissues appropriately. Prognosis is generally good after treatment of most prolapses, and a return to normal breeding function is encountered in most birds as long as underlying predisposing factors are identified and eliminated.

Excessive Egg-laying

Excessive or chronic egg-laying occurs when a hen has a larger than normal clutch size or has repeated clutches, regardless of the presence of a suitable mate or the breeding season.[45] Commonly predisposed pet bird species include budgerigars, lovebirds, and cockatiels. Predisposing factors may include imprinting on humans or possibly a genetic lack of hormonal balance in controlling egg-laying. Excessive egg-laying can result in a depletion of the nutritional body stores of the hen, and ultimately may predispose the bird to egg binding, osteoporosis, and malnutrition.

Preventative management is done in several stages, with behavior modification techniques as well as medical and surgical options—all of which should be discussed and explained at the time of the initial examination of the bird. Behavior modification options should include (1) improving the dietary plan of the hen to decrease the severity of her nutritional and metabolic drain; (2) avoiding removal of eggs from her laying site (this can trigger the double-clutch phenomenon and magnify the problem); (3) decreasing the photoperiod of the hen to a maximum of 8 to 10 hours per day; (4) removing the hen's preferred nesting sites; (5) removing toys or other cage items toward which the bird has a sexual affinity; and (6) changing cages and cage location in the home to a different or "new" environment.

Medical therapy should include nutritional or vitamin and mineral supplementation to correct nutritional imbalances detected at the time of initial examination. Options for medical therapy that can be considered include (1) medroxyprogesterone injections to interrupt the ovulatory cycle (however, the adverse effects such as polyuria, polydipsia, depression, obesity, diabetes mellitus, liver damage, and immunosuppression need to be discussed); (2) oral testosterone supplementation to interrupt the ovulatory cycle (it is contraindicated in the presence of liver disease); and (3) leuprolide acetate to prevent egg-laying in cockatiels.[46] Human chorionic gonadotropin (hCG) has recently been suggested as another therapeutic option to suppress ovulation in chronic egg layers (Teresa Lightfoot, personal communication, 1995). Numerous clinical reports of favorable response with no identified adverse effects are encouraging. The specific mode of action of hCG and the dose and frequency of its use are currently anecdotal. It should not be used as the sole therapy in birds with egg yolk peritonitis or other reproductive tract–associated inflammatory abdominal disease. Salpingohysterectomy may be used as a definitive solution to overproduction of eggs in a companion bird with no breeding intent.

Careful and detailed education of owners of the susceptible pet bird species during annual examinations, telephone reminders by well-educated receptionists, and discussion of available options at the time of the initial presentation will result in a more complete understanding of this problem. Prevention is preferable to presentation of the bird in an advanced state of nutritional depletion with secondary problems and a guarded prognosis. Aviculturalists need to be counseled on the possibility of overproduction of some species, resulting in potentially serious reproductive and systemic health compromise. Careful veterinary review and monitoring of the records of breeding birds and egg and chick hatch quality and viability reveal early indicators of nutritional depletion in excessively producing hens.

Abdominal Distention Associated with Reproductive Tract Disorders

Abdominal distention is a nonspecific sign frequently attributed to reproductive system disease in avian species (Fig. 36–20). Many of the specific diseases capable of producing this visible abnormality are fairly well advanced and, as a result, abdominal distention should be viewed as a serious sign warranting prompt and accurate diagnosis. All of the diseases in this section may feature abdominal distention as a clinical sign (Table 36–3).

Egg Yolk Peritonitis

Egg yolk peritonitis is a catch-all diagnostic term used to describe peritonitis associated with the presence of egg yolk material. Actually internal laying, ectopic ovulation, and septic and nonseptic

Table 36–3

REPRODUCTIVE DISORDERS THAT MAY BE ASSOCIATED WITH ABDOMINAL DISTENTION

Female	Male
Egg yolk peritonitis	Testicular neoplasia
Cystic ovaries	Orchitis
Ovarian neoplasia	
Oophoritis	
Uterine torsion	
Oviduct impaction	
Uterine rupture	
Ectopic eggs	
Salpingitis	

yolk-related peritonitis all can occur. In addition, these may be seen in conjunction with concurrent metabolic, nutritional, or other systemic diseases. Egg yolk peritonitis is thought to be caused by general factors such as ectopic ovulation or oviductal disease. Potential causes of ectopic eggs include a normal reverse peristalsis of the oviduct, trauma, or stress. Ectopic ovulation alone does not necessarily result in peritonitis, and it has been described as a frequently occurring disorder of several taxonomic orders of birds. Oviductal diseases resulting in secondary yolk peritonitis include infectious salpingitis, rupture of the oviduct, neoplasia, and cystic hyperplasia.

The clinical signs of egg yolk peritonitis include gradual weight loss, intermittent depression, and ascites with an accompanying history of recent egg-laying or broodiness. Not all hens with egg yolk peritonitis have ascites. Hens of some species, such as waterfowl, more frequently show abdominal distention.

Egg yolk peritonitis is diagnosed through a combination of physical examination and supportive laboratory findings. Birds with ascites may demonstrate septic or nonseptic inflammation on cytologic examination of abdominal fluid; frequently, yolk or fat globules may be seen. Leukocytosis with relative heterophilia is a common hematologic finding, and many hens have peripheral hypercalcemia, hypercholesterolemia, and hyperglobulinemia compatible with their pre- and immediate postovulatory status. Some cockatiels may actually have egg yolk visible in their peripheral blood smears and above the buffy coat in separated blood samples.

Treatment of egg yolk peritonitis depends on the

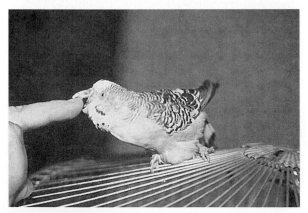

Figure 36–20

Abdominal distention includes a fairly large differential diagnosis at presentation. This budgerigar had a unilateral testicular seminoma that was successfully removed.

severity of clinical signs. Many birds improve with supportive care alone and no further intervention. Birds that are clinically unstable because of the severity of the ascites may require abdominocentesis and supportive care such as broad-spectrum antibiotics, fluid and shock therapy, and warmth. Surgical exploration and removal of inspissated eggs, yolk, and other material may be indicated for birds in stable condition if significant pathology is present. The return of the reproductive tract to functional normalcy remains questionable, however, even after the bird is clinically normal. Preventive treatment with medroxyprogesterone has been suggested as a means to prevent further ovulation and aid in the resolution of ascites in some cases, but its use is not a uniformly accepted practice among avian veterinarians. Waterfowl and Galliformes frequently have severe pathologic changes and, in my experience, salpingohysterectomy is required more frequently in these species than in most psittacines.

Cystic Ovarian Disease

Ovarian cysts have been mentioned to occur in canaries, budgerigars, and pheasants,[45] and occur frequently in cockatiels. Although the specific cause of this disorder is not known, it is believed to be endocrine in origin. In advanced cystic ovarian disease, abdominal distention and related signs are commonly noted. Radiographically, an increase in soft tissue density in the area of the ovary and hyperostosis may be observed. Ultrasonographic examination may easily delineate fluid-filled cysts in the region of the ovary. Cystic ovarian disease has been observed on routine laparoscopic examination in asymptomatic hens, and it has been assumed that these hens have impaired reproductive performance capabilities. Fluid aspirate of the cysts at surgery or endoscopy reveal a clear to yellowish straw-colored fluid of low cellularity.

Treatment has included transabdominal aspiration of cysts, surgical removal of the ovarian cysts or ovary, testosterone, and human chorionic gonadotropin. The long-term resolution of this problem after therapy is questioned, and it is believed that reproductive performance of these hens should be regarded as suboptimal at best.

Ovarian Neoplasia

Of the psittacine species, ovarian neoplastic disease is most commonly reported in the budgerigar.[31, 32] Gallinaceous species are the avian taxonomic group most frequently diagnosed with ovarian neoplasia. When seen with abdominal distention as a clinical sign, most ovarian neoplastic disease is fairly advanced, and prognosis for successful therapy is generally poor. Diagnosis is supported by radiography, ultrasonography, exploratory laparotomy, and biopsy. Egg retention, oviductal impaction, cystic ovarian disease, abdominal hernias, and ascites may be seen in conjunction with neoplastic ovarian disease. Lymphomatosis, adenocarcinomas, leiomyosarcomas, leiomyomas, adenomas, and granulosa cell tumors have been reported.[32, 45, 47]

Oophoritis

Infectious causes of clinical oophoritis have been most commonly mentioned in the literature, with pathogens including *Salmonella* species and other bacterial agents.[45] In advanced septic oophoritis, peritonitis and secondary abdominal distention are common. Other advanced signs of disease include anorexia, cachexia, septicemia, and sudden death. Earlier signs of disease suggestive of infectious oophoritis may include infertility, egg binding, and an inordinate incidence of infectious embryonic mortality in breeding hens or infectious omphalitis in neonatal chicks. Therapy includes appropriate antimicrobials as indicated by the suspected or confirmed pathogen. Prognosis for return to normal reproductive performance is guarded, because complete resolution of bacterial oophoritis is not easily accomplished.

Uterine Torsion

Uterine torsion is infrequently diagnosed in its early stages. It is associated with abdominal distention, usually resulting from peritonitis. Early clinical signs may include depression and anorexia following recent oviposition. Diagnosis is established at exploratory laparotomy. Frequently, severe vascular compromise requires salpingohysterectomy, and loss of future reproduction ensues if the bird was intended as a breeding animal.

Oviduct Impaction

Impaction of the oviduct is most frequently seen as a consequence of dystocia, infectious metritis, or salpingitis.[45] In more advanced stages of disease, abdominal distention may be noted, resulting from accumulated eggs and egg material or peritonitis.[48] Early clinical signs may include a cessation of egg-laying in the presence of "broodiness" or other normal reproductive behaviors, cachexia, or general ill health. In general, large bird species tend to show fewer severe clinical signs until disease is quite advanced. Diagnosis is supported by history, physical examination, radiography, and ultrasonography. Surgical exploration and removal of impacted eggs and material is both diagnostic and curative. Advanced cases may require salpingohysterectomy. Some demonstrate adhesions or peritonitis. At the time of surgery, obtaining oviduct culture and biopsy specimens should be considered as an aid in identifying a primary cause.

Uterine Rupture

Uterine rupture can occur as a result of dystocia or oviductal disease. Administration of oxytocin or prostaglandins to birds with dystocia may sometimes be responsible for rupture of the oviductal wall. Abdominal distention, when noted, is usually the result of peritonitis or the deposition of eggs and oviductal contents in the coelomic cavity. Diagnosis is supported as in oviductal impaction and confirmed at surgery. Frequently, when more advanced stages of disease are present at the time of diagnosis, the reproductive tract may require removal. Even if not removed, prognosis for return to normal oviductal function is guarded at best.

Ectopic Eggs

Ectopic eggs are seen occasionally in birds, and they require surgical removal. Causes of ectopic eggs include uterine rupture or reverse peristalsis of the oviduct. Reverse peristalsis may be triggered by physiologic stress, nutritional imbalances, obstruction of the oviduct, or salpingitis. A diagnosis of ectopic eggs is aided by palpation, radiology, and ultrasonography, and is confirmed at surgery or by endoscopy. Large species of birds such as ratites generally benefit more from diagnosis with ultrasonography than smaller species because of the ability to visualize oviduct around the egg in a bound hen versus failure to see oviduct in a bird with an ectopic egg.

Salpingitis

Salpingitis is generally described as an infectious disease process associated with airsacculitis, liver disease, pneumonia, or ascending infections of the oviduct.[45] Infectious agents may not necessarily be involved with salpingitis, although documentation of these cases is comparatively rare. Some of the more commonly identified infectious bacterial agents include *Escherichia coli,* and *Mycoplasma, Salmonella, Pasturella,* and *Streptococcus* species. Newcastle virus infection is associated with salpingitis in many bird species.[45] In ground-nesting species such as Anseriformes and emus, non–lactose-fermenting gram-negative bacterial infections such as *Pseudomonas aeruginosa, Proteus mirabilis,* and *Proteus vulgaris* are encountered. Noninfectious causes of salpingitis include mechanical trauma and inflammation resulting from difficult oviposition and nutritional imbalances in the hen. Clinical signs of salpingitis are vague and difficult to detect in many birds and include infertility, abnormally shaped eggs, abnormally colored eggs, and mild depression. More advanced signs include abdominal distention, anorexia, and cachexia. Diagnosis is supported by history, physical examination including ultrasonography in large bird species, radiography, and egg culture testing. Definitive diagnosis is established by culture results of a specimen from the oviduct or biopsy of oviductal tissue. Treatment of salpingitis is based on the suspected underlying cause. Birds that have been treated medically or surgically should have careful followup through the next breeding season to ensure complete resolution of the problem and return to breeding performance. Advanced cases may require salpingohysterectomy, which results in a loss of future breeding capability.

Reproductive Disorders of the Male

Neoplasia

Most testicular neoplasms are unilateral.[31] Abdominal distention is the most commonly reported clinical sign, and this is usually noted in fairly advanced stages of disease. Specific neoplasms reported include Sertoli cell tumors, seminomas, interstitial cell tumors, and lymphosarcoma.[31, 32] Leiomyosarcoma and carcinoma have been reported to arise from the epididymis and ductus deferens.[49, 50] Treatment, if the neoplasm is detected early, includes orchiectomy.

Orchitis

Infectious orchitis can originate from adjacent organ systems, hematogenous spread, or ascending infections. Early signs of disease are vague unless associated with more severe and multisystemic signs of septicemia. Infertility may be an early sign that warrants the consideration of infectious orchitis in the differential diagnosis. Diagnosis of infectious orchitis is supported by endoscopic examination, and cytology, culture, and biopsy examinations of lesions. Therapy is based on the infectious agents identified.

Phallic Prolapse

Avian species with large phalluses occasionally have prolapse. Primary causes of phallic prolapse are believed to be trauma, infection, or weather fluctuations.[45] In chronic prolapse, amputation of the phallus may be indicated if the tissues are deemed no longer viable. In waterfowl and ostriches, the birds are sometimes sedated; the cloaca and phallus are carefully examined, evaluated, and cleansed; and the everted tissues are gently and anatomically replaced. Pursestring sutures of the cloaca or two vertical stay sutures may be placed to temporarily hold the phallus in place until swelling and secondary inflammation are resolved. If the phallus is severely traumatized or becomes avascular, amputation may be indicated, resulting in a loss of potential breeding capacity.

Reproductive Disorders of Both Male and Female

Papillomatous Disease

Cloacal papillomatous disease may result in secondary infectious cloacitis that may seed infectious uro-genital system disease (Fig. 36–21). The cause is unknown. This disease is believed to be either a neoplastic disorder or caused by an infectious agent. Infertility may be attributed to mechanical obstruction as well as bacterial infection resulting from papillomatous disease of the cloaca.[51] Cloacal papillomas have also been associated with bile duct carcinomas in Amazon parrots[52] (see also Chapter 34). Some believe that the presence of papillomatous disease poses no real threat or impingement on breeder performance.

Cloacitis

Cloacitis can result from infectious as well as noninfectious causes in bird species, and can result in secondary urogenital disease because the urodeal outlets of the male and female reproductive and urinary systems are in that location. Treatment of cloacitis is based on identification of the specific cause. Appropriate antibiotic and anti-inflammatory therapy may be indicated, and careful and regular swabbing of the cloaca with petroleum jelly will prevent secondary fecal or urate accumulation and irritation of the inflamed tissues.

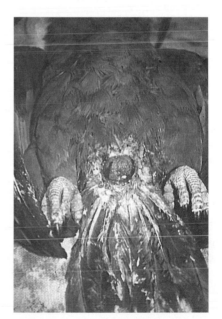

Figure 36–21

Cloacal papillomatosis may be manifested as mechanically induced infertility, recurrent cloacitis, or potentially seed secondary infectious bacterial urogenital system disease.

Cloacalithiasis

Cloacalithiasis is infrequently seen in caged bird species. This condition may result from prior egg binding, infectious cloacitis, or neurologic abnormalities of the cloaca. Although most stones are removable with medical or surgical therapy, long-term prognosis remains guarded, and prognosis for return to normal breeding performance is poor. Once a cloacalith has been removed, treatment as for cloacitis is appropriate, with careful monitoring to ensure that neurologic function of the cloacal wall is present.

Cloacal Neoplasia

Papillomatous disease is described as a neoplastic disease as well as a potentially infectious disease of psittacine species. Cloacal carcinomas are infrequently seen in avian species.

Infertility

The existing literature predominantly reflects documented end-stage reproductive tract disease, and comparatively low rates of early diagnosis, treatment, and return to normal function for individual birds and flocks. As our diagnostic abilities and techniques in preventive management improve, we should become more effective as veterinarians in early detection, therapy, and preventive management of reproductive diseases and disorders of avian species. Focus will likely shift toward subclinical disease throughout a flock and will require a closer relationship between attending veterinarian and aviculturalist than that established in the examination rooms of veterinary practices. Record review and analysis, discussion of production goals, and active involvement in the financial plan of the aviculturalist are required for the profession to better serve the serious production-oriented aviculturalist in the future. Simple documentation of end-stage reproductive disease alone for a flock or an individual bird without offering effective plans for prevention should not be viewed as optimal veterinary service.

Infertility is a particularly common clinical complaint (Fig. 36–22). Unlike some of the specific medical diseases of the reproductive tract mentioned previously, managing the clinical problem of infertility frequently crosses the line from companion or individual bird medicine into production-oriented medicine. As a result, flock management techniques, in addition to those techniques used in the individual bird, are important to the diagnostic and therapeutic approach.

Infertility is defined as sterility, or the absence of the ability to conceive or induce conception. Therefore, clinical infertility in psittacine species should be manifested as infertile eggs or the inability to produce eggs at all. In addition, infertility may be either a permanent or transient problem, and many of the specific causes of infertility do not require direct veterinary intervention. In many of the more advanced or severe individual reproductive tract diseases previously discussed, infertility is an early clinical sign.

Any disease process that directly or indirectly affects the anatomy or function of the reproductive tract can result in clinical infertility. Infertility can also be created by many normal physiologic mechanisms as well as management flaws. As a result, without actually visiting an aviary and reviewing

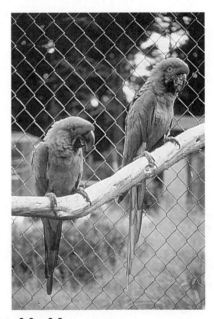

Figure 36–22

Infertility is a particularly common and complex problem that avian practitioners are asked to address.

T a b l e 3 6 – 4

FLOW CHART FOR INFERTILITY ASSESSMENT

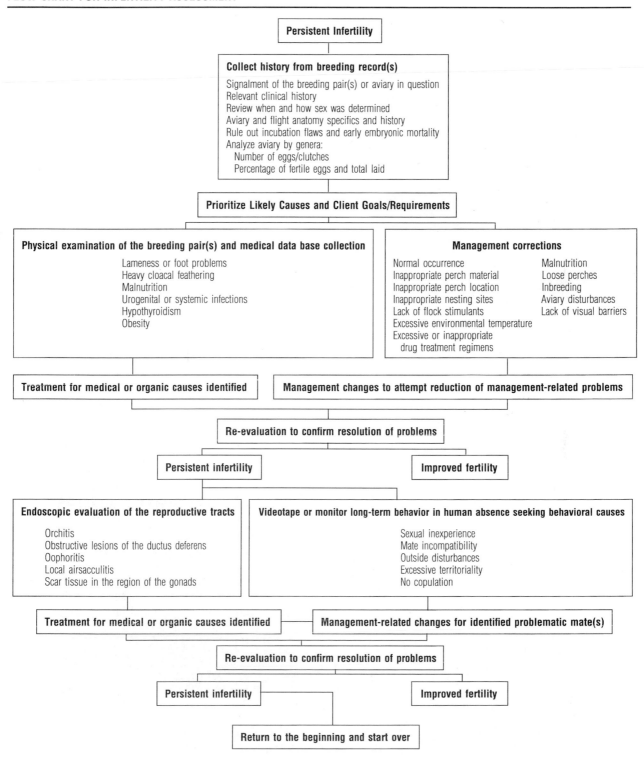

Persistent Infertility

Collect history from breeding record(s)

Signalment of the breeding pair(s) or aviary in question
Relevant clinical history
Review when and how sex was determined
Aviary and flight anatomy specifics and history
Rule out incubation flaws and early embryonic mortality
Analyze aviary by genera:
  Number of eggs/clutches
  Percentage of fertile eggs and total laid

Prioritize Likely Causes and Client Goals/Requirements

Physical examination of the breeding pair(s) and medical data base collection

Lameness or foot problems
Heavy cloacal feathering
Malnutrition
Urogenital or systemic infections
Hypothyroidism
Obesity

Management corrections

Normal occurrence
Inappropriate perch material
Inappropriate perch location
Inappropriate nesting sites
Lack of flock stimulants
Excessive environmental temperature
Excessive or inappropriate
  drug treatment regimens

Malnutrition
Loose perches
Inbreeding
Aviary disturbances
Lack of visual barriers

Treatment for medical or organic causes identified

Management changes to attempt reduction of management-related problems

Re-evaluation to confirm resolution of problems

Persistent infertility

Improved fertility

Endoscopic evaluation of the reproductive tracts

Orchitis
Obstructive lesions of the ductus deferens
Oophoritis
Local airsacculitis
Scar tissue in the region of the gonads

Videotape or monitor long-term behavior in human absence seeking behavioral causes

Sexual inexperience
Mate incompatibility
Outside disturbances
Excessive territoriality
No copulation

Treatment for medical or organic causes identified

Management-related changes for identified problematic mate(s)

Re-evaluation to confirm resolution of problems

Persistent infertility

Improved fertility

Return to the beginning and start over

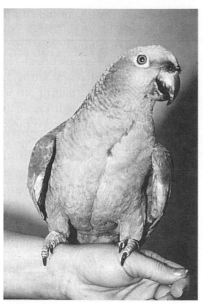

Figure 36–23

Obesity, particularly in Amazon parrots, still remains fairly under-recognized and is a significant contributor to infertility and other reproductive problems.

the records, the attending veterinarian will have little ability to definitively narrow the differential diagnosis for flock fertility problems. Even with facility inspection, record review, and medical workup of problematic pairs or groups, infertility evaluations pose a significant challenge to the attending veterinarian (Table 36–4). Often, a flock management program for a sizeable collection requires several years to effectively identify breeding histories and performance parameters of pairs and address production problems.

The major causes of psittacine infertility are separated into two major groups for diagnostic purposes: medical and nonmedical causes.[51] The most prevalent and common causes of infertility lie in the nonmedical category. The nonmedical causes of infertility include immaturity, normal variation for the species, sexual inexperience, loose perches, inappropriate perch material, aviary disturbances, inappropriate nesting site and materials, lack of flock stimulants, inbreeding or other genetic flaws, excessive or inappropriate drug therapies, mate incompatibility, homosexual pairs, malnutrition, and heavy cloacal feathering. Medically linked causes of infertility may include obesity, visual problems,

malnutrition, reproductive tract infections, airsacculitis or scar tissue in the area of the gonads, cloacal abnormalities, systemic disease, hypothyroidism, and various toxic effects (Fig. 36–23).

The diagnostic tools used in the clinical approach to infertility include the entire spectrum available to the avian practitioner. Physical examination and visual evaluation of the individual birds are mandatory. Hematologic tests, biochemical profiles, bacterial culture and sensitivity tests, and Gram's stains provide information to screen the systemic health status of individual birds and are readily available to practitioners. Radiography is indicated if airsacculitis or gonadal function deficits related to local disease processes are suspected. In some species such as ratites, ultrasonography is a particularly valuable diagnostic tool in the routine pre- or postbreeding season workup as well as in the infertility examination. Ultrasonography can also be helpful in the early recognition of oviductal disease in waterfowl. Endoscopy is invaluable in many species to visually determine the sex and assess gonadal activity and morphology. Biopsy of identified lesions or aspiration of cystic structures can provide invaluable diagnostic input.

Aviary or breeding site evaluation is realistically the only means for an experienced practitioner to accurately assess nonmedical causes of infertility. Videotape monitoring of the bird's behavior and aviary conditions can provide input regarding mate

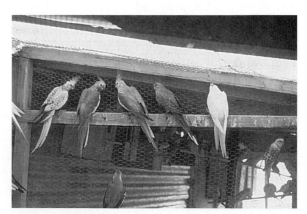

Figure 36–24

Infertility frequently is detected by flock production record analysis rather than individual bird examination. Appropriate flock management, through careful record review, can lead to progressive and successful veterinary services for the individual birds in the collection as well as the owner.

compatibility, aviary disturbances, sexual inexperience, or design flaws that interfere with the perceived biosecurity of breeding pairs (Fig. 36–24).

Record review and analysis, and comparison with anticipated production goals of the client are mandatory in the infertility examination. Unfortunately, this is also the most frequently overlooked portion of the infertility examination. Data collected by the aviculturalist should be collated by the attending veterinarian and scrutinized with care for patterns that may indicate need for investigation or managerial intervention. Some of the common record calculations that I recommend include fertility rates, embryonic mortalities, pediatric mortalities, saleable chicks produced per egg laid, and saleable chicks produced per fertile egg laid. These calculations should be made each year for each breeding pair, and by species group as well as by the location of the building in the breeding aviary. Overall aviary statistics should be calculated as well. Without records to analyze and evaluate, there is comparatively less ability for the practitioner to effectively focus on a well-prioritized differential diagnosis. This can result in unnecessary expense to and disillusionment of the client, and ultimately loss to the client, the veterinarian, and most importantly, the birds themselves.

References

1. Lumeij JT: Nephrology. In Ritchie BW, Harrison GJ, Harrison LR (eds): Avian Medicine: Principles and Application. Lake Worth, FL, Wingers Publishing, 1994, pp 539–555.
2. Gill FB: Ornithology, ed 2. New York, WH Freeman and Company, 1994.
3. James FC, Shugart HH: Robin phenology study. Condor 6:159–168, 1974.
4. Speer BL: Stunting in the large macaws. In Rosenthal K, Fudge AM (eds): Noninfectious Disease in Exotic Animals. Semin Avian Exotic Pet Med 4(1):9–14, 1995.
5. Hochleithner M: Biochemistries. In Ritchie BW, Harrison GJ, Harrison LR (eds): Avian Medicine: Principles and Application. Lake Worth, FL, Wingers Publishing, 1994, pp 223–245.
6. Chou ST: Relative importance of liver and kidney synthesis of uric acid in chickens. Can J Physiol Pharmacol 50:936–939, 1972.
7. Lumeij TJ: A Contribution to Clinical Investigative Methods for Birds, With Special Reference to the Racing Pigeon (*Columbia livia domestica*). Utrecht, Proefshrift, 1987.
8. Bell DJ, Freeman BM: Physiology and Biochemistry of the Domestic Fowl. New York, Academic Press, 1971.
9. Lewandowski AH, Campbell TW, Harrison GJ: Clinical chemistries. In Harrison G, Harrison L (eds): Clinical Avian Medicine and Surgery. Philadelphia, WB Saunders, 1986, pp 192–200.
10. Phalen DN, Ambrus S, Graham DL: The avian urinary system: Form, function, diseases. Proc Assoc Avian Vet, Phoenix, 1990, pp 44–57.
11. Bernier GM, Morin, G, Marsolais, G: A generalized inclusion body disease in the budgerigar (*Melopsittacus undulatus*). Avian Dis 25:1083–1092, 1981.
12. Davis RB: A viral disease of fledgling budgerigars. Avian Dis 25:179–183, 1981.
13. Lowenstein LJ, Fry DM: Adenovirus-like particles associated with intranuclear inclusion bodies in the kidney of a common murre (*Uria aalge*). Avian Dis 29:208–213, 1985.
14. Mori F: Inclusion bodies containing adenovirus-like particles in the kidneys of psittacine birds. Avian Pathol 18:197–202, 1989.
15. Cavill JP: Viral diseases. In Petrak ML (ed): Diseases of Cage and Aviary Birds, Philadelphia, Lea & Febiger, 1982, pp 515–519.
16. Speer BL: The eclectus parrot: Medicine an avicultural aspect. Proc Assoc Avian Vet, Seattle, 1989, pp 239–247.
17. Gerlach H: Viruses. In Ritchie BW, Harrison GJ, Harrison LR (eds): Avian Medicine: Principles and Application. Lake Worth, FL, Wingers Publishing, 1994, pp 863–948.
18. Gerlach H: Bacterial diseases. In Harrison GJ, Harrison LR (eds): Clinical Avian Medicine and Surgery. Philadelphia, WB Saunders, 1986, pp 434–453.
19. Gray ML: Listeriosis in fowls—a review. Avian Dis 2:146–314, 1985.
20. Halliwell WH, Graham DL: Bacterial diseases of birds of prey. In Fowler ME (ed): Zoo and Wild Animal Medicine. Philadelphia, WB Saunders, 1986, pp 449–457.
21. Dorrestein GM: Diseases of pigeons with emphasis on racing pigeons. Proc Assoc Avian Vet, Boulder, 1985, pp 181–203.
22. Olsen GH, Shane SH, Harrington KS: Investigation of the pathology of *Klebsiella* pneumonia in psittacine birds. Proc Assoc Avian Vet, Miami, 1986, pp 237–239.
23. Gerlach H: *Chlamydia*. In Harrison GJ, Harrison LR (eds): Clinical Avian Medicine and Surgery. Philadelphia, WB Saunders, 1986, pp 457–463.
24. Helman RG, Jensen JM, Russel RG: Systemic protozoal disease in zebra finches. J Am Vet Med Assoc 185:1400–1401, 1984.
25. Gardiner GH, Imes GP: Cryptosporidium sp in the kidneys of a black-throated finch. J Am Vet Med Assoc 185:1401–1402, 1984.
26. Nobila MN, Kwapien RP: Microsporidian infection in the pied peach-faced lovebird. Avian Dis 2:198–204, 1977.
27. Randall CJ: Microsporidian infection in lovebirds (*Agapornis* sp). Avian Pathol 15:223–231, 1986.
28. Ratcliffe HL: Incidence and nature of tumours in captive wild mammals and birds. Am J Cancer 17:116–135, 1933.
29. Lumeij JT, Redig PT: Hyperuricemia and visceral gout induced by allopurinol in red-tailed hawks (*Buteo jamaicensis*). Proc Dtsch Vet Gessellshaft, Munchen, 1992.
30. Kinde H: A fatal case of oak poisoning in a Double-Wattled Cassowary (*Casuarius casuarius*). Avian Dis 32:849–851, 1988.
31. Latimer KS: Oncology. In Ritchie BW, Harrison GJ, Harrison LR (eds): Avian Medicine: Principles and Application. Lake Worth, FL, Wingers Publishing, 1994, pp 641–672.
32. Leach MW: A survey of neoplasia in pet birds. In Schmidt RE, Fudge AM: Neoplasia. Semin Avian Exotic Pet Med 1(2):52–64, 1992.
33. Bauck LA: Renal disease in the budgerigar. Proc Assoc Avian Vet, Toronto, 1984, pp 1–9.
34. Siller WG: Kidney diseases in the fowl. In Gordon RF, Jordan, TTW (eds): Poultry Diseases, ed 2. London, Balliere Tindall, 1982, pp 247–259.

35. Ekstrom DD, Degernes L: Avian gout. Proc Assoc Avian Vet, Seattle, 1989, pp 130–138.

36. Bauck L: Diseases of the foot in cage and aviary birds. Proc First Intl Conf Zool Avian Med, Oahu, 1987, pp 109–115.

37. Altman RB: Noninfectious diseases in parrots, cockatoos, macaws, and perching birds (Psittaciformes and Passeriformes). In Current Veterinary Therapy VI, Small Animal Practice. Philadelphia, WB Saunders, 1977, pp 703–705.

38. Gandal CP: Anesthetic and surgical techniques. In Petrak, ML (ed): Diseases of Cage and Aviary Birds, 2nd ed. Philadelphia, Lea & Febiger, 1982, pp 304–328.

39. Harrison GJ: Endoscopy. In Harrison GJ, Harrison LR (eds): Clinical Avian Medicine and Surgery. Philadelphia, WB Saunders, 1986, pp 234–244.

40. Halliwell WH: Toxic and metabolic conditions in birds of prey, raptors (Falconiformes and Strigiformes). In Fowler, ME (ed): Zoo and Wild Animal Medicine, ed 2. Philadelphia, WB Saunders, 1986, pp 431–432.

41. Austil RE, Cole RK: Impaired renal clearance of uric acid in chickens having hyperuricemia and articular gout. Am J Physiol 223:525–530, 1972.

42. Lowenstine LJ: Diseases of excess in nutritional disorders of birds. In Fowler ME (ed): Zoo and Wild Animal Medicine, ed 2. Philadelphia, WB Saunders, 1986, p 203.

43. Humphreys PN: Noninfectious diseases. Ducks, geese, swans and screamers (Anseriformes). In Fowler ME (ed): Zoo and Wild Animal Medicine, ed 2. Philadelphia, WB Saunders, 1986, p 355.

44. Takeshita K: Hypervitaminosis D in baby macaws. Proc Assoc Avian Vet, Miami, 1986, pp 341–345.

45. Joyner KL: Theriogenology. In Ritchie BR, Harrison GJ, Harrison LR (eds): Avian Medicine: Principles and Application. Lake Worth, FL, Wingers Publishing, 1994, pp 748–804.

46. Millam JR, Finney H: Leuprolide acetate can reversibly prevent egg laying in cockatiels. Proc Assoc Avian Vet, Nashville, 1993, p 46.

47. Nath R, Singh CM: Studies on pathology of uro-genital tract of poultry. 1. Pathology of the Genital Tract. Haryana Agricult Univ J Res pp 1106–1111, 1971.

48. Degernes LA: Chronic oviduct obstruction and salpingitis in an African grey parrot. Proc Assoc Avian Vet, New Orleans, 1992, pp 156–157.

49. Petrak ML, Gilmore CE: Neoplasms. In Petrak ML (ed): Diseases of Cage and Aviary Birds, ed 2. Philadelphia, Lea & Febiger, 1982, pp 606–637.

50. Reece RL: Observations on naturally occurring neoplasms in birds in the state of Victoria, Australia. Avian Pathol 21:3–32, 1992.

51. Speer BL: A clinical approach to psittacine infertility. Proc Assoc Avian Vet, Chicago, 1991, pp 173–187.

52. Hillyer EV, Moroff S, Hoefer H: Bile duct carcinomas in two out of ten Amazon parrots with cloacal papillomas. J Assoc Avian Vet 5:91–95, 1991.

37

Immune System

A detailed consideration of the structure and the function of the avian immune system is beyond the scope of this text, and this chapter will give a brief overview. Birds have both primary and secondary lymphoid organs. Primary lymphoid organs are the thymus and the bursa of Fabricius.[1] Secondary lymphoid organs include the spleen; lymph nodes, which are found only in some waterfowl; and disseminated lymphoid tissue in the hardian glands, the alimentary tract, the bone marrow, and solitary nodules in all organs.[2] Most of the experimental work referred to in this chapter has been done in chickens and may not be completely applicable to other species in all cases.

PRIMARY LYMPHOID ORGANS

Thymus

The thymus originates with the parathyroid glands from the third and fourth pharyngeal pouches.[3] It is found in the neck of birds, and there may be multiple lobules consisting of epithelial cells with each lobule covered by a connective tissue capsule (Fig. 37–1). Each lobule has a cortex and medulla. During development of the thymus, the epithelial cells become a loosely arranged reticulum, and lymphocyte progenitor cells from the bone marrow invade this reticulum. Lymphocytes become most dense in the cortex of the thymus. Thymic (Hassal's) corpuscles are present in the medulla.[4] The thymic mass is largest in the sexually immature bird, with a decreased weight accompanying the onset of sexual maturity. In most birds there is persistence of some thymic tissue throughout life. The thymus processes

and serves as a source of T lymphocytes, which are circulating cells responsible for cell-mediated immune responses. Thymic epithelial cells produce unrelated polypeptide hormones such as thymosines and thymoproteins.

Four systems of T-cell differentiation alloantigens have been reported in chickens.[5] Approximately 65% of the mononuclear cells in the spleen and 80% of those in the blood of chickens are T-cells. T-cells function in delayed hypersensitivity reactions that include the reaction in tuberculin skin testing and a portion of the response to mycobacterial infection in birds. T-cells also function in allergic contact dermatitis, in which protein-chemical com-

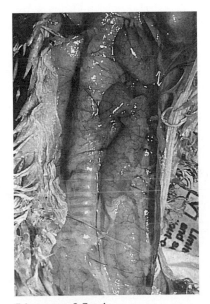

Figure 37–1

Normal thymus in a macaw chick.

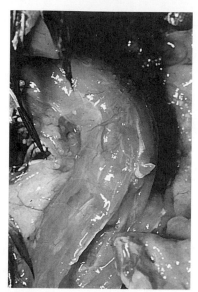

Figure 37-2

Thymic degeneration and hemorrhage due to polyomavirus infection in a conure.

plexes bind to Langerhans cells in the dermis and form foci that trigger a T-cell response. In chickens, T-cells also play an important part in the resistance to parasites and probably to viral-induced tumors.[5]

Veterinarians making a differential diagnosis of premature thymic loss should weigh a variety of stress factors including viral infections, muscular fatigue, cold, restraint, and high levels of testosterone. Viral infection of the bursa may lead to compromise of cell-mediated functions. Although the exact mechanism is not known,[6] avian viral particles may interact with macrophages to stimulate suppression factors. As a result, there are decreased numbers of cytotoxic T-cells, a lowered resistance to intracellular bacterial infection such as mycobacteriosis, increased susceptibility to some unusual infectious diseases, and reduction of the previously mentioned antitumor defense mechanisms. At necropsy, reduced size and number of thymic lobules are noted (Fig. 37–2). The gross appearance of the thymus reflects the age and species of bird. No experimentally verified correlation of psittacine age and thymic size is available, making evaluation of thymic change difficult. Histologically, lymphoid cell depletion and loss of corticomedullary differentiation are seen. A definitive diagnosis of some viral infections (polyoma virus and circovirus) may be possible if inclusion bodies are present.

In pet avian species, few reports are available on specific diseases leading to enlargement of the thymus. Those reported include congenital cyst formation, epithelial thymoma, and thymic lymphosarcoma.[7] Cyst formation may be obvious grossly, but a definitive differential diagnosis depends on microscopic examination of the lesion. Keratinized cysts associated with vitamin A deficiency have also been seen.

Bursa of Fabricius

The bursa of Fabricius is a dorsal median diverticulum of the proctodeal region of the cloaca. Its shape varies with species of bird. In psittacine birds, it is oval or pear-shaped and has a central cavity (Fig. 37–3). In ratites, the bursa is composed of pedunculated projections containing lymphoid follicles. The wall of the bursa is folded and covered by simple columnar or pseudostratified columnar epithelium. Lymphoid nodules are located between epithelial folds. Each of these nodules contains a cortex and medulla, separated by a basement membrane (Fig. 37–4). Follicle-associated epithelium separates the cortex from the medulla. Bursal development in chickens begins on the fourth day of embryonic development as a cluster of mesenchymal cells that are gradually surrounded by epithelium.[8, 9] Controlled studies on growth and development of the bursa of Fabricius have not been done in psittacine birds; however, in the author's experience, well-developed bursal tissue is present in psittacines at an older age than has been reported for chickens.[10]

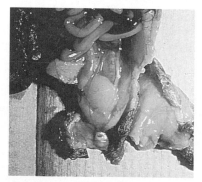

Figure 37-3

Normal psittacine bursa of Fabricius. The cloaca has been dissected away.

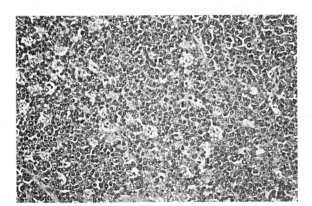

Figure 37-4

Histologic appearance of normal psittacine bursa of Fabricius in a 4-month-old eclectus parrot.

Within the bursa, there is a stepwise differentiation of B-lymphocytes. These cells are responsible for humoral immunity. The bursa of Fabricius serves as a source of these cells to seed secondary lymphoid organs, with the seeding beginning as early as day 17 of incubation, and the bursa is necessary for normal thymic development. The bursa of Fabricius produces hormones including bursapoietin, which induces maturation of bone marrow cells in bursa sites, and lymphocyte and thrombocyte inhibiting factors.[9] In chickens, IgM, IgG, IgA, and possible IgG analogues have been described, as have IgG and IgM allotypes.[10]

Bursal Diseases and Lesions

Bursal lymphocyte depletion can occur during fetal life or after hatching. Regression of the bursa because of stress is mediated by the hypothalamic-pituitary-adrenal axis. Production of steroid hormones occurs in interrenal cells (cortex) of the adrenal gland, which leads to lymphocytolysis. The result may be an immunosuppressed or immunodeficient bird, particularly one deficient in humoral immunity. Immunosuppression is most severe in chickens experimentally when there is loss of cells prior to the seeding of B-cells into the secondary lymphoid organs.[10] If adequate numbers of B-cells have invaded these organs, there can be severe bursal hypoplasia without severe immunodeficiency. The loss of humoral immunity under various circumstances makes young birds more susceptible to many bacterial diseases, as well as some fungal infections.

Specific causes of bursal necrosis or depletion include environmental stress such as abnormal temperature, humidity, and excessive noise during incubation or after hatching, as well as poor nutrition. Some toxins, such as excessive vitamin D, can lead to similar lesions. Bacterial or parasitic infections are potential causes of bursal depletion, as is an excess of testosterone. A lack of triiodothyronine (T_3) may result in lowered bursal weight.[11] A number of viral infections are potential causes of bursal lymphoid depletion in pet avian species. These include circovirus infection,[12] polyomavirus infection,[13] avian poxvirus infection, adenovirus infection, and herpesvirus infection.

Gross morphologic changes include a reduction in bursal size and various levels of edema and hemorrhage, depending on the underlying cause (Fig. 37-5). Normal bursal involution appears to be more prolonged in psittacines than in chickens, with well-developed follicles present in some psittacines at 18 to 20 months of age. Both gross and histologic changes in suspected bursal disease must be correlated with the age of the bird. Histologically, the change is dependent in some degree on the time of exposure and on whether the change is

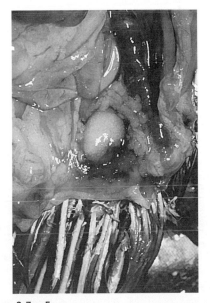

Figure 37-5

Conure with polyomavirus infection. The bursa is smaller than normal and hemorrhagic.

acute or chronic. Small irregularly shaped follicles with minimal numbers of lymphocytes indicate chronic disease or application of the stress either during fetal organogenesis or immediately after hatching. Active necrosis of remaining lymphoid cells may occur. Bursal follicles of normal size with severe acute necrosis indicate more acute stress during neonatal life (Fig. 37–6). Histologically, there is a variable loss of lymphoid cells with accumulation of necrotic debris. In the case of bacterial or fungal infections, heterophil infiltration may be evident and the causative organisms may be seen. In severe cases, abscess formation is noted. Diagnosis of the underlying disease process is possible in some viral diseases because of the formation of specific inclusion bodies (Fig. 37–7).

Secondary Effects and Lesions in Birds with Inadequate Bursal Development or Bursal Disease

As a result of failure to seed secondary organs with lymphocytes, splenic hypoplasia may occur, with the spleen being small and pale, but because of the thymic contribution, the degree of hypoplasia is variable. In many birds, death can occur with no other apparent gross or histologic lesion. There appears to be a correlation between bursal disease and presumed immune system deficiencies and aspiration of foreign material. Perhaps infected birds are weak or have poor reflexes; however, the exact pathogenesis is not known. Many birds with histor-

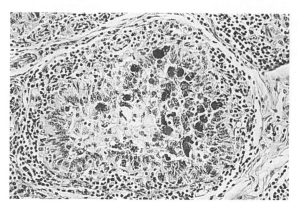

Figure 37–7

Severe lymphoid depletion and inclusion body formation in an African grey parrot with systemic circovirus infection.

ies of doing poorly or being undersized die as a result of severe acute inhalation and/or inhalation pneumonia.

Severe secondary bacterial infections are seen; the liver is the primary organ involved. Affected livers are usually enlarged, mottled, and pale. Histologically, there is often necrosis and marked bacterial proliferation with little inflammatory response. Differential diagnosis includes primary bacterial infections or possibly metabolic liver disease. Histologic examination results showing the presence of little or no inflammatory response are more important in making a proper diagnosis than culture results, because bacteria are present whether bacterial disease is primary or secondary. In young psittacines (or any avian species) it is important to evaluate gross specimens and submit the bursa for histologic examination, or the true cause of the problem may not be determined.

Fungal infections are another frequently encountered problem. Mycotic pneumonia and/or airsacculitis due to organisms morphologically consistent with *Aspergillus* are seen. These infections may be the result of immunosuppression, or may result from the same stress factors that cause bursal lesions and immunosuppression. Although no gross changes are usually noted, there is usually a lack of disseminated lymphoid tissue, and diseases such as cryptosporidiosis are noted histologically, with organisms present on various epithelial surfaces.

Proliferative Changes in the Bursa of Fabricius

Occasionally, young birds with disseminated histiocytic, plasmacytic, and lymphoid proliferation are

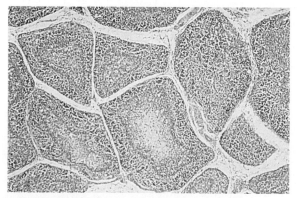

Figure 37–6

Histologic appearance of the bursa from a cockatoo with polyomavirus infection. There is depletion of lymphoid cells with proliferation of reticular cells. The follicle-associated epithelium is easily seen. (Compare with Figure 37–4.)

found. This change usually involves the bursa as well as the spleen and other lymphoid organs, and the cause is often not determined; however, the changes are suggestive of some chronic antigenic stimulation. Lymphosarcoma in young birds may also involve the bursa of Fabricius. Affected bursas are enlarged, white, and somewhat firm. Histologically, there is effacement of bursal follicles by the neoplastic lymphoid cells (Fig. 37–8).

SECONDARY LYMPHOID ORGANS

Spleen

The spleen is present on the right side of the junction between the proventriculus and the ventriculus, and it varies in size and shape, depending on the species of bird. It may be round and elongated or slightly triangular. The spleen has a thin capsule and no well-defined trabeculae, with a basic network of reticular fibers and cells. Lymphoid tissue surrounds arteries, and there are numerous venous sinuses. In birds, the spleen functions as a site of phagocytosis of aged erythrocytes, in lymphopoiesis, and in antibody production. The spleen of birds is not a significant blood reservoir.[8]

Localized or systemic disorders affecting the spleen can result in either a small spleen or a large spleen. Small spleens are either hypoplastic or atrophic. In young birds, variable splenic hypoplasia is the result of bursal disease and a lack of

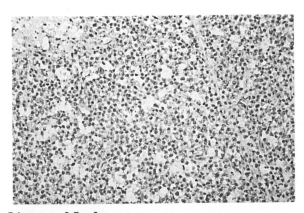

Figure 37–8

Lymphosarcoma in a young Amazon parrot. There is effacement of normal bursal architecture by a monomorphic sheet of immature lymphoid cells.

seeding of the spleen by B-lymphocytes, even though T-lymphocytes are still present. In older birds, splenic lymphoid atrophy may be present because of various stresses and chronic stress adaptation. Splenic lymphoid necrosis has been associated with viral disease, other infectious disease, and environmental or nutritional stress. With aging, there is a normal amount of splenic atrophy.

Splenic enlargement is associated with various conditions. The amount of splenic enlargement varies, and affected spleens may be congested or pale and are diffusely affected, or may contain multiple foci that grossly vary in color and consistency. Acute viral disease is a potential cause of splenic enlargement, with polyomavirus and herpesvirus being two primary problems in psittacine birds.[14, 15] Histologically, there is necrosis of lymphoid tissue. Specific diagnosis is made by the finding of characteristic inclusion bodies.

Systemic bacterial disease, caused by both gram-negative and gram-positive bacteria, results in a large spleen that usually has multiple pale foci. These are areas of necrosis and fibrin deposition, often associated with heterophil infiltration. Specific diagnosis histologically is not possible; however, either gram-negative or gram-positive bacteria can be identified by appropriate histochemical methods. Splenic enlargement is also a feature of chlamydial infection.[16] Histologic examination reveals histiocytosis as the predominant lesion. Although the histologic lesion may be suggestive of chlamydiosis, unless organisms are present, a specific diagnosis cannot be made. Acid-fast infections often are noted in the spleen. In psittacine birds, there is usually a diffuse infiltration by large macrophages containing acid-fast organisms. In other avian species caseated foci may be found surrounded by macrophages and numerous giant cells. The diagnosis is made by appropriate histochemical methods.

Disseminated mycotic infections can induce splenic enlargement. Histologic examination is necessary to differentiate these cases from bacterial infections. A variety of protozoal diseases can affect the spleen in pet avian species. Systemic sarcosporidiosis is not uncommon in psittacine birds, particularly in warmer climates, and it leads to an enlarged spleen that histologically is infiltrated by numerous plasma cells and macrophages.[17] Plasmodial infections in raptors and canaries also lead to marked splenic enlargement with the accumulation of macrophages and plasma cells as well as reactive lymphocytes. In raptors, there is often production of malarial pigment, a gray-black pigment produced by the parasite, which leads to a characteristic diffusely black spleen on gross examination.

Noninfectious causes of splenic enlargement include amyloidosis, which leads to a pale, homogeneous, enlarged spleen. Histologically, there is variable amyloid deposition. Neoplastic disease can produce a markedly enlarged spleen. Both myeloproliferative disease and lymphosarcoma are reported. Primary fibrosarcoma and leiomyosarcoma may also occur in the spleen. Although not common, metastasis of various neoplasms can cause splenic enlargement. Differentiation of the various splenic neoplastic diseases is done histologically.[7]

Disseminated Lymphoid Tissue

Disseminated lymphoid tissue occurs in the harderian gland, alimentary tract, bone marrow, and as solitary nodules in some organs. Those organs containing the disseminated lymphoid tissue vary with different species of bird. In some waterfowl, structures morphologically consistent with lymph nodes are seen.[2] These organs and structures respond in a fashion similar to that of the spleen and are affected by the same conditions.

PRIMARY DISORDERS OF THE IMMUNE SYSTEM

Autoimmune Diseases

Autoimmune conditions are suspected in birds; however, with the exception of autoimmune thyroiditis in chickens, none has been proved. In chickens, there is autoantibody formation against thyroglobulin.[10] This condition has been considered to be a B-cell–mediated disease in the obese strain of chickens, with a pathogenesis similar to autoimmune diseases in man. A positive correlation exists between antithyroglobulin antibody levels and lymphoid infiltration of the thyroid gland. The inflammation can be reduced if affected birds are bursectomized. The pathogenesis of the condition has also been described as thyroid autoantigens presented to T-helper cells, with autoantigen-binding B-cells entering the thyroid from the circulation with proliferation. The latter cells differentiate into antigen-producing cells and may finally appear as mature plasma cells.[18] Although not proved to be an autoimmune disease, a morphologically similar disease has been seen in a young African grey parrot. The histologic changes are typical of the changes noted in chickens (Fig. 37–9). There is some indication that autoimmune skin disease and hemolytic anemia may also occur in psittacine birds; however, as with thyroiditis, no definitive proof has yet been established.

Immune-Mediated Diseases

Allergic dermatitis has not been definitively proved to exist in psittacine or other pet avian species; however, clinical disease and histologic lesions consistent with probable allergic dermatitis are seen in birds that are pruritic and engage in feather picking. Until specific tests for allergens are developed for birds, the condition will remain difficult to document. Skin biopsy may be of some value in the differential diagnosis of clinical dermatitis.

A severe pneumonitis considered to be the result of allergy is seen in psittacines, particularly in blue and gold macaws. This condition usually occurs as a medical emergency, with affected birds having severe difficulty with breathing and death often resulting shortly after presentation. The sensitizing allergens are believed to be endotoxin fragments, powder down, and feather particles from other psit-

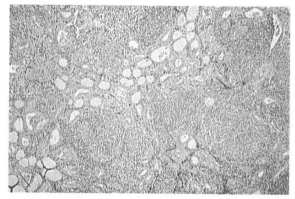

F i g u r e 3 7 – 9

Lymphocytic thyroiditis in a young African grey parrot. The lesion is morphologically similar to that of autoimmune thyroiditis in chickens.

tacine birds, and organisms such as *Aspergillus*.[19] Before the acute and often fatal episode, birds may have mild attacks that result in some histologic changes; however, these are often not clinically noticeable. On gross examination, the lungs are usually red and wet. Histologically, the affected birds have collapsed lungs with diffuse congestion and edema as well as possible hemorrhage. There may be hypertrophy of atrial muscles depending on the frequency of previous attacks. A mild nonsuppurative inflammatory infiltrate may be seen.

Another possible immune-mediated condition in psittacine birds is proventricular dilatation syndrome. This disease is considered to be the result of a virus that affects both the central and peripheral nervous system, with resultant loss of tone of the proventriculus and ventriculus, and subsequent clinical signs and lesions. Although the disease is considered to be of viral etiology, the morphologic lesions involving the nervous system (which include a primarily nonsuppurative inflammatory infiltrate in the central nervous system, dorsal root, and autonomic ganglia) may represent an immune-mediated disease that occurs even in the absence of viral activity. This type of lesion is similar to that noted in various viral diseases of mammals resulting in immunopathologic processes.[20]

VACCINATION AND IMMUNOTHERAPY

Vaccines have been introduced for Pacheco's disease and psittacine pox.[21] Although these vaccines can provide an acceptable level of immunity, side effects including sudden death and chronic granulomatous cellulitis have been reported. Experimental vaccines for psittacine beak and feather disease and polyomavirus infection have also been developed.[22] These vaccines represent a beginning in the development of means to control infectious diseases. New developments in experimental immunology[23] may lead to specific vaccines against diseases controlled by cell-mediated immunity.

Therapy for immune-mediated and autoimmune diseases in animals has been associated with steroidal and nonsteroidal anti-inflammatory drugs that are effective in some inflammatory conditions. Other treatment modalities may be more readily available, based on ongoing research. Blockage of the proinflammation effects of endotoxin by altering the binding of endotoxin with specific cell membrane receptors or serum proteins may be possible. Inhibition of cytokines to affect the initiation of inflammation may eventually be possible, but the cost and timing of treatment precludes use of currently available commercial preparations.[24]

Acknowledgment

The author wishes to thank Drs. David Graham and Victoria Joseph for their review and helpful comments.

References

1. Tizard I: Veterinary Immunology, An Introduction, ed 4. Philadelphia, WB Saunders, 1992.
2. King AS, McLelland J: Birds: Their Structure and Function. London, Bailliere Tindall, 1984.
3. Payne LN, Powell PC: The lymphoid system. In Freeman, BM (ed): Physiology and Biochemistry of the Domestic Fowl, vol. 5. New York, Academic Press, 1981.
4. White RG: The structural organization of avian lymphoid tissues. In Rose ME, Payne LN, Freeman BM (eds): Avian Immunology, 16th Poultry Science Symposium. Edinburgh, Clark, Constable Ltd, 1981, pp 21–44.
5. Chi DS, Galton JE, Thorbecke GJ: Role of T-cells in immune responses of the chicken. In Rose ME, Payne LN, Freeman BM (eds): Avian Immunology, 16th Poultry Science Symposium. Edinburgh, Clark, Constable Ltd, 1981, pp 21–24, 103–134.
6. Sharma JM, Frederickson TL: Mechanisms of T-cell immunosuppression by infectious bursal disease virus of chickens. In Weber WT, Ewerti DL (eds): Avian Immunology, Proc 2nd Intl Conf Avian Immunology. Philadelphia. Alan R. Liss. 1980, pp 283–294.
7. Schmidt RE: Morphologic diagnosis of avian neoplasms. Semin Avian Exotic Pet Med, 1:73–79, 1992.
8. Toivanen A, Toivanen P, Eskola J, Lassila I: Ontogeny of the chicken lymphoid system. In Rose ME, Payne LN, Freeman BM (eds): Avian Immunology, 16th Poultry Science Symposium. Edinburgh, Clark, Constable Ltd, 1981, pp 45–62.
9. Glick B: Bursa of Fabricius. In Farner DS, King JR, Parkes KC (eds): Avian Biology, vol VII. New York, Academic Press, 1983, pp 443–484.
10. Ivanyi J: Functions of the B-lymphoid system in chickens. In Rose ME, Payne LN, Freeman BM (eds): Avian Immunology 16th Poultry Science Symposium. Edinburgh, Clark, Constable Ltd, 1981, pp 21–44, 63–101.
11. Haddad EE, Mushady MM: Effects of thyrotrophic-releasing hormone, triiodothyronine and chicken growth hormone on plasma concentrations of thyroxine, triiodothyronine, growth hormone and growth of lymphoid organs, and leukocyte populations in immature male chickens. Poult Sci 69:1094–1102, 1990.
12. Latimer KS, Rakich PM, Niagro FD, et al: An updated review of psittacine beak and feather disease. J Assoc Avian Vet 5:211–220, 1991.

13. Graham DL, Calnek BW: Papovavirus isolation in hand-fed parrots: Virus isolation and pathology. Avian Dis 31:298–410, 1987.

14. Ritchie BW, Niagro FD, Latimer KS, et al: Avian polyomavirus: An overview. J Assoc Avian Vet 5:147–153, 1991.

15. Gaskin JM: Psittacine viral diseases: A perspective. J Zoo Wildl Med 20:249–264, 1989.

16. Graham DL: A color atlas of avian chlamydiosis. In Fudge, AM (ed) Semin Avian Exotic Pet Med vol 2:184–189, 1993.

17. Page GD, Schmidt RE, English JH, et al: Antemortem diagnosis and treatment of sarcocystosis in two species of psittacines. J Zoo Wildl Med 23:77–85, 1992.

18. Wick O: Autoimmune disease in an avian species: The obese strain (os) of chickens as a model for human Hashimoto thyroiditis. In Toivanen A, Toivanen P (eds): Avian Immunology: Basis and Practice, vol. II. Boca Raton, CRC Press, 1987, pp 169–184.

19. Taylor M: Personal communication, 1992.

20. Nathanson N, Martin J, Peterson G, et al: Experimental virus-induced immunopathology of the central nervous system. In Mieschen P, Bolis L, Garini S, et al (eds): Second symposium on immunopathology of the central and peripheral nervous system. Basel, Schwabe & Co, 1979, 95–112.

21. Fudge AM: Psittacine vaccines. Proc Assoc Avian Vet, Phoenix, 1990, pp 292–300.

22. Ritchie BW, Niagro FD, Latimer KS, et al: A polyomavirus overview and evaluation of an experimental polyomavirus vaccine. Proc Assoc Avian Vet, New Orleans, 1992, pp 1–4.

23. Scott P: IL-12: Initiation cytokine for cell-mediated immunity. Science 260:496–497, 1993.

24. Breiden MA: Endothelium and inflammation. J Am Vet Med Assoc 203:300–306, 1993.

Christine Davis

38

Behavioral Problems

BASIC CONSIDERATIONS OF BEHAVIOR MODIFICATION

Behavioral problems in psittacines are as diverse and as intricate as those of any other intelligent creature. To employ mere "shotgun" techniques for modifying undesirable behavior would be as irresponsible as doing so for the majority of medical problems incurred throughout the animal's lifetime. There are certain specific behavioral guidelines that can, in *some* cases, make it possible to circumvent, or even eliminate, some undesirable behaviors.

AGGRESSION AND BITING

Etiology

As with most behaviors, aggression can be the result of myriad factors; however, some of the more prevalent causes seen in the domestic environment are described.

Jealousy

Most psittacines are naturally monogamous and favor one person in the household. If the bird is taught *at the very outset* to be handled by all of the primary adult members of the household, aggressive displays due to jealousy can be greatly decreased. Favoring one person is often unavoidable, but resultant aggressive behavior can be significantly diminished and often eliminated completely.

New humans, especially infants, or new animals of any species can also be the source of jealousy and must be introduced carefully into the bird's environment. An area considered neutral by the primary bird can be chosen for the introduction. The primary bird *should be held by its favorite person* and praised with treats and tickles during the first introduction to the new individual. After a few minutes of familiarization, the new individual is then taken (preferably by another family member) into the primary bird's area of the house at the same time that the primary bird is returned to that area.

New birds should not initially be placed in the primary bird's cage or on its play areas, nor should the primary bird be relocated by the new bird's presence.

Territorial Behavior

In the wild, protection of the nest is essential to the welfare of the mate and young. Whatever space the bird occupies on a regular basis becomes the bird's territory and it *must* be defended, especially if the bird is, by nature, an aggressive individual. Whether the area is a cage or a favorite spot within the home is irrelevant.

Baby birds do not protect their territory; protection is the job of the parent. If a bird is kept in the "child" role and the owner is perceived as the "parent," defense of territory no longer becomes necessary and aggression diminishes or disappears completely.

Threats, Real or Perceived

In the wild, the bird is preyed upon. By nature, the bird is not a fighter and usually depends on a

653

"flight" response as its primary option. In captivity, that option is usually eliminated, and the bird must resort to a "fight" or aggressive reaction.

The first and most obvious question is whether the bird was tame initially. Is the bird wild-caught and untamed, or is it an unsocialized, hand-fed, domestically bred individual? In either case, such a bird exhibits aggressive displays when it feels threatened. Surprisingly, the client often fails to consider the possibility that the bird is untamed.

Quick or unfamiliar movements, sudden loud sounds, strange individuals (human or animal), or unfamiliar objects in the bird's visual field can all be perceived as threatening. If a bird is pursued across the floor or around the inside of the cage, this also is perceived as threatening (i.e., predatory) behavior, and the bird may acquire a dislike of the person involved in the episode. Examine the cage or perch location from the bird's perspective and rectify any "threatening" situations.

Often, birds with crippled or missing toes, or baby birds with poor balance (especially African grey parrots) bite because they do not feel secure. This behavior should not be punished because it results from the owner's interacting improperly with the bird. The clumsy bird should be held close to the body so that its beak rests against the person's chest or abdomen. This allays feelings of insecurity and eliminates the need to bite.

Sexual Maturity

The idea that aggression is linked to sexual maturity is greatly overemphasized. Most birds, if well behaved to begin with, do not become unmanageable during times of hormone flux. There may be a slight increase in aggression, but this is usually manageable. Sudden aggressive displays during sexual maturity are usually seen in birds that are wild or undisciplined from the outset.

Care must be taken that the owner does not stimulate the bird sexually. Rubbing the hindquarters or engaging in long periods of body contact may alter the bird's perception of the person. The person may then be perceived as a mate, which can contribute to hormone fluctuations.

Providing the bird with dark "nesting" areas, whether intentional or not, alters its hormone production and stimulates reproductive behavior.

Pain

Often, a bird that is sick or in pain strikes out to avoid being handled. This is an aspect that *must* be considered and pursued, especially by the veterinarian.

Clinical Signs

Displays of aggression vary with the different species of birds and their individual personalities; however, certain signs are common in aggressive displays. Signs of aggression are usually visual and include lunging, striking, biting, pupillary constriction, tail flaring, arching of the neck, or violent play (i.e., tearing and ripping papers or toys while exhibiting the aforementioned behavior). Often there are vocal displays as well.

In crested species such as cockatoos, raising of the crest and a forward flaring of the feathers around the beak is also displayed. Wings are raised and extended. The bird may lunge or strike openmouthed at the individual being threatened or at other objects in the area, while pointedly staring at the individual being threatened. Stalking individuals being threatened is common. Screaming can also be a display of aggression.

Diagnosis

Psittacine behavior can be confusing when described by the client and usually must be examined within the context of the situation. Sometimes, what is construed by the person to be aggressive activity may actually be harmless mating displays. Do not always accept the client's assessment of the behavior, especially if clients are not familiar with normal avian behavior. If the bird is becoming less manageable, avoiding interaction previously welcomed from the owner, or actually biting people, the behavior is usually interpreted as problem behavior.

Corrective Techniques

The following general hints are conducive to tempering aggressive tendencies. If they fail, an avian behavior counselor should be contacted.

The height of the bird as it relates to its environment is directly correlated to its feelings of dominance. Keeping the bird's head at a level in which it is midchest to the owner will do much to lessen or eliminate aggressive displays. Ignoring the bird by not looking at it, talking to it, or interacting with it during its display behavior will help to discourage it. Covering the cage for a period of 10 minutes during an aggressive display will show the bird that it is being "banished" for its undesirable behavior. Most sociable birds desire interaction and do not like this.

Prevention

Do not allow the bird free run of the household. Teach it to remain on a play gym or inside its cage until it is invited to interact. Bird owners should avoid situations that put the owner in a submissive or mate role.

SCREAMING

Screaming is a natural vocalization for most large hookbill species in the wild. Vocalization is especially pronounced at dawn and dusk, and may aid flock members in determining the location of their companions. However, loud displays of screaming do not have to be tolerated in the domestic environment. Playful chattering can replace raucous screeching without psychological damage to the bird.

Etiology

Noise is an important stimulus. It is natural for the bird to match the level of noise in the environment. The "jungle" screaming of other birds at dawn and dusk or other noise in the domestic environment, such as loud music, garbage disposals, lawn mowers, and vacuum cleaners, stimulates loud vocalizations. Aggression and territorial behavior lead the bird to scream to alert all others in the area that the screamer is dominant. Seeking attention or attempting to control the owner can also lead to screaming behavior.

Separation anxiety is another cause of screaming.

As with other intelligent creatures, birds can suffer separation anxiety when their "flock" members, human or otherwise, are out of sight. Fear of abandonment by the flock is a very real threat. In the wild, birds do not experience abandonment unless they are too ill or injured to join their companions.

There are species differences in screaming behavior. Most birds can learn to be quiet; however, some species (e.g., *Aratinga* species) are predisposed to vocal displays. This tendency needs to be considered prior to purchase.

Clinical Signs

Screaming or excessive vocalizations that are inappropriate or intolerable to other inhabitants of the environment signal a behavioral problem.

Diagnosis

Correction of the behavior should begin with assessing the type of vocalization the bird is exhibiting. What is an ear-splitting vocal display to some people may be perfectly tolerable to others. If the screaming is intolerable to the individuals in the environment or their neighbors, it can be considered a problem.

Corrective Techniques

Corrective techniques vary widely with the disposition and situation of each bird and are determined by the history. Each contributing factor must be determined and addressed.

Covering the cage, isolation from the "flock" (in a room by itself or in a carrier), or being ignored by principal household members for a period of 10 minutes can show the bird that the behavior is undesirable and will not be tolerated. Elimination, if possible, of environmental stimuli can be effective in the early stages, if it is done before the behavior becomes habitual.

Prevention

The etiology must be considered and all contributing factors reduced or eliminated. With temporary outbursts, such as screaming in response to lawn mowers or garbage disposals, the bird should be ignored until the activity is over and the behavior stops.

Care must be taken not to inadvertently reinforce the screaming behavior. The bird should not be looked at, talked to, or touched while screaming. Any interaction, even if it is intended by the person as negative, is positive reinforcement of the behavior. As with most behavior problems, having a well-adjusted bird that can occupy its time in a healthy manner is an extremely important aspect in the prevention of undesirable behaviors.

FEATHER PICKING AND MUTILATION

Of all undesirable behaviors, feather picking and mutilation are the most heartbreaking and difficult to treat. These are very frustrating problems, and it is imperative that clients be counseled with extreme patience and compassion.

Etiology

Medical

In birds that engage in feather picking, a complete physical examination and indicated diagnostic tests are necessary before a diagnosis of a behavioral problem is made. Many subclinical infections can cause or exacerbate feather picking.

Environmental

Changes in weather (i.e., heat, cold, humidity, dryness, and possible allergens) should be taken into consideration as possible factors. New members of the household (human or animal), changes in the home environment, or changes in any aspect of the life of the primary "flock" member, whether emotional, personal or work-related, can all contribute to the behavior. In extremely young birds, it can be a learned behavior if there is already a feather-picking bird in the environment.

Fear, Nervousness, Separation Anxiety

Extremely heavy activity or movement, a high level of noise, or large numbers of animals in the immediate environment can make the bird nervous.

Birds can see colors and some have distinct preferences. Some colors can elicit strong behavioral reactions; red can be a color that elicits pleasure or fear, depending upon the bird.

Often feather picking can be traced to changes in the owner's life (i.e., absences, vacation, change in work schedule, family emergency). Do not underestimate the client's emotional state as a possible contributing factor. Birds are flock creatures and may interpret any situation that does not feel "right" or safe within that "flock" as possibly life-threatening.

Sexual

As with humans, shifts in hormone levels can make a bird nervous and irritable. Some aspects of hormone production in psittacines are contingent upon environmental factors. Situations that may stimulate hormone changes must be examined. These include exposure to long photoperiods, usually occurring in the summer when there are long daylight hours; other sexually mature or nesting birds in the environment, especially if there is direct interaction with the bird in question; and dark places or nest boxes that may stimulate nesting behavior. Certain toys, which the bird treats as "babies" or "eggs," may stimulate nesting behavior and increase sexual feather picking. Prolonged periods of cuddling, with close body contact, or rubbing the tail area or the backs of females can also contribute to hormone shifts. Any of these situations can also promote excessive egg-laying in unmated birds.

Control or Attention

Birds may engage in feather picking to seek attention. If the bird is feather picking and the client proceeds to scold it, examine the areas in question, sweetly admonish the bird, or even just look at the bird, the behavior is reinforced and the bird will continue to pick.

Boredom

Most birds are flock creatures that are accustomed to vigorous activity in the wild. Chewing is a natural part of their behavior and, if toys and objects for chewing are not available, the bird may pick at its feathers out of boredom.

Species Predisposition

Some birds appear to be predisposed to feather picking and do so as a response to any environmental or physiological stress. In some species, such as cockatoos, there is liberal social preening. Individual birds of these species may be predisposed to feather picking when kept as single pets.

Clinical Signs

Signs vary widely, from ruffling areas on the wing tops, to complete denuding of the trunk, wings, and legs. Partial or complete feathers may be damaged or missing. In birds that engage in self-mutilation the effect may range from simple dermal laceration to severe soft tissue wounds, such as the chewing off of toes and tearing of breast muscle.

Diagnosis

Diagnosis can often be difficult; some people may misinterpret the bird's condition. Frequently, first-time bird owners mistake normal preening and molting behavior for feather picking. In addition, birds who play roughly on cages that have extremely thin bars frequently damage or break their tail feathers; the feather barbs will be missing from that area, with just the central shaft evident. Young, playful birds often have poor feathering prior to their first molt.

Corrective Techniques

Correction takes some detective work and is directly contingent upon the etiology of the condition. Often, there is more than one cause, and each one must be examined and eradicated to achieve suc-

cess. Mutilation of the flesh may result in neuropathy and is not easily cured with simple behavior modification. Medical intervention is advised in birds that engage in self-mutilation. (See Chapter 32, Dermatology.)

Removing the bird from environmental sources that induce nervousness or fear is important. Often, owners must be aware of and control their own stress levels. Limiting activity that may stimulate the bird sexually or increase hormone production is necessary, especially during the bird's normal breeding period. Owners must take care not to inadvertently reinforce the feather-picking behavior by giving the bird inappropriate attention.

In acute or chronic cases, a collar can be used to temporarily restrain the bird. Collaring in behavioral feather picking will work only if it is used in conjunction with a customized behavior modification program. If the bird is not retrained during the period when it is wearing a collar, the behavior will return after it is removed.

Birds use their feet to grip, climb, and eat; therefore, most birds adapt better to a tube-type collar than a wide collar. This allows them to see their feet and to use them for limited normal functions. However, with a tube collar, most birds can still reach their wings and legs to feather pick. Tube collars work best in birds that pick only the chest area.

Owners should offer toys that duplicate the sensation of feather picking and reinforce the behavior when the bird chooses to play with them. Wooden ice cream sticks, plastic or paper straws (in the wrapper), paper towel and toilet paper rolls (unscented), wooden scrub brushes with natural fiber bristles, whisk brooms, and toothbrushes all duplicate the sensation of feather picking.

Prevention

Some species of birds, including cockatoos, African grey parrots, and eclectus parrots, are predisposed to feather picking. Regardless of the species, most negative behaviors can be greatly reduced or eliminated by teaching the bird to play by itself, with or without toys. "Clingy" birds need to be taught to be independent, yet interactive. Avoid any of the situations that may increase hormone production and exacerbate subsequent behaviors. Reward the bird for chewing on toys instead of its feathers.

There is no prescription for behavior modification. For success, each situation must be assessed according to its unique components, and a program devised in which all deviant behaviors are corrected.

A background in human psychology as well as psychology of animal behavior is helpful. Negative behaviors commonly result from the way people interact with a bird. Providing clear behavioral boundaries in a consistent manner is required for successful behavioral modification.

Pharmacology and Therapeutics

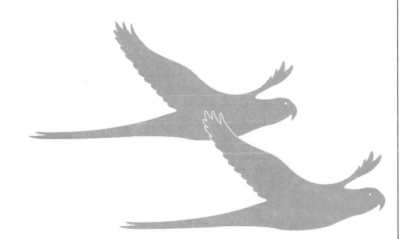

39A

Gerry M. Dorrestein

Metabolism, Pharmacology, and Therapy

The basis for the successful management of avian patients is knowledge of the principles and techniques of supportive care and emergency medicine.[1] And, although the basic concepts of therapy of small animal medicine apply to birds, adaptations must be made to compensate for their unique anatomy and physiology.

Especially in a critically ill bird, stabilization of the patient's condition is essential. It is not sufficient to start "an antibacterial therapy." Other major components may include additional medical and surgical components such as fluid therapy, tube feeding, debridement of inflammatory tissue, or drainage of exudate.[2] The physiology of metabolism, body temperature, temperature regulation, heat loss, heat stress, and the role of water economy are essential elements to understand in order to correct the derailments of normal function.

Knowledge of the principles of therapy in birds is rapidly expanding. Large interspecies differences in metabolic elimination, drug distribution, anatomy, and physiology of the digestive and respiratory system do exist. As in mammals, formulation of the dosage form and the presence of disease conditions may influence drug efficacy.[3]

In many instances, drug products are indicated that are not licensed for use in birds. Preparations that have not been clinically tested can be dangerous to birds because of the active compound or the galenic composition, even if they are highly effective against the isolated agent or compatible in other animals.

PHYSIOLOGY OF METABOLISM AND BODY TEMPERATURE

The High Body Temperature of Birds

Birds have a high rate of metabolism. Flight and maintenance of high body temperature (endothermia) use large amounts of energy. In general, the rates of physiologic processes increase with temperature. Transmission speed of nerve impulses increases 1.8 times with every 10°C increase in temperature. The speed and strength of muscle fiber contractions triple with each 10°C rise in temperature.[4]

The maintenance of high body temperatures through endothermia, however, is energetically expensive; birds expend 20 to 30 times more energy than do similar-sized reptiles. Both the circulatory and respiratory systems have evolved exceptional capacities for the delivery of energy and oxygen to the body's cells as well as rapid removal of poisonous metabolic waste products.

Birds regulate their body temperatures at 40° to 42°C by adjusting plumage insulation, by increasing heat production through shivering when cold, and by evaporative water loss through panting and gular fluttering when hot. Regulation of blood flow through the feet aids heat loss or retention. To save energy, some birds, notably hummingbirds, swifts, and nightjars, can lower body temperature and become torpid. Birds can also elevate body temperature a few degrees to reduce the need for evapora-

661

tive water loss and to store body heat for cold nights. Heat production during flight can be lost quickly with little loss of water. However, birds have little latitude for higher body temperatures; 46°C is lethal.

Levels of Metabolism

Basal Metabolism

All birds have a high basal metabolic rate (BMR), and, for their various sizes, passerine birds have the highest rates of any group of vertebrate animals. The average BMR of a passerine bird is 50 to 60% higher than that of nonpasserines of the same body size. There are, however, exceptions in both directions.

Basal metabolism relates directly to mass, although not in a 1:1 relationship. The relationship, in most cases, is given by the formula

$$BMR = K(W^{0.75})$$

K is a theoretical constant for kilocalories required per 24 hours and varies with the species of bird. K is 129 for passerines and 78 for nonpasserines. W is weight in kilograms.

The formula reflects the relationship between metabolism and mass in the context of the surface area from which heat is lost.

This formula is essential for calculating the daily energy needs of a bird in case of illness and stress associated with decreased nutritional intake. The BMR is also sometimes used for extrapolating a dose regimen from one species to another.

Activity Metabolism

Basal metabolism represents the expenditure of minimal energy. A bird usually spends only a fraction of its day at this low metabolic level, most of its time being spent in activities that require more energy and oxygen. Just being awake or resting increases the metabolic rate 25 to 80% above the basal rate.

The increased metabolism of birds resting in a small cage without temperature stress reflects only increased muscle tension and mental activity; this is measured as a 25% increase. For clinical use the maintenance energy requirement (MER) is used and is defined as the BMR plus additional energy (approximately 1.5 times the BMR in adult animals) needed for normal physiologic activity, digestion, and absorption.[1] With growth, disease, or stress, animals are in a hypermetabolic state with daily energy needs that surpass the MER. The amount of increased demand depends on the type of injury or stress and varies from one to three times the MER.

Although it costs more per unit time, flight is generally a more efficient form of locomotion than running. To fly 1 km, a 10-g bird uses less than 1% of the energy that a 10-g mouse uses to run the same distance. The energy expended in power flight per unit time generally exceeds that of other modes of locomotion, but estimates of flight metabolism range from two to 25 times the BMR, with variations that reflect flight mode, flight speeds, wing shape, and/or laboratory constraints. Hovering in one place is extremely expensive, depending on body size; for example, seven to 17 times the BMR in hummingbirds.[4]

Peak reproductive activities increase total daily energy expenditures by as much as 50%. At the beginning of the breeding season, courtship, territoriality, and nest building demand significant effort. Only minor amounts of productive energy are channelled into growth of the gonadal tissues, but subsequent egg formation and egg-laying by females impose new demands on energy and nutrition.

Incubation can create an energy shortage because it limits the amount of time a bird can forage for its own maintenance. The parents then face another surge of demands on their time and energy when the chicks hatch and require food and brooding.

The complete moult is a major undertaking. Moult draws significantly on protein and energy reserves to synthesize feather structure and to offset the effects of poorer insulation and flight efficacy. The increase in daily metabolism during peak periods of feather production can be as high as 15 to 25%.

Insulation and Heat Loss

A bird's thermal relationship with its environment is central to its survival. Endothermia is part of a dynamic relationship between internal heat production and external heat loss to the environment. The rate of heat loss from the body is proportional to the absolute difference between body temperature and the environmental temperature, and the rate of heat transfer across the surface layers.

Contour feathers in the plumage contribute to a bird's insulation, but the true down feathers underneath the contour feathers are of primary importance. Insulation increases with the amount of plumage. Birds adjust the position of their feathers to enhance either heat loss or heat conservation. Fluffing the feathers in response to cold creates more air pockets and increases the insulation value of the plumage. Birds continuously adjust the position of their feathers in relation to air (room) temperature. Holding the wings out from the body and extreme elevation of the back (scapular) feathers enhance heat loss by exposing the bare apterial skin to convection. Metabolism and heat production of dark-plumaged birds decrease as a result of exposure to strong radiant energy (heat lamp), but those of white-plumaged birds do not, unless the bird erects its feathers and orients its body so that the warmth (radiation) touches its skin directly.

The net thermal effect of plumage, however, is influenced by wind (draft, ventilation). Metabolism may need to increase to compensate for such heat loss due to convection, even when the air temperature is in the thermoneutral zone. Small birds are particularly vulnerable to convective heat loss because they have more surface area relative to mass than do large birds.[4] These cooling effects of "wind" are most pronounced on black feathers, which concentrate radiant heat near the surface of the plumage and can increase the amount of heat a bird's body absorbs from the environment when there is no "breeze."

The potential for excessive heat loss by evaporative cooling is highest in small individuals with more heat-losing surface area relative to mass, and in poorly feathered birds and unfeathered babies with no plumage insulation at all. They, therefore, favor most hot humid climates, like a warm room, 25° to 30°C, with high humidity (greater than 70%). Conversely, cool, dry air is favored by larger, well-plumaged, white or light-colored birds (like white swans and gulls) with reduced surface areas that conserve heat. Large body sizes also increase potential energy stores and ability to fast.

Small or poorly feathered birds, therefore, quickly

go into a negative metabolic balance that depletes their energy stores, especially when they are under disease or stressful states, and they often need additional nutritional support even though they are still eating.

Temperature Regulation

The model of endothermia, developed by Scholander and coworkers,[5] is one of the foundations of avian thermobiology. In the thermoneutral zone, the amount of oxygen consumed by resting birds does not change with the temperature. At lower and higher temperatures outside the thermoneutral zone, temperature regulation requires increases in metabolism (Fig. 39A–1). This model is oversimplified, but it provides the basis for an orderly consideration of the processes that are involved in the control of body temperature. As we have seen, most birds do not have to change their rates of heat production to maintain an average body temperature of 40°C in the thermoneutral zone. Birds can control the rates of heat loss by changing feather positions, by varying rates of return of venous blood flow from the skin, by manipulating blood circulation in their feet, and by changing the exposure of their extremities, all of which require little direct energy expenditure.

Responses to Cold Stress

A cooling bird first tenses its muscles and begins to shiver, a response that increases oxygen consumption. The pectoral muscles are the major source of heat production by shivering, supplemented by leg muscles in some species.

The lower critical temperature of large birds is lower than that of small birds. In absence of special adaptations, therefore, small birds are more sensitive to cold than are large birds; they shiver at a higher temperature. Birds also select microclimates that reduce their rate of heat loss. Roosting in holes or protected sites such as evergreen trees greatly reduces heat loss, which is especially important during cold winters for small passerine birds. Natural physical adjustment to seasonal changes in temperature, acclimatization, reduces on a daily basis the costs of thermoregulation. This process may go

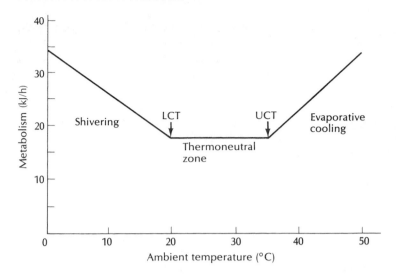

Scholander's model of endothermy. Metabolism increases below the lower critical temperature (LCT), primarily as a result of shivering heat production. Metabolism increases above the upper critical temperature (UCT) because of active loss of heat through panting and evaporative cooling as well as the direct effects of higher temperatures on cellular functions. Metabolism is relatively insensitive to changing ambient temperature in the zone of thermoneutrality. (From Gill FB: Ornithology, ed 2. New York, WH Freeman and Company, 1995, p 131.)

over a period of weeks or months. However, in nature, ambient temperatures decrease and metabolic costs increase with distance from the equator. For example, a house sparrow in Panama expends 58 to 67 KJ per day in summer and winter, whereas house sparrows in Manitoba expend 117 KJ in summer and 151 KJ per day in winter, twice as much as the Panamanian counterparts.

Hypothermia and Torpor

As an energy-saving measure, avian body temperatures fluctuate a few degrees during the day and may drop 2° to 3°C at night (hypothermia). Some small birds can lower their body temperature even further and enter a state of torpor in which they are unresponsive to most stimuli and incapable of normal activity. The oxygen consumption of a hummingbird drops by 75% when it allows its body temperature to drop 10°C. They can even allow their nighttime body temperature to drop 20° to 32°C below normal.

Warming up is the main difficulty with hypothermia, especially with deep torpor. Birds waking from torpor begin to show good muscular coordination at 26° to 27°C, but require body temperatures of at least 34° to 35°C for normal activity. A small hummingbird requires about 1 hour to arouse from torpor at 20°C, but a medium-sized bird such as an American kestrel would require 12 hours to warm up from a hypothermic body temperature of 20°C.[4]

Responses to Heat Stress

Birds generally respond to externally imposed heat loads through avoidance behaviors, physiologic defenses, and controlled elevation of body temperature (hyperthermia). Simple heat avoidance behaviors include reduced activity at midday, seeking shade, bathing, or thermal soaring to cooler air. Desert-adapted birds also tend to have low metabolic rates, which foster lower rates of water turnover and lower food requirements.[6]

Panting increases evaporative cooling from the upper respiratory tract and is a highly effective method of heat loss. Birds typically ventilate faster during heat stress, when body temperatures rise from 41° to 44°C and above. Not only does it increase metabolism, but also it will induce a shift in blood acidity (carbon dioxide [CO_2] loss, pH increase). It also presents additional risk in the form of water loss (dehydration).

To supplement panting when they are hot, some birds rapidly vibrate the hyoid muscles and bones in their throats (gular fluttering); this action increases the rate of heat loss through evaporation of water from the mouth lining and upper throat.

Birds do not have sweat glands but evaporate water directly through the skin. Evaporative water loss through the skin is especially well developed in certain pigeons and doves and involves dilatation of blood vessels in the skin of the neck.[7]

When necessary, birds, especially large-footed water birds such as herons and gulls, can lose most of their metabolic heat through their feet. Alternatively, when heat conservation is important, they can control flow by blood shunting to reduce this loss by more than 90%. In addition, a mechanism called "countercurrent heat exchange" conserves body heat at low air temperatures.

Heat produced during flight could cause lethal increases in body temperature. The body temperature of budgerigars flying at 35 km per hour (in 37°C air) rises to 44°C; they store 13% of the heat they produce. However, flight itself increases convective heat loss. The airstream compresses the plumage to the skin, and extension of the wings exposes the thinly feathered ventral base of the wing. As a result, the rate of heat loss by flying parakeets increases to 3.1 times the resting value at 20°C. Direct nonevaporative heat loss from these bare skin areas account for 20% of a bird's total heat loss at low and medium temperature.

PHYSIOLOGY OF WATER ECONOMY

Satisfying daily energy requirements is only one side of the physiologic coin.[4] Water economy is equally important, especially in arid environments. Enhanced evaporative heat loss is essential to avoid heat stress during strenuous activity. Water is used and replaced at high rates as a result of high evaporative water losses and the limited capacity of birds for concentrating electrolytes in the urine. Birds replace water from several sources.

Water present in food satisfies the fluid needs of many birds, particularly nectar-eating or fruit-eating birds and meat-eating raptors. Likewise, insect-eating birds get most of the water they need from the body fluids of consumed insects; unlike seed-eating birds, they rarely visit water supplies. Because they specialize in dry foods, seed-eating birds experience the greatest need for "free" water.

Metabolic water, which is produced as a byproduct of the oxidation of organic compounds containing hydrogen molecules, supplements ingested water. The metabolism of 1 g of fat yields 1.07 g of water; 1 g of carbohydrate or protein produces about 0.56 and 0.40 g of water, respectively.[4] Small birds (those weighing less than 40 g) can replace less of their evaporative water loss with metabolic water than can large birds,[8] but certain exceptional seed-eating birds, primarily small desert passerines

such as zebra finches, can survive, drinking not a drop, on a diet of air-dried seeds containing less than 10% water, which they supplement with metabolic water.

Much water potentially lost by evaporation is conserved by countercurrent cooling in the nasal and respiratory passages, a general function of the nares and pharynx of small birds. The respiratory passages are cooled by the evaporation of water from the nasal passages during inhalation. During exhalation, the warm, humid air from the lungs comes in contact with the cool respiratory passage, causing water vapor to condense on the nasal passages before the air is finally exhaled. The condensed water then evaporates and is recovered by the cool, dry air that is inhaled when the bird takes its next breath. This recovery system reduces evaporative water losses, especially at colder ambient temperatures, to levels closer to that replaced by metabolic water production.

For the role of the kidneys in the water metabolism see also Chapter 36, Urogenital Disorders.

BASIC PRINCIPLES OF PHARMACOTHERAPY

Medicating birds is accomplished by the same methods of administration used in mammals, but with several special considerations.[3] In pet avian medicine, many dosage regimens have been designed largely on an empirical basis. However, as the knowledge of drug disposition and metabolism in various avian species expands, it is increasingly evident that differences exist in dosage, dosage interval, and organ distribution, not only between birds and mammals but between individual avian species.[9] It is not possible to speak of "the pet bird," in view of the large number of totally different species. It is clear that, except for poultry, there is almost no drug formulation available that has been designed for pet birds.

Optimal use of drugs, including the treatment of infectious diseases, depends on diagnosis, sensitivity to the drug, potential toxicity, pharmacokinetics and pharmacodynamics of the drug, husbandry practices, anatomic and physiologic differences between the species, and many other considerations. Furthermore, it should be realized that the pharmacokinetics of drugs can be substantially changed by disease, especially when organs that play a major role in the absorption, biotransformation, and excretion of drugs (e.g., intestine, liver, and kidney) are involved. This becomes especially important when the excretion of drugs with low therapeutic index is impaired. Another important point is that it is not only the plasma (blood) concentration that is clinically relevant but especially the concentration at the site of action.

The relationship between bacterial identification and the need for antibiotic therapy is a tenuous one. The identification and isolation of potential bacterial pathogens is not a "green light" for the recommendation of antibiotic administration. Rather, it should act as a signal that further consideration is necessary to reach a therapeutic plan if it is deemed necessary.[10] In addition, the finding of coccidia in a fecal sample does not alone signal need for anticoccidial therapy. The clinical evaluation of the patient should support the laboratory findings.

Environmental evaluation and manipulation coupled with good hygiene, husbandry, and nutrition should always be considered as part of a therapeutic plan to aid in correcting a potential infectious problem.[11]

SENSITIVITY TESTS AND INTERPRETATION

Whether to begin antibiotic therapy before culture and sensitivity test results are available depends on the clinical situation (see also Chapter 18, Bacteriology). Some antibiotics, such as chloramphenicol, chlortetracycline, and doxycycline, are known to suppress the immune system and may actually make the situation worse when a fungal infection rather than a bacterial infection is present. However, birds are often critically ill when they suffer from bacterial infections, and postponing antibiotic therapy until culture results are available could be fatal. When appropriate samples are taken before treatment is started, however, this may help the practitioner to correct the therapy when remission of clinical signs does not occur.[2]

Under optimal conditions the sensitivity test is important in selecting antimicrobial therapy. It is becoming more obvious that the breakpoints between sensitive and insensitive in avian medicine may be different from the accepted standard in human and mammalian medicine. This may occur because the attainable blood levels for many drugs might be lower in birds than in mammals because of short elimination half-lives, different bioavailability, and different administration routes.[12, 13]

Therefore, if a test indicates that an organism is susceptible, the treatment may only be successful if drug concentrations similar to those in humans are achieved. The sensitivity of the microorganism in avian medicine ideally should be reported as a minimum inhibiting concentration (MIC) in a broth dilution technique. When the pharmacokinetics of the drug of choice are known (especially the concentration at the site of action) effective therapy can be expected.

Even when the drugs are reported as sensitive in vitro, treatment failure may occur. Reasons include inappropriate drugs, failure to reach the effective MIC in blood or tissues, inadequate treatment intervals or length, compromised tissues, inadequate host immune system, and persistent exposure to environmental sources of the organism. If no clinical response is seen within 48 hours, a change to an antibiotic from another group should be considered,[2] and the diagnosis and therapeutic approach should be reevaluated.

ROUTE OF ADMINISTRATION

The medication of birds may be accomplished either by individual bolus dosing or by treating on an individual or flock basis by mixing with feed or drinking water. Although the desired formulation of drugs for avian species is often dictated by the most practical or economical method of administration, the route of administration is often limited by the drug formulation available. In general, medicated food and drinking water are traditionally favored routes for poultry but seldom achieve therapeutic drug concentrations in companion and aviary birds. Most serious microbial infections must be treated by the direct oral or a parenteral route.[13]

Factors influencing the route of administration and dosage regimen in pet birds are[3, 13]:

- Severity of the disease or infection
- Flock versus individual treatment
- Tame or domesticated versus wild birds
- Large versus tiny birds
- Seed-eating versus meat(fish)-eating birds

- So-called food specialists
- Anatomic differences
- Behavioral or environmental differences
- Availability of drug formulations
- Frequency of administration
- Ability of the owner to complete the treatment regimen
- Economics (and registration demands)

These factors not only influence the choice of the route of administration but also limit the utility of the drugs available.

DOSE EXTRAPOLATION

The most common dose regimens for pet birds based on information available from empirical and experimental data are given in the Formulary (Chapter 39B).

For other drugs or other species the dosage must be extrapolated from available data. Although species are sometimes considered to be similar in their metabolism of drugs, this belief may lead either to inadequate therapy or to toxicity. Therefore, when this information is not available, extrapolation is best based on metabolic extrapolation (allometric scaling). Allometric scaling is a method that can be used to predict dosages of pharmaceuticals for nontraditional animals.[14] Basically, the metabolic rate rather than body weight is used for dose estimation. Allometric scaling allows translation of a dosage from mg/kg to mg/kcal units.

As we have seen above, the metabolic rate is more closely related to body surface area than to body mass. Indeed, half-life of a drug that is metabolized and eliminated by the body decreases as the metabolic rate increases. The basal metabolic rate is sometimes also called the minimum energy cost (MEC) in kilocalories utilized per day and may be calculated from the formula

$$MEC = K \times W^{0.75}$$

Another way of expressing the metabolic rate is to divide the BMR by the body weight to obtain the specific MEC (SMEC) in units of kcal/kg/day. The allometric scaling equation is then

$$SMEC = K \times W^{0.75}/W$$

where K is the constant equal to the kilocalories used in 1 day by a hypothetical 1-kg animal in resting state, determined for different taxonomic groups, and W is the weight (mass) in kg.[14]

The BMR, however, in birds (K = 78) does not differ significantly from mammals (K = 70) as a class, with exception for Passeriformes (K = 129). Therefore, differences found in pharmacokinetics between endothermic animals are often predominantly related to differences in body surface area or metabolic weight and sometimes to differences in metabolic pathways.

The fate of a drug in the body (protein binding, volume of distribution, biotransformation, and excretion) can differ between species (sometimes strains of a species), because the relationship between transformation and excretion is determined by BMR and heredity (different metabolic pathways or metabolites). In general, there is little variation among species in the manner by which polar compounds (like gentamicin) are excreted. This is in contrast to the wide interspecies variations and unpredictability associated with biotransformation of extensively metabolized drugs (like chloramphenicol and sulfonamides).

Allometric scaling can be used to help tailor drug dosages to varied body size; however, it does not take into account variations in metabolic pathways for drugs between species. However, these limitations are mostly valid also for the direct extrapolation. Consequently, when enough information is available, the therapeutic regimens should be adapted for each species.

COMPARATIVE ANATOMY IN RELATION TO DRUG ADMINISTRATION

The oral route is often used for administration of drugs to avian species. When the drug preparation is a suspension, capsule, or tablet, release from the dosage form is frequently the rate-limiting step in the overall absorption process. Because of marked differences in the anatomy of the digestive system of birds, variations can be expected in both rate and extent of drug absorption from an oral formulation.[3] Availability and absorption are influenced by the crop flora, crop pH, gizzard function and morphology, the presence of grit, intestinal function, the presence of a functional ceca, and an indigenous microflora.

The differences between birds and mammals in their response to nebulization are the result of the unique anatomy and physiology of the avian respiratory system. Anatomic differences in lung structure (neo- and paleopulmo) and the lack of physical activity of the sick bird during treatment, even under optimal technical conditions, reduce drugs' access to only 20% of the lung tissue in many bird species. The cranial air sacs are not reached at all. At rest there is no air exchange in most of the respiratory tract.[15] Nevertheless, therapeutic levels in the lungs and air sacs are reported after nebulization in several birds.[16, 17] To establish local drug levels in the lungs and air sacs, the particles or drops should be between 1 and 3 μm. In chickens, aerosolized particles between 3 and 7 μm are generally deposited on the mucosal surface of the nasal cavity and trachea.[18] The primary benefit of nebulization is to humidify the air and locally treat respiratory tract infections. Nebulization is an excellent method to prevent dehydration of a patient, when respiratory distress increases evaporative water loss in a heated hospitalization cage.

Local therapeutic levels of drugs in the respiratory tract (e.g., amphotericin B) can be attained by intratracheal application or using an air sac tube.[1]

METHODS OF DRUG ADMINISTRATION

Flock Versus Individual Treatment

Pet and zoo birds are often kept in flocks, breeding colonies, or large numbers of breeding pairs confined to separate flight pens (e.g., backyard poultry, pigeons, canaries and other finches, budgerigars, parakeets and, more recently, many parrot species). Many pet birds are housed individually or in pairs in households (e.g., canary, budgerigar, cockatiel, parrot, mynah bird, Turkish dove). The approach to medication depends on the situation presented for treatment.

Flock treatment regimens for poultry have been fairly extensively researched and are often, but not always, applicable when treating flocks of pigeons or pet birds.[19] When dealing with individual birds the drug administration techniques differ from those commonly used in individual mammals. Techniques differ when dealing with the individual tame bird or wild bird, a large flock of recently imported

birds, a breeding flock, or a hand-feeding baby bird. Because many drugs are rapidly eliminated in birds, the maintenance of therapeutic levels requires frequent dosing, which necessitates excessive handling of the birds. Individual handling and physical restraint are stressful and must be minimized. The value of frequent administration of drugs must then be weighed against the stress caused by handling.

Individual Oral Dosage Forms

Tablets are not popular for birds because the administration can be both time-consuming and uncertain. In addition, tablets available for humans or mammals contain too much drug. Administering part of a tablet makes the dose uncertain. Many birds have a crop that forms a storage organ. The unpredictable emptying time of the crop, the lack of a large volume of fluid, and the relative high pH make the crop incomparable to the mammalian stomach. Administration in an empty crop improves the uniformity of the pharmacokinetics. The problems can be overcome by grinding the tablet, making a suspension, and feeding it by gavage.

Several antiparasitic drugs (carnidazole, clazuril, levamisole, and praziquantel) are marketed in tablet form for pigeons. Those drugs need to be given only once to be effective, and the onset of activity after administration is less important. Most of these tablets do not need to be administered in an empty crop and do not disintegrate before arriving in the gizzard, resulting in a bolus delivery.

Capsules are a good alternative to tablets. They are preferably administered into an empty crop. Capsules are especially useful for the treatment of individual pigeons and chickens. In avian medicine the capsule is used also as a container for drugs to be applied to the food or drinking water. It allows an exact measure for medication of a small volume of water.

Solutions and suspensions are seldom used on a flock basis for direct administration to birds. A disadvantage of all liquid drug forms is that the administration may result in regurgitation or inhalation, and either some of the dose may be lost or aspiration pneumonia may occur. These preparations can be mixed with food and administered by gavage, especially in hand-fed baby birds or sick birds requiring fluids and nutrients.

In individual birds (like parrots) the addition of drugs to a favorite food increases the chance of acceptance. Oral suspensions, ground tablets, or the contents of capsules may be applied to fruits, yogurt, peanut butter, sandwiches, fresh corn, cooked sweet potatoes, monkey biscuits, or other relished items.

Parenteral Dosage Forms

Parenteral administration is the most exact and effective method for administering drugs to pet birds. This route is primarily used in individual birds that are difficult to handle and in critically ill birds. An exception to this is the treatment of chlamydiosis with doxycycline or long-acting oxytetracycline. The parenteral preparations are most commonly administered intramuscularly (IM) in the pectoral or leg muscles. The venous plexus, which lies between the superficial and deep pectoral muscle, should not be punctured. A disadvantage is the relatively large volume that may have to be injected. Therefore, individual birds should be carefully weighed and appropriate dilutions and syringes should be used to enable accurate dosing. Repeated injections in the same side of the breast or the use of irritating drugs intramuscularly may result in muscle necrosis or atrophy. Intramuscular injection of irritating formulations increases the activity of creatine phosphokinase (CK), alanine-aminotransferase (ASAT), and aspartate-aminotransferase (ALAT). Drugs administered in the posterior pectoral muscle or legs may pass through the renal portal system prior to entering the general circulation. Sympathetic stimulation tends to open the valves in the renal portal system, resulting in a direct flow of the blood from the caudal part of the bird to the vena cava caudalis.[20]

The subcutaneous route in the neck region or the groin is often a preferable alternative, but because of minimal amounts of dermis and the low elasticity of the skin, part of the fluid may flow out. Irritating drugs may cause skin necrosis and ulceration.

Air spaces may be effectively reached by intratracheal or air sac injections. Joints and sinuses are other sites in which direct injection of drugs may be useful.

Intravenous injections should be reserved for emergencies and one-time drug administration. Veins may also be needed for blood withdrawal for diagnostic tests. If repeated drug administration is required, the intraosseous route allows stable access to the intravascular space.[13]

Topical Medications

Topical medications include skin application, eye drops and ointments, nasal flushes, infraorbital sinus injections, and intratracheal and intra air sac administration.

External applications should be used carefully and sparingly because they can mat the feathers. These drugs can be toxic if ingested while the bird preens

Medication in Feed or Water

The major methods of administering drugs to poultry and other birds are via feed and water. This is largely based on convenience and the difficulties associated with individual administration to large numbers of birds. For most drugs, however, water-administered medication is unreliable in psittacines and pigeons and should not be used.

Medication in feed is a reliable way of medicating pet birds, as long as the birds are still eating normally. The total daily intake of drug mixed with food should be equal to the desired daily dose calculated on an individual basis. However, the interactions between a drug and food cannot be entirely predicted, and the dosage forms need to be evaluated. The only proof of bioavailability is pharmacokinetic study in various species.

Most pet birds are seed-eating (dehusking their seeds) or grain-eating birds; neither type of food is suitable for mixing homogeneously. In those cases the medication needs to be given through mashes, pellets, and impregnated seeds. Unfortunately, some species are very reluctant to accept mashed feed or pellets, if unaccustomed to them.

Because of the negative influence of calcium and magnesium on the bioavailability of tetracyclines, grit-mineral administration has to be discontinued during treatment. During egg production and breeding, this can result in soft-shelled eggs and rickets in the chicks.

A practical method of adding drugs to a grain mixture is by coating a moist food, which is then added to the mixture. This method is often used for pigeons and backyard poultry. Yogurt as a base for administering drugs is often readily accepted by psittacines.

In contrast to the use of tablets, the storage of medicated food in the crop of many birds is an advantage. From this reservoir there is a continuous delivery of drug. Pharmacologically, food medication can simulate a slow-release system, which provides decreased fluctuations in drug concentrations in tissues.

Drug concentrations for medicated feed cannot be extrapolated from one diet to another without knowing the energy content and palatability of the diets.[13] Both factors influence feed intake.

Medication in water is controversial in pet avian medicine but is often the only practical means of drug administration. It is the least stressful method for medicating birds, especially with drugs that are palatable. Theoretically, the bird frequently self-doses during the day. However, studies in parrots, pigeons, and chickens showed that therapeutic blood levels for many drugs were not attained via the drinking water, because of factors such as unacceptance, poor solubility, and day length. As a guide, the volume of water consumed by the bird needs to contain the calculated daily dose in milligrams per kilogram. Many drugs are stable for only a short time in water, which necessitates frequent changes.

Although therapeutic blood levels may not be achieved with many drugs, levels in the intestine may be sufficient to control enteric infections. The use of medicated water can be valuable for reducing the spread of diseases that have arisen through contaminated water.

Medicated water may be rejected because of color or taste. Xerophilic birds, that are adapted to dry and hot climates (e.g., budgerigars, zebra finches, and Australian parakeets) may not consume any water containing dissolved medications. In breeding flocks, the male bird may consume large amounts of water to feed the female in the nest, resulting in toxic drug levels in the male.

References

1. Quesenberry KE, Hillyer EV: Supportive care and emergency therapy. In Ritchie BW, Harrison GJ, Harrison LR (eds): Avian Medicine: Principles and Application. Lake Worth, FL, Wingers Publishing, 1994, pp 382–416.
2. Lumeij JT: Psittacine antimicrobial therapy. In Antimicrobial Therapy in Caged and Exotic Pets. Int Sympos, Trenton, NJ, Vet Learn Serv, 1995, pp 38–48.
3. Dorrestein GM: Antimicrobial drug use in pet birds. In Prescott JF, Baggot JD (eds): Antimicrobial Therapy in Veterinary Medicine, ed 2. Ames, Iowa State University Press, 1993, pp 490–506.
4. Gill FB: Ornithology, ed 2. New York, WH Freeman and Company, 1995.
5. Scholander PF, Hock R, Walters V, et al: Heat regulation in some arctic and tropical mammals and birds. Biol Bull Woods Hole Mass 99:237–258, 1950.
6. Dawson WR: Physiological studies of desert birds: Present and future considerations. J Aid Environ 7:133–155, 1984.
7. Marder J, Arieli Y, Ben-Asher J: Defendence strategies against environmental heat stress in birds. Isr J Zool 36:61–75, 1989.
8. Bartholomew GA: Body temperature and energy metabolism. In Gordon MS (ed): Animal Physiology: Principles and Adaptations, ed 4. New York, Macmillan, 1982, pp 333–406.
9. Quesenberry KE: Avian antimicrobial therapeutics. In Jacobson ER, Kollias GV (eds): Exotic Animals. New York, Churchill Livingstone, 1988, pp 177–207.
10. Worell AB: Pediatric bacterial diseases. Semin Avian Exotic Pet Med 2:116–124, 1993.
11. Fudge AM, Reavill DR, Rosskopf WJ: Clincal aspects of avian Pseudomonas infections: A retrospective study. Proc Assoc Avian Vet, New Orleans, 1992, pp 141–155.
12. Dorrestein GM: Infectious diseases and their therapy in Passeriformes. In Antimicrobial Therapy in Caged and Exotic Pets. Int Sympos, Trenton, NJ, Vet Learn Serv, 1995, pp 11–27.
13. Flammer K: Antimicrobial therapy. In Ritchie BW, Harrison GJ, Harrison LR (eds): Avian Medicine: Principles and Application. Lake Worth, FL, Wingers Publishing, 1994, pp 434–456.
14. Sedgwick CJ, Pokras MA: Extrapolating rational drug doses and treatment periods by allometric scaling. Proc 55th Annual Meeting Am Anim Hosp Assoc, 1988, pp 156–157.
15. Duncker H-R: The air sac system of birds. A contribution to the functional anatomy of the respiratory apparatus. Ergebnisse der Anatomie und Entwickelungsgeschichte 45, 1971.
16. Locke D, Bush M: Tylosine aerosol therapy in quail and pigeons. J Zoo Anim Med 15:67, 1984.
17. Spink RR: Aerosol therapy. In Harrison GJ, Harrison LR (eds): Clinical Avian Medicine and Surgery. Philadelphia, WB Saunders, 1986, pp 376–379.
18. Hayter RB, Besch EL: Airborne-particle deposition in the respiratory tract of chickens. Poultry Sci 53:1507, 1974.
19. Clubb SL: Therapeutics, individual and flock treatment regimens. In Harrison GJ, Harrison LR (eds): Clinical Avian Medicine and Surgery. Philadelphia, WB Saunders, 1986, pp 327–355.
20. Skadhauge E: Osmoregulation in birds. Berlin, Springer Verlag, 1981.

Thomas N. Tully, Jr.

39B

Formulary

Numerous articles and book chapters have been published on avian therapeutics and drug dosages.[1-4] Many published therapeutic protocols list a wide range of drug dosages to be administered to the avian patient. Therapeutic protocols for dogs, cats, and common domesticated farm animals are usually based upon pharmacologic studies. But unlike veterinarians who treat domestic animals, the avian practitioner must care for many different species. Drugs that perform well in certain avian species may be inappropriate or even toxic in others. In this chapter the accumulated data from published avian formularies are presented in a straightforward, concise form that will enable the practitioner to make knowledgeable judgements when treating an ill patient.

Treatment regimens are most successful when a specific diagnosis has been made. An informed client and a complete understanding of disease processes allow the veterinarian to make the correct prognosis and therapeutic choices.

The dosages in this chapter are taken from published reports and pharmacokinetic studies. There are separate sections on pigeon and ratite therapeutics and emergency avian medications. Few species-specific pharmacodynamic studies have been performed, therefore dosages are often based on experience. All information on side effects and treatment protocol should be expressed to the client to prevent misunderstandings or complications.

FLUID AND NUTRITIONAL THERAPEUTICS

Stabilizing the condition of an ill avian patient is critical. Before diagnostic tests or treatments are initiated, the bird's health status should be evaluated. The hydration status and condition of the bird determine if fluid therapy and nutritional supplementation are needed.

EVALUATION OF AVIAN HYDRATION STATUS[6]

1. Skin elasticity (featherless areas)
2. Ocular pressure
3. Corneal hydration
4. Packed cell volume
5. Plasma protein

In some cases one or more of the parameters may not be good indicators of hydration status (i.e., young bird packed cell volume), but in general these parameters should be followed. Intravenous (IV) fluid therapy is the fastest way to rehydrate the critically ill patient, with subcutaneous and oral routes offering alternative, slower distribution.[6]

Avian Fluid Replacement

1. Maintenance is 50 ml/kg/day (neonates require 2–3 times the maintenance fluid of adults)[7]

2. Dehydration deficit is estimated normal weight × percent dehydration

The deficit should be replaced over a 48-hour period in bolus dosages, divided into four doses daily. Maintenance fluid levels should be maintained until the bird is drinking and eating on its own for 2 to 3 days.[6]

VOLUMES OF IV BOLUS FLUIDS[6]

Canary	1 ml
Budgerigar	1–2 ml
Cockatiel	2–3 ml
Conure	4–6 ml
Amazon	8–10 ml
Macaw	15–25 ml

Nutritional supplementation is important for birds that are anorexic and in poor physical condition. Hospitalized birds may be anorexic for psychological reasons (stress, fever), even if they are not affected by illness. Care must be taken to evaluate and maintain the patient's hydration status if hyperosmolar formulas are fed. All supplements must be highly nutritious, readily digested and absorbed.

FEEDING VOLUME CALCULATIONS[8]

A. Basal metabolic rate (BMR) = K ($W^{0.75}$)

   K = kilocalories in a 24-hour period

      K = 78 psittacines

      K = 129 passerines

   W = weight of bird in kilograms

B. Calculation for nutritional maintenance (1.5 × BMR = maintenance/day) in kcal/day

C. Trauma nutritional adjustment (1.2 × maintenance) = kcal/day

D. Milliliters of formula per day

   Kcal required/day ÷ kcal/ml of formula = ml of formula required

TUBE FEEDING VOLUMES[6]

Canary	0.5–1 ml
Budgerigar	1.3 ml
Cockatiel	3–8 ml
Conure	10–12 ml
Amazon	15–20 ml
Macaw	20–40 ml

ANTIMICROBIAL THERAPY

Antibiotics may be the most abused or most useful class of drugs available to the veterinary practitioner. The use of over-the-counter antibiotic treatments can perpetuate illness and delay appropriate diagnosis and treatment. Making the proper diagnosis and antibiotic selection (through culture and sensitivity testing) and using the appropriate treatment protocol increase the success rate of avian practitioners treating bacterial infections. The source of the bacterial contamination should be identified and removed.

ANTIMICROBIAL DRUG MECHANISMS OF ACTIONS[9]

Mechanism	Drug
A. Target DNA gyrase	Quinolones
B. Inhibition of cell wall synthesis	Cephalosporins, penicillins
C. Alteration of cell wall permeability	Polymyxin B
D. Reversible inhibition of ribosomal function	Chloramphenicol Clindamycin Macrolides Lincomycin Tetracyclines
E. Irreversible inhibition of ribosomal function	Aminoglycosides
F. Antimetabolites	Sulfonamides Trimethoprim

Antimicrobial Drug Classification[9]

Bactericidal	**Bacteriostatic**
Aminoglycosides	Chloramphenicol
Cephalosporins	Clindamycin
Penicillins	Erythromycin
Polymyxins	Lincomycin
Quinolones	Macrolides
	Sulfonamides (primarily bacteriostatic, although bacteriocidal concentration may be reached in urine)
	Tetracyclines (sometimes bacteriocidal)

With any therapeutic protocol, handling of birds should be minimized to reduce stress. Flock treatment with water- or food-based medication *may* work, but extremely ill birds may not ingest enough medication to maintain therapeutic blood levels. If medications are administered via drinking water, fruits and vegetables that have high water content should be limited to prevent hydration through foodstuffs.[1]

Antifungal Therapy

Some of the most frustrating avian infections to treat and diagnose are fungal diseases. Chronic fungal diseases involving *Aspergillosis* species and/or *Candida albicans* are often the result of immunosuppression and may include bacterial infections. If vascular supply to affected tissue is reduced by tissue necrosis, achieving therapeutic tissue levels of antifungal agents is unlikely, thereby decreasing treatment success.[10] Treatment of fungal infections in companion birds usually is prolonged, expensive, and in the past was often ineffective.[11] The general health status of a patient on antifungal therapy must be monitored as much as possible because of the potential side effects of these drugs.

ANTIPARASITIC DRUG MECHANISMS OF ACTIONS[12]

A. Fumarate reductase inhibitors — Fenbendazole
Thiabendazole
Cambendazole
Mebendazole
Oxfendazole

B. Cause paralysis by stimulating cholinergic receptors — Levamisole

C. Gamma aminobutyric acid-interfering drugs — Ivermectin

D. Adenosine triphosphate synthesis blockers — Niclosamide
Rafoxanide

E. Alteration of parasite defense mechanism — Praziquantel

F. Neuromuscular blocking agent — Piperazine

G. Depolarizing neuromuscular blocking agents — Pyrantel tartrate
Pyrantel pamoate

H. Damage DNA strands — Carnidazole
Ronidazole
Metronidazole
Dimetridazole
Ipronidazole tinidazole

I. Competitive antagonism against PABA, resulting in inhibition of folic acid synthesis — Sulfonamides used as coccidial medication

Because of the misuse of antiparasitic and antiprotozoal drugs, especially in poultry species, many efficacious drugs have been removed from the market. Only proper usage under veterinary supervision will keep many of the antiparasitic drugs we now have available in the years to come. Most drug dosages were developed for poultry species, and thus close observation of the patient during therapy and rechecking of the stool to determine if the bird is free of parasites are important.[12]

Management is as important as drug therapy in the control of parasites. Reduction of vermin and vector contact with the birds, a clean aviary, quarantine, and a post-purchase physical examination are imperative to maintaining an aviary free of parasites.

Acknowledgment

The author thanks Beth Wilson and Dr. Marvene Augustus for patience and technical assistance in preparing this manuscript.

References

1. Flammer K: Antimicrobial therapy. In Ritchie BW, Harrison GJ, Harrison LR (eds): Avian Medicine: Principles and Applications. Lake Worth, FL, Wingers Publishing, 1994, pp 434–456.
2. Ritchie BW, Harrison GJ: Formulary. In Ritchie BW, Harrison GJ, Harrison LR (eds): Avian Medicine: Principles and Appliations. Lake Worth, FL, Wingers Publishing, 1994, pp 457–478.
3. Clubb SL: Special species: Birds. In Johnston DE (ed): The Bristol Veterinary Handbook of Antimicrobial Therapy, ed 2. Evansville, IN, Veterinary Learning Systems Co., 1987, pp 188–199.
4. Bauck L: Therapeutics. Semin Avian Exotic Pet Med 2(1):2–7, 1993.
5. Baggot JD: Principles of Drug Disposition in Domestic Animals. Philadelphia, WB Saunders, 1977.
6. Huff OG: Avian fluid therapy and nutritional therapeutics. Semin Avian Exotic Pet Med 2(1):13–16, 1993.
7. Calnek BW: Disease of Poultry, ed 9. Ames, IA, Iowa State University Press, 1993, pp 49–51.
8. Quesenberry KE: Nutritional support of the avian patient. Proc Assoc Avian Vet, 1989, pp 11–18.
9. Rivieve JE: Basic principles of antibiotic use. In Johnston DE (ed): The Bristol Veterinary Handbook of Antimicrobial Therapy, ed 2. Evansville, IN, Veterinary Learning Systems Co., 1987, pp 9–16.
10. Van Cutsein J: Experimental fungal diseases and treatment. J Assoc Avian Vet 2:15, 1988.
11. Prus SE: Avian antifungal therapy. Semin Avian Exotic Pet Med 2(1):30–32, 1993.
12. Marshall R: Avian anthelmintics and antiprotozoals. Semin Avian Exotic Pet Med 2(1):33–41, 1993.
13. Ritchie BW: Emergency care of avian patients. North Am Vet Conf Proc 8:806–808, 1994.
14. Taylor MT: Avian anesthesia—A clinical update. Scientific Proc First Int Conf Zoo Avian Med, Oahu, Assoc Avian Vet, 1987, pp 519–524.
15. Clubb S: Therapeutics. In Harrison GJ, Harrison LR (eds): Clinical Avian Medicine and Surgery. Philadelphia, WB Saunders, 1986, pp 327–355.
16. Rosskopf WJ: Therapeutic agents for raptors. Assoc Avian Vet Today 1:146, 1987.
17. McDonald S: Summary of medications for use in psittacine birds. J Assoc Avian Vet 3(3):120–127, 1989.
18. Mautino M: Lead intoxication. Proc Assoc Avian Vet, Phoenix, 1990, pp 245–247.
19. Ritchie BW: Avian therapeutics. Proc Assoc Avian Vet, Phoenix, 1990, pp 415–431.
20. Bauck L: Analgesics in avian medicine. Proc Assoc Avian Vet, Phoenix, 1990, pp 239–244.
21. Perelman B: Evaluation of azole antimycotic agents using an experimental model of aspergillosis in turkey poults. Proc Eur Conf Avian Med Surg, 1993, pp 120–126.
22. Hines RS, Sharkey P, Friday RB: Itraconazole treatment of pulmonary, ocular and uropygial aspergillosis and candidiasis in birds. Proc Am Assoc Zoo Vet, Padre Island, TX, 1990, pp 322–326.
23. Okamoto MP, Nakhiro RK, Chin A, et al: Cefepime: A new fourth-generation cephalosporin. Am J Hosp Pharm 51:463–477, 1994.
24. Flammer K: An update on psittacine antimicrobial pharmacokinetics. Proc Assoc Avian Vet, Phoenix, 1990, pp 218–220.
25. Parrot T: New clinical trials using acyclovir. Proc Assoc Avian Vet, Phoenix, 1990, pp 237–238.
26. Bauck L, Hoefer HL: Avian antimicrobial therapy. Semin Avian Exotic Pet Med 2(1):17–22, 1993.
27. Dorrestein GM: Avian chlamydiosis therapy. Semin Avian Exotic Pet Med 2(1):23–29, 1993.

28. Cannon MJ: Parasites. Proc 178 Avian Med, Proceedings of General Conference of Veterinary Science, Sydney, Australia, University of Sydney, 1991, pp 47–53.

29. Dorrestein GM: Diseases of passerines. Proc Assoc Avian Vet, Boulder, CO, 1985, pp 53–71.

30. George JR: Parasitology for Veterinarians. Philadelphia, WB Saunders, 1980.

31. Westerhof I, Lumeij JT: An introduction to avian therapeutics. Proc Second Eur Sympos Assoc Avian Vet, 1989, p 71.

32. Schepkens E: Ivermectin treatment of ascaridiasis and capillariosis in pigeons. Ann Med Vet 129(7):475–485, 1985.

33. Dorrestein GM: Examination, diagnosis and therapy of disease in aviary birds. Proc Sympos Bird Dis, Beerse, Belgium, 1987, pp 123–154.

34. Vanderheyden N: Psittacine papillomas. Proc Assoc Avian Vet, Houston, 1988, p 23.

35. Fudge AM: Avian giardiasis—syndromes, diagnosis and therapy. Proc Assoc Avian Vet, Miami, 1986, pp 119–124.

36. Clubb SL: Sarcocystosis in psittacine birds. In Schubot RM, Clubb KJ, Clubb SL (eds): Psittacine Aviculture. Loxahatchee, FL, Aviculture Breeding and Research Center, 1992, pp 20–24.

37. Greve JH: Parasitic diseases. In Fowler ME (ed): Zoo and Wild Animal Medicine. Philadelphia, WB Saunders, 1978, p 374.

38. Ramsey EC: Trichomoniasis in a flock of budgerigars. Proc Assoc Avian Vet, Phoenix, 1990, pp 308–311.

39. Altman RB: Parasitic diseases of birds. In Kirk RW (ed): Current Veterinary Therapy VI. Philadelphia, WB Saunders, 1966, p 683.

40. Harlin RW: Pigeons. Vet Clin North Am 24(1):157–173, 1994.

41. McGruder ED, Jensen J, Johnson JH: Zoo Dose (2.0). College Station, TX, Wildlife and Exotic Animal Tele Consultants, 1994.

EMERGENCY DRUGS

	Drug	Form	Species	Route	Dosage	Comments
1.	Activated[13] charcoal, kaolin (Toxiban) Vet-A-Mix	Suspension (104 mg/ml activated charcoal and 62.5 mg/ml kaolin)	Most	Oral	0.02–0.08 mg as needed	For absorption of ingested toxins Mix with sodium sulfate to form lead complexes Can be mixed with hemicellulose to function as a bulk laxative
2.	Atropine[14] Butler, Vedco	0.5 mg/ml injectable	Most	IM	0.01–0.02 mg/kg	Not recommended for preanesthetic in avian species Thicker respiratory secretions which may block endotracheal tube Used in organophosphate poisoning Does not dilate pupils in avian species
3.	Avipro[2] Vetark Animal Health	Lactobacillus powder	Psittacines	Oral	4 g/200 ml of water	Used as a supplement in debilitated birds. In drinking water or given orally or by gavage
4.	Bismuth Subsalicylate[2] (Pepto-Bismol)	Oral suspension 1.75% subsalicylate	Most	Oral	2 ml/kg BID	For gastrointestinal irritation May help remove ingested toxins
5.	Blood, whole[13]		Most	Slow IV	5% of recipient's body weight	Use heparin anti-clotting agent For anemia, clotting factor problems
6.	Butorphanol[2, 20] tartrate (Stadol) Bristol	Injectable solution Torbutrol (10 mg/ml) Tablets Torbugesic (1, 5 or 10 mg)	Psittaciformes	IV Oral	3–4 mg/kg	Anti-tussive effects, may control abdominal pain Use with caution in liver-compromised patients
7.	Calcium disodium[17] Versonate calcium EDTA 3M Pharmaceuticals	Injectable solution (200 mg/ml)	Most	IM	35 mg/kg	Chelate lead and zinc May cause renal tubular necrosis and should be discontinued if polyuria/polydipsia occur
8.	Calcium gluconate[15] Vedco Phoenix, Butler	Solution 23 mg/ml injectable solution 5 mg (Ca glycerophosphate and 5 mg Ca lactate/ml)	Most Most Most Most	Water IM, SC IV Feed	1 ml/30 ml of water to effect 5–10 mg/kg BID as needed 50–10 mg/kg slowly to effect 1/8 tsp/kg	For emergency situation nutritional deficiencies, egg binding. May chelate some tetracyclines if given orally
9.	Dexamethasone[17] (Azium) Schering Plough Health	Injectable solution 2 or 4 mg/ml	Most Raptors	IM or IV IM or IV	2–4 mg/kg SID–TID 1 mg/kg	Anti-inflammatory Treatment of shock and endotoxemia from gram-negative bacterial infection May be used as adjunct therapy for treating goiter in budgerigars
10.	Dextrose 50%[15]	Injectable solution	Most	IV	50–100 mg/kg slowly	Hypoglycemia
11.	Diazepam[15] (Valium) Roche	Injectable solution 5%–50 mg/ml 50%–500 mg/ml	Most Psittacines	IV Oral	0.5 mg/kg BID–TID 2.5–4 mg/kg as needed	Anticonvulsants Feather picking (sedation) Analgesia

EMERGENCY DRUGS *Continued*

	Drug	Form	Species	Route	Dosage	Comments
12.	Diethylene triamine penta-acetic acid[18]	Injectable solution	Most	IM	30 mg/kg BID	Lead chelation
13.	Digoxin[2] (Cardoxin) EVSCO	Oral solution Cardoxin 15 mg/ml Lanoxin 0.05 mg/ml	Conures Parakeets	Oral	0.02–0.05 mg/kg SID	Limited avian research
14.	Dimercaprol[13] (Bal) Becton Dickinson	Injectable solution 100 mg/ml	Most	Oral	25–35 mg/kg BID 5 days per week for 3–5 weeks	Painful injections IM Less toxic than calcium EDTA Better at reducing blood lead levels than CaEDTA
15.	Dimercaptosuccinic[13] (DMSA) acid	Injectable solution 100 mg/ml	Most	PO	30–90 mg/kg	Lead chelation
16.	Dinoprostone, PGE[2]	Gel	Psittacines	Topical application into cloaca	0.5 mg	For vaginal sphincter relaxation and egg binding
17.	Doxapram HCL[15] (Dopram) Fort Dodge	Injectable solution 20 mg/ml	Most	IM, IV or SC	5–10 mg/kg once	Respiratory stimulant
18.	D-penicillamine[18] (Cuprimine) Merck (Depen) Wallace	Capsules 125–250 mg Tablets 250 mg	Most	Oral	52 mg/kg BID	Carefully monitor patients Chelating agent Gastrointestinal irritation and blood dyscrasias possible
19.	Epinephrine (1:1000)[16] Webster, Vedco Butler, Phoenix	Injectable solution	Most	IV, Intraosseous IT, IC	0.1 mg/kg	Dilute with 10 parts lactated Ringer's solution Use only in extreme emergencies Easy to overdose
20.	Lactated Ringer's solution[16]	Injectable solution	Most	IV, IM, SC IV, IM, SC	50 ml/kg/day (maintenance dose) + 1/2 fluid deficit first day	Maintenance Dehydration Emergency treatment
			Lovebird	IV, IM, SC	3 ml/IV	Maximum amount to be given over 5–10 minute period
			Cockatiel	IV, IM, SC	5 ml/IV	Maximum amount to be given over 5–10 minute period
			Amazon	IV, IM, SC	25 ml/IV	Maximum amount to be given over 5–10 minute period
			Cockatoo	IV, IM, SC	40 ml/IV	Maximum amount to be given over 5–10 minute period
			Macaw	IV, IM, SC	60 ml/IV	Maximum amount to be given over 5–10 minute period
21.	Mannitol[13] Webster Vedco	Injectable solution 20 mg/ml 180 mg/ml	Most	Slow IV	0.5 mg/kg SID	Reduces intraocular and intracranial pressure
22.	Mineral oil[2]		Most	Oral (by gavage)	6–10 ml/kg as needed	For impaction and foreign body removal
23.	Oxytocin[17] Butler (Lextron) Vedco	20 units/ml	Most	IM	0.025 ml/100 g body wt	For uncomplicated uterine stasis only Used in combination with calcium gluconate for dystocia
24.	2-PAM[13]	Injectable solution	Most	IM	10–100 mg/kg	Antidote for short-term organophosphate toxicities
25.	Phenobarbital[13] Lilly Rugby	Elixir 3 mg/ml Oral solution 4 mg/ml	Most	Oral	1–2 mg/kg BID	May cause gastrointestinal side effects Do not use on patient with gastrointestinal blockage Mild sedative effect
26.	Potassium chloride[19]	Injectable solution	Most	IV	0.1–0.3 mg/kg	May cause cardiac irregularities
27.	Prednisolone[15] (Cort-Sol) Butler	Sodium succinate Tablet 5 mg Injectable	Most	Oral IM or IV	6 mg/kg BID 0.5–1 mg/kg once 2.4 mg/kg	Anti-inflammatory in shock or trauma cases Avoid long-term treatment Mix one 5 mg tablet in 2.6 ml or water for 2 ml suspension
28.	Propranolol[2] (Inderal) Wyeth-Ayerst	Tablet 20, 40, 60, 80 mg Injectable solution 1 mg/ml	Most	IM IV	0.2 mg/kg 0.04 mg/kg	Used in cases of tachycardia Monitor patient carefully for side effects

Table continued on following page

EMERGENCY DRUGS *Continued*

	Drug	Form	Species	Route	Dosage	Comments
29.	Sodium bicarbonate[13]	Solution	Most	IV	1–4 mEq/kg slowly over 15–30 minutes, do not exceed 4 mEq/kg	Indications in severe metabolic acidosis
30.	Sodium sulfate[2] (Golytely) Braintree Laboratories		Large birds	Oral	2 g/kg slowly for 2 days	Do not use in dehydrated patients or with poor gastrointestinal function Osmotic cathartic Indication—to form insoluble complexes in heavy metal poisoning cases within GI tract

AVIAN ANTIMICROBIAL THERAPY

	Drug	Form	Species	Route	Dosage	Comments
1.	Acyclovir[25] (Zovirax) Burroughs Wellcome	IV solution powder 50 mg/ml 200 mg cap 40 mg/ml suspension	Most	PO IM IV	80 mg/kg TID up to 240 mg/kg of food	Muscle necrosis if given IM Phlebitis and neurologic signs if given IV Has been shown to affect sperm development and fetal development in mammals

2.	Amikacin sulfate[13] (Amiglyde) Aveco (Amikin) Bristol Labs	50 mg/ml 240 mg/ml	Most	IV IM	10–15 mg/kg BID	Nephrotoxicity increased with dehydrated patients
						Synergistic effect when used with third generation penicillins
						Risk factors predisposing to aminoglycoside nephrotoxicosis:
						    Prior renal insufficiency
						    Advanced age
						    Increased dose or frequency
						    Hepatic disease
						    Hypovolemia, dehydration
						    Metabolic acidosis
						    Exposure to other nephrotoxins
						    Severe sepsis, endotoxemia

3.	Amoxicillin[5] (Amoxi-drops) (Amoxi-Inject) SmithKline	50 mg/ml Amoxi-drops 250 mg/ml Amoxi-Inject	Most Columbiformes	PO IM	150–174 mg/kg QID 150 mg/kg q4h	Not a very effective drug against common avian pathogens Better gastrointestinal absorption than ampicillin
4.	Ampicillin[3] (Polyflex) Fort Dodge	100 mg/ml	Psittaciformes Psittaciformes Galliformes	PO IM PO	100–200 mg/kg QID 100 mg/kg q4h 250 mg/8 oz of drinking water	Poor gastrointestinal absorption High gastrointestinal specificity based on antibiotic sensitivity of organism
5.	Azithromycin[2] (Zythromax) Pfizer	250 or 500 mg cap	Most	PO	One drop 30 mg/ml suspension to 1 g body weight BID	A 30 mg/ml suspension is made by mixing a 250 mg capsule contents in 8 ml of lactulose Give on empty stomach
6.	Carbenicillin[17] (Geocillin) Roerig	382 mg tablets	Psittaciformes	IM IV Intratracheal	100–200 mg/kg/BID or TID 100–200 mg/kg BID or TID 100 mg/kg SID	Synergistic with aminoglycosides Has been used intratracheal with severe *Pseudomonas* sp. infections once a day Bad taste
7.	Cefepime[23] (Maxipime) Bristol-Myers Squibb	Pending FDA approval	Psittaciformes	IM or IV	———	Penetrates blood-brain barrier A new fourth generation cephalosporin with excellent activity against gram negative organisms in vitro especially the Enterobacteriaceae and *Pseudomonas* sp. possible dosage similar to other 3rd generation cephalosporins
8.	Cefotaxime[24] (Claforan) Hoechst-Roussel	Injectable solution Variable concentration	Most	IM, IV	75–100 mg/kg	Penetrates blood-brain barrier For best results QID therapy is recommended
9.	Cefoxitin[2] (Mefoxitin)	Injectable solution Variable concentration	Most	IM, IV	50–75 mg/kg	———

AVIAN ANTIMICROBIAL THERAPY *Continued*

	Drug	Form	Species	Route	Dosage	Comments
10.	Ceftriaxone[24] (Rocephin) Roche	Injectable solution Variable concentration	Most	IM, IV	75–100 mg/kg QID or every four hours	Can be reconstituted into 10–250 mg/ml concentrations When reconstituted into lower concentrations the Rocephin should be administered IV Cannot be thawed and refrozen
11.	Ceftazidime[17] (Fortaz) Glaxo Pharmaceuticals	Injectable solution Variable concentration	Most	IM, IV	75–100 mg/kg TID, QID	Penetrates blood-brain barrier For best results QID therapy is recommended
12.	Ceftiofur (Naxcel) Upjohn	Injectable solution Variable concentration	Most	IM	50–100 mg/kg QID	Similar treatment regimens to other third generation cephalosporins
13.	Cephalexin[17] (Keflex Pediatric) Suspension Vista	Oral suspension 10–250 mg/ml	Most Cranes Emus	PO PO	50–100 mg/kg QID 35–50 mg/kg QID	Low efficacy for many gram (−) Good for staph dermatitis
14.	Cephalothin[2] (Keflin) Lilly	Injectable solution	Most	IM, IV	100 mg/kg QID	Not absorbed from the GI tract Painful injection
15.	Cephradine[2] (Velosef) Squibb	Suspension 25 or 50 mg/ml	Most	PO	35–50 mg/kg	See Cephalexin
16.	Chloramphenicol[17] Parke-Davis; Fort Dodge	a) Injectable solution 100 mg/ml b) Suspension 30 mg/ml	Psittaciformes Most Galliformes	IV, IM IM PO	50 mg/kg TID or QID 80 mg/kg BID or TID 50 mg/kg TID or QID	May cause blood dyscrasias in humans Caution should be used when prescribing to debilitated patients Oral suspension may be difficult to obtain, but effective in gastroenteritis cases
17.	Chlortetracycline[17] (Aureomycin) American Cyanamid	Feed additive 100 g/lb Tablet 25 mg Powder 200 mg/tsp	Psittaciformes	PO	Treated millet 0.5% Formulated diets 1% 0.25–1.0% for 45 days	Not the most effective drug against *Chlamydia psittaci* infections May have immunosuppressive effect Only approved treatment
18.	Ciprofloxacin[26] (Cipro) Miles	Tablets 250, 500, or 750 mg Injectable solution 200 or 400 mg/ml Ophthalmic solution 3 mg/ml	Psittaciformes Most	PO, IM	15–20 mg/kg BID	Oral suspension made by crushing 500 mg tablet in 10 ml distilled water for 50 mg/ml suspension Very effective broad-spectrum antibiotic
19.	Clindamycin[2] (Antirobe) Upjohn	Suspension 25 mg/ml Capsule 24, 75 or 150 mg	Pigeons	Oral	100 mg/kg SID	Monitor renal and hepatic function during long-term use and for secondary yeast infections—has been noted in mammals Good for bone and joint infections
20.	Doxycycline[27] Pfizer; Henry Schein	Suspension 5 mg/ml	Cockatiels Amazons	Oral	40–50 mg/kg SID or BID	Macaws sensitive to doxycycline and may regurgitate following oral administration Monitor for secondary yeast infection IM use causes muscle necrosis and bleeding with subsequent infections
		Vibramycin monohydrate syrup 10 mg/ml Vibramycin calcium syrup Capsules 100 mg Henry Schein	African greys Cockatoos	Oral	25 mg/kg SID or BID	
		U.S. Injectable solution 10 mg/ml Vibramycin Hyclate Europe, Canada Injectable solution 20 mg/ml Vibravenös	Other Psittaciformes	IV	25 mg/kg SID for 3 days	
			Psittaciformes	IM Vibravenös	(Macaws) 75–100 mg/kg every 5–7 days for 45 days (Other Psittaciformes) 25–50 mg/kg every 5–7 days for 45 days	

Table continued on following page

AVIAN ANTIMICROBIAL THERAPY *Continued*

	Drug	Form	Species	Route	Dosage	Comments
21.	Enrofloxacin[26] (Baytril) Itave/Diamond	Tablet 5.7, 22.7, or 68 mg Injectable solution	Amazons African greys Cockatoos Psittaciformes	IM, PO IM, PO SC, Oral (food)	7.5–15 mg/kg SID/BID 5 mg/kg BID 250–1000 ppm	Injectable solution may be administered orally Poor taste Monitor birds with renal damage or in a debilitated state Very little evidence of joint problems developing in young avian species
22.	Erythromycin[15] (Sanofi) Lextron	Injectable solution 100 or 200 mg/ml Tablets 250 or 500 mg	Most Most Psittaciformes	Oral Powder Nebulize Injectable	500 mg/gallon of drinking water 1 ml/10 ml saline for 15 min TID 10–20 mg/kg BID	May be effective against *Mycoplasma* infections
23.	Ethambutal[2] hydrochloride (Myambutol) Lederle	Tablets 100 or 400 mg	Most	Oral suspension	15 mg/kg BID	For combination treatment of *Mycobacterium avium* infections
24.	Gentamicin[26] (Gentamicin sulfate) Butler, Schering	Injectable 50 mg/ml Ophthalmic solution 3 mg/ml	Most	IM Ophthalmic solution	2.5 mg/kg BID 2–3 drops intranasal TID	Gentamicin should be used parenterally as last resort. Extreme danger to many avian species because of nephrotoxicity
25.	Isoniazid[2] (INH) IBA Pharmaceutical	300 mg tablet	Most	Oral	5–10 mg/kg BID	For avian tuberculosis treatment, side effects include GI problems (regurgitation, anorexia) and neurologic disorders
26.	Lincomycin HCL[3] (Lincocin) Upjohn	Oral solution 50 mg/ml Injectable 100 mg/ml	Budgerigars Amazon parrots Raptors Most	Oral Oral Oral Water	1 drop BID 75 mg/kg BID 100 mg/kg SID 1/8–1/4 tsp/pint of water	Use carefully, side effect of overdose is death. Useful in dermatitis cases
27.	Nitrofurazone[17] (Furacin) SmithKline Beecham	Soluble powder 9.2%– 92 mg/ml Ointment 0.2%–2 mg/ml	Most Lories Lorikeets Mynahs	Water Water	1 tsp/gallon 0.5 tsp/gallon water *Do not mix in food/nectar	Coccidiostat in some birds Toxic if overdosed To fruit and nectar eating birds Soluble powder not available in US
28.	Oxytetracycline[26] (Liquamycin-LA200) Pfizer	Injectable solution 200 mg/ml	Pheasants Raptors Psittaciformes Cockatoos	IM IM IM IM, SC	43 mg/kg SID 16 mg/kg SID 58 mg/kg SID 50–100 mg/kg every 2–3 days	IM administration may cause muscle necrosis
29.	Piperacillin[26] (Pipracil) Lederle	Injectable solution 200 mg/ml	Most Amazon parrots	IM, IV IM	200 mg/kg TID, QID 75–100 mg/kg QID to every 4 hours	Excellent for synergistic use with aminoglycosides against multiresistant *Pseudomonas* infections
30.	Procaine-penicillin G[3] (Ambi-pen) Butler Penicillin benzathine (Benza-pen) SmithKline Beecham	Injectable solution 150,000 units penicillin G procaine and 150,000 units penicillin benzathine	Galliformes Anseriformes	IM	200 mg/kg every 24 hours	Should not be used on birds less than 1 kg in weight because of toxic effects
31.	Rifampin[2] (Rifadin) Marion Merrel Dow	150 or 300 mg capsule	Most	Oral	10–20 mg/kg BID	Used for avian tuberculosis treatment Observe for toxic side effects (In humans, causes urine to be red in color)
32.	Streptomycin[3] (Streptomycin sulfate) Pfizer	400 mg/ml injection	Most Columbiformes Galliformes	IM	10–30 mg/kg BID, TID	Good treatment in larger birds Use extra caution due to toxicity hazard
33.	Spectinomycin[17] (Spectam) Sanofi, Syntex	Injectable solution 50 or 100 mg/ml Water soluble solution 50 mg/ml	Galliformes	Water IM	150–250 mg/l water	Flock treatment for enteritis caused by bacterial pathogens
34.	Sulfachlorpyridazine (Vetisulid) Solvay	Water soluble powder	Most	Water	0.25–1 tsp/gallon 5–10 days	Excellent flock treatment for *E. coli* infections Check sensitivity

AVIAN ANTIMICROBIAL THERAPY *Continued*

	Drug	Form	Species	Route	Dosage	Comments
35.	Tetracycline[17] (Panmycin Aquadrops) Upjohn	Capsules 150 mg Suspension or solution 100 mg/ml	Most Psittacines	Water PO or by gavage	1/4 tsp/liter 5–10 days 200–250 mg/kg BID	May be immunosuppressive in avian species May have developmental side effects in avian species, particulary toucans Change 2 or 3 times daily if used in drinking water
36.	Ticarcillin[15] (Ticar) SmithKline Beecham	Injectable solution Variable concentration	Most	IM, IV	150–200 mg/kg TID, QID	Good synergistic affect with aminoglycosides
37.	Tobramycin[3] Nebcin	Injectable solution 40 mg/ml	Pheasants Cranes Psittaciformes	IM	25–5 mg/kg BID	For highly resistant *Pseudomonas* sp. strains
38.	Trimethoprim[2] and Sulfamethoxazole (Bactrim) Roche (Tribrissen) Coopers	Suspension 8 mg trimethoprim and 40 mg sufamethoxazole/ml	Psittaciformes Pigeons	Oral IM PO	16–24 mg/kg BID or TID 8 mg/kg BID 50 mg/kg SID 25 mg/kg BID	Regurgitation has been described as a potential side effect Injectable tribrissen not available in US Patients suffering from liver disease or bone marrow suppression should not be treated with this drug
39.	Tylosin[17] (Tylan) Butler; Elanco	Injectable 50 mg/ml or 200 mg/ml Soluble powder with vitamins 250 g/8.81 oz	Most	IM Water Nebulization	10–40 mg/kg TID, QID 2 tsp/gallon 1 hour BID 100 mg/0m saline for 1 hour BID	Useful in *Mycoplasma* upper respiratory and ocular injections in psittacines especially cockatiels *Eye spray*—soluble powder mixed 1:10 with sterile water

AVIAN ANTIPARASITIC THERAPY

	Drug	Form	Species	Route	Dosage	Comments
1.	Albendazole (Valbazen) SmithKline Beecham	113.6 mg/ml suspension	Ratites	Oral	1 ml/50 lb body weight BID, for 3 days. Repeat in 2 weeks	For protozoal infection in ratites, rheas
2.	Amprolium[28] (Corid, Amprol plus) MSD, Ag Vet	Solution 9.6%– 96 mg/ml	Most	Drinking water	2–4 ml/gallon for 5–7 days repeat	Management control of coccidia is important for total treatment efficacy May be good treatment for coccidia in flock outbreak Monitor flock for recurrence
3.	Carbaryl[15] (Sevin) Southern Agricultural Insecticides, Inc.	5% powder	Most	Topical	Light dusting on feathers	Good ectoparasite control when lightly dusted into bird's feathers Add 1 to 2 teaspoons to nesting material to control insects depending on size of box
4.	Carnidazole[29] (Spartrix) Wildlife Labs Janssen	Tablet 10 mg	Pigeons	Oral	Adults 200 mg/kg once Newly weaned 100 mg/kg once 20–30 mg/kg single oral dose	Primarily for *Trichomonas* sp., good antiprotozoal drug, wide margin of safety
5.	Chloroquine[29] (Reschin R) Bayer (Arlen) Winthrop	Tablet 500 mg	Penguins	Oral	10 mg/kg once then 5 mg/kg at 6, 18, 24 hours	Primarily used to treat *Plasmodium* usually in combination with primaquine Overdose may result in death
6.	Chlorsulon[2] (Curatrem) MSD Ag Vet	Oral suspension 8.5%, 8.5 mg/ml	Psittaciformes	Oral	20 mg/kg, 3 times, 2 weeks apart	Tapeworms and liver flukes
7.	Clazuril[2, 30] (Appertex) Janssen	Tablet 2.5 mg	Pigeons Poultry	Oral	5–10 mg/kg once daily times 3 days on, 2 days off	Coccidiostat in pigeons and poultry High efficacy
8.	Crotamiton[15] (Eurax) Westwood Squibb	Cream 10% Lotion 10%	Psittaciformes	Topical	Apply to affected areas	Knemidokoptic mite infestation

Table continued on following page

AVIAN ANTIPARASITIC THERAPY *Continued*

	Drug	Form	Species	Route	Dosage	Comments
9.	Dimetridazole[15] (Emtryl/d) Jense/Salsbery (Emtryl/R) Rhone/Merieux	Soluble Powder 182 g/6.42 oz	Budgerigars	Oral (gavage)	Stock solution 1 tsp 1 pint water Dose: 0.5 ml/30 g repeat in 12–24 hours	Not available in US Use lower dosages for softbills, lories, and birds with young *Not to be used on Peking robins and finches* Overdose in hot weather—seizures/death
10.	Febendazole[17] (Panacur) Hoechst-Roussel	Oral suspension 10%–100 mg/ml	Anseriformes Most	Oral Oral Water Feed	5–15 mg/kg daily for 5 days 10–50 mg/kg SID for 3–5 days 125 mg/L × 5 days 50 mg/L × 5 days 100 mg/kg of feed × 5 days	Low margin of safety with softbills. Do not use during molting May not be the most effective agent to treat finches for nematodes and some trematodes
11.	Ipronidazole[17] (Ipropan) Roche	Soluble powder 61 g/2.65 oz	Most Psittaciformes	Water Oral	500 mg/gallon for 7–21 days 0.25 tsp/gallon	Antiprotozoal drug Not available in the US
12.	Ivermectin[32] (Ivomec) Eqvalan Merck, Ag Vet	Injectable solution 10 mg/ml Oral suspension	Most Pigeons Raptors	IM, Oral Oral/subcutaneous Subcutaneous	200 µg/kg repeat in 10–14 days 3 mg/kg single dose 0.4 mg/kg single dose	Dilute in propylene glycol Low dose threshold for finches and budgies Treats nematodes, mites, and lice Propylene glycol may be toxic in large doses
13.	Levamisole[33] (Levasole) Pitman-Moore (Tramisole) American Cyanamid (L-Spartakon) Janssen	Injectable 13.65% 136.5 mg/ml Tablets 20 mg	Anseriformes Australian parakeets Most Most	Oral (gavage) Oral (gavage) Oral (drinking water) IM, SC	20–50 mg/kg 15 mg/kg repeat 10 days 5–15 ml/gallon 1–3 days 5 mg/kg repeat 10–14 days	Immunostimulant 2 mg/kg IM every 14 days for three dosages Low therapeutic index—follow dose regimens carefully
14.	Mebendazole[15] (Telmintic, Telmin) Pitman-Moore	Soluble powder Telmintic 40 mg/g Suspension Telmin 33.3 mg/ml	Psittaciformes Canaries Anseriformes	Oral Oral Oral	25 mg/kg SID for 5 days 10 mg/kg BID for 5 days 5–15 mg/kg daily for 2 days	Do not use during breeding season Capillaria is sensitive For nematodes, some cestodes, trematodes Toxic in pigeons, cormorants, pelicans and raptors
15.	Mepacrine HCl[34] Bayer	Tablet 100 mg	Canaries	Oral	0.24 mg/g body weight twice daily	*Plasmodium* in canaries
16.	Metronidazole[35] (Flagyl) Searle Feagnase 400 Liomont	Tablets 250 or 500 mg Injectable solution 5 mg/ml	Psittaciformes	Oral IM	50–60 mg/kg BID for 10 days 10 mg/kg SID for 2 days	Liquid from Mexico Not in finches Some preparations have adverse reaction to aluminum
17.	Monensin sodium[2] (Coban) Elanco	Feed additive 45 or 60 g/lb	Galliformes Cranes Quail Pigeons	Feed	90 g/ton feed	Not in guinea fowl or turkeys Coccidiostat
18.	Niclosamide[12] (Nicloside) Miles	Tablet 500 mg	Most Finches	Gavage Gavage	50 mg/kg repeat in 10–14 days 500 mg/kg weekly for 4 weeks	Possible toxicity in pigeons, geese, and other Anseriformes For tapeworms
19.	Oxfendazole[12] (Synthic) (Benzelmin) Syntex	Suspension 90.6 or 225 mg/ml	Most	Oral	10–40 mg oral single dose range	Nematode treatment Do not use in breeding season
20.	Piperazine[15] Agri-labs	Suspension 17%– 170 mg/ml 34%–340 mg/ml	Galliformes Anseriformes Raptors Psittacines	Oral Oral Oral	100–500 mg/kg repeat 10–14 days 45–200 mg/kg 100 mg/kg single dose 250 mg/kg single dose	May not be effective against nematodes in psittacine species and finches
21.	Praziquantel[17] (Droncit) Bayvet Haver/Diamond	Tablets 23 or 34 mg Injectable solution 56.8 mg/ml	Most	Oral IM	10–20 mg/kg repeat 10–14 days 9 mg/kg (Flukes: SID for 3 days then oral for 11 days, tapeworms: once, then repeat in 10 days)	For tapeworms especially in greys and cockatoos May not be effective against liver flukes May not eliminate adult tapeworms Injectable may be toxic to finches

AVIAN ANTIPARASITIC THERAPY *Continued*

	Drug	Form	Species	Route	Dosage	Comments
22.	Primaquine[34] (Phosphate) Winthrop	Tablets 26.3 mg	Penguins	Oral Oral	0.03 mg/kg SID for 3 days 0.3–1.0 mg/kg orally TID for 1 to 3 days	Used to treat *Plasmodium* sp. usually in combination with chloroquine
23.	Pyrantel pamoate[15] (Strongid T, Nemex) Pfizer	Oral suspension 4.5 mg/ml	Most	Oral	4.5 mg/kg repeat 10–14 days	For nematodes, poultry feed mixes also available
24.	Pyrethrins[3]	Spray/mist solution	Most	Topical	Lightly mist feathers	For ectoparasites that are resistant to carbaryl Treat under wing
25.	Pyrimethamine[36] (Daraprim) Burroughs Welcome	Tablet 25 mg; one tablet can be mixed to formulate suspension with 21 ml of distilled water, 4 ml K-Y jelly	Most	Oral	0.25–0.5 mg/kg orally twice daily for 30 days	For toxoplasma, *Sarcocystis* and *Leukocytozoan* Used in combination with sulfamethoxazole/ trimethoprim to treat Sarcocystis
26.	Quinacrine HCl[37] (Atabrine, Sanofi, Mepacrine) Winthrop	Tablet 100 mg	Psittaciformes	Oral	5–10 mg/kg SID for 10 days	Low therapeutic index
27.	Ronidazole[38] (Ronivet-S) Vetafarm (Ridzole)	4% powder	Passerines	Oral Water	400 mg of 10% powder per liter water for 7 days 6–10 mg/kg orally SID for 6–10 days	For protozoal parasites
		10% powder	Psittaciformes Pigeons	Water	1–2 g of 105 powder per liter water for 7 days	Not available in the US
28.	Sulfamethazine[12] (Albon)	Liquid	Most	Oral	0.5 ml (of 250 mg/ml liquid) per liter for 3 days on, 2 days off, repeat	Coccidiostat
29.	Thiabendazole[39, 15] (Equizole) MSD agent	Suspension 4 mg/30 ml	Most	Oral	Ascarids 250–500 mg/kg repeat 10–14 days *Syngamus trachea* 100 mg/kg SID for 7–10 days	For treatment of helminth parasites especially *Syngamus trachea* May be toxic to cranes, ratites, and diving ducks

ANTIFUNGAL DRUGS

	Drug	Form	Species	Route	Dosage	Comments
1.	Amphotericin B[15] (Fungizone) Squibb	Injectable solution 5 mg/ml Lotion 3%	Most	IV Intratracheal Nebulize	1.5 mg/kg BID, TID 1 mg/kg BID to TID 1 mg/ml saline for 15 min BID	Possible nephrotoxicity and may cause blood dyscrasias Subcutaneous efficacy is unknown
2.	Caprillic acid[2] (Kaprycidin A) Ecological Formulas	Capsule 325 mg	Most	Oral	1/4 capsule/300 g	Adjunct treatment of antifungal treatment using imidazole
3.	Chlorhexidine[17] (Nolvasan) Fort Dodge	Solution 20 mg/ml	Most	Oral Topical	10–30 ml/gallon drinking water 0.5% as a wound cleanser	Toxic to finches Use properly May help prevent or treat mild gastrointestinal candidiasis Disinfectant
4.	Enilconazole[21] (Clinafarm) Sterwin	Solution 138 mg/ml	Most	Aerosol spray	———	For disinfecting equipment for aspergillosis problems May cause irreversible ocular damage
5.	Fluconazole[19] (Diflucan) Roerig	Tablets 50, 100, or 200 mg Injectable solution 2 mg/ml	Most	Oral	2–5 mg/kg SID for 7 days 2 mg/kg–100 mg tablet crushed in 20 ml Nystatin	Passes into cerebrospinal fluid Agglutination possible

Table continued on following page

ANTIFUNGAL DRUGS *Continued*

	Drug	Form	Species	Route	Dosage	Comments
6.	Flucytosine[17] 5-Fluorocytosine	Capsule 250 mg and 500 mg	Most	Oral	30–50 mg/kg BID for 21 days	Use with amphotericin B for *Aspergillus* sp. infections. Blood dyscrasias have been noted
7.	Gentian violet[15] Unavailable in US now	Powder or solution 16 mg/ml	Psittaciformes	Topical	Apply to affected area with cotton swab	Topical application as drying agent. Excellent for crop candidiasis and skin fold candidiasis in hyacinth macaw babies
8.	Itraconazole[22] (Sporanox) Janssen	Capsules 100 mg	Most	Oral	5–10 mg/kg BID for 4–5 weeks	Seems to be very effective against in vivo *Aspergillus* infections. Less toxic than other antifungals. Expensive
9.	Ketoconazole[19] (Nizoral) Janssen	Tablet 200 mg can be dissolved in 0.8 ml one M HCl acid and 3.2 ml of water	Most	Oral Water Feed	20–30 mg/kg BID for 21 days 200 mg/l 10–20 mg/kg	Possible liver damage. Elevated liver enzymes during treatment. No published reports in birds of liver damage
10.	Miconazole[2] (Monistat) Janssen	Injectable solution 10 mg/ml Ointment 1 or 2%	Psittaciformes	IV Topical	20 mg/kg TID Ointment	Good for use in systemic *Candida* or *Cryptococcus* infections. Give slowly IV to prevent adverse cardiac reactions. Ointment for dermal infections
11.	Nystatin[17] (Mycostatin) Apothecon (Mycozo) Squibb	Oral suspension 100,000 units/ml Feed premix Myco 20	Most Most	Oral Feed	1 ml/300 g BID to TID for 7 days	Must come into contact with *Candida* organisms. For gastrointestinal *Candida* infections only
12.	STA solution[2]	Salicyclic acid (3 g) Tannic acid 3 g in ethyl alcohol to 100 ml	Most	Topical	As needed	For fungal dermatitis

MISCELLANEOUS DRUGS

	Drug	Form	Species	Route	Dosage	Comments
1.	Acetylcysteine[15] (Mucomyst) Bristol	Solution 20% mucomyst 10% mucomyst 10	Psittaciformes	Nebulization	2–5 drops per treatment in nebulizer	Neonates may be sensitive when nebulized
2.	Acetaminophen (Tylenol) McNeil Consumer Products	Regular strength tablets Acetaminophen 325 mg Elixir Concentration	Most	Oral	0.15 ml elixir/liter water 160 mg/5 ml	
3.	Acetylsalicylic acid[15] (Aspirin) Butler, Vedco	Tablets 5 or 60 grain	Most	Oral	1 tablet in 250 ml water	Pain anti-inflammatory used as an anticlotting agent
4.	ACTH[2] (Adrenal corticotrophic hormone) (adrenomone) Burns Biotech	Injectable solution 40 or 80 IU/ml	Psittaciformes	IM	16 IU	For ACTH stimulation test
5.	Allopurinol[17] (Zyloprim) Burroughs Wellcome	Tablet 100 or 300 mg	Psittaciformes	Drinking water	Stock: 1 tablet (100 mg) in 10 ml water—20 drops of stock suspension in 1 oz water daily	For articular gout. Keep patient hydrated
6.	Aminopentamide[2] Hydrogen sulfate (Centrine) Aveco	Injectable solution	Most	IM, SC	0.05 mg/kg BID 5 doses maximum	Antiemetic. Antidiarrheal, slows GI motility
7.	Aminoloid[2] Schering	————	Raptors	IM	0.25–0.75 mg/kg repeat 10–14 days	Induction of molt in raptors

MISCELLANEOUS DRUGS *Continued*

	Drug	Form	Species	Route	Dosage	Comments
8.	Amitriptyline HCl[2] (Elavil) Stuart (Endep) Roche	Tablet 10, 25, 50, 75, 100, 150 mg Injectable solution 10 mg/ml	Psittaciformes	Oral	1–2 mg/kg SID–BID	Many adverse side effects Used for feather picking Do not use with monoamine oxidase inhibitors
9.	Chlorine bleach	100 mg/ml	Most	Water Topical	Disinfect water 8 drops/gallon	Corrosive to metal, undiluted causes respiratory irritation
10.	Cisapride (Propulsid) Janssen	Tablets 10–20 mg	Psittacines	Oral	1 mg/kg BID	Use in cases of gastroepithelial irritation; has been used with no side effects
11.	Clomipramine HCl[2] (Anafranil)	Capsule 25, 50, or 75 mg	Psittaciformes	Oral	0.5–1 mg/kg SID or BID	Antidepressant numerous metabolic side effects used for self-mutilating patients
12.	Colchicine[2] Merck, Lilly	Tablet containing 0.5 mg colchicine and 0.5 mg probenecid	Psittaciformes	Oral	0.04 mg/kg/day BID	Discontinue if vomiting or diarrhea occur Antigout activity May potentiate gout in some cases
13.	Copper sulfate (Caustic powder) Phoenix Butler	Powder 51%	Most	Topical	Applied to affected areas as needed	Treating cases of ulcerative dermatitis
14.	Desoxycortisone[15] (Acetate) Ciba-Geigy Animal Health	Injectable solution 25 mg/ml 4 cc vial	Psittaciformes	IM	4 mg/kg SID	May cause hypoadrenocorticism
15.	Dioctyl sulfosuccinate (DSS)[17] (Colase) Mead-Johnson Warner-Chilcott	Tablets 50, 240, 250, 1000 mg Syrup 50 mg/15 ml 60 mg/15 ml 150 mg/15 ml 50 mg/15 ml	Psittaciformes	Drinking water	1 ml/30 ml water	Laxative, expelling lead from GI tract
16.	Diethylstilbestrol[15] diphosphate (Stilphostrol) Miles	Tablet 50 mg Injectable solution 0.25 mg/ml	Most	IM Oral	0.1–0.3 ml/kg 1 drop/30 ml water	Low therapeutic index
17.	Dimethylsulfoxide[2] (Domoso) Syntex	Liquid or gel 900 mg/ml	Most	Topical	1 ml/kg BID as needed for swelling	Avoid contact with human skin. May cause anorexia
18.	Dinoprost[2] Tromethamine (Lutalyse) Upjohn	Solution 5 mg/ml	Most	IM	0.02–0.1 mg/kg once	May facilitate egg passage. Contains prostaglandin F2 alpha For egg binding
19.	Diphenhydramine HCl[2] (Benadryl) Parke-Davis	Capsule 24 or 50 mg Injectable solution 10 to 50 mg/ml	Psittaciformes	Oral	0.5 tsp/8 oz water or 2–4 mg/kg BID	For feather pickers or highly stressed birds Toxic side effects
20.	Doxepin HCl[2] (Sinequan) Roerig	Capsules 10, 25, 50, 75, 100 or 150 mg Suspension 10 mg/ml	Psittaciformes	Oral	0.5–1 mg/kg BID	May cause severe lethargy Antidepressant
21.	D-tubocurarine[2]	Solution 3 mg/ml	Raptors	Ophthalmic drops	Every 5 minutes for three times	Mydriatic
22.	Echinacea[2] Biobotanica	Solution	Psittaciformes	Oral Water	2.5 drops/kg 5 days/cup of water	Immunostimulant especially in viral infections Holistic use
23.	EDTA-TRIS[2] Lysozyme solution	Solution mix 3.07 g Trizma HCl 3.17 g Trizmabase 1.12 g disodium EDTA in 100 ml water	Most	Topical	Used intratracheally, intranasally, or wound lavage	Help antibiotics penetrate bacterial cell wall
24.	Ergonovine maleate[15] Ergotrate maleate	Solution 0.2 mg/ml	Most	IV, Intraosseous IT, IC	0.1 mg/kg single dose	Causes firm contractions of the uterus. Do not use if egg may be adhered to uterine wall
25.	Ferric subsulfate Monsel's solution	Liquid or powder	Most	Topical	As needed to stop bleeding especially after nail trim	May cause feather cysts if used into damaged follicles

Table continued on following page

MISCELLANEOUS DRUGS *Continued*

	Drug	Form	Species	Route	Dosage	Comments
26.	Flunixin-meglumine[15] (Banamine) Schering	Injectable solution 50 mg/ml	Most	IM	1–10 mg/kg	Anti-inflammatory, may cause diarrhea or vomiting
27.	Furosemide[17] (Lasix) Hoescht-Roussel	Injectable solution 50 mg/ml Syrup 10 mg/ml	Most	IM, SC Oral	0.15–2 mg/kg SID/BID	Used as a diuretic Some avian species are sensitive and may exhibit neurologic signs before death
28.	Haloperidol[2] (Haldol) Henry Schein	Oral solution 2 mg/ml Injectable solution 50 or 100 mg/ml	Psittaciformes	IM Oral	1–2 mg/kg every 2 to 3 weeks 0.2 mg/kg BID for birds <1 kg 0.15 mg/kg BID for birds >1 kg	Used for feather picking and self-trauma in birds Some psittacine species may be sensitive. May have to regulate dosage
29.	ImmunoRegulin[2] ImmunoVet Inc.	Injectable solution 0.4 mg/ml 5 ml vial	Most			Immunostimulant May cause death in some avian species
30.	Iodine[17]	Solution 50 mg/ml free iodine 100 mg/ml potassium iodine	Budgerigars	Water IM	Stock mix 2 ml of Lugol solution in 30 ml of water Mix one drop of stock in 250 ml of drinking water	For goiter in budgerigars
31.	Hydrocortisone[15] (Sodium succinate) Huffman	100 mg/2 ml vial 250 mg/2 ml vial	Most	IM	10 mg/kg SID	Hypoadrenocorticism
32.	Insulin NPH[15] (NPH-ILETIN-I) Lilly	Injectable solution 100 units/ml 10 ml vial	Most	IM	0.5–3 units/kg	Diabetes
33.	Kaolin/pectin[15] (Kaopectate) Roxane	Oral suspension 30 ml	Most	PO	2 ml/kg BID–TID	Diarrhea
34.	Lactobacillus[2] (Probiocin) Pioneer (Benebac) Pet Ag	Powder or gel	Psittaciformes	Oral	1 pinch/day/bird 1 tsp/quart hand feeding formula	Inoculation of GI tract Young and debilitated birds
35.	Lactulose[17] (Cephulac) Marion Merrell Dow	Oral suspension 667 mg/ml	Most	Oral	0.3 ml/kg	Used in cases of hepatitis and liver disease May act as appetite stimulant Discontinue or reduce dosage if diarrhea occurs
36.	Lipoform Tabs[25] Vet-A-Mix	Chewable tablet	Most	PO	500 mg SID	Prevent liver damage in face of viral infection
37.	Levothyroxine sodium[17] (Thyroxine L) Butler	Tablet 0.1, 0.2, 0.3, 0.5 or 0.8 mg Suspension 0.4 mg/ml	Most	Oral	20 µg/kg SID/BID	May induce molt and other adverse side effects Long-term therapy should be monitored
38.	Leuprolide[2] (Lupron) TAP Pharmaceutical	Lyphilized microspheres 7.5 mg/vial	Psittaciformes	IM		Causes a reduction of ovarian activity May be able to reduce levels of testosterone Works short-term
39.	Lorelco[2] (Probacoll) Marion Merrell Dow	Tablets 250 or 500 mg	Psittaciformes	Oral	0.25 tsp/day for 2–4 months	Used in birds to control lipemia and suppress the growth of lipomas
40.	Medroxyprogesterone acetate[17] Upjohn	Tablets 2.5, 5, or 10 mg (Provera promone) injectable suspension 100 mg/ml (Pepoprovera)	Pigeons Most	Oral (feed) IM, SC	0.1% of ration continuous 5–25 mg/kg every 4–6 weeks	Used to inhibit ovulation; cockatoos and Quaker parrots appear to be very sensitive Feather picking in male psittacines PU/PO, polyphagia, weight gain, increase liver enzymes
41.	Methylprednisolone acetate[2] (Depo-medrol) Upjohn	Injectable solution 20 or 40 mg/ml	Most	IM	0.5–1 mg/kg	Adrenal cortical insufficiency Allergic disorders, immune disorders
42.	Methocarbamol (Robaxin)	———	Most	IM	130 mg/kg	Muscle relaxation

MISCELLANEOUS DRUGS *Continued*

	Drug	Form	Species	Route	Dosage	Comments
43.	Metoclopramide HCl[2] (Reglan) Robbins	Tablets 10 mg Syrup 1 mg/ml Injectable solution 5 mg/ml	Most	IM, IV Oral	0.5 mg/kg	Indicated for GI motility problems Rule out foreign body ingestion
44.	Naloxone hydrochloride[2] Quad	0.4 mg/ml multidose vial	Most	IV	2 mg SID	Narcotic and tranquilizer antagonist
45.	Neomycin[16] (Biosol) Upjohn	Solution 50 mg/ml	Most	Water	1–8 drops/30 ml water 5 g/gallon water	Do not use Biosol M product. Possible toxicity
46.	Neomycin ointment Schering		All	Topical	BID or QID as needed	Good for abrasions and skin infections
47.	Nortriptyline HCl[2] (Aventyl HCl) Lilly	Tablet 25 mg/ml Syrup 2 mg/ml	Psittaciformes	Oral	1 ml/4 oz drinking water	Antidepressant used in feather picking and self-mutilation cases
48.	Pancreatic enzymes[2] (Viokase V) Fort Dodge (Hi-Vegi-Tip) Freeda Vit	2400 g Tablets	Most	Oral (food)	1/8 tsp/kg	May be used to aid in food digestion in birds suffering from GI disorders
49.	Phenylbutazone[2] (Butazolidin) Coopers	Injectable solution 200 mg/ml Tablet 100 or 400 mg	Psittaciformes Raptors	Oral	3.5–7 mg/kg BID 20 mg/kg TID	Do not give SC or IM Anti-inflammatory
50.	Stanozolol[17] (Winstrol V) Upjohn	Tablet 2 mg Injectable solution 50 mg/ml	Most	IM	25 to 50 mg/kg	Increase weight gain in anorectic cases Monitor patients with hepatic or renal problems May not achieve desired results
51.	Sucralfate[2] (Carafate) Marion Merrell Dow	Tablet 1 g	Psittaciformes	Oral	25 mg/kg TID	Protective coating formed in proventriculus
52.	Testosterone[15, 17] (Cypionate) Henry Schein, Upjohn	Methyltestosterone tablet 10 or 20 mg Injectable solution 200 mg/ml Depo-testosterone	Most	IM	8 mg/kg weekly as needed	Do not use in cases of liver and renal diseases May be used in cases of reproductive-associated feather picking and chronic egg-laying
53.	TSH[2] Tytropan Armour	Injectable solution 10 IU/vial	Psittaciformes	IM	1–21 IU/kg	Used for thyroid stimulation testing
54.	Triamcinolone[2] (Vetalog)	Ointment	Most	IM	0.5 mg/kg once	Ointment
55.	Yeast cell derivatives (Preparation H) Whitehall Laboratories	Ointment	Most	Topical	As needed	Stimulate epithelial healing especially abrasions and lacerations

NUTRITIONAL SUPPLEMENTS

	Drug	Form	Species	Route	Dosage	Comments
1	Ascorbic acid[15] (Vitamin C) Phoenix, Vedco	Injectable solution 250 mg/ml	Most	IM	20–40 mg/kg daily to weekly	———
2.	Avipro[2] Vetark Animal Health	Powder 50 g jar	Psittaciformes	Oral	4 g/200 ml water	Lactobacillus Supplementation in critical patients
3.	Cyanocobalamin[15] (Vitamin B$_{12}$) Butler	Injectable solution 1 or 3 mg/ml	Most	IM	250–500 µg/kg once/week	Urates may turn pink
4.	Iron dextran[17] Butler, Lextron, Vedco	Solution 100 mg/ml	Most	IM	10 mg/kg repeat in 7–10 days if needed	Deficiency Care must be taken when used in birds, subject to hemochromatosis Following hemorrhage

Table continued on following page

NUTRITIONAL SUPPLEMENTS *Continued*

	Drug	Form	Species	Route	Dosage	Comments
5.	Vitamin[17] A, D$_3$, E Mortar & Pestle Pharmacy	Aqueous emulsion	Most	IM	0.1–0.2 ml/300 g weekly	Calcium deficiencies Debilitated patients Supplementation Epithelial disorders at injection sites, especially in cockatiels Large animal preparations too high in vitamin D for birds
6.	Vitamin B complex[15] Butler, Lextron, Vedco	Thiamine 50 mg/ml solution	Most	IM	1–3 mg thiamine/kg weekly	May be difficult to obtain
7.	Vitamin E/Selenium[17] (Seletoc) Schering	Injectable solution 1 mg Se and 50 mg Vit E/ml	Most	IM IM or SC	0.05 to 0.1 mg/kg every 14 days	———
8.	Vitamin K$_1$[17]	Injectable solution 10 mg/ml Tablets 25 mg	Most	IM	0.2–2.5 mg/kg as needed	For cases of extreme blood loss, anemia Warfarin toxicity, hemorrhagic disorders

PIGEON THERAPEUTICS[40]

	Drug	Dose	Route
1.	Aminoglycosides (Ophthalmic solution only)	1 drop QID	Topical ophthalmic treatment
2.	Amoxicillin	100 g/kg BID 2 to 3 g/gallon drinking water	PO
3.	Amoxicillin with clavulanic acid	125 mg/kg BID	PO
4.	Amprolium	1 tsp/gallon of 20% powder 8 ml/gallon of 9.64% solution for 3–5 days	Oral
5.	Carbenicillin	100 mg/kg BID or TID	IM
6.	Carnidazole	20 mg/kg	PO
7.	Cefadroxil	100 mg/kg BID	PO
8.	Cefotaxime	100 mg/kg BID/TID	IM
9.	Ceftazidime	100 mg/kg BID/TID	IM
10.	Cephalexin	100 mg/kg BID/TID	PO
11.	Chloramphenicol	60 to 100 mg/kg TID 250 mg/kg QID Ophthalmic drops TID/QID	IM PO Topical
12.	Chlortetracycline/Oxytetracycline (Mix fresh twice a day)	50 mg/kg TID or QID 1000 mg to 1500 mg/gallon drinking water	PO Oral
13.	Clazuril	5 mg/kg	PO
14.	Dimetridazole	¼ to ½ tsp/gallon for 3–5 days in drinking water	Oral
15.	Doxycycline	25 to 50 mg/kg BID	PO
16.	Enrofloxacin	12–15 mg/kg BID 150 to 160 mg/gallon drinking water	PO Oral
17.	Erythromycin	125 mg/kg TID 2–3 g/gallon drinking water for 7–14 dys	PO
18.	Fenbendazole	10–12 mg/kg SID for 3 days	PO
19.	Ivermectin	0.5 mg to 1 mg/kg	PO, IM, SC
20.	Levamisole	40 mg/kg once 1000 to 1500 mg/gallon drinking water for 24 hours	PO
21.	Lincomycin	25–50 mg/kg	IM
22.	Mebendazole	5–6 mg/kg for 3–5 days ¼–½ tsp/gallon drinking water 3–5 days (Dog wormer prep)	Oral Oral
23.	Metronidazole	200–250 mg/kg for 3–7 days 4000 mg/gallon drinking water from 3–7 days	PO Drinking water

PIGEON THERAPEUTICS[40] *Continued*

	Drug	Dose	Route
24.	Nystatin	100,000 units/kg BID	PO
25.	Piperacillin	100 mg/kg BID/TID	IM
26.	Piperazine	35 mg/kg for 2 days 300 mg/gallon drinking water for 2 days	PO
27.	Primaquine/phosphate	1–2 26.3 mg tablets/gallon drinking water For 10–21 days before race season Then 1–2 days weekly	Oral
28.	Pyrantel pamoate	20–25 mg/kg	PO
29.	Pyrethrin, permethrin	Powder (under wings, dorsal aspect, and vent area) Dip (a) 2 oz dip (cat dip prep) (b) 3 gallons water (c) 6 drops dishwashing detergent	Topical Submerge bird to neck level on warm days Do not repeat for 7 days
30.	Quinacrine	1–3 tablets/gallon drinking water for 10–21 days	Oral
31.	Ronidazole	(½–¾ tsp) 400 mg/gallon for 3–5 days	Oral
32.	Spectinomycin	25–35 mg/kg BID/TID 600–1000 mg/gallon drinking water	IM Oral
33.	Sulfachlorpyridazine	1200 mg/gallon for 7–10 days in drinking water	Oral
34.	Sulfadimethoxine	1250–1500 mg/gallon drinking water on first day followed by 750–1000 mg for four days Supplement B vitamins for 5 days then retreat	Oral Oral
35.	Sulfamethazine	1500 mg/gallon drinking water on first day followed by 750–1000 mg per gallon for 4 days Supplement B vitamins for 5 days then retreat	
36.	Trimethoprim/sulfadiazine or sulfamethoxazole	60 mg/kg BID 1800–3600 mg/gallon drinking water for 7–10 days	PO Oral
37.	Tylocin	25–50 mg/kg BID (2 tsp, soluble powder 250 g/8.81 oz) = 3 g/gallon drinking water	IM, SC Drinking water

RATITE THERAPEUTICS,[41] ANTIBIOTICS/ANTIFUNGALS

	Drug	Dose	Route
1.	Amikacin	11 mg/kg BID	IM, SC
2.	Amoxicillin	10 mg/kg TID	PO, IM
3.	Ampicillin	15 mg/kg QID	PO
4.	Ampicillin	7 mg/kg QID	IV, IM, SC
5.	Carbenicillin	15 mg/kg TID	IV
6.	Cefazolin	16 mg/kg QID	IM, IV
7.	Cephalexin	22 mg/kg TID	PO
8.	Cephalothin sodium	32 mg/kg QID	IM, IV
9.	Chloramphenicol	50 mg/kg TID	PO, IV, IM, SC
10.	Chlortetracycline	20 mg/kg TID	PO
11.	Ciprofloxacin	6 mg/kg BID	PO
12.	Clavamox	13.75 mg/kg BID	PO
13.	Dicloxacillin	35 mg/kg TID	PO
14.	Doxycycline	35 mg/kg SID	PO
15.	Enrofloxacin	2.5 mg/kg BID	PO, SC, IM
16.	Erythromycin	10 mg/kg TID	PO
17.	Flucytosine	100 mg/kg BID	PO
18.	Gentamicin	2 mg/kg TID	IM, SC
19.	Griseofulvin	50 mg/kg SID	PO
20.	Itraconazole	5 mg/kg SID	PO
21.	Ketoconazole	10 mg/kg SID	PO
22.	Metronidazole	25 mg/kg BID	PO
23.	Norfloxacin	5 mg/kg BID	PO
24.	Polymyxin B	2 mg/kg BID	PO, SC
25.	Trimethoprim sulfa	15 mg/kg BID	PO, SC
26.	Tylosin	10 mg/kg TID	PO
27.	Tylosin	5 mg/kg BID	IV, IM

MISCELLANEOUS DRUGS

	Drug	Dose	Route
1.	Aminophylline	10 mg/kg TID	PO, IM, IV
2.	Atropine	0.05 mg/kg QID	IV, SC, IM
3.	Cimetidine	5 mg/kg TID	PO, IV
4.	Cimetidine	10 mg/kg BID	IM
5.	Dipyrone	25 mg/kg TID	SC, IM, IV
6.	Doxapram	7 mg/kg every hour	IV
7.	Flumethasone	1.5 mg/kg SID	PO, IM, IV, SC
8.	Hydrocortisone (shock)	50 mg/kg SID	IV
9.	Hydrocortisone	4.4 mg/kg BID	PO
10.	Lomotil	2.5 mg/kg QID	PO
11.	Mannitol	1500 mg/kg QID	IV
12.	Phenylbutazone	14 mg/kg BID	PO
13.	Prednisolone (immune suppression)	2 mg/kg BID	PO, IM
14.	Prednisolone (prolonged therapy)	1.25 mg/kg every 48 hours	PO
15.	Prednisolone (shock)	8.5 mg/kg every hour	IV

Surgery

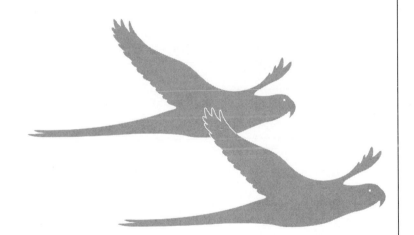

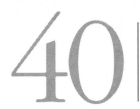

Robert B. Altman

General Surgical Considerations

The introduction of isoflurane to avian surgery has made possible prolonged anesthetic and surgical periods and has afforded the avian surgeon the ability to perform more intricate procedures with a greater margin of safety. Technologic advances such as endoscopy, electrosurgery, magnification, and microsurgery have also added a dimension that broadens the scope of surgical procedures that can be safely and successfully performed. The avian surgeon requires greater surgical skill than his or her mammalian surgeon counterpart because of the small size of most avian patients and the anatomic variations compared with mammals. Gentle handling of fragile tissues, the need to work in small tight spaces, the requirement of total hemostasis, and the necessity to work rapidly place additional demands on the avian surgeon.

One of the most important factors in enhancing the bird's ability to survive a surgical procedure is to perform as complete and comprehensive a presurgical evaluation as possible. Accurate assessment of the patient's physiologic and pathophysiologic state allows the surgeon to take measures to counteract deficits such as nutritional deficiencies, hypoglycemia, hypothermia, hypotension, hypovolemia, anemia, and dehydration.

With pre-, intra-, and postoperative monitoring and support, it is possible to stabilize the patient's physiologic condition and greatly increase the bird's chances of survival.

PRESURGICAL EVALUATION

It is essential that a physical examination be as comprehensive as possible. Careful, painstaking history-taking is important because most pet owners are unfamiliar with normal parameters and can often fail to recognize or overlook abnormal behavior or physical signs pertinent to the bird's physical state.

Assessment of the bird's nutritional state[1, 2] is important to determine deficiencies in blood calcium and calcification of skeletal tissue, which are relevant to bone quality. Decalcified, thin, long bone cortices are more susceptible to fracture and often fail to heal. Therefore, careful handling and positioning are essential to avoid iatrogenic fracture, particularly of the humerus. Bone quality is also important when determining the technique of fracture repair.

Both obesity and emaciation are conditions that can significantly increase the anesthetic and surgical risk. Obese birds may have large visceral fatty deposits that can compromise the respiratory effort by infringing upon the air sacs, thereby decreasing tidal volume.[1] Because most of the anesthetic agents in current use are detoxified in the liver, impaired liver function from fatty infiltration or fatty degeneration can affect anesthetic tolerance.

Nutritionally debilitated birds with low glycogen levels cannot always handle the stress associated with anesthesia and surgery. They may become hypoglycemic and succumb during or after the surgical episode. Debilitated birds also have difficulty responding to normal wound healing.

During the physical examination it is important to discover cardiopulmonary abnormalities. Observation of the bird's resting breathing pattern can reveal abnormalities. Open-mouth breathing and increased thoracic excursions associated with rhythmic tail bobbing can be an indication of cardiopulmonary impairment.

Stressing the bird by handling (examination) for at least 2 minutes or permitting the bird 2 minutes of free flight in an enclosed room and then observing any exaggerated breathing patterns is a simple cardiopulmonary function test. Normal recovery time should be no longer than 3 to 5 minutes.[1-3] If recovery time exceeds 5 minutes, cardiopulmonary compromise should be considered. Auscultation of the air sacs can reveal gross irregularities.

It is important to develop the most comprehensive data base feasible to identify and correct physiologic abnormalities before or during the surgical procedure. Considerations such as the size and physical condition of the patient, the economic constraints of the owner, and the length and urgency of the procedure can be limiting factors.

After the physical examination has been completed and evaluated, the clinical pathology workup should be undertaken.

CLINICAL PATHOLOGY EVALUATION

A complete clinical pathology workup offers the most comprehensive data base possible[1-5] (Table 40–1). This presurgical evaluation is not always practical or possible. Although not as informative, a minimal data base should include tests for packed cell volume (PCV), total solids, and serum glucose concentration.

Patients with blood glucose levels below 200 mg/dl should be supported with 2.5% dextrose in half strength saline or 5% dextrose and saline administered preferably by the intravenous route pre- and/or intraoperatively.

Birds with a hematocrit level above 55 to 60% should be given lactated Ringer's solution or glucose in saline to combat dehydration pre- and intraoperatively. Anemic birds with PCV levels below 20% are extremely poor surgical risks and have a much greater chance of survival if given whole blood transfusions.

There is controversy as to the safety and efficacy of blood transfusions. In a study done in 1983,[6] this author found a high percentage of transfusion reactions by cross-matching after a second transfusion of heterologous blood. In another study in 1995[7] investigators indicated that cross-matching of blood from different species resulted in agglutination or hemolysis in 66% of the cases. Cross-matching of blood from birds of the same species did not result in agglutination.

In a study in pigeons, Sandmeier and coworkers[8] found that with homologous transfusions, red blood cell survival was only 7 days, compared with the normal survival time of 27 days. With heterologous transfusions, red blood cells had a half-life of less than 1 day. Ideally, blood donors should be of the same species or at least of the same genus. It is this author's opinion that although the ideal blood donor is species-related, genus-related transfusions and even non–genus-related transfusions are of value in supporting the anemic patient during a surgical procedure as long as cross-matching is done before giving the transfusion. The survival benefits of heterologous transfusions have been apparent when compared with giving only fluid support. Cross-matching is simply performed by mixing serum of the recipient with whole blood of the donor. Agglutination occurs immediately with positive reactors (Fig. 40–1).

Assessment of liver function can be extremely important when evaluating surgical patients. Liver dysfunction can affect detoxification of anesthetic gases and blood clotting. Elevated bile acid, aspartate aminotransferase (AST), and serum cholesterol concentrations[9] appear to put the patient at greater risk.

Radiographic evaluation of the respiratory system, gastrointestinal system, and skeletal structures of the bird often reveals information essential to the surgical procedure.

A physiologic imbalance found after examination of the patient should be addressed, treated, and rectified whenever possible, before the surgical procedure is undertaken. If postponement of the pro-

Table 40–1

IDEAL CLINICAL PATHOLOGY WORKUP

1. CBC and chemistry profile
2. Estimated thrombocyte count or clotting time[5]
3. Survey radiographs
4. Choanal or cloacal bacterial culture and sensitivity test
5. Body temperature
6. Heart rate (ECG)

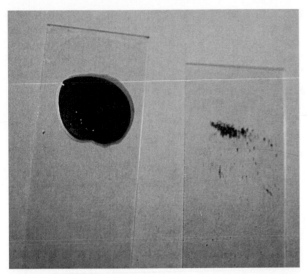

Figure 40-1

One drop of the serum of the recipient is on a slide mixed with one drop of whole blood from the donor. The slide at the right shows lysis from a cross-matching reaction.

cedure is not possible, pre- and intraoperative support are essential.

MONITORING THE PATIENT

For procedures exceeding 10 minutes, careful monitoring of the bird's body temperature and heart rate and rhythm is as important as anesthetic monitoring (see Chapter 46). Determining baseline parameters before induction of anesthesia will make monitoring of the surgical patient meaningful.

Body Temperature

In 1979, a study on body temperature and heart rate[10] during avian anesthesia demonstrated a rapid and, in some cases, precipitous drop in body temperature during the first 10 minutes of anesthesia. Heat loss can occur from patient contact with cold surfaces through conduction and radiation; from expired respiratory and anesthetic gases; from exposed featherless areas plucked during surgical preparation; from evaporation of liquids such as alcohol used in preparation of the surgical site; and through exposure of visceral organs and air sac

surfaces.[1] Core body temperature loss can exceed 12 to 15°F within the first 10 minutes of induction and maintenance of anesthesia. The temperature loss usually continues as long as the depth of anesthesia is not adjusted. Gas anesthetic agents depress muscular activity and centers of thermoregulation. By reducing the anesthetic gas concentration, muscle activity (quivering) causes an almost immediate rise in body temperature.

Temperature loss exceeding 10°F[1, 11] can cause arrhythmias resulting in anesthetic death. Body temperature can be monitored throughout the surgical procedure using an electronic thermometer (Electro Therm, Veterinary Specialty Products, Inc., Boca Raton, FL) with a cloacal temperature probe (Fig. 40–2).

Heat conservation can be achieved in a number of ways. (1) When preparing the surgical site, do not pluck feathers in excess of that which is necessary for surgical exposure; (2) if using alcohol, use it sparingly to avoid evaporation resulting in heat loss; (3) work as rapidly as possible to reduce anesthetic time; (4) insulate cold tabletops and use a circulating hot water jacket (Water Blanket, Gaymar, Orchard Park, NY) or heating platforms (Vari Temp Heating Platform, Veterinary Specialty Products, Inc.) to supply supplemental heat (Fig. 40–3). In a 1988 study,[12] these heat sources seem to be the most efficient in reducing heat loss. (5) Warm parenteral fluids to 96°F before administration. (6) Warming anesthetic gases may also have a heat-conserving effect on the anesthetized patient.

Despite all measures of thermal support, it is

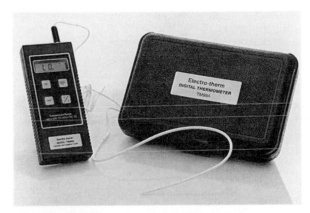

Figure 40-2

An electronic thermometer and cloacal temperature probe. (Courtesy Veterinary Specialty Products, Inc.)

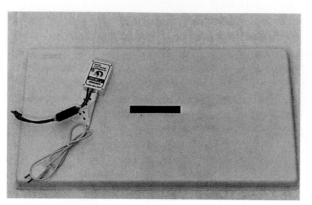

Figure 40–3

An electronic heating platform with adjustable thermostat. (Courtesy Veterinary Specialty Products, Inc.)

not possible to maintain normothermia. However, supplemental heat minimizes heat loss and is therefore a necessity during a surgical procedure.

Cardiac Monitoring

Heart rate and cardiac function should be monitored with a standard or esophageal stethoscope, an ultrasonic Doppler flow apparatus, a pulse oximeter, or a cardiac monitor or electrocardiogram (ECG) tracing throughout a surgical procedure exceeding 10 minutes in duration. A pulse oximeter or Doppler sensor can be placed on the cranial tibial or medial metatarsal arteries.

Bradycardia is a consequence of inhalation anesthesia. Prolonged surgical procedures potentiate the risk of life-threatening bradycardia and arrhythmias with resultant hypotension. If these cardiac changes go unnoticed, anesthetic death can be a consequence.

Heart rate can decrease as much as 223 beats per minute in as short a time as 10 minutes.[10] As anesthesia deepens, changes in the ECG indicate pending danger. T waves become smaller, the R waves increase, and the S wave is reduced.[9, 13] If unchecked, arrhythmias progress if the anesthetic level is not decreased. Reduction of anesthetic level is indicated in cases of dramatic decreases in heart rate or cardiac arrhythmias.

Atropine helps to stabilize a decreasing heart rate, but the consequence of increased viscosity of respiratory secretions must be considered.

PATIENT PREPARATION

All materials needed for patient preparation should be gathered in advance of induction of anesthesia. Presurgical handling and stress should be minimized by performing all patient preparation after the bird has been anesthetized. Anesthesia also reduces pain associated with feather plucking. It is important to defeather the surgical area to afford an adequate sterile field; however, excessive plucking increases the surface area for heat loss. Contour and covert body feathers grow in definitive feather tracks, and in some areas of the body these feather tracks are separated by wide apterylous areas. Therefore, spreading of the feathers in some instances can offer an adequate surgical field, avoiding feather plucking.

Before plucking, a conservative amount of alcohol should be sprinkled or spread on the feathers to be plucked. This prevents feathers from floating around the operating room while being plucked and discarded. Feathers should be plucked parallel to their growth and follicle direction.[2, 4] Plucking feathers at an angle to their growth direction increases the potential for tearing the skin. Contour and down feathers can be removed three or four at a time.[10] Large feathers, particularly wing and tail feathers, should be grasped at the base of the follicle and pulled in the direction of the feather growth. Grasp the feather shaft gently at its base with slight pressure exerted against the skin surrounding the follicle. This supports the integument surrounding the follicle and prevents injury to the area as the feather is being pulled. Large flight and tail feathers should be grasped as close to the skin as possible and pulled parallel to the growth pattern with a hemostat or a pair of pliers. Flight feathers should be plucked only if necessary. This technique decreases the chance of the feather breaking, leaving the shaft in the follicle. In some instances, it may be prudent to cut the primary wing feathers if many feathers are involved. This diminishes soft tissue trauma and hemorrhage to the skin, muscles, and periosteal attachments. Aggressive feather plucking not only increases the risk of tearing surrounding skin, but also increases the risk of hemorrhage and postoperative tissue reaction seen as edema and swelling. Plucking wing and tail feathers appears to be painful to the unanesthetized bird. Plucking

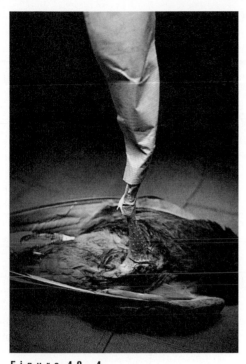

Figure 40-4

Steri-Strip placed on the leg for surgical draping.

flight feathers may also damage follicles and cause feather cysts or ingrown feathers.

It is extremely disconcerting to have feathers surrounding the surgical site encroach on the sterile field during the surgical procedure. By placing a sterile, water-soluble surgical lubricant on the feathers surrounding the incision site, feathers are prevented from encroaching onto the surgical field. Excessive amounts of lubricant can unnecessarily involve feathers well beyond the surgical site and can interfere with adhesives used with surgical drapes to isolate the incisional area.

A functional way of aseptically wrapping appendages, particularly for orthopedic surgery, is to wrap the limb with a nonadhesive bandage material (Vetrap, 3M Animal Care Products, St. Paul, MN) and then cover this material with a sterile adhesive drape strip (Steri-Strips, Econo-Tape-Strips, General Econopak, Inc., Philadelphia, PA). The sterile strip can be applied directly to the appendage, making the wrapped area less bulky. This strip sticks to the area tenaciously, is easily applied, and is moderately easy to remove (Fig. 40–4). It can maintain a sterile field on an area in which plucking feathers

is undesirable or impossible, or on an area that cannot be aseptically prepared.

Draping the avian patient presents a problem not encountered in mammalian surgery. Because it is essential to observe the patient's respirations to monitor anesthesia, the surgical drape must be either tented over the patient·or transparent. Tenting does not afford the anesthetist adequate visualization of thoracic excursions. In addition, tenting makes it more difficult to maintain a sterile field and interferes with the surgeon's working area. Clear plastic drapes (Transparent Surgical Drape, Veterinary Specialty Products, Inc.), which afford total visual exposure, are ideal (Fig. 40–5). These drapes have the added advantage of sticking to the surgical field with a medical-grade skin adhesive, which is easily removed at the termination of the procedure.

Skin preparation for creating and maintaining a sterile field is as important in the avian patient as it is in mammalian surgical preparation. Although skin pathogens appear to be less likely to cause wound infections, perhaps because of the bird's high body temperature, strict aseptic technique is essential.

In an unpublished study, this author found granuloma formation and infection in pigeons undergoing abdominal and thoracic laparoscopic examination in which a nonsterile laparoscope was used. In several cases, it took many weeks for granuloma formation to occur.

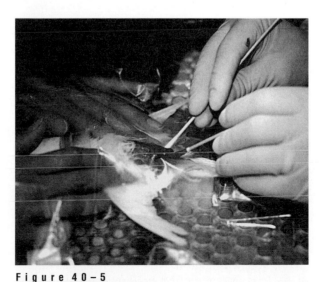

Figure 40-5

Transparent surgical drape in use.

Povidone-iodine 1% (Betadine solution, Purdue Frederick Co., Norwalk, CT) and chlorhexidine diacetate 0.05% (Nolvasan solution, Fort Dodge Labs, Inc., Fort Dodge, IA) are the two most commonly used skin sterilizing agents in veterinary medicine. In a study by Osuna and coworkers,[14] povidone-iodine appeared to produce more skin reactions such as edema, erythema, and wheals in a high percentage of dogs as compared with reactions in dogs similarly treated with chlorhexidine.

Chlorhexidine possesses qualities such as a broader antibacterial spectrum with longer residual effect than povidone-iodine and is not inactivated in the presence of blood or organic material. When applying the surgical scrub solution, gently wash the skin from the center area of the incision site out toward the feathers at least three times. In so doing, the skin in the plucked area is sterilized and the feathers surrounding this area are cleansed.

After the iodine or chlorhexidine scrub, many surgeons wipe the area with alcohol. If this is done, alcohol should be used sparingly to reduce heat loss from evaporation. Alcohol should be given ample time to evaporate before using electrosurgery to avoid ignition of the alcohol. If a water-soluble gel is applied to the surrounding feathers, it should be used sparingly to avoid negating the adhesive effect of the surgical drape.

POSITIONING

Positioning the patient is dependent upon the location of the surgical site. The lateral and ventrodorsal (VD) position are the two basic positions affording access to the vast majority of surgical sites (Table 40–2). Birds should never be placed in a dorsoventral (DV) position because the bird's body weight can inhibit normal thoracic movement during anesthesia. When the bird is positioned in the VD position, care should be taken to avoid pressure on the thorax by the drape, instruments, or the surgeon's hands. Some clinicians are more comfortable positioning the patient on an elevated platform. Restraint apparatuses (Avian Restraint Device, Veterinary Specialty Products, Inc.; Miami Vice, Henry Shein, Port Washington, New York) are also appropriate for positioning and holding the patient (Fig. 40–6).

Table 40–2

ACCESS TO SURGICAL SITES FROM A LATERAL OR VD POSITION

	Lateral	VD
Lateral and dorsal head	+	0
Lateral neck and crop	+	+/−
Ventral crop	+/−	+
Thorax	+/−	+
Lateral abdominal	+	+/−
Ventral abdominal	+/−	+
Dorsum and uropygial gland	+	0
Wings	+	+
Legs	+	+
Tail	+/−	+

+ = accessibility; +/− = partial accessibility; 0 = inaccessible

TISSUE HANDLING

The characteristics of avian tissues differ considerably from those of mammalian tissues.[15–16] Avian skin is thin, relatively dry, has less tensile strength, is high in dermal and epidermal lipids, and is more delicate than mammalian skin, particularly in the neonate and pediatric patient. In obese birds with fatty deposition in the skin, tensile strength is further decreased and the skin tears easily, affecting suture placement. It is essential to manipulate the tissue gently to avoid sutures from tearing out. Large bites should be taken, sutures should not be

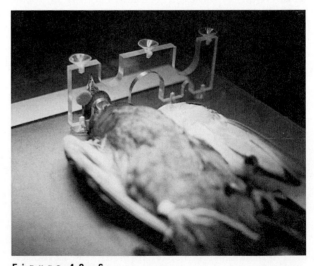

Figure 40–6

Avian restraint device restraining patient in ventrodorsal position.

cinched down tight, and excessive skin tension should be avoided.

Avian skin, partially because of the lack of subcutaneous tissue, has little elasticity and stretchability. Therefore, to accomplish closure, it is necessary to bluntly separate the skin from its underlying tissue. Skin elasticity over the ventral body surface is two to three times that of the dorsal body surface. Much of the skin covering the appendages has little to no elasticity, making closure difficult. It is sometimes necessary to make releasing incisions on either side of an incision to approximate skin closure.

Muscle fibers can split and tear with excessive manipulation. The abdominal musculature and peritoneum are thin, friable, and easily torn and traumatized with improper instrumentation. When handling viscera, a steady gentle hand is necessary, because these tissues have little tensile strength and tear easily. Because the quality of avian and mammalian tissues differs, the instrumentation used must be small, atraumatic, and gentle to the tissues. Rat-toothed forceps are traumatic to all avian tissues and should only be used if the teeth are very small.

The use of radiosurgery (see Chapter 43) permits rapid, gentle handling of avian tissue. Magnification and microsurgical instrumentation also ensure gentle atraumatic tissue handling.

EQUIPMENT AND INSTRUMENTATION

Because avian tissues require gentle, careful instrumentation, the most appropriate instruments are those used for delicate tissues in human and small animal surgery. Ophthalmic instruments are the most suitable for this purpose. Small Brown-Adson thumb forceps or iris forceps with very small teeth, and micro-mosquito hemostats are ideal for avian tissues. Tissue elevation can be accomplished with moist sterile cotton-tipped applicators or a fine tissue spatula (Castroviejo cyclodialysis spatula, Spectrum Surgical Instruments, Cleveland, OH) (Fig. 40–7A, B). Tissue and organ retraction can be accomplished with sterile cotton-tipped applicators; however, these applicators are drying to visceral tissue unless they have been freshly presoaked in

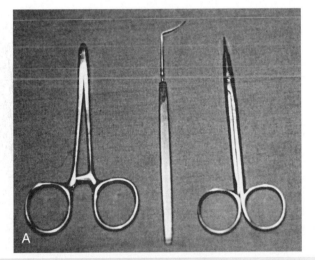

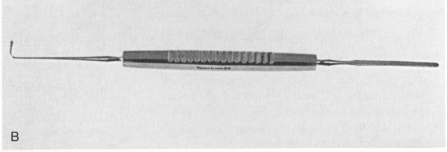

Figure 40–7

(A) (left to right) Small ophthalmic needle holder; Castroviejo cyclodialysis spatula; small straight iris scissors. *(B)* Knapp iris spatula and squint hook. (Courtesy Spectrum Surgical Instruments.)

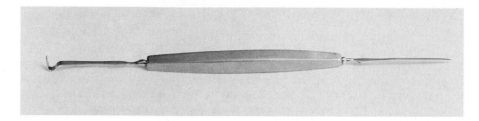

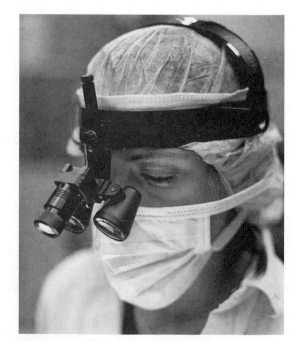

F i g u r e 4 0 – 8

Tissue retractor and tissue elevator. (Courtesy Veterinary Specialty Products, Inc.)

saline. A single instrument that can be used for blunt dissection, tissue elevation, and tissue retraction (VSP Tissue Retractor/Tissue Elevator, Veterinary Specialty Products, Inc.) minimizes changing instruments and is time-saving (Fig. 40–8).

Various styles of eyelid retractors are excellent retractors for intraabdominal and thoracic procedures. For small birds (budgerigars and cockatiels), Heiss retractors work well. For medium-size birds (conures and Amazon parrots), Alm retractors can be used, and for large birds (macaws), mini-Balfour retractors are appropriate.[2]

Various sizes and shapes of iris scissors (Fig. 40–7A) are the most appropriate for use as cutting instruments. Most tissue cutting should be performed with radiosurgical transsection (see Chapter 43). Hemostasis is effectively accomplished with radiosurgery. The use of a ball electrode or bipolar forceps offers the most practical hemorrhage control and decreases the need to ligate blood vessels. Maintaining a visual field by sponging should be performed with sterile cotton-tipped applicators or ophthalmic surgical spears (Microsponge, Alcon Surgical, Inc., Ft Worth, TX).[17] A simple atraumatic means of ligation is the use of Hemoclips (Weck Hemoclips, Solvay Animal Health, Inc., Mendota Heights, MN). Hemoclips are effective for ligating blood vessels and resected ends of organ tissue such as in the removal of the oviduct. Small and medium-size Hemoclips are the most suitable for avian surgery. An applicator is necessary for their placement. This type of tissue ligation places the least amount of tension on the tissues being ligated and is simple to apply, particularly when working deep in the body cavity.

Small ophthalmic and microsurgical needle holders are the most appropriate for suturing. Microsurgical needle holders are very well balanced with rounded handles so that they can be used with fingertip efficiency. Magnification permits more gentle tissue manipulation and offers the surgeon the best field of vision to accomplish surgical repair.

An operating microscope with a lens objective in the vicinity of 150 mm and a 12.5-mm binocular objective is the most practical.[18] A quality ocular loupe with a light source (Fig. 40–9) (Surgitel, General Scientific Corp., Ann Arbor, MI) can also be used for magnification in lieu of an operating microscope. Operating microscopes are indispensable and essential for use in surgical cases in which vascular and nerve damage has occurred, and in patients in which it is mandatory to restore normal function. The disadvantages of microsurgical technique are the increased surgical time required for a procedure, the need for microsurgical training and

F i g u r e 4 0 – 9

Magnification using an ocular loupe and halogen light. An ocular loupe offers a wide range of vision.

experience, the prerequisite of abstaining from alcohol and caffeine products, the expense of microsurgical equipment, and the space requirement for the operating microscope itself.

Good ocular loupes with an attached light source offer the surgeon more flexibility of movement and light direction. Using loupes does not necessitate the training required for microsurgical techniques or the length of surgical time required of an operating microscope, and are considerably less costly. For pinpoint lighting, when magnification head lamps are not available, light from an endoscopic light source can be used.[2, 19]

Suction is occasionally required in avian surgery. An excellent suction tip that can be used for both suction and coagulation is the Ellman suction coagulator (Ellman Suction Coagulator, Ellman International Corp., Hewlett, NY), which is supplied with interchangeable suction tips from 1/16-inch to 1/8-inch diameter. A hole in the handle permits fingertip control of the vacuum pressure and permits simultaneous coagulation.

TISSUE HEALING AND WOUND MANAGEMENT

Tissue healing results in a direct and immediate response to the tissue insult. Healing is dependent upon many factors, and the sequence of events determining wound healing occurs in stages. Mammalian wound healing was described in five stages[2, 20–21]: inflammatory, fibroplastic, epithelization, contraction, and remodeling stages. Others have reported wound healing in a three-phase sequence of events: inflammation, fibroplasia, and remodeling.[22–24] The inflammatory phase has been well documented in chickens.[25–29] Within the first 12 hours, mammalian and chicken skin respond similarly. Initially, hemorrhage is controlled by vasoconstriction, and then within 30 minutes vasodilatation occurs.[25] Within the first 2 to 5 hours, heterophils and monocytes infiltrate the margins of the traumatized tissue.[22, 25–26] Throughout this period, phagocytosis of bacterial, necrotic, and cellular debris occurs. Mononuclear cells (lymphocytes, monocytes, macrophages, and plasma cells) shift to the predominant cell type by the end of 12 hours and heterophils decrease.

Macrophages and multinucleated giant cells phagocytize the necrotic leukocytes that have accumulated at the margins of the necrotic tissue during their phagocytic activity. During this period and throughout the next few days, fibroblasts appear. This terminates the first phase of wound healing.

The next stage of wound healing, the fibroplastic phase, begins on the third or fourth day in chickens.[25] Fibroblasts synthesize collagen in the form of microfibrils. The microfibrils aggregate into larger fibers over a period of time.[22] Capillaries developing from surrounding vessels infiltrate the wound, and wound contraction occurs. Epithelial cells proliferate and migrate across the wound surface.[22, 30] The fibroplastic phase develops over a period of 14 to 15 days.

In the third and final stage of wound healing, there is a decrease in the number of fibroblasts, with remodeling of the collagen bed by thicker and stronger collagen fibers.

The last two stages of avian wound healing have not been documented, as has the first. It is thought that the final stage may take weeks to several months, as has been seen in mammalian studies. The quality of wound healing is based on the degree of bacterial contamination and the amount of tissue damage sustained. Surgical wounds created by scissor, scalpel, or electrosurgical incision in which strict asepsis has been maintained heal by primary intention in the shortest period of time. Factors influencing surgical wound healing are postsurgical contamination, reactivity to suture materials, motion, and tension at the incision site.

The rate of wound healing in traumatic injuries is affected by many factors. Traumatic injuries in wild and pet birds include lacerations, abrasions, punctures such as bite wounds or gunshot wounds, and thermal burns such as crop burns in baby birds. Treatment of wounds should include cleansing and debridement where possible, wound closure, and wound protection and covering.

Nonsurgical wounds should be debrided and all foreign material removed from the injury site. The wound should be cleansed with a dilute Betadine or a chlorhexidine solution. In wounds in which there is a considerable amount of necrotic tissue, a modified Dakin solution can be used as a mild oxidizing solution to clean up necrotic tissue.[31] Modified Dakin solution is a 1:10 dilution of household bleach and water, buffered to a pH of 7. This solution can mildly irritate normal tissue and can be used as a less expensive alternative to proteolytic enzymes.

Wound closure should have the least amount of tension possible. It is sometimes necessary to make releasing skin incisions to reduce tension. Covering both open and closed wounds acts as a barrier to microorganisms, as well as promotes healing and prevents scab formation, which impedes epithelial cell migration across the wound. Two products that have been used effectively in birds, particularly in wounds with large epithelial defects that have to granulate over large areas to heal, are a moisture and vaporpermeable dressing (Tegaderm, 3M Animal Care Products)[22–32] and an occlusive hydrocolloidal bandage (Dermaheal [DuoDerm], Squibb, Princeton, NJ).[33–34]

SUTURE MATERIALS AND PATTERNS

Selecting the suture material most appropriate for a specific procedure is dependent upon many factors.[35] This choice can be made by establishing a definitive set of criteria.

1. The nature of tissue into which the sutures are placed is a determining factor. As previously discussed, tissues have different qualities and tensile strengths, and therefore accommodate some suture materials better than others.

2. The degree of contamination and infection of the incision or wound is an important factor in the choice of suture material.[2, 36] Braided suture material has a wicking effect, potentially transporting microbes from infected to healthy tissue, and is therefore less suitable than monofilament.

3. Tying quality of suture material can be a factor, particularly when working in very small areas (body cavity, mouth) or working with fragile and friable tissue. Manipulation of the suture material can affect the tension placed on the tissue during the knot-tying process and, in some cases, can cause tearing of the tissue.

4. The amount of tissue reaction caused by the suture material should be minimal and is a factor in making a choice of material desired. The amount of tissue and inflammatory reactivity of the suture material is proportional to the ability of the suture material to potentiate infection.[2, 36]

5. The number of throws for tying the suture material is a factor. Some suture materials require three throws whereas others require five or six. Loosely tied knots are more easily picked opened and chewed by a bird's beak.

6. The absorption time of suture material is important, particularly when working in contaminated wounds. Too-rapid absorption of suture material in slow-healing wounds can predispose to wound dehiscence. The necessity or desire for suture removal also affects the surgeon's choice.

7. The final decision is the personal preference of the surgeon. Individual surgeons find working with some material uncomfortable, thus increasing suture placement time. Therefore, suture material qualities coupled with individual tissue requirements and the surgeon's confidence and experience with the suture material are factors influencing the material chosen.

Suture Material

Polyglactin 910 (Vicryl, Ethicon, Inc., Somerville, NJ) is a synthetic braided material. It produced the most intense inflammatory reaction in a study in noninfected wounds in pigeons,[37] causing separation of fiber strands with an influx of fibroblasts and phagocytic cells. However, the suture material had disappeared within 60 days of placement.[37] This reaction, however, is not found in mammals. This suture material has the best tying qualities, requiring three ties.

Polydioxanone (PDS, Ethicon, Inc.) created the least amount of tissue reaction,[37] but took 120 days for degradation. PDS is a monofilament with moderate to poor tying quality and requires four to five throws for knot tying.

Medium chromic catgut is a monofilament product creating a marked inflammatory reaction with delayed absorption (in excess of 120 days). This material has moderate to poor tying quality and requires three ties.

Of the nonabsorbable materials, *monofilament wire* and *mono- and multifilament stainless steel* are nonreactive and create minimal tissue reaction. *Nylon* has good tying quality and requires three ties whereas multifilament stainless steel has poor tying quality and requires two throws for knot tying.

In choosing suture materials, all of the characteristics described must be considered, as well as personal preference. Because of its tying quality, which permits gentle tissue handling, the relatively few throws required for knot tying, and moderately rapid absorption rate, this author's preference for sterile or noncontaminated wounds or incisions is Polyglactin 910, even though it was shown to have tissue reactivity. In grossly contaminated wounds, a nonreactive, slow-absorbing, monofilament material like PDS or a nonabsorbing material like nylon or stainless steel is preferred. Some surgeons[2] have a preference for stainless steel; however, this author finds that it has a tendency to cut through tissue, is more difficult to tie, and requires removal.

Suture Patterns

Suture patterns should be kept as simple and uncomplicated as possible. The primary aim of suture placement is to achieve closure of the wound or incision, using the least amount of suture material, minimizing tissue reaction, taking the least amount of time for placement, and creating the least amount of tension on the incision. Therefore, suture bites should be made far enough away from the incision margins to avoid their tearing out, far enough apart to decrease the amount of suture material used, but close enough to get good closure.

A simple continuous pattern is the pattern of choice, requires the least amount of suture material, can be placed in one-half the time of an interrupted pattern, and is the simplest to remove if nonabsorbable material is used. An interrupted pattern should be used in viscera for lumen closure; in a tissue where leakage is a possibility; or in areas in which the bird is more apt to scratch, pick, or chew at the incision site. Examples of such sensitive areas are the feet distal to the tarsometatarsal area, the cere, and face.

POSTOPERATIVE CARE

Although the immediate anesthetic and operative period is the most crucial, the postoperative period is of equal importance. It is essential during the postoperative period to monitor, support, and assist the patient to regain physiologic "normalcy" altered by the anesthetic and surgical period.

It is necessary to reestablish normal fluid balance,

which is altered by the stress from pain, anesthesia, blood loss, hypothermia, and hypotension caused by the release of epinephrine and norepinephrine.[38] The postoperative period extends from the time the anesthetic is discontinued to the point when the bird is perching, eating, and drinking, and when physiologic changes resulting from the anesthesia and surgery have been corrected.

Extubation should occur as soon as the swallowing reflex returns and the bird starts chewing on the endotracheal tube. After extubation, clearance of tracheal mucous plugs or regurgitated crop contents should be ensured. The patient should be positioned so that there is minimal movement to avoid orthostatic hypotension potentiated by hypothermia, hypovolemia, hypoglycemia, and postoperative pain. Many clinicians wrap the patient in a towel to conserve body heat and prevent excessive movement during recovery. Ambient temperature should be maintained at 85°F by a heating device until core body temperature approaches normal. Excessive heat can result in dilatation of vasoconstricted peripheral vessels in hypovolemic birds, and can increase the metabolic demand for glucose in hypoglycemic birds with the potential of creating acute death during recovery (see Chapter 46).

All monitoring devices should remain attached as long as possible to acquire postoperative data. The patient should be kept in an oxygen-enriched environment by the endotracheal tube or facemask as long as possible.

The clinician should prioritize correcting fluid and electrolyte imbalances created by the associated anesthetic and surgical stress. The body fluids are shifted away from the gastrointestinal tract, kidneys, and extremities and are redistributed to the heart and brain.[38] With surgically induced tissue trauma or moderate-to-severe blood loss, a release of epinephrine and norepinephrine can create further shifts in body fluids.[39] Blood flow away from the kidneys into the central circulation can result in reduced urine output, resulting in sodium and water retention.[38] If presurgical glucose levels were borderline or low (<200 mg/dl), monitoring postoperative blood glucose levels should be considered.

Pain is usually not a major problem in postoperative patients. If experienced, it is manifested by picking at the incision, continually shifting weight from one leg to the other, or general restlessness. Analgesics can be administered (see Chapter 46).

Rarely is there the necessity to collar a bird to prevent picking at the suture line. Procedures most likely to be associated with postoperative pain or discomfort are surgery of the beak, cere, and extremities, and orthopedic procedures. The patient should be allowed to recover in a small, quiet, semidarkened environment until it is capable of perching. Small plastic heated recovery tanks are suitable for this purpose.

When able to perch, the bird should be returned to its cage with food and water offered. The bird should be observed during this period to ensure that it is eating and drinking. Most birds take food and water shortly after recovery. It is essential to maintain adequate nutrition to restore the energy demands depleted during the surgical procedure and to nourish wound repair.[40]

When the bird is perching, moving about the cage freely and eating and drinking, the postoperative period has ended.

References

1. Murray MJ: Pre-Anesthetic evaluation and support of the avian patient. American Avian Vet Surgical Symposium, 1994, pp 7–11.
2. Bennett RA: Surgical considerations. In Ritchie, Harrison GJ, Harrison LR (eds): Avian Medicine: Principles & Application. Lake Worth, FL, Wingers Publishing, 1994, pp 1081–1095.
3. McCluggage DM: Surgical principles in birds. Avian and Exotic Animal Medicine Symposium, School of Veterinary Medicine, University of California, Davis, January, 1992, pp 27–31.
4. Altman RB: General principles of avian surgery: Comp Cont Ed Prac Vet 3:177–183, 1985.
5. Campbell TW: Selected blood biochemical tests used to detect the presence of hepatic disease in birds. Proceedings of the AAV, Miami, FL, 1986, pp 43–51.
6. Altman, RB: Heterologous blood transfusions in avian species. Proc Assoc Avian Vet, 1983, pp 28–32.
7. Stauber E, Washizuka A, Wilson E, Wardrop J: Crossmatching reactions of blood from various avian species. Proc 3rd Conference of the European Committee of the Association of Avian Vets, 1995, pp 142–144.
8. Sandmeier P, Stauber EH, Wardrop KJ, Washizuka A: Survival of pigeon red blood cells after transfusion into selected raptors. J Am Vet Med Assoc 204:427–429, 1994.
9. Harrison GJ: Evaluation and support of the surgical patient. In Harrison GJ, Harrison LR (eds): Clinical Avian Medicine and Surgery. Philadelphia, WB Saunders, 1986, pp 543–549.
10. Altman RB, Miller MS: Effects of anesthesia on the temperature and electrocardiogram of birds. Ann Proc Am Assoc Zoo Vet, Denver, 1979, pp 61–62a.
11. LaBonde J: Preparation and monitoring of the avian surgical patient. Avian Surgical Symposium, 1994, pp 36–38.
12. Jenkins JR: Evaluation of thermal support for the avian surgical patient. Proc Assoc Avian Vet, Houston, 1988, pp 153–157.
13. Ritchie BW: Anesthesia in birds. AAV Introduction to Avian Medicine and Surgery, 1991, pp S1–5.
14. Osuna DJ, DeYoung, DJ, Walker, RL: Comparison of three skin preparation techniques in the dog. Part 1: Experimental trial. Vet Surg 19:14, 1990.
15. Altman RB: Electrosurgery and tissue handling techniques. AAV Proc Avian Surgical Symposium, 1994, pp 18–19.
16. Altman RB: Introduction to avian surgery. AAV Practical Lab Proceedings and Manual, 1995, pp 39–43.
17. Curtis-Velasco M: Surgical instrumentation. Proc AAV Surgical Symposium, 1994, pp 1–6.
18. Doyle JE: Introduction to microsurgery. In Harrison GH, Harrison LR (eds): Clinical Avian Medicine and Surgery. Philadelphia, WB Saunders, 1986, pp 568–576.
19. Lupu C: Instrumentation. Proc AAV Surgical Symposium, 1994, pp 43–44.
20. Probst CW, Bright RM: Wound healing. In Slatter DH (ed): Textbook of Small Animal Surgery. Philadelphia, WB Saunders, 1985, pp 28–37.
21. Peacock EE: Wound Repair, ed 4. Philadelphia, WB Saunders, 1984, pp 1–140.
22. Degernes LA: Soft tissue wound management in avian patients. Proc Assoc Avian Vet, New Orleans, 1992, pp 476–483.
23. Bojrab MJ: A Handbook on Veterinary Wound Management, Boston, Kendall, 1981.
24. Fowler D: Principles of wound healing, In Harari J (ed): Surgical Complications and Wound Healing in the Small Animal Practice. Philadelphia, WB Saunders, 1993, pp 1–32.
25. Carlson HC, Allen JR: The acute inflammatory reaction in chicken skin: Blood cellular response. Avian Dis 13:817–833, 1969.
26. Awadhiya RP, Vegad JL, Kohle GN: Test studies on acute inflammation in the chicken using mesentery as a system. Res Vet Sci 29:122–180, 1980.
27. Degernes LA, Redig PT: Soft tissue wound management in avian patients. Proc Assoc Avian Vet, Phoenix, 1990, pp 182–190.
28. Jortner BS, Adams WR: Turpentine-induced inflammation in the chicken. A light- and electron microscope study with emphasis on the macrophage epithelioid cell, and multinucleated giant cell reaction. Avian Dis 15:533–550, 1971.
29. Jain NK, Vegad JG, Awadhiya RP: Studies on acute inflammation in the chicken using turpentine induced pleuroperitonitis as a test system. Vet Rec 110:421–422, 1982.
30. Johnston DE: The processes in wound healing. J Am Animal Hosp Assoc 13:186–196, 1977.
31. MacCoy D: Topical treatment of wounds. Am Avian Vet Today 2:99, 1988.
32. Degernes L: Wound management in avian patients. J Assoc Avian Vet 3:131, 1989.
33. Aguilar RF, Redig TP: The use of occlusive hydrocolloidal bandages in raptor wound management. Proc Am Assoc Zoo Vets 1991, pp 266–267.
34. Cambre RC: Use of DuoDerm hydroactive dressing (Convatec, Squibb) for wound healing in zoo animals. Proc Am Assoc Zoo Vets, 1984, pp 27–28.
35. Altman RB: Introduction to avian surgery. AAV Practical Lab Procedures Manual, 1995, pp 39–44.
36. Smeak DD, Wendelburg KL: Choosing suture material for use in contaminated or infected wounds. Comp Cont Ed Pract Vet 11:467–475, 1989.

37. Bennett RA, Yeager M, Trapp A, Cambre RC: Tissue reaction to five suture materials in pigeons. Proc Assoc Avian Vet, New Orleans, 1992, pp 212–218.

38. Jenkins JR: Postoperative care. Proc AAV Avian Surgical Symposium, 1994, pp 45–49.

39. Sturkie PD: Heart and circulation: Anatomy, hemodynamics, blood pressure, blood flow. In Sturkie PD (ed): Avian Physiology, ed 4. New York, Springer-Verlag, 1986, pp 130–166.

40. Layton CE: Nutritional support of the surgical patient. In Harari J (ed): Surgical Complications and Wound Healing in the Small Animal Practice. Philadelphia, WB Saunders, 1993, pp 89–121.

Robert B. Altman

41

Soft Tissue Surgical Procedures

For many years avian surgery remained one of the enigmatic aspects of avian practice. Only the most skilled, most adventuresome, or most foolhardy would attempt it.

The size of many patients, anatomic variations from mammalian species, friability of avian tissue, inaccessibility of organs in small body cavities, and sparsity of avian surgical literature discouraged many practitioners from performing even simple procedures. A major limiting factor was the anesthetic risk, particularly with prolonged procedures. Technical advances have reduced the surgical risk and have made avian surgery a reality for the average practitioner.

The introduction of isoflurane was a major step in decreasing surgical risk as well as making prolonged surgical procedures feasible. The introduction of radiosurgery, magnification, cryosurgery, and endoscopy has opened doors for the avian surgeon, and the availability of educational seminars and surgical workshops has made surgery possible for the beginning as well as the experienced avian practitioner.

Surgery is a modality requiring experience. Therefore, the practitioner should take every opportunity for practice before attempting a procedure on a client's bird. Working on dead birds offers experience in surgical anatomy; however, performing procedures on live specimens gives the surgeon the true feeling of avian tissue handling and hemostasis.

Wildlife cases requiring surgery provide an excellent way to become experienced in surgical technique as well as performing a public service and assisting conservation.

SURGERY OF THE HEAD

Ophthalmic Surgery

Eyelid, conjunctival, corneal, and eye globe problems requiring surgical intervention are frequently encountered. Eyelids can become deformed as the result of trauma, avian pox infection (Fig. 41–1), and rarely congenital atresia (Fig. 41–2), agenesis[1] and ankyloblepharon.[2]

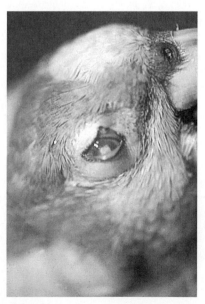

Figure 41–1

Notching of the upper eyelid of a blue-fronted Amazon parrot *(Amazona aestiva)* as the result of lid necrosis from psittacine pox. Surgical reconstruction of the lid was necessary.

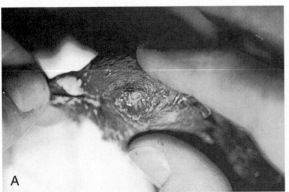
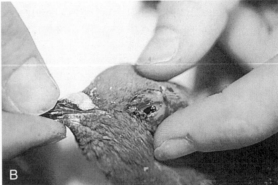

Figure 41-2

(A) Pigeon with congenital atresia of the eyelids. *(B)* Postoperative reconstruction of the eyelid.

Eyelid lacerations and deforming defects should be debrided and sutured with 5–0 or 6–0 absorbable suture material. The placement of the first suture is important for the recreation of the lid margins. Split thickness sutures prevent abrasions of the cornea by the suture material.[3]

A fairly common cause of corneal ulceration and epiphora resulting from exposure keratitis is ectropion of the lower eyelid. This idiopathic paresis is seen in cockatiels and umbrella cockatoos.[4] To correct the drooping of the inferior lid, a lateral canthoplasty can be performed. The margins of the eyelids at the lateral canthus are removed using scissors. A longer strip of eyelid is removed from the inferior lid to stretch and accommodate for the drooping eyelid. The length of lid removed depends on the laxity of the lower lid. A 5–0 to 6–0 absorbable suture is placed at the remaining ends of the lid margins using a split-thickness technique. The skin is then sutured, with sutures extending from the newly constructed lateral canthus laterally, closing only skin and not conjunctiva. A slight excess of skin remains ventrally that requires careful suture placement to avoid puckering of the suture line.

Another technique[4] requires removal of a thin strip of eyelid margin from the inferior and superior lids at the lateral and medial canthus. Approximately one-fourth of the eyelid length is excised. The eyelids are sutured together with 8–0 to 10–0 nylon in an interrupted pattern starting at the lateral extent of the incision and extending medially.

Problems of the ocular adnexa are uncommon. Obstruction of the lacrimal duct can occur from oxyspirurids and from an exudative plug resulting from a sinus infection. Occasionally, a large exudative plug lies under the nictitans (see Color Fig. 41–3) at the medial canthus. After removal of the exudative plug, the lacrimal puncta can be seen under the lower eyelid near the medial canthus. Using a lacrimal duct cannula or a microhematocrit pipette (Fig. 41–4), the lacrimal duct can be flushed.

Conjunctival masses forming on the nictitans are seen in cockatiels, sometimes causing irritation to the cornea. These masses are moderately vascular, and radiosurgery should be employed to excise them to avoid excessive hemorrhage. Conjunctival papillomas (see Color Fig. 41–5) are also readily excised with radiosurgical instrumentation.

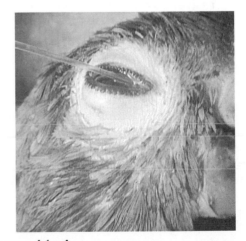

Figure 41-4

Cannulation and irrigation of the lacrimal duct obstructed with exudate.

Corneal ulceration is probably the most common lesion encountered in the avian eye. The associated keratitis can cause corneal edema with opacity of the cornea, lacrimation, epiphora, and rubbing of the eye. Trauma, eyelid abnormalities, and foreign bodies are the primary causes.

Corneal ulcers that do not respond to antibiotic therapy often respond to gentle debridement and a temporary tarsorrhaphy. If there is lipping of the margins of the corneal ulcer, gentle teasing of the ulcer margin with a moist cotton-tipped applicator frees the margins and then permits trimming of the ulcer margin with a number 11 or 15 scalpel blade. Because it is not possible to create a conjunctival flap or suture the nictitans because of its constant motion and friability, a tarsorrhaphy protects the cornea while it is healing. One or two horizontal mattress sutures using 4–0 to 6–0 nylon[5] can be used to keep the eyelid margins together. Alternatively, three to four simple interrupted sutures can be placed into the lid, exiting at the lid margins so that there is no rubbing of the cornea by the suture material.

Corneal and scleral lacerations can be sutured using 6–0 to 10–0 nylon. Although nylon necessitates removal under anesthesia, there is less reactivity to the suture material.

Lens removal is required as a consequence of cataract formation or lens luxation resulting from trauma. For large birds such as large raptors, ultrasonic phacoemulsification has been reported.[6] For smaller birds, extracapsular extraction[4, 7, 8] is the preferred surgical technique. Lens removal requires magnification using an operating microscope or ocular loupe. A small incision is made at the limbus at about five o'clock (Fig. 41–6) using a cataract knife or a number 11 scalpel blade.

The tip of a 26-gauge 1-inch needle is bent at an angle to form a small spur or hook. The needle is inserted into the anterior chamber through the incision opening. The spur is pulled across the anterior lens capsule, tearing it. The needle is then withdrawn and another needle is inserted into the lens through the torn lens capsule, and the lens material is flushed out through the anterior chamber with lactated Ringer's solution. The posterior lens capsule is left intact. The incision in the cornea is sutured with 6–0 to 10–0 nylon using an interrupted pattern.

Postoperative care requires cage rest with appli-

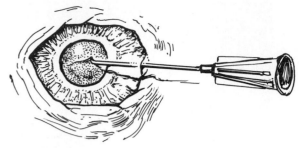

F i g u r e   4 1 – 6

After incision through the cornea at the limbus, the spur at the end of a hypodermic needle is inserted through the corneal incision and is pulled across the anterior lens capsule to lacerate the capsule, so that the lens material can be flushed out of the anterior chamber.

cation of an antibiotic-steroid ophthalmic ointment for a minimum of 14 days.

Eye Enucleation

Eye enucleation may be indicated because of trauma that does not respond to medical or surgical intervention, generalized bulbar infection, glaucoma, and neoplastic lesions.

Several methods of enucleation have been cited in the literature.[4, 9, 10] Karpinsky[9] advises evisceration of the eye for a more cosmetic appearance. The cornea and the lens and uvea are removed and the lids are trimmed and sutured, leaving the remnant of the globe within the orbit. This technique allows residual secretory tissue to remain within the orbit as a potential source of future infection. This author prefers to remove the entire globe.[10]

A circumferential incision is carefully made through the skin of the eyelids approximately 2 to 3 mm from the lid margins, with care to include all glandular tissue (Fig. 41–7A, B). Care must be taken to maintain the integrity of the palpebral conjunctiva. The palpebral conjunctiva and the skin of the eyelids are carefully bluntly dissected apart. The medial canthus has a fibrous attachment that must be dissected to completely isolate the lid margins. The lid margins are either sutured or clamped together with two Allis tissue forceps, and slight tension is placed on the dissected eyelids in a direction away from the globe. The palpebral conjunctiva is attached at the limbus (Fig. 41–8A, B) and gentle tension slightly changes the contour of the eyeball,

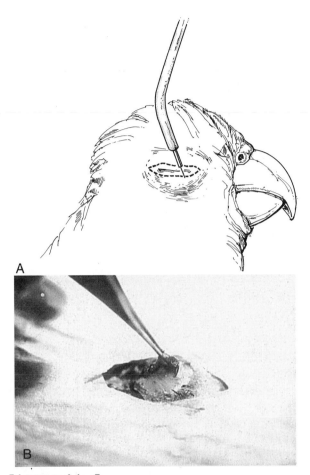

A

B

F i g u r e   4 1 – 7

(A) and *(B)* A circumferential skin incision encircling the eyelids is made 2 to 3 mm from the lid margins. Care must be taken to avoid incising through the palpebral conjunctiva.

possibility of hemorrhage from the neurovascular stump. Sealing the blood vessels using radiosurgical coagulation maintains hemostasis. Avoid excessive application of the coagulation electrode to the neurovascular stump to avoid excessive lateral heat buildup on the optic nerve. The stump should not be grasped with a hemostat in an attempt to curtail bleeding because of the risk of excessive tension on the optic chiasma. In instances in which hemorrhage cannot be adequately controlled, a piece of sterile gel foam can be used to pack off the socket. The eyelids are sutured with a simple interrupted pattern using 5–0 to 7–0 Vicryl. By leaving as much nonsecretory tissue as possible within the orbit, the

permitting access behind the eye yet not creating excessive tension on the optic nerve and the optic chiasma. Because the optic nerve is so short, excessive tension can affect the contralateral nerve, causing blindness.

The muscles and fat posterior to the eyeball are transected and a curved hemostat or hemoclip is placed around the optic nerve and accompanying blood vessels close to the eye globe. With a curved scissors, the neurovascular bundle is then incised as close to its attachment at the base of the eye as possible. If there is insufficient space to insert a hemostat or hemoclip applicator, the neurovascular bundle can be cut with a curved scissors, and the globe and surrounding fat and glandular tissue are removed. Clamping the blood vessels decreases the

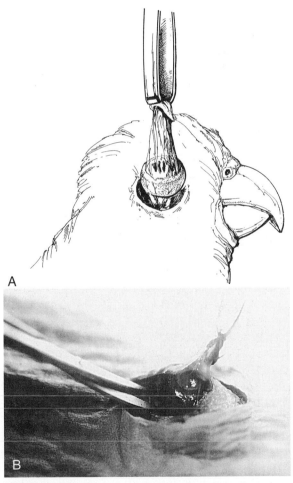

A

B

F i g u r e   4 1 – 8

(A) The separated lid margins and palpebral conjunctiva attached at the limbus are drawn away from the eye, placing tension at the limbus. *(B)* A curved scissors is placed behind the eye to transect the optic nerve and accompanying vascular supply.

sutured eyelids develop less concavity with a more cosmetically acceptable result.

If any secretory tissue is retained within the orbit, a draining fistula can result postoperatively (see Color Fig. 41–9). If this occurs, the eyelids should be reopened and the tissue removed.

Another technique[4] partially collapses the eye globe by incising the cornea and expressing the lens and vitreous. The eye does not totally collapse because of the scleral ossicles. Partial collapse of the eye globe permits easier access behind the eye to the optic nerve.

For cosmetic purposes, an ocular prosthesis can be implanted to prevent sinking in of the sutured eyelid.[4]

Surgery of the Ear

Few problems require surgical intervention pertaining to the ear. This author has seen otitis externa with exudative plugs that required curettage. Occasionally, hard beads of dried exudate must be removed from the ear to treat the ear topically. Both benign[11] and malignant tumors (see Chapter 33) of the ear have been reported. Tumors of the avian ear can be difficult to reach because of the small size of the ear canal. Both radiosurgical and cryosurgical techniques have been employed to remove these masses.

Surgery of the Mouth

Surgical problems of the beak are well detailed in Chapters 44A and 44B. Surgery of the mouth includes lancing and curetting abscesses found on the surface of the tongue and along the choana and palate. These abscesses are most frequently associated with hypovitaminosis A. Lancing and curetting of these abscesses, most of which are sterile inclusion cysts if associated with vitamin A deficiency, usually enhance healing and offer the bird relief of discomfort. If the condition has progressed to the point where many large inclusion cysts are present, these cysts can interfere with eating and, if severe enough, with breathing.

Occasionally, a single large abscess develops at the base of the tongue, interfering with tongue function. This abscess can be seen at the ventral depression of the mandible as a white nodule. By incising over the central aspect of the abscess and curetting out the exudative content of the nodule, the tongue returns to normal with correction of the diet and vitamin supplementation. When incising and curetting the abscess, care should be exercised not to injure any of the vital structures of the tongue.

Lacerations of the tongue are seen with moderate frequency. A simple interrupted suture using 5–0 to 6–0 Vicryl after careful debridement of the epithelial margins results in rapid uneventful healing. The tongue of birds, particularly psittacine birds, is such a vital structure for the bird's ability to eat that it is important to conserve as much tissue as possible after severe trauma.

Papillomas of the mouth are easy to remove using radiosurgery.

SURGERY OF THE GASTROINTESTINAL SYSTEM

Extraabdominal surgical procedures, aside from problems of the oral pharynx already addressed, include problems associated with the crop and esophagus.

Crop

Lacerations of the crop, necrotizing lesions such as those caused by ingestion of caustic material (biting off the tip of a silver nitrate stick), thermal burns from the ingestion of hot microwaved food in hand-fed babies, crop fistulas from trauma, ingestion of foreign bodies, and crop calculi may require a surgical approach to the crop. In instances in which the crop must be entered, all attempts should be made to remove foreign objects via endoscopy through the mouth before ingluviotomy is attempted.

Ingluviotomy

The size of the incision into the crop is based on the size of the instruments being inserted or the foreign body to be removed. The tissues of the crop have the capacity to stretch; however, the incision should be of sufficient length that the foreign material can be removed without force. This minimizes trauma to the crop.

A skin incision is made over the left side of the crop near the thoracic inlet. Care should be taken to avoid incising the wall of the crop, particularly when radiosurgery is employed. The skin is bluntly separated from the crop and an incision of sufficient length made into the crop. If an endoscopic approach is needed, a simple stab wound into the crop will suffice. If endoscopic examination of the proventriculus is desired, the endoscope can easily be passed into the esophagus to reach the proventriculus.

Closure of the crop is made with a simple interrupted pattern using 3–0 to 5–0 absorbable sutures. The sutures should be close enough to prevent leakage of fluid.

When repairing a crop fistula from thermal burns, it is mandatory to permit the burned tissue enough time to demarcate before surgical debridement is attempted. As a result of the burn, sclerosing vessels can cause tissue necrosis beyond the debrided wound margins, causing wound dehiscence.

Closure is in two layers, as described in the section on ingluviotomy. If the area of necrosis is large and the skin and crop cannot be dissected apart, a single-layer closure is possible after thorough debridement of the fistula margins extending to healthy tissue. A simple interrupted pattern of 5–0 to 7–0 nylon should be used.

Esophagus

Esophageal Stricture

Strictures of the esophagus have been reported in a duck[12] and in a hyacinth macaw.[13] Both strictures were in the thoracic esophagus and required three bougienage treatments. The etiology was unknown and both birds recovered and were able to eat normally following treatment.

A lubricated rubber feeding tube slightly larger than a tube that was previously introduced without resistance was passed down the esophagus and, at the point of resistance, was gently forced through the strictured area. Several weeks[12] to several months[13] later, another tube slightly larger than the first was passed through the strictured area. A third bougienage treatment was repeated at an equal

interval. The birds started eating after the first tube was passed and continued to eat thereafter.

Esophageal Laceration and Perforation

Trauma to the anterior esophagus occurs as the result of excessive force while using a rigid or rubber feeding tube when feeding baby birds. Even experienced aviculturists puncture through the esophagus while attempting to feed many birds or as the result of aggressive head-bobbing by a hungry chick. If the laceration is recognized when it occurs, immediate attempts at repair should be made. However, the problem is usually not discovered until days after the incident occurs. Food material is deposited or leaks into the extra-esophageal subcutaneous space. A severe inflammatory response soon becomes infected, causing toxic effects.

For immediate repair, incision into the cervical subcutaneous area around the laceration should be followed by thorough irrigation of the area to remove all food particles, debridement of necrotic tissue, and debridement of the margins of the lacerated esophagus. Closure is accomplished with 5–0 to 7–0 polydioxanone (PDS) using an inverted mattress suture placed close together to prevent leakage.

If the lesion is not discovered until abcessation has taken place, the area should be irrigated and debrided, and the necrotic subcutaneous tissue and fascia should be removed. Placement of a proventricular feeding tube[4] bypasses the perforation and should be kept in place until surgical repair of the esophagus can be undertaken 5 to 7 days later. Fourteen to 21 days of antibiotics should be administered to prevent abcessation.

Foreign bodies lodged in the anterior esophagus should be removed through the mouth using endoscopic grasping forceps. If the foreign body is lodged and cannot be brought out through the mouth, attempts should be made to push it into the crop after lubrication. A simple ingluviotomy incision then facilitates its removal. For foreign bodies lodged in the posterior esophagus, retrieval should be attempted through an incision in the crop, or attempts should be made to push the foreign body into the proventriculus and its removal facilitated by a proventriculotomy or ventriculotomy.

Approaches to the Abdominal Cavity

Transabdominal Laparotomy (Celiotomy)

Several abdominal approaches are possible with the patient restrained in a ventrodorsal position: (1) ventral midline; (2) transabdominal; (3) abdominal flap.

The choice of incisional approach to the coelomic cavity depends upon the location of the lesion within the abdominal cavity. Five basic incisional approaches have been described[4, 10, 11, 14] and are illustrated in (Fig. 41–10).

A ventral midline incision (see Fig. 41–10) extending from the caudal border of the sternum to just cranial to the cloaca offers limited exposure to the anterior abdomen. Exposure to the caudal abdomen permits visualization of the cloaca. Retraction of the incisional opening is restricted because of the limitations of the length of the incision. The only advantage of this approach is that it offers exposure to the caudal aspect of the cloaca.

A partial- or full-flap incision (Fig. 41–10) offers better access to the anterior abdominal cavity but can cause weakness in the abdominal wall and permit exposure to only one side of the cavity. A double abdominal flap offers access to the entire

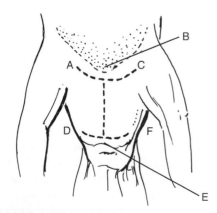

F i g u r e 4 1 – 1 0

Ventral approaches to the abdominal cavity. B-E: Ventral midline incision; A-B-E: partial-flap incision; A-B-E-D: full-flap incision; A-B-E-D + C-B-E-F: double abdominal flap incision; A-B-C: transabdominal incision.

caudal abdomen but further weakens the abdominal wall.

A transabdominal incision (Fig. 41–10) offers access to both sides of the abdomen with full visualization of the posterior abdomen and offers the least potential for abdominal wall weakening.

A lateral approach offers the greatest exposure to the cranial abdomen and the posterior thoracic region. Its limiting disadvantage is that it permits access to only one side of the abdomen (coelomic cavity).

Surgical Approaches to the Abdomen and Thorax

All ventral abdominal approaches into the abdomen require simple linear incisions through both the skin and abdominal musculature.

The abdominal skin should be grasped with forceps and tented off the abdominal musculature. A small stab incision is made in the skin and the incision is extended to the desired length (Fig. 41–11*A*). The abdominal musculature is then elevated off the abdominal viscera. A stab incision through the abdominal muscles and peritoneum is followed by incision of these structures in one direction, and then in the opposite direction (Fig. 41–11*B*). By tenting the skin and muscles, the surgeon avoids inadvertently lacerating underlying viscera. Particular care should be taken with a patient exhibiting abdominal distension. A tumor or enlarged organ can elevate the abdominal viscera against the abdominal wall, increasing the risk of visceral laceration.

For a *transabdominal approach,* the length of the incision should be sufficient to offer adequate exposure within the abdominal cavity. It is possible to extend the incision from the groin of one leg to the groin of the opposite leg, extending across the entire abdomen.

It is important when making a transabdominal incision that the incision be made parallel and 2 to 4 mm distal to the caudal margin of the sternum to allow for adequate closure of the abdominal muscles.

On entry into the abdominal cavity the supraduodenal loop containing the pancreas is found in the bird's right quadrant. The right liver lobe can be visualized in some birds. The ventriculus is found in

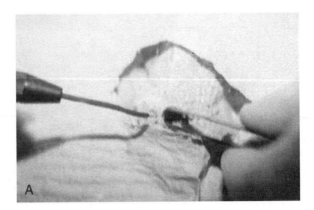

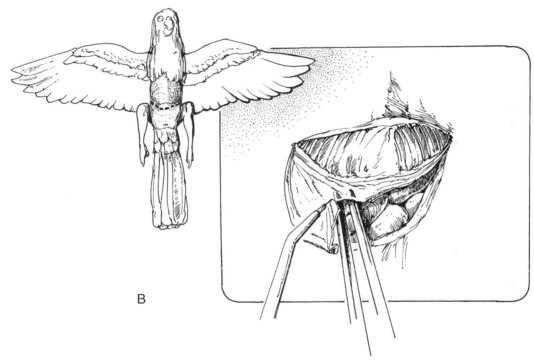

Figure 41-11

(A) The skin is elevated off the abdominal muscles and a small stab incision is made in the skin. A pair of forceps is placed into the opening; the skin is elevated off the abdominal muscles and is incised. *(B) (Left)* The skin incision for a transabdominal laparotomy should be made 2 to 4 mm distal to the caudal border of the sternum. *(Right)* The abdominal muscles are tented off the abdominal viscera with forceps and the muscles are incised.

the left abdominal hemisphere distal to the sternal border. By entering the left side of the abdomen to reach the abdominal organs, the air sacs are compromised. An incision must be made in the air sac of sufficient size to offer adequate exposure. Upon opening the air sacs, anesthetic gas escapes into the operating room, and frequently the bird's anesthetic level decreases and the patient can start to awaken from anesthesia. Momentarily holding

the incision closed or increasing the gas flow can bring the bird back to a satisfactory anesthetic plane. Closure of the skin and muscles should be accomplished using a two-layer technique with a continuous pattern of absorbable suture material. A transabdominal incision is this author's preferred approach for ventriculotomy and other procedures when access to both sides of the abdomen is necessary.

When performing intraabdominal surgery, magnification enhances visualization of the operative field.

Approach to the left lateral abdomen requires an oblique skin incision in the paralumbar fossa just caudal to the last rib, extending from the proximal end of the pubis to the sixth rib dorsal to the uncinate process.[14] Intercostal vessels run along the cranial border of the ribs and are vulnerable to transsection and hemorrhage, particularly at the dorsal portion of the rib. Proper coagulation of these vessels is necessary to avoid excessive hemorrhage. The left leg should be pulled and held caudally.

Incision through the lateral abdominal muscles may be extended across the distal end of the seventh and eighth ribs. Some authors advocate removal of these ribs[4, 11, 14] in species larger than conures. This author prefers to avoid removal of these ribs because closure is less difficult, particularly with larger birds. Retraction is necessary to maintain adequate exposure. Small mini-Balfour, Heiss, Alm,[4] Graefe, or other ophthalmic lid retractors can be used.

On entering the coelomic cavity the thoracic air sacs can be visualized. These air sacs can be seen as two thin clear semiopaque membranes merging at an acute angle to each other. To reach the gonads and caudal abdominal viscera, these air sacs must be incised. The left lobe of the lung can be visualized in the anterior aspect of the thoracic cavity.

Closure using a simple continuous pattern often suffices. Occasionally, it may be necessary to place a few interrupted sutures around the last rib to pull the incision together. The abdominal wall under the cranial aspect of the anterior thigh muscle is often thin and has poor suture-holding quality. Good closure of the lateral abdominal wall ensures an adequate seal and avoids air leakage with the potential for subcutaneous emphysema. This approach offers good access to the proventriculus, gonads, adrenal gland, oviduct, and cranial lobe of the kidney.

Proventriculotomy

Indications for proventriculotomy include removal of foreign material including food impaction, heavy metal and other ingested material that could not be removed via endoscopy, removal of foreign bodies from the ventriculus, and biopsy for confirmation

of myenteric ganglioneuritis (psittacine proventricular dilatation syndrome PPDS).[4, 15, 16]

In psittacines, the left lateral approach offers the greatest exposure of the proventriculus. The ventral suspensory ligaments are carefully bluntly dissected to permit elevation of the proventriculus to the opening of the incision.

The proventriculus varies in different species and in many is thin-walled and friable. The blood vessels of the proventricular wall are readily visualized. Stay sutures should be placed in the ventriculus, just distal to the isthmus (junction of proventriculus and ventriculus) and, with gentle traction, the proventriculus is elevated to the incision opening. The proventricular wall is fragile in many species, particularly carnivorous birds. Care should be taken when applying traction to this organ. An incision is made into the proventriculus from the isthmus cranially, avoiding as many surface blood vessels as possible (Fig. 41–12).

Before entering the proventriculus, the surgical area should be packed off with saline-soaked sponges to avoid leakage of proventricular and ventricular fluid into the coelomic cavity. Proventricular contents should be gently removed using atraumatic scoops or forceps with suction. Care should be taken to avoid removal of large objects through too small a proventricular incision, because the tissue tears easily. The proventriculus is closed with a simple continuous pattern using a fine monofila-

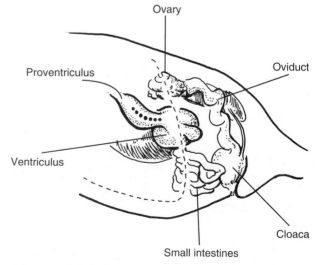

F i g u r e   4 1 – 1 2

The incision into the proventriculus is started at the isthmus and extended cranially *(dotted line)*.

ment long-lasting absorbable suture (PDS) with a small swedged-on atraumatic needle. Bites in the proventricular wall should be fairly close together to obtain good apposition of the incision margins. Placement of a second inverting suture pattern oversewing the first suture line can be an interrupted or continuous pattern and should extend beyond both ends of the first suture line to avoid leakage. By maintaining good apposition on the first suture line, and oversewing with fairly close bites on the inverting suture pattern, there is less chance of leakage, which is reported with moderate frequency.[15]

Carefully infusing saline into the proventriculus via a feeding tube can aid in detecting incisional leakage. Leakage is more likely to occur on the third to fifth postoperative day, because wound strength is diminished from the immediate postoperative period.[4] The bird should be permitted to eat immediately after surgery; however, the food should be offered in frequent small portions to avoid overdistension.

Because the omentum is lacking in birds, it has been postulated that the increased potential for leakage results from the lack of an omental seal.[4, 15]

Surgical complications are seen with greater frequency in birds than mammals. Therefore, all attempts of endoscopic-guided emptying of the proventriculus from the crop should be exhausted before proventriculotomy is attempted.

The approach to proventriculotomy in the ostrich chick[17] is through a ventral midline incision. The ventriculus can be exposed by blunt dissection just caudal to the sternum (xiphoid process). The ventral serosal surface of the exposed proventriculus is sutured to the skin to minimize leakage and contamination into the coelomic cavity. The surgical field is packed off with saline-soaked gauze and the proventriculus is incised. The impacted material is removed after the proventricular flush is suctioned off, and the proventriculus is closed as previously described.

Ventriculotomy

Several surgical approaches for ventriculotomy have been described. Some surgeons prefer a lateral abdominal approach[4] and incise through the proventriculus by extending a proventricular incision caudally through the isthmus and dilating the open-

ing adequately to remove the ventricular contents by instrumentation (Fig. 41–12). This technique eliminates the necessity to incise the ventriculus, which is felt to be more difficult to seal.

This author has been successful using a transabdominal approach and isolating the ventriculus (Fig. 41–13A). It is necessary to break through the abdominal air sacs to reach the ventriculus. The small fatty ligament attached to the ventriculus should be carefully dissected off the surface of the ventriculus, while attempting to maintain the integrity of the gastric blood vessels. The lighter colored, thin-muscled elliptical area of the ventriculus can then be visualized (Fig. 41–13B). This area often pouches out from the ventricular surface. These muscle fibers course in a different direction from the heavily muscled ventriculus and can be palpated by running a finger down the medial surface of the ventriculus (Fig. 41–13B) and finding the soft depression of this muscle in the thick-walled ventriculus.

A stab incision is made transversely across the ellipse (Fig. 41–13C) and the foreign material is removed. Care should be taken to avoid traumatizing the margins of the ventricular incision. Usually, only a single-layer, noninverting simple interrupted suture pattern can be placed in this area; 5–0 to 7–0 PDS with a small atraumatic swedged on needle is used. The sutures should be placed close together to avoid leakage. One author[18] suggests a two-layer simple interrupted closure of the ventriculus after making an incision into the heavily muscled wall of the distal ventriculus. It is difficult to get full access into the ventriculus with this technique.

Gastrointestinal Alimentation

In some instances, areas of the upper gastrointestinal tract require bypassing for periods of time exceeding 24 to 48 hours. Injuries to the oral pharyngeal area, proximal esophagus, or crop may necessitate placement of a pharyngostomy feeding tube.[4] Disease processes such as severe trichomoniasis or candidiasis causing damage to the mucosa of these organs or surgical intervention in which time is needed for healing require placement of a pharyngostomy tube.

This simple procedure takes only a few minutes to accomplish. The feathers from the right cervical area are plucked and the area is surgically prepared. A feeding tube is placed into the esophagus just

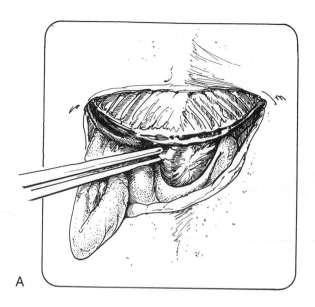

A

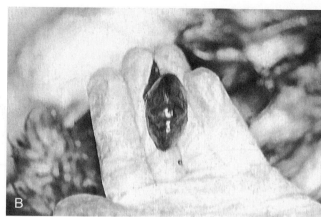

B

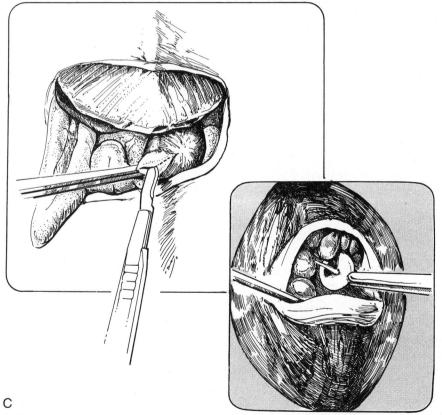

C

Figure 41-13

(A) Reflecting the fatty ligaments attached to the ventriculus, the ventriculus can be grasped and elevated to the opening of the abdominal incision on the left side of the abdomen. Note the duodenal loop encircling the pancreas on the right abdominal quadrant. *(B)* The elliptical thin-muscled area of the ventriculus pouches out from the surface of the ventriculus with muscle fibers coursing in a horizontal direction. *(C)* A stab incision is made into the proventriculus, and the foreign material is removed without stretching or traumatizing the margins of the incision.

distal to the mandible. A small skin incision reveals the esophagus distended by the feeding tube. A 1-mm to 2-mm incision is made in the esophagus and as one tube is slowly withdrawn, a second is passed through the skin incision into the esophageal incision and passed down into the crop or distal esophagus. The feeding tube is sutured to the skin incision, and the feeding tube is folded and bandaged to the dorsal neck area to prevent the bird from picking at it. After removal of the pharyngostomy tube, the skin and esophagus are allowed to granulate and heal.

Totally bypassing the oral pharyngeal area, anterior esophagus, and crop can be accomplished by placement of the feeding tube directly into the crop and distal esophagus,[18] using an ingluviotomy incision previously described.

When it is necessary to bypass the distal esophagus, proventriculus, or ventriculus, a duodenostomy tube can be inserted. This procedure was described in pigeons.[19] A ventral midline incision exposes the duodenal loop in the right posterior abdominal quadrant. The pancreas separates the ascending from the descending duodenum.

An indwelling jugular catheter is passed through the left abdominal wall and into the descending duodenum and advanced along the ascending loop approximately 4 to 6 cm. The jugular catheter should not have a diameter greater than one-third the diameter of the duodenum. After the needle is withdrawn from the catheter, the duodenum is sewn to the body wall with one or two 5–0 Prolene sutures to stabilize the duodenum and seal the opening of the duodenum and the body wall. The abdominal incision is closed with a standard two-layer technique. The catheter is secured to the body wall and sutured in place to the skin. The catheter is brought cranial to the leg, and the excess is coiled and sutured to the left lateral body wall under the wing. The catheter should be flushed with saline and capped off with an injection cap. Formula should be fed four to six times daily at a rate of 1 ml per 15 seconds. The catheter should be flushed with saline or sterile water before and after each feeding to prevent clogging of the feeding tube. The catheter should not be removed until the fifth day to allow the duodenum to adhere to the body wall and seal off. After removal of the catheter, the wound into the duodenum should be allowed to close on its own.

With some birds, it is necessary to use a restraining collar to prevent the bird from pulling at the catheter.

Intestinal Surgery

Surgery of the intestinal tract is required as the result of lodged foreign bodies, penetrating abdominal wounds, iatrogenic lacerations of loops of bowel created during laparotomy approach, and biopsy.

For cage birds, it is essential to perform these procedures with magnification, because the diameter of the intestines is small and the suture material required for repair is 7–0 to 10–0, requiring microsurgical instrumentation. Using larger diameter suture material potentiates stricture and occlusion. For larger species, ophthalmic instrumentation will suffice; however, magnification is beneficial.

Cloacal Surgery

The three problems requiring cloacal surgery are cloacal papillomas, cloacal mucosal inflammation and hypertrophy, and cloacal prolapse.

Cloacal papillomas present as cherry-like clusters of red mucosal tissue often prolapsing from the vent. Some papillomas are pedunculated and intermittently extrude from the cloaca and then retract back into the cloaca. These papillomas can be resected using radiosurgery or removed with cryosurgery. Because of the vascularity, scissor or scalpel blade removal results in a great deal of bleeding, which is frequently difficult to control.

Inflammation and hypertrophy of the cloacal mucosa at the mucocutaneous junction result in the appearance of a cherry-red mass of tissue protruding intermittently or continuously from the cloacal opening. The etiology of this condition is unknown and can probably be equated to hemorrhoids in mammals.

The primary concern for both cloacal conditions is that the mucosa becomes inflamed, ulcerates, and bleeds. This condition can cause discomfort to the bird and can initiate tenesmus, which exacerbates the problem. The sooner surgical intervention takes place, the better the prognosis. This author has seen chronic mucosal infection lead to ascending infections to the ureters and kidneys.

Radiosurgical reduction of hypertrophied mucosa or cryosurgical freezing of the tissue offers the least amount of blood loss, which is substantial with scalpel blade resection. Packing off the cloaca with gauze sponges often controls bleeding. It is essential to be sure to resect only the mucosal layer, leaving the muscularis intact.

After cryosurgery, the affected tissue usually necroses and sloughs by the sixth to ninth postoperative day. Some clinicians use antibiotic steroidal ointments postoperatively to decrease inflammation, infection, and discomfort.

Cloacapexy

The etiology of cloacal prolapse is unknown. It appears that there is a neuromuscular deficit of the cloacal wall and often the cloacal sphincter, with loss of sphincter tone. This condition is seen most frequently in Old World psittacines, particularly cockatoos. It has been postulated that a chronic gram-negative enteritis may be the initiating factor[20]; however, many cases are seen in which repeated cloacal cultures revealed no gram-negative bacteria.

Because of the loss of muscle tone of the cloacal wall and cloacal sphincter, innervation to this structure seems to be the problem; however, this has not been confirmed histopathologically. A breakdown of cloacal attachment has been reported.[21]

It is essential to differentiate between cloacal prolapse, hypertrophy, and papilloma. On physical examination, the cloaca should be visually explored without anesthesia to evaluate muscle tone and visualize the mucosa. Differentiation and identification of these three diseases are not difficult.

Many practitioners have employed the use of either pursestring[18] or transverse stay sutures[4, 18] in the cloaca to treat this condition. The only advantage in using this technique is to prevent the prolapsing tissue from drying out and becoming traumatized, ulcerated, and infected, and allowing enough time for treatment to reduce inflammation, swelling, and infection prior to surgery.

Two simple interrupted sutures are placed[21] equidistant across the cloaca at approximately one-third and two-thirds the distance across the cloacal opening (Fig. 41–14).

It is critical to permit adequate passage of fecal material when using a pursestring or interrupted sutures or a mattress suture to prevent prolapse. This can be done by placing a feeding tube of suitable size into the cloaca and tying a pursestring suture gently down to the feeding tube and then withdrawing the feeding tube. One author[4] has experienced cloacal atony as a result of nerve damage after application of a pursestring suture; however, this author has used this technique without untoward results.

Small shallow parallel bites passing only through the skin are placed near the point at which the sphincter extends from the body wall. Three–0 to 5–0 nylon suture material with a fine-curve cutting edge needle is used. There should be from five to six bites, depending upon the size of the bird. When tying the knot, both ends of the suture material should be pulled with equal tension, but not cinched down tight on the sphincter.

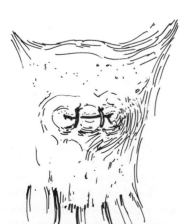

F i g u r e 4 1 – 1 4

Two simple interrupted sutures or a mattress suture is placed across the cloacal opening, leaving a sufficient opening for urine and feces to pass.

A number of techniques and modifications are used to permanently stabilize and reduce cloacal prolapse. The goal of this procedure is to prevent recurring partial or complete prolapse by suturing the cloaca to intraabdominal structures.

One technique described[21] approaches the cloaca via a ventral abdominal incision. The cloaca is pushed forward by inserting a gloved finger or an atraumatic probe into the cloacal orifice and distending the cloaca cranially and ventrally toward the incision opening. It is essential to remove any fat attached to the cloacal wall.

Stay sutures penetrating the cloacal mucosa are placed at the cranial lateral aspect of the cloaca at 10 and 2 o'clock. The sutures are passed around the last rib on each side and tied with enough tension to slightly invert the cloacal opening.

If the cloaca extends far enough anteriorly that the rib stay sutures are not sufficient to create enough tension, the stay sutures can be fixed to the cranial border of the sternum. Sutures are then placed in the lateral and ventral cloacal wall and sutured to the abdominal musculature. The author suggested using Vicryl; however, the degradation of Vicryl is too rapid and a longer-lasting material such as PDS should be used.

This author used a technique[10] employing a transverse abdominal approach combining the use of four stay sutures that were placed through the lateral cloacal margins and were passed around the pubis (Fig. 41–15; see also color figure). The cloaca was distended craniad with a lubricated gloved finger or an atraumatic probe (lubricated cotton-tipped applicator) and a transabdominal incision was made just cranial to the cranial border of the distended cloaca. This incision usually bisected the abdomen halfway between the sternal border and the cloacal orifice. After placement of the stay sutures, the cranial aspect of the cloacal serosa is incised and the cloacal submucosa is sutured to and incorporated into the abdominal wall closure. It is felt that a transverse abdominal incision provides even distribution of tension compared with a ventral midline approach.[20] A transabdominal incision without the benefit of stay sutures has had equally rewarding results.

A technique described by Jenkins[22] uses a ventral midline incision. A small (2–5 mm) vertical incision is made in the wall through the cloacal serosa 5 to 10 mm from the midline. A paramedian incision is

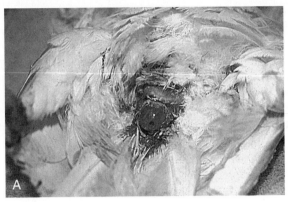

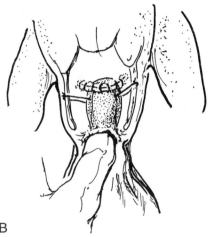

Figure 41–15

(A) Prolapsed cloaca in a cockatoo. Note the rectal opening. *(B)* Performing a cloacopexy. Stay sutures are placed around the pubis and through the lateral cloacal wall. The subserosa at the cranial border of the cloaca is sutured to the abdominal incision during closure.

then made into the peritoneum and the body wall corresponding to the cloacal incision so that the serosal surface of the peritoneum and the cloaca can be sutured together. A second similar incision is made 5 to 10 mm to the opposite side of the midline, and these serosal surfaces are apposed and sutured. Jenkins' approach appears to have equally good results but is more difficult and time-consuming.

Regardless of the technique used, it is essential to place enough cranial tension on the cloaca to prevent recurrence, and it is necessary to develop a subserosal seal between the cloaca and the peritoneal surface.

A percutaneous technique,[23] although noninvasive, has inherent risks. Two to three sutures are passed through the abdominal wall into the cloaca and back out through the abdominal wall. Because this technique is used only to get the bird through a temporary period (2 to 4 weeks), the risk of perforating or lacerating a visceral organ or entrapping the ureters makes this technique too risky to be practical. It is essential to digitally push the cloaca up against the abdominal wall when placing the sutures to avoid the hazards described earlier. The sutures are removed in 2 to 4 weeks.

Another technique described[4] to permanently keep a flaccid cloaca from prolapsing is to remove one-half to three-quarters of the margin of the cloacal sphincter and then suture the remaining sphincter to permanently reduce the size of the cloacal opening. Complications associated with this technique include the bird's inability to pass feces and the potential for adhesions and stricture.

Adhesions of the cloaca can also occur as the result of surgical correction of cloacal hyperplasia or cloacal papillomatosis. Successful treatment of such a case employed a combination of manual dilation and nutrition rehabilitation.[24]

SURGERY OF THE RESPIRATORY SYSTEM

The cere of birds, particularly psittacine birds, is a sensitive vascular structure. Trauma to this structure is infrequent; however, severe distortion to the cere and nostril can result from the formation of a rhinolith.[4] Secretions from a chronic sinus infection or rhinitis become caseous and harden to a firm mass that is dry and hard on the surface. As the infection progresses, the rhinolith becomes larger and can cause a huge disfiguring crater in the nostril. These bead-like rhinoliths must be gently separated from the wall of the nasal cavity. Care must be taken as the caseous mass is removed from the nasal cavity, because trauma to the operculum or nasal conchae results in bleeding that can be difficult to control. It is often possible to elevate the entire caseous mass out of the nasal cavity using a small ear curet (Fig. 41–16*A*). In other instances, the mass must be removed piecemeal and the soft exudate under the mass must be gently debrided and removed from the cavity using a small loop ear curet or a small cup curet.

To visualize the inside of the nostril after the rhinolith has been removed, a focal light source and magnification are necessary. After the rhinolith has been removed and the nasal cavity well cleaned, the nostril should be flushed with a saline antibiotic solution, and a water-based antibiotic ointment should be infiltrated into the opening daily for several days to keep the nasal mucosa from drying.

It is essential to perform bacterial and fungal cultures from the exudate removed for followup systemic therapy.

Occasionally, if severe bleeding is encountered, the nostril should be packed off with gauze for 24 to 48 hours. Hypertrophy of the cere[25] in female budgerigars can result in the development of a dry, hard, brown growth of cornified epithelial tissue growing out from the surface of the cere often giving a unicorn appearance. The preferred treatment is daily application of a softening ointment until the cornified tissue softens and peels off the surface of the cere. If this regimen is unsuccessful, careful surgical separation should be attempted. Care must be taken to avoid excessive hemorrhage.

Sinusitis

One of the most common respiratory problems encountered in birds, particularly psittacine birds, is infection of the sinuses. The infraorbital sinuses in birds is a series of cavities and diverticula partially surrounding the eye. There is variation from species to species. The lateral walls of the sinuses are formed by the facial muscles and have no bony covering. The sinuses communicate with each other through a central nasal sinus. The infraorbital sinuses communicate with the rhinal cavity and the oral cavity through the infundibular cleft.[26]

Bacterial, fungal, and yeast infections usually cause chronic infection with caseous exudate filling and often distending the sinuses. Long-term infection can cause tissue necrosis.

Isolation and identification of the infectious agent are essential and can be accomplished by flushing the sinuses to culture the organisms. If the nasal sinuses are involved, a sterile blunted 18-gauge needle is inserted into the opening of the nostril and sterile saline is flushed into the nasal sinus. The fluid is then aspirated into the syringe and transferred to culture media. It is essential to surgically

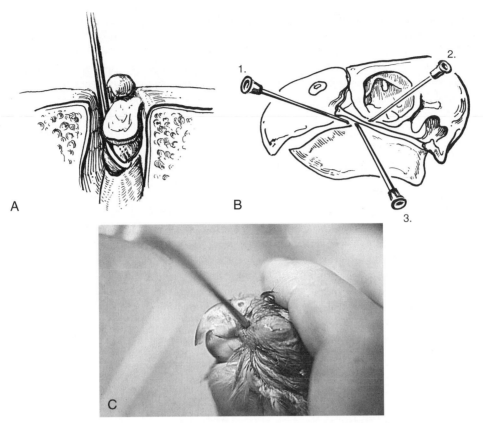

Figure 41-16

(A) A loop curet is used to gently tease the exudate out of the nostril, without traumatizing the operculum. *(B)* Needle 1 passes under the zygomatic arch into the infraorbital diverticulum of the infraorbital sinus. Needle 2 is directed rostrally and passes over the zygomatic arch into the infraorbital diverticulum beneath the eye. Needle 3 enters through the commissure of the beak and passes under the zygomatic arch, then enters into the suborbital diverticulum of the infraorbital sinus. *(C)* The cannula passes into the infraorbital diverticulum beneath the eye.

cleanse the cere or nostril before the flush to avoid contamination of the sample.

Flushing the rhinal cavity with an antibiotic saline mixture assists in treating infections in this area by forcing the flush solution into the nasal sinus with gentle moderate pressure. It is sometimes possible to recreate patency from the sinus through the palatine opening in the choanal cleft. This can be confirmed by observing the fluid passing through the palatine opening into the mouth.

Aspiration from the infraorbital diverticulum of the infraorbital sinus can be accomplished by directing a needle toward a point midway between the external nares and the eye. The needle is inserted through the skin of the commissure of the beak and held parallel to the side of the head. The needle should pass under the zygomatic arch into the infra-

orbital sinus[27] (Fig. 41–16*B, C*; see also color figure).

Aspiration of the infraorbital diverticulum beneath the eye is accomplished by directing the needle over the zygomatic arch and then directing it rostrally. By directing the needle caudally, entering from the commissure of the beak and passing the needle under the zygomatic arch, the diverticulum of the infraorbital sinus can be entered. Care should be taken with all of these procedures to avoid puncturing the globe of the eye. Necrotic bony plates protecting the eye can easily be punctured.

These approaches can be used to flush the sinuses, but care must be taken not to infuse the saline antibiotic solution with excessive pressure and overdistend the sinus. For chronic infection of the supraorbital sinuses in which access to the sinuses is difficult, a radical procedure of sinus trephination[28] offers access to the sinus to permit flushing and treatment of the dorsal and caudal area of the sinus. By creating an opening into the sinus, treatment can be continued over a long enough period of time to eliminate the infection. The surgical approach differs from species to species because of anatomic variations. A skin incision is made in a plane between the nares and the medial commissure of the eyelids approximately two-fifths to one-half centimeters from the rostral-most plane of the eye and nares (Fig. 41–17). With a sterile drill, a hole is made in the frontal bone angled toward the midline. A second hole is drilled on the opposite side. Cultures are taken from the sinuses, and the area is irrigated and treated with appropriate antibiotics. The opening closes fairly rapidly unless attempts are made to keep it open. This is generally a bloody procedure and extreme care must be taken to avoid damage to the globe of the eye. Although infrequently needed, this procedure may be the only successful means of treating a supraorbital infection.

Inflation of the Cervicocephalic Air Sacs

This condition can be seen as a generalized or localized area of subcutaneous emphysema around the head, neck, and thorax. The etiology is unknown, but trauma is thought to be the most likely cause.

Some birds display localized areas of inflated skin

that can be restricted to one side of the face or an eyelid, whereas other birds can have gross distension of the cervical and cephalic region.

Many surgical approaches have been suggested, including the placement of air sac release tubes[4] and the placement of a cutaneous stent.[29]

In this author's experience, maintaining stents and air release tubes is difficult and requires restraint devices and constant monitoring of the aperture of the device.

By incising the ballooned skin after surgical scrub and spreading the incision to create a large opening, the air is forced out, deflating the ballooned area. The skin heals in from 3 to 6 days, and often the procedure has to be repeated several times before air leakage no longer occurs. Results with this technique have been rewarding in a majority of cases.

Tracheotomy

Entry to the lumen of the trachea is necessary for the removal of tracheal or syringeal foreign bodies or granulomas that could not be removed by endoscopy.[4, 30] With the bird in ventrodorsal recumbency, a 3- to 5-cm midline incision is made in the skin from the thoracic inlet cranially. With blunt dissection, the crop is freed from its attachments and reflected to one side. The clavicular air sac that surrounds the trachea, syrinx, and primary bronchus is bluntly dissected and the trachea is isolated. The trachea is grasped, and with blunt dissection

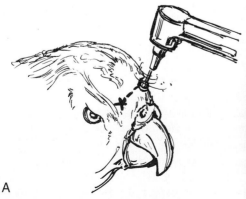
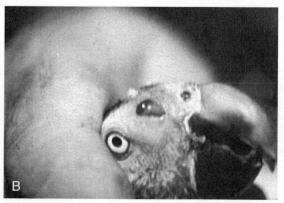

F i g u r e   4 1 – 1 7

(A) Landmarks for sinus trephination. The site of entry into the frontal sinus is in a plane on a line connecting the nostril and the medial canthus of the eye. *(B)* An African grey parrot *(Psittacus erithacus)* after sinus trephination and infiltration of an antibiotic ointment into the sinus opening.

the sternotracheal muscles that anchor the trachea within the thoracic inlet are isolated, clamped off, and transected. With gentle tension, the trachea and syrinx can be retracted cranially. Extreme care should be taken or the primary bronchus can be torn away from the syrinx. An incision is made between the tracheal rings, halfway across the annular ligament, allowing access to the lumen for retrieval of foreign bodies or granulomas. Closing the trachea requires placement of sutures through the annular ligament, encompassing at least one tracheal ring on each side of the tracheal incision. Fine monofilament absorbable suture material should be used, and at least four to five simple interrupted sutures should be placed (Fig. 41–18). Tracheotomy should be attempted only if all other attempts at retrieval are exhausted.

Devocalization

Inhibiting vocalization in birds may be one of the most controversial, difficult, and unrewarding avian surgical procedures performed. The purpose of devocalizing birds is to prevent the loud and untimely noise created by such birds as roosters and peacocks. These birds are kept as ornamental pets and the loud vocalization is disturbing to neighbors. Local ordinances often preclude the keeping of

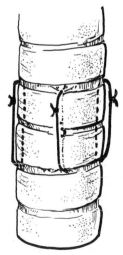

Figure 41–18

Sutures are placed around two annular rings, one on each side of the incision through the annular ligament to close the tracheotomy incision.

these birds, and owners are unable to find alternative housing for them. The owners are therefore faced with the alternative of devocalization or euthanasia. Because of the emotional attachment to the bird, many people choose the surgical procedure even though the risks are great and the cost is high.

Many pet owners and veterinarians are greatly concerned regarding the ethical implications of this procedure. These ethical ramifications must be resolved by both the owner and the surgeon before a decision on surgery or euthanasia can be made.

The issue of devocalization in psittacine birds, however, is not controversial because the outcome of this surgical procedure has profound psychological effects on the birds, and placement and relocation of psittacine birds are not the problems as in barnyard species. As a result, this procedure should not be performed in psittacine species.

Devoicing of the domestic fowl was first described in 1953.[31] The pessulus was cauterized through the lumen of the trachea. This procedure was unsuccessful because many of the birds regained vocalization. In 1964, a technique was described, which bonded a stainless steel wire mesh bent to a **V** form to the cauterized tympaniform membrane with a tissue adhesive.[32] This method met with limited success. Another technique[11] described the use of phenol swabbed on the surface of the syrinx to create scar tissue and prevent resonance of the tympanic membrane.

This author uses a modification of the technique described by Bougerol.[33] The surgical approach is the same as previously described for tracheotomy. When the trachea is isolated, the sternal tracheal muscles can be visualized when the veterinarian is looking into the thoracic inlet (Fig. 41–19). The muscles are clamped with a hemostat as close to their lateral attachments to the trachea as possible and transected. If the hemostats are maintained for a few minutes after transection, there is rarely any bleeding.

The syrinx and the bifurcation of the primary bronchus can be visualized lying just cranial to the heart. The syrinx is anatomically different and its depth within the thoracic inlet varies in each species. Therefore, care should be taken in identifying the tympaniform membrane. Very little tension should be placed on the trachea and syrinx because the primary bronchial attachments to the syrinx are

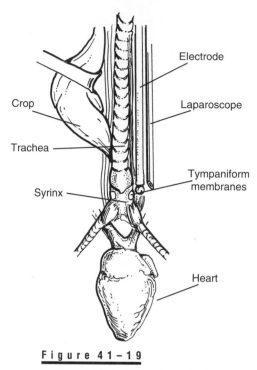

Figure 41–19

Approach to the syrinx for devocalization.

very friable and can tear, causing avulsion of the syrinx.

A 1.9-mm to 2.7-mm rigid endoscope with a 30° offset angle is passed beside the lateral side of the trachea to the syrinx. The membranes of the lateral syrinx can be visualized and identified. A long insulated radiosurgical ball electrode is passed along the barrel of the endoscope until the ball comes into the field of vision. The membrane should then be coagulated sufficiently to create the formation of scar tissue to inhibit the resonance of the syringeal membranes, thereby dulling or eliminating vocalization. The procedure is less difficult using a video camera on the endoscope because the surgeon can work unencumbered while viewing the monitor.

The procedure is then repeated on the opposite side. Inadequate coagulation of the syringeal membranes creates only temporary or partial devocalization. Excessive coagulation necroses the membranes, causing sloughing and death. Skin closure is accomplished with a simple continuous pattern.

This procedure frequently results in a high mortality rate (as high as 20–25%) and a moderately high rate of either partial or complete revocalization. It is therefore a procedure that should be performed only as a last resort in lieu of euthanizing the bird and should never be attempted on psittacine birds. Castration may be a viable alternative to devocalization (see Genitourinary Surgery).

Lung Biopsy

Biopsy samples of lung tissue can be used for diagnosing respiratory disease in which tissue samples are used primarily for bacterial and fungal isolation and infrequently for histologic or cytologic examination.

Lung tissue can be sampled using endoscopic-guided biopsy forceps via a cranial air sac approach.[34] Two sizes of biopsy forceps (5 French and 2.7 French) were used, with the 2.7 French forceps offering a better biopsy sample. Post-sampling hemorrhage was significant but localized. A surgical approach through the third intercostal space offered good visualization of the lung through the incision site. For biopsy of diseased lung tissue, sampling can be achieved by gently teasing the lung from its attachment to the ribs and inserting biopsy forceps through an intercostal or caudal air sac approach.

Because the avian lung is more vascular and clotting is less efficient than in mammals, vascular clips placed across the lung in a pie-shaped wedge permit removing a wedge-shaped sample contained within the vascular clips with little to no bleeding.

SURGERY OF THE GENITOURINARY TRACT

Biopsy of the kidney is the only specific surgical procedure performed on the urinary system. Indications for renal biopsy are chronic polyuria and polydipsia, persistent elevation of uric acid, or undiagnosed clinical signs of kidney disease.

Biopsy of the cranial pole of the kidney via a lateral abdominal approach offers the greatest visibility and access to the site. Although an endoscopic-guided biopsy from this approach is neither difficult nor excessively stressful to the patient, controlling hemorrhage from the biopsy site can be difficult.

The lateral laparotomy approach offers a larger field of vision of the kidney and permits more reliable hemostasis via radiosurgical coagulation. Approach to the caudal pole of the kidney via a transabdominal incision offers access to both kidneys.

A simple dorsal pelvic approach to the caudal lobe of the kidney was developed by W.K. Sudemeyer (personal communication). An area of skin from the point of the femoral head to the pelvic midline and laterally to the origin of the iliotibialis lateralis muscle is surgically prepared, and a flap incision is made within this area with the base of the flap attached on the lateral aspect of the area. The skin is dissected and reflected laterally. A 3- to 5-mm hole is drilled through the cranial lateral margin of the levator cordae muscle in the post-acetabulum ilium with a sterile rotary drill. The bone is brush-drilled away until the caudal abdominal air sac and the renal tissue are visualized. The opening can be enlarged with a small rongeur forceps. A biopsy sample is taken from the exposed kidney, and the skin flap is closed and sutured. Gel foam can be incorporated into the closure to control bleeding.

Surgical Reproductive Problems in the Female Bird

Peritonitis associated with egg-laying is a common problem in cockatiels, lovebirds, budgerigars, macaws, ducks, and barnyard fowl.[4, 35] Peritonitis can occur when the ovum escapes the infundibulum and falls into the coelomic cavity or yolk material leaks from a ruptured oviduct or uterus. A severe inflammatory response is reflected in the bird's hemogram as a toxic heterophilia and leukocytosis.[36] Large amounts of abdominal fluid can accumulate in the abdominal cavity (Fig. 41–20). Abdominocentesis can reveal from a modified almost acellular transudate to a thick exudate with toxic degenerative and mononuclear cells. Cultures rarely reveal bacterial involvement. The severe inflammatory response results from a reaction to the foreign protein of the yolk material.

In most cases antibiotic therapy is of little value, and only mild localized cases can be expected to respond to medical therapy. Early surgical intervention offers a greater chance of success than attempting to treat the bird medically and losing valuable time.

A transabdominal approach offers the greatest exposure to the abdominal cavity. The bird should be positioned at an angle with the head slightly elevated to prevent abdominal fluid from infiltrating the air sacs. The fluid should be aspirated and the abdominal cavity carefully explored for granulomas frequently associated with this condition. Usually a substantial amount of fibrinous material is deposited throughout the abdominal cavity causing many adhesions, particularly to loops of bowel and ovi-

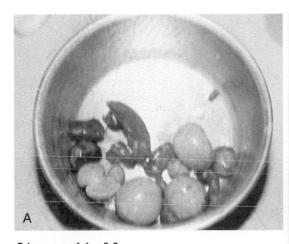
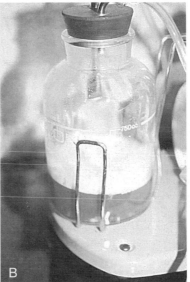

Figure 41–20

(A) Soft-shelled eggs, yolks, and granulomas surgically removed from the abdomen of a Peking duck with peritonitis. *(B)* Abdominal fluid suctioned during exploratory surgery in this duck.

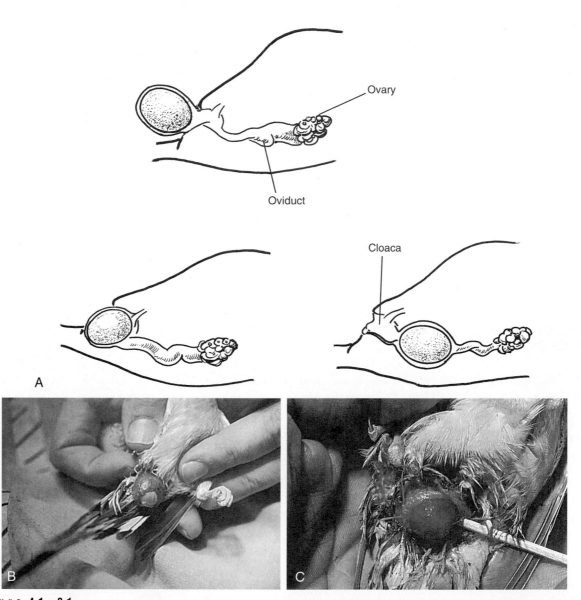

Ovary

Oviduct

Cloaca

A

B

C

Figure 41-21

(A) Three positions of egg binding. (Top) Position 1: The egg is wrapped in the prolapsed oviduct, external to the cloacal opening. (Bottom left) Position 2: The egg wrapped in the oviduct is retained in the cloaca and pelvic canal. (Bottom right) Position 3: The egg is in the vagina, within the coelomic cavity, unable to pass the vaginal-cloacal orifice. (B) Egg-bound budgerigar (Melopsittacus undulatus) as seen in position 1. (C) The egg is in the pelvic canal and cloaca as seen in position 2.

duct and uterus. If possible, the oviduct should be carefully isolated and checked for tears. Unless the bird is a valuable breeding bird, removal of the oviduct is advised. The abdominal cavity should be flushed with warm saline and closed with a standard two-layer closure. Because of the severe inflammatory response, a guarded prognosis must be given.

Dystocia (Egg Binding)

Egg binding is a common problem, particularly in ducks and psittacine birds, and has been associated with malformations including oversized, soft-shelled, rough surfaced, or irregularly shaped eggs. Uterine atony, poor nutrition, genetic predispositions, and compression of the reproductive tract from abdominal masses have also contributed to this condition.[4, 35, 37-41]

Birds can present with eggs retained in one of three positions (Fig. 41–21A). Common to budgerigars and less frequently to cockatiels, the egg can be present hanging from the cloacal opening wrapped within the prolapsed uterus or oviduct[21, 35] (Fig. 41–21B; see also color figure). With this presentation, the removal of the egg is rapid and simple, but the damage to the oviduct or uterus can be extensive as the result of drying and necrosis of the tissues, loss of vascular supply from torsion, or trauma to the exposed surface of the oviduct. Severe tissue alteration can result in as little as 30 to 60 minutes.[4] Rapid surgical intervention can be critical.

If an opening in the uterus permits visualization of the eggshell, gentle teasing of the uterine wall from the surface of the egg and aspiration of the egg contents followed by compression and compacting of the eggshell facilitates retrieval through the uterine opening. If the eggshell cannot be visualized or the uterine tissue is dry and tightly adhered to the egg, an incision must be made in the prolapsed tissue to present the egg (Fig. 41–22). If the uterine tissue is viable, the incision can be sutured with 5–0 to 8–0 absorbable monofilament suture material, using a simple continuous appositional pattern. If the tissues are devitalized and suturing is not possible, the dry necrotic tissue should be dissected away, the egg removed, and the incision closed, assuming that there is enough tissue remaining. If suturing is not possible, the prolapsed

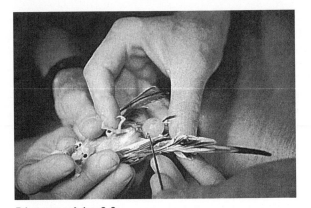

Figure 41–22

The prolapsed uterus is incised and the egg is removed.

tissue should be reduced through the cloacal vaginal orifice. Occasionally, tenesmus causes continued tissue prolapsing, requiring pursestring sutures (see Fig. 41–14). Systemic antibiotics should be given for a minimum of 7 to 14 days.

In the second presentation, the egg is wrapped within the prolapsed tissue in the pelvic canal (Fig. 41–21C; see also color figure). By dilating the cloacal opening and making an incision into the wall of the uterus, the egg contents can be evacuated by ovocentesis and the compressed eggshell removed through the incision. Preplacing absorbable monofilament stay sutures before making the incision makes closure of the incision rapid and simple. In most instances both of the described procedures can be accomplished without the need for anesthesia.

An episiotomy in the ventral midline through the cloacal sphincter has been used to deliver eggs from the pelvic canal.[23] However, attempts at removal by ovocentesis should be exhausted before this approach is attempted.

In the third presentation, the egg has not passed through the vaginal-cloacal orifice and is retained within the uterus in the coelomic cavity. The bird must be anesthetized and the cloacal orifice dilated. If the eggshell is visible through the vaginal cloacal orifice, a syringe with an 18-gauge needle attached can be used to bore a hole in the exposed eggshell and aspirate the entire contents of the egg. By gentle digital pressure over the caudal abdomen, the egg can be compacted and then removed with forceps through the vaginal cloacal opening. Irrigating the uterus with warm sterile saline assists removal of residual shell fragments.

All egg-bound birds should be radiographed before surgery to ensure that there is not more than one egg present. Postoperative radiographs reveal retained shell particles.

If the egg cannot be visualized through the cloaca, an exploratory laparotomy using a transabdominal approach (see Color Fig. 41–23) permits removal of the egg. Unless the bird is a breeding hen, a hysterectomy should be performed to prevent recurrences.

When a bird is presented in good physical condition with typical signs of egg-laying and the egg has not been presented, it is advisable to place the bird in a heated environment (85 to 90°) for 24 hours before contemplating surgery. Frequently the egg passes and averts the need for surgical intervention.

Hysterectomy (Salpingohysterectomy)

Removal of the oviduct and uterus is required for problems associated with egg peritonitis, prolapsing of the oviduct and uterus, persistent egg-laying, and for birds with abnormal egg production or pyometra-like conditions of the uterus (see Color Fig. 41–24).

The anatomy of the female reproductive tract includes the ovary, infundibulum, oviduct, uterus (shell gland) and vagina, which joins the cloaca at the vaginal cloacal orifice.

Hysterectomy can be performed from either a transabdominal[42] or a lateral approach.[4, 38, 39] The lateral approach offers excellent access to the entire reproductive tract but is restrictive to the left coelomic cavity. The transabdominal approach provides access to both the left and right side of the coelomic cavity, but offers poor exposure to the ovary and oviduct.

Using a lateral laparotomy approach, the fimbria of the infundibulum, which lies just caudal to the ovary, is elevated and the dorsal suspensory ligament is exposed. A branch of the ovarian artery can be found within this ligament. A hemoclip is placed across the ligament close to its ovarian attachment. If the ovarian artery is not included within the vascular clip, it retracts under the ovary and continues to bleed.[4] As the suspensory ligament is transected, care must be taken to avoid the ureter. If there is bleeding from any of the blood vessels within the suspensory ligament, radiosurgical coag-

ulation quickly controls the hemorrhage. Slight tension should be placed on the oviduct when the avascular dorsal ligament is incised to permit the convolutions of the uterus to straighten out. A hemoclip should be placed across the vagina as it attaches to the cloaca, with care not to incorporate the ureter. For large birds, ligating the vagina ensures adequate closure. The oviduct and uterus are then removed and the incision is closed with a standard two-layer closure. Because of their friability, it is essential to place little to no tension on these tissues.

Using a transabdominal approach, the first hemoclip is applied to the vagina, and as the ventral ligament is incised, the oviduct uncoils. It is not always possible to remove the entire oviduct. The proximal ovarian vascular clip is more difficult to apply because the ovary is located deep within the abdominal cavity and should be placed as close to the ovary as possible. Care should be taken to avoid tension on the uterus and oviduct as it uncoils.

Rarely after hysterectomy, an ovum is deposited into the coelomic cavity[38, 39] with resultant yolk peritonitis. It is postulated that there is a phenomenon in which hormonal feedback from the uterus to the ovary[4, 11, 23, 35] inhibits follicular release. However, there has been a report of yolk peritonitis after hysterectomy in a duck and quail,[35] and this author has had a similar experience in two ducks.

Ovariectomy

The surgical removal of the left ovary in birds has been a difficult and unrewarding procedure. Complications leading to mortality are ever-present, and this procedure is rarely attempted. From a lateral approach, Bennett[4] has reported two procedures with unfavorable results. The use of carbon dioxide laser to destroy the ovary was impractical, and the placement of vascular clips across the ovarian vascular supply is a difficult, high-risk procedure. With magnification, vascular clips are placed blindly under the ovary and secured with an angled applicator to clamp off the ovarian vessels without entrapping the aorta or nerves. In small birds, a single hemoclip will suffice. This clip should be applied from a caudal to a cranial direction. In larger birds, one vascular clip is applied from a cranial direction and a second from a caudal direction.

This author has used a technique employing radiosurgical ablation of the ovary (unpublished study). This procedure is not difficult but should be performed with magnification. After a standard left lateral laparotomy approach, the ovary is isolated by breaking through the surrounding air sac. If the bird is very immature and there are few to no follicles on the ovary, the ovary is coagulated using a ball electrode. Care must be taken when coagulating the anterior pole of the ovary to avoid contact with the adrenal gland. In mature birds with active ovarian follicles the follicular contents are aspirated using a suction coagulator (Ellman International Corp., Hewlett, NY), and the ovary is coagulated while the follicles are being aspirated. The considerable amount of smoke generated during the coagulation procedure can be evacuated with the suction electrode. This procedure has been effective with immature females; however, mature hens with active follicles have had regeneration of ovarian tissue with subsequent ovulatory activity. This technique shows promise; however, in mature birds, a considerable amount of time is required to coagulate the ovary.

Orchidectomy

Caponization in poultry is a procedure that has been successfully performed for many years. The mortality rate is very low considering the number of birds that have been caponized. This procedure is done on cockerels that are between 1 and 2 weeks of age.

The purpose of caponization is to reduce aggression in growing roosters and to add body fat until the bird is marketable.

In ratites, the procedure is used to control aggressive behavior, thereby reducing risk to other birds and to keepers.[43] The testicles are approached via an incision through the costal notch and lumbar fossa. This incision should be of sufficient size to introduce a hand into the body cavity to grasp the testicle and twist it until it tears away from its attachment. It is easier to locate the testicle during the breeding season when the testicles are large; however, at that time there is greater risk of postoperative hemorrhage. In large birds it may be possible to reach the opposite testicle from the one side and repeat the procedure through a single surgical entry incision. However, with smaller birds it is necessary to grasp the testicle from an incision on each side.

Orchidectomy in peacocks and roosters is a means of muting vocalization, negating the necessity of undergoing a devocalization procedure. The use of vascular clips has been suggested for these species.[4] Application of the clips is less difficult in the male than it is in the female. A transabdominal approach eliminates the need for an incision on both sides. This approach in psittacines is very difficult and results in too high a mortality risk.

In galliformes and psittacine birds, a procedure was developed in which the testicles are exposed from a lateral approach[44] and the avascular portion of the testicular tunic is incised after the tunic has been opened. The parenchymal testicular tissue is expressed and suctioned away. This technique met with partial success because a high percentage of the testicular tissue regenerated.

This author has coagulated the testicles of pigeons and one aggressive blue-fronted Amazon parrot *(Amazona aestiva)*. The parrot was bilaterally sterilized by using the same coagulating technique as previously described for ovariectomy. In immature pigeons, ablation of the testicle by radiosurgical coagulation was uncomplicated and in many birds the gonads were absent 6 months after the procedure. In mature birds, particularly birds with hypertrophied testicles, the rate of testicular regeneration was much higher.

Refinement of the coagulation procedure by incorporating a planing technique appears to be more efficacious (see Chapter 43). In the single psittacine in which this procedure was performed, endoscopic examination revealed no apparent testicular regeneration 5 months after surgery, and the bird displayed significantly modified behavior.

SURGERY OF THE INTEGUMENT AND MISCELLANEOUS PROCEDURES

Split Sternum

This condition is seen in free-flying birds that collide with objects and split the skin over the sternum on impact. In companion birds, this condition occurs when the birds either collide with objects or fall to the ground as a result of the inability to obtain lift because of trimmed primary wing feathers. The impact causes laceration and necrosis of the skin directly over the keel. Contamination and drying of the subcutaneous tissues prevent the lacerated skin margins from healing. The periosteum over the sternal margin is often dry and necrotic, and incisional breakdown is common and wound dehiscence is frequent. Simple suturing of debrided wound margins are often ineffective and the wound keeps dehiscing.

The skin over this area has very little elasticity, and therefore closure without tension is difficult to achieve. The wound margins and dry or necrotic subcutaneous tissue must be debrided, and the skin over the pectoral muscles must be undermined to the extent that the wound can be closed with very little tension.

If the periosteum of the sternal border is dry or necrotic, this tissue must be curetted down to healthy bone. The undermined skin is sutured with interrupted 5–0 absorbable suture material using a mattress suture pattern. Good incisional apposition is essential. Large bites prevent the suture from tearing out. If tension on the suture line is excessive or wound closure is not possible, a parallel releasing incision on one or both sides of the wound relieves the tension. These incisions should be allowed to heal as open wounds.

Feather Cysts

Feather cysts of primary wing and tail feathers are seen in canaries and several species of psittacine birds. Possible etiologic factors influencing these feather cysts include heredity; malformed cystic feathers; nutritional deficiencies; trauma; and viral, bacterial, and parasitic infections.[45]

Multiple feathers growing from a single follicle are commonly seen in canaries and occasionally psittacine birds. These cysts are very vascular, and all blood vessels must be sealed and the entire cyst lining excised. For single feather cysts, radiosurgical excision eliminates postoperative bleeding. Care must be taken to avoid damaging surrounding structures during excision. With multiple cysts on the torso of the bird, radical excision of the entire feather track was suggested to prevent recurrence.[45]

Amputation of the Uropygial Gland

Pathology requiring removal of the uropygial gland includes impaction, obstruction of the papilla, ab-

scess, tumors, and chronic dermatitis of the skin covering and surrounding the gland. Abscesses have been seen in many avian species and should be approached medically before removal is attempted. Gentle pressure over the gland occasionally dislodges an obstructed papilla and permits manual expression of the infected lobe. The application of hot compresses two to three times daily for 24 to 48 hours can aid in manually expressing debris from the gland. If debris cannot be expressed or does not respond to medical treatment or the gland ruptures, it is better to perform excisional surgery before chronic inflammation compromises the surgical procedure. Surgery is always indicated when tumors and chronic dermatitis involves the gland. Adenomas, adenocarcinomas, and papillomas of the uropygial gland[46] have been reported.

Excision of the uropygial gland in penguins was described.[47] Because the skin over the synsacrum is tightly adhered to the underlying fascia and elasticity is minimal, conservation of as much skin as possible facilitates closure. A midline straight linear incision is made over the bifurcation of the two lobes from the cranial toward the caudal pole of the gland. The incision circumscribes the papilla and is extended to the end of the caudal pole, and the papilla is excised. With blunt dissection, the skin over the gland is undermined while coagulating blood vessels as the skin is reflected off the dorsal aspect of the gland. The vascular supply to the gland comes from a paired vessel feeding the cranial base of the gland and then sending two additional branches to the midpoint and caudal end of the gland. The glands are attached to the deep areolar fascia over the synsacrum.[47]

As blunt dissection continues, the vessels are identified and ligated or coagulated with bipolar forceps. The gland is dissected circumferentially starting at the cranial pole until it can be lifted off the synsacral surface.[4] As the caudal pole is dissected, care must be taken to avoid compromising the blood supply to the tail feathers lying just beneath the caudal pole. Closure of the fascia helps to reduce tension on the skin sutures.

The skin is closed with a simple interrupted pattern. If the gland has ruptured or is severely chronically infected, dissection and conservation of skin becomes difficult. Cases exist in which total skin closure is not possible and the incision must heal by granulation. In psittacine birds, it is sometimes necessary to use restraining devices to inhibit post-surgical plucking at the incision.

Amputation of the Tail (Pygostyle)

Tail amputation is indicated for chronic nonresolving dermatitis in which discomfort results in self-mutilation, in cases of severe trauma with avulsion of part of the tail, and in cases of disfiguring recurring feather cysts. All feathers must be plucked from the surface of the tail and the long tail feathers should be cut. The area is prepared for surgery and a semicircular skin incision is made on the dorsal surface of the tail starting at the cranial aspect of the tail base where the tail starts to widen. The incision is extended from one side of the tail to the other with the convex part of the skin flap directed toward the end of the tail. The tail is flexed dorsally and a similar incision is made through the skin on the ventral surface. Care should be taken to avoid structures associated with the cloacal sphincter. The two incisions should join at the lateral margins of the tail base. The skin flaps are undermined, exposing the muscular attachments of the tail.

The levator caudae and depressor caudae muscles along with the remaining muscle groups are ligated and transected as close to the tail as possible. The blood vessels are easily identified and ligated, and the tail is disarticulated at the sacrococcygeal junction. The two skin flaps are apposed and sutured with a simple interrupted pattern. Creating skin flaps permits easy closure without tension (Fig. 41–25).

The tail is used for flight and balance; however, tailless birds display no balance problems following surgery.

Tumors

Tumors involving the skin and subcutaneous tissue include lipomas, myelolipomas, xanthomas, liposarcomas, fibromas, fibrosarcomas, squamous cell carcinomas, adenocarcinomas, and papillomas.[46, 48]

Surgical excision of these tumors requires meticulous dissection and controlled hemostasis. One of the most frequently seen avian tumors is the lipoma. In the budgerigar, rose-breasted cockatoo, and sev-

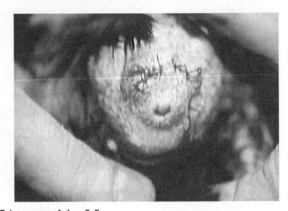

Figure 41–25

An African grey parrot *(Psittacus erithacus)* immediately after a tail amputation.

eral species of Amazon parrots, these fatty masses can grow rapidly.

Lipomas in the budgerigar are found in the subcutis around the sternum and caudal abdomen. These tumors are well encapsulated and usually vascular. The tumor capsule is usually tenaciously adhered to the surface of the pectoral muscles. In large fast-growing lipomas, central fat necrosis can be extensive.

An elliptical skin incision over the tumor mass leaves enough skin to maintain a tensionless closure. The skin is carefully bluntly dissected off the capsule of the tumor and tissues adhered to the tumor capsule, and blood vessels are incised and coagulated using radiosurgery. Care must be taken during dissection to avoid tearing the tumor capsule and permitting the necrosed fat to leak into the incision site. When the tumor has been dissected free of its attachment to the skin and subcutaneous tissue, the capsule is teased off the muscle surface by blunt dissection. It is sometimes necessary to tear some pectoral muscle fibers to remove the tumor capsule. Strict total hemostasis is essential to avoid life-threatening postoperative hematomas after skin closure. Small vessels and torn muscle fibers can start to ooze when the bird recovers from anesthesia and blood pressure returns to normal.

Lipomas in cockatoos and parrots are less well defined, and they spread across the caudal abdomen (Fig. 41–26). Because this tumor is more diffuse, total surgical removal is more difficult. These masses have many blood vessels infiltrating the fatty tissue, and in many cases, total excision is impossi-

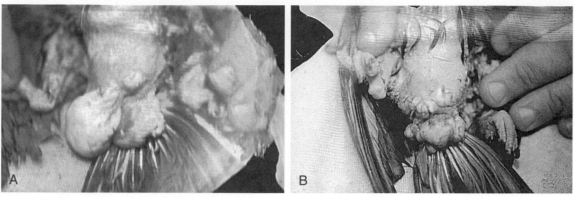

Figure 41–26

(A) Two large lipomas extending from the caudal abdomen in an Amazon parrot. The skin covering these masses has been traumatized and ulcerated. *(B)* Postoperative resection of fatty tissue. Note generalized fat infiltration around the tail.

ble. Debulking reduces the extra body weight and eliminates the threat of skin ulceration and hemorrhage caused when the bird drags this enlarged posterior abdominal mass on the perch or cage floor.

Obese birds with fatty tumors should be placed on a strict low-fat diet and an exercise program to reduce the fatty tissue as much as possible before surgery.

Surgical removal of most intraabdominal tumors is unrewarding. These tumors are difficult to remove; surgery requires magnification and usually result in the bird's demise.

Abdominal Hernias

The etiology of abdominal hernias is unknown. These hernias may be related to a hormonal imbalance causing a weakening of the abdominal muscles in budgerigars and cockatiels[4] (Fig. 41–27; see also color figure). In chronic egg-laying hens, changes in calcium metabolism are thought to contribute to muscular atony and distension of the caudal abdomen.[48] This author has seen this condition in budgerigars, cockatiels, and Amazon parrots that have never laid an egg. Surgical intervention should be undertaken if the distended abdomen is

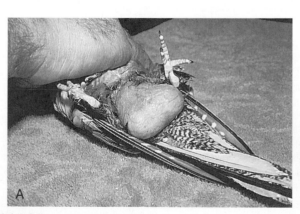
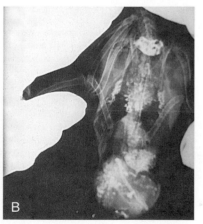

Figure 41–27

(A) Abdominal hernia in a cockatiel *(Nymphicus hollandicus).* *(B)* Ventrodorsal radiograph of a parrot with a large abdominal hernia. A contrast medium was given prior to taking the radiograph. The entire visceral content is in the hernial sac. Note the aspirated barium in the lungs.

being traumatized by rubbing on the cage floor, or if the bird displays respiratory distress, has difficulty expressing urates and feces from the cloaca, or has the entire abdominal viscera within the hernial sac.[49]

Abdominal hernias in birds are not true hernias because there is no opening in the aponeurosis of the abdominal muscles and typically there is no hernial ring. Therefore, entrapment and strangulation of abdominal viscera do not occur. Atony and breakdown of abdominal musculature appear to occur. As the condition progresses, increased muscle relaxation and abdominal distension take place. It is necessary to perform contrast radiography in these birds to ensure that there are no predisposing abdominal masses or cysts and to determine if the viscera is contained within the hernial sac.

Corrective surgery involves a "tummy tuck" procedure in which an elliptical transabdominal incision through the skin and abdominal muscles reduces the size of the distended hernial sac by removing part of the abdominal wall. Before an incision is made, the abdominal viscera should be palpated and reduced back to their normal abdominal positions. It is necessary to be sure that there are no adhesions of the abdominal wall to loops of bowel to ensure that iatrogenic laceration of the abdominal viscera does not result. The amount of tissue removed determines the degree of reduction of the hernial sac.

The abdominal muscles and skin are closed in a standard two-layer closure using a simple continuous pattern. By decreasing the amount of abdominal musculature, this procedure reduces intraabdominal space.

The procedure is safe and uncomplicated, but abdominal distension frequently recurs as the muscles continue to become atonic and stretch.

Large hernial repairs have been reenforced with surgical mesh.[4]

References

1. Kern TJ, Murphy CJ, Heck WR: Partial upper eye lid agenesis in a peregrine falcon. J Am Vet Med Assoc 187:1207, 1985.
2. Greenwood AG, Barnett KC: The investigation of visual defects in raptors. In Recent Advances in the Study of Raptor Diseases. West Yorkshire, England, Chiron, 1981, pp 131–135.
3. Murphy CJ: Ocular lesions in birds of prey. *In* Fowler ME (ed): Zoo and Wild Animal Medicine, Current Therapy 3. Philadelphia, WB Saunders, 1993, pp 213–218.
4. Bennett RA: Soft tissue surgery. In Ritchie BW, Harrison GJ, Harrison LR (eds): Avian Medicine: Principles and Application. Lake Worth, FL, Wingers Publishing, 1994, pp 1097–1136.
5. Williams D: Ophthalmology. In Ritchie BW, Harrison GJ, Harrison LR (eds): Avian Medicine: Principles and Application. Lake Worth, FL, Wingers Publishing, pp 676–689.
6. Kern TJ, Murphy CJ, Riis RC: Lens extraction by phacoemulsification in two raptors. J Am Vet Med Assoc 185:1403–1406, 1984.
7. Moore CP, Pickett JP, Beehler B: Extracapsular extraction of a senile cataract in an Andean condor. J Am Vet Med Assoc 187:1211–1214, 1985.
8. Hacker DV, Shitrinm: Cataract extraction in a mandarin duck. J Am Anim Hosp Assoc 24:679–682, 1988.
9. Karpinski L, Clubb S: Clinical aspects of ophthalmology. In Care Birds. Proc Assoc Avian Vet, 1983, pp 216–227.
10. Altman RB: Specific surgical techniques. Practical Lab Proc and Manual Assoc Avian Vet, 1994, pp 93–95.
11. Harrison GJ: Selected surgical procedures. In Harrison GJ, Harrison LR (eds): Clinical Avian Medicine and Surgery. Philadelphia, WB Saunders, 1986, p 381.
12. Altman RB: Esophageal stricture in a duck. J Am Vet Med Assoc 143(1):46, 1963.
13. VanSant F: Resolution of an esophageal stricture in a hyacinth macaw. Proc Assoc Avian Vet, 1992, pp 177–179.
14. Jenkins JR: Approaches to the abdominal cavity. Assoc Avian Vets Avian Surgical Symp, 1994, pp 20–23.
15. McCluggage D: Proventriculotomy: A study of select cases. Proc Assoc Avian Vet, 1992, pp 195–198.
16. Stewart JS: Husbandry, medical and surgical management of ratites: Part II. Proc Am Assoc Zoo Vets, 1989, pp 119–122.
17. Stewart JS: A simple proventriculotomy technique for the ostrich. J Assoc Avian Vets 5(3):139–141, 1991.
18. Rosskopf Jr WJ: Surgery of the avian digestive system. Proc Mid Atlantic Assoc Avian Vet, 1991, pp 160–168.
19. Goring RL, Goldman A, Kaufman K, et al: Needle catheter duodenostomy: A technique for duodenal alimentation of birds. J Am Vet Assoc 189:1017–1019, 1986.
20. Avgeris S, Rigg D: Cloacapexy in a sulphur-crested cockatoo. J Am Anim Hosp Assoc 24:407–410, 1988.
21. Rosskopf WJ, Woerpel RW: Cloacal conditions in pet birds with a cloaca-pexy update. Proc Assoc Avian Vet, 1989, pp 156–163.
22. Jenkins JR: Avian soft tissue surgery: Part I. Proc Am Coll Vet Surgeons, 1992, pp 631–633.
23. Martin HD: Avian reproductive emergencies, surgical management. Vet Med Rep 2(3):250–253, 1990.
24. VanSant F: Resolution of a cloacal adhesion in a blue-fronted Amazon. Proc Assoc Avian Vet, 1995, pp 155–164.
25. Rosskopf WJ: Surgery of the avian respiratory system. Proc Mid Atlantic Assoc Avian Vet, 1991, pp 149–158.
26. Walsh M: Upper respiratory disease in avian species: The rhinal cavities, sinuses, and cervicocephalic air sac system. Proc Assoc Avian Vet Int Conf Avian Med, 1984, pp 151–154.
27. Campbell TW: Cytology. In Ritchie, Harrison GJ, Harrison LR (eds): Avian Medicine: Principles and Application. Lake Worth, FL, Wingers Publishers, 1994, pp 200–222.
28. Rosskopf WJ, Woerpel RW: Sinus trephination of the supraorbital sinuses in psittacine birds: An aid in the treatment of chronic sinus infections. Proc Mid Atlantic States Assoc Avian Vet, 1994, pp 170–176.
29. Harris JM: Teflon dermal stent for correction of subcutaneous emphysema. Proc Assoc Avian Vet, 1991, pp 20–21.

30. Bennett RA: Avian soft tissue surgery wet lab. Practical Lab Proc Assoc Avian Vet, 1994, pp 77–81.

31. Durant AJ: Removing the vocal cords of the fowl. J Am Vet Med Assoc 122:14–17, 1953.

32. Gross WB: Devoicing the chicken. Poult Sci 43:1143–1144, 1964.

33. Bougerol C: A new technique for devocalization in birds. Proc Eur Committee Assoc Avian Vet, 1991, pp 143–145.

34. Hunter DB, Taylor M: Lung biopsy as a diagnostic technique in avian medicine. Proc Assoc Avian Vet, 1992, pp 207–210.

35. Rosskopf WJ, Woerpel RW: Pet avian obstetrics. Proc First Int Zoo Avian Med, 1987, pp 213–231.

36. Fudge AM: Criteria for surgical intervention to treat egg yolk peritonitis. AAV Today, 2(2):91, 1988.

37. Altman RB: General principles in avian surgery. Comp Contin Ed Pract Vet 3(2):177–183, 1981.

38. Harrison GJ: Reproductive medicine. In Harrison GJ, Harrison LR (eds): Clinical Avian Medicine and Surgery. Philadelphia, WB Saunders, 1986, pp 625–626.

39. McCluggage D: Hysterectomy: A review of selected cases. Proc Assoc Avian Vet, 1992, pp 201–206.

40. Hochleithner M, Lechner C: Egg binding in a budgerigar (Melopsittacus undulatus) caused by a cyst of the right oviduct. AAV Today 2(3):136–138, 1988.

41. Wissman MA: Unusual C-section and hysterectomy in the Isle of Pines amazon. Proc Assoc Avian Vet, 1991, pp 265–266.

42. Smith RE: Hysterectomy to relieve reproductive disorders in birds. Avian Exotic Pract 2:40–43, 1985.

43. Sikarski JG: Ostrich castration for behavioral control. Proc First Int Conf Zoo Avian Med, 1987, p 416.

44. Orr MG: Avian castration technique without testicular ligation. Proc Assoc Avian Vet, 1994, pp 23–26.

45. Bauck L: Radical surgery for the treatment of feather cysts in the canary. AAV Today 1:No(5)200–201, 1987.

46. Petrak ML, Gilmore CE: Neoplasms in diseases of cage and aviary birds. In Petrak ML (ed): Diseases of Cage and Aviary Birds. Philadelphia, Lea & Febiger, 1982, pp 606–637.

47. MacCoy D, Campbell TW: Excision of impacted and ruptured uropygial glands in the Gentoo Penguins (pygoscelis papua). Proc Am Assoc Zoo Vet, 1991, pp 259–260.

48. Latimer KS: Oncology. In Ritchie BW, Harrison GJ, Harrison LR (eds): Avian Medicine: Principles and Application. Lake Worth, FL, Wingers Publishing, 1994, pp 240–245.

49. Martin HD: Abdominal hernia with formation of a urate concretion in a cockatiel. J Am Vet Med Assoc 189(10):1332–1333, 1986.

42

Orthopedic Surgery

Great advances have been made in the treatment of fractures in birds. Methods of stabilization that were previously thought not applicable to avian fracture repair have been used successfully with modifications, taking into account the delicate nature of avian bone. Virtually all orthopedic techniques developed for use in mammals have application in avian fracture stabilization.

The bones of birds are relatively brittle and have thin cortices. They have a higher calcium content than mammalian bone, making them more brittle and prone to developing comminutions.[1-7] The bones of the pelvic girdle, some ribs, the humerus, and the femur of flighted birds are pneumatic with large air-filled medullary canals that are involved in the respiratory cycle during flight. Pneumatic bone also decreases the skeletal mass, making flight easier but increasing the risk of fragmentation during trauma. Distal to the tibiotarsus and the proximal half of the humerus there is little soft tissue covering the bones. As a result, avian fractures are frequently open and comminuted with loose or missing fragments. When a pneumatic bone is involved, subcutaneous emphysema is common but usually resolves quickly (within 24 hours) without consequence. Iatrogenic fractures during repair attempts may result from excessive manipulation of fracture fragments.

The principles of fracture stabilization in birds are analogous to those of fractures in mammals. The goal of accurate anatomic alignment involves restoration of the bone's original length, axial alignment, and rotational orientation. Rotational alignment is especially important in free-ranging birds with wing fractures, because even a slight degree of malalignment may result in a significant alteration in flight.[8] Rotational, bending, shearing, and compressive forces must be addressed when stabilizing a fracture. The more complex the fracture, the more forces must be neutralized to achieve rigid stabilization for the best healing potential. Minimizing soft tissue dissection and disruption of the vascular and muscular support of the bone is also important.

The bird's intended function must be taken into account in deciding the method of fixation to be used. Complete return to function must be achieved for release when working with free-ranging birds. In some birds, limb function is critical for breeding as well as for flight and capturing prey. Some loss of limb function in companion birds is usually acceptable. When leg dysfunction is involved, there may be concern regarding the development of pododermatitis (bumblefoot). Psittacines use their beak as a tool for ambulation, and many softbill birds are very lightweight and are not prone to the development of pododermatitis. In these species, even leg amputation should be considered a viable salvage procedure.

BONE HEALING

Limited information is available on bone healing in birds. The degree of displacement, amount of motion at the site, presence of infection, and the amount of damage to the blood supply are believed to influence the rate of fracture healing.[9] Primary bone healing is characterized by the direct growth of Haversian systems across the fracture gap with minimal callus production. Primary bone healing occurs under conditions of rigid stabilization with minimal fracture gap. This type of bone healing has been described in birds with fractures stabilized with bone plates.[10]

Avian fractures more commonly heal by secondary bone healing or callus healing because of the presence of a larger fracture gap or micromotion. The cellular events occurring during secondary healing in birds are similar to those of mammals.[3, 6] Even in pneumatic bones where the endosteum is difficult to identify histologically, endosteal callus production provides the major and early support for fracture healing. Periosteal callus production is less extensive and provides only secondary support.[3]

The blood supply to bone arises from the periosteal soft tissues, the medullary supply (nutrient artery), and metaphyseal and epiphyseal vessels.[11] Many avian fractures are comminuted with fragments that are detached from all soft tissue support. If they are not grossly infected and they can be rigidly and anatomically reconstructed, these fragments should be incorporated into the fracture repair because they provide structural support and precursors and cells for bone production, and they are usually incorporated into the healing callus.[12]

In general, avian bones heal faster than mammalian bones.[3, 6, 11, 13, 14] A simple, closed fracture is often clinically stable after 2 or 3 weeks. Radiographic union often lags behind clinical union, requiring 3 to 6 weeks for the development of radiographically visible callus. Fixation devices may be removed before radiographic evidence of healing is present if the fracture is palpably stable and early implant removal is indicated.

Osteomyelitis is not usually characterized by signs of systemic illness.[12, 15] The site fills with caseous, purulent material and the ends of the bone become sclerotic, arresting the healing process.[12] In some cases, the callus may be able to bridge around the caseous material and stabilize the fracture. The abscess site then serves as a nidus for systemic illness if the patient's condition becomes compromised for other reasons. All necrotic and infected debris should be removed and culture and sensitivity testing performed. Implants that do not provide rigid stabilization should be avoided in fractures that are open, contaminated, or infected.

Both viable and nonviable nonunion fractures occur in birds, and the principles for treatment are the same as those described for mammals.[16] Surgical intervention is required and should include rigid stabilization with compression at the fracture site, appropriate treatment of infection, and autogenous bone grafting.

BONE GRAFTS

Bone grafts[1, 7, 17, 18] promote fracture healing by osteogenesis, osteoinduction, and osteoconduction. When a graft is harvested and transferred, a small percentage of donor cells survive and produce new bone, completing the process of osteogenesis. A series of proteins within the graft (bone morphogenic proteins or BMPs) recruit mesenchymal cells to become chondroblasts and osteoblasts, which then produce cartilage and bone—osteoinduction. The spicules and fragments of bone act as a scaffold for the ingrowth of new bone—osteoconduction. Cancellous grafts are usually preferred because of the larger surface area and higher concentration of cells.

Sources for autogenous bone grafts in birds are limited. Cortical grafts provide mechanical support, but acceptable donor sources are lacking.[10, 12, 19] Allografts or xenografts of cortical bone may be alternatives. In a study of the effects of cortical allografts and xenografts in pigeons, grafts were associated with a higher incidence of incisional dehiscence, sequestrum formation, and foreign body reaction.[19] Cancellous bone may be harvested for grafting from the proximal tibiotarsus or ulna in large birds. The humerus, pelvis, and femur are usually not applicable as sources for cancellous bone in flighted birds because they are pneumatic. Autogenous corticocancellous bone grafts are often the most applicable grafts for avian fracture repair.

The keel and ribs may be harvested for corticocancellous bone. The last two ribs (17th and 18th) are easily approached for collection.[17] The section from the uncinate process (dorsal) to the junction between the sternal and vertebral ribs (ventral) may be collected. Care is taken to preserve the inner periosteum, preventing invasion of the coelomic cavity; however, in small birds this cannot be avoided. The sternum provides a larger amount of corticocancellous bone.[20, 21] The pectoral muscles are elevated off each side of the carina sterni (keel) and the central portion of the keel is removed, creating a bucket handle configuration (Fig. 42–1). The pectoral muscles are reattached to the keel

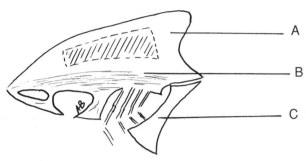

To collect a corticocancellous bone graft from the sternum, the pectoral muscles are elevated from both sides of the carina sterni (keel). The central portion of the keel is removed using an osteotome as outlined. The pectoral muscles are sutured to the ventral portion of the carina sterni once the graft has been harvested. *A*, Keel; *B*, sternum; *C*, coracoid. (Ventrodorsal position.)

during closure. Once harvested, the graft may be split through the medulla and used in an onlay fashion or cut into fragments with rongeurs to be used in or around the fracture site.

METHODS OF FRACTURE FIXATION

Many factors determine the best type of fixation to use for repair of a fracture, including the patient's natural behavior and activity level, the functional requirements placed on the affected limb, the type of injury, and the bone involved. The surgeon must have knowledge of the basic anatomy and surgical approaches, particularly the location of the major arteries, veins, and nerves. These approaches have been described.[5, 20–24] During the approach to a fracture, if it is necessary to transect a muscle for appropriate exposure, it should be transected as close as possible to its origin or insertion to optimize limb function. The flight feathers attach to the periosteum of the ulna (secondary feathers) and the major metacarpus (primary feathers). In these locations, periosteal elevation should be avoided to prevent damage to the follicles, which could result in abnormal feather growth. When treating fractures of pneumatic bones, the end of the proximal fracture should be covered prior to wound irrigation to prevent fluid from entering the air sac and lung, potentially causing air sacculitis, pneumonia, or asphyxiation.

It is vital to minimize intraoperative soft tissue

trauma and keep the tissues moist and aseptic. Aggressive tissue manipulation results in additional vascular compromise and scarring. Gentle manipulation of soft tissue is mandatory. During closed reduction, it is often difficult to achieve accurate reduction, resulting in soft tissue trauma from repeated attempts to apply traction. During open reduction, traction is applied directly to the bone and the fracture can be directly visualized, facilitating accurate reduction with less soft tissue damage.

Frequently, soft tissue injury associated with a fracture is more likely to result in loss of function and delayed healing than the fracture itself. Birds are particularly prone to the development of fracture disease associated with limb immobilization, which occurs with the use of transarticular external skeletal fixation (ESF) or external coaptation. Damage is characterized by the development of joint ankylosis, muscle atrophy, tendon contracture, and entrapment of tendons and ligaments within the callus.[3, 4, 6, 7, 9, 10, 13, 15, 17, 25–30]

A fracture associated with a skin wound, regardless of how minor, should be treated as an open, contaminated fracture. This may influence the decision on what type of fixation is most appropriate for fracture stabilization. In some cases, infection is obvious because of the presence of caseous, purulent material. All devitalized, necrotic, and purulent material should be surgically debrided. Culture samples should be taken from the wound and the patient treated with appropriate systemic antibiotic therapy. The wound should be copiously irrigated with physiologic saline. There is no objective evidence that irrigation solutions containing antibiotics or antiseptics are advantageous. In fact, many are irritating to tissues and delay healing.[5] Drains usually function poorly in birds because birds do not degrade proteins well, and they form caseous rather than liquid pus. In cases when infection is likely to persist, it is best to perform open surgical debridement every 1 to 7 days until all necrotic debris has been removed and the remaining tissues are healthy, as confirmed by culture results. This may be accomplished either by treating the tissues as an open wound or by reopening the incision for debridement.

External Coaptation

External coaptation[41, 48, 49, 53, 64, 69, 80] refers to the use of bandages, slings, and splints for fracture stabilization. It is most often considered if some decrease in limb function is acceptable or if there is minimal fracture displacement and soft tissue damage. In birds with pathologic fractures resulting from metabolic bone disease, the bone is usually too soft to hold most fixation devices, making external coaptation the treatment of choice.[1, 5] Other indications for the use of external coaptation include fractures of bones that are too small for other methods of fixation and patients with metabolic abnormalities, making the risk of anesthesia and surgery of more concern than accurate fracture alignment.

In some situations, cage rest alone may be considered adequate for fracture management; however, external coaptation should immobilize the fracture. Although alignment may be poor, pain is diminished by stabilizing the fracture. External coaptation is simple, generally inexpensive, requires little equipment and expertise, carries minimal risk of inducing infection, and can be applied with only a short anesthesia time.

Muscle atrophy, joint ankylosis, tendon contraction or entrapment within callus, shortening of the bone, and fracture malalignment are common consequences of treating fractures with external coaptation. In birds requiring normal limb function, fracture disease is second only to osteomyelitis as a cause of poor clinical outcome and failure of patient release.[8]

External coaptation is often associated with a prolonged convalescence because it is difficult to achieve complete immobilization. This may predispose the patient to other problems, such as stress death and bumblefoot of the contralateral limb with leg fractures.[20, 31] Coaptation should be removed as early as possible to minimize the potential for the development of fracture disease, stress death, and other complications.

When applying external coaptation, the joints proximal and distal to the fracture should be immobilized to adequately stabilize the fracture site.[12, 17, 28, 30] The bandage should be monitored at least weekly for evidence of soiling, vascular compromise, slippage, or other problem that may be an indication for replacement of the coaptation. When applying coaptation, care must be taken to avoid covering the vent, thus preventing elimination, and compressing the sternum, thus preventing normal respiration. It is best not to use especially sticky adhesives such as those on adhesive tape. The glue sticks to the feathers, making them easily soiled and interfering with normal preening.[17, 20, 22] In addition, avian skin is very delicate, and when adhesives are removed they often damage the underlying skin or cause a dermatopathy. Masking tape, drafting tape, paper tape, and self-adhesive tapes work well with avian patients because their adhesives are mild. Red materials should be avoided when bandaging raptors because the bird may be attracted to the bandage. Gauze should be avoided with psittacines because the bird may pull at individual strings. The strings may then tighten and cause occlusion of vessels underlying the site.

In general, the following steps should be used for applying external coaptation for fracture management. Stirrups may be useful when bandaging legs to prevent the device from slipping off. They are not generally required with fractures of the wing. The primary layer should be a light layer of soft conforming cast padding. It is important to use only a light layer and a width appropriate to the size of the patient. Using a wide roll of padding on a small limb results in a bandage that is lumpy and does not properly immobilize the fracture. Over the padding a light layer of conforming gauze is applied with enough compression to provide support for the fracture but not so much that the vascular supply to the extremity is compromised. In psittacine birds, gauze may be replaced with self-adhesive tape (Vetrap), which will not unravel.

Some form of splint material may be incorporated into the secondary layer to provide additional fracture support. Wood applicator sticks, tongue depressors, aluminum rods, lightweight casting material, or other material that will provide bending support may be incorporated into the bandage. Orthoplast (Johnson & Johnson Products, Inc., New Brunswick, NJ), Hexcelite (Hexcel Medical, Dublin, CA), and Veterinary Thermoplastic (VTP; Imex Veterinary, Inc., Longview, TX) are solid at room temperature but become soft and malleable when immersed in hot water. Orthoplast is supplied as a solid sheet that is somewhat difficult to mold and bend to conform to the bird's extremity. Hexcelite is a wide mesh that conforms well but has less bending stability than Orthoplast. VTP is a solid sheet of thermoplastic material impregnated with a gauze mesh. This material is more malleable than Orthoplast and stronger than Hexcelite. The tertiary layer should help keep the bandage clean and dry. Self-adhesive tape works well for this layer.

The type of external coaptation most appropriate varies with the bone fractured. Different types of external coaptation are discussed under methods of fixation for various bones.

Internal Fixation

Internal fixation provides the best chance to obtain accurate anatomic alignment and reduction of the fracture for a good functional outcome. The surgical approaches to the long bones of birds have been described.[5, 8, 20–24, 32] When closing, if there is concern regarding the viability of a portion of bone, it is helpful to cover that segment with healthy soft tissues. If this may compromise function in a free-ranging bird, only the skin need be closed over the fracture site.

Internal fixation requires general anesthesia, which may be prolonged with difficult fractures. When dealing with closed fractures, a lengthy anesthesia period introduces the potential for osteomyelitis. Some degree of surgical expertise is essential, the degree depending upon the type of fixation selected. In addition, depending upon the type of fixation, some implants are quite expensive.

Stainless Steel Intramedullary Pins

Intramedullary (IM) pins for internal fixation are familiar to most veterinarians, are relatively inexpensive, require little surgical exposure, provide axial alignment, and counteract bending forces.[15, 17, 28, 33–35] IM pins do not counteract rotation and shear forces.[7, 10, 12, 13, 15, 17, 24, 25, 28, 31, 34, 36] If the fracture is unstable, excessive callus may form, resulting in fracture disease that may prevent release of free-ranging birds. The cortices of avian bones are thin, providing little purchase for IM pins. Whether or not the weight of these implants affects flight or carriage of the extremity, their proximity to joints and tendency to cause periarticular fibrosis require that they be surgically removed as early as possible. Fortunately in most cases, the exposure required for pin removal is minimal and the pins slip out easily through a stab incision under local anesthe-

sia. Orthopedic wires do not require removal in most cases.

Inserting an IM pin in avian bone must be done very gently. The bone is thin and brittle. If excessive force is applied, iatrogenic fracture and soft tissue injury from the pin may result. The trochar point of the pin easily cuts through the bone with minimal pressure and gentle back and forth rotation of the wrist. It is important to prevent wobbling that may create iatrogenic fractures and an excessively large hole, predisposing the bone to collapse and motion at the fracture site. Once through the cortex, the pin is easily advanced through the medullary canal with gentle pressure and rotation. When resistance is encountered it indicates that the other cortex has been engaged. The pin should be seated by advancing it with one or two twists of the wrist. Farther advancement risks penetration into the joint.

Partially threaded pins do not increase resistance to pullout when used as IM pins.[37] It has been suggested that if partially threaded pins exit the cortex, they will prevent collapse at the fracture site.[23, 24] Although the threads may engage one cortex, the other fracture fragment is free to slide along the smooth portion of the pin, resulting in collapse. IM pins provide little resistance to rotation, compression, and shear forces, and additional means of fixation may be required to counteract these forces.

Cerclage, hemicerclage, or interfragmentary wires; external skeletal fixation; or stack pinning may be used to provide rotation and shear stability.[1, 9, 23, 24] Stack pinning is most applicable to fractures of the humerus and femur. It is best not to use external coaptation in conjunction with internal fixation to counter these forces because the disadvantages of both techniques are combined[1, 10, 29]; however, in some situations a combined approach may be necessary. Because of their tendency to stimulate periarticular fibrosis and joint ankylosis, it is best not to insert pins through or near a joint. If external coaptation is used in conjunction with IM pins, the repair should be gradually stressed as early as possible by removing the pin or the external coaptation as early as 2 weeks following repair. With most fractures this is adequate for the formation of fibrous callus that will eventually support the fracture. External coaptation may be added to internal fixation to prevent weight-bearing, but coaptation should not be expected to prevent motion.

The diameter of the pin used should be approximately 50% of the diameter of the bone. This will allow the formation of endosteal callus, minimize the weight of the implants, decrease the risk of damaging the nutrient artery, minimize the risk of creating iatrogenic fractures, and yet provide adequate bending stability and axial alignment.

The fracture should be examined for the presence of fissures, which should be treated using cerclage wires before the pin is inserted. The direction of pin insertion is defined by where the insertion begins. *Normograde* insertion describes insertion of the pin beginning at a natural end of the bone and advancing the pin toward the fracture site. *Retrograde* insertion refers to insertion of the pin from the fracture site and advancing the pin out either the proximal or distal end of the bone. These terms do not indicate whether the pin is inserted in a proximal or distal direction.[38]

Cross pins are usually indicated for fractures of the metaphysis. The ends of the pins should be cut flush with the surface of the bone because they are inserted very close to the joint. Alternatively, they may be countersunk below the surface of the bone. This makes removal more difficult, but it may not be necessary to remove the pins, especially if they are countersunk. The Rush technique for pin insertion is based on a specific type of pin designed for stabilization of metaphyseal fractures (Rush pins). They are inserted in a manner similar to that for the insertion of cross pins; however, they do not exit the cortex but bounce off the inner cortex and travel as intramedullary pins toward the other end of the bone. This provides a spring-loaded, three-point fixation for additional stability (Fig. 42–2).[38]

Orthopedic Wires

Principles for using orthopedic wires are well described.[35] Orthopedic wire is available in many sizes appropriate for use in even very small patients. In very small birds, suture material may be substituted for orthopedic wire, affording the advantage of be-

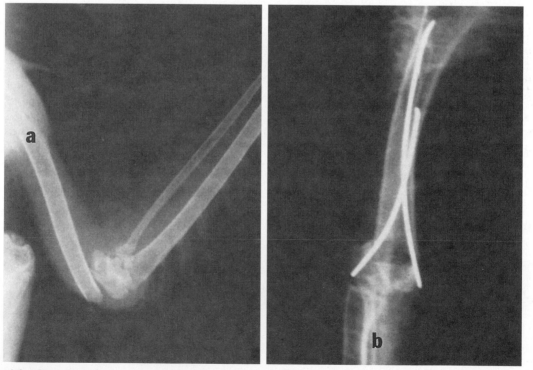

F i g u r e 4 2 – 2

(a, b) A fracture of the distal humerus in a red-tailed hawk *(Buteo jamaicensis)* was treated with Rush-type pins. This bird was released following pin removal. (From Bennett RA, Kuzma AB: Fracture management in birds. J Zoo Wildl Med 23:5–38, 1992.)

ing absorbable. Wire suture material may also be used but is suitable only for small avian patients.

It is important to recognize that orthopedic wires are an adjunct to other forms of fracture stabilization and are not to be used as a sole means of fixation because they are not stable against bending force. Cerclage wires are applicable to oblique fractures in which the length of the obliquity is at least twice the diameter of the bone. At least two wires should be used for oblique fractures or to hold butterfly fragments in place. A single wire may be used to stabilize fissure fractures.

Hemicerclage wires may be used for stabilization against rotational forces especially with short oblique fractures. They stabilize only against rotation and shear forces in one direction because they consist of only one strand of wire. Interfragmentary figure eight wires stabilize against rotation in both directions and are applicable to transverse and short oblique fractures (Fig. 42–3).[35]

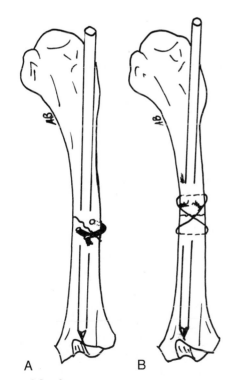

Figure 42–3

(A) Hemicerclage wires are used for stabilizing short oblique fractures against rotation. The wires counteract rotation only in one direction and rely on cortical contact to prevent rotation in the other direction. *(B)* Interfragmentary figure eight wires are used to stabilize transverse fractures against rotation. They counteract rotation in both directions.

Absorbable IM Pins

Polydioxanone (PDS) pins (Ortho-Sorb; Johnson & Johnson) have been evaluated for use in avian humeral fractures.[39] These pins are used in human orthopedic surgery and are reported to be completely absorbed by 6 months following implantation. PDS pins are not as stiff as stainless steel pins. Humeral osteotomies in pigeons were stabilized with PDS pins and stainless steel pins. Those stabilized with PDS pins healed with a larger callus than those stabilized with steel pins, which was thought to be the result of their being less rigid.[39] External coaptation was recommended as adjunct support because of the concern that the PDS pins were not sufficiently rigid. The major advantage of PDS pins is that surgical removal is not required, and their use may be indicated where pin removal would be difficult; however, they are technically difficult to insert.

Polypropylene Rods

Polypropylene welding rods[20, 22, 34] are available at plastic supply companies (sizes include $3/32$, $1/8$, $5/32$, $3/16$ inches). They are biologically inert, can be sterilized in an autoclave, are lightweight compared with stainless steel pins, and are relatively inexpensive (approximately $5.00/lb). They are easily cut to an appropriate length and are inserted using a shuttle technique that does not damage joint surfaces. Used with various adjunct techniques, they allow early return to function so that rehabilitation can begin as early as 7 days postoperatively.

These rods are best suited to diaphyseal fractures that have little or no contamination or comminution. The length of the rod used is limited to the length of the longer fracture segment. The depth of purchase within the bone is limited to the length of the shorter segment; if the segment is small, only a short portion can be shuttled into it (Fig. 42–4). A stress riser effect may be created at the ends of the pins, predisposing to fracture at that location. Because only relatively large-diameter rods are available, they are not appropriate for use in birds weighing less than 75 g. These rods are not as rigid as steel pins; when used without additional support, micromotion at the fracture may delay healing. Once inserted it is difficult to remove the rods,

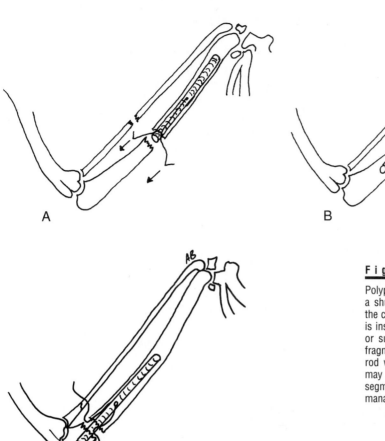

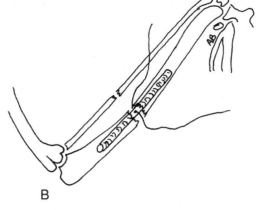

F i g u r e   4 2 – 4

Polypropylene rods are inserted into the medullary canal using a shuttle technique. *(A)* A wire or suture is passed through the center of the rod and the entire rod with the attached wire is inserted into the longer fragment. *(B)* The ends of the wire or suture are pulled so that the rod shuttles into the other fragment. *(C)* If one bone segment is short, the polypropylene rod will not gain significant purchase in that segment. This may limit its usefulness for treating fractures with a short segment. (*A and B* from Bennett RA, Kuzma AB: Fracture management in birds. J Zoo Wildl Med 23:5–38, 1992.)

making them inappropriate for use with open fractures where they may serve as a nidus for infection and bring a significant risk of development of osteomyelitis.

Like IM pins, polypropylene rods provide no resistance to axial and rotational forces. Several techniques have been used to provide rotational stability. Kirschner wires or small pins may be inserted transversely through one cortex, the rod, and the other cortex on both sides of the fracture. An external skeletal fixator may be added to prevent rotation. Intramedullary polymethylmethacrylate may be used to fill the medullary interstices to prevent rotation.

The shuttle technique requires some degree of experience to perform proficiently. The rod is cut to the length of the longer fracture segment by inserting it into the medullary canal until it contacts the metaphyseal cancellous bone and can no longer be advanced (see Fig. 42–4). The rod is removed and a hole drilled near its center using a small Kirschner wire or hypodermic needle (see Fig. 42–6). Suture material is passed through the hole and the rod is inserted into the longer segment, allowing the fracture to be reduced. Traction is applied to the suture to pull the rod into the shorter segment. If possible, the rod should be advanced to its midpoint so that equal lengths of rod are within each segment.

Threaded Steel Shuttle Pins

A technique was developed for using fully threaded steel IM pins as shuttle pins because polypropylene is not as rigid as steel (Fig. 42–5). The pin is cut to

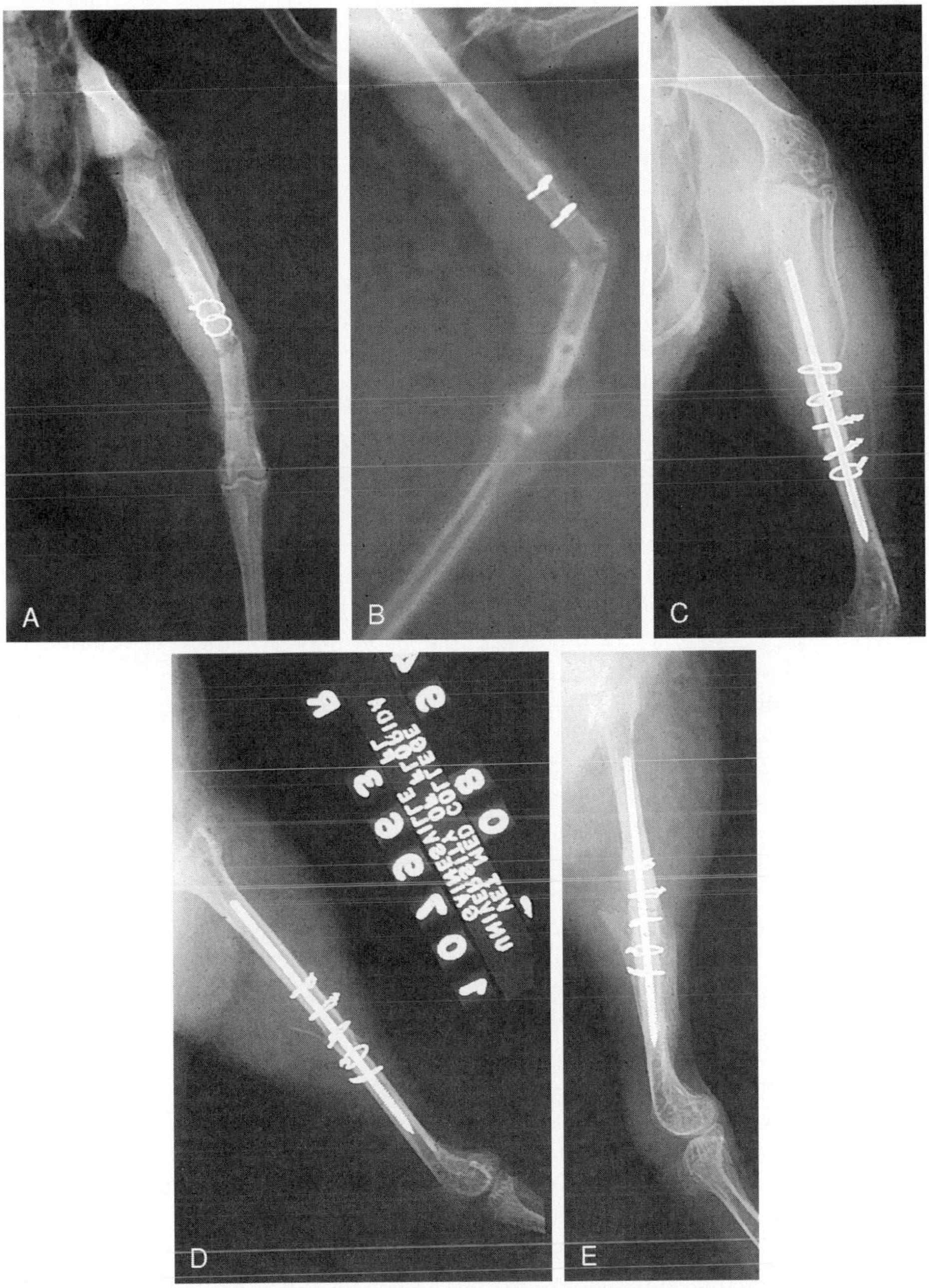

Figure 42–5

(A, B) An IM polypropylene rod with IM PMM was used to stabilize a fracture of the tibiotarsus in this barn owl *(Tyto alba)*. The rod bent and the implants had to be removed. *(C, D)* This fracture of the tibiotarsus in a muscovy duck was stabilized using a threaded IM shuttle pin with IM PMM. It was a long oblique fracture, and cerclage wires were used for rotational stability. *(E)* The fracture was healed 3 weeks postoperatively.

the length of the longer segment as described earlier. The pin should be cut so that when it is inserted into the longer segment the end extends slightly beyond the edge of the fracture. The pin is inserted into that segment and the fracture reduced. A hypodermic needle is inserted through the fracture gap to engage the threads extending beyond the fracture edge. The needle is used to advance the threaded pin into the other segment of bone. It should be advanced to the approximate midpoint of the pin or, if the other segment is short, until it reaches the end of the bone (see Fig. 42–5). Fully threaded or partially threaded positive-profile pins should be used to avoid pin failure at the threaded-nonthreaded junction.

Intramedullary Polymethylmethacrylate

Polymethylmethacrylate (PMM) is a bone cement marketed as a liquid monomer (20 ml) to be mixed with a powdered polymer containing barium sulfate, which makes the mixture radiopaque (40 g) (Surgical Simplex-P, Howmedica, Inc. Rutherford, NJ; LVC Bone Cement, Zimmer, Warsaw, Indiana).[1] The liquid and powder may be separately aseptically divided into 10 aliquots for use in avian fracture repair where only a small volume is needed. It is vital that asepsis be maintained because if the PMM becomes contaminated it can serve as a nidus for infection when placed within the bone. Because the liquid is sensitive to light, it must be stored in a light-protected container or maintained in a dark place. This material does not have adhesive properties; however, when mixed the exothermic polymerization reaction results in a 3% volume expansion, aiding in the formation of a cohesive bond.[8] Cooling both components to 3°C before mixing increases both the working time and shear strength of the cement. PMM does not adhere to itself when an attempt is made to join two aliquots. Instead, lamination occurs, and fracture of the PMM is likely at this location.[7, 40, 41]

PMM may be used alone for fracture stabilization or in combination with other forms of fixation. It is lightweight, rapidly stable, and does not interfere with joint function, allowing for early return to function. Once placed in the medullary canal PMM cannot be removed. If osteomyelitis develops, it may act as a nidus for infection making its use inappro-priate for contaminated or infected fractures. Heat-stable antibiotics may be added to help prevent infection. Cephalothin at 1 g per packet or 100 mg per aliquot is commonly recommended.[10, 29, 42] The bacteriostatic effects have been shown to last up to 5 years.[7, 43, 44] PMM is brittle and may break at the fracture site if used as the only means of fixation in birds weighing over 500 g.[29] Filling the medullary canal completely does not appear to interfere with healing.

Three techniques can be used to place PMM in the medullary canal. The medullary canal should be prepared by cleaning and drying it with cotton-tipped applicators. The PMM may be mixed to a doughy consistency and packed into each fracture segment. Once each segment is filled, the fracture is reduced and held in reduction while the cement polymerizes. Lamination of the PMM is likely with this method, making the repair susceptible to re-fracture at the site where the PMM in each segment was to bond together. To avoid this problem the cement may be mixed to a liquid consistency and placed into a syringe. Holes are created in each end of the bone, the fracture is reduced and held in reduction, and the liquid cement is injected into one of the holes while the other serves as a vent for air within the medullary cavity to escape. Alternatively, the liquid cement may be injected into each segment using a "back-fill" technique. In birds weighing less than 1 kg, a 16-gauge needle may be used or for larger birds a section of polyvinyl chloride intravenous tubing may be used. Red rubber tubing should not be used because it accelerates the reaction, causing the PMM to set up within the tubing. The needle or tubing is inserted as far as possible into the medullary canal and the liquid cement is injected while the tubing is withdrawn. Once both segments are back-filled with cement, the fracture is reduced and held in reduction while the cement cures. With all methods, care should be taken to ensure that cement has not seeped between fracture fragments because its presence acts as a physical barrier to callus bridging.[7, 45]

Intramedullary PMM With a Pin or Rod

IM PMM may be used in conjunction with IM steel pins or polypropylene rods to improve rotational stability and enhance resistance to bending. This technique requires precise timing and coordination. Each fracture segment must be at least 1 to 2 cm long to achieve adequate stability.[26]

The threaded pin or polypropylene rod should fill approximately one-half the diameter of the medullary canal to allow space for the PMM. Barbs are cut into the polypropylene rod to create an irregular surface into which the cement may bond (Fig. 42–6). A scalpel is used to slice the surface, creating barbs pointing toward the ends of the rod; they must point away from the fracture when placed within the medullary canal. The threads of threaded pins act in a similar fashion. The rod or pin is inserted using a shuttle technique and the PMM is injected around the pin using a back-fill technique. The limb should be supported for 7 to 10 days to allow for soft tissue healing. In many cases, patients treated with this method of fracture stabilization are able to begin rehabilitation in 2 to 6 weeks.

External Skeletal Fixation (ESF)

There are many types of ESF[7, 13, 14, 17, 20, 22, 23, 27, 31, 46] used in fracture management, with the Kirschner-Ehmer splint (Osteotech INT., Timonium, MD) being one type. Because of this, the Kirschner device or K-E apparatus refers only to the commercially available splint consisting of steel clamps and connecting bars. Biphasic fixators use an acrylic cement column instead of connecting bars and clamps. Fixation pins are inserted through stab incisions in the skin transversely through both cortices of the affected bone. Steinmann pins, Kirschner wires, hypodermic needles, or spinal needles may be used as fixation pins. Positive-profile threaded fixation pins (IMEX Interface and IMEX Centerface Pins; Imex Veterinary, Inc.) probably provide better bone-holding power and are available in sizes as small as 0.035 inches in diameter. Devices called Half-Pins For Acrylic Fixators are also available and have positive profile threads near the point as well as a roughened surface on the shaft to improve cement bonding (Imex Veterinary, Inc.).

External fixators are well tolerated by birds and may be applied to almost any bone, including bones of the distal extremities. They do not interfere with joint function or stimulate periarticular fibrosis, allowing for early return to function. External fixators can be maintained for long periods of time with minimal morbidity to allow stabilization of fractures that are slow to heal. Minimal surgical dissection is required to obtain good fracture alignment. ESF is stable against all fracture forces. Fixators are ideal for open fractures because soft tissue injuries may be treated without interfering with the fixation. Fixators can often be removed without general anesthesia.

Metal fixators such as the K-E apparatus are heavy. The connecting system that extends beyond the body surface may traumatize other parts of the body by rubbing on them or it may catch on something and pull out. Avian bones have thin cortices and fixation pins loosen quickly, which may predis-

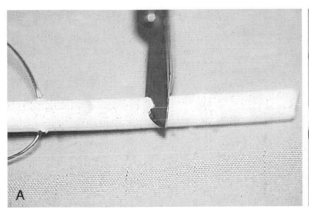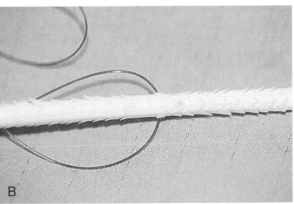

Figure 42–6

(A) A scalpel is used to cut barbs into the polypropylene rod to improve its bonding with the PMM cement. *(B)* A suture or small-gauge wire is passed through a hole in the rod to be used to shuttle the rod.

pose the bird to fractures at the pin-bone interface.[7, 9, 14, 34] Fixation pin purchase can be improved by using threaded pins. It is best to use pins with threads laid onto the pin shaft (positive profile). The core diameter of the pin with positive-profile threads is uniform throughout its length. Negative-profile pins have threads cut into the shaft. The core diameter in the threaded portion is less than that of the nonthreaded portion, decreasing the bending strength and creating a stress riser effect at the threaded-nonthreaded junction. Positive-profile fixation pins have been reported to remain stable in avian fractures for 3 months, as compared with 3 to 6 weeks for nonthreaded and other types of threaded pins.[5] Iatrogenic fractures occur during insertion if fixation pins are not inserted gently and carefully. Predrilling has been suggested as a means of obtaining more secure pin placement with less chance of creating iatrogenic fracture during insertion.[5] Although no studies confirm the reported benefit of predrilling, it may be most beneficial when placing positive-profile threaded pins.

ESF is best used for stabilizing fractures of bones where other methods of fixation would result in periarticular fibrosis, for open and contaminated fractures, highly comminuted fractures, corrective osteotomies, metaphyseal and epiphyseal fractures, and luxations. Type I fixators penetrate both cortices but only one skin surface (Fig. 42–7). Type II fixators penetrate both skin surfaces as well as both cortices with two connecting systems. Type III fixators combine types I and II in different planes, creating a three-dimensional frame. The stability of the fixator increases as the complexity increases. Other modifiers may be used to describe the number of fixation pins, type of clamps, and number of connecting systems used.[47]

Principles for application of ESF have been described.[9, 20, 22, 47–49] Fixation pins should be inserted through a stab incision in intact skin, not into wounds or incisions. Large muscle masses should be avoided because contraction moves the fixation pin, causing premature loosening and patient discomfort. Fixation pins should penetrate both cortices even with type I fixators to achieve maximal pin purchase. To prevent lateral sliding of the bone along fixation pins, at least one pin in each segment should be inserted at an angle of 35 to 55° to the long axis of the bone. If positive-profile threaded pins are used, it may not be necessary to place the

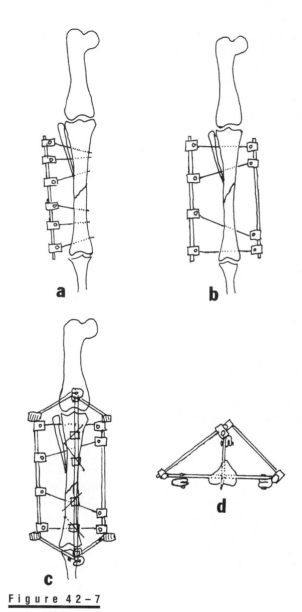

Figure 42–7

(A) Type I external skeletal fixator. *(B)* Type II fixator. *(C, D)* Type III fixator. (From Bennett RA, Kuzma AB: Fracture management in birds. J Zoo Wildl Med 23:5–38, 1992.)

pins at an angle because the threads will prevent lateral movement of the bone with respect to the pins. At least two fixation pins should be placed in each segment. When used as additional stabilization for other methods of internal fixation, one pin in each segment may be used. The most proximal and distal fixation pins should be placed as close to the ends of the bones as possible to distribute the forces along the entire bone. Yet, the farther from the fracture site the pins are placed the less stable the device. Therefore, as many pins as the length of the bone can accommodate should be inserted along as much of the length of the bone as possible. The connecting system should be placed as close as possible to the skin surface for the best stability, but space must be provided for postoperative soft tissue swelling. An IM polypropylene shuttle rod may be used to improve fixation pin purchase in avian bones but should not be used with open, contaminated fractures.[23, 27]

K-E Splints

Kirschner-Ehmer splints are familiar to most veterinarians. The components are ready to apply and easy to connect. K-E splints are quite heavy and, although three sizes are marketed, only two are appropriate for avian patients. Even the small size is too large for most companion birds. The splints are relatively expensive, approaching the cost of bone plates and screws. The fixation pins must be inserted in a linear configuration to be able to apply the connecting system. This is best accomplished by first determining the total number of fixation pins to be used. The most proximal and distal pins are placed, the total number of clamps added to the connecting bar, and the connecting system attached to the first two pins. The subsequent pins are then passed individually, first through the clamp, then the skin, soft tissue, and bone. Using this technique, all pins are in line with the connecting bar and clamps. All sharp points should be padded to avoid traumatizing adjacent surfaces.[23, 50]

Biphasic Fixators

This type of ESF uses stainless steel fixation pins and another type of material for the connecting system. Many materials used are lightweight and can be connected to very small pins, hypodermic needles, or spinal needles making them applicable to even very small avian patients. The connecting materials are generally inexpensive and can be applied even if the pins are not in a linear configuration.

Nonsterile PMM (Technovit; Jorgensen Labs, Loveland, CO) or dental acrylic cement may be used to connect fixation pins.[1, 27] The pins should be notched or bent over to improve the cohesive cement bond. Half-pins For Acrylic Fixators have a roughened shaft surface to improve the cement bond.

Pins may be bent over to act as reinforcing bars within the cement by holding the base of the pin with a snubnosed wire twister to ensure that the bending force is not transferred to the bone, which might result in iatrogenic fracture. Using a second wire twister, the pin is bent over parallel to the bone at a distance from the bone sufficient to allow room for soft tissues and the PMM connecting system (Fig. 42–8). Once the fixation pins are prepared, the PMM is mixed to a dough consistency and molded around the fixation pins. Fracture reduction is maintained until the cement has cured.

Another technique uses flexible tubing such as a Penrose drain. The fixation pins are passed through the tubing, the fracture is reduced, and the cement is injected into the tubing while still in a liquid form as the fracture is maintained in reduction until curing is complete. Fixation pins are usually inserted at an angle to prevent the cement from pulling off the pins; however, the angle makes it difficult to slide the tubing over the pins. Latex tubing (Technical Products of Georgia, Decatur, GA) is much easier to work with and comes in a variety of sizes.

Hexcelite[23, 50] and VTP may be used for the connecting system, especially in small patients. The material is softened in hot water, applied to the fixation pins, and allowed to cool while the fracture is maintained in reduction. VTP is more firm than Hexcelite when cool. Both materials are easily trimmed with bandage scissors. Sharp points should be padded to avoid causing dermal injury.

For very small birds (<300 g), epoxy resin may be used to connect the fixation pins.[46] A small card such as a portion of an index card is folded to form a V-shaped trough and placed over the fixation pins, which are placed in linear alignment. The trough is then filled with epoxy, which is allowed to cure while the fracture is maintained in reduction. Care should be taken to ensure that epoxy does not drop onto the skin. Additional pins may be placed into the trough to act as reinforcing bars. This type of connecting system can weigh as little as 3 g.

An even smaller connecting system can be fashioned from a Kirschner wire.[46] Each fixation pin is glued to this connecting bar using epoxy. Cyanoac-

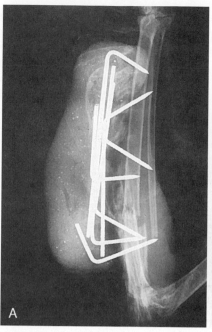
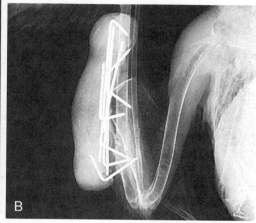

Figure 42–8

(A) This fracture of the radius and ulna was treated with a type I fixator with the fixation pins bent over and incorporated into the connecting system of PMM. *(B)* The fracture healed uneventfully.

rylate glue may be used to temporarily adhere the fixation pins to the connecting bar while the epoxy is mixed, applied, and allowed to cure.

Bone Plates

In the past, relatively few attempts[4, 10, 17, 27, 51, 57] were made to stabilize avian fractures with bone plates, because it was felt that the thin avian cortices would not hold bone screws.[9, 13, 15, 17, 34, 52–55] Plate fixation was limited to large terrestrial birds with thick cortices. New equipment and techniques have demonstrated that bone plating has a place in avian fracture management.

Bone plates allow anatomic alignment with rigid stabilization, avoid interference with joint motion, and allow early return to function. Some fractures treated with bone plates appear to heal by primary bone healing with little or no callus production.[10] The fixation lies completely within the body and does not attract the patient's attention or cause injury to adjacent structures as external coaptation and ESF do.

Plating is relatively expensive, technically difficult to implant, and requires specialized equipment and surgeon training. Extensive soft tissue dissection is required for implantation and removal, necessitating long sessions under anesthesia. Properly applied plates may be used in open, contaminated fractures; however, if improperly applied, they can become a nidus for continued infection. Other disadvantages of plating in birds are not well documented but include the potential for stress protection, cold sensitivity, and delayed fracture healing.[5]

Finger plates, semitubular plates, dynamic compression plates (DCP), and veterinary cuttable plates have been used successfully to treat avian fractures. Standard ASIF (American Society of Internal Fixation) techniques are used.[56] Semitubular plates conform well to round avian bones. This is a modified application because these plates were designed to rest on top of the bone, their stability being a function of their semicircular configuration. If the plate is bent in such a manner that the curve is lost, it becomes weaker. Semitubular plates are thin, making it easier to close soft tissues over them. In general they are not as strong as dynamic compression plates and are available only in sizes that are relatively large for most avian patients.

Veterinary cuttable plates (VCP) (Synthes, Paoli, PA) are 30 cm long with 50 holes and may be cut to an appropriate length. The smaller size may be used with 1.5-mm or 2.0-mm screws and the larger size with 2.0-mm or 2.7-mm screws. Cuttable plates are small and lightweight with holes placed close together. They may be stacked to improve their strength.

The technique for proper screw insertion has been described for avian bone and is different from that used in mammals because of the thin cortices of avian bone.[1, 51] If a screw is stripped, a nut may be fashioned from a small piece of a polypropylene syringe case, drilled, and tapped to hold screw threads.[51] IM PMM may be used to improve screw purchase.[4, 10, 27, 57] The medullary canal is back-filled as previously described. It is important that the PMM extend at least 1 cm beyond the ends of the plate to prevent creating a stress riser effect. The plate should span as much of the bone as possible to increase the flexural strength of the system.

External coaptation should be applied for 24 hours following bone plate application to help reduce soft tissue swelling. The patient should be confined to a small cage with only limited exercise for 2 weeks. Flight training can begin as early as 2 weeks following surgery.

Plate removal is rarely necessary. It appears that cold sensitivity, stress protection, and the weight of the implants are not of major concern in birds.[4, 10, 27, 57] A low incidence of implant-associated osteosarcoma is reported in mammals but has never been documented in birds. A plate causing a problem should be removed. Timing for plate removal is based on physical and radiographic evaluation of fracture healing.

The Doyle Technique

It is well recognized that compression at the fracture site aids in bone healing. In an effort to accomplish this goal, the Doyle technique was developed.[5] This technique combines the IM support of the Rush technique with external fixation. The ends of the pins extending outside the skin are connected with a dental impact rubber band to provide compression at the fracture site and improve the rotational stability. The Doyle system is a lighter system than the traditional ESF devices because the Rush-type

pins used are somewhat smaller than those used with external fixators and fewer pins are used.

It is important to note that some type of IM support is required with this type of fixation. If external fixation pins are connected with an impact rubber band, compression is achieved along the cortex closest to the rubber band (the cis cortex). This compressive force results in distraction of the fracture at the opposite cortex (the trans cortex). It is also imperative that a buttress be achieved on the compression side. If there is a gap, the fracture collapses as a result of the compressive force.

The Doyle technique involves placing an IM pin using the Rush technique from the metaphysis of the bone. The pin should enter the medullary canal, bounce off the trans cortex, and move toward the cis cortex again. Two pins are placed in this manner, one at the distal metaphysis and one at the proximal metaphysis. These pins are then bent to be perpendicular to the long axis of the bone, and a small hook is created at the end of each pin. The two hooks are then connected with a dental impact rubber band (Fig. 42–9). In most cases, 0.025- to 0.062-inch Kirschner wires are used. The pin must be inserted as far from the fracture as possible to obtain the most secure system. The external apparatus is then padded and bandaged. In most cases the rubber band is removed in 10 to 21 days and the IM pin approximately 1 to 3 weeks later, based on radiographic evidence of bone healing.

A modification of this technique involves placing the first pin as described earlier. The second pin is inserted at a 45° angle to the long axis of the bone and perpendicular to the angle at which the initial pin was inserted. This pin is inserted in a cross pin fashion and penetrates the far cortex.

An additional modification may be made by using a single IM pin to provide axial support. Two pins are then inserted at 45° angles to the long axis of the bone and connected in a similar fashion using a dental impact rubber band. The disadvantage of this is the IM placement of the pin, which risks causing periarticular fibrosis.

FRACTURES OF THE THORACIC LIMB

Fractures of the Pectoral Girdle

Fractures of the pectoral girdle usually occur when a bird flies into an object or is hit by a moving

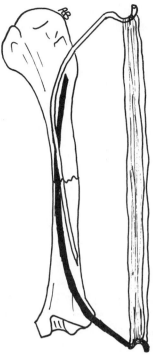

F i g u r e   4 2 – 9

The Doyle technique uses two pins inserted in a Rush pin fashion, one in each metaphysis. The pins are then connected with a rubber band to achieve compression at the fracture site.

vehicle. Fractures of the scapula or the clavicle are generally treated by cage rest or external coaptation. In one study, coracoid fractures accounted for 86% of avian fractures at a raptor facility.[58] Because of the intricate anatomy of the avian shoulder joint (Fig. 42–10), fractures of the coracoid are frequently undiagnosed.[58] Many birds with coracoid fractures are able to fly but only for a short distance. Fractures of the coracoid bone are treated by cage rest or external coaptation in companion birds or when fracture displacement is minimal. Displaced fractures of the coracoid should be treated by internal fixation in birds that require the ability to achieve precision flight. A single IM pin is usually adequate to provide axial alignment and bending stability. Following IM pinning, the affected wing should be supported with external coaptation.

The surgical approach to the coracoid bone involves transection of the cranial portion of the pectoral and supracoracoid muscles.[32] The initial skin incision is made along the clavicle on the affected side and extended along the lateral edge of the keel approximately one-fifth the length of the keel. The pectoral muscle is incised along the border of the clavicle and the keel, as described for the skin incision. The clavicular artery is located within this muscle mass and its transection often results in hemorrhage, which can be controlled with electrosurgery. It is located near the midpoint of the clavicle. A corresponding incision is made in the insertion of the supracoracoid muscle, and the coracoid bone is located immediately below.

The coracoid bone courses at an angle of approximately 45° from the shoulder joint to the keel. In most cases it is best to pass the pin retrograde from the fracture site out the shoulder joint, reduce the fracture, and seat the pin into the proximal fragment of the coracoid bone. If the pin is advanced too far it may penetrate the sternum and heart. To avoid penetrating the heart it is best to preset the distance on the pin chuck to the desired depth of pin insertion.

For closure, the muscles are sutured to their insertions on the keel and the clavicle. It is best to add external coaptation on the affected wing for 7 to 10 days postoperatively to allow soft tissues to heal. The end of the pin at the shoulder should be left long enough to facilitate removal following fracture healing. It is important to note that the distal end of the coracoid articulates with the humerus. Because of this the pin is removed as soon as possible to minimize the degree of periarticular fibrosis and shoulder joint ankylosis.

Fractures of the Humerus

In most cases, fractures of the humerus are best treated by internal fixation. The strong pectoral, supracoracoid, and biceps brachii muscles pull the distal segment toward the shoulder joint, creating severe overriding. This is less of a problem with fractures of the proximal humerus. With such fractures the surrounding muscle mass may provide adequate stability to prevent severe displacement of the fractures (Fig. 42–11). Treatment with external coaptation may result in malunion and diminished flight capability.[58]

When treating fractures of the humerus with external coaptation it is important to immobilize the shoulder joint by bandaging the wing to the body. This can be accomplished by using one of several

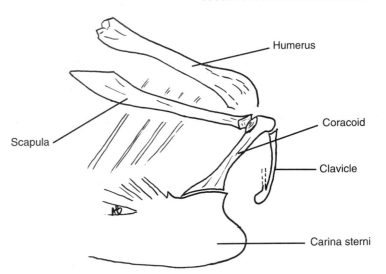

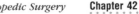

Figure 42-10

The osseous anatomy of the pectoral girdle. The humeral head is not shown. Note that the scapula and the coracoid both articulate with the head of the humerus.

techniques. The wing may be bandaged to the body using a figure eight configuration around the bird such that the bandage crosses over the back of the bird and encircles both shoulders and carpi within the cranial loop of the figure eight and both elbows with the caudal loop of the figure eight (Fig. 42–12). In most cases it is best to incorporate only one wing, leaving the other wing free for the bird to use for balancing.

The second technique uses two encircling bandages connected over the back. The first loop stabilizes both shoulders and carpi and the second loop stabilizes both elbows. These two encircling wraps are then connected along the dorsal midline with a

tape band preventing the bandage from being displaced either cranially or caudally (see Fig. 42–12).

An alternative method of immobilization involves placing a wrap on the wing as described for fractures of the radius and ulna. This immobilizes the elbow and carpus. The wrapped wing is then bandaged to the body, thus immobilizing the shoulder joint.

Most techniques for internal fracture fixation are applicable to fractures of the humerus in birds, including bone plates, IM devices with or without IM PMM and orthopedic wires, and ESF. The primary limitation when using ESF for fractures of the

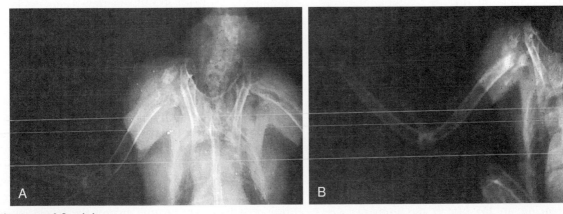

Figure 42-11

(A) This comminuted fracture of the humerus in a sharp-shinned hawk (Accipiter striatus) was treated using cage rest only. The bird regained the ability to fly and was released. (B) Radiographs made prior to release showed that a pseudoarthrosis had developed; however, the ventral and dorsal tubercles had not healed to the humerus.

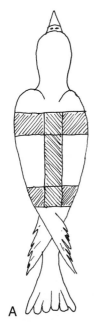

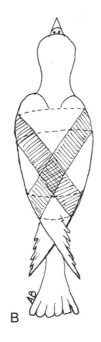

Figure 42–12

(A) A fractured humerus can be immobilized by wrapping the wing to the body using two encircling wraps—one at the shoulders to stabilize the carpi and one at the elbows. These are joined by a single band of tape dorsally to prevent the wraps from slipping. *(B)* A figure eight bandage encircling both carpi cranially and both elbows caudally may also be used to immobilize a fractured wing. (From Bennett RA, Kuzma AB: Fracture management in birds. J Zoo Wildl Med 23:5–38, 1992.)

humerus is that through-and-through fixation pins, as would be used with a type II or type III fixation device, cannot be applied. The humerus lies in close proximity to the chest wall of the bird, and devices placed on the medial aspect of the humerus interfere with and cause traumatic abrasions of the pectoral region. Type I ESF or biplanar skeletal fixation with two type I fixators applied at approximately 90° angles are applicable for fractures of the humerus (see Fig. 42–18). This type of ESF may be used with or without IM support. When treating open fractures of the humerus, ESF is often the treatment of choice. ESF allows the surgeon to treat soft tissue injuries and monitor for evidence of infection while maintaining fracture stability. Even with open fractures, IM pins may be used in conjunction with the ESF.

When placing an IM pin in the humerus it is generally in a retrograde fashion, exiting the pectoral crest of the proximal humerus. Normograde insertion initiated at the pectoral crest for closed pin-ning techniques is also applicable. It is best not to penetrate the distal cortex of the humerus because this predisposes the bird to periarticular fibrosis at the elbow and limited wing function. Techniques have been described for retrograde and normograde placement of pins penetrating the dorsal or ventral epicondylar region of the humerus. A pin may also be inserted in a normograde direction beginning in the caudodistal humerus.[58] The tendon of insertion of the triceps muscle is identified and retracted so that the pin may be inserted through the caudal cortex. The pin is then advanced across the fracture and into but not through the cancellous bone of the pectoral crest of the proximal humerus.

When treating distal metaphyseal fractures of the humerus, a cross pin or a Rush-type pin technique is applicable. When the fracture is very distal, a type I transarticular ESF device may be appropriate.[58]

Fractures of the Radius and Ulna

External coaptation is applicable to some fractures of the radius and ulna, especially if only one of the two bones is fractured. In such cases the intact bone serves as an internal splint so that with external coaptation the functional outcome is generally good. In cases where there is severe distraction, synostosis may occur between the radius and ulna, indicating a need for internal fixation.

A figure eight bandage may be applied to the wing to immobilize the elbow and the carpus, thus stabilizing the radius and the ulna (Fig. 42–13*A*). One loop of the figure eight encircles the carpus and the other encircles the elbow. Generally, the bandage is started by encircling the carpus and crossing over the lateral surface of the radius and ulna. It then proceeds around the lateral side of the wing, encircling medially to engage the distal humerus, thus immobilizing the elbow joint. Once the initial figure eight configuration has been started, additional wraps may be applied to provide a more stable immobilization of the wing. When treating fractures of the proximal radius and ulna, this type of bandage may potentiate fracture over-riding, which may in turn disrupt the basilic artery and vein and the radial nerve.[5]

The braille sling has been used by falconers for many years (Fig. 42–13*B*). It consists of a strip of

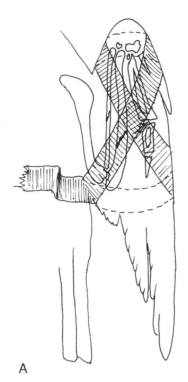
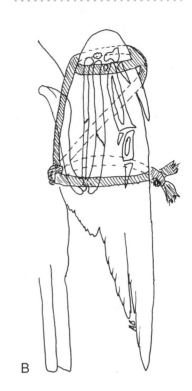

Figure 42–13

(A) A figure eight bandage applied to stabilize a fracture of the radius and ulna should encircle the carpus cranially and the elbow caudally and should cross on the lateral surface of the wing. *(B)* A braille sling may also be used to immobilize a fractured radius and ulna. A long strip of cloth or leather with a slit at the approximate midpoint is placed with the slit over the carpus and then tied medial to the distal humerus, wrapped around the elbow, and tied again. (From Bennett RA, Kuzma AB: Fracture management in birds. J Zoo Wildl Med 23:5–38, 1992.)

A

B

bandaging material with a longitudinal slit at the approximate midpoint. Many falconers use soft leather for this type of external coaptation. The slit is placed over the carpus to immobilize that joint. The two strips are brought together medial to the elbow and tied at the level of the distal humerus. The remaining length of material is then crossed over the distal manus to incorporate the flight feathers and encircle the elbow joint, and it is tied a final time. Many falconers modify this sling by adding a covering over the carpus to prevent trauma from the cage walls.

ESF is the type of fixation most appropriate for treating fractures of both the radius and ulna in birds requiring precision flight. When treating open fractures it allows the surgeon to manage the soft tissues during fracture healing. Even with closed fractures of the radius and ulna, an ESF is appropriate because it does not invade articular or periarticular structures, thus minimizing the risk of fracture disease. Type II or type III fixators are not applicable to radius and ulna fractures because they may cause trauma to the body of the bird from the medial connecting system. The flight feather follicles are attached to the periosteum of the ulna.

Careful insertion is required to avoid damaging the feather follicles, which could result in abnormal feather growth. When using ESF on the ulna, fixation pin purchase may be improved and IM support added by using a shuttled polypropylene rod (Fig. 42–14).

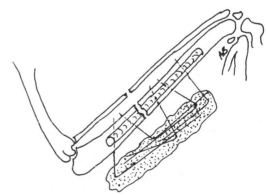

Figure 42–14

Fixation pin purchase can be improved by inserting an intramedullary polypropylene rod through which the fixation pins pass. The fixation pins may be bent over and incorporated into the cement of a biphasic fixator. (From Bennett RA, Kuzma AB: Fracture management in birds. J Zoo Wildl Med 23:5–38, 1992.)

In most cases, the ulna is stabilized and no stabilization of the radius is required; however, if there is significant displacement of the fracture fragments of the radius, internal stabilization of the radius may be required to prevent synostosis. If synostosis develops it may be treated surgically by removing the osseous bridge and placing a fat graft in the interosseous space created to prevent recurrence.[58] Because of the small size of the radius, it is difficult to apply an external fixator. The radius fracture may be stabilized with an interfragmentary orthopedic wire, such as a figure eight wire, or a shuttle pin, providing axial alignment and bending stability. This is generally all that is required to prevent the formation of synostosis. A technique for retrograde placement of an IM pin in the radius exiting at the carpus has also been described.[58]

For simple closed fractures of the radius and ulna, an IM pin with external coaptation is frequently adequate to allow fracture healing. In such cases, the IM pin will likely be left in place only 2 to 3 weeks, minimizing the periarticular fibrosis associated with the IM pin. In many free-ranging birds, this can still cause significant periarticular damage and inhibit flight; however, for most pet birds and birds that do not require precision flying this is frequently a very successful method of immobilization.

An IM pin in the ulna should be placed in a normograde fashion from a point distal to the elbow. The insertion is generally initiated between the second and third flight feather follicles distal to the elbow. The initial cut in the bone is made by inserting the pin perpendicular to the long axis of the bone. Once the surgeon can feel the trochar of the pin cutting through the bone, the angle is changed to a very acute angle so that the pin enters and follows the medullary canal of the ulna. Careful insertion is required to avoid penetrating the distal ulna and carpus, predisposing the bird to periarticular fibrosis. In order to avoid penetrating the distal ulna, some prefer to create a guide hole at the point of pin insertion. The next size larger pin with its trochar tip removed is inserted into the guide hole and advanced to the distal metaphysis of the ulna. Because the point has been removed, it is less likely to penetrate the epiphysis and invade the joint.[58] If the pin must be inserted in a retrograde fashion from the fracture out the proximal ulna, it is vital that it be directed out the caudal aspect of the ulna as far from the elbow joint as possible.

Fractures of the radius and ulna are also very amenable to treatment with IM shuttle pin and PMM. IM PMM must be used with caution when treating open fractures because the results of infection can be disastrous.

Fractures of the Carpometacarpus

Fractures of the carpometacarpus are susceptible to avascular necrosis distal to the point of injury because there is a single artery (the superficial ulnar artery) supplying the distal wing in birds. If this vessel is damaged, avascular necrosis distal to the point of injury occurs. This must be kept in mind when surgically treating fractures of the carpometacarpus because the surgeon can cause iatrogenic injury to this vessel.

Fractures of the carpometacarpus may be treated with external coaptation using either a figure eight bandage or a braille sling. In some cases it may be deemed necessary to perform internal fixation. IM pins placed in the carpometacarpus are generally placed in the medullary canal of the major metacarpus portion. Because of the anatomy, pins generally invade either an articular or periarticular surface, predisposing to periarticular fibrosis. ESF may be the most appropriate form of stabilization for this type of fracture in large birds when precision flight is required. Very small pins or hypodermic needles may be used as fixation pins.

If some periarticular fibrosis may be tolerated, an IM pin may be inserted into the major metacarpus portion by either normograde or retrograde insertion. The pin is best inserted to exit the carpus rather than the carpometacarpophalangeal joint. When placed in normograde fashion, the pin should be inserted through the extensor process of the carpometacarpus. This requires that the pin make a rather sharp bend for it to migrate along the medullary canal of the major metacarpus. Alternatively, the insertion may be initiated between the radial carpal bone and the extensor process of the carpometacarpus, providing a more direct angle for insertion into the major metacarpus. The wing should then be bandaged in flexion so that the pin exiting the carpus does not damage the radial carpal bone or the articular surfaces of the distal radius and ulna. This also provides some rotational stability.

FRACTURES OF THE PELVIC LIMB

Fractures of the pelvic limb in birds (see Fig. 42–10) occur less frequently than fractures of the thoracic limb. They are also less common in free-ranging birds than in companion birds.[58] It should be noted that most companion birds function well following leg amputation. The light weight of passerine birds allows them to function without the development of pododermatitis. Psittacines use their beak as a crutch and function well when a leg has been amputated.

Fractures of the Femur

As with fractures of the humerus, fractures of the femur are not generally amenable to treatment with external coaptation. External coaptation may be used if some limb shortening is acceptable. If the alignment is adequate, if the animal is still able to prehend with the affected foot, and if there is no change in weight-bearing capacity that would predispose to arthritis or pododermatitis, external coaptation may be used. In most cases the pull of the musculature causes overriding of the fracture when external coaptation alone is used.

The best method for external coaptation of femur fractures is a spica splint (Fig. 42–15). The spica splint is applied to immobilize the hip joint. The splint is molded to the contour of the curvature over the dorsum of the bird and down the leg to the level of the tibiotarsus or tarsometatarsus, with the leg being maintained in a normal standing position. The abdomen and affected leg are adequately padded, and the splint is applied and secured in place. This type of splint does not overcome the muscular tension that results in overriding of the fracture fragments; however, it does maintain the axial alignment of the limb. In some cases it may be used as an adjunct to an IM pin, providing rotational stability while relying on the IM pin for axial alignment. Some fractures of the distal femur are amenable to stabilization using Schroeder-Thomas splints (Fig. 42–16).

Femoral fractures may also be treated using a

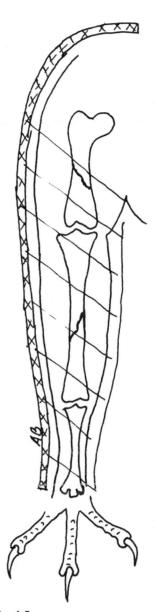

F i g u r e 4 2 – 1 5

A spica splint can be used to immobilize fractures of the femur or tibiotarsus. The splint extends to the dorsal midline and is bandaged around the abdomen to immobilize the coxofemoral joint. (From Bennett RA, Kuzma AB: Fracture management in birds. J Zoo Wildl Med 23:5–38, 1992.)

stirrup–encircling-bandage technique. Tape is used to create a stirrup around the foot. The tape is then wrapped along the lateral surface of the leg to pull the leg into flexion. The tape should pass over the dorsum at the level of the synsacrum and then around the abdomen and across the foot again (Fig.

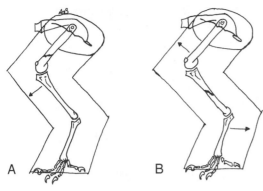

F i g u r e　4 2 – 1 6

A Schroeder-Thomas splint is formed with the limb in a normal standing position. Traction is achieved by applying tension to the joints proximal and distal to the fracture. To apply traction to the distal femur *(A)*, the tibiotarsus is taped to the cranial bar, applying tension to the stifle joint. For a fracture of the tibiotarsus *(B)*, the femur is taped to the cranial bar and the tarsometatarsus is taped to the caudal bar, applying tension to the stifle and hock, respectively. (From Bennett RA, Kuzma AB: Fracture management in birds. J Zoo Wildl Med 23:5–38, 1992.)

42–17). This technique does not overcome the pull of the muscles and the resulting overriding of the fracture fragments. It is best used for fractures that are minimally displaced or as an adjunct to an IM pin.

Internal fixation of femur fractures is the treatment of choice in most cases. Such fractures may be stabilized with a variety of internal fixation methods; however, as discussed with fractures of the humerus, type I external fixators are most appropriate for use on the femur because the type II and type III fixators cause damage to the body wall medial to the leg. External fixators may be used with or without IM support. For added stability, two type I fixators may be placed on the femur at 90° angles and away from the medial aspect of the thigh (Fig. 42–18). IM pins and orthopedic wires are also appropriate for use with fractures of the femur. Bone plates have also been used with success.

Normograde insertion of IM pins is generally recommended. Insertion is initiated at the trochanteric fossa. This technique can also be used for closed pinning techniques and may be less likely to cause damage to the sciatic nerve. Distal metaphyseal fractures of the femur may be treated with a cross pin or Rush-type pin technique.

Fractures of the Tibiotarsus

As with fractures of the femur, most fractures of the tibiotarsus are best treated with internal stabilization. External coaptation is most appropriate if there is good anatomic alignment and some compromise in limb length is not likely to affect the weight-bearing capacity of the limb, predisposing the bird to pododermatitis and arthritis.

Schroeder-Thomas splints serve well to immobilize fractures of the tibiotarsus as well as the tarsometatarsus. They may also be used as an adjunct to IM pinning to prevent rotation while allowing some weight-bearing to minimize the tendency to develop pododermatitis on the contralateral limb. The construction and method for applying these splints have been described and illustrated.[1, 23, 59, 60] It is important to emphasize that the Schroeder-Thomas splint is not an extension splint; however, it is a traction splint. The splint should be fashioned to conform to the angles of the leg in a normal standing position. Tapes are then placed to apply traction to the joints proximal and distal to the fracture, allowing the fracture fragments to be separated and pulled into alignment (see Fig. 42–16). If improperly constructed or applied, pressure in the inguinal area can result in tissue necrosis and self-mutilation.[59]

Tape splints are generally used in birds weighing less than 200 g.[61] The feathers are removed from the limb and the skin is cleansed with alcohol. Porous adhesive tape is applied across the tibiotarsus to include the stifle and the hock on both the medial and lateral sides (Fig. 42–19). The tape along the cranial and caudal aspects of the leg is pinched together as close to the skin as possible using a hemostat. This immobilizes the fracture. Excess tape is trimmed along the cranial and caudal aspects of the splint. The number of layers of tape applied varies with the patient's size. Cyanoacrylate glue may be applied to the outer surface of the tape to increase its stiffness.[59] In most birds it is difficult to include the stifle in the splint, making this type of coaptation most applicable to fractures of the middle to distal tibiotarsus.

IM pins and orthopedic wires, bone plates in large birds, and ESF have been used to treat fractures of the tibiotarsus with success. With fractures of the tibiotarsus, a type II ESF device may be applied because the medial connecting system will not interfere with the bird's body. ESF is often used

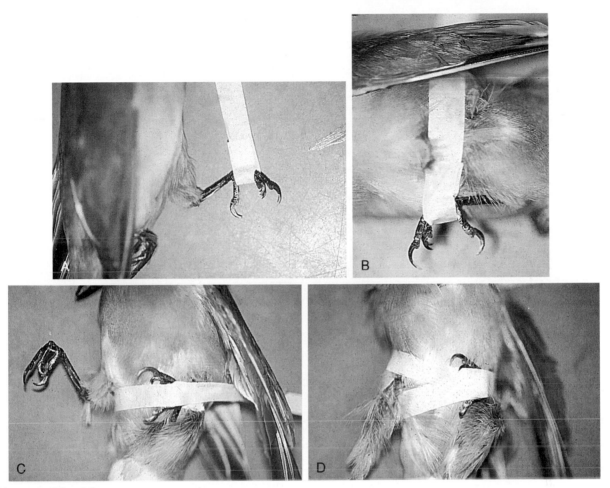

Figure 42-17

To construct an off–weight-bearing sling for the leg, *(A)* the tape is placed from medial to lateral to create a stirrup effect. *(B)* The tape is then brought around the lateral surface of the leg, over the dorsum, and caudal to the contralateral limb. *(C)* The tape continues over the bottom of the foot, along the lateral aspect of the leg again, over the dorsum, and cranial to the contralateral leg, ending across the bottom of the foot again. *(D)* Having one strip of tape cranial to the contralateral limb and the other strip caudal to it prevents the sling from slipping.

for open and comminuted fractures of the tibiotarsus to allow treatment of the soft tissues during the healing process.

Normograde insertion is recommended for placing an IM pin in the tibiotarsus because the surgeon has more control over the location of the pin within the stifle joint. The pin should be placed through the craniomedial aspect of the proximal tibiotarsus. This portion of the plateau is little affected by pin penetration because when the bird perches or flies the stifle is generally maintained in flexion. In the flexed position this portion of the joint is not articular. Normograde insertion also provides the advantage of inserting the pin using a closed technique.

Proximal and distal metaphyseal fractures of the tibiotarsus may be treated using a cross pin or Rush-type pin technique.

Fractures of the Tarsometatarsus

As with fractures of the carpometacarpus, fractures in this location may result in avascular necrosis distal to the site of trauma. In addition, both the proximal and distal ends of this bone are intimately involved in articulations with the adjacent bones. The tarsometatarsus does not have a medullary canal and thus a pin must be drilled the entire length of the bone.[59] There is no good entry point for IM

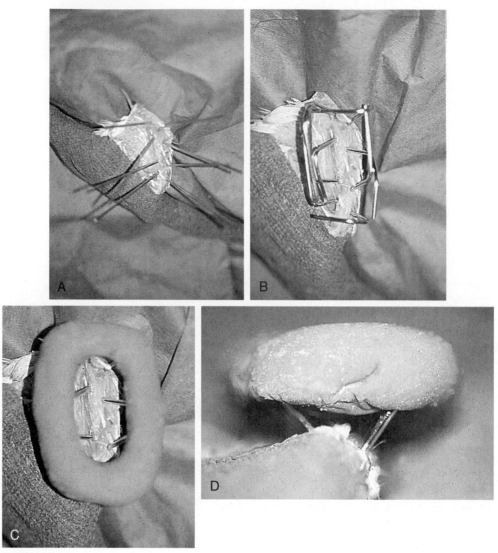

Figure 42–18

For fractures of the humerus and femur, two type I fixators can be placed at 90° degrees to each other and connected at the proximal and distal pins as demonstrated on this diaphyseal fracture of the humerus in a cockatoo. *(A)* The fixation pins are inserted along the humerus in two rows at 90° to each other. *(B)* The pins are bent over to act as reinforcing bars, and the most proximal and distal pins are bent over to connect to the opposite fixation system. *(C)* PMM is used for the connecting systems uniting the fixation pins of each type I fixator as well as uniting the two systems at the proximal and distal ends. *(D)* The two fixators constructed at 90° degrees to each other and connected are significantly stronger than one type I fixator.

pin insertion with most of these fractures. ESF has some application in certain instances.

It is best to use a type II ESF device on the tarsometatarsus. The bone has a somewhat horse-shoe configuration on cross section with the tendon running along the plantar surface and the artery and vein running along the cranial surface of the bone. These structures must be avoided during pin placement. It is best to get good purchase within the bone by placing them through the thickest portion of the bone.

External coaptation is frequently the treatment of choice for fractures of the tarsometatarsus. Schroeder-Thomas splints, tape splints, and reinforced plantar splints are appropriate for treating this type of fracture (Fig. 42–20).

pin or Kirschner wire molded to conform to the plantar surface of the affected digit. It is important to immobilize the joints proximal and distal to the affected bone. Phalangeal fractures may also be immobilized using a ball type of bandage. Placing a ball of gauze in the grasp of the bird's foot, the toes are bound around the surface of the ball with conforming gauze and tape. With such a ball bandage the bird is able to bear weight on the ball while the fracture fragments are immobilized by the tape.

Another type of splint for fractures of the digits is made by cutting a piece of flat material such as lightweight casting material or x-ray film to the shape of the foot (e.g., **X**-shaped for psittacines). The plantar surface of the foot is placed on the splint and secured (Fig. 42–21). This type of splint is flat and allows earlier return to function following splint removal than a ball bandage.

LUXATIONS

There are few reports of methods for managing luxations in birds. Coxofemoral luxations are frequently the result of trauma during restraint or the bird getting its leg caught within the cage structure or a fence. Elbow luxations occur in raptors primarily from trauma occurring during flight. It is crucial to reduce the luxation as early as possible to minimize the formation of periarticular fibrosis. Within a period of as little as 3 days, significant fibrosis

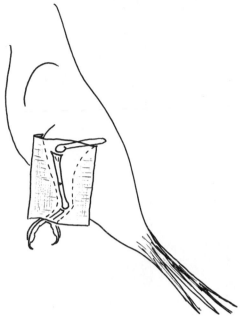

Figure 42–19

For small birds, a tape splint can be used to stabilize a fracture of the tibiotarsus. The tape is applied to immobilize the stifle and hock joints. (From Altman RB: Disorders of The Skeletal System. In Petrak ML [ed]: Diseases of Cage and Aviary Birds. Philadelphia; Lea & Febiger, 1982, © Waverly Press.)

Fractures of the Digits

Fractures of the digits are best treated with external coaptation. Reinforced plantar splints are applicable using a lightweight casting material, or a Steinmann

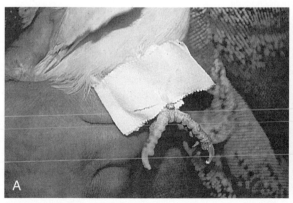
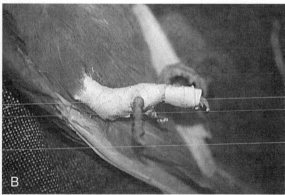

Figure 42–20

(A) This distal tarsometatarsus fracture was initially treated with a tape splint (the black line on the tape indicates the location of the fracture). *(B)* The splint did not immobilize the tarsometatarsophalangeal joint and was replaced with a plantar splint, which effectively immobilized the joints proximal and distal to the fracture.

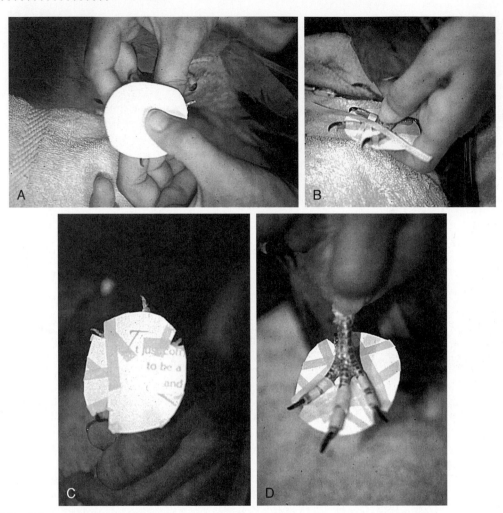

Figure 42–21

For fractures of the digits a snowshoe splint works well. *(A)* The splint material is cut to fit the foot so that the digits are maintained in extension. *(B)* Strips of tape are applied to the top side of the splint to immobilize the digits in a normal position. *(C)* The strips are wrapped around and secured to the bottom of the splint. *(D)* Additional tape is added to immobilize the digit.

occurs, inhibiting reduction of the luxation and predisposing to joint ankylosis.

Luxation of the Shoulder

Luxations of the shoulder usually involve avulsion of the ventral tubercle of the proximal humerus.[5] These may be treated by bandaging the wing to the body to immobilize the shoulder joint for 10 to 14 days. If precision flight is required, an open reduction and reattachment of the ventral tubercle may be beneficial. The shoulder joint is not a very stable joint, and reluxation is common.

Elbow Luxations

Luxation of the elbow is usually the result of severe blunt trauma strong enough to disrupt the ligamentous support.[62] This type of injury occurs infrequently in companion birds but has been reported to occur in 12% of raptor patients.[62] Because of the anatomy, luxation occurs in a dorsal, caudal, or caudodorsal aspect (Fig. 42–22). Ventral luxation occurs only in association with fracture of the radius.

The wing is held with the elbow extended (drooped) and externally rotated. Pain, crepitus, and swelling are noted on palpation of the affected

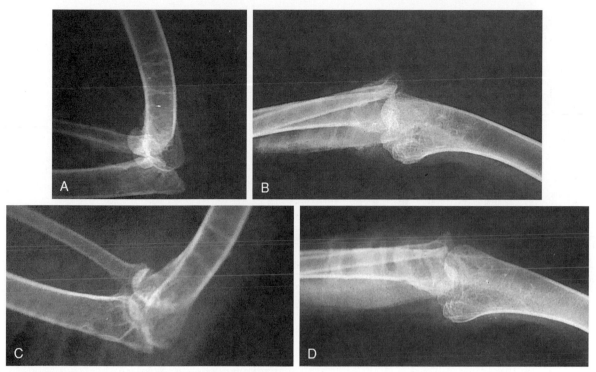

Figure 42–22

(A) Elbow luxation, lateral view. Note that the condyles overlie the radius and ulna, which is diagnostic for luxation. *(B)* Elbow luxation, anteroposterior view. Note that the radius and ulna are displaced dorsally (laterally) with respect to the humerus. *(C, D)* The luxation has been reduced. The articulation between the humerus and the ulna is normal; however, the radial head remains subluxated.

elbow. The wing should be examined for concomitant soft tissue injury, which may affect prognosis. The presence of open wounds and fractures has been associated with a poor prognosis for return to normal function.[62]

Reduction is accomplished by flexing the elbow, which counteracts the force of the scapulotriceps muscle pulling the ulna caudally. Maintaining flexion, the radius and ulna are internally rotated while pressure is applied to the dorsal (lateral) aspect of the radial head to force it into apposition with the dorsal (lateral) humeral condyle. As the elbow is gently extended, a "pop" is often palpable as reduction is completed. In cases with severe ligamentous damage, the pop may not be palpable.

If the joint is stable following reduction, it may be supported with a figure eight bandage for 7 to 12 days. When there is severe ligamentous damage, as evidenced by laxity following reduction, a transarticular ESF device may be applied to maintain reduction. Controlled physical therapy is initiated following removal of the support. Four of eight

raptors with elbow luxations in one study were subsequently released.[62]

Luxation of the Carpus

Luxations of the carpus are generally ventral. The bird holds the wing with the carpus extended and externally rotated at the carpus (Fig. 42–23). Reduction is accomplished by applying traction and abduction (dorsal) to the distal extremity. The carpometacarpus is then toggled into reduction and the carpus is flexed and adducted (ventrally). With the carpus in flexion, a figure eight bandage is applied to maintain reduction for 7 to 12 days. With large birds or those with chronic luxations, open reduction may be indicated. In cases when there is significant laxity following reduction, a transarticular pin or ESF device may be placed to maintain reduction. The pin is placed with the carpus in a normal degree of flexion through the main body of the carpometacarpus and into the ulna, immobilizing

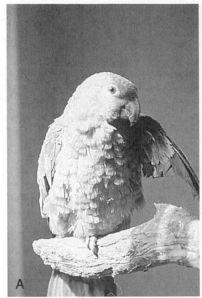
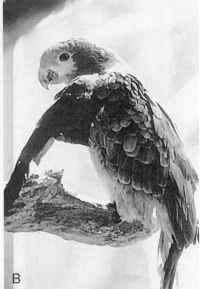

Figure 42–23

A bird with a ventral luxation of the carpus holds the wing extended and externally rotated at the carpus.

the carpus. After support devices are removed, controlled physical therapy is initiated.

Coxofemoral Luxations

In most psittacine birds and raptors, the coxofemoral joint is not a tight-fitting ball and socket joint but is one with a significant amount of cranial to caudal gliding motion with little abduction and adduction.[5, 63] It is a diarthrodial joint supported by a round ligament as well as collateral ligaments.[64] The ventral ligaments (pubofemoral and iliofemoral ligaments) and the round ligament are primarily involved in maintaining the femoral head within the acetabulum. To create luxation, both of these structures must be disrupted (Fig. 42–24).[64] In many species the dorsal rim of the acetabulum is well developed and extends as the antitrochanter to articulate with the broad, flat femoral neck and trochanter.[32, 63, 64] This inhibits limb abduction.

Coxofemoral luxations are generally the result of traction and rotational trauma such as that which occurs when the leg is caught.[63, 64] Most luxations are craniodorsal in birds, although cranioventral luxation has also been reported.[5, 63] Closed reduction and stabilization with slings, splints, and casts have been recommended.[17, 64, 65] In some cases, the luxation may be reduced and maintained using a transarticular pin. The pin is inserted through the trochanter into the head of the femur and across the acetabulum. This pin must be inserted carefully to avoid injuring the kidney, which lies on the medial side of the acetabulum (see Fig. 42–25). The chuck should be set on the pin at a predetermined length. If inserted too deeply, the pin penetrates the kidney, resulting in excessive intracoelomic hemorrhage. The limb should be supported using an off–weight-bearing sling or spica splint to prevent pin migration. In most cases, there is sufficient production of scar tissue by 5 to 7 days postoperatively that the pin may be safely removed. Long-term maintenance of a transarticular pin predisposes the bird to development of degenerative joint disease.

Surgical reduction and stabilization are considered the treatment of choice for acute coxofemoral luxations. For chronic luxations, a femoral head and neck excision arthroplasty is often indicated. The surgical approach for both of these is the craniolateral approach, which also allows for the placement of support sutures. Other approaches including ventral[66] and caudolateral[64] have also been used.

A curved skin incision is made from the cranial aspect of the ilium to the trochanter, then along the femur about ⅓ of its length. The bodies of the iliotibialis (cranialis and lateralis) and the iliofibularis are separated, exposing the iliotrochantericus

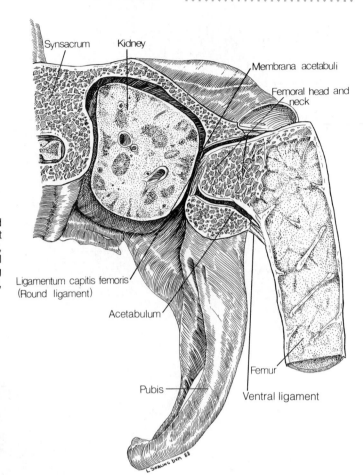

Figure 42-24

To create luxation of the coxofemoral joint, both the round ligament of the femur and the ventral collateral ligament must be disrupted. There is no bone at the medial acetabulum; rather, there is a membrana acetabuli. The kidney lies directly medial to the membrana acetabuli. (From Martin HD, Kabler R, Sealing L: The avian coxofemoral joint. J Assoc Avian Vet 1:22–30, 1989.)

caudalis and iliofemoralis externus, which are transected near their insertions on the trochanter (Fig. 42–25).[32, 63] This allows access to the joint capsule, which should be incised, allowing enough tissue on each side for closure. Following reduction of the luxation, stabilization sutures are placed from the trochanter to the dorsolateral iliac crest caudal to the central axis of the femur, and from the trochanter to the cranial rim of the acetabulum. The sutures are placed through the bone, and while the stifle is maintained in a normal standing position, the sutures are tightened. These sutures prevent excessive external rotation of the leg in the recovery period. The joint capsule is closed and the iliotrochantericus caudalis and iliofemoralis externus are reapposed. The remainder of the closure is routine.

When performing a femoral head and neck excision arthroplasty, the same approach is used. The head and neck of the femur are removed with appropriate-sized rongeurs, ensuring that no rough or sharp edges remain. Following femoral head and neck excision arthroplasty, there is a tendency for external rotation of the limb. This can be countered using the support sutures described earlier. Because polydioxanone suture remains for over 4 months in birds but is eventually absorbed, it is an appropriate choice for these antirotational sutures.[67]

Postoperatively the limb should be supported in a spica splint or off–weight-bearing sling for 1 to 2 weeks. It is best to maintain the bird in a cage with smooth walls and a perch near the floor to discourage attempts to climb.

Luxation of the Stifle

Luxation of the stifle with damage to the collateral ligaments occurs in companion birds following trau-

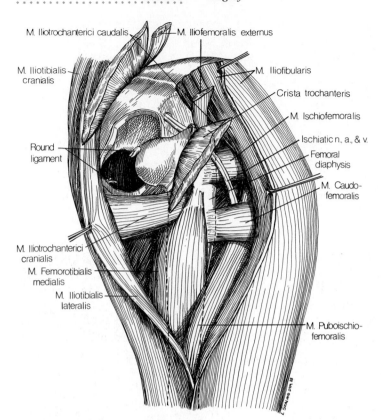

M. Iliotrochanterici caudalis

M. Iliofemoralis externus

M. Iliotibialis cranialis

M. Iliofibularis

Crista trochanteris

M. Ischiofemoralis

Ischiatic n., a., & v.

Round ligament

Femoral diaphysis

M. Caudo-femoralis

M. Iliotrochanterici cranialis

M. Femorotibialis medialis

M. Iliotibialis lateralis

M. Puboischio-femoralis

Figure 42–25

The surgical approach to the coxofemoral joint involves separation of the iliotibialis and iliofibularis. The iliotrochantericus caudalis and the iliofemoralis externus are transected near their insertion on the trochanter. (From Martin HD, Kabler R, Sealing L: The avian coxofemoral joint. J Assoc Avian Vet 1:22–30, 1989.)

matic episodes. Frequently, multiple ligamentous injury to the stifle occurs. Not only is a positive drawer sign elicited but also medial and/or lateral collateral instability exists. Surgical repair of the ligaments may be attempted especially in large birds; however, in most small companion birds the size of the ligaments precludes surgical apposition. In such cases transarticular ESF may be used to maintain the stifle in reduction, allowing periarticular fibrosis to stabilize the joint. This technique has been used with positive results, whereas more traditional techniques using external coaptation have not been used.[68]

At least two fixation pins should be placed in the femur and in the tibiotarsus. With the limb in a normal standing position, the pin in the proximal femur is connected to the pin in the distal tibiotarsus, and the distal femoral pin is connected to the proximal pin in the tibiotarsus (Fig. 42–26). Alternatively, a type II fixator may be placed in a cranial to caudal plane[68]; however, this results in more muscle trauma and decreased patient acceptance.

The device is maintained for 3 to 6 weeks to allow scar tissue to mature and stabilize the joint.

LIMB DEFORMITIES

Angular deformities of the legs of birds have been described in a variety of species including Psittaciformes, Falconiformes, and Stringiformes, as well as ratites. A causal relationship has been established between nutrition, genetics, trauma from parents, malposition within the egg, inappropriate exercise, nest substrate, and other factors.[68] Various techniques have been used to correct angular deformities of the legs, including electrocautery to inhibit bone growth, periosteal stripping especially in ratites, and corrective osteotomy with application of various stabilization devices. Splints, foam supports, hobbles, braces, and other devices have been used with variable success in young, actively growing patients with acute injuries. In general, the younger the patient the better and quicker the response to therapy.

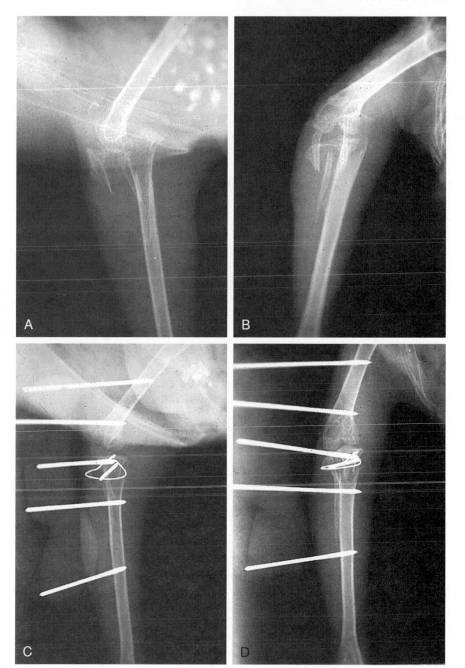

Figure 42–26

(A, B) This proximal metaphyseal fracture of the tibiotarsus in a cockatoo was reduced and maintained in reduction with an interfragmentary pin and wire. *(C, D)* The repair was supported with a transarticular ESF device. A similar approach would be used to stabilize a stifle with multiple ligamentous injury. (Photo courtesy of Dr. Steve Gilson, Sonora Veterinary Surgery and Oncology, Scottsdale, AZ.)

Mild deformities may respond to placing the infant in a deep cup with a rough base such as a paper towel lining. The diameter of the cup should restrict lateral slipping of the limbs and force them to be maintained under the bird. Splay leg may respond to tape hobbles placed between the tarsometatarsi. The bird must then be placed in a cup to maintain the head elevated, because hobbled chicks tend to fall forward.

Foam rubber blocks may be used to redirect limb alignment. A foam block may be cut to fit between the legs when they are in a normal orientation. A groove is created on each side to accommodate the limbs. The limbs are placed in a normal position within these grooves and secured in place. Alternatively, an **X** or hole may be cut for each leg in a block of foam thick enough to allow the legs to be pulled through the foam while the sternum rests comfortably on the block. The legs are pulled through and secured to the bottom of the block with the feet in a normal orientation. These types of support may need to be maintained for 7 to 10 days, but the patient should be closely evaluated and sustained until correction is achieved.

Many cases of angular limb deformity in birds are related to displacement of the digital flexor tendons along the plantar surface of the hock joint. Generally there is medial luxation of the tendons, resulting in external rotation of the distal tibiotarsus and proximal tarsometatarsus. This is a result of tension generated across the tarsal joint. The condition is somewhat analogous to medial patellar luxation of dogs. The degree of severity is usually a function of duration and stage of development at which the tendon slips. If identified early, splinting, taping, and fitting foam devices are effective in correcting the malalignment; however, when there is permanent displacement as a result of long-term tendon luxation, conservative methods usually fail.

As in dogs with medial patellar luxation, the indicated surgical therapy varies with the case. The surgeon's approach should be to do whatever is necessary to correct the alignment. In most cases this involves deepening of the tendon groove on the plantar aspect of the distal tibiotarsus and imbricating the lateral tendon sheath to maintain the tendon in reduction. When there is bone deformation, corrective osteotomies are indicated. The goal of surgery is to realign the bones and the tendon mechanism to reestablish the orientation of the foot. The earlier the alignment is reestablished, the better the long-term outcome.

Transverse, oblique, wedge, and dome osteotomies have been used to correct angular bone deformities. A modified dome osteotomy technique appears to be the most valuable.[5, 69] It allows three-dimensional manipulation of the bone to correct deformities in more than one plane. The manipulation is easy to plan and perform and does not result in limb shortening. There is good bone-to-bone contact, which results in better bone healing.

The radiographic view that demonstrates the most severe angle should be used for planning the osteotomy. Lines are drawn along the medullary canal of the proximal and distal segments to determine the point of intersection. It is at this location that the osteotomy is performed. A series of holes is drilled transversely through the bone at this location in a curved (dome) configuration. The holes may then be connected, allowing the bone to be realigned. In cases where thick cortices are involved, it may be necessary to connect the drill holes using a high-speed burr with a side-cutting bit. When the alignment is corrected, the osteotomy is stabilized using appropriate fixation devices, such as an ESF or a bone plate.

POSTOPERATIVE MANAGEMENT

When managing the postoperative avian orthopedic patient, the clinician must not only assess the bone healing but must also monitor the patient's general physical condition, evaluate for the occurrence of secondary complications, and institute physical therapy for the affected limb.[70] If the fracture was open, a culture sample of the bone should be taken at surgery and serial complete blood counts evaluated during the recovery period. Birds prone to fungal infections such as aspergillosis and candidiasis should be monitored for evidence of these infections, especially if they are maintained on long-term antibiotic therapy. Radiographic assessment should be made first at 3 weeks postoperatively, then every 2 weeks until radiographic evidence of union is present. In most cases clinical union occurs prior to radiographic evidence of union. In the early stages of bone healing, it is often difficult to distinguish osteomyelitis from periosteal bone callus. Both appear radiographically as periosteal proliferation and sclerosis with increased medullary bone density.[5]

Staged destabilization of the fracture may be indicated if fracture healing appears to be progressing normally. In cases when two forms of stabilization are used—for example, an IM pin and ESF for a humeral fracture—one may often be removed at 3 weeks postoperatively while the other is maintained until a stronger union is present.

In most cases, some type of restricted activity is required following fracture stabilization. This may be afforded by external coaptation or simply by placing the bird in a confined environment that does not allow it to use the affected limb excessively. Controlled physical therapy is beneficial by improving the vascular flow through the affected region. In addition, the controlled stress applied promotes bone healing.[5] Methods of controlled physical therapy depend on the type of injury and the stability of the repair, as well as the required function of the affected limb. The goals are to improve the range of motion in muscle tone and strength of the affected limb, restore circulatory and neurologic function, and recover cardiovascular endurance.[26, 70] In the early phases of healing, therapy should be conducted under general anesthesia. Each joint that is immobilized is individually exercised through its range of motion. The range of motion is monitored using a goniometer. Therapy is provided at least twice weekly. After the fracture has healed, more aggressive passive and active therapy may be initiated. Secondary complications include osteomyelitis, sequestration of bone, reduced joint function, muscle and patagium damage, nerve and vascular dysfunction, and delayed and nonunion fracture.[70]

Prognosis varies with the required function of the patient, which may be different for companion and aviary birds compared with free-ranging birds. Companion birds frequently do very well postoperatively because the majority of their fractures are not open or comminuted. Free-ranging birds, especially birds of prey, require precision flight. Even slight rotational malalignment, especially at the distal wing, may result in diminished ability to fly with precision. Furthermore, radioulnar synostosis limits the ability to supinate and pronate the limb properly by preventing the sliding motion between these two bones. This can inhibit precision flight. Fractures located at or near a joint commonly heal with joint ankylosis affecting the long-term prognosis. Osteomyelitis occurs with some degree of frequency in birds with open fractures. This results in delayed fracture healing and significantly increases the occurrence of fracture disease. Leg fractures in companion birds generally carry a good prognosis; however, in birds of prey requiring the ability to grab and kill prey items, leg fractures may result in dysfunction and decreased ability to hunt.

References

1. Bennett RA, Kuzma AB: Fracture management in birds. J Zoo Wildl Med 23(1):5–38, 1992.
2. Borman ER, Putney DL, Jessup D: Use of acrylic bone cement in avian orthopedics. J Am Anim Hosp Assoc 14:602–604, 1978.
3. Bush M, Montali RJ, Novak GR, James AE: The healing of avian fractures: A histologic xeroradiographic study. J Am Anim Hosp Assoc 12:768–773, 1976.
4. Kuzma AB, Hunter B: Osteotomy and derotation of the humerus in a turkey vulture using intramedullary polymethylmethacrylate and bone plate fixation. Can Vet J 30:900–901, 1989.
5. Martin HD, Ritchie BW: Orthopedic surgical techniques. In Ritchie BW, Harrison GJ, Harrison LR (eds): Avian Medicine: Principles and Applications. Lake Worth, FL, Wingers Publishing, 1994, pp 1137–1169.
6. Montali RJ, Bush M: Avian fracture repair, radiographic and histologic correlation. Annu Proc Am Assoc Zoo Vet, 1975, pp 150–154.
7. Putney DL, Borman ER, Lohse CL: Methylmethacrylate fixation of avian humerus fractures: A radiographic, histologic study. J Am Anim Hosp Assoc 19:773–782, 1983.
8. Redig PT, Roush JC: Orthopedic and soft tissue surgery in raptorial species. In Fowler ME (ed): Zoo and Wild Animal Medicine. Philadelphia, WB Saunders 1987, pp 246–253.
9. Gandal CP: Anesthetic and surgical techniques. In Petrak ML (ed): Diseases of Cage and Aviary Birds. Philadelphia, Lea & Febiger, 1982, pp 304–328.
10. Kuzma AB, Hunter B: A new technique for avian fracture repair using intramedullary polymethylmethacrylate and bone plate fixation. J Am Anim Hosp Assoc 27:239–248, 1991.
11. Milton JL: Principles of fracture treatment and bone healing. 13th Annu Vet Surg Forum—Avian Surg, 1985, pp 91–96.
12. Newton CD, Zeitlin S: Avian fracture healing. J Am Vet Med Assoc 170:620–625, 1977.
13. Bush M: External fixation of avian fractures. J Am Vet Med Assoc 171:943–946, 1977.
14. Williams RJ, Holland M, Milton JL, Hoover JP: A comparative study of treatment methods for long bone fractures. Companion Anim Pract 1(4):48–55, 1987.
15. Withrow SJ: General principles of fracture repair in raptors. Compend Cont Ed Pract Vet 4:116–121, 1982.
16. Kaderly RE: Delayed union, nonunion, and malunion. In Slatter DH (ed): Textbook of Small Animal Surgery, 2nd ed. Philadelphia, WB Saunders, 1993, pp 1676–1685.
17. Roush JC: Avian orthopedics. In Kirk RW (ed): Current Veterinary Therapy VII. Philadelphia, WB Saunders, 1980, pp 662–673.
18. Stevenson S: Bone grafting. In Slatter DH (ed): Textbook of Small Animal Surgery, 2nd ed. Philadelphia, WB Saunders, 1993, pp 1694–1703.
19. MacCoy DM, Haschek WM: Healing of transverse humeral fractures in pigeons treated with ethylene oxide sterilized, dry-stored, onlay cortical xenografts and allografts. Am J Vet Res 49:106–111, 1988.
20. MacCoy DM: Techniques of fracture treatment and their indications: External and internal fixation. Proc 1st Intl Conf Zool Avian Med, 1987, pp 549–562.
21. MacCoy DM, Redig PT: Surgical approaches to and repair of wing fractures. Proc 1st Intl Conf Zool Avian Med, 1987, pp 564–577.
22. MacCoy DM: Techniques of fracture treatment and their indications: External and internal fixation. 13th Vet Surg Forum—Avian Surg, 1985, pp 97–109.
23. Redig PT: A clinical review of orthopedic techniques used in the rehabilitation of raptors. In Fowler ME (ed): Zoo and Wildlife Animal Medicine, 2nd ed. Philadelphia, WB Saunders, 1986, pp 388–401.

24. Redig PT: Basic orthopedic surgical techniques. In Harrison GJ, Harrison LR (eds): Clinical Avian Medicine and Surgery. Philadelphia, WB Saunders, 1986, pp 596–598.

25. Bush M: Avian orthopedics. Annu Proc Am Assoc Zoo Vet, 1974, pp 111–113.

26. Degernes LA, Lind PJ, Olson DE, Redig PT: Evaluating avian fractures for use of methylmethacrylate orthopedic technique. J Assoc Avian Vet 3(2):64–67, 1989.

27. Kuzma AB: Avian orthopedics: An update and review of new techniques. Proc Am Assoc Zoo Vet, 1990, pp 159–162.

28. Levitt L: Avian orthopedics. Compend Cont Ed Pract Vet 11:899–929, 1989.

29. Lind PJ, Gushwa DA, VanEk JA: Fracture repair in two owls using polypropylene rods and acrylic bone cement. Assoc Avian Vet Today 2(3):128–132, 1988.

30. MacCoy DM, Milton JL: Treatment of fractures of the leg. 13th Vet Surg Forum—Avian Surg, 1985, pp 117–126.

31. Bush M, James AE: Some considerations of practice of orthopedics in exotic animals. J Am Anim Hosp Assoc 11:587–594, 1975.

32. Orosz SE, Ensley PK, Haynes CJ: Avian Surgical Anatomy: Thoracic and Pelvic Limbs. Philadelphia, WB Saunders, 1992.

33. Elkins AD, Blass CE: Management of avian fractures, Part 2—pins and wires. Vet Med Small Anim Clin 77:825–828, 1982.

34. MacCoy DM: High density polymer rods as an intramedullary fixation device in birds. J Am Anim Hosp Assoc 19:767–772, 1983.

35. Pardo AD: Methods of internal fracture fixation—cerclage wiring and tension band fixation. In Slatter DH (ed): Textbook of Small Animal Surgery, 2nd ed. Philadelphia, WB Saunders, 1993, pp 1631–1640.

36. Rowley J, Pshyk BW: Repair of a fractured humerus in a red-tailed hawk. Vet Med Small Anim Clin 76:1180–1181, 1981.

37. Howard PE, and Brusewitz GH: An in vitro comparison of the holding strength of partially threaded vs. nonthreaded intramedullary pins. Vet Surg 12:119–122, 1983.

38. DeYoung DJ, Probst CW: Methods of internal fracture fixation—general principles. In Slatter DH (ed): Textbook of Small Animal Surgery, 2nd ed. Philadelphia, WB Saunders, 1993, pp 1610–1631.

39. Wan PY, Adair HS, Patton CS, Faulk BS: Comparison of bone healing using polydioxanone and stainless steel intramedullary pins in transverse, midhumeral osteotomies in pigeons (Columba livia). J Zoo Wildl Med 25(2):264–269, 1994.

40. Anderson GI: Polymethylmethacrylate: A review of the implications and complications of its use in orthopedic surgery. Vet Comp Orthop Trauma 2:74–79, 1988.

41. Astleford WJ, Asher MA, Lindholm US, Rockwood CA: Physical and mechanical factors affecting the shear strength of methylmethacrylate. J Bone Joint Surg 55A(3):661, 1973.

42. Marks KE: Antibiotic-impregnated acrylic bone cement. J Bone Joint Surg 58A:358–364, 1976.

43. Schurman DC, Trindale C, Hirshman HP: Antibiotic-acrylic bone cement composites. J Bone Joint Surg 60A:978–984, 1978.

44. Wahlig H, Dingeldein E: Antibiotics and bone cement. Experimental and long term observations. Acta Orthop Scand 51:49–56, 1980.

45. Hubbard MJS: The effect of acrylic cement on the union of internally fixed experimental fractures of the femoral shaft in the rabbit. Injury 11:325–331, 1980.

46. MacCoy DM: Modified Kirschner splints for application to small birds. Vet Med Small Anim Clin 76:853–856, 1981.

47. Egger EL: External skeletal fixation—general principles. In Slatter DH (ed): Textbook of Small Animal Surgery, 2nd ed. Philadelphia, WB Saunders, 1993, pp 1641–1656.

48. Brinker WO, Flo GL: Principles and applications of external skeletal fixation. Vet Clin North Am Small Anim Pract 5:197–208, 1975.

49. Brooker AF: Principles of External Fixation. Baltimore, Williams & Wilkins, 1983.

50. Satterfield WC, O'Rourke, KI: External skeletal fixation in avian orthopedics using a modified through-and-through Kirschner-Ehmer splint technique (the Boston technique). J Am Anim Hosp Assoc 17:635–637, 1981.

51. Howard PE: The use of bone plates in the repair of avian fractures. J Am Anim Hosp Assoc 26:613–622, 1990.

52. Bauck L, Fowler JD, Cribb P: Tibial osteotomy in an emu. Companion Anim Pract 1:26–30, 1987.

53. Bush MJ, Hughes JL, Ensley PK, James AE: Fracture repair in exotics using internal fixation. J Am Anim Hosp Assoc 12:746–751, 1976.

54. Leeds EB: Tibial fracture repair in a double-waddled cassowary. J Vet Orthop 1:21–27, 1979.

55. Wingfield WE, DeYoung DW: Anesthetic and surgical management of eagles with orthopedic difficulties. Vet Med Small Anim Clin 67:991–993, 1972.

56. Brinker WO, Hohn RB, Prieur WD: Manual of Internal Fixation in Small Animals. New York, Springer-Verlag, 1984.

57. Kuzma AB, Hunter B: Avian fracture repair using intramedullary bone cement and plate fixation. Proc Conf Assoc Avian Vet, 1989, pp 177–181.

58. Howard DJ, Redig PT: Orthopedics of the wing. Semin Avian Exotic Pet Med 3(2):51–62, 1994.

59. Hess R: Management of orthopedic problems of the avian pelvic limb. Semin Avian Exotic Pet Med 3(2):63–72, 1994.

60. Redig PT, Roush JC: Surgical approaches to the long bones of raptors. In Fowler ME (ed): Zoo and Wild Animal Medicine. Philadelphia, WB Saunders, 1978.

61. Altman RB: Fractures of the extremities of birds. In Kirk RW (ed): Current Veterinary Therapy VI. Philadelphia, WB Saunders, 1977.

62. Martin HD, Bruecker KA, Herrick DD, Scherpelz J: Elbow luxations in raptors: A review of eight cases. In Redig PT, Cooper JE, Remple JD, Homer DB (eds): Raptor Biomedicine. Minneapolis, University of Minnesota Press, 1993, pp 199–206.

63. Martin HD, Kabler R, Sealing L: The avian coxofemoral joint. J Assoc Avian Vet 1(1):22–30, 1989.

64. MacCoy DM: Excision arthroplasty for management of coxofemoral luxations in pet birds. J Am Vet Med Assoc 194(1):95–97, 1989.

65. Altman RB: Disorders of the skeletal system. In Petrak ML (ed): Diseases of Cage and Aviary Birds, 2nd ed. Philadelphia, Lea & Febiger, 1982, pp 386–387.

66. Campbell TW, Rudd RG: Excision arthroplasty in a Toco toucan (Rhamphastos toco toco) for the correction of an osteoarthritis of the right coxofemoral joint. Proc 1st Conf Zool Avian Med, 1987, pp 227–278.

67. Bennett RA, Yeager M, Trapp A, Cambre RC: Tissue reaction to five suture materials in pigeons (Columbia livia). Proc Conf Assoc Avian Vet, 1992, pp 212–218.

68. Clipsham RC: Correction of pediatric leg disorders. Proc Conf Assoc Avian Vet, 1991, pp 200–204.

69. Greenacre CB, Aron DN, Ritchie BW: Dome osteotomy for successful correction of angular limb deformities. Proc Conf Assoc Avian Vet, 1994, pp 39–44.

70. Cooney J, Mueller L: Postoperative management of the avian orthopedic patient. Semin Avian Exotic Pet Med 3(2):100–107, 1994.

43

Radiosurgery (Electrosurgery)

Radiosurgery performed skillfully, using the correct current combined with proper technique, offers the avian surgeon a modality that fulfills the two most important requirements of avian surgery —decreased anesthetic and surgical time, and total hemostasis. Because these two elements are critical to avian surgical success, a detailed discussion of radiosurgical theory and proper current selection and technique is included in this text.

Radiosurgery, frequently called electrosurgery, uses high-frequency radiowaves to alter or destroy tissue for therapeutic purposes.

In 1892, Arsene d'Arnsonval[1] studied the effects of high-frequency current on humans. With frequency above 10,000 cycles per second, heat was produced, but there was no neuromuscular response. Using d'Arnsonval's solenoid, Ovidin in 1899 described the destructive effect of sparks on tissues. In 1907 Deforest patented a triode radio tube with which he could make tissue incisions using a frequency above 2 MHz. In 1926, the surgeon Wyeth[2] used the newly invented pentode tube and achieved incisions that healed by third intent.

In 1969, Dr. Irving Ellman, a dentist and electrical engineer, designed a compact solid state radiosurgical dental unit using fully rectified current. Four years later, Ellman redesigned and patented the unit with a fully rectified filtered current allowing only a pure frequency signal of 3,800,000 cycles per second. At this optimal frequency, this instrument offered fully rectified filtered and unfiltered current, partially rectified current, and unfiltered sparking current (fulguration). Except for a few modifications, such as increased power and a broader range

of accessories, this is the same instrument now in use (Fig. 43–1).

In 1974, Friedman, Margolin, and Piliero[3] found that epithelium and connective tissue incised with fully rectified filtered current showed less tissue alteration than tissue incised with a nonfiltered rectified or spark gap current.

Harrison and Kelly[4] found that an electrosurgical instrument using partially rectified current produces

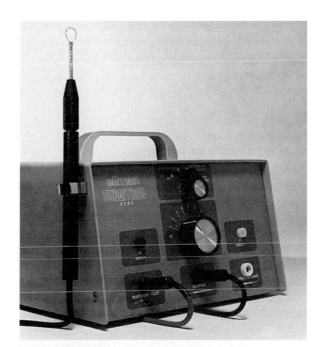

Figure 43–1

Radiosurgical unit showing alternating current, radiofrequency lights, jack openings, power dial, and current selector switch and electrode handle with a loop electrode. (Courtesy Ellman International Corp.)

more heat at the surgical site than an instrument delivering fully rectified current.

In 1978, Maness, Roeber, Clark, and Cataldo[5] proved that 3.8 MHz was the optimal oscillating current for incising soft tissue when they published "Histological Evaluation of Electrosurgery With Varying Frequency and Wave Form." Other investigators found that lower frequencies produced greater tissue alteration with delayed and poor quality healing (Figs. 43–2 and 43–3).

The radiosurgical unit is composed of a high-frequency amplifier. Alternating current is converted to direct current within the electrosurgical unit and passed into a tuned coil capacitator that generates the electrosurgical signal. The radiofrequency wave is passed through a high-frequency wave form adapter that alters the shape and magnitude of the radiowaves, creating the available wave forms. The wave forms are then passed through a high-frequency amplifier to increase the power level of various wave forms. After the wave forms are passed through coupling circuits, the radiofrequency current is passed through the active electrode tip.[6] The electrode tip is the active electrode transmitting the radiofrequency wave to the tissue.

The passive electrode or ground plate acts as an antenna by focusing the radiofrequency waves emitted by the active electrode. The ground plate does not have to be in direct contact with the tissue but should be as close to the incision site as practically possible. The ground plate increases the efficiency of radiosurgical technique and decreases

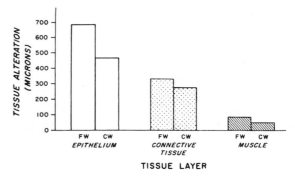

FW - Full Wave Rectification Fully Rectified Current
CW - Continuous Wave   Fully Filtered Current

F i g u r e   4 3 – 3

The comparative tissue alteration of epithelium, connective tissue, and muscle using fully rectified filtered and fully rectified nonfiltered current. (Courtesy Ellman International Corp.)

lateral heat. The ground plate should be well insulated.

Electrosection is accomplished by the application of high-frequency radiowaves to tissue. This high-frequency radiowave produces alternating electric fields of electromagnetic waves. These radiowaves result in heat production that causes volatilization of intracellular fluids at the point of active electrode contact. The heat production is created by the resistance of the tissues to the alternating fields of electromagnetic waves. Radiosurgical incision occurs by controlled internal volatilization of the cells along the path of the electrode while the electrode tip remains cool. This high-frequency energy causes molecular heat in each cell and is known as lateral heat.[7]

Becoming proficient in electrosurgical technique requires understanding of the four types of generated current. It is essential to know the function and use of each current to master the techniques necessary to minimize lateral heat.

Four wave forms can be used by the electrosurgeon.[6] Fully rectified filtered current is the purest current in avian surgery and produces approximately 90% cutting and 10% coagulation. It is used primarily for taking biopsies as well as making skin incisions. This current is the *only* current that should be used for taking biopsy samples.

Fully rectified unfiltered current is used for most incisions and dissection in avian surgery because of

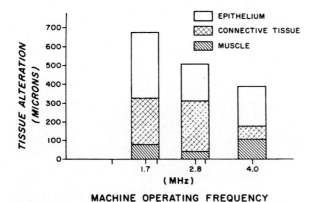

MACHINE OPERATING FREQUENCY

F i g u r e   4 3 – 2

The effects of tissue alteration at higher radiofrequency on epithelium, connective tissue, and muscle. (Courtesy Ellman International Corp.)

its coagulating capability. This current offers approximately 50% cutting and 50% coagulation.

Partially rectified current has no cutting quality and is used exclusively for coagulation, desiccation, and hemostasis. This wave form offers 10% cutting and 90% coagulation.

Fulguration is a spark gap generator and operates on the principle of a condenser discharging across a spark gap. There is a concentration of heat energy at the site of contact of the electrode, causing marked dehydration of the tissue. This current is used for superficial coagulation of tissue, has no cutting quality, and has little use in avian surgery.

Pure radiosurgical technique minimizes lateral heat. Lateral heat (LH) can be expressed by the formula[6]

Lateral heat = Time during which electrode contacts tissue
× intensity of power × frequency of unit
× waveform of the radio signal
× electrode size

Proper tuning of radiosurgical equipment is essential.[8] The electrosurgical unit is a radio transmitter and as such must be fine-tuned for good reception, as a radio would be. Many fixed environmental factors at the operative location must be compensated for by proper tuning of the equipment. These variables include

1. Manufacturer's specification; even units from the same manufacturer differ in wave form and output characteristics
2. Electric current output, which varies with local demand
3. Building construction (wood, metal, etc.)
4. Tissue impedance
5. Proximity of the passive electrode to the active electrode.

Once the equipment is tuned within a specific location, retuning needs to be done only if the operative location is changed.

To fine-tune an electrosurgical instrument, the unit should be set to either fully rectified filtered or fully rectified unfiltered current and the power dial turned to full power. Using the passive electrode (ground plate) placed under a piece of tissue (beefsteak), the current should be initiated and an incision made. The result will be a great deal of sparking, smoke, and blanching of tissue. The power should be gradually reduced until there is a slight amount of drag on the electrode tip, with shreds of tissue adhering to the electrode. The resulting incision shows blanching at the incision margins. At this point, the power should be slightly increased to eliminate the drag. When ideally tuned, the tip should produce no drag, no sparking, and minimal smoke with no blanching of tissue. It is better to have slightly too much than too little current.

Many advantages are attributed to radiosurgery, and relatively minor disadvantages are cited. The most important function of radiosurgery for avian surgery is that it permits the degree of hemorrhage control desired. The fine wire electrodes are flexible and can be bent, shaped, or lengthened to accommodate any incision size or shape. The electrode requires no pressure for cutting or for coagulating. Because the electrodes are self-sterilizing, seeding of bacteria into the incision site is always avoided.

As a result of the hemostatic capabilities and ease of use, surgical time is greatly reduced, thus reducing anesthetic time.

The disadvantages of radiosurgery are few and of little consequence. By using proper technique, the majority of these disadvantages can be avoided. Because of the interference with unshielded cardiac pacemakers (pacemakers manufactured prior to 1976), this equipment should not be used in the presence of a person with an unshielded pacemaker.

Radiosurgery does not function well in fields in which there is pooling of fluids (e.g., blood, saliva, or ascitic fluid). Sponging or suction is necessary with the accumulation of these fluids. Electrosurgery cannot be used in the presence of explosive or volatile fluids or gases such as ether or alcohol. If alcohol is used for surgical preparation, complete evaporation must be permitted before electrosurgery is performed.

Electrocardiogram (ECG) monitoring electrodes should be placed as far away from the passive electrode as possible to avoid interference and burns. At high frequencies above 4 MHz, the current can travel along blood vessels and nerve paths, causing coagulation at distant points from the surgical site.[9] This occurs because the narrow channel of tissue is more conductive than the surrounding tissue. This phenomenon is called "channeling."

Thermoelectric burns can occur when current from a radiosurgical unit using a monopolar electrode grounds through a point of high-current density rather than the low-current density of the ground plate.[10] Thermoelectric burn occurrence is rare, and the incidence can be reduced by using an insulated ground plate positioned on the body surface to dissipate heat. It is important to use the greatest possible area of contact between the patient and the ground plate. Using the lowest functional power setting and decreasing tissue contact time also decrease the potential for tissue burns.

Interference with electronic monitoring devices and computer and telephone systems can occur during activation of the radiofrequency (RF) current. This phenomenon occurs as the result of RF leakage emitted from all electrosurgical equipment. This problem can most frequently be solved by plugging the electrosurgical unit into a different circuit line or by placing an RF filter between the wall outlet and the radiosurgical unit. This RF filter is available in most electronic equipment stores.

TECHNIQUE

The following considerations are directed toward reducing lateral heat and are necessary to achieve sound radiosurgical skills.

The finer the electrode tip, the less energy is required. The fine wire electrode is the most suitable for avian surgery (Fig. 43–4).

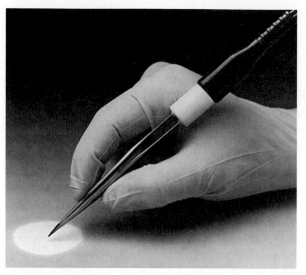

Figure 43–5

Bipolar forceps used for pinpoint coagulation. (Courtesy Ellman International Corp.)

Energy is distributed along the entire noninsulated surface of the electrode. Therefore, it is essential during electrosection to keep the electrode tip perpendicular to the tissue being incised to minimize lateral heat.

When incising tissue, the electrode tip should be moved across the tissue as rapidly as possible at a minimum rate of 7 mm per second.

During the surgical procedure, the electrode must be kept clean for the highest efficiency.

When making an incision, the current should be initiated before the electrode touches the tissue to dispel the initial current surge. The electrode should be lifted off the surface of the tissue at the end of the incision stroke to prevent excessive contact time with resultant lateral heat. Restrict electrode-to-tissue contact to 2 to 3 seconds. If an incision is incomplete or requires lengthening or deepening, 8 seconds should elapse between electrode strokes using a fine wire electrode, and 15 seconds should elapse between incisions using a loop electrode (see Fig. 43–4) to allow for cooling of the tissue.

When using the ball electrode for hemostasis, it is necessary to have light contact between the electrode and the tissue surface. Pressure on the electrode interferes with proper tissue coagulation.

The use of bipolar forceps (Fig. 43–5) for rapid, precise hemostasis is an important timesaving tech-

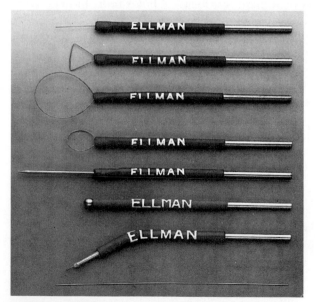

Figure 43–4

Various sizes and shapes of fine wire, loop, and ball electrodes used for avian surgery. (Courtesy Ellman International Corp.)

nique for avian surgery. Bipolar forceps are small, fine-pointed forceps in which one jaw of the forceps acts as the active electrode and the opposite jaw as the passive electrode. Coagulation takes place between the two points of the electrode. The surgeon has the ability to coagulate small defined segments with pinpoint precision, thereby permitting rapid, precise coagulation of blood vessels or tissue, with minimal lateral heat and without affecting surrounding tissue.

Bennett[11] and Harrison[12] describe a technique of incising tissue using the Harrison Modified Bipolar Forceps.* This author does not use this technique because it is contrary to the basic principle of using the smallest electrode to perform the necessary function. Considerably more lateral heat is generated. When small pieces of tissue are grasped with a bipolar forceps, pressure on the forceps should be minimal. This permits a small space between the jaws holding the tissue.

CARE OF ELECTROSURGICAL EQUIPMENT

Electrode tips are made of surgical-grade tungsten wire, which eventually volatilizes and breaks. If abused and misused, they carbonize and wear out. Although autoclaving is recommended, it reduces the functional lifespan of the electrodes. The electrodes can be placed in cold sterilization for 25 minutes or can be gas sterilized. Choice of sterilization is based on manufacturer's specifications.

Preventing Electrode Breakage

1. The correct wave form should be used. Never try to cut using partially rectified current.
2. The ground plate should be in close proximity to the operative site. The ground plate does not need to have contact with skin.
3. Electrodes should be handled by the insulated shafts only.
4. Bend electrodes only at their insulated shaft.
5. Tissues should be moist.
6. Always activate the unit before making contact with the tissue.

7. Never apply pressure. This will bend electrodes.
8. If there is resistance, drag, or tissue adhering to the electrode, the power setting is too low. This will cause bending and breakage.
9. If there is sparking, the power setting is too high, which will cause carbonization.
10. Electrode loops require slightly higher power than straight wire electrodes and are more fragile.

Cleaning the Electrodes During Surgery

Set the radiosurgical instrument on fully rectified filtered or nonfiltered wave form. Slightly increase the power and place the electrode between folds of a gauze pad soaked in saline. Activate the unit for 1 to 2 seconds while moving the electrode back and forth within the gauze. Volatilization of water molecules steam-cleans the electrode. Gentle scraping of the electrode on an electrode cleaning pad or gentle scraping with a scalpel blade removes the adhered tissue particles.

Care and Cleaning of the Electrode After Use

Electrodes should not be scrubbed with a brush or an abrasive. Electrodes should be placed in a hydrogen peroxide solution or, preferably, in an ultrasonic cleaner for 3 to 5 minutes.

Most hand pieces and cords can be subjected to the pressure, temperature, and humidity of steam sterilization; however, hand pieces that contain electronic activation switching mechanisms are generally not made to tolerate this procedure.

Cold sterilization is suitable for electrode tips and many cords and electrode handles, other than handles with switching mechanisms. Prolonged immersion in chemical solution may damage plastic and insulating materials.

It is essential that the operator know which attachment parts of the equipment can be autoclaved. Suitability for autoclaving varies from manufacturer to manufacturer. Many manufacturers recommend that the equipment be tested and evaluated for safety and effectiveness every 2 years.

When problems or inefficient function occurs while using the electrosurgical equipment, a sys-

*Ellman International Manufacturing, Hewlett, New York.

Table 43–1
TROUBLESHOOTING FLOW CHART FOR RADIOSURGERY*

1. If the red alternating current (A/C) power light does NOT go on, there is no current to the unit or the fuse in the unit has blown.
   If the A/C power light goes on, proceed to Step 2.
2. If the white radiofrequency (RF) light does NOT go on
   a. The unit is not generating RF waves
   b. The foot pedal is not functioning
      (Either a or b indicates a problem with the unit.)
   c. The current selector switch is in the OFF position
   If the RF light goes on, proceed to Step 3.
3. If there is NO current generating from the end of the electrode
   a. The electrode is not seated properly in the hand piece
   b. The wire to the electrode handle is broken
   c. The jacks may not be properly plugged into the unit
   d. There is an improper power setting
   If the above are functioning properly, proceed to Step 4.
4. If there is INSUFFICIENT current generating from the electrode
   a. Check to see if the ground plate is positioned properly or if the jack is plugged in
   b. Check to see if the current selector is in the proper position
   c. Check to see if the tissue is too dry

Ninety-five percent of problems can be solved by the above procedure. If all of the above functions seem to be normal and there is still a problem, call the manufacturer for assistance.

*Applicable to the Surgitron FFPF, Ellman International, Hewlett, NY.

tematic approach to overcome the problem quickly can be implemented by following the troubleshooting flow chart (Table 43–1). Ninety-five percent of problems encountered result from improper operator use.

The skills necessary to become an accomplished electrosurgeon can be developed quickly by paying attention to detail. Once it is mastered, the surgeon will find that electrosurgery is a modality that increases the veterinarian's surgical capabilities and increases the survival rate of avian patients.

References

1. White WF: Radiosurgery and advancement over the scalpel in many procedures. Podiatry Products Rep Jan:16–17, 1986.
2. Wyeth GA: Surgery of Neoplastic Disease by Electrothermic Method. New York, Paul B. Hoeber, 1926.
3. Friedman J, Margolin J, Piliero S: A preliminary study of the histological effects of three different types of electrical currents. NY State Dent J 40:349, 1979.
4. Harrison JD, Kelly WJ: Tissue response to electrosurgery. In Oringer MJ (ed): Electrosurgery in Dentistry, ed 2. Philadelphia, WB Saunders, 1975, pp 186–190.
5. Maness WL, Roeber ES, Clark RE, et al: Histological evaluation of electrosurgery with varying frequency and waveform. J Prosthet Dent 40:304–312, 1978.
6. Sherman JA: Oral Electrosurgery, An Illustrated Clinical Guide. London, Martin Dunitz, 1992, pp 7–11.
7. Kiser GC: Electrosurgery in fixed partial dentures. Laboratory Manual, The University of Texas Dental School at San Antonio, Dept Restorative Dentistry, Div Crown and Bridge.
8. Altman RB: Principles and applications of electrosurgery: 1994. Assoc Avian Vet Annual Conference Practical Labs Proceedings and Manual, 1994, pp 85–92.
9. Fucci V, Elkins AD: Electrosurgery: Principles and guidelines in veterinary medicine. Contin Ed 13(3):407–414, 1991.
10. Coyne BE, Bednarski RM, Bilbrey SA: Thermoelectric burns from improper grounding of electrocautery units: Two case reports. J. A. Aminal Hosp. 29:7–9, 1993.
11. Bennett RA: Surgical considerations. In Harrison G, Harrison L, Ritchie B (eds): Avian Medicine: Principles and Applications. Lake Worth, FL, Wingers Publishing, 1994, pp 1081–1095.
12. Harrison GJ: Surgical instrumentation and special techniques. In Harrison GJ, Harrison LR (eds): Clinical Avian Medicine and Surgery. Philadelphia, WB Saunders, 1986, pp 560–567.

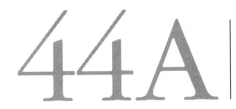

Beak Repair, Rhamphorthotics

Success with beak repair has been elusive despite obvious need; many species require maxillofacial repair and reconstruction. Beak repair is necessary to return the bird to normal alimentary function and self-sufficiency, especially wild birds destined for release. New synthetic skin adhesives and dental bonding agents allowed development of satisfactory protocols for beak reconstruction and correction.

Orthognathia is "the branch of oral medicine dealing with the cause and treatment of malposition of the bones of the jaws,"[1] but this definition denotes limitations because it refers solely to orthopedic disorders. Rhamphorthotics translates into the use of appliances to support, align, prevent, or correct deformities in, or improve the function of, moving parts of the beak. The term more properly defines the goals of the discipline.

The scope of the discipline of rhamphorthotics and avian orthognathics is massive. Avian taxonomy is largely based on variations in head and beak anatomy.[1a, 2] The functions of the beak include[36]: food procurement; protection; sexual display and courtship; nest making, egg turning and feeding of chicks; communication; grooming/preening; evaporative heat loss (panting); and locomotion (hookbills).

The demands put on beak performance require precise corrective measures and an understanding of the differences and similarities in orthodontics, orthopedics, and soft tissue repair.

GLOSSARY

The following terms are important for properly identifying surgical landmarks and understanding the final goal of correction, and for accurate communication with fellow practitioners.

appliance. Device used to apply force to oral structures for intentional movement or stabilization

abutment. Oral structure or implant used for anchorage or support for device or prosthesis

attrition. Wearing away of keratin by beak-to-beak contact

beak (aka "bill"). Horn-covered projection of the face that forms the mouth parts

cere.[1a, 14] Basal part of the beak that has remained soft and lies above the nasal opening. It is not present in all species.

culmen.[1a] Dorsal midline of the upper beak

epignathous.[1a] Hookbilled

eponychium.[1a] Corneous, epidermal ridge or extension at the base and sides of rhinothecal keratin and commonly confused with the cere, although the location may be the same. Generally seen in species with hard rhamphotheca more than soft types. Archtype presentation is seen in Columbiformes.

gape.[1a] Mouth slit (oral opening)

gnathotheca.[33] Mandibular keratin tissues

gonys.[1a] Ventral midline curve of the lower beak

holorhinal.[38] Position when the external nares do not extend caudal to nasofrontal hinge (e.g., Anseriformes and Galliformes)

773

malar regions.[33] Soft tissues that cover the jaws where keratinization does not form a beak

mentum[1a] **(aka "chin").** Line where right and left halves of the lower beak are united

operculum.[1a] Cartilaginous scale overhanging the external nares

prokinesis.[1a, 14] Type of cranial kinesis with movement of the upper jaw in relation to the braincase (e.g., parrots, Galliformes, Anseriformes). May be absent in species with fusion of the frontal and nasal bones (e.g., ostriches and raptors)

prosthesis. Artificial part that replaces a natural body part

prosthodontics. Branch of dentistry concerned with construction of appliances to replace missing oral structures

rhamphotheca.[33] Keratin layers of the entire beak

rhinotheca.[33] Premaxillary keratin tissues

rhynchokinesis.[14] Condition when the elevation of the upper jaw is in the midbody of premaxilla rostral to the kinetic joint because of flexible bone cortex. Does not depend on sliding action of the joint quadrate mechanism. Seen in waterfowl

rictus.[1a] Soft triangle of tissue found at the junction of the upper and lower beak (oral commissure)

rostrum mandibularis.[33] Mandibular beak

rostrum maxillaris.[33] Premaxillary beak

schizorhinal.[38] Long external nares and canals that terminate in the slit caudal to the nasofrontal hinge (e.g., terns, pigeons, shorebirds)

splint. Apparatus designed to prevent motion or displacement

thermoplastic adhesive. An exothermic synthetic liquid monomer that polymerizes into a solid, inert material. Usually a cyanoacrylate (CA) that is activated by moisture. Degree of exothermia is variable, but generally is greater when an accelerator substance is added

tomium.[1a] Working (cutting) edges of the beak

zygomatic arch. Bony structure composed of the maxilla, jugal and quatrojugal bones[11]

ANATOMIC AND PHYSIOLOGIC CONSIDERATIONS

The bones of the face are derived from the first two embryonic pharyngeal arches and the structures of the mouth are largely deviations of the first arch.[4] The beak is barely visible in the chicken embryo at 5½ days and becomes a recognizable structure by day 7. Beak cornification begins by day 10 and a hard surface structure is present by day 14.[16, 50]

Altricial species have increasing rates of embryonic growth and metabolism continuously throughout incubation, whereas precocial chicks have a growth plateau shortly before hatching. Beak development may be accelerated in these species at comparative dates of development. The skull is composed of a greater number of bones that fuse early in life, giving the appearance of a single bone.[35] Many species such as Amazon parrots, owls, and Rhamphastidae have extensively pneumatized skulls to lighten the skeleton for flight but are lacking in species-sustaining force to the skull (e.g., woodpeckers and diving birds).[20, 35, 40] Pneumatization may take up to 1 to 2 years for completion in some species and includes extensive diverticula of the beak and periorbital region, especially noted in psittacines.[1a, 11, 14, 20, 34, 35, 38]

The bones involved in jaw motion are the quadrate, articular, pterygoid, jugal, palatine, frontal and nasal.[11, 14, 20, 38] The muscles of mastication and their actions are[39]

Action	Muscle
1. Lower jaw depression. Assists upper jaw elevation	Depressor mandibulae
2. Lower jaw elevation	Adductor mandibulae externus Adductor mandibulae caudalis Pseutotemporalis superficialis
3. Upper jaw depression. Retracts ptyergoid and palatine bones. Assists elevation of lower jaw	Pseudotemporalis Profundus
4. Upper jaw elevation. Moves quadrate and palate forward	Protractor Quadrapterygoidei

The mandibular nerve (V3) is the primary motor innervation for the masticatory muscles, with the facial nerve (VII) supplying the depressor mandibulae.[11, 42] Motor innervation for the tongue is provided by the hypoglossal nerve (XII) via its lingual ramus branch. Sensory innervation is supplied by the trigeminal nerve (V) and its three main branches:[42]

V1 (deep ophthalmic nerve) Tip of the premaxilla

(bill tip organ), deep layers of the rhinotheca and rostral palate. Bony canals exist in the premaxilla for its exit

V2 (maxillary nerve) Floor and wall of the nasal cavity, palatine mucosa

V3 (mandibular nerve) Skin and gnathotheca, intermandibular skin, mucosa of the rostral lower jaw and palate near the rictus. Mental rami exist in the mandibula for its exit

The blood supply to the oral structures consists of a complex network of microvasculature containing numerous arteriovenous anastomoses that also serve for thermoregulation. Venous plexi often surround arteries, especially branches of the oral cavity where countercurrent heat exchange may occur. The external carotid artery is the primary supplier and its two main branches, the mandibular and maxillary arteries, give rise to other significant sources, such as:[41]

Maxillary Artery Origin	
Branch	**Supplies**
Facial artery	Muscles of mastication, quadrate bone, quadrojugal bar
Submandibular artery	Found medial to the ventral mandibular artery, supplies rostral intermandibular skin and its appendages, mandible, and deep layers of gnathotheca
Palatine artery	Upper jaw mucosa of the pharynx and palate, premaxilla, and rhinotheca
Mandibular Artery Origin	
Branch	**Supplies**
Lingual artery	Tongue, mucosa of floor of mouth, submandibular salivary gland, deep layer of gnathotheca, mandibular symphysis
Tomial arteries	Found parallel to tomium of gnathotheca

The bones of the beak are covered by several horny plates that vary in number and shape according to the specific species.[1a, 2] The suture lines are no longer visible in most modern birds, but a few species show vestiges (e.g., ostriches, skuas) or obvious plate anatomy, such as shearwaters and petrals. Coues (1903) identified seven names for various plates and gave locations for each in Procellariiformes (albatrosses and fulmars). Bureau[58] described nine plates for the puffin, where the superficial layers of the beak are shed every fall in an annual, postbreeding "moult."[1a, 2] These plates have been referred to in previous publications as growth centers.[22, 30, 33, 48] The theory of the plates being discontinuous has been contested by most modern investigators, because most birds have no identifiable sutures or landmarks. However, fossil bird remains clearly show their origins and the remnants in the species named above give evidence of an evolutionary precedence.

Beaks are covered by a dermis and a keratinized epidermis (horn), which is a dynamic tissue that constantly grows, migrates, and desquamates. The dermis is an extremely thin, highly vascular layer sandwiched between two hard substances. Epithelial integrity depends upon an intact vascular dermis. The maxillary beak is connected to the skull via a kinetic joint, which may become fused in some species, and a series of articular joints on the ventral aspects of the maxilla.[1a, 14, 34, 35, 38] The quadrate mechanism (quadrate bone and zygomatic arch) allows the upper jaw to rotate upward and depress the mandible to create a relatively greater gape with faster closing ability than is possible with a single temporomandibular joint. The quadrate and zygomatic arches are equivalent to the mammalian malleus (articular portion) and incus (quadrate).

The bone of the upper beak is the result of fusion of the premaxilla and nasal bone. Ducks and parrots also have a fusion to the maxillaries, which is called the "prosopium."[1a, 14] Large diverticula of the infraorbital sinus and/or external nares cause the premaxilla to be very thin and lightweight.[20, 34, 35] The mandible is the fusion of five bones. The largest and most rostral forms a mandibular symphysis, called the "dentary," and the suture line is fully ossified.[38] Regeneration of avulsed bony jaw tissues is extremely limited in the advanced juvenile and adult when full growth potential is reached.[53] Specific jaw pressures and kinetics differ between orders and genera. No specific cephalometric studies are available for birds to date. Reconstruction and rhamphorthotics require keen observation of normal jaw use, normal behavior, behavior prediction during recovery, and no small amount of artistic creativity.[18, 21, 22, 25, 33, 45, 48]

Keratin is present in two forms. A weight-bearing (working) horn is found on the tips and tomia of both beaks and extends as far as the palatine ridge of the rhinotheca.[1a] A second type (covering horn) lies on the outer noncontact surfaces of both beaks. Keratin is produced from the stratum germinativum at all sites and migrates to the surface. Keratin also migrates as the result of underlying transitional cells directed at various angles in columns toward the tomial edges. In some places, keratin migrates inward to become part of the internal rhamphotheca as a localized event. This disproves the theory of sliding, discontinuous keratin sheets (Lüdicke)[1a, 59] and theories proposed in previous publications where continuous growth advancing from base to tip has been reported.[22, 33, 55] Beak keratin growth rates have been reported as being ¼ to ½ inch per month in various psittacine species.[11, 33]

A cere may or may not be present and may be naked or partially or fully feathered. It is defined as the base of the rhinotheca that has remained soft.[1] It does not contribute significantly to the production of keratin, as has been previously reported.[22, 33] The boundaries between cere and the base of the rhinotheca can be determined with a metal probe in that the membranous keratin of the cere yields to pressure, whereas the hard keratin of the beak does not.[1a]

SURGICAL REPAIR

Acquired Defects

Trauma is the most common patient presentation. Punctures, crush wounds, lacerations, fractures, avulsions, and thermal burns are routinely sustained from blunt contact injuries and attacks from cage mates, other pet species, and owners.[8, 22, 33, 48]

Beak pathology and malocclusion may also have an underlying etiology that results in abnormal wear, development, growth, or susceptibility to trauma. Malnutrition, vitamin deficiency and excess, liver disorders, infectious disease (e.g., psittacine beak and feather disease [PBFD]), tuberculosis, mycosis, poxvirus, knemidocoptic), diabetes mellitus, hormonal disorders, neoplasia, toxins, reproductive activity, and genetics have all been reported as causes of beak pathology in a wide range of avian species.[12, 13, 16, 20, 23, 26–29, 31, 32, 48, 56, 57] Diagnosis should be vigorously pursued to identify underlying disease processes that may mimic primary beak pathology before corrective procedures are undertaken. Seasonal proliferation of keratin may be related to normal breeding behaviors and should not be confused with acquired or congenital defects.

Subluxation

Forcible hyperextension of the nasofrontal hinge occurs most commonly when the weight of the body is thrust onto the opened rostrum maxillaris. The resulting clinical appearance is a bird with mild to marked discomfort, an inability to close the mouth to some degree, and reticence or refusal to eat. Radiographs reveal the maxilla resting on or above the dorsal edge of the frontal bone. It is important to review the location and integrity of the zygomatic arc because its articulations may not be intact and fractures have been noted in a few cases. High-detail radiography is essential for this diagnosis.

Therapy requires general anesthesia and reduction of the subluxated joint into its normal position.[10] It is important to check the palatine area for the presence of bone fragments because the vomer and rostral portion of the frontal bones may penetrate the choanal mucosa. Visible fragments penetrating the mucosa should be removed and the wounds flushed with a disinfectant. Large wounds may be sealed with tissue glue (*N*-butylcyanoacrylate) and antibiotic therapy started when appropriate. Dilute chlorhexidine solution (Nolvasan, Fort Dodge) oral flushes administered four times a day (qid) for 3 to 5 days assist in minor wound healing without the need for tissue adhesives (Fig. 44A–1).

Fractures of the quadrate mechanism require a mandibular-premaxillary splint. The only clinical sign noted on presentation in one case was a persistent clawing at the oral cavity. Radiographs should be taken to identify the fracture.

The jaw should be placed in a slightly opened position under general anesthesia or heavy sedation. Secure a wire mesh impregnated with an

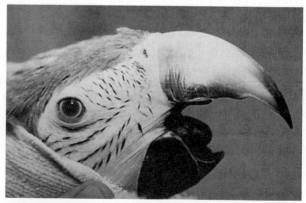

F i g u r e 4 4 A – 1

Subluxation of the premaxilla in a hybrid macaw. The condition was successfully reduced under anesthesia.

acrylic cement at the lateral aspects of the rhinotheca and gnathotheca in a vertical fashion to stabilize the zygomatic arch. It should be applied in a manner similar to an interdental bridge in human or small animal orthodontics.[36]

It is crucial to leave the gape open enough for the expulsion of vomitus and to allow ad libitum water intake. A soft diet or forced feedings should be instituted. The cage environment should be devoid of furniture or bars to prevent climbing. Bilateral appliance application may be necessary for heavy-billed patients. Two weeks is required for callus formation (Fig. 44A–2).

Mandibular Fractures

Beak fractures are significant emergencies because of the inherent power during contraction of most pet avian jaws, especially in psittacines. Continued pressure on damaged jaw tissues and desiccation of deep tissues exposed via keratin defects quickly lead to irreparable damage. Beak pressure is in proportion to the size of the bird. Welty[5] reported a Maxentford hawfinch bite pressure (body weight 2 oz) at 159 lb per square inch, powerful enough to crack olive pits. Macaw jaw exertions are reported at over 200 lb per square inch.[6]

The principal efforts for fracture management are debridement and disinfection; systemic antimicrobial therapy; salvage and restoration of vascular supply to soft and bony tissues; reapposition of the jaw bones; coverage of the bony structures with soft tissue; and rigid stabilization of the jaw.

Flush wounds with copious amounts of warm saline and disinfectant solution, such as a tamed iodophor (betadine solution, Purdue Frederick) or chlorhexidine solution (Nolvasan).

Gently prepare the wound with a surgical scrub and rinse thoroughly to remove residual detergent from the pockets between bony and soft tissues. Great care must be taken not to destroy the delicate vasculature at the wound margins, especially major vessels such as the tomial arteries.

Minor defects may be reapposed and cemented back into place using appropriate acrylic thermoplastics such as ethylcyanoacrylate (Cyano-Veneer, Ellman Co., Hewlett, NY) or methoxyethylcyanocrylate (Sincomet, Henkel Adhesive Co., Kankakee, Ill).[1a] *N*-isobutyl cyanoacrylates (Tissue-Glu, Ellman Co.; Vet-Bond, 3M Co., St. Paul, MN; Nexaband, Tri Point Medical, Raleigh, NC) are adequate for minor keratin defects but are rarely strong enough for use as a splint or at the tomium.[43] Methylcyanoacrylate (Crazy Glue) is too irritating and exothermic and is not approved for tissue application.

Fractures of the mandibular ramus and lateral dentary bone[38] often heal after splinting with multiple layers of dental acrylic adhesives allowed to dry in succession over contoured wire or nylon mesh strips. Wrap the materials over the tomial edges along transverse planes of the jaw and incorporate the body of the mandible and gnathotheca in a solid but lightweight cast on all three surfaces. Light-sensitive acrylics (Sunschein, Henry Schein, Port Washington, NY; Triad VLC, Dentsply, York, PA) may be used as an additional overlay for added strength on top of a thermoplastic acrylic coat applied as a foundation layer.[31] Do not allow acrylic adhesives to fill gaps between the vascular dermis or bone because they create an impermeable barrier to cell migration. Increasing the viscosity of the synthetic adhesives in these cases is a preferred approach because the acrylic polymerizes over the wound surface, not within it.

Extensive multiple fractures and symphyseal fractures of the mandible often require the use of stainless steel wire to achieve stabilization. The prognosis is always guarded because of the frequent incidence of osteomyelitis, avascular necrosis, nonunion, and tissue avulsion for these injuries.

At least two wires should be placed in such a

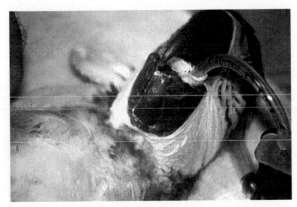

F i g u r e   4 4 A – 2

One or two mesh strips are used for vertical stabilization. Bilateral application may be required.

fashion that fracture compression is achieved. Because of the path of motion and the muscular pull on the mandible, many fracture sites tend to separate and disrupt cellular bridging of both soft and ossified tissues during the healing phase.[36] Use one or preferably two mattress-pattern hemicerclage wires or figure-eight cerclage wires at each end of the fracture. The temptation to tunnel the wires around the bone under the keratin in a cerclage fashion should be avoided because of the resulting massive vascular disruption. Pass the wires directly through the lateral and labial aspects of the gnathotheca. Predrill holes with a sterile burr or hypodermic needle, which also is an excellent wire guide. Wire holes should be flushed of debris with a disinfectant or antibiotic and the area coated with an appropriate cyanoacrylic (Figs. 44A–2, 44A–3).[52]

Adding wire mesh strips into the overlay increases splint rigidity. Ultraviolet-sensitive acrylic overlays or wires passed through the rami of both mandibles act as anchor points for external wires or adhesive splints, which are alternative techniques for strengthening the splint or cast. The choice of cerclage or K-wires depends on the patient size. Slightly depressing the internal aspects of the wires allows for less tongue obstruction during mastication and better patient cooperation during recovery. The final configuration has the metal supports closely adhered to both the internal and external gnathothecal surface, and the entire structure rests under the tongue. Great delicacy must be employed in deforming the wire down into the mouth to

avoid tearing the keratin penetration sites during mastication. The ends of the wires should be turned down at right angles and incorporated into an acrylic cast to prevent rotation and debris buildup. The internal or lingual aspects should be coated and incorporated into an intra-oral splint, much like a mandibular dental splint for canine patients.[36] Be aware that each additional invasion into the dermal and bony tissues represents a possible disruption of the vascular supply and a potential route for infection. In small patients, use external fixation in preference to steel and surgical invasion to reduce the likelihood of a compromised healing site.[37]

Pay particular attention to oral hygiene, adequate feed intake (independently or via tube feeding), balanced diet consumption, nutritional supplementation for vitamin- and calcium–deficient patients, and restricted activity via smooth-sided holding cages, such as an acrylic chamber.

Analgesia is important for success because disintegration of beak appliances leaves little chance for a successful second procedure if tissue damage is further aggravated by the patient. Sedation using diazepam (Valium, Roche) or butorphanol (Torbutrol, Bristol) and inflammation reduction using flunixine (Banamine, Schering) are valuable in returning the patient to health, especially during the critical first few postoperative days.[33, 48] Sedation using injectable agents may be required to augment analgesics for proper postoperative patient recovery.

Postoperative radiographs should be taken 2 or 3

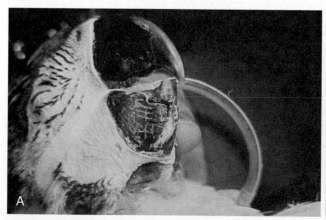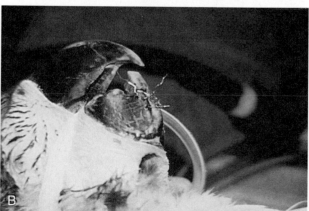

F i g u r e   4 4 A – 3

(A) Traumatic puncture and fracture of the mandible by the parents. The wound was debrided and prepared for closure. *(B)* Mandibular fracture closed with stainless steel wire and ready for a thermoplastic cast.

weeks after fixation to evaluate healing. The surgical site is generally exposed by controlled debridement for assessment every 20 to 30 days using a steel cutting wheel or burr. Wounds are debrided, flushed, and resealed until epithelial integrity is restored or secondary intention fibrosis has covered the injured surface and radiographs indicate good internal callus formation without evidence of osteomyelitis.

Bilateral fractures of the mandibular rami carry a poor prognosis, especially in small species and birds with slender mandibles (i.e., passerines and softbills). The blood supply dermal layers are delicate and often completely disrupted, resulting in avascular necrosis.

Periacute trauma may respond to rapid repair with good apposition and stabilization. In psittacines and large zoologic specimens (e.g., cranes, ratites) that have a heavier mandible and associated cortices, use cerclage wire, pins, and acrylic splints or casts.[19, 24, 46] Species with membranous-type keratin of the beak and mostly cancellous bone (e.g., ducks, geese) respond poorly to invasive hardware. External whole-beak acrylic casts are recommended. Smaller birds, passerines and songbirds, and small psittacines also suffer insult from the insertion of internal fixation.[51] Bilateral hemimandibulectomy may be the only salvage procedure possible. Prosthetic replacement for partial rostrum mandibularis avulsions has been used with variable success, but it is generally not recommended.[21, 24, 46]

Mandibular symphyseal splits warrant special mention because the recovery rate is unexpectedly low in comparison with the success rate in other small pets.[36, 53] Rapid local necrosis and desiccation of the thin vascular dermis results in a high incidence of nonunion fractures. The symphysis of the mandible is also nonchondrus with a slower rate of primary cell regeneration at the injury site in comparison with osteoblastic migration.

Vigorously debride the split area in wounds older than several hours and immediately close the wound. In smaller species use a lightweight, external acrylic jaw cast rather than an internal rigid (e.g., steel wire or pin) fixation apparatus. In larger birds, especially parrots and macaws, use cerclage wire in a simple interrupted or cruciate pattern. Wire guide holes must be flushed, disinfected, and sealed over using a sterile, nonirritating acrylic thermoplastic splint or cast.

External casts of visible-light–cured (VLC) acrylics are indicated for birds with powerful bite capacities. Transverse mandibular pins and/or mesh splints can be incorporated into the casts so that jaw integrity is not compromised.[53]

Congenital Defects

Malocclusive beak disorders are seen with regularity in avicultural and pet avian practice. Congenital beak deformities in poultry, cormorants, and a few psittacine species have been associated with numerous etiologies, including folacin and biotin deficiency[7–10, 16, 56] (brachygnathism); calcium deficiency[7–10, 12, 16] (soft beak and skull); manganese deficiency[7–10, 16] (mandibular pragmethism); selenium toxicity[54] (wry face); incubation hyperthermia[7–11] (variable); aflatoxins[7–10, 16]; egg malpositioning[7–11, 56] (scissors beak); genetics[5–9, 16]; and chemical toxins.[57]

Orthodontic research shows that malocclusion is not simply the result of independent inheritance of facial characteristics. The precise role of heredity as an etiologic agent for malocclusion has not been clarified.[36]

Management appears to play a significant role in the appearance of congenital beak defects.[7–10, 12, 33, 56] A revision of management practices in one large commercial psittacine aviary reduced beak deformities in weaned chicks from an 8% severe defect incidence to a 4% slight to imperceptible deviation rate over a 3-year period through improved egg and chick care, despite a 250% increase in total chick production.[56]

Scissors Beak

Scissors beak is a lateral deviation of the rhinotheca, which reduces proper occlusion and effective use of the internal rhinothecal keratin ridge. Deviation may be to the left or right but has been noted by the author to be predominantly rightsided. The incidence was found to be nearly equal in another independent survey.[56] The defect is seen predominantly, but not exclusively, in psittacines.

The deformity may affect only the keratin of the rhinothecal tip (majority of cases), the premaxilla or the entire rostrum maxillaris and nasofrontal hinge (a small minority of cases). High-detail radiography is recommended prior to correction as a prognostic aid. In all cases, the placement of the upper beak off the sagittal plane leads to excessive wear on the ipsilateral aspect and a proliferation of uninhibited keratin on the contralateral corner of the gnathotheca. Cockatoos and macaws are the most commonly affected species, but various large and small psittacines have been documented with the exception of Eclectus parrots.[33, 34, 48, 52, 56]

Correction may be as simple as finger pressure and frequent daily manipulations in very young chicks. Self-corrections have been noted in a few cases. The majority of cases presented to clinicians require surgical intervention for permanent correction (Fig. 44A–4).

A rhamphorthotic appliance passively encourages redirection of the premaxilla through keratin and/or bony remodeling. Construct a steeply sloped ramp, which applies increasing resistance to the rhinotheca as the mouth is closed, similar to the inclined plane devices used in human and small animal orthodontics for moving teeth through bite pressures.[37] Attempts to use beak stalls, halo devices, dental brackets, or buttons with masal (rubber) chains have all been less successful because of

insecure anchorage at tension sites, increased labor intensity, patient handling, client noncompliance, and a prolonged treatment period.[10, 33, 48, 49] Isoflurane is the anesthetic agent of choice, but a ketamine-diazepam combination can be used. Gas delivery has traditionally been via endotracheal tubes; however, the use of abdominal air sac intubation has eliminated the problems of unpredictable apnea, airway mucus obstruction, excessive intrathoracic pressures, and surgical site interference.

Grind the beak into its normal shape with a grinding wheel (Dremel, Racine, WI) and trim the contralateral mandibular corner down below the occlusal plane to enhance bite correction at approximately a 30° angle. Score the keratin in a grid-like fashion near the tip of the maxillary beak to enhance adherence of the cement. The grid pattern should extend to the intermandibular keratin (if present in that species) and onto the internal aspects of the rostral gnathotheca. Remove loose keratin, rinse the area, disinfect, and dry. Do not penetrate the basal layer of keratin and expose the underlying dermis. Experience and a light touch help to differentiate tissue density while grinding. Areas with hemorrhage produced by overzealous grinding should be disinfected and sealed with tissue glue (CA).

Cast the entire work area with a light layer of thin methyl- or methoxycyanoacrylate or composite acrylic to create a foundation intimately adhered into the keratin grid. Hold a strip of stainless steel mesh to the external face of the rostral gnathotheca in a vertical position so that it lies between the midline of the beak and the ipsilateral corner on the affected side of the face. This will become the framework for the inclined ramp that forces the upper beak medially back to the midline. Some placement discretion is required in smaller species (Fig. 44A–5).

Cement the upright mesh to the foundation layer with liquid CA and angle the dorsal aspect of the mesh toward the midline at 45°. Stiffen the entire mesh with adhesive and allow it to dry. Additional coats of acrylic incorporate the framework and beak, including the lingual aspects. The entire structure should be level with the medial canthus on the affected side of the face (Fig. 44A–6).

Use a fine drill bit to drill guide holes through the mandible along the lateral edges of the mesh strip. Three pairs of holes equally placed in the space between the occlusal surface and the mucous

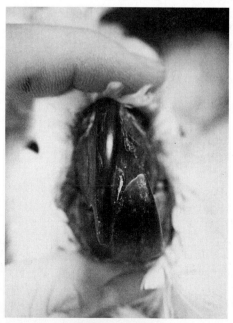

Figure 44A–4

Classic scissors-beak presentation, rostral view.

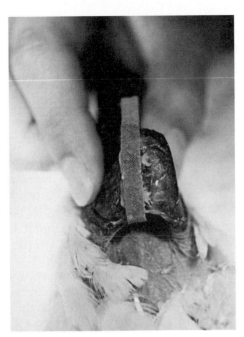

Figure 44A–5

Vertical mesh splint cemented to the gnathotheca prior to drilling wire holes.

membranes of the oral cavity are desirable, but four provide greater rigidity for the final appliance. Only two holes may be possible in smaller patients. Pass a sterile stainless steel wire through the mandible, encompassing the upright mesh, and tighten the wire carefully to avoid breakage. The wires must

be secure to prevent the appliance from loosening under repeated jaw pressure. A hypodermic needle serves as an excellent wire guide, if needed.

Hemorrhage is controlled; the wire holes are flushed, disinfected, and dried; and an overcoat of acrylic or composite resin is laid over the wires to create a smooth surface. The mesh, CA foundation, and anterior gnathotheca are incorporated into one structure by layering the surfaces with a VLC acrylic paste or sheet. The VLC acrylic can be laid down on sectional sheets or as balls of syringed or provisional material. It is smoothed into place by finger pressure to create the appliance shape. Harden the acrylic by using a special ultraviolet light designed to activate the polymerization of the dental material.

Add additional portions until sufficient acrylic is present to create a ramp with a steep curve that is continuous from the lateral occlusal edge of the far side of the gnathotheca to the dorsal tip of the appliance (Figs. 44A–7, 44A–8). The opposite side should have a 45° angle formed by a moderately thin wall of acrylic from the dorsal point of the mesh to the angle of the gape. Insufficient height or total bulk posterior to the appliance on the affected side allows the patient to slip the tip of the beak over the acrylic point and aggravate the condition by becoming caught. The ventral aspects should envelope the front of the gnathotheca, inside and out, to prevent cracking of the base under jaw pressure. The lateral aspects should wrap distally enough to provide resistance to forward motion when the bird grips a stationary object during climbing or in an attempt to remove the appliance.

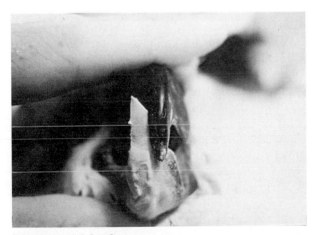

Figure 44A–6

Vertical mesh frame impregnated with acrylic and ready to receive the visible-light-cure acrylic overcoat.

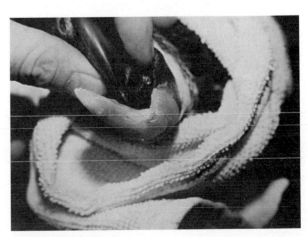

Figure 44 A–7

Rostral view of a scissors-beak corrective appliance.

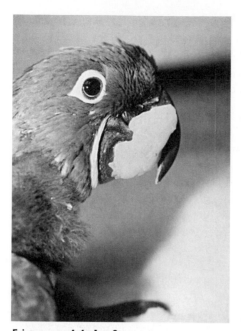

Figure 44 A–8

Lateral view of a scissors-beak corrective appliance.

Evaluate the device for surface smoothness (against debris retention), overall weight, functional architecture, beak closure, and lateral pressure against the rhinotheca. Close air sac tube entry sites with tissue glue and administer analgesics plus anti-inflammatory medications to reduce postoperative discomfort. Systemic antibiotics are not needed with proper surgical technique. Owners should clean the device several times daily. The appliance should be rechecked at least once a week for progress, slippage, and sanitation. Thirty days appears to be a good overall average for correction, but some young macaws have achieved correction in as little as 5 days, and some adult cockatoos have required 60 to 90 days. A juvenile hyacinth macaw required 12 weeks because of the inherently slower growth rate.[10] The acrylic loosens about every 20 days from normal keratin exfoliation and use. Applying a thin layer of cyanoacrylic around and under the device recements it to the new keratin.

Remove the appliance under anesthesia with a cutting burr along the rostral and lingual midline until the keratin and wires are just exposed. A line along the occlusal surface should be cut and the appliance gently removed in sections. Remove excess keratin retained under the device and clean the surface and wire holes with iodine chlorhexidine or another antibacterial and antifungal solution. Seal the wire holes with cyanoacrylic. If the final appearance and beak manipulations are normal, recurrence is unlikely.

Mandibular Prognathism

This debilitating deviation of the upper beak is also referred to as "parrot beak." The condition can vary from a "lazy beak" condition in which the tip of the rhinotheca rests on or just inside the gnathotheca, to severe malformations in which the upper beak is curled under at 180° or more and is pressing on the tongue.

Correction via the use of a beak appliance is preferable to dependency on cutting, grinding, and trauma to the sensitive bill tip organ of the rhinotheca.

Species susceptibility is widespread but most common in cockatoos.[33, 49, 56] It is suspected that very mild cases may be the equivalent to results of thumb-sucking behaviors in children.

The anatomic analysis in a case of true mandibular prognathism (MP) is a shortened premaxilla and/or nasal and frontal bones. Be aware that the mandible of the normal hatchling chick is longer than the premaxilla and that the growth of both jaws occurs in spurts.[4, 36, 56] Temporary length imbalance may be beneficial for assisting parents in feeding chicks, and it is suggested that parents assist normal beak development by hooking onto the rhinotheca.[56] Only very rare instances of this condition have been documented in wild-hatched and parent-fed chicks (Fig. 44A–9).

The acrylic appliance is designed to achieve the same effect that the parents are believed to contribute. The artificial extension of the rhinotheca out and over the lower jaw directs its growth in the chick or remodeling in the older bird. At the same time, the ligaments of the nasofrontal hinge are stretched to prevent permanent contracture of this joint. Obviously, this system works most effectively for epignathous species.

The patient is placed under general anesthesia. Abdominal air sac anesthetic tube placement is advantageous. Grind away any overgrowth of the rhamphotheca but not to a point of reducing the occlusal surface to less than normal.

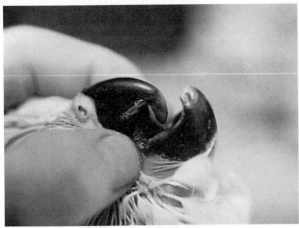

Figure 44 A-9

Severe mandibular prognathism with rhinothecal compression.

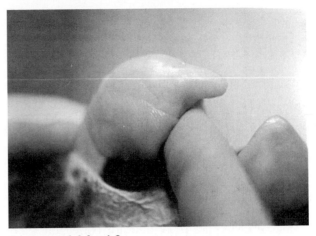

Figure 44A-10

Finger-mold technique for visible-light-cure acrylic application.

Cut a full-circumference groove into the hard keratin of the rhinothecal tip halfway between the tip and the inner keratin ridge. The chick must be old enough to have developed sufficiently hard keratin to avoid injury. Repeat the circular groove once or twice above the first cut, as allowed by the length of the beak. These indentations allow prolonged bonding with the acrylic. Clean, disinfect, and seal evidence of dermal invasion with tissue glue.

The superficial layer of keratin is roughened over all surfaces of the rhinotheca back to at least 50 to 75% of the upper beak. The area is then sealed with a low-viscosity CA and allowed to dry.[22, 52]

VLC acrylics are rolled into a conical shape, and the tip of the rhinotheca is inserted centrally into the flattened base. Gloved hands reduce material drag and sticking. Cooling the acrylic (sheet, tube, or provisional) material in a cup of refrigerated water until use also reduces handling difficulties. Push the softened acrylic upward and back along all three facets of the rhinotheca in a uniform layer, spreading it until more is needed. Additional balls of the hand-warmed plastic are pressed onto the leading edge of the already applied layer to form the cone. The acrylic may be light-cured in sections as it is added or as a final cast, according to the surgeon's preference. Extend the cone rostrally at approximately a 60 to 90° angle in a gentle curve. The tip of the cone should be uniformly tapered and long enough to prevent it from reentry into the oral cavity (Fig. 44A–10).

The appliance should be of uniform thickness with sufficient thickness to prevent fracture but not enough to add excess weight. The surface should be smooth and the edges confluent with the beak to prevent food retention. Smooth hardened rough spots with a grinding wheel. The critical contact areas are at the inner rhinothecal keratin ridge, where the greatest pressures are exerted, and along the sides. The farther up the beak body the device is applied, the greater the distribution of work force and the reduction of risk of loss (Fig. 44A–11).

It should be impossible or difficult to place the appliance tip into the gnathotheca while the bird is still under anesthesia. If impossible or very difficult, anesthesia should be reversed.

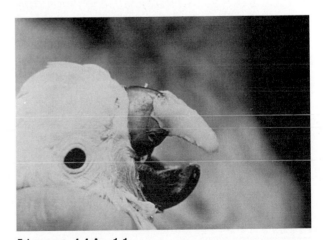

Figure 44A-11

Finished mandibular prognathism corrective appliance.

Some transient discomfort should be expected during the first few hours to days as the nasofrontal joint is forcibly extended and the associated ligaments stretched. Light sedation should be considered in adults that persist in trying to remove the appliance because of discomfort or aversion.

Aftercare involves routine sanitation and checking the periphery of the appliance for loosening. Schedule weekly rechecks for progress and to reseal loose edges with a low-viscosity CA. Generally, 14 to 30 days are sufficient to correct most defects, particularly in unweaned birds. Normal activities may be allowed as soon as the patient arrives home. Adults may require more time for correction. One adult bare-eyed cockatoo required 6 months of appliance reattachment and correction because of age, appliance intolerance, and sporadic client compliance before success was achieved.

Removal is usually accomplished with digital manipulation, especially if significant growth has occurred (Fig. 44A–12). If growth has been minimal, exceptionally deep notches were present, or correction was achieved quickly, cut the cone carefully with a cutting burr or wheel as the density of the beak is less than the cured acrylic (Fig. 44A–13).

Avulsion

Upper and lower beak loss is most often caused by attack by a cage mate or another trauma.[21, 24, 30, 33, 44–47, 49, 57]

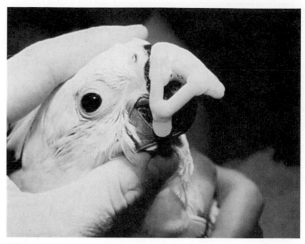

Figure 44A–13

Modified mandibular prognathism appliance to control secondary scissors beak.

Attempts to reattach amputated beaks have been uniformly unsuccessful. Prosthetic replacement has been successful for variable periods of time, but no lifelong permanent implantations have been reported.[18, 19, 21, 24, 45–47, 54]

Radical bilateral hemimandibulectomy at the level of the rictus and excision of the rostrum maxillaris just proximal to the nasofrontal hinge has been successful in psittacines, despite concerns to the contrary.

After shock, hemorrhage, and infection are con-

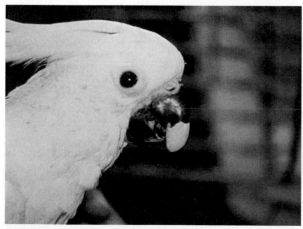

Figure 44A–12

Corrected mandibular prognathism with appliance migration due to growth.

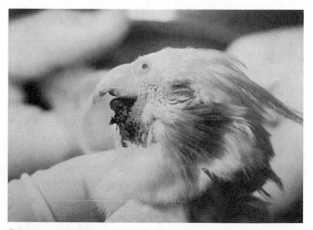

Figure 44A–14

Bilateral mandibulectomy as a result of severe trauma and avascular necrosis. Self feeding is accomplished in a deep cup in which soft table foods are placed.

trolled, assess the tissue for viability. Remnants of functional beak (upper or lower) should be retained whenever possible. The patient must undergo forced feedings for several days to weeks until new feeding behaviors are learned. Offer soft diets, soaked pelleted diets, hulled seeds, and cooked table foods in various dish shapes until an effective trapping technique is perfected. Deep cups that allow the patient to stand within them to shovel food into a corner, and paper cups with the front quarter cut down halfway are helpful for retraining. Aftercare involves intermittent trimming of the remaining beak (Fig. 44A–14).

References

1. Dorland's Illustrated Medical Dictionary, 28th ed. Philadelphia, WB Saunders Co, 1994, p 1193.
1a. Lucas AM, Stettenheim PR: Avian Anatomy: Integument. Agriculture Handbook 362. Washington, DC, Agriculture Research Service, US Department of Agriculture, 1972.
2. Freethy R: Secrets of Bird Life. New York, Blandford Press, Sterling Publishing, 1990, pp 1–23.
3. Steiner C, Davis R: Caged Bird Medicine. Ames, IA, Iowa State University Press, 1981.
4. Langman J: Medical Embryology, ed 3. Baltimore, Williams & Williams, 1975.
5. Welty JC: Life of Birds, ed 2. Eastbourne, UK, Saunders, 1975.
6. Cunningham M: Personal communication, Los Angeles, 1993.
7. Clipsham R: Prenatal medical management, part I. Am Fed Avicult Watchbird 18(5):20–23, 1992.
8. Clipsham R: Prenatal Medical Management, part II. Am Fed Avicult Watchbird 19(6):14–20, 1993.
9. Clipsham R: Prenatal medical management, part III. Am Fed Avicult Watchbird 20(7):44–46, 1993.
10. Clipsham R: Noninfectious diseases of pediatric psittacines. Semin Avian Exotic Pet Med 1(1):22–33, 1992.
11. Petrak ML: Diseases of Cage and Aviary Birds, ed 2. Philadelphia, Lea & Febiger, 1982.
12. Perry R, Gill J: Disorders of the avian integument. Vet Clin North Am Small Anim Pract 21(6):1307–1325, 1992.
13. Clipsham R: Introduction to psittacine pediatrics. Vet Clin North Am Small Anim Pract 21(6):1361–1392, 1991.
14. McLelland J: A Color Atlas of Avian Anatomy. Philadelphia, WB Saunders, 1991.
15. Vleck CM, Vleck D: Metabolism and Energetics of Avian Embryos. J Exp Zool [Suppl] 1:341–345, 1987.
16. Calnek BW, Barnes JH, Beard CW, et al: Diseases of Poultry, ed 9. Ames, IA, Iowa State University Press, 1991.
17. Clipsham RC, Murray MJ: Small Pets; Birds, Rabbits and Exotics. Santa Cruz, CA, Veterinarian Postgraduate Institute, 1993.
18. Coles BH: Avian Medicine and Surgery. Oxford, UK, Blackwell Scientific Publications, 1985.
19. Sleamaker T, Foster W: Prosthetic device for a salmon crested cockatoo. J Am Vet Med Assoc 183(11):1300–1301, 1983.
20. Harrison G, Harrison L: Clinical Avian Medicine and Surgery. Philadelphia, WB Saunders, 1986.
21. Hansen E: Personal communication, Tuscon, AZ, Reid Park Zoo, 1991.
22. Clipsham R: Surgical beak correction. J Assoc Avian Vet 3(4):188–189, 1989.
23. Dustin L: Clinical conditions in a pet canary practice. J Assoc Avian Vet 4(2):80–82, 1990.
24. Morris P, Weigel J: Methacrylate beak prosthesis in a maribou stork (Leptoptilos Crumeniferus). J Assoc Avian Vet 4(2):103–107, 1990.
25. Hildebrand M: Analysis of Vertebrate Structure. New York, John Wiley & Sons, 1974.
26. Ritchie B, Harrison G, Harrison L: A review of psittacine beak and feather disease. J Assoc Avian Vet 3(3):143–149, 1989.
27. Greenacre C, Latimer K, Niagro F, et al: Psittacine beak and feather disease in a scarlet macaw. J Assoc Avian Vet 6(2):95–98, 1992.
28. Leach M: Survey of neoplasms in pet birds. Semin Avian Exotic Pet Med 1(2):52–64, 1992.
29. Campbell T: Neoplasia. In Harrison G (ed): Clinical Avian Medicine and Surgery. Philadelphia, WB Saunders, YEAR, pp 500–508.
30. Clipsham R: Surgical beak restoration and correction. Proc Assoc Avian Vet, Seattle, 1989, pp 164–176.
31. Speer B: The Eclectus parrot: Medical and avicultural aspects. Proc Assoc Avian Vet, Seattle, 1989, pp 239–247.
32. Ritchie B, Harrison G, Harrison L: Advances in understanding the PBFD virus. Proc Assoc Avian Vet, Phoenix, 1990, pp 12–24.
33. Clipsham R: Surgical correction of beaks. Proc Assoc Avian Vet, Phoenix, 1990, pp 325–333.
34. Rubel GA, Isenbugel E, Wolvekamp P (eds): Atlas of Diagnostic Radiology of Exotic Pets. Philadelphia, WB Saunders, 1991.
35. Smith S, Smith B: Atlas of Avian Radiographic Anatomy. Philadelphia, WB Saunders, 1992.
36. Harvey C, Emily P: Small Animal Denistry. St. Louis, Mosby-YearBook, 1993.
37. Holmstrom S: Veterinary Dental Techniques for the Small Animal Practitioner. Philadelphia, WB Saunders, 1992.
38. Feduccia A: Aves Osteology. In Getty R (ed): The Anatomy of the Domestic Animals, ed 5, vol II. Philadelphia, WB Saunders, 1975.
39. Vanderberge JC: Aves myology. In Getty R (ed): The Anatomy of the Domestic Animals, ed 5, vol II. Philadelphia, WB Saunders, 1975.
40. King AS: Aves respiratory system. In Getty R (ed): The Anatomy of the Domestic Animals, ed 5, vol II. Philadelphia, WB Saunders, 1975.
41. Baumel JJ: Aves heart and blood vessels. in Getty R (ed): The Anatomy of the Domestic Animals, ed 5, vol II. Philadelphia, WB Saunders, 1975.
42. Baumel JJ: Aves nervous system. In Getty R (ed): The Anatomy of the Domestic Animals, ed 5, vol II. Philadelphia, WB Saunders, 1975.
43. Harrison G: IME 211: Some suggested uses for surgical glue. Assoc Avian Vet Newsletter 3(2):34, 1982.
44. Ryan T: IME 228: Tocotoucan bill repair. Assoc Avian Vet Newsletter, 3(2):44, 1982.
45. Fagan D: IME 225: Beak repair in a South American black eagle. Assoc Avian Vet Newsletter 3(2):41, 1982.
46. Morris P, Weigel J: Mandibular fracture repair in a marabou stork (Leptoptilos crumeniferus) with a methyacrylate prosthesis. Proc Assoc Avian Vet, Miami, 1986, pp 303–305.
47. Wolf L: Prosthetic bill technique in a Canada goose. Proc Assoc Avian Vet, Boulder, CO, 1985, pp 177–179.
48. Clipsham R: Surgical beak restoration and correction. Proc Am Fed Avicult, San Diego, 1991, pp 81–98.

49. Clipsham, R: Psittacine pediatrics: Medicine, surgery and management. Proc Midwest Avian Res Expo, Lexington, KY, 1992, pp 17–36.

50. Romanoff AL: The Avian Embryo: Structural and Functional Development. New York, Macmillan, 1960.

51. Clipsham R: Rhamphorthotics: Surgical correction of maxillofacial defects. Semin Avian Exotic Pet Med 3:2, 92–99, 1994.

52. Clipsham R: Surgical correction of beaks: Wet lab protocol. Proc Assoc Avian Vet Lab Manual, Chicago, IL, 1991.

53. Withrow S: Principles and application of cerclage wires. In Bojrab J (ed): Current Techniques in Small Animal Surgery, ed 2. Philadelphia, Lea & Febiger, 1983, pp 757–762.

54. Lowenstein L: Personal communication, Davis, CA, 1993.

55. MacDonald S: Anatomical and physiological characteristics of birds and how they differ from mammals. Proc Assoc Avian Vet, Phoenix, 1990, pp 372–389.

56. Schubot R, Clubb K, Clubb S: Psittacine Aviculture. Loxahatchee, FL, Aviculture Breeding and Research Center, 1992.

57. Coniff R: Why catfish farmers want to throttle the crow of the sea. Smithsonian 22(2):44–55, 1991.

58. Bureau L: De La Mue du bec et des ornements palpébraux du Marcareux arctique, Fratercula arctica, Steph. après La saison des amours. Soc Zool de France Bull 2:377–399, 1877.

59. Lüdicke M. Wachstum und Abnutzung des Vogelschabels. Zool Jahrb (Abt. 2. Anat U Ontog) 57:465–533, 1933.

44B

Beak Repair, Acrylics

The primary functions of the avian beak are the procurement of food and water and preparation of food for ingestion. The beak is used variably to crack and hull seed, and for carrying, tearing, crushing, and shearing food. The beak, in many species of birds, is used for defense and protection as well as an adjunct to locomotion by holding and climbing. It is also used for routine grooming, preening, mating, communication, feeding young, and habitat exploitation. Names synonymous with "beak" are "bill" and "rostrum." Beak anatomy, size, and shape are related functions.

ANATOMY AND PHYSIOLOGY

To make an accurate assessment of beak abnormalities and their repair, it is essential to understand the anatomic and physiologic influences affecting beak repair.

The rostrum includes the upper beak, or rostrum maxillare, and the lower beak or rostrum mandibulare. The rhamphotheca, the horny covering of the beak, is a keratinized thickening of the corneum of epidermis.[1-5] The rhamphotheca of the rostrum maxillare is called the rhinotheca, and of the rostrum mandibulare, the gnathotheca.[1, 6]

Most species of birds have a prokinetic, streptostylic skull.[4, 7] According to Evans,[8] as the zygomatic arch is forced rostrally, it exerts force on the ventrolateral margins of the premaxilla. A similar force is transmitted from the quadrate to the pterygoid bone to the palatine bones, which forces the caudoventral margins of the upper jaw forward and upward, thereby raising the upper jaw (Fig. 44B–1).

The degree of flexibility and motion of the maxil-

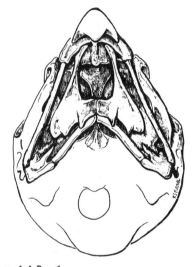

Figure 44B–1

Ventral aspect of a budgerigar skull with the mandible removed.

lary beak varies among different avian species. Psittacines, in which the frontal maxillary joint is a synovial joint, have the highest degree of movement and flexibility of the maxilla.[2, 3] The lower jaw articulates with the quadrate bone (see Fig. 44A–1). In species such as the budgerigar and other psittacines, this articulation is relatively loose, permitting considerable anterior and posterior movement to adapt with normal occlusion. The lower beak slips inside the upper beak when the jaws are closed and fits into the notch in the roof of the mouth. The medial side of the notch is part of the palatine ridge.

The hard keratin of the beak adjoins the cere, a membranous tissue surrounding the nares. The cere is softer keratin and may be naked or feathered. Waterfowl have a naked fleshy cere. The cere of

Amazon parrots is partially feathered with filoplumes, and the cere is completely feathered in Eclectus parrots.[3] The junction of the beak to the soft skin of the head may be gradual or abrupt.[9]

The dorsal medial line of the upper beak is called the "culmen" and the midventral line of the lower beak is called the "gonys." This is the line of the mandibular symphysis. The strength and rigidity of the beak comes primarily from the underlying bone. It is important to realize that the structure of the beak varies in different species of birds.

It is essential to be familiar with the physiology of beak growth to understand the dynamics of beak restoration. Histologically, the germinative layer has epidermal papillae that interdigitate with the dermal papillae.[9] Each papilla has a capillary close to the basal surface of the epidermis. The rhamphotheca or cornified keratin layer of the upper beak grows from the dermis, which covers the premaxilla (Fig. 44B–2). The rhamphotheca grows in sheets away from the dermis in a cranioventral plane (Fig. 44B–3). The growth rate varies with the various anatomic surfaces as well as from the normal wear resulting from demands placed upon the specific growth areas. As the keratin sheets migrate outward and toward the beak tip, normal beak function chips off the outermost layers as the keratin layers approach the tip of the beak. It is not clearly understood what

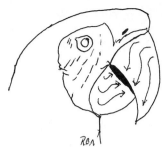

F i g u r e 4 4 B – 3

The rhamphotheca grows in migrating sheets. The rhinotheca grows away from the dermis and in a plane toward the beak tip. The gnathotheca grows away from the dermis toward the beak margin.

controls beak growth rate or why some areas of the rhamphotheca grow faster than others.

Rostrally, the rhamphotheca changes to hard keratin. The cutting edge of the upper and lower beak is called the "tomis." The tomis is composed of hard keratin.

The keratin of the lower beak (gnathotheca) grows craniodorsally at a more rapid rate than that of its upper counterpart[3]; however, there is an even contact surface of the mandibular beak in most species. Subsequently, the gnathotheca wears more uniformly than the rhamphotheca. The growth rate of immature adolescent birds is more rapid than that of adult birds.

The rictus is a triangular area of soft skin joining the upper and lower beak. The tissue of the rictus forms another transition from the hard keratin of the beak to a soft thin corneum of skin.

Consideration of the growth rate and direction is necessary to determine the potential ejection time of the repair implant or prosthesis resulting from contour changes. Clipsham[3] indicated that complete replacement of the rhamphotheca averages about 6 months. Replacement of keratin in nonpsittacine species appears to be much slower. Birds that exert great beak pressure and have highly functional beaks appear to have more rapid keratin replacement.

It is important to estimate the degree of dermal damage to offer an accurate prognosis. Destroyed dermal tissue does not regenerate keratin. In crush-type injuries, areas of dermal destruction and capillary disruption can cause uneven patterns of keratin replacement and growth rate.

Unless there is partial to total loss of beak struc-

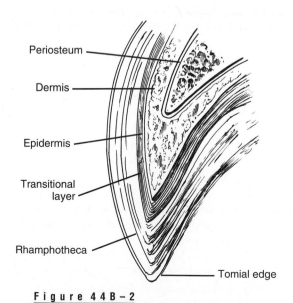

Periosteum

Dermis

Epidermis

Transitional layer

Rhamphotheca

Tomial edge

F i g u r e 4 4 B – 2

Cross-section of the upper beak of a psittacine bird.

ture requiring a prosthesis, beak repair is a temporary measure taken to secure unstable fragments, fill defects, afford normal function, and eliminate potential infection of the nasal sinus during the healing period.

BEAK ABNORMALITIES

Most abnormalities of the beak are traumatic in origin. Other causes are parasitic; viral (pox), bacterial, and fungal infections; nutritional deficiencies; and congenital deformities.

Traumatic injuries include cracks and fissures, punctures, lacerations, fractures, and avulsions. These injuries are commonly caused by impact as the result of the bird flying into solid objects or into mirrors or windows when depth perception becomes distorted.

Bite wounds from parents, cage or aviary mates, and other household pets are also common traumatic injuries.

Birds that are permitted free flight through the house often have doors and drawers closed on their heads or fly into ceiling fans. Occasionally, hookbilled birds wedge their beaks in a cage or on cage toys and cause injury during frantic attempts to free themselves.

The goals of beak repair and reconstruction are to return the beak, as much as possible, to normal function and structure for as long as possible. In instances in which time is needed for healing, an ideal result would be a repair that lasts throughout the healing phase and creates a barrier against the entry of infectious agents. For injuries and deformities in which there is loss of structure with no hope of regeneration, prosthetics are applied to restore function and appearance. The prosthesis should remain as long as possible to permit the bird to acclimate to alternate feeding and locomotion methods.

Although not essential to function, aesthetics are very important to many bird owners. The restoration should therefore appear similar to the natural beak. With care and some artistic skill it is possible to accomplish a repair invisible to anything less than close scrutiny. Although restoring normal preening, courtship, and vocalization is not always essential, for endangered species and breeding birds these considerations can be of great importance.[2]

ACRYLIC BONDING AGENTS

For the majority of abnormalities, cyanoacrylic is used as a bonding agent to repair the injured beak until the injury heals with a new keratin layer.

Of the cyanoacrylates tested by this author (Table 44B–1), ethylcyanoacrylate (Cyano-Veneer, Ellman International Corp., Hewlett, NY) is the most functional, economical, and safest product available for beak repair. The bonding quality of ethylcyanoacrylate is the result of intermolecular adhesion of the

Table 44B–1

ACRYLIC BONDING AGENTS

	Grade	Function
Cyanoacrylates		
Cyanodent	Ethylcyanoacrylate	Beak repair/prosthesis
Tissu-Glu	Isobutylcyanoacrylate	Bonding soft tissue
Crazy Glue	Methylcyanoacrylate	Commercial grade; do not use
Methylacrylates		
Temp-Plus	Isobutylmethylacrylate	Prosthesis
Hoof Repair	Methylmethacrylate	Commercial grade; do not use
Light-curing Composite *Resin*		
Sunschein		Beak repair/prosthesis
Jet Repair		Beak repair
Fiberglass		
Delta-Lite "S"		Prosthesis for hollow beak

cyanoacrylate with the biologic tissue to which it bonds.[10]

Cyano-Veneer liquid combines the adhesive bonding capacity of cyanoacrylate with a white powder that can be color-matched when combined with a pigmented shade powder, producing a cold-curing resin that is fast-setting. This product is made without amine accelerators, giving it color stability.[11]

Cyano-Veneer is uncomplicated to work with, has excellent bonding quality, and can easily be mixed for color matching. It requires no external device for curing (ultraviolet light), is bacteriostatic, and is relatively inexpensive. Cyano-Veneer is available in a veterinary kit (Ellman Cyano-Veneer Repair Kit) containing all of the components necessary for the majority of reconstructive repairs.

Visible-light–curing composite has been successfully used for beak repair.[12] Sunschein (Henry Schein, Port Washington, NY) is a light-sensitive synthetic that is easily shaped and can be molded like clay. It is easy to work with. The advantages of light-curing composites are that they are easily molded and shaped and can be used to fill large defects or to create beak prostheses, and they have a short curing process. The primary disadvantage of light-curing composites is that they cannot be color-matched with natural beak color[12, 13] and require use of a costly ultraviolet curing light.

Triad II (Dentsply International Inc., York, PA) is a resin sheet visible-light–curing composite[12, 13] with advantages and disadvantages similar to those of Sunshein.

Methyl methacrylate (Hoof Acrylic, Technovit, Jorgensen Laboratories, Loveland, CO) has been used for beak repair and beak prostheses; however, the curing process is exothermic, the material is toxic to tissues, and the product cannot be color-matched.

Jet Repair (Jet Repair Acrylic, Lang Dental Products, Wheeling, IL), a cold-cured methacrylate, does not reach the high temperatures during polymerization that Hoof Acrylic does,[7] but it has the same disadvantages as methacrylate.

Ethylcyanoacrylate (Cyanodent) has a mild exothermic curing process and forms a very hard durable material that is excellent for beak restoration.

Materials such as Hoof Acrylic, Crazy Glue, and other household bonding agents have properties that are unsuitable for beak repair and should not be used (see Table 44B–1).

Working with Acrylics

The technique for mixing Cyano-Veneer for color matching is uncomplicated and requires little artistic skill. The colors included in the repair kit are clear and white powder shades. The stain kit shades are yellow, black, pink, and blue.

The color shades necessary to develop the correct color match should be mixed on a waxed paper surface with the white shade powder using a flat toothpick or a dental plastic filling instrument. Small quantities of the color shade should be mixed with three to five times the amount of the white powder to attain a matching color with the beak to which it is being applied (Fig. 44B–4A). This ratio depends upon the color to be matched. When matching black or gray color, very small amounts of the gray color shade are required. The two powders should be uniformly mixed on a mixing pad. Note that the color of the mixed powder shades is much lighter than the final color of the combined mixed powder and Cyanodent liquid.

Two to three drops of Cyanodent liquid should be placed on the mixing pad adjacent to the mixed powder (Fig. 44B–4B). A small amount of the powder mix is brought over and mixed rapidly with the Cyanodent liquid (Fig. 44B–4C) to attain a thick, smooth, syrupy consistency (Fig. 44B–4D). This mixture must be applied quickly because the Cyano-Veneer hardens rapidly (in 30 to 90 seconds).

Most psittacine and passerine birds require a shade of yellow, gray, or black; however, some species such as toucans that have combinations of black, brown, yellow, red, orange, and blue colors to their beaks require more artistic ability to achieve careful color and pattern matching.

Technique for Cyano-Veneer Repair

Abraded surfaces of the traumatized beak should be cleaned and all loose particles of keratin should be debrided and removed (Fig. 44B–5A). The margins of the defect should be etched by grinding or sanding with a dental or Dremel drill (Emerson Electric Co., Racine, WI) (Fig. 44B–5B). The surface should then be washed and dried thoroughly.

A thin mix of the color-matched acrylic is applied in layers using a flat toothpick or a dental plastic

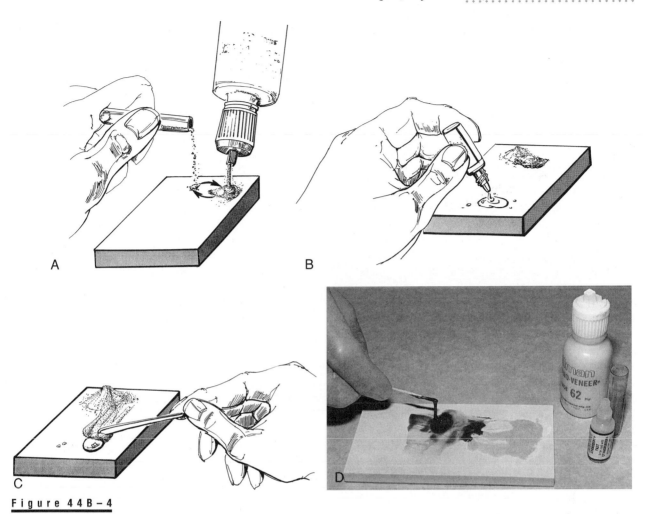

F i g u r e 4 4 B – 4

(A) Mixing the white powder shade with the stain kit shade. Powders should be homogeneously mixed. *(B)* Cyanodent liquid to be mixed with the powder mixture. *(C)* Small quantities of powder are brought to the drops of liquid and quickly and homogeneously mixed. *(D)* The color-mixed powders are combined with the Cyanodent liquid and mixed to the consistency of a thick syrup.

filling instrument to the margins of the defect until the defect is covered (Fig. 44B–5C). The Cyano-Veneer should be applied evenly, with the veneer rising slightly above the surface of the rhampho-theca (Fig. 44B–5C, inset). Complete hardening takes 5 to 7 minutes. The curing time can be increased by using a drop of Cyanodent retarder or decreased by using a drop of Cyano-Veneer Quick-Set.

The bonded acrylic is ground and shaped to the level of the beak surface using a fine grinding stone or sanding disk set at low speed (Fig. 44B–5D). The bonded area is then wiped with a damp cloth and allowed to dry. If desired, a glaze can be produced by applying a thin coat of Cyanodent liquid or Cyano-Veneer Quick-Set.

Ethylcyanoacrylate does not generate heat when curing and can be used anywhere on the beak; however, the resulting fumes are irritating to the sclera. Precautions should be taken to protect the bird's eyes. An ophthalmic ointment protects the eyes sufficiently and should be routinely applied before using the cyanoacrylate.

If the diameter of the defect being filled is in excess of 2.0 cm, it is difficult to impossible to fill this gap as described with this technique. By bonding a precut piece of nylon or stainless steel splint-grid (included in the repair kit) (Fig. 44B–5E), over

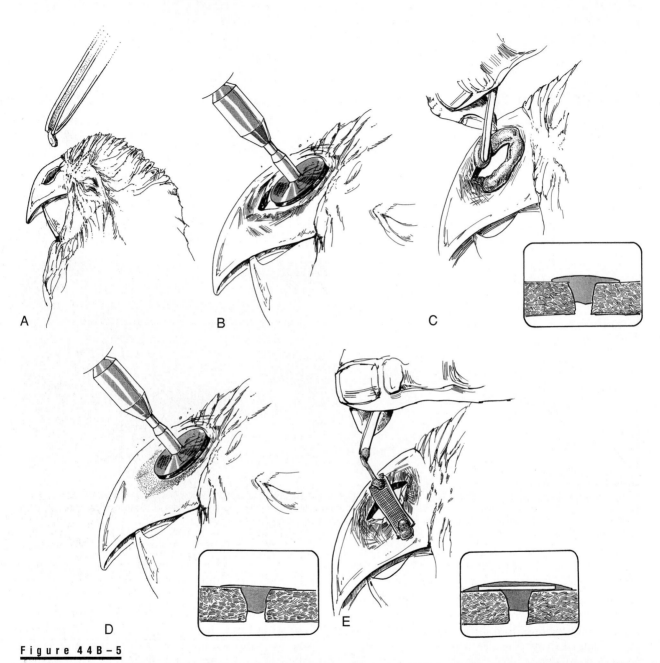

(A) Loose keratin particles are removed from the wound margins and the beak is cleaned. *(B)* The keratin around the margin of the wound is etched in preparation for the bonding material. *(C)* The Cyano-Veneer is applied to the margins of the wound defect until the defect is covered. *(Inset)* Cross-section of a defect showing how the acrylic fills the defect opening and is slightly elevated from the surface of the rhamphotheca. *(D)* The acrylic is ground smooth and even. *(Inset)* The acrylic is ground to the level of the rhamphotheca and blended in. *(E)* Stainless steel or nylon mesh splint grids are used to bridge the gap and build up the acrylic repair. *(Inset)* When ground smooth, the acrylic repair will blend smoothly with the beak surface.

the opening of the defect with Cyanodent, the Cyano-Veneer can then be used to repair the defect. This type of defect is easily filled with light-curing acrylic.

Cracks and Fissures

All penetrating fissures or cracks require acrylic repair to prevent infection of the dermis or nasal sinus.

Beak cracks and fissures occur in birds as a result of trauma. Simple cracks or fissures can be bonded with a small amount of acrylic placed over the defect and sanded smooth. If the crack extends through the rhampthotheca and there is instability on either side of the crack, stabilization by bonding permits the crack to heal without further splitting or breaking off. The strongest repair is achieved by tying stainless steel wire sutures across the crack and incorporating the wire into a color-matched acrylic, bonding the beak and the wire.

Stabilization can also be achieved by bonding nylon or wire mesh across the crack and perpendicular to it.

Punctures

As with penetrating cracks and fissures, punctures require closure with dental acrylics. During the growth of the beak, as the result of keratin sheet migration, the acrylic implant is ejected as the contour of the puncture changes. Ejection can occur as quickly as 2 to 3 weeks from the time of repair.[2]

If bacterial contamination is present, it is essential to treat the wound prior to bonding to avoid sealing in the offending organisms. Petroleum-based ointments interfere with acrylic bonding. Therefore, all topical antifungal agents and antibiotics should be water-soluble.

Fractures

Fractures of the mandible and maxilla require fixation and stabilization to permit the fracture site to heal. Fixation usually affords immediate return to function, enabling the bird to eat and drink. If a beak fracture occurs horizontal to the nasomaxillary

frontal joint, and the fracture is close to this joint, repair is difficult, recovery time is prolonged, and the prognosis is guarded. For stabilization, stainless steel suture wires must be placed through the facial bones to draw the wound edges into apposition. This can interfere with normal function of the kinetic joint.

If the fracture is 3 to 4 mm cranial to the junction of the rhamphotheca and the facial skin, stainless steel wire sutures should be placed across the fracture line to stabilize the fracture. Ideally, at least three sutures should be used. If there is insufficient space to permit the placement of three sutures, two will suffice (Fig. 44B–6A, B). Having only one suture allows excessive torque and motion at the suture hole, and the suture can pull away from the beak.

Placement of sutures across the mandibular or maxillary fracture is accomplished by drilling holes with a 20- or 22-gauge hypodermic needle in small species, and a K-wire in large species.

When using a needle, the needle should be drilled through the fragment from the lateral to the lingual surface. The suture wire is passed into the hub and through the bore of the needle to the lingual side. It is then grasped with a hemostat or needle holder as it emerges through the bore of the needle. The needle is withdrawn, leaving the wire threaded through the hole. A second hole is drilled in the opposite fragment in alignment with the first hole. The end of the suture wire is passed into the bevel of the needle from the lingual to the lateral side and the needle is withdrawn, pulling the wire with it (Fig. 44B–6C). The wire is firmly tied or twisted, reducing the fracture (Fig. 44B–6D).

Three wires should be placed in this manner. The color-matched dental acrylic is then placed across the fracture line, thereby covering the fracture and incorporating the wire sutures into the bonded area (Fig. 44B–6E). It is essential that the surface of the beak be thoroughly clean and dry before application of the acrylic. The bonding area is then ground smooth with a dental or Dremel drill, leaving a strong, aesthetically pleasing restoration.

Perfect stability of the fracture site should be achieved. Patient acceptance is excellent, and most birds eat and drink immediately after the repair.

In large species, the holes are drilled with a K-wire and are usually large enough to permit simple passage of the wire, negating the need to use the

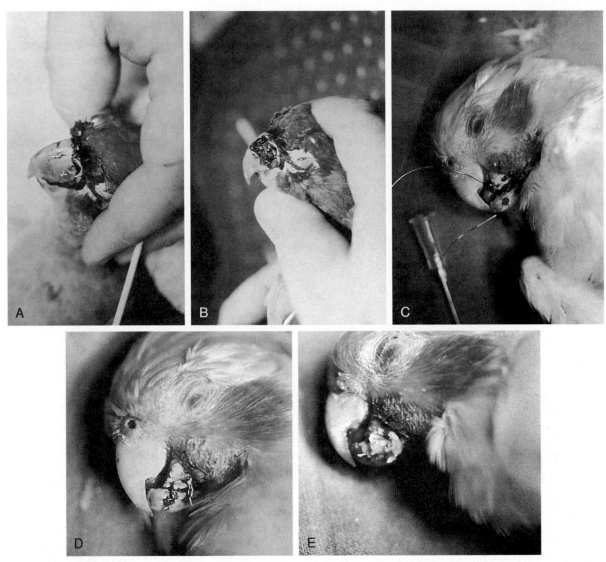

F i g u r e 4 4 B – 6

(A) Two wires have been placed across the fracture of the maxilla. *(B)* Application of acrylic (not color-matched) over the wires and fracture. *(C)* Wire placed through holes drilled with a hypodermic needle across the fracture of the mandible. *(D)* Wires secured to reduce mandibular fracture. *(E)* Acrylic placed over the stainless steel wires and fracture before grinding and finishing.

hypodermic needle as a guide. This technique is applicable to mandibular symphyseal (gonys) fractures as well. In fractures of the mandible and maxilla with severe trauma and damage to the dermis, growth changes occur and fracture segments can grow in diverging directions, creating major beak disfigurement (Fig. 44B–7A, B).

AVULSION AND BEAK PROSTHESIS

Information applicable to beak prosthesis is becoming more widely reported in the veterinary literature.[3, 4, 7, 13–18]

Avulsion of the rostrum can be partial or complete. Loss of the rostrum mandibulare is of greater consequence than loss of the maxilla because the ability to eat and drink is severely to completely compromised. Total loss of the mandible leads to the demise of the bird because replacement is not possible. Some birds have been able to adapt to loss of the maxilla.

Partial avulsion in passerine birds offers greater possibilities for successful prosthetic replacement than in psittacines because of the differences in pressure dynamics. Replacement of a partially avulsed maxilla in psittacines is difficult. In passerines, a partially avulsed maxilla or mandible is amenable to a prosthesis, and success is achieved in a sufficient number of cases to warrant attempts at replacement. In instances in which partial loss of the maxilla has left the bird disfigured but still able to prehend and ingest food, it is better to allow the bird enough time to see if any growth of the rhamphotheca occurs (2–3 months).

In most instances after injury, modification in feeding is necessary because the bird will not be able to hull and eat seeds. Most birds can adapt to soft foods, pelleted foods, or hulled seed. If the bird adapts well to its disability, exhibits no regrowth of the rhamphotheca, and the owner is not concerned with the aesthetics of the defect, a prosthesis should not be considered.

A prosthesis should be considered if function must be restored to allow essential use of the beak (i.e., eating or drinking) when the bird is engaged in display as a zoologic specimen, feeding young, diving, or using the beak tips to prehend and swallow food. Long-term maintenance of function is not realistic in birds in which high stresses are applied to the prosthesis.[7]

Understanding skull biomechanics and the forces and stresses applied during beak function is essential when contemplating the application of a pros-

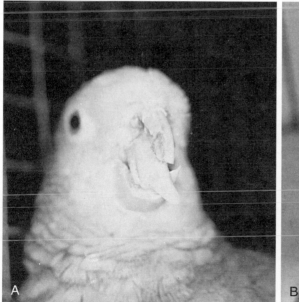
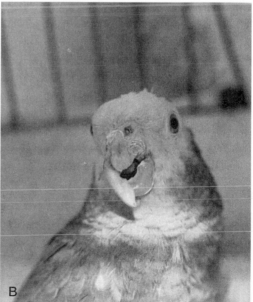

Figure 44B–7

(A and B) Reattached avulsed beak 20 weeks after surgery. Note divergent patterns of growth.

thesis. The prokinetic skull articulates and moves at the junction of the nasal and frontal bones.[19] The extent of the forces exerted during mastication and locomotion determine the failure rate of the prosthesis. When a bird closes its upper and lower beak on an object, three external forces act on the maxilla.[7] The force applied by the pterygoideus muscle is transferred caudally and rostrally to the maxilla by the palatines. The second force results from the material being bitten and is perpendicular to the beak. The final force is an angular force at the nasofrontal hinge.[7] The combination of all three forces must equate to zero for the maxilla to maintain its structural stability.[7] To increase the force on the bitten object, increased pressure must be applied by the pterygoideus muscle or the distance from the object to the base of the beak must be shortened.[20] When a bird bites down on an object, a compressive force is applied to the maxilla. That force is resisted by an opposing force from the pterygoideus and other muscles. The sum of all the forces applied is at the nasofrontal hinge. This hinge acts as a fulcrum when forces are applied. A second fulcrum is exerted at the junction of the beak and the prosthesis.

Surgical Management of Avulsion

Avulsion can result from trauma as well as necrosis from an infection. The type of trauma is important. Crushing injuries create a great deal of trauma to the remaining stump. Shearing injuries such as bite injuries create much less trauma to the beak remnant. Assessment of the degree of trauma to the stump as well as evaluation of the patient's general physical condition help determine when prosthesis application should be contemplated. Oral trauma can result in injury to the dermis with vascular compromise and gross contamination of the remaining portion of the beak.

These factors must be considered before application of a prosthesis. In addition, the bird's general physical condition must be stable. Mycotic and bacterial contamination of the injured area must be completely eliminated. Laboratory testing is the only way to ensure that infection has been eliminated.

The stump should be thoroughly cleansed by flushing with warm saline. All fragmented particles of rhamphotheca and bone should be removed and traumatized tissue gently debrided. During the recovery period, the bird must be supported by parenteral fluids and hyperalimentation. When the tissues of the stump have completely healed, application of a prosthesis can be considered.

If alternate feeding techniques have been successfully implemented during treatment of the stump, and if aesthetics and beak functions other than feeding and drinking are not a concern, a beak prosthesis is not necessary. However, if a prosthesis is indicated, the earlier mentioned stresses and torque factors must be assessed.

Prosthetic Materials

In small species such as budgerigars, cockatiels, and small passerine birds, the prosthesis can be fashioned from a ethylcyanoacrylate or light-curing acrylic resin. For beak replacement in larger birds, the use of Cyano-Veneer as a prosthetic is expensive and difficult because only small amounts can be worked with at a time. A temporary dental bridge acrylic Temp-Plus (Ellman International Corporation, Hewlett, NY) is an isobutylmethacrylic that hardens in approximately 5 minutes, does not shrink, can be carved and shaped, and is inexpensive. Temp-Plus can be colored to any desired color by adding Cyanodent Stain Kit Shades. After mixing and while curing, Temp-Plus heats to about 108 to 110°F and cools quickly as it hardens. During the curing process, this product becomes clay-like in consistency and can be molded into a desired shape before it hardens. After mixing Temp-Plus powder and liquid, a strong acrylic odor permeates the area. Adequate ventilation is desirable. Other methacrylate products are available but are exothermic and cannot be color-matched. Light-cured acrylics are easy to mold and work with, are nonexothermic, and harden quickly. The primary drawback to light-cured materials is that they are excellent for constructing the prosthesis but cannot be color-matched and therefore do not produce an aesthetic repair.

When molding a beak from Temp-Plus, the stump of the beak to which the prosthesis will be attached should be pressed into the molded prosthetic material while the material is soft enough to create an impression. This process ensures a perfect fit of the prosthesis onto the stump of the rostrum. This also creates a lip that extends around the stump and beyond the rostral aspect of the stump.

Concurrently, an impression of the opposing beak should be formed on the occlusal surface to match normal occlusion. This can be done by closing the beak with a little pressure while the material is still of a clay-like consistency. The hardened, molded prosthesis should be carved with a dental or Dremel drill to the proper size and shape and then attached to the stump.

The most difficult part of the procedure is attaching the prosthesis to the stump. The fractured end of the mandible or maxilla must be completely healed before attempting to attach the prosthesis.

Mandible Prosthesis

For prosthesis repair of a partial avulsion of the mandible in small nonpsittacine birds, it is necessary to drill holes into the exposed edges of the right and left mandibular bone and pass a stainless steel wire antegrade into each drilled hole. The bone is used as an anchor base for the wire, which acts as a strong matrix upon which the acrylic can be built (Fig. 44B–8A–C). Cyano-Veneer is applied to the wire matrix and built up to the size and shape desired. Carving and sanding are done to shape the acrylic to form a perfect fitting prosthesis.

In large species such as storks,[15] it is better to thread Steinmann pins bilaterally into the ventral mandibular bodies and dorsally along the occlusal border. These four pins offer a strong, rigid foundation for the acrylic, resist rotational forces, and eliminate stresses on all fulcrum points at the prosthesis-beak junction (Fig. 44B–9A, B).

Maxilla Prosthesis

To replace an avulsed maxilla, the prosthesis can be attached in one of three ways. If there is beak deformity and the deformed part can be incorporated into the prosthesis (Fig. 44B–10A–C), the prosthesis can be bonded to the existing beak to achieve an aesthetically acceptable, normally functioning replacement. This technique is not suitable for psittacine birds because there is excessive pressure and torque on the prosthesis.

If possible, it is best to secure a prosthesis without using pins, wires, or screws. Metal implants have the potential of loosening, creating pressure areas that result in necrosis and form a matrix for infection.

The second method is the placement of stainless steel pins, K-wires, hypodermic needles, and/or screws into the maxillary bone or palatine process, depending on the species. The implants are used as a matrix upon which the prosthesis is built. This

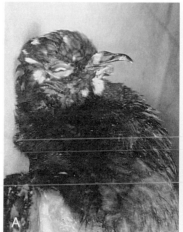
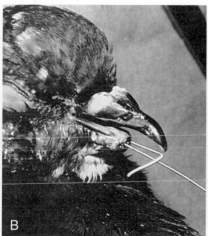
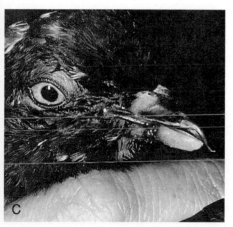

Figure 44B–8

(A) Repair of an avulsion of the anterior half of a pigeon mandible. *(B)* Stainless steel wires are implanted into holes drilled into the mandible. The wires are bent to form a matrix for a mandibular prosthesis. *(C)* Completed mandibular prosthesis without color-matching.

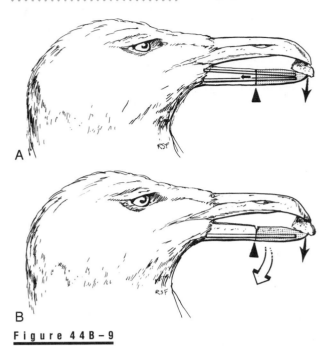

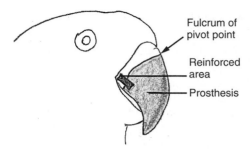

Figure 44B–11

Prosthetic maxilla showing pivot point and area to be reinforced.

Figure 44B–9

(A) Two-pin insertion. The insertion of two pins into the ventral mandibular body resists rotation forces, as well as eliminating stressors on the fulcrum of the prosthesis. The triangle represents the fulcrum and the arrows, the stressors. *(B)* One-pin insertion demonstrates instability at the point opposite the fulcrum.

The third technique requires a perfect fit of the stump onto the opposing end of the prosthesis, allowing at least 1 cm of overlap of the prosthesis on the stump. The artificial beak is then attached by bonding strips of nylon mesh splint-grids to the prosthesis and the beak stump with Cyano-Veneer. It is necessary to evaluate the pressure forces on the prosthesis and reinforce the surface opposite the pivot point (Fig. 44B–11). This technique must be used if wires cannot be implanted into the bone. For birds such as toucans with a long, hollow, light maxilla, an orthopedic fiberglass bandage such as Delta-Lite "S" (Johnson & Johnson Orthopaedics Inc., Raynham, MA) can be used to form the avulsed portion of the maxilla. It is often necessary to make impression molds using dental alginate impression material to form and shape the prosthesis (Fig. 44B–12A, B).

method is the least acceptable because considerable wear can occur at the pin placement site, creating the potential for infection and irritation of the soft tissues.

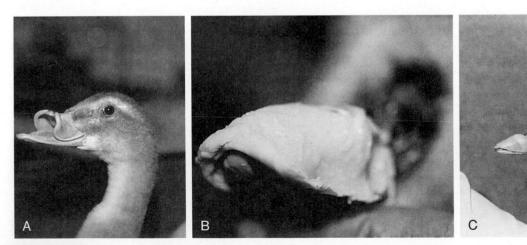

Figure 44B–10

Prosthetic repair of a congenital deformity of the upper beak of a duck. *(A)* Deformed upper beak of a juvenile mallard duck. *(B)* Adding the molded Temp-Plus to the maxilla to form the prosthesis. *(C)* Completed prosthesis after shaping and grinding.

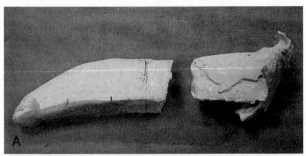

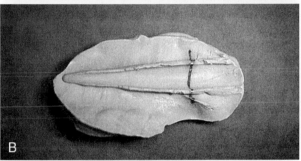

Figure 44B–12

(A) Delta-Lite hollow prosthesis *(left)*. An Algenate impression of the maxillary stump *(right)*. *(B)* Algenate impression of the mandible.

If the maxilla is partially avulsed and attachment of any vascular structure remains, attempts should be made to reattach the beak with the hopes that enough collateral circulation and healing will take place to restore beak function. Wires and dental acrylics are used to reattach the partially avulsed maxilla.

Because every injury is different, the method of repair must be left to the skill and ingenuity of the surgeon. It is important to consider the vector forces on the maxilla and to minimize their effect as much as the injury will allow. The owner should be advised that the resulting repair may not be successful, depending on the vascular disruption and destruction of dermis. In a high percentage of cases, particularly those beaks that are partially avulsed and have linear fractures, the repaired beak will be functional but with a great deal of distortion and disfigurement.

In the event of total avulsion and complete loss of vascular supply, attempts at replacement of the natural beak will be futile because the avulsed portion will undergo necrosis.

Repair of simple cracks, fissures, and punctures using dental acrylics is simple, functional, and aesthetic. Usually, repair can be accomplished without anesthesia in minor injuries, and in the majority of cases the prognosis is excellent. Injuries that result in large defects, particularly amputations and avulsions, always have a guarded prognosis. The technique of repair of these defects is much more complicated and requires a higher level of skill on the part of the surgeon.

References

1. Altman RB: Acrylic beak repair. Proc 1st Conf Eur Committee Assoc Avian Vet, Vienna, Austria, 1991, pp 399–401.
2. Clipsham R: Rhamphorthotics and surgical corrections of maxillofacial defects. Semin Avian Exotic Pet Med 3(2):92–99, 1994.
3. Clipsham R: Surgical beak restoration and correction. Proc Assoc Avian Vet, Seattle, WA, 1989, pp 164–176.
4. Lawton MPC: An approach to surgical repair of beaks. Proc 1993 Eur Conf Avian Med Surg, Utrecht, The Netherlands, 1993, pp 86–90.
5. Lucas AM, Stettenheim PR: Avian Anatomy, Integument, Part II. Agriculture Handbook 362, Washington DC, US Govt Printing Office, pp 579–580.
6. Thomas AL (ed): A New Dictionary of Birds. London, Nelson, 1964.
7. Greenwell M, Robertson JJ, Constantinescu GM: Avian Beak Prosthesis. Compendium, Exotic Animal Medicine, vol. 2, 1991, pp 50–55.
8. Evans H: Anatomy of the budgerigar. In Petrak (ed): Diseases of Cage and Aviary Birds. Philadelphia, Lea & Febiger, 1982, pp 119–130.
9. Lucas AM, Stettenheim PR: Avian Anatomy, Integument, Part II, Agriculture Handbook 362, Washington DC, US Govt Printing Office, 1972, p 585.
10. Mitrosky MJ Jr: Cyanoacrylate used as a Bonding Agent Beneath Amalgam and Composite Restorations. Quintessence International, vol. 9. Chicago, IL, Quintessence Pub, 1981, pp 871–874.
11. Feinberg E, The acrylic veneer crown. Dent Clin North Am 19(2):291–298, 1976.
12. Clipsham R: Surgical correction of beaks. Proc Assoc Avian Vet, Phoenix, AZ, 1990, pp 325–333.
13. Rupiper DJ: Application of visible light-curing composite splints to fractured avian legs. J Assoc Avian Vet 7(3):147–149, 1993.
14. Frye FL: Prostheses enhance quality of life. Vet Med 79(7):931–935, 1984.
15. Morris PJ, Weigel JP: Methacrylate beak prosthesis in a marabou stork. J Assoc Avian Vet 4(2):103–106, 1990.
16. Sleamaker TF: Prosthetic beak for a salmon crested cockatoo. J Am Vet Med Assoc 183(11):1300–1301, 1983.
17. Vollmar VA: Benhandlung eines Unterschnabelabrisses bei einem Graupapagei durch Angringen einer Kunstharprosthese. Kleintier Praxis 30:165–168, 1965.
18. Wolf L: Prosthetic bill technique for a Canada goose. Proc Assoc Avian Vet, 1985, pp 177–180.
19. Bock WJ: Kinetics of the avian skull. J Morphol 114:1–42, 1964.
20. Bock WJ: An approach to the functional analysis of bill shape. Auk 83:10–51, 1966.

Manfred Hochleithner

45

Endoscopy

Endoscopy enables the veterinarian to examine the internal organs of birds for diagnostic purposes using a minor surgical procedure. New optical systems with advanced viewing capability, manufactured as human arthroscopes, cystoscopes, and laparoscopes, adapt well for use in avian patients. The use of modern, safe anesthetics makes endoscopy possible not only for sex determination in healthy birds but also as a valuable diagnostic aid in sick birds. Internal organs and tissues as well as the choana, oral cavity, upper gastrointestinal tract, and trachea can be directly observed and pathologic changes can be diagnosed. Today, clinical endoscopy is a very useful diagnostic procedure that enhances clinical examination.

HISTORY

Endoscopes have been used in avian medicine since 1970. Initially, endoscopy was used to sex monomorphic birds. Many sexing techniques were inaccurate, leading to improperly paired birds with resultant economic loss and frustration to the breeder. Internal examination of the abdomen provided a reliable method of sex differentiation and has the added advantage of allowing examination of other organs and tissues for diagnostic purposes.[1-9]

TECHNIQUE AND PROCEDURE

Before Starting the Procedure

Diagnostic endoscopy of birds is not without risk. The patient may have an underlying medical problem that could be potentiated by anesthesia and endoscopy. To be most effective, endoscopy should be used in association with other diagnostic procedures such as clinical examination, radiology techniques, and/or blood chemistry. Before starting the procedure certain questions have to be answered: Can a potential problem be localized using another diagnostic technique? Will the endoscopic procedure enhance pathophysiologic knowledge? Does the general condition of the bird preclude the anesthetic risk, or should the patient receive supportive care before the procedure? Will the patient's suspected problem cause procedural difficulties during the examination? For example, ascites increases tremendously the potential risk of the procedure.

If a bird undergoes anesthesia for any other diagnostic procedure (e.g., radiology), endoscopic examination of the upper respiratory or gastrointestinal tract can be included as a useful diagnostic procedure with minimal additional manipulation. Endoscopic examination is particularly useful in birds displaying clinical signs of inappetence, vomiting, or respiratory difficulty.

Complications

Probably the most dangerous moment during laparoscopy is when the abdominal wall is pierced with the forceps. Internal organs can easily be damaged, especially if they are enlarged (e.g., in proventriculus-proventriculus dilatation syndrome). Proper control of the instruments is very important, and increased stability can be achieved by placing the elbows on the operating table. The effects of damage or rupture of an organ can be serious. Puncture of the gastrointestinal tract requires surgical correction. If considerable hemorrhage occurs during endoscopy, the unaesthetized bird should be positioned with its head up at a 45° angle. In this position, the blood will remain in the caudal portion of the air sac and will not enter the lungs. Occasionally postoperative subcutaneous emphysema develops. The subcutaneous air can be aspirated and the bird's movements restricted by cage rest until the incision is healed.

Anesthesia

Isoflurane is the anesthetic of choice.

Prelaparoscopic Fasting

Food should be withheld for 3 hours before endoscopy to prevent regurgitation and distention of the proventriculus. In small birds (those weighing <100g) and birds of prey, fasting for 24 hours simplifies visualization of the abdominal organs because the gastrointestinal tract is empty.

Equipment

The basic equipment for avian endoscopy is a light source, a fiberoptic cable, and a small-diameter endoscope. Significant advantages have been seen since the development of the Hopkins rod lens optical system, which was designed using special glass rods instead of small lenses placed in certain intervals. Although these endoscopes have a smaller diameter than their predecessors, the image is much brighter and the viewing angle is larger; therefore, a much larger portion of the object can be seen in a single viewing field. This decreases the time required for examination and manipulation.

Light Source, Fiberoptic Cable

The light source supplies illumination and generates a significant amount of heat. The fiberoptic cable therefore separates the patient and operator from the source of heat, while transmitting light and maintaining maneuverability. The cable is composed of many special glass fibers that transmit light via internal reflection. It is flexible, allowing the veterinarian relative freedom of movement.

Endoscope

Various diameters and viewing angles of telescopes are used by veterinarians. The telescope should have a diameter useful for most species seen in avian practice and a suitable viewing angle employed during laparoscopy and upper gastrointestinal and respiratory tract examination.

The diameter that seems most useful is 2.7 mm. This size of telescope can be used in birds as small as 25 g (*Phyrrhura* species) and still allow photographs with an external flash. It can also be used to examine the trachea, choana, esophagus, and crop, whereas a larger diameter can make the examination of the trachea impossible. A larger diameter endoscope (4 mm) is required for video documentation and high-quality photographs.

Two viewing angles are used in avian practice. The 0° straightforward telescope, with a larger viewing angle, provides good orientation of the area visualized. The 0° telescopes allow a more natural approach that permits the veterinarian to use the normal perspective as the eye would visualize the field looking straight ahead. In avian practice, this scope is preferred for the trachea, crop, and choana. With the 30° forward oblique telescope, a larger area can be observed by rotating the telescope. By the use of this scope, the veterinarian can slide over internal organs and inspect their upper surface.

For general use, a length of 170–180 mm and a 30° forward oblique telescope with a 2.7-mm diameter is recommended for avian practice (see Color Fig. 45–1).

Cleaning and Sterilization of the Endoscope

Endoscopic examinations should always be performed using sterile instruments because diseases can easily be transmitted by the endoscope. This is especially true during routine sexing, when many birds are handled within a short time frame.

To prevent blood and other contaminants from drying on the endoscope, it should be placed in a container filled with a cleaning/disinfectant solution immediately after use. Most instruments should not be cleaned in an ultrasonic bath. Before sterilization, the endoscope must be carefully cleaned, and any organic material (blood) must be removed. Only a clean surface can be reached by the sterilization medium. Gas sterilization or chemical disinfection can be used. Disinfectant solutions that are specifically made for endoscopes such as Alhydex, Gigasept, Kohrsolex, i.D., or Sekusept should be used. Soaking for too long can result in corrosion; therefore the manufacturers' instructions and recommendations have to be carefully followed.

Checking the Endoscope

Before starting any procedure, the fiberoptic light carriers should be examined. The end of the fiber surface has to be held against the light source and checked on the opposite end. Black spots or dark surfaces indicate broken optical fibers.

Anatomic Positioning and Technique

Laparoscopy

The unique anatomy of the avian air sac system is the primary reason that laparoscopy is such an important diagnostic procedure in the avian patient. The peritoneal cavities in *Gallus domesticus* have been well described in anatomic literature for many years,[10, 11] but their clinical significance during endoscopic examinations is seldom discussed.[12]

The intestinal peritoneal cavity is the most important and largest of the peritoneal cavities. The gonads are suspended within the intestinal peritoneal cavity. During laparoscopy, the gonads are clearly visible, although they are covered by a thin, transparent, and conforming layer composed of air sac and peritoneum. On close examination, small blood vessels within the air sac wall cover the gonads with peritoneal effusion. In some disease processes (e.g., ascites), the intestinal peritoneal cavity can become distended with fluid, and puncture during endoscopic examination can lead to death as the result of inhalation of fluid.

During a routine endoscopic examination two air sacs are visualized. After puncturing through the abdominal wall, the tip of the endoscope is within the caudal thoracic air sac. Examination of the lung is possible craniodorsally. Occasionally, the air sac

wall between the caudal thoracic air sac and the abdominal air sac is transparent enough to visualize the gonad, and during routine sexing the air sac wall does not have to be punctured.

To visualize the kidney, adrenal gland, spleen, intestine, and gonad, the endoscope enters into the abdominal air sac through the described air sac wall. The tip of the endoscope is positioned close to the air sac wall in a location devoid of blood vessels, and by gentle pressure the air sac membrane is punctured.

Positioning the Bird

The side in which the endoscope is inserted depends on the area and organs to be examined or biopsied. Because sexing is a primary reason for endoscopic examination, the same approach is usually used for diagnostic laparoscopy as well. The bird is placed on its right side and the wings are reflected dorsally. The wing can be restrained using strips of adhesive tape. Because the bird may need to be moved during the examination, restraining the bird manually gives greater flexibility. Standardization of positioning is important to obtain reproducible results in individual patients.

The bird's left leg is pulled caudally. The muscle mass of the femur (m. iliotibialis) is reflected caudally and the endoscope enters between the last two ribs or just behind the last rib, approximately 5 to 10 mm ventral to the acetabulum.[1–7]

If the leg is drawn forward, the posterior point of the sternum is followed dorsolaterally until a notch is felt. This notch lies between the sternum and the last rib. A skin incision has to be made just caudal to the muscle where the semitendinosus muscle (m. flexor lateralis) passes over the rib. The shape of the notch and its relative position vary greatly with the species of bird.[5–7]

The preferred approach for examination and biopsy of the liver is through the ventral midline, immediately posterior to the sternum.[4, 5, 9, 13]

A direct approach to the intestinal peritoneal cavity has been described.[5] Blunt entry is made just caudal to the pubis and ventral to the ischium. The endoscope enters the caudal portion of the intestinal peritoneal cavity but can be directed cranially to view the kidney and gonads. The advantage of this method is that the air sac wall is not penetrated. The caudal portion of the kidney can be biopsied from there.

As few feathers as possible are plucked in all positions, exposing an area approximately 1 cm in diameter. Special care must be taken if continuous bleeding from the feather follicles is observed. Excessive bleeding when plucking the feathers may indicate potential coagulopathy, which is a contraindication for performing endoscopy. The skin is swabbed with disinfectant and the surrounding feathers are moistened with a water-soluble sterile gel to avoid contamination of the operating field by encroaching feathers.

A small incision is made in the skin using a scalpel. The muscle layer is bluntly dissected by means of a small mosquito forceps. A distinct "pop" indicates penetration into the air sac. The forceps is opened slightly to enlarge the hole, and the endoscope is inserted under visual control. Visualization should begin as soon as the scope is introduced into the incision. Superficial skin bleeding must be controlled before the endoscope is inserted. A drop of blood can obscure the field of view directly or, when exposed to airflow from the air sacs, can produce a foam that may render the examination impossible. Vision may also be impaired by fat or membranes that adhere to the top of the endoscope. The front element of the endoscope can be cleaned by touching it gently to the intestine. When the endoscope is removed, the various layers through which the stab incision has been made slide over each other and close the wound. If sterile technique has been observed, routine antibiotic therapy is unnecessary. If bleeding occurs from the wound at the end of the operation, slight digital pressure for 1 minute or a single suture can be used for hemostasis.

Biopsies

The diagnostic potential of endoscopy is greatly enhanced by the histologic examination of tissue samples achieved by biopsy. Several biopsy techniques with particular emphasis on the liver have been described.[3, 13, 14, 15] A rigid biopsy forceps can be introduced alongside the endoscope through a single puncture. The forceps has to be brought carefully into position along the shaft of the endoscope. It is advantageous to use a larger diameter

trocar sleeve, which facilitates the introduction of a telescope and a biopsy instrument through the single puncture (e.g., 14.5 French sheath with 5 French instrument channel—67065 C, Karl Storz GmbH, Tuttlingen, Germany).[5, 15] Usually hemostasis during tissue biopsy is not a significant problem.[5, 15]

Choana, Trachea

Endoscopy of the upper respiratory and gastrointestinal tract is a useful, fast, and safe procedure. The inner beak, choana, tongue, and larynx can be easily examined using an endoscope. For endoscopy of the upper respiratory tract, the bird is placed in sternal recumbency with its neck fully extended. In smaller birds or those with severe respiratory disorders, it is much safer to insert an abdominal air sac tube to allow respiration during tracheal endoscopy. Depending on the size of the bird and the length of the endoscope, the tracheal bifurcation may be examined.

Esophagus, Crop

For endoscopy of the esophagus and crop, the neck is fully extended, so that the esophagus is as straight as possible. Usually, the field of view is much clearer as the endoscope is withdrawn from the crop because mucus and ingesta can cover the tip of the endoscope on entry. All manipulations are done very gently. Visualization of the crop and esophagus can be enhanced by insufflation of the crop using a soft rubber feeding tube.

Proventriculus

Examination of the proventriculus is possible using a rigid endoscope entering the gastrointestinal tract from a midline ingluviotomy. A small incision is made in the skin and crop, and the endoscope is gently introduced through the opening and passed into the distal esophagus and proventriculus (see Color Fig. 45–2). Foreign bodies can be removed by passing a grasping or biopsy forceps alongside the endoscope or using a 14.5 French sheath with 5 French instrument channel.

DESCRIPTION OF ORGANS AND COMMONPLACE LESIONS

Lungs

Upon entering the abdominal air sac, the pink lung can be seen cranially with its ostium into the abdominal air sac. Granulomas often can be seen around this ostium and are common. This is predominantly because of infections with aspergillosis. Pigment spots due to anthracosis may be seen but are usually not associated with clinical signs. Inflammation of the lung normally can be recognized by color change from pink to red (see Color Figs. 45–3 to 45–5).

Air Sacs

Normal air sacs are clear with a few visible small surface vessels. Varying degrees of opaqueness can be seen in clinically normal birds. Fat infiltration and air sacculitis resulting from different etiologic agents are commonly found during endoscopy. Granulomas resulting from infectious agents such as *Aspergillus, Mycobacterium,* or *Salmonella* species can be seen in birds with respiratory disorders (see Color Figs. 45–6 to 45–9).

Proventriculus

The proventriculus is a smooth, elongated white organ at the midventral aspect of the abdominal air sac. The size of the proventriculus can easily be assessed during the examination. With experience, the normal size and appearance of the proventriculus as seen through the endoscope enables the clinician to diagnose enlargements such as those seen with neuropathic gastric dilation (see Color Fig. 45–10).

Kidney

The kidney is a multiple, lobulated red organ. Discoloration due to anemia or urate stasis is sometimes found during routine sexing in birds showing no clinical signs. This is common in recently imported African grey parrots. Tumors are more common in budgerigars than in larger psittacines, and therefore are seldom diagnosed by endoscopy (see Color Figs. 45–11, 45–12).

Adrenal Gland

The adrenal gland is variable in shape and color and can be confused with a gonad. In mature psittacines, the view of the adrenal gland may be obscured by the gonad, especially in females.

Gonads

The gonads are located at the anterior pole of the kidneys. The testicle is usually elliptic in shape, and blood vessels traverse its smooth surface. It can be partly or totally pigmented, depending on the species. Its size varies, depending on age, species, and stage of the reproductive cycle (can increase up to 500 times).[16] Avian testes are paired.

The ovary of a mature hen has grapelike clusters of prominent follicles. Pigmentation is present in different species. Differentiation of an immature ovary from a testicle can sometimes be difficult because large follicles are absent in immature females. This difficulty can be resolved by locating the supporting ligament of the infundibulum of the oviduct as it crosses the cranial division of the kidney. This ligament is found only in females (see Color Fig. 45–11).[17]

Evaluation of nonproductive breeding birds may reveal gonadal abnormalities.

Spleen

The spleen is usually rounded, purple to brownish-red in color, and often speckled in psittacines (see Color Fig. 45–13). In pigeons and finches, the organ is more elongated. Enlargement is the predominant pathologic finding. Enlargement can be seen with various infectious diseases, especially psittacosis.

Liver

Changes in size and color of the liver can be observed during endoscopic examination. Liver biopsies are recommended in suspected cases of liver abnormalities to confirm a specific diagnosis (see Color Figs. 45–14, 45–15).[5]

Choana

The choana is visible as a V-shaped cleft in the roof of the mouth. Papillae can be seen lining the border of the cavity. Entering the choanal slit, the nasal septum and the dorsal part of the choana can be observed.

Oral Cavity, Tongue, Esophagus, Crop

The large muscular tongue with attendant salivary glands can be examined. Inspissation of keratinized debris due to squamous metaplasia can be seen in psittacines suffering from hypovitaminosis A. Pigeons, birds of prey, and sometimes psittacines have caseous yellow membranes resulting from trichomoniasis. *Aspergillus* granulomas are white in color and cannot be displaced with the scope, as is possible with trichomoniasis lesions. In hand-fed baby birds suffering from crop stasis, foreign bodies or plaques associated with candidiasis can be found.

Trachea

The ability to examine the trachea depends on the size of the bird and the diameter and length of the endoscope. The trachea may be examined for parasites (gapeworms, air sac mites), foreign bodies, and bacterial or fungal plaques. In cases of severe aspergillosis, the trachea can be partially or completely obstructed by a granuloma. Tracheitis can be recognized by the red discoloration of the tracheal epithelial linings (see Color Figs. 45–16, 45–17).

Cloaca

Endoscopic examination of the cloaca may be useful in birds with egg binding, cloacal bleeding, or tissue protrusion. Insufflation using a soft rubber feeding tube may be used with digital pressure applied around the scope barrel to retain air for enhanced viewing. After the cloaca is entered, the rectum, vaginal prominence, and sometimes a retained egg or papillomas can be seen.[3]

References

1. Bailey RE: Surgery for sexing and observing gonad condition in birds. Auk 70:497–500, 1952.
2. Gylstorff I, Grimm F: Vogelkrankheiten. Stuttgart, Verlag Schattauer, 1987, pp 509–510.
3. Harrison GJ: Anesthesiology. In Harrison GJ, Harrison L: Avian Medicine and Surgery. Philadelphia, WB Saunders, 1986, pp 549–559.
4. Lumeij JT, Westerhof I: Clinical endoscopy in birds. Proc 2nd Eur Sympos Avian Med Surg, Utrecht, 1989, pp 154–163.
5. Lumeij JT: Endoscopy. In Lumeij JT: A Contribution to Clinical Investigative Methods for Birds with Special References to the Racing Pigeon (*Columbia livia domestica*). Utrecht, Poefschrift, 1987, pp 151–166.
6. Taylor M: Endoscopy. Proc Assoc Avian Vet, Houston, 1990, pp 319–324.
7. Hochleithner M: Endoscopy. Proc 1993 Eur Conf Avian Med Surg 1993, pp 162–166.
8. Eaton TM: Surgical sexing and diagnostic laparoscopy. In Price CJ: Manual of Parrots, Budgerigars and Other Psittacine Birds. West Sussex, UK, British Small Animal Veterinary Association, 1989.
9. McDonald SE: Endoscopic examination. In Burr EW: Companion Bird Medicine. Ames, Iowa State University Press, 1987, pp 166–174.
10. Goodchild WM: Differentiation of the body cavities and air sacs of *Gallus domesticus* post mortem and their location in vivo. Br Poult Sci 11:209–215, 1970.
11. McLelland J, King AS: The gross anatomy of the peritoneal coelomic cavities of *Gallus domesticus*. Anatomischer Anzeiger 127:480–490, 1970.
12. Taylor M: Ventral hepatic and intestinal peritoneal cavities: An endoscopic perspective. Proc 1993 Eur Conf Avian Med Surg, 1993, pp 132–136.
13. Kolias GV: Liver biopsy techniques in avian clinical practice. Vet Clin North Am 14(2):287–298, 1984.
14. Satterfield W: Early diagnosis of avian tuberculosis by laparoscopy and liver biopsy. In Cooper, JE, Greenwood AG: Recent advance in the study of raptor diseases. Proceedings of the London International Symposium on Diseases of Birds of Prey. Keighly, Chiron Publications, 1981.
15. Taylor M: Diagnostic application of a new endoscopic system for birds. Proc 1993 Eur Conf Avian Med Surg, 1993, pp 127–131.
16. King AS, McClelland J: Birds: Their Structure and Function. London, Baillière Tindall, 1984.
17. Taylor M: A morphologic approach to the endoscopic determination of sex in juvenile macaws. J Assoc Avian Vet 3(4):199–201, 1989.

Darryl J. Heard

46

Anesthesia and Analgesia

The ability to safely restrain and anesthetize a wide range of bird species is essential for the avian veterinarian. Furthermore, the level of skill required increases as more complex and lengthier procedures are performed in critical patients. In some instances anesthesia is the major limiting factor for a procedure. Successful avian anesthesia requires understanding of anatomy and physiology, knowledge of available anesthetic regimens, preparation, perioperative stabilization and support, appropriate equipment, attentive monitoring, and practice.

PREANESTHETIC PREPARATION

History and Physical Examination

Although a comprehensive history and physical examination ideally are obtained before anesthesia is induced, chemical restraint is necessary for a complete examination of some birds. Additionally, in some debilitated patients anesthesia is used to avoid stress and struggling associated with physical restraint. Preoperative assessment is primarily directed at evaluating cardiopulmonary function and reserve. The patient is observed in a quiet environment for evidence of tachypnea, abnormal breathing patterns (e.g., open-mouth breathing), and tail bobbing. Exercise tolerance is assessed by how fast respiration returns to normal after brief restraint. The nares are examined for obstruction that may interfere with mask induction. The heart is auscultated for abnormal rate and rhythm, and murmurs. Hydration is evaluated by examining the mouth for dryness and the peripheral veins for turgidity, and

by rolling the skin between fingers to assess turgor. The crop and ventriculus are palpated to detect distention.

Diagnostics

A minimal clinicopathologic data base includes packed cell volume (PCV), total protein, and blood glucose. Further diagnostic tests (e.g., hematologic and clinical chemistry panels and radiographs) are performed as indicated by the condition of the bird. Many common infectious and toxic diseases impair hepatic and renal function, the primary excretion routes for parenteral anesthetics.

Fasting

Fasting decreases regurgitation and passive reflux and proventricular and ventricular distention that interferes with normal respiratory airflow. A distended proventriculus also increases the chances for perforation during laparoscopy. Fasting duration is related to size and clinical status; large birds (>500 g) are fasted 12 hours or longer, whereas for smaller birds the period is proportionately less (budgerigars and canaries 6–12 hours). One author recommends overnight fasting for all birds, regardless of size.[18] The author has observed sunflower kernels in the proventriculus of some parrots after 24 hours of fasting. Patients with paralytic ileus and gastrointestinal obstructions are fasted, and fluids, electrolytes, and glucose are administered either intravenously (IV) or intraosseously (IO). Fluid-distended crops are emptied by gavage. Grit, toys, and paper and wood chips are removed from the cage

during the perianesthetic period to prevent ingestion. Water is offered up to 2 to 3 hours before
induction. Vultures actively regurgitate when restrained and may have passive reflux of large volumes of fluid under anesthesia. Perianesthetic regurgitation has also been observed by the author in
other raptors, and in sea birds, crows, and mynah
birds. Deep inhalant anesthesia promotes passive
gastrointestinal reflux by decreasing smooth muscle tone.

Stabilization

Ideally the condition of all patients is physiologically stable before anesthesia. If not, stabilization is
an immediate postinduction priority. Severe anemia
and fluid and metabolic disorders are corrected.
Intravenous access is established in critically ill patients and in those anticipated to have extensive
hemorrhage. Patients with cardiopulmonary compromise are preoxygenated either in an oxygen
cage or by mask, avoiding struggling that increases
oxygen consumption and cardiac work.

PREMEDICATION

Premedication is not commonly used because it
prolongs recovery, and its effects are often variable.
The phenothiazine tranquilizers (e.g., acepromazine, chlorpromazine) are long-acting, and ineffective and produce peripheral vasodilation and hypotension.[15, 24] The α_2-adrenoceptor agonist xylazine
([Rompun], Haver/Diamond Scientific, Shawnee,
KS) (5–100 mg/kg) alone produces excitement and
occasionally convulsions, prolonged induction and
recovery, inadequate surgical analgesia, and hypoventilation resulting in respiratory acidemia.[31, 52]

Benzodiazepines

Benzodiazepines (e.g., diazepam, midazolam, zolazepam) produce dose-dependent sedative-hypnosis
and muscle relaxation.[7, 20] They are used for anxio-
lysis in wild-caught or aviary birds, and to facilitate
handling during general anesthesia induction and
for minor nonpainful procedures. Benzodiazepines
are combined with the dissociative anesthetics keta-

mine and tiletamine to improve muscle relaxation
and duration. They also have anticonvulsant properties and produce amnesia, but they are not analgesics.[20] Disadvantages of benzodiazepines include
unpredictable effect, dysphoria, struggling, and incoordination and ataxia.

Diazepam (Lemmon Co., Sellersville, PA) is dissolved in propylene glycol, which can produce hypotension and cardiac collapse when given rapidly
IV in dehydrated and hypovolemic patients.[5] In
chickens, diazepam (2.5 mg/kg IV) produced mild
sedation, hypotension, bradycardia, bradypnea, and
hypothermia.[7] Midazolam (Hoffman-LaRoche, Nutley, NJ) is water-soluble, short-acting (15–30 minutes), and slightly more potent than diazepam.[20] In
Canada geese, midazolam (2 mg/kg IM) induced
moderate sedation adequate for radiographic positioning in 15 minutes and lasting 20 minutes or
less.[61] The only cardiopulmonary effect observed
was a moderate tachypnea.[61] Zolazepam, (Zolazepam-Tiletamine [Telazol], Fort Dodge Laboratories, Fort Dodge, IA) a potent long-acting benzodiazepine, is combined with tiletamine in the
commercial preparation Telazol.

Parasympatholytics

Parasympatholytics (e.g., atropine and glycopyrrolate) inhibit respiratory and salivary secretion, gastrointestinal motility (including that of the crop),
and bradyarrhythmias.[40, 58] Their routine use is not
indicated in birds. Glycopyrrolate ([Robinul-V] Fort
Dodge Laboratories) (0.01–0.03 mg/kg) is more potent, has a longer effect, and is a more selective
antisecretory agent than atropine.[5, 41] Conversely,
atropine (0.04–0.1 mg/kg) (Fort Dodge Laboratories), with its faster onset, is indicated in cardiac
emergencies associated with bradyarrhythmias.[5, 41]

LOCAL ANESTHESIA

Local anesthesia is not often used because of potential adverse drug effects and the stress associated
with physical restraint. It is most useful in tame or
sedated large birds (e.g., pigeons, poultry, ratites,
waterfowl). Small-volume syringes (tuberculin or
insulin) with either 25- or 27-gauge needles are
essential for administration, and the lowest concen-

tration available is used. Care is taken to avoid vessels or highly vascular areas. Volumes are calculated to avoid overdosage, and epinephrine solutions are not used. Adverse effects are usually the result of overdosage; for example, if 0.2 ml 2% lidocaine is used in a 200-g bird, the dose is 20 mg/kg, which is greater than the toxic dose of 4 to 10 mg/kg reported in mammals.[5] The lethal dose$_{50}$ (LD$_{50}$) of procaine in budgerigars is reported to be as low as 200 mg/kg.[27] Clinical signs of lidocaine toxicity are dose-dependent, ranging from initial excitement and seizures to depression, respiratory arrest, and cardiovascular collapse.[58] Seizures are controlled with diazepam (0.1–1 mg/kg IV), whereas ventilatory and cardiovascular collapse are treated with intubation, ventilation, and fluids (10–20 ml/kg IV), respectively. Longer-acting local anesthetic agents (e.g., bupivacaine) are more potent than lidocaine and affect the cardiovascular system at lower doses.[58]

PARENTERAL ANESTHESIA

Parenteral anesthesia is reserved by the author for short procedures to avoid prolonged recovery and mortality. An accurate weight of the bird and appropriate-sized syringe are essential for small volume injection. Furthermore, a means of ventilation and a source of oxygen should always be available.

Routes of Administration

Intramuscular. IM injections are made into either the pectoral or thigh muscles. Although a theoretical consideration, the renal portal system[59] does not clinically appear to affect either duration or quality of anesthesia produced by hindleg injection.

Intravenous. IV injections are administered into either the basilic, medial metatarsal, or right jugular veins. The basilic vein is usually avoided because it is difficult to provide good hemostasis in a struggling bird. Injections into the jugular vein are made slowly to avoid marked myocardial depression and retroperfusion of the brain with high drug concentrations. Intravenous doses are 50 to 70% of the IM dose.

Intraosseous. IO catheterization is indicated when IV access is impossible or too time-consuming.[40] The most accessible and easily maintained

site for IO catheter placement is the distal end of the ulna (see later).[47] The proximal tibiotarsus can also be used.

Parenteral Drugs

Metabolic Drug Scaling

Metabolic scaling of parenteral drug doses between species and diverse body sizes has been evaluated and described by Sedgwick and coworkers.[54] In general, the parenteral drug dose required to produce a given anesthetic level varies nonlinearly with size; the smaller the bird the greater the dose/unit of body weight. Sedgwick and coworkers, however, have demonstrated that many drug doses are uniform when related to the metabolic size of an animal.[54] To calculate such a dose the daily minimum energy cost (MEC) is first determined using the equation

$$MEC = K \times M_b^{0.75}$$

where M_b = body weight (kg) and K = 129 and 78 for passerines and nonpasserines, respectively.

The total dose of a drug is then calculated and divided by the MEC value to give an MEC dose (mg/kcal).[54] This MEC dose can then be used to calculate drug dose in larger or smaller birds by first calculating MEC for that bird and multiplying by the MEC dose. For example, the MEC for a 30-g budgerigar is

$$78 \times 0.03^{0.75} = 5.6 \text{ kcal/day.}$$

If the MEC dose of ketamine is 0.2 mg/kcal, this bird would require 1.1 mg or 36 mg/kg.

Propofol

Propofol is an ultrashort-acting, noncumulative IV anesthetic. In pigeons (14 mg/kg, 0.15 mg/kcal IV) it produced a smooth and rapid induction, good muscle relaxation of short duration (2 to 7 minutes), marked respiratory depression, and a very narrow safety margin in spontaneously breathing birds.[11] In mammals, propofol induces dose-dependent cardiopulmonary depression similar to that caused by thiopental.[58]

Ketamine

The dissociative anesthetic ketamine ([Ketaset], Fort Dodge Laboratories) produces a cataleptoid state with open eyes, occasional purposeful skeletal movements, and hypertonus independent of stimulation.[51, 58] Water-soluble ketamine HCl is administered either IM or IV. When given IM it initially produces incoordination and opisthotony followed by relaxation within 1 to 3 minutes, and in large birds manual restraint may be necessary to avoid neck and leg trauma.[52] Duration of maximal effect is dose-dependent, and recovery is characterized by incoordination, excitement, head shaking, and wing flapping.[52] Recovery from ketamine immobilization is in part related to redistribution followed by hepatic biotransformation and/or renal excretion.[5] Consequently, repetitive dosing and presence of renal disease and severe dehydration result in prolonged recoveries. A short duration of effect is achieved using a moderate IV dose. If it is necessary to prolong a procedure, 30 to 50% of the original dose is given to effect. Commercial preparations of ketamine are a racemic mixture of two optical isomers (D+ and L−).[58] The D+ isomer is a more potent analgesic and less likely to cause emergence reactions.[58] In great horned owls, the L− isomer produced inadequate muscle relaxation, cardiac arrhythmias, and marked excitatory behavior during recovery compared with the D+ form.[45]

Although blood pressure and cardiac output are generally maintained because of increased sympathetic activity and catecholamine release, ketamine directly depresses myocardial contractility and may cause cardiac collapse in birds with marginal cardiovascular reserve.[58] In Pekin ducks (20 mg/kg, 0.3 mg/kcal IV) and white leghorn chickens (30–120 mg/kg, 0.4–1.6 mg/kcal IM) ketamine did not significantly affect respiration,[31, 51] while in red-tailed hawks (30 mg/kg, 0.4 mg/kcal IM) it produced mild hyperventilation.[28] In budgerigars, death from high-dose ketamine appeared to be due to respiratory arrest followed by cardiac arrest.[35]

In chickens, the median effective dose of IV ketamine for 15 minutes of anesthesia or longer was 14 mg/kg (0.18 mg/kcal), median lethal dose was 67.9 mg/kg (0.85 mg/kcal), and surgical analgesia was not apparent at doses less than 60 mg/kg (0.74 mg/kcal).[38] In budgerigars, the ketamine lethal dose was approximately 500 mg/kg IM (2.7 mg/kcal),

whereas an adequate anesthetic dose was estimated to be within 50 to 100 mg/kg IM (0.3–0.5 mg/kcal).[35] Avian ketamine MEC doses (see earlier) were determined by Sedgwick and coworkers[54] using data reported by Samour and coworkers.[52] These doses corresponded well with those in the cat in which 0.2, 0.4, and 0.6 mg/kcal were low, moderate, and high doses, respectively.[54] Guidelines for avian ketamine doses based on these MEC dosages are given in Table 46–1. In the penguin, gallinule, water rail, golden pheasant, turaco, and hornbill, IM ketamine produced only light sedation and excited recovery.[52]

Diazepam-Ketamine

Diazepam improves muscle relaxation, anesthetic duration, and recovery. Surgical anesthesia is not as good as with xylazine-ketamine, but adverse cardiopulmonary effects are less. In chickens, diazepam-ketamine (2.5 mg/kg IV–75 mg/kg IM; 0.03 mg/kcal IV–1.0 mg/kcal IM) resulted in rapid tranquilization and loss of the righting reflex, with recovery in 90 to 100 minutes.[7] Opisthotonus was common, short-term myotonic limb contractions were present in all birds, and pain reflexes were elicited at all times.[7] Although bradycardia was observed, blood pressure, respiration rate, and body temperature remained stable.[7] In raptors diazepam-ketamine IV (1 to 1.5 mg/kg–30 to 40 mg/kg; 0.010 to 0.019 mg/kcal–0.10 to 0.5 mg/kcal) was successfully used for various surgical procedures.[44] However, too-rapid injection produced prolonged apnea, cardiac arrhythmias, and increased risk of death.[44] Hence the recommendation is to administer divided doses at intervals of 2 to 3 minutes. In raptors apparent overdose was observed in fat birds.[44]

Xylazine-Ketamine

The addition of xylazine to ketamine improves muscle relaxation, duration of surgical analgesia, and recovery. However, recovery is prolonged and adverse cardiopulmonary effects are increased.[31, 52] Eyes still remain open and palpebral reflex is preserved.[52] In Pekin ducks xylazine-ketamine IV (1 mg/kg–20 mg/kg; 0.02 mg/kcal–0.3 mg/kcal) produced respiratory depression and acidemia, and hy-

Table 46-1

GUIDELINES FOR THE DETERMINATION OF KETAMINE DOSE* IN NONPASSERINES AND PASSERINES

Weight (kg)	Nonpasserines						Passerines					
	Low Dose		Medium Dose		High Dose		Low Dose		Medium Dose		High Dose	
	MG/KG	TOTAL MG	MG/KG	TOTAL MG	MG/KG	TOTAL MG	MG/KG	TOTAL MG	MG/KG	TOTAL MG	MG/KG	TOTAL MG
0.03	33	1	67	2	100	3	67	2	133	4	200	6
0.10	30	3	60	6	80	8	50	5	90	9	140	14
0.20	25	5	45	9	70	14	40	8	75	15	115	23
0.30	20	6	43	13	63	19	33	10	70	21	103	31
0.40	20	8	40	16	60	24	33	13	65	26	98	39
0.50	18	9	38	19	56	28	30	15	62	31	92	46
0.60	18	11	35	21	53	32	30	18	58	35	88	53
0.70	17	12	34	24	51	36	29	20	56	39	84	59
0.80	16	13	33	26	50	40	28	22	55	44	81	65
0.90	16	14	32	29	48	43	27	24	53	48	80	72
1.00	16	16	31	31	47	47	26	26	52	52	77	77
1.50	14	21	28	42	42	63						
2.00	13	26	26	52	40	79						
4.00	11	44	22	88	33	132						

*Based on MEC dosages of 0.2 mg/kcal (low dose), 0.4 mg/kcal (medium dose), and 0.6 mg/kcal (high dose).[54] MEC (Minimum Energy Cost) calculated from $K \times M_b^{0.75}$ where K = 78 and 129 for nonpasserines and passerines, respectively, and M_b = body weight (kg). For short periods of immobilization use the low dose, and decrease the dose when combining with either diazepam or xylazine.

poxemia.[31] Additionally, moderate hyperthermia was observed.[31] In red-tailed hawks, xylazine-ketamine IV (2.2 mg/kg–4.4 mg/kg; 0.03 mg/kcal–0.06 mg/kcal) also induced bradypnea, as well as bradycardia.[9] In turkey vultures, xylazine-ketamine IM (1 mg/kg–10 mg/kg; 0.01 mg/kcal–0.1 mg/kcal) rapidly induced a consistent level of anesthesia (induction time 5.4 ± 1 minute and duration 109.8 ± 25.4 minutes).[1] For convenience, equal volumes of xylazine (20 mg/ml) and ketamine (100 mg/ml) are combined (final concentration 10 mg/ml–50 mg/ml) and a dose based on ml/kg is calculated.[17, 25] The MEC dose using this technique is reported to be 0.002 to 0.004 ml/kcal.[25] Guidelines for xylazine-ketamine doses are given in Table 46–2.

α_2-Adrenoceptor Antagonists

Although either partially or completely successful in reversing the effects of xylazine, α_2-adrenoceptor antagonists do not reverse the effects of ketamine. Yohimbine ([Antagenil] Wildlife Laboratories, Ft. Collins, CO) shortened recovery when administered 40 to 45 minutes after xylazine-ketamine in budgerigars[21] (0.275 mg/kg, 0.0015 mg/kcal, IV; xylazine 10 mg/kg, 0.054 mg/kcal, IM; ketamine 40 mg/kg, 0.2 mg/kcal, IM), guineafowl[60] (1 mg/kg, 0.014 mg/

kcal, IV; xylazine 1 mg/kg, 0.014 mg/kcal, IM; ketamine 25 mg/kg, 0.3 mg/kcal, IM), and red-tailed hawks[9] (0.1 mg/kg, 0.0013 mg/kcal, IV; xylazine 2.2 mg/kg, 0.030 mg/kcal, IV; ketamine 4.4 mg/kg, 0.06 mg/kcal, IV). Yohimbine (0.125 mg/kg, 0.005 mg/kcal, IV) has also been used to reverse xylazine (1 mg/kg, 0.04 mg/kcal, IM) in ostriches.[43] Similarly, in turkey vultures, tolazoline ([Priscoline] Ciba, Summit, NJ) (15 mg/kg, 0.2 mg/kcal, IV) hastened recovery when administered 45 minutes after xylazine-ketamine (1 mg/kg–10 mg/kg; 0.01–0.1 mg/kcal).[1] In red-tailed hawks, yohimbine was observed to exert no profound cardiopulmonary changes.[9] However, the author has observed excitement and mortality in mammals at yohimbine doses greater than 1 mg/kg.

Zolazepam-Tiletamine

The dissociative anesthetic tiletamine is combined with the potent benzodiazepine zolazepam in the commercial combination Telazol. Tiletamine is approximately three times as potent as ketamine, and recovery is much prolonged.[5] In Pekin ducks, Telazol (13 mg/kg, 0.2 mg/kcal, IM) produced adequate anesthesia in 15 minutes for liver biopsy and recovery in 3 to 5 hours.[6] Occasionally, additional doses

Table 46–2

RECOMMENDED VOLUMES* (MLS) OF A XYLAZINE-KETAMINE COMBINATION (EQUAL VOLUMES OF XYLAZINE 20 MG/ML AND KETAMINE 100 MG/ML)

Weight (kg)	Parrots		Passerines		Nonpasserines	
	IV Dose	IM Dose	Low Dose	High Dose	Low Dose	High Dose
0.03	0.005	0.01	0.02	0.04	0.01	0.02
0.10	0.01	0.02	0.05	0.09	0.03	0.06
0.20	0.025	0.05	0.08	0.15	0.05	0.09
0.30	0.025–0.05	0.05–0.1	0.10	0.21	0.06	0.13
0.40			0.13	0.26	0.08	0.16
0.50	0.04–0.05	0.08–0.1	0.15	0.31	0.09	0.19
0.60	0.06–0.07	0.12–0.15	0.18	0.35	0.11	0.21
0.70			0.20	0.39	0.12	0.24
0.80	0.075–0.10	0.15–0.20	0.22	0.44	0.13	0.26
0.90			0.24	0.48	0.15	0.29
1.00			0.26	0.52	0.16	0.31
1.50					0.21	0.42
2.00					0.26	0.52
4.00					0.44	0.88

*Based on an MEC dosage of 0.002 to 0.004 ml/kcal.[25] MEC calculated from K × $M_b^{0.75}$, where K = 78 and 129 for nonpasserines and passerines, respectively, and M_b = body weight (kg). Doses for parrots are from Harrison.[17] Administer 50–70% of recommended dose, then wait 5–10 min before giving the rest to effect. Always have a source of oxygen and ventilation available.

(3 mg/kg) were required. Telazol has also been used in ostriches (see later).

INHALATION ANESTHESIA

Inhalation Anesthetic Potency

Minimum anesthetic concentration (MAC) or dose (MAD) is a measure of inhalant anesthetic potency in birds. It refers to the anesthetic concentration (vol%) that produces immobility in 50% of an anesthetized population subjected to a noxious stimulus (Table 46–3).[30, 32, 33] A potent inhalation anesthetic has a low MAC value. MAC is similar within and across species, and is decreased by hypothermia.[42] Maintenance surgical anesthesia vaporizer settings are approximately 25% higher than MAC, for example:

halothane MAC = 0.85 ± 0.09% in chickens, maintenance = 1–1.5%[30, 58]

In spontaneously breathing large birds, discrepancies between vaporizer setting and anesthetic effect are overcome by controlled ventilation and increased flow rate.

Inhalation Anesthetic Agents

The four inhalation anesthetic agents that are commonly available to practitioners include methoxy-

Table 46–3

AVIAN INHALATION ANESTHETIC MAC VALUES AND RECOMMENDED AVIAN INDUCTION AND MAINTENANCE VAPORIZER SETTINGS*

Inhalation Anesthetic	Species	MAC (vol %)	Induction (%)	Maintenance (%)
Nitrous oxide	Not determined		50–66	50–66
Methoxyflurane			≥3.0	0.25–0.5
Halothane	Chicken	0.85 ± 0.09	≤2.0	1.0–1.5
Isoflurane	Pekin duck	1.30 ± 0.23	≤3.0	1.5–2.5
	Sandhill crane	1.34 ± 0.14		

*Published values.[30, 32, 33]

flurane, halothane, isoflurane, and nitrous oxide. Ether is not indicated for use in the modern avian practice because of its high flammability and the availability of other agents.

Methoxyflurane

Methoxyflurane is the most potent (low MAC) of the available inhalation agents. However, it has high tissue solubility resulting in prolonged induction and recovery.[58] Methoxyflurane has a very low saturated vapor pressure, decreasing the potential for attaining lethal concentrations.[58] This is an advantage only when using nonprecision vaporizers. Methoxyflurane is inexpensive and a good analgesic and muscle relaxant, and it produces no myocardial sensitization.[58] It does produce a dose-dependent decrease in cardiopulmonary function.[41, 58] Induction vaporizer settings are often greater than 3%, whereas maintenance is 0.2 to 0.5%.

Halothane

Until the arrival of isoflurane, halothane was the preferred avian anesthetic. Halothane has the advantages of being inexpensive, potent, nonexplosive, having relatively low tissue solubility, and producing moderate muscle relaxation.[58] Dose-dependent cardiopulmonary depression, myocardial sensitization to catecholamine-induced arrhythmias, and potential hepatotoxicity are the major disadvantages of halothane use.[30, 58] In adult Pekin ducks, halothane (2–2.5%) produced a moderate tachycardia (60–100%), hypotension (10–15%), and bradypnea (50–70%).[13] Observed arrhythmias included ventricular fibrillation, ventricular bigeminy, and multifocal ventricular rhythms.[13] Induction vaporizer setting should not exceed 2%, and maintenance is 1 to 1.5%.

Isoflurane

Isoflurane ([AErrane] Anaquest, Madison, WI) is the preferred avian inhalant anesthetic because it offers very rapid induction and recovery, less depression of cardiac output than other agents, apparent absence of sensitization to myocardial-induced ar-

rhythmias, lower incidence of hepatotoxicity, and reasonable muscle relaxation.[41, 58] Its major disadvantages are dose-dependent cardiopulmonary depression, decreased blood pressure, and cost. Isoflurane (2.0–3.0%) produced less tachycardia, hypotension, and bradypnea in Pekin ducks, and no arrhythmias when compared with halothane (2–2.5%).[13] Although isoflurane in Pekin ducks and sandhill cranes at MAC and 1.5 MAC had few effects on cardiovascular function, it was associated with significant hypoventilation.[32, 33] In Pekin ducks, neither respiration rate nor tidal volume was a good determinant of adequacy of ventilation.[33] In mechanically ventilated chickens, isoflurane anesthesia (end-tidal 2.1%) resulted in a significantly lower threshold for electrical fibrillation of the heart when compared with halothane (end-tidal 1.2%) or pentobarbital (30 mg/kg, IV).[14] Induction vaporizer setting should not exceed 3% and maintenance is 1.5 to 2%.

Nitrous Oxide

The use of nitrous oxide gas (N_2O) in birds has been controversial, mainly because of misunderstanding of avian respiratory anatomy. Although N_2O expands closed gas-filled spaces within the body, it does not cause air sac expansion because air sacs communicate with the outside.[58] However, some diving birds (e.g., pelicans, gannets) have subcutaneous air pockets that do not communicate with the respiratory system, and therefore N_2O can result in expansion and possible rupture.[46] Nitrous oxide is the least potent inhalation anesthetic, and it is recommended that an inspired concentration between 50 and 66% be used. This decreases the inspired oxygen concentration, and nitrous oxide is therefore not used in birds with marginal respiratory reserve. Nitrous oxide has the advantages of being odorless and having very low tissue solubility, which results in very rapid uptake as well as excretion. Nitrous oxide decreases the anesthetic requirement of concurrently administered anesthetic agents because of its analgesic effect and facilitates the uptake of other inhalation anesthetics through the second gas effect.[41, 58] The author has found N_2O to be a useful adjunct to inhalation anesthesia in ratites. The major disadvantages of N_2O are its low

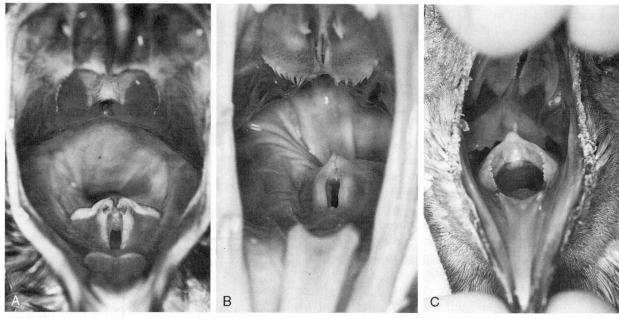

Figure 46–5

Oral cavities of *(A)* a sharp-shinned hawk, *(B)* a ring-billed gull, and *(C)* a pigeon. Note the presence of the glottis at the base of the tongue.

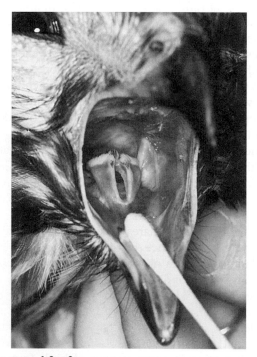

Figure 46–6

Visualization of the glottis is facilitated by the use of a good light source, opening the mouth wide, and pulling the tongue forward with either a cotton-tipped swab or a gauze square.

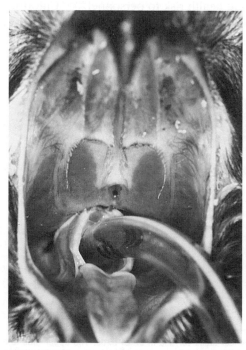

Figure 46–7

Correct placement of an endotracheal tube is assessed by direct visualization and by the detection of exhaled air as condensation in the tube.

increase the rate of anesthetic uptake, because doing so may prove fatal. Induction using an aquarium is easy, but the anesthetic concentration is variable, and there is a potential for injury as the bird struggles. Injectable anesthesia (ketamine IV or IM) is used to facilitate handling in difficult patients during gaseous induction and/or intubation.

Intubation

Intubation is performed for controlled ventilation, to protect against aspiration, to allow lower respiratory tract suction, and to minimize fresh gas flow and deadspace. Tracheal mucosal trauma, caused by inflated cuffs and rough intubation, is promoted by complete tracheal rings that prevent expansion. Severe trauma results in tracheal stenosis. The largest diameter endotracheal tube possible is selected to provide an adequate seal and reduce airway resistance. Tube length extending from the patient is limited to reduce mechanical deadspace.

The avian glottis is readily identified at the base of the tongue (Fig. 46–5). Observation is facilitated by grasping the tongue with gauze or a cotton-tipped applicator and pulling it forward (Fig. 46–6). For intubation, the bird's mouth is opened by an assistant with gauze placed around the upper and lower beak. This exposes the glottis, and the tube bevel is turned sideways to pass through into the trachea (Fig. 46–7). In some species of birds (e.g., flamingos) the glottis is not easily seen. The tube is passed blindly by palpating the trachea externally with the head and neck in extension. Unlike mammals, birds can still vocalize when intubated because of the presence of the syrinx at the tracheal bifurcation. Furthermore, vocalization can occur on both inhalation and exhalation, and can be induced by mechanical ventilation.

Light sources used to illuminate the glottis include penlights, laryngoscopes with small straight blades, head lamps, goose neck lamps, and examination lights. In awake birds, 1% lidocaine is applied topically to the glottis before the lubricated tube is placed. In birds that may chew the endotracheal tube, a roll of gauze squares is taped in the mouth. Tubes are taped in place and lubricant is placed in the eyes. The down eye should be protected because the avian cornea protrudes from the head.

Muscle Relaxants

The use of a muscle relaxant during inhalation anesthesia is indicated to provide good muscle relaxation, prevent movement during ophthalmic surgery, and reduce inhalant anesthetic requirement. The major disadvantages are the need for ventilatory support and the absence of analgesia when muscle relaxants are used alone.

Atracurium

In chickens, the ultra–short-acting nondepolarizing muscle relaxant atracurium besylate has been evaluated as an adjunct to isoflurane anesthesia.[39] Muscle relaxation was monitored with a nerve stimulator. The effective dose to result in 95% twitch depression in 50% of birds was calculated to be 0.25 mg/kg, IV.[39] At this dose the total duration of action was around 30 to 40 minutes, increasing to 45 to 55 minutes when the dose was increased to 0.45 mg/kg. Small increases in heart rate and blood pressure were observed. The administration of edrophonium (0.5 mg/kg, IV) greatly hastened return of normal muscle strength.

PERIANESTHETIC MONITORING AND SUPPORT

Perianesthetic monitoring and support are a major determinant of anesthetic success, particularly in critically ill patients. The level of monitoring and support is determined by patient status and the procedure to be done. Monitoring should include regular assessment of depth and cardiopulmonary function.

Depth

The stages of narcosis and anesthesia in birds have previously been classified based on those used in mammals (Table 46–5).[3, 34] The most useful guides to anesthetic depth are response to painful stimuli, muscle tone, palpebral reflex, and respiratory rate and depth. Jaw tone is used to subjectively assess muscle tone. The palpebral reflex is usually present until light surgical anesthesia is effected, whereas

T a b l e   4 6 – 5

GUIDELINES FOR DETERMINATION OF AVIAN ANESTHETIC DEPTH

System	Response Variable	I	II	III Light	III Medium	III Deep	IV Brainstem Hypoxemia, Ischemia
Nervous	Cere reflex	+ + + +		+ + +	0	0	0
	Feather plucking	+ + + +		+ + +	±	0	0
	Pedal reflex	+ + + +		+ + +	0	0	0
	Surgical stimulation	+ + + +		+ +	±	0	0
Cardiovascular	Blood pressure	Hypertension		Normal	Increasing hypotension		Shock level
	Dysrhythmia potential	+ + +		+ +	+	+ +	+ + + +
	Heart rate	Tachycardia		Progressive bradycardia			Weak or imperceptible
Gastrointestinal	Reflux potential	0		+	+ +	+ + +	+ + + +
	Salivation	+ + + +	+ + +	+		0	
	Vomiting probability	+ + +		+		±	
Musculoskeletal	Abdominal muscle tone	+ + + +		+ +	+		0
	Jaw tone	+ + + +		+ +	+	0	
	Limb muscle tone	+ + + +		+ +	+	0	
	Cloacal sphincter	May void		Progressive relaxation		Atonic	
Ocular	Corneal reflex	+ + + +		+ + +	+ +	±	
	Palpebral reflex	+ + + +		+ +	±	0	
	Pupil size	Variable, often dilated, may see hippus		Usually constricted			Dilated
Respiratory	Cough	+ + + +	+ + +	+		0	
	Depth	Irregular or increased		Progressive decrease		Irregular	Apnea
	Intubation	No		Yes			
	Mucous membrane, skin color			Normal		Pale to white ± cyanosis	
	Pattern	Occasional breath holding		Normal		Irregular	Apnea ± agonal gasping
	Rate	Tachypnea		Progressive bradypnea			
Other							Piloerection

*Data from Arnall, Vet Rec, 1961[3]; Lamb, Veterinary Anesthesia, 1984.[34]

the corneal response persists to deeper levels. At medium planes of anesthesia respiration rate is regular. Sudden piloerection and pupillary dilation usually occur with cardiac arrest. Anesthetic level should be appropriate to the procedure; some procedures are likely to be more painful than others and depth is adjusted accordingly. Some of the more painful stimuli to birds are removal of feathers, manipulation of bone, and visceral traction.

Allometric Scaling of Physiologic Variables

Reference ranges for physiologic variables vary with animal size. For most variables this relationship is not linear and is described by an allometric equation of the general form

$$y = a \times x^b \,^{[53]}$$

The use of allometric equations for determination of expected variable reference ranges during anesthesia has been described by Sedgwick,[55] and serves as guidelines for the anesthetized avian patient. Changes of 20% above or below the calculated value are considered abnormal.[55]

Cardiovascular Monitoring

Resting avian heart rate (beats/minute) is estimated from the allometric equation

$$f_h = 155.8 \, M_b{}^{-0.23}$$
$$(M_b = \text{body weight in kg})^{[53]}$$

Auscultation

Auscultation is used to determine rate and rhythm. Cardiac sounds are muffled by the sternum and pectoral musculature, whereas sounds with the greatest intensity are heard below the sternum and at the thoracic inlet. Although continuous auscultation is not possible during a surgical procedure, a good quality stethoscope should always be available. Esophageal stethoscopes are used in some species but are difficult to position in birds with crops.

Electrocardiography

Heart rate and rhythm are continuously monitored by electrocardiograms (ECG) during long and complex procedures with an ECG machine with an oscilloscope. The ECG machine must be capable of monitoring high heart rates, have a freeze function for interpretation, and allow a printout. Avian ECG quality is maximized using electrode paste, needles, or stainless steel suture to improve lead contact. The author usually monitors leads I or II.

Ultrasonic Doppler Flow Apparatus

The Doppler flow apparatus (Parks Medical Electronics, Aloha, OR) gives an audible signal of arterial flow, allowing continuous monitoring of heart rate and rhythm as well as sudden changes in pressure. A pediatric probe is placed over either an ulnar or metatarsal artery (Fig. 46–8). It can also be placed under the tongue or against the carotid ar-

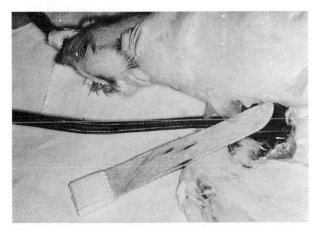

F i g u r e   4 6 – 8

The Doppler flow apparatus gives an audible signal of arterial flow. A pediatric probe is placed over either an ulnar or a metatarsal artery.

tery in the neck. The pencil probe attachment is used to check cardiac and peripheral blood flow in emergencies.

Arterial Blood Pressure

Indirect blood pressure is determined in large birds in the same manner as mammals.[59] However, the appropriate size of cuff (width = 70–80% of circumference) must be used or the values will be too high or too low.[59] Alternatively, intra-arterial catheters are placed for direct blood pressure measurement. Appropriately sized over-the-needle catheters (18–24 gauge) are placed in either the ulnar or metatarsal arteries and connected through heparinized saline-filled pressure tubing to a pressure transducer placed at the level of the heart. The catheter is secured by either suturing or using tissue glue. Besides providing a constant assessment of blood pressure, an arterial line allows blood sampling for arterial blood gas measurement. Normal arterial blood pressures vary between avian species, sexes, age, and breed.[59] In many birds the arterial pressures are higher than those expected for mammals.[59] Apparent hypertension has been described in an ostrich.[36]

Orthostatic Hypotension

During the perianesthetic period, rapid changes in body position are avoided to prevent the development of orthostatic hypotension. This effect is exacerbated by dehydration, hypovolemia, and anesthesia.[58] Severe orthostatic hypotension decreases venous return and induces cardiac arrest. A common time for this to occur is at the end of a surgical procedure when the drapes are removed and the recovering bird is rapidly picked up before being returned to recovery.

Cardiovascular Support

Intravenous Catheterization

In those birds in which it is possible, IV catheters are placed in either the ulnar or jugular veins. In large birds, the medial metatarsal vein may also be used. In very small birds, veins are temporarily catheterized with small-gauge butterfly catheters (25 or 27 gauge). In larger birds, over-the-needle catheters are preferred. The basilic vein is most easily entered proximal to the elbow joint where it straightens out along the humerus. Catheters are secured with either sutures or tissue glue.

Intraosseous Catheterization

An 18- to 22-gauge spinal needle is used in patients weighing 500 g or more, whereas in smaller birds and neonates, 25- to 30-gauge hypodermic needles are used.[47] The cannula should be long enough to penetrate to the midpoint of the ulna. After feather removal and aseptic preparation, the lateral notch on the distal ulna is palpated and the needle positioned at its center and parallel to the median plane of the bone. The needle is advanced with a slightly rotating movement into the supported ulna, and should pass without resistance into the marrow cavity. The needle is aspirated to check for bone marrow and flushed with heparinized saline to prevent occlusion and check for free flow. The cannula is flushed twice daily with heparinized saline. In pigeons, lactated Ringer's solution infused into an IO catheter reached the systemic circulation in 30 seconds, and an infusion rate of 20 ml/kg/hr was achieved.[29] An alternate site for intraosseous catheterization is the proximal tibiotarsal bone.

Fluids

A fluid delivery line should be established before beginning major surgical procedures to provide a slow infusion (5–10 ml/kg/hr) of balanced electrolyte solution. Dextrose is added as indicated. Commercial small-volume syringe infusion pumps are used for accurate fluid administration. Guidelines for rate of avian fluid infusion have not been established and should be extrapolated from those for mammals.

Blood Transfusion

Although birds are better able to tolerate severe blood loss than mammals, excessive hemorrhage is a common cause of avian anesthetic mortality. Land and nonflying birds (chickens, pheasants) are less tolerant to blood loss than flying species (pigeons, ducks).[59] Avian total blood volume ranges from 6 to 11% of body weight.[59] Estimated hemorrhage of 5 to 10% of blood volume is treated with three times the volume in balanced electrolyte solution. A blood transfusion is indicated when hemorrhage exceeds 20 to 30% of circulating blood volume. Other indications for transfusion include decreases in hemoglobin concentration below 8 g/dl and PCV 15% or less. Factors that further effect the decision to transfuse include hemoglobin saturation and adequacy of cardiac output. Sources of blood donation include siblings, same species, and same order, in decreasing desirability. Because approximately 10% of a donor's blood is collected, it is usually necessary to have two donors available. Blood is collected into a heparinized syringe using a 23- or 25-gauge butterfly catheter, gently mixed, then immediately transfused. The syringe and catheter are heparinized by drawing heparin (1000 IU/ml) into the syringe and then expelling it. Blood is not collected into either citrate phosphate dextrose or lithium ethylenediaminetetraacetate (EDTA) because they can produce a calcium-responsive tetany. Lithium EDTA also produces hemolysis in some species.

RESPIRATORY MONITORING

Respiration Rate

Resting respiration rate (breaths/min) is estimated from the allometric equations

$$f_{resp} = 17.2\, M_b - 0.31\ (M_b = \text{body weight in kg})[53]$$

Respiration rate is calculated by either watching thoracic movement or expiratory condensation in a clear endotracheal tube. Commercial respiratory monitors that attach to the end of the endotracheal tube are very helpful in monitoring respiration.

Ventilation

Adequacy of ventilation is difficult to visually assess. Although there are devices available to measure ventilation, they are not accurate for small birds and they increase mechanical deadspace and resistance. The most accurate method of assessing ventilation is by determination of arterial partial pressure of carbon dioxide ($PaCO_2$). Tidal volume (ml) and minute ventilation (ml/min) are estimated from the allometric equations

$$V_t = 13.2\ M_b^{1.08}\ \text{(tidal volume) and}\ V = 284\ M_b^{0.77}$$
(minute ventilation)[53]

Blood Gas Analysis

The measurement of blood gas values and pH is useful for the evaluation of ventilation, oxygen transport and delivery, and metabolic status. Blood gas values in birds are corrected to body temperature for easy interpretation. Blood gas values are similar to those obtained in mammals, and the interpretation is the same.[59]

Respiratory Support

Birds have a slower rate of breathing (1/3) and increased tidal volume ($4\times$) when compared with a mammal of the same size.[59] Small changes in respiration rate therefore have a greater effect on overall minute ventilation in birds than in mammals. In addition, absence of a diaphragm and dependence on thoracic wall movement, for both inspiratory and expiratory movement of air, make birds very susceptible to the respiratory depressant effects of anesthetics. This potential for hypoventilation is further exacerbated by hindrance of normal thoracic movements (e.g., from heavy surgical drapes or leaning hands on the bird) and pathologic conditions such as obesity and intra-abdominal masses. For the above reasons the author routinely assists ventilation of birds under anesthesia. This has the added effect when using inhalation anesthetics of providing more even ventilation.

Although the lungs are fixed to the thoracic wall, atelectasis may still be a problem in anesthetized birds. The author has had several dorsally recumbent patients die under anesthesia, and subsequent histologic examination has shown collapse and obstruction of the small airways. The development of atelectasis may be partially prevented with ventila-

tion. Additional causes of ventilatory difficulties may include the accumulation of blood and fluids in the air sacs with subsequent migration to the lungs. When suspected, the bird should be held vertical until it recovers. Furthermore, hemostasis should be meticulous during surgery, and flushing the coelomic cavities should be avoided. It has been shown in chickens that dorsal recumbency results in a 40 to 50% decrease in tidal volume and 20 to 50% increase in respiratory rate, with an overall 10 to 60% decrease in minute ventilation.[26] This is thought to be the result of visceral compression of the air sacs.[26]

Temperature Monitoring and Support

Maintenance of normal body temperature is important for normal metabolic rate. Hypothermia results in peripheral vasoconstriction, bradycardia, hypotension, and when severe, ventricular fibrillation. As body temperature returns to normal, peripheral vasodilation occurs, and oxygen and glucose requirements increase, unmasking hypovolemia, hypoglycemia, and hypoxemia. In general, avian deep body temperatures are higher than those in mammals; in large flightless and diving birds and species that are capable of torpor, they tend to be low.[59] In addition, deep body temperature of birds fluctuates during the course of a day; the smaller the bird, the greater the fluctuation.[59] Fasting also decreases body temperature.[59] Birds that become dehydrated (e.g., ostriches and turkeys) are not able to prevent hyperthermia as well because of decreased evaporative cooling.[59] Respiratory evaporative cooling is extremely important in birds.[59] Temperature is monitored continuously or intermittently. Esophageal probes, although optimal for core body temperature measurement, are difficult to place in birds with crops.

Hypothermia is reduced by decreasing anesthetic time, using limited surgical preparation solutions, using warm fluids, wrapping the bird in plastic bubble wrap, and using circulating water blankets and heat lamps. Electric heating pads produce severe burns, as do heat lamps if placed too close.

Glucose Monitoring and Support

Most avian patients are small and consequently their glucose and glycogen reserves are small. Hence, blood glucose is assessed preoperatively in debilitated animals, and it is monitored intermittently during prolonged procedures and recovery. Under anesthesia, hypoglycemia may be manifested as nonresponsive bradycardia, hypotension, and pupillary dilation. Glucose is administered when blood levels fall below 200 mg/dl. Although a bolus of 50% dextrose (1–2 ml/kg, IV) is given in emergencies (glucose ≤60 mg/dl), it is better to use an infusion to prevent rebound hypoglycemia. Hypertonic solutions of subcutaneous dextrose produce dehydration.

RESUSCITATION

Avian resuscitation follows the mammalian protocol (airway, breathing, circulation, and drugs).[48] Time between detection and initiation of resuscitation is critical; most avian patients are small, and consequently tissue oxygen reserves are rapidly exhausted during cardiopulmonary arrest. Cardiopulmonary arrest is best prevented with perioperative stabilization and attentive monitoring. Successful resuscitation is facilitated by intubation, ventilatory support, and replacement of vascular access lines. If necessary, all drugs required during resuscitation can be administered IO.[40] If it is not possible to intubate a bird, flapping of the wings appears to provide some air movement, and may also facilitate venous return to the heart from the pectoral musculature. The author has successfully resuscitated several small birds using this technique.

RECOVERY

Recovery is a critical period in avian anesthesia, during which the patient should be carefully restrained in a warm, quiet environment and monitored. The duration and quality of recovery are primarily determined by the anesthetic agents used, the duration of the procedure, and the magnitude of physiologic dysfunction incurred during the procedure. Causes of prolonged recovery include hypothermia, hypoglycemia, and anesthetic overdose. Care should be taken in rewarming a bird that is hypovolemic and/or hypoglycemic, because warming results in dilation of vasoconstricted peripheral vessels, as well as increased metabolic demand for

glucose. These phenomena may explain some of the sudden deaths that occur a few hours into recovery.

ANALGESIA

Principles

Birds may express pain with clinical signs of anorexia, depression, lameness, or vocalization on palpation. Protracted pain adversely affects the well-being of the avian patient in the perianesthetic and postoperative periods.[56] Unfortunately, avian analgesia has been neglected through ignorance, the belief that birds do not experience pain, and the difficulty in assessing pain by behavioral clues. Further research is necessary to assess the pharmacology of analgesics in birds.

Analgesics

Avian analgesia has been reviewed by Bauck.[4] There are four major groups of analgesics available: glucocorticoids, nonsteroidal anti-inflammatories, α_2-adrenoceptor agonists, and opioids.[56] Glucocorticoids and nonsteroidal anti-inflammatory agents produce analgesia by inhibition of prostaglandin synthesis. They are of most value for alleviation of moderate soft tissue pain and pruritus. Flunixin meglumine (0.5 mg/kg) has been used by the author with moderate success to alleviate pain in birds with crop burns, muscle trauma, and other soft tissue injuries. Prolonged use results in adverse effects such as gastrointestinal ulceration and renal damage. The mechanism of analgesia produced by α_2-adrenoceptor agonists is controversial, and the level and type of analgesia produced appears to vary between species.[56] A combination of xylazine and ketamine does appear to improve the surgical analgesia produced by the latter. Opioid analgesics produce analgesia through opioid receptors present primarily in the central nervous system. There are several opioid receptor subtypes. Pure μ opioid receptor agonists (e.g., morphine, meperidine) are used for severe pain. Mixed agonist-antagonists (e.g., butorphanol, pentazocine) and partial agonists (e.g., buprenorphine) are used for moderate pain. In budgerigars, butorphanol ([Torbugesic],

Fort Dodge Laboratories) (3–4 mg/kg, 0.02 mg/kcal, IM) produced no change in heart and respiration rates, and induced regurgitation and cloacal straining at high dosages (10 mg/kg, 0.06 mg/kcal, IM).[4] In mammals, opioids produce ventilatory depression, bradycardia, and hypotension.[5] Avoid their use in hypotensive birds and those with respiratory compromise. Guidelines for analgesic drug dosages based on metabolic scaling from mammalian dosages are given in Table 46–6.

ANESTHESIA FOR SPECIFIC PROBLEMS

Neonatal and Pediatric Anesthesia

There are two broad types of avian neonate—altricial and precocial. Altricial neonates hatch at an earlier stage of maturity than precocial neonates. Regardless of neonate type it is assumed that hepatic and renal function is immature, and parenteral drug excretion is therefore likely to be prolonged. In addition, glycogen reserves are small, and hypoglycemia may develop perioperatively. All neonates develop hypothermia rapidly because of their large surface area-to-volume ratio. Furthermore, altricial neonates have very poor thermoregulatory ability.[59]

It is therefore very important to provide adequate warmth for neonates during the perianesthetic period, minimize the period of anesthesia, and aim for rapid return to normal function.

Avian neonates are likely to become dehydrated during prolonged procedures because of their high water requirements and loss of water from the respiratory system when subjected to inhalant anesthesia. Placement of an IO catheter is lifesaving in some procedures. Regurgitation is common during the perianesthetic period in birds with full crops, and fasting is recommended to reduce the crop volume. However, sufficient food may still remain in the proventriculus and ventriculus for reflux. Air sac volume is smaller in neonates because of high gastrointestinal volume. For anesthesia of avian neonates the author mask-induces with isoflurane, intubates, and ventilates (Fig. 46–9).

Ophthalmic Surgery

For intraocular surgery it is necessary to have a dilated, centrally fixed, nonmoving eye. This cannot be achieved by increasing the depth of anesthesia without endangering the patient. The use of a muscle relaxant (see earlier) can be used to provide

T a b l e 4 6 – 6

GUIDELINE DOSES* (MG) OF ANALGESICS FOR USE IN PASSERINE (P) AND NONPASSERINE (NP) BIRDS

| Weight (kg) | Nonsteroidal Anti-inflammatory | | Opioid Analgesics | | | | | |
| | Flunixin | | Morphine | | Meperidine | | Butorphanol | |
	P	NP	P	NP	P	NP	P	NP
0.03	0.1	0.1	0.3	0.2	3	2	0.2	0.1
0.10	0.2	0.1	0.7	0.4	7	4	0.5	0.3
0.20	0.3	0.2	1.2	0.7	12	7	0.8	0.5
0.30	0.5	0.3	1.6	0.9	16	9	1.0	0.6
0.40	0.6	0.4	1.9	1.2	19	12	1.3	0.8
0.50	0.7	0.4	2.3	1.4	23	14	1.5	0.9
0.60	0.8	0.5	2.6	1.6	26	16	1.8	1.1
0.70	0.9	0.5	3.0	1.8	30	18	2.0	1.2
0.80	1.0	0.6	3.3	2.0	33	20	2.2	1.3
0.90	1.1	0.6	3.6	2.2	36	22	2.4	1.4
1.00	1.2	0.7	3.9	2.3	39	23	2.6	1.6
1.50		1.0		3.2		32		2.1

*Doses for flunixin, morphine, and meperidine are scaled from moderate to high dosages used in a 20-kg dog (flunixin = 0.3 mg/kg = 0.009 mg/kcal, morphine = 1 mg/kg = 0.03 mg/kcal, meperidine = 10 mg/kg = 0.3 mg/kcal).[5, 41, 54] Butorphanol dosage scaled from that found to be safe in budgerigars (0.1 mg/35 gm = 0.02 mg/kcal).[4] Minimum daily energy cost (MEC) calculated from K × $M_b^{0.75}$, where K = 129 and 78 for passerines and nonpasserines, respectively, and M_b = body weight (kg).[54] For IV administration, halve the dose and give slowly. Prolonged high-dose administration of flunixin may result in gastrointestinal and renal damage.[5] Opioids produce sedation, respiratory depression, and bradycardia and hypotension at high dosages.[5]

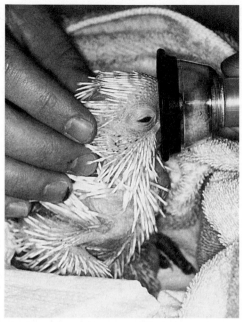

Figure 46–9

For anesthesia of avian neonates, the author uses mask induction with isoflurane, then intubates and ventilates.

relaxation without deep anesthesia. The author has not observed or heard of the oculocardiac reflex (vagally induced bradycardia caused by manipulation of the globe) in birds. Enucleation often results in much hemorrhage, and it may be necessary to preoperatively prepare for a transfusion.

Radiography

Many avian radiographs are taken on an outpatient basis, and for diagnostic quality it is necessary to provide good relaxation. Ketamine alone provides inadequate relaxation and prolonged recovery. The addition of either midazolam or diazepam reduces the dose of ketamine required and provides better relaxation. However, the author prefers an inhalation agent, usually isoflurane, for good relaxation and short duration of effect.

Respiratory Impairment—Upper Airway Obstruction

Avian patients with severe respiratory compromise are given oxygen before handling. The use of

isoflurane to provide restraint is often preferable to physical restraint alone.

The unique design of the avian respiratory system allows oxygen and inhalation anesthetics to be delivered through the air sacs.[50] In an emergency, oxygen is insufflated directly into the air sacs through a line connected to a large-gauge needle. If the airway obstruction is complete, a large tube is rapidly placed. An abdominal air sac tube is placed either behind the back leg or through the paralumbar fossa, as for surgical sexing.[50] A skin incision is made with a scalpel, and small forceps are then used to penetrate the muscle and peritoneum. The largest tube possible is used; for medium to large birds sterile endotracheal tubes can be used, whereas small catheters work well in smaller birds. A technique for placement of a tube in the clavicular air sac has been described and evaluated in phenobarbital-sedated ducks.[49] Cannulation of the clavicular air sac resulted in a significant increase in tidal volume and minute ventilation, whereas PaO_2, $PaCO_2$, heart rate, and mean arterial blood pressure remained unchanged from control values.[49] Air sac cannulas can be used for administration of inhalant anesthetics in spontaneously breathing birds. Cannulas are periodically checked for partial or complete occlusion.

Surgical Sexing

Some form of analgesia should always be used during surgical sexing. Isoflurane is excellent for this procedure because it allows rapid induction and recovery. Alternatively, low-dose IV ketamine in the medial metatarsal vein gives approximately 10 minutes of surgical analgesia and restraint, with a shorter recovery than with the use of a drug combination. In restrained large birds, some veterinarians infiltrate the laparoscopy site with local anesthetic. Care should be taken to avoid overdosage (see earlier).

ANESTHESIA FOR SPECIFIC AVIAN GROUPS

Parrots (Psittaciformes)

Anesthesia in parrots is mask-induced with an inhalation agent; parrots are intubated and maintained on a non-rebreathing system. Birds that are difficult to restrain are given ketamine IV (medial metatarsal vein) or IM. The use of a xylazine-ketamine combination has been described (see Table 46–2).[17]

Penguins (Sphenisciformes)

Anesthesia in penguins is induced with either ketamine or inhalation agents. Hyperthermia can be a problem, particularly in struggling obese animals. The trachea bifurcates early, and care is therefore taken to prevent placement of the endotracheal tube into a major bronchus. Ketamine alone produces poor restraint.[52]

Pigeons (Columbiformes)

Anesthesia for pigeons is the same as for parrots, except awake endotracheal intubation is possible.

Poultry (Galliformes)

Anesthesia for poultry is the same as for pigeons, and has been reviewed by Hartsfield and coworkers.[19]

Raptors (Falconiformes and Strigiformes)

Raptors require firm and quiet restraint, with control of the head and talons always to avoid injury to the holder. A towel wrapped around the body prevents wing flapping. The talons of raptors can be wrapped during the perioperative period to prevent trauma to personnel. Large raptors often require chemical restraint (ketamine, diazepam-ketamine) before induction of inhalation anesthesia.[44] In African vultures, ketamine alone (18–42 mg/kg, IM) produced marked salivation, excitation, and convulsions, inadequate surgical anesthesia, and a prolonged recovery.[52] Strigiformes (owls) are more sensitive than Falconiformes (hawks, eagles, etc.) to ketamine.[44] In addition, barred, long-eared, and short-eared owls require only one-half the dose of great horned, screech, and saw-whet owls.[44]

Ratites (Struthioniformes, Rheiformes, Casuariiformes, Apterygiformes, Tinamiformes)

Ratites (ostriches, emus, rheas, cassowaries) are difficult to restrain and anesthetize. Struggling is common and may be very violent, causing trauma to the animal and veterinarian. Physical restraint of ratites has been reviewed by Jensen.[23] All ratites kick forward, and placing a cover over the eyes facilitates handling of some animals, as does darkness. Keeping the bird's head lowered discourages it from kicking and jumping. Sitting on a restrained ratite interferes with the bird's respiration. At the University of Florida, all ratites are hospitalized in padded stalls. For examination and drug administration the stall is darkened, a hood placed, and the bird compressed against a wall using a covered foam pad. Intramuscular injections are given in the thigh, and IV injections are given into the basilic vein.

It is unsafe to induce anesthesia with inhalant anesthesia alone, except in young or moribund ratites.[8, 22] In the emu, ketamine (25 mg/kg, 0.8 mg/kcal, IM, + 5 mg/kg IV every 10 min) produced adequate restraint for minor procedures.[16] Disadvantages of this regimen include prolonged and difficult recovery and large induction volume. Combination of ketamine with either xylazine or diazepam improves induction and recovery and decreases ketamine dosage. The author has had good success in difficult ostriches using a modification of a technique used at Texas A&M—xylazine 2.2 mg/kg IM, wait 15 minutes, then give ketamine 2 to 4 mg/kg IV to effect, intubate, and maintain with isoflurane in oxygen and N_2O.[8, 22] Xylazine produces sedation and wing drooping. Although zolazepam-tiletamine (4–12 mg/kg IM, 2–8 mg/kg, IV) offers the advantages of rapid smooth induction and small injection volume, recoveries are prolonged and excitatory, and apnea has been observed.[8, 22, 57, 62] Carfentanil ([Wildnil] Wildlife Laboratories, Ft. Collins, CO) and etorphine have been used in ratites, but they produce a period of excitement during induction and occasional apnea.[8, 43] They do offer the advantages of rapid reversal with diprenorphine and small injection volume. Acepromazine and xylazine have been used in combination with these drugs to improve immobilization.[43]

During anesthesia the legs are secured to prevent

injury if the animal should lighten during a procedure. However, it is important that prolonged struggling does not occur with the legs restrained because it may induce exertional rhabdomyolysis. The head and neck should be padded and placed in extension, and abnormal body positions avoided. Arteries are readily identified on the lateral and dorsal tarsometatarsus and ulna. Arteries provide access for direct blood pressure measurement and arterial blood gas analysis during major or prolonged procedures.

Recovery of ratites is a critical period. At the University of Florida, ratites are placed in sternal recumbency, and the head and neck are supported until the bird is able to hold it up itself. The bird is prevented from rising until it is fully awake by a heavy foam pad tented over the top of it. It is important to have a quiet, darkened environment to prevent unnecessary struggling.

Sea and Shorebirds (Charadriiformes, Spheniciformes, Gaviiformes, Podicipediformes, Procellariiformes, Pelecaniformes)

Anesthesia of sea and shorebirds is the same as for most other birds. Some diving birds have closed nares (e.g., gannets), preventing mask induction. The trachea of the pelican is small, and the glottal opening is deep within the pouch. As discussed above, N_2O expands the subcutaneous air cells in some diving birds. Perianesthetic regurgitation is common.

Wading Birds (Ciconiiformes, Gruiformes)

Long-legged wading birds must be carefully restrained to prevent trauma. Large cranes and storks are dangerous to handle and restrain, and eye protection should be worn. Awake intubation and inhalation anesthesia with isoflurane is the anesthetic technique of choice.

Waterfowl (Anseriformes)

As for most avian species, inhalant anesthesia is preferred. However, inhalant anesthesia is reported to be more difficult in waterfowl.[25] Furthermore, longer induction times with both inhalant and injectable anesthetics have been observed, possibly because of large fat deposits.[25] When intubating waterfowl and other long-necked birds it is important to keep the neck and head extended to prevent kinking of the tube against the tracheal wall. Large subcutaneous fat deposits may be present, and they interfere with IM injections.

References

1. Allen JL, Oosterhuis JE: Effect of tolazoline on xylazine-ketamine-induced anesthesia in turkey vultures. J Am Vet Med Assoc 189(9):1011–1012, 1986.
2. Altman RB: A method for reducing exposure of operating room personnel to anesthetic gas. J Am Assoc Avian Vet 6(2):99–101, 1992.
3. Arnall L: Anesthesia and surgery in cage and aviary birds (I). Vet Rec 73:139–142, 1961.
4. Bauck L: Analgesics in avian medicine. Proc Am Assoc Avian Vet, 1990, pp 239–244.
5. Booth NH, McDonald LE (eds): Veterinary Pharmacology and Therapeutics, ed 6. Ames, Iowa State University Press, 1988.
6. Carp NZ, Saputelli J, Halbherr C, et al: A technique for liver biopsy performed in Pekin ducks using anesthesia with Telazol. Lab Anim Sci 41(5):474–475, 1991.
7. Christensen J, Fosse RT, Halvorsen OJ, et al: Comparison of various anesthetic regimens in the domestic fowl. Am J Vet Res 48(11):1649–1657, 1987.
8. Cornick JL, Jensen J: Anesthetic management of ostriches. J Am Vet Med Assoc 200(11):1661–1666, 1992.
9. Degernes LA, Kreeger TJ, Mandsager R, et al: Ketamine-xylazine anesthesia in red-tailed hawks with antagonism by yohimbine. J Wildl Dis 24(2):322–326, 1988.
10. Dorsch JA, Dorsch SE: Understanding Anesthesia Equipment. Construction, Care and Complications, ed 2. Baltimore, Williams & Wilkins, 1984.
11. Fitzgerald G, Cooper JE: Preliminary studies on the use of propofol in the domestic pigeon (*Columba livia*). Res Vet Sci 49:334–338, 1990.
12. Franz DR, Dixon RS: A mask system for halothane anesthesia of guinea pigs. Lab Anim Sci 38(6):743–744, 1988.
13. Goelz MF, Hahn AW, Kelley ST: Effects of halothane and isoflurane on mean arterial blood pressure, heart rate, and respiratory rate in adult Pekin ducks. Am J Vet Res 51(3):458–460, 1990.
14. Greenlees KJ, Clutton RE, Larsen CT, Eyre P: Effect of halothane, isoflurane, and pentobarbital anesthesia on myocardial irritability in chickens. Am J Vet Res 51(5):757–758, 1990.
15. Grono LR: Anesthesia of budgerigars. Aust Vet J 37:463, 1961.
16. Grubb B: Use of ketamine to restrain and anesthetize emus. Vet Med Small Anim Clin 78:247–248, 1983.
17. Harrison GJ, Harrison LR (eds): Clinical Avian Medicine and Surgery. Philadelphia, WB Saunders, 1986.
18. Harrison GJ: Pre-anesthetic fasting recommended. (In My Experience.) J Am Assoc Avian Vet 5(3):126, 1991.
19. Hartsfield SM, McGrath CJ: Anesthetic techniques in poultry. Vet Clin North Am Food Anim Pract 2(3):711–730, 1986.
20. Harvey SC: Hypnotics and sedatives. In Gilman AG, Good-

man LS, Rall TW, et al (eds): The Pharmacological Basis of Therapeutics. New York, Macmillan, 1985, pp 339–371.

21. Heaton JT, Brauth SE: Effects of yohimbine as a reversing agent for ketamine-xylazine anesthesia in budgerigars. Lab Anim Sci 42(1):54–56, 1992.

22. Jensen JM, Johnson JH, Weiner ST: Husbandry and Medical Management of Ostriches, Emus and Rheas. College Station, TX Wildlife and Exotic Animal Teleconsultants, 1992.

23. Jensen JM: Ratite restraint and handling. In Fowler ME (ed): Zoo and Wild Animal Medicine. Current Therapy III. Philadelphia, WB Saunders, 1993, pp 198–200.

24. Jordan FTW, Sanford J, Wright A: Anesthesia in the fowl. J Comp Pathol 70:437–448, 1960.

25. Kaufman E, Pokras M, Sedgwick C: Anesthesia in waterfowl. (In My Experience.) Am Avian Vet Today 2(2):98, 1988.

26. King AS, Payne DC: Normal breathing and the effects of posture in *Gallus domesticus*. J Physiol 174:340–347, 1964.

27. Klide AM: Avian anesthesia. Vet Clin North Am 3(2):175–186, 1973.

28. Kollias GV Jr, McLeish I: Effects of ketamine hydrochloride in red-tailed hawks *(Buteo jamaicensis)*. I. Arterial blood gas and acid base. Comp Biochem Physiol 60:57–59, 1978.

29. Lamberski N: Fluid dynamics of intraosseous fluid administration in birds. J Zoo Wildl Med 23(1):47–54, 1992.

30. Ludders JW, Mitchell GS, Schaefer SL: Minimum anesthetic dose and cardiopulmonary dose response for halothane in chickens. Am J Vet Res 49(6):929–932, 1988.

31. Ludders JW, Rode J, Mitchell GS, et al: Effects of ketamine, xylazine, and a combination of ketamine and xylazine in Pekin ducks. Am J Vet Res 50(2):245–249, 1989.

32. Ludders JW, Rode J, Mitchell GS: Isoflurane anesthesia in sandhill cranes *(Grus canadensis)*: Minimal anesthetic concentration and cardiopulmonary dose-response during spontaneous and controlled breathing. Anesth Analg 68:511–516, 1989.

33. Ludders JW, Mitchell GS, Rode J: Minimal anesthetic concentration and cardiopulmonary dose response of isoflurane in ducks. Vet Surg 19(4):304–307, 1990.

34. Lumb WV, Jones EW: Veterinary Anesthesia. Philadelphia, Lea & Febiger, 1984.

35. Mandelker L: A toxicity study of ketamine HCl in parakeets. Vet Med Small Anim Clin 68(5):487–488, 1973.

36. Matthews NS, Burba DJ, Cornick JL: Premature ventricular contractions and apparent hypertension during anesthesia in an ostrich. J Am Vet Med Assoc 198(11):1959–1961, 1991.

37. Mauderly JL: An anesthetic system for small laboratory animals. Lab Anim Sci 25(3):331–333, 1975.

38. McGrath CJ, Lee JC, Campbell VL: Dose-response anesthetic effects of ketamine in the chicken. Am J Vet Res 45(3):531–534, 1984.

39. Nicholson A, Ilkiw JE: Neuromuscular and cardiovascular effects of atracurium in isoflurane-anesthetized chickens. Am J Vet Res 53(12):2337–2342, 1992.

40. Otto CM, McCall Kaufman G, Crowe DT: Intraosseous infusion of fluids and therapeutics. Compend Cont Educ 11(4):421–431, 1989.

41. Paddleford RR (ed): Manual of Small Animal Anesthesia. New York, Churchill Livingstone, 1988.

42. Quasha AL, Eger EI, Tinker JH: Determination and application of MAC. Anesthesiology 53:315–334, 1980.

43. Raath JP, Quandt SKF, Malan JH: Ostrich *(Struthio camelus)* immobilisation using carfentanil and xylazine and reversal with yohimbine and naltrexone. J S Afr Vet Assoc 63(4):138–140, 1992.

44. Redig PT, Duke GE: Intravenously administered ketamine HCl and diazepam for anesthesia of raptors. J Am Vet Med Assoc 169(9):886–888, 1976.

45. Redig PT, Larson AA, Duke GE: Response of great horned owls given the optical isomers of ketamine. Am J Vet Res 45(1):125–127, 1984.

46. Reynold WT: Unusual anesthetic complication in a pelican. Vet Rec 113:204, 1983.

47. Ritchie BW, Otto CM, Latimer KS, Crowe DT: A technique of intraosseous cannulation for intravenous therapy in birds. Compend Cont Educ 12(1):55–58, 1990.

48. Robello CD, Crowe DT Jr: Cardiopulmonary resuscitation: Current recommendations. Vet Clin North Am Small Anim Pract 19(6):1127–1149, 1989.

49. Rode JA, Bartholow S, Ludders JW: Ventilation through an air sac cannula during tracheal obstruction in ducks. J Am Assoc Avian Vet 4(2):98–101, 1990.

50. Rosskopf WJ, Woerpel RW: Abdominal air sac breathing tube placement in psittacine birds and raptors, its use as an emergency airway in cases of tracheal obstruction. Proc Am Assoc Avian Vet, 1990, 215–217.

51. Salerno A, Van Tienhoven A: The effect of ketamine on heart rate, respiratory rate and EEG of white leghorn hens. Comp Biochem Physiol 55:69–75, 1976.

52. Samour JH, Jones DM, Knight JA, et al: Comparative studies of the use of some injectable anaesthetic agents in birds. Vet Rec 115:6–11, 1984.

53. Schmidt-Nielsen K: Scaling. Why Is Animal Size So Important? New York, Cambridge University Press, 1984.

54. Sedgwick C, Pokras M, Kaufman G: Metabolic scaling: Using estimated energy costs to extrapolate drug doses between different species and different individuals of diverse body sizes. Proc Am Assoc Zoo Vet, 1990, pp 249–254.

55. Sedgwick C: Allometrically scaling the data base for vital sign assessment used in general anesthesia of zoological species. Proc Am Assoc Zoo Vet, 1991, pp 360–369.

56. Short CE, Poznak AV (eds): Animal Pain. New York, Churchill Livingstone, 1992.

57. Stewart JS: Husbandry, Medical and Surgical Management of Ratites: Part II. Proc Am Assoc Zoo Vet, 1989, pp 119–122.

58. Stoelting RK: Pharmacology and Physiology in Anesthetic Practice. Philadelphia, JB Lippincott, 1987.

59. Sturkie PD (ed): Avian Physiology. New York, Springer-Verlag, 1986.

60. Teare JA: Antagonism of xylazine hydrochloride-ketamine hydrochloride immobilization in guineafowl *(Numidia meleagris)* by yohimbine hydrochloride. J Wildl Dis 23(2):301–305, 1987.

61. Valverde A, Honeyman VL, Dyson DH, et al: Determination of a sedative dose and influence of midazolam on cardiopulmonary function in Canada geese. Am J Vet Res 51(7):1071–1074, 1990.

62. Van Heerden J, Keffen RH: A preliminary investigation into the immobilising potential of tiletamine/zolazepam mixture, metomidate, a metomidate and azaperone combination and medetomidine in ostriches *(Struthio camelus)*. J S Afr Vet Assoc 62(3):114–117, 1991.

David M. McCluggage

47

Bandaging

Bandaging includes the application of splinting materials for sprains and fractures as well as conventional and acrylic bandaging of wounds. This chapter also presents a discussion of collars. Anesthesia should be administered during the application of bandages to decrease stress to the patient and to facilitate application.

For this discussion, small birds are those weighing less than 130 g, medium-sized birds are 130 to 600 g, and large birds are more than 600 g. Larger birds such as ratites, eagles, and cranes require very special techniques and are not covered in this chapter.

MATERIALS

Bandage Materials

Nonadhesive bandage materials are preferred to protect the feathers from damage when bandaging is removed. Gauzes that have some stretch (Kling, Johnson & Johnson, Arlington, TX) are often the best choice for the first bandage layer. Because stretch gauze is easily shredded by a bird's beak with fibers becoming dangerously entwined around the body parts, it must always be covered by a layer of nonfibrous material.

Bandages that stick to themselves without the use of adhesives (Vetwrap, 3M Company Animal Care Products, St. Paul, MN) are effective. They are lightweight, often requiring only one layer, and do not shred easily.

Semiocclusive bandages (Tegaderm, 3M Company, St. Paul, MN) have proved to be particularly effective in birds, but they are very thin and trans-

parent, making application difficult. They are supplied as thin rectangular sheets sandwiched between two layers of paper. The rectangular sheets are cut into strips before removing the backing from the sticky side and rolled onto or around the affected appendage while removing the opposite backing paper. Semiocclusive bandages are useful for abrasions and self-induced traumatic lesions. Two or three layers are applied around the appendage. The bandage is left on for several days.

Isobutyl acrylic bandages (Tissue Glu, Ellman International, Inc., Hewlett, NY) can be applied by painting the affected skin with the acrylic material. It is used in areas where other bandages are not appropriate or where large gaps in the skin cannot be sutured. The wounds can be debrided, cleaned, and rebandaged with the acrylic as needed.

Dressings

Water-miscible ointments are applied to the skin to promote healing and prevent infections. Oil-based products should be avoided because they spread through the feathers during preening and inhibit the normal thermoregulatory function of the feathers. Ointments containing corticosteroids must be cautiously applied because of their potential for inducing iatrogenic hyperadrenocorticism.

PELVIC GIRDLE AND HINDLIMB

Tibiotarsal Fractures

Tibiotarsal fractures are perhaps the most common fractures seen. They are often found in smaller birds that have suffered attacks by animals, falls, or another trauma to the leg. Metabolic bone disease also causes pathologic fractures of the tibiotarsal bone.

Following fracture, the bird becomes acutely lame with moderate swelling at the fracture site. The tibiotarsus is an easily palpable long bone. With any of these techniques the tibiotarsal-tarsometatarsal joint in psittacines must be positioned at a 90° angle, with the plantar surface of the tarsometatarsus almost resting on the ground. Radiographs may be indicated to assess location of the fracture and type of fixation needed; however, diagnosis can be made by palpation.

A tape splint (Fig. 47–1) is the repair method of choice in small birds (Table 47–1). Medium and large birds can be splinted using a modified Thomas splint (Fig. 47–2). As an alternative, the tibiotarsus may be splinted using a moldable thermoplastic material (Thermoplast, IMEX Veterinary Inc., Longview, TX). After padding the leg heavily, mold the material around the leg, leaving an opening along one side of the splint (clam shell). Apply a pressure wrap around the splint material, producing an effect similar to that of a Robert Jones bandage.

Tibiotarsal fractures often heal in 3 weeks. The prognosis is usually excellent. The practitioner need not be concerned with the tattered appearance of the splint, which is seen after a couple of weeks.

Tarsometatarsal Fractures

Tarsometatarsal fractures are easily diagnosed by palpation. Many are open fractures because of the lack of muscles surrounding the tarsometatarsus.

Tape splints, when modified by adding a stirrup passing longitudinally down the lateral tarsometatarsus under the foot and back up the medial side, are appropriate for small birds. For medium-sized and larger birds, or if the fracture is severely comminuted, a more rigid support is needed. Thomas splints work well in this situation. Most fractures heal in 3 weeks. Open fractures and comminuted fractures must be given a guarded prognosis.

Digital Fractures

Psittacine and passerine birds have four digits with from two to five phalanges, depending on the digit. Ball splints have been used to treat digital fractures, but "snowshoe splints" appear to be more effective. Moldable plastics are cut to approximate the shape

Figure 47–1

(A) A tape splint is used for fractures of the tibia and proximal metatarsus. The tape is wrapped around the bird's leg using three to four layers while tension is applied to the leg to keep the fractured segments in apposition. The tibiotarsal-tarsometatarsal joint is flexed in the normal standing position for the species, and the tape is crimped with a needle holder or hemostat. *(B)* The tape is crimped as close as possible to the muscles surrounding the tibia. With proper angulation of the tibiotarsal-tarsometatarsal joint, the bird can perch in a normal standing position.

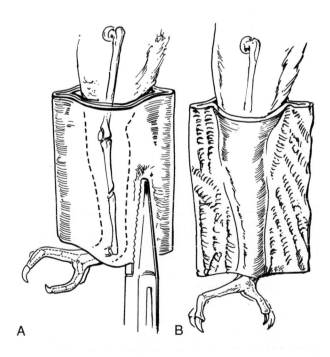

A   B

T a b l e 4 7 – 1

TECHNIQUES OF BANDAGING OR SPLINTING EXTREMITY FRACTURES OR LUXATIONS

Problem	Tape Splint	Figure-of-Eight	Thomas Splint	Spica Splint	Snowshoe	Other Method
Sprain/luxation of the wing		Wing bound to body if lesion at or above elbow				
Tibial fractures	In birds <130 g		In birds >130 g			Robert Jones; moldable plastics
Femoral fractures				May at times work well		Internal fixation best
Tarsometatarsal fractures	Include ankle stirrup; birds <130 g		Best in birds >130 g			
Digital fractures	Tape two toes together				Digit distal to fracture site may necrose	
Radial/ulnar fractures		Synostosis may result				Internal fixation
Carpometacarpal fractures		Effective, but flight often impaired				
Hip luxation				May work but reluxation possible		Surgical fixation

of the foot and are attached to the foot with bandage materials. The toes are wrapped with padding and the "snowshoe" is attached with gauze wraps followed by adhesive bandages. The phalanx distal to the fracture site can sustain necrosis from an avascular condition. Nonunion of the fracture is uncommon, although diminished function may be seen following healing. Tape splints tend to fall off by the time the toe is healed.

Pododermatitis

Pododermatitis (bumblefoot) is an infection of the plantar surface of the foot that can progress to deeper infections, including tendon necrosis and osteomyelitis of the digital bones. Improper husbandry is the major cause of the disease. Malnutrition and hypovitaminosis A are suspected in many cases.[1] Improper perch or floor design also contributes to the disease. Other pathologic conditions, such as *Knemidokoptes* mites, pox virus infections, traumatic injuries, and frostbite, can lead to pododermatitis.

Pododermatitis is first seen as a thinning of the skin of the plantar surface of the foot or hock. Progression to severe dermal thickening, ulcerated and necrotic areas, marked cellulitis, osteomyelitis, and tenosynovitis can lead to loss of part or all of the foot from infection.[2]

Treatment is often difficult, and thus prevention is vital. The goal of treatment is to reduce inflammation and swelling, establish drainage if needed, and provide antibacterial therapy and wound management to allow healing.[3] Halliwell has proposed a classification of raptor bumblefoot into four categories.[4] Redig has detailed a protocol for treating raptor bumblefoot using these four categories.[5]

Radiographs are indicated to determine the severity of infection. All cases require repeated cleaning and soaking in a disinfectant solution.

Birds with mild cases with moderate swelling and no osteomyelitis need nutritional supplementation and modifications to perch design. Antimicrobials may be used but will likely have only a marginal effect in the absence of improved husbandry.

More severe cases need bandaging or surgical debridement followed by bandaging. The goal is to eliminate the infection through drainage and relieve pressure on the plantar surface of the foot to allow healing. Use of dental acrylic shoes[6] appears to be the method of choice in reducing pressure on the foot during healing. The toes are padded, a wire frame with **U**-shaped bends at each toe is fashioned in a circular mode around the toes, and the wire and toes are encased in the acrylic. Once completed, there is a ring of acrylic that prevents the plantar surface of the foot from contacting the ground. The acrylic splint is left on the foot for 2 weeks. Frequent debridement is often needed for

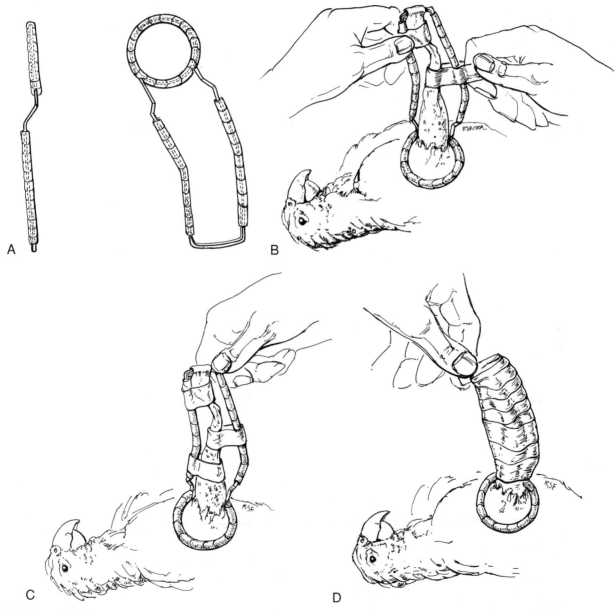

Figure 47-2

Modified Thomas splint. *(A)* The wire is bent, shaped, and padded to conform with the bird's leg. *(B and C)* The leg is placed through the loop of the splint. The distal end of the foot is transfixed to the splint. Gauze or tape is wrapped around the leg to maintain proper alignment of the fracture fragments. *(D)* Tape or Vetrap is placed around the splint, covering the leg.

the most severe lesions. Once healed, the foot is very susceptible to reinjury for 2 or more months. Carefully pad the perches for 26 to 28 weeks after bandage removal.

Dislocation of the Hip

Diagnosis of hip luxation is usually achieved by palpation of the affected leg. Birds are presented with acute, severe lameness or total inability to use the involved leg. Partial return to normal function can occur over a period of time.

Following reduction of a coxofemoral luxation, a spica splint should be applied to the leg for 3 weeks. If the joint again sustains luxation following removal of the splint, the prognosis is poor. A surgical method for repair has been described.[7]

THORACIC GIRDLE AND WING

Fractures of the Wing

Trauma from impact injuries, wing entrapment in cage bars and toys, and gunshot wounds often leads to fractures of the wing. The patient is always presented with a dropped wing. The fractures can usually be diagnosed through palpation. Radiographs are indicated to assess severity of fracture and method of repair.

Many fractures heal well after treatment with external coaptation, with return to full function (see Table 47–1). The wing is especially amenable to splinting because the body provides an accurate mold allowing for healing to take place in a physiologically normal position.[8] Because of the complications inherent in internal fixation and the fact that a return to full flight is often not essential for cage and aviary birds, many wing fractures are best managed by the application of splints.

Fractures for which a good prognosis[9] can be anticipated employing external coaptation include those of the (1) coracoid, scapula, furcula; (2) humerus (proximal, closed); (3) radius (midshaft to distal, closed or open); (4) ulna (proximal to distal, closed); (5) radius and ulna (midshaft to distal, closed); and (6) carpometacarpus (closed).

Figure-of-Eight Bandage Splint

A figure-of-eight splint provides adequate stabilization for fractures of the radius and ulna, carpometacarpus, and digits. It is also effective for some fractures of the pectoral girdle and humerus. When used in conjunction with a body wrap, it can be effective as a support for internal fixation of wing fractures.

With the wing folded against the body in a normal flexed position, the bandage is applied in a figure-of-eight pattern (Fig. 47–3). Start by wrapping gauze around the ventral aspect of the humerus and over the dorsal aspect of the wing. Then pass the gauze over and around the carpus, and then back across the dorsum of the wing, and finally back under the humerus. An excessively bulky bandage is a detriment. Only two layers of bandage material are used, first a gauze wrap followed by a nonadhesive self-adhering bandage.

With fractures of the humerus or shoulder girdle, the wing needs to be secured against the body. The opposite wing is always left free. Fractures distal to the humeroulnar joint should not have the wing bound to the body. Leaving the wing free allows for better and more comfortable bandaging.

WOUND REPAIR

Dog and Cat Scratch Wounds

Dog and cat scratches or bites must be vigorously treated for infection. All dog- and cat-induced wounds, regardless of severity, should be treated as an emergency. Bacteria, especially *Pasteurella* species,[10] commonly infect these wounds, causing a potentially fatal bacterial septicemia. Small wounds should not be sutured. Deep puncture wounds should be left open to drain and granulate because of their potential for infections. Larger lacerations that are only a few hours old can be vigorously flushed with chlorhexidine solutions and sutured closed. Older wounds should be debrided, cleaned, and bandaged. Rebandaging and debriding twice daily can prepare an infected wound for closure in a few days.

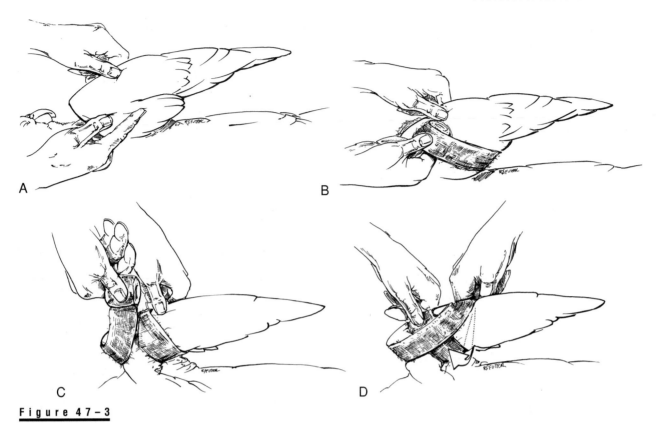

Figure 47-3

A figure-of-eight bandage splint. *(A)* The wing is held in its normal flexed position. *(B)* Gauze is wrapped around the ventral aspect of the humerus and brought over the dorsal aspect of the wing. *(C)* The gauze is then wrapped over the humero-radioulnar joint and around the carpus. *(D)* The gauze is then brought under the wing and wrapped back over the dorsum and under the humerus.

Wounds of the Head and Eye

The etiology of these lesions is usually trauma, including hitting ceiling fans, getting the head caught in the cage or toys, and mutilation from cage mates. Wounds can be bandaged by fashioning a hood bandage over the head with a nonstick dressing underneath (Telfa Pads, 3M Corp., St. Paul, MN).

Wing Tip Trauma

Wing tip trauma is most commonly seen in the cockatiel from repeated hitting of the wing on hard surfaces. This is most frequently observed in birds that have wing trims and those that chew off their primary flight feathers. Damaged primary flight feathers can be plucked, allowing new feathers to grow in safely while the bird is in a body shirt.

Collars

Before applying a collar, the patient should be tested for the presence of subclinical illness (e.g., by complete blood count, radiographs) and observed closely following application. This author always observes the bird for at least 6 hours after application to determine proper fit and to see whether the bird adapts to the presence of the collar. Collars are often very stressful for a bird and should not be applied frivolously. There are three types of collars available: Elizabethan collars, modified reversed Elizabethan collars, and tube collars.

Tube Collar

A tube collar is a cylindrical splint that is padded and placed around the neck, maintaining the neck in extension. By keeping the bird from bending its

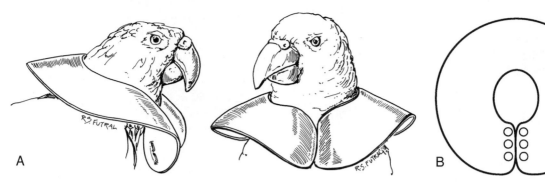

Figure 47 – 4

(A and B) A modified and reversed Elizabethan cervical collar is placed around the neck; the ends of the collar are bent under and fastened with a staple.

head, it prevents the bird from biting at its body. It can be fashioned out of radiograph film. Another method is to cut an appropriately sized syringe case in a spiral shape that can then be pulled open to place around the neck and allowed to gently spring back into shape, while encircling the neck. The tube collar looks very uncomfortable to the owner and decreases the movement of the neck for eating and drinking. If improperly fit, the neck can be extended excessively, causing severe pain and deformity. Some self-mutilation problems are best handled with a tube collar.

Modified and Reversed Elizabethan Collar

In the author's experience, a modified and reversed Elizabethan collar is effective in most situations. They are comfortable to wear, allow freedom of movement, and appear reasonably humane to the owner.

The best materials to construct a collar are semi-rigid clear plastic and vinyl. Many hardware stores carry appropriate thicknesses. Because this material is clear, the bird can see its body and know where to place its feet. Used radiograph film can also be employed to construct the collar. Larger birds can have two or more layers glued together before cutting the collar. Once formed, the collar can be secured using staples. With screw-type rivets as closures, the owner can easily remove and reattach the collar.

The size of the collar varies significantly based on the size of the bird and parts of the body needing

protection. The collar must be particularly long when its purpose is to preclude self-mutilation of the feet. A common error when constructing the collar is to cut the neck hole too large; it should be barely large enough to comfortably fit around the neck (including room for a thin layer of padding). The collar is placed in a conical shape spreading down around the bird's shoulders, with two ends bent under and stapled (Fig. 47–4).

A rigid plastic collar that is a combination of the tube collar and the Elizabethan collar (Avian Restraint Collar, Veterinary Specialty Products, Inc.,

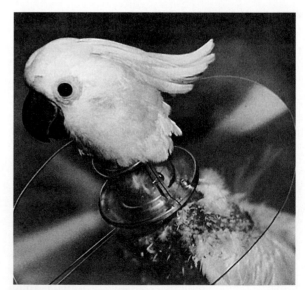

Figure 47 – 5

An avian restraint collar and extension on a sulfur-crested cockatoo.

Boca Raton, FL) (Fig. 47–5) is commercially available. It has proved to be particularly effective and atraumatic to the patient and is the author's preference.

References

1. Harrison GJ, Harrison L, Disorders of the integument. In Harrison GJ, Harrison LR (eds): Clinical Avian Medicine and Surgery. Philadelphia, WB Saunders, 1986, pp 362–375.
2. McCluggage DM: Surgery of the integument. Semin Avian Exotic Pet Med 2(2):76–82, 1993.
3. Degernes LA, Talbot BJ, Mueller LR: Raptor foot care. J Assoc Avian Vets 4(2):93–95, 1990.
4. Halliwell WH: Bumblefoot infections in birds of prey. J Zoo Anim Med 6(4):8–10, 1975.
5. Redig PT: Treatment of bumblefoot and the management of aspergillosis and various other problems commonly seen in raptors. Proc 1st Intl Conf Zoo Avian Med, Hawaii, 1987, pp 309–321.
6. Hess RE Jr: The use of dental acrylic shoes for the treatment of bumblefoot. Proc Assoc Avian Vet, Nashville, 1993, pp 135–137.
7. Martin HD, Kabler R, Sealing L: The avian coxofemoral joint: A review of regional anatomy and report of an open-reduction technique for repair of a coxofemoral luxation. J Assoc Avian Vet 1(1):22–30, 1989.
8. Ward FP: Repair of wing fractures in a red-shouldered hawk. Vet Med/Small Anim Clin 65(6):550–552, 1970.
9. Redig PT: Evaluation and nonsurgical management of fractures. In Harrison GJ (ed): Clinical Avian Medicine and Surgery. Philadelphia, WB Saunders, 1986, pp 382–383.
10. Harrison GJ, Woerpel RW, Rosskopf WJ, et al: Symptomatic therapy and emergency medicine. In Harrison GJ, Harrison LR (eds): Clinical Avian Medicine and Surgery. Philadelphia, WB Saunders, 1986, pp 362–375.

Emergency Medicine

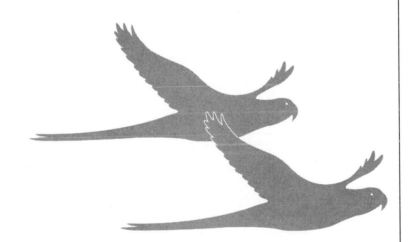

Jeffrey R. Jenkins

48

Avian Critical Care and Emergency Medicine

Much of avian medicine is emergency medicine because of the rapid metabolism of birds and their ability to "hide" symptoms. This ability or behavior is thought to be a preservation response allowing the bird to compensate for disease. As with all creatures, a crisis arises when the animal can no longer compensate for illness, and signs of a problem become evident. Critically ill birds are often presented in an advanced state of decompensation. Successful treatment depends on the orchestration of supportive care, diagnosis, and treatment. Often the diagnosis lies in the signalment. Neonates reach a state of decompensation much earlier than adults and suffer from a larger variety of management-related problems.

The majority of traumatic incidents seen in pet birds involve interactions between cage mates or the immediate environment (caging). Rarely are pet birds subjected to vehicular trauma.[1] Wild birds are frequently presented with traumatic injuries ranging from gunshots and electrocution to wounds inflicted by predators and prey.

As with all animals, including humans, it is important to initiate therapy of the traumatized avian patient within the "golden period." The golden period is defined as the period of time following the injury in which appropriate therapy will result in the most satisfactory outcome (Fig. 48–1). Not only survival but also return to normal function are the goals.[2] This time period varies, and may span only a few hours in birds with serious injuries. Adequate preparation is important in emergency situations. Equipment and drugs should be prepared and accessible and a triage of treatment should be formulated to deal with critical cases.

Preparation for the avian emergency begins with personnel, including the veterinarian, followed by equipment, supplies, and facility. Preparation of the veterinarian begins in education and an understanding of physiology, pathophysiology, and pharmacology. The physiologic changes pertaining to avian critical care are reviewed in this chapter, but a deeper knowledge will greatly aid the clinician. In addition, a knowledge of social and behavioral habits of the avian patient will be of great benefit.

Preparation of hospital personnel also begins in training, and involves the establishment of a system

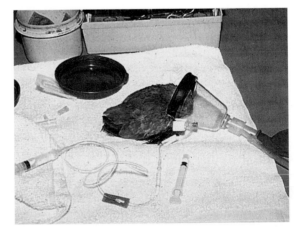

Figure 48-1

An immature red-winged parrot *(Aprosmictus erythropterus erythropterus)* attacked by a dog is given oxygen by face mask while fluids are administered through an intraosseous catheter. It is important to initiate therapy of the traumatized avian patient within the "golden period" or the period of time following the injury in which appropriate therapy will result in the most satisfactory outcome. Not only survival but also return to normal function are goals of treatment.

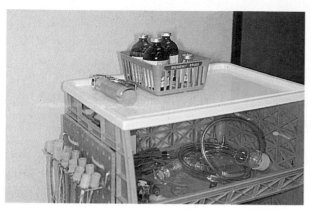

Figure 48–2

Emergency drugs, supplies, and equipment should be preassembled in a central location known to all hospital staff. Treatment rooms or anesthesia induction areas are often used for emergency supplies, because these are areas where much of the required equipment and therapeutics are used during planned procedures.

of triage and hospital standard operating procedures for emergency and critical situations. In this chapter, triage criteria and standard operating procedures for a number of emergency situations are reviewed. Triage techniques and standard operating procedures should be updated periodically. Emergency drugs, supplies, and equipment should be preassembled in a central location known to all hospital staff (Fig. 48–2). Items should be maintained and inventoried regularly. Equipment operation should be tested at regular intervals, especially those items not used on a daily basis. Treatment or anesthesia induction areas are often storage sites for emergency supplies, because these are areas where much of the required equipment and therapeutics are used.

PHYSIOLOGY OF AVIAN CRITICAL CARE

Metabolic Rate

The rate that disease progresses in an animal is often proportional to the animal's metabolic rate. The metabolic rate of nonpasserine birds, including psittacines, ratites, and pigeons, is proportionally the same as eutherian mammals; however, the size of the average avian patient is significantly smaller than that of the average mammalian patient. Passer-

ine birds are thought to have a metabolic rate twice that of mammals of equal size.

Body Fluids, Hypovolemia (Blood Loss and Hemorrhage), and Hypotension

Research on the fluid compartment of birds shows that it is similar in many ways to that of mammals. The fluid component of birds is divided into intracellular and extracellular compartments. The total liquid volume of birds has been calculated to be approximately 60% of the (adult) body weight. This value varies from species to species. It appears to be inversely proportional to water turnover (metabolic rate, drinking rate, and evaporation). The liquid content of males and young animals is slightly more than that of females and older animals; this is because of their lower fat content. The extracellular compartment is composed of plasma and interstitial fluids. Extracellular water is reported to be between 17.5% and 23.9%.[3] As with total water content, extracellular water varies with sex and age and is proportional to total body water. Blood volume (cells and plasma) measured in chickens ranges between 4.4% and 8.3% of body weight.[3] It is higher in young birds (6.6–8.3%) than in adults (4.4–5.2%), and is also higher at high elevations or in low oxygen conditions. Table 48–1 shows some known blood volume values. Avian blood is more viscous than mammalian blood at a given hematocrit because of the lower rate of deformity of nucleated cells. Birds make up for this greater viscosity with greater capillary density. The specific gravity of avian blood is most influenced by plasma proteins, although other substances play a role. Osmotic pressure of birds is lower than that of mammals. This is because of the low level of albumins in

Table 48–1

BLOOD VOLUME VALUES

Species	Blood Volume (Percent Body Weight)
Pheasant	4.8
Turkey	7.8
Pigeon	9.2
Red-tailed hawk	6.2
Great horned owl	6.4
Ostrich	4.5

birds, which have a greater effect on osmotic pressure than globulins.[3]

The control of erythropoiesis in birds differs from that in mammals. Control is primarily hormonal. Erythropoietin and erythropoiesis-stimulating factor are the primary hormones involved. Avian erythropoietin is stimulated by hypoxia and suppressed by induced polycythemia. Erythropoiesis is also stimulated by androgens and adrenal cortical hormones. The avian erythrocyte (RBC) has a short life span (coturnix quail 33–35 days, pigeons 35–45 days, ducks 42 days) compared with that of mammals (humans 90–120 days, rats 45–50 days, and mice 20–30 days). The life span of the avian RBC is proportional to the bird's metabolic rate.[3]

Birds react to hypovolemia and hypotension in much the same manner as other animals. Reduced blood pressure causes an increase in precapillary resistance. This is associated with an increase in catecholamines, primarily norepinephrine. This change (in the chicken) is not associated with a carotid sinus baroreceptor as it is in mammals. Birds tolerate blood loss better than most mammals. In a study of animals bled at a rate of 1% body weight per hour, mammals and nonflying avian species were outperformed by flying birds. Some pigeons survived removal of blood equal to 9% of their body weight (equal to their total blood volume) before significant mortality occurred.[4] This illustrates the degree that fluids move from the interstitial space into the circulation in birds. The movement of these fluids results in hemodilution. Decreases in hematocrit, hemoglobin, and plasma proteins affect osmolarity and osmotic pressure.

Arginine vasotocin (AVT), the avian antidiuretic hormone (ADH), is released in response to low blood pressure. AVT has been shown to cause a rise of free fatty acids and growth hormone. It does not cause vasoconstriction or increased precapillary resistance as does ADH in mammals. Free fatty acids, which are the major source of energy for avian tissues, are similarly stimulated by catecholamines. There is little breakdown of adipose tissue for this purpose. During fasting, nearly 90% of the mobilized lipids are stored in the liver. Paradoxically, the liver converts free fatty acids into keto-acids rather than triglycerides. Whether this is the result of a fatty acid overload or is a preferred metabolic pathway is yet to be determined. Prostaglandins, which play an important role in hemorrhage in mammals, have not been shown to be involved in the bird's (e.g., chicken's) reaction to hypovolemia or hypotension.[5]

Avian renal function decreases (oliguria) or stops (anuria) with hypovolemia and hypotension. This change is thought to be the result of the renin-angiotensin system, aldosterone, and AVT. Increased AVT levels result in increased urine osmolality, decreased urine volume, and decreased water clearance. This change is caused by a change in collecting duct permeability and a drop in the number of reptilian-type nephrons filtering urine, which decreases the volume flowing through collection ducts. Reabsorption occurs mostly in the cloaca of birds. Cloacal stasis, seen in severely ill birds, may be a mechanism for storing and reabsorbing water. Decreased urine production helps expand blood volume.

Hypovolemia and hypotension may result in acidosis in birds. Poor oxygenation can be assumed to occur, but lactic acidosis because of the anaerobic formation of lactate from pyruvate does not occur, glycogen stores are not depleted, and lipolysis does not take place. In critically ill patients, acidosis may result as a consequence of free fatty acids' use of energy, rather than incomplete lipid oxygenation or anaerobic formation of lactate resulting from the poor oxygenation of tissues. As with mammals, acid-base levels affect avian respiration and renal function. Carbon dioxide (CO_2) and oxygen (O_2) levels influence chemoreceptors in carotid bodies and other locations. Suppressing these hypoxic drives results in hypoventilation and acidosis. Therapy may cause a decrease in blood pH (acidemia) in the critically ill patient. An abrupt change causes cardiac dysrhythmias, leading to decreased cardiac output or failure. Decreased cardiac output may exaggerate the acidemic state. Because CO_2 crosses the blood-brain barrier more rapidly than bicarbonate, a subsequent decrease in cerebrospinal fluid pH results from acidemia, depressing the central nervous system. Treatment of acid-base imbalance is based on returning circulation, respiration, and energy balance to normal. Details of treatment are covered later.

Like mammals, birds use volume control mechanisms to preserve organ function in response to hypovolemia. After the initial response these mechanisms may have a deleterious effect. Compensative mechanisms are often inadequate, and both peripheral and central blood flow may be insufficient. Poor oxygen delivery to peripheral organs causes cellular hypoxia, a shift to anaerobic metabolism, or ischemic injury, resulting in the release of potentially toxic substances. Poor blood flow perpetuates the tissue injury. Shock, as it is defined in mammals, does not occur in birds; birds do not develop lactic acidosis caused by cellular hypoxia that progresses to peripheral circulatory failure and the pooling of blood in terminal circulatory beds in small vessels. General failure of the circulation does occur, however, because of hypovolemia (hypovolemic shock) and heart failure (cardiogenic shock), and is thought to occur because of sepsis (septic shock). It is the pathogenesis at the tissue and cellular level that appears to differ. Continued clinical research into hemorrhage, hypovolemia, and hypotension, and their effects in birds on a cellular level, is needed, as is research on the role of catecholamines, glucocorticosteroids, and free fatty acids in the treatment of shock in birds.

Acid-base Balance

Changes in acid-base levels affect avian respiration and renal function, as they do in other animals. CO_2 and O_2 concentrations influence chemoreceptors in carotid bodies and other locations. Suppressing this hypoxic drive results in hypoventilation and acidosis. Some species are resistant to the effects of hypoxia, including barr-headed geese and rheas, which make no response to hypoxia, and burrowing owls, which are resistant to the effects of both hypoxia and hypercapnia.[6] This resistance may prevent hyperventilation in situations when the bird will not benefit from an increased respiratory rate. Hydrogen ion excretion occurs in superficial cortical collecting ducts in the avian kidney. The mechanism is not well defined. This differs from mammals, where hydrogen ion excretion occurs in the proximal tubules. Bicarbonate transport is similarly not well studied or understood in birds; however, birds can produce urine that is less acid than plasma.

Coagulation and Hemostasis

The basic physiology of coagulation in birds is similar to that of mammals. When a vessel is injured,

a cascade of events takes place—vasoconstriction occurs, a plug is formed by thrombocytes, and soluble plasma proteins are transformed from fibrinogen to fibrin to form a stable clot. This process is mediated by thrombin, which also activates factor X (fibrin stabilizing factor). Avian thrombin is derived from prothrombin and catalyzed by calcium (Ca^{++}) ions. An intrinsic pathway exists but plays a minor role. Coagulation, therefore, depends especially on the extrinsic clotting system, and involves the release of tissue thromboplastin.

Vitamin K is essential for normal blood coagulation in birds, as it is in mammals. It is supplied by diet and bacterial synthesis (lower intestinal tract); however, bacterial synthesis alone will not meet the bird's needs. Therefore, birds depend on exogenous sources of vitamin K. Vitamin K plays a vital role in the synthesis of prothrombin and accessory factors VII, IX, and X, where it acts as a cofactor in post-ribosomal protein modification that allows proteins to participate in a specific protein-Ca^{++}-phospholipid interaction. Birds have been shown to be less sensitive to coumarin-type anticoagulants than mammals.[3] This may be the result of low concentrations of factor VII. Vitamin K antagonist effects may be overcome by feeding vitamin K. Daily dietary requirements are normally less than 1 mg/kg.

Thermoregulation

Resting thermoneutral temperatures vary with species between 38.1°C (emu) and 42°C (pigeon) (100.6°F and 107.9°F).[7] Heat balance determines body temperature. Heat produced in deep-seated organs is transferred to skin and mucous membranes by conduction and vascular convection. The conduction of heat through tissues is significantly affected by fat because of fat's lower rate of conduction. With the exception of some sea birds and waterfowl, fat plays a small role in birds because of its location deep in the abdomen.

Vascular convection is the most important means of heat transfer in thermoneutral situations when there is normal circulation to the skin of the bird. It is reduced in situations when the bird is cold or in a state of "shock" resulting in reduced blood flow to the skin from precapillary vasoconstriction. Heat is lost at a rate proportional to the ratio of surface area to volume. Small birds face an enormous task in maintaining their body temperature, especially in a cold environment.

Nonevaporative and evaporative heat loss occurs in birds, as with other animals. Nonevaporative heat loss consists of radiation, convection, and conduction of heat. *Radiation* is the transfer of heat in the form of electromagnetic waves from the surface of the bird to the surfaces in the environment that are lower in temperature than that of the bird. Heat gain by radiation also occurs. Feathers, especially the color of the plumage, may affect the "emissivity" or the ability of the surface of the bird to radiate heat. Air is not involved in this process. *Convection* involves the actual movement of molecules on the air. Air in contact with the surface of the bird takes energy from the bird and is warmed. This causes the air to become less dense and rise, being replaced by cooler, denser air. More heat is lost if air is moving past the bird or if the bird is moving through the air. *Conduction* involves the transfer of energy from molecule to molecule, but unlike convection there is no translocation of molecules. Conduction is greatest at points where the bird contacts surfaces with a high conductive index, such as metal. Respiratory neural heat loss consists of air warmed by convection and conduction in the upper respiratory tract. Much of this heat is recovered when it is exhaled.

The bird's plumage provides an effective barrier to heat loss. Body contour and down feathers trap air and allow little convective movement to occur. Fluffing feathers increases insulation and decreases thermal conductance. The thin covering of oil and sebaceous secretions, originating from the skin and uropygial gland,[7] on the surface of feathers makes them resistant to wetting and reduces conduction. Evaporative heat loss occurs when moisture evaporates from skin or mucous membranes. It is important because it is the only way the bird may lose heat when air temperature equals body temperature. *Cutaneous evaporation* is limited by the lack of sweat glands in avian skin. Even so, cutaneous water loss occurs and may be greater than respiratory evaporation.

Respiratory evaporation, in the form of panting, is the most important thermoregulation mechanism of birds. The extensive air sac system allows birds the means to direct increased ventilation during panting to parts of the respiratory tract that are not involved with the exchange of gas between blood and air. The amount of air that a bird may dissipate by panting is considerable, in some species equal to all the heat they produce, the cooling occurring mainly from the upper respiratory tract. Control of body temperature involves peripheral temperature receptors and temperature-sensitive neurons in the central nervous system. Shivering, panting, and behavioral responses to changes in temperature are regulated by the anterior hypothalamus-preoptic region. Birds develop a fever in response to some bacterial infections and respond to antipyretic drugs such as acetylsalicylic acid (aspirin) with reduction of fever. Fever may be induced by the injection of prostaglandin E_1 in pigeons. These observations suggest that the febrile response of birds is similar to that of mammals.[8]

Thermal support of the critically ill avian patient is essential. Supportive environments and treatment modalities that minimize heat loss should be used. Body temperature may be profoundly affected by the metabolic failure associated with critical illnesses. Heat balance is affected both by decreased production and increased loss. Some treatment techniques may contribute to heat loss. A bird that is unable to stand may lose profound amounts of heat by conduction if it is in contact with an unheated surface. Cleansing a wound with cold liquid or with alcohol may contribute to heat lost by conduction and evaporation, respectively. Unpublished studies in the author's practice have shown that a subcutaneous injection of crystalloid fluids given to a budgerigar at room temperature (21°C, 70°F), and in a volume equal to 3% of body weight, resulted in a drop of core temperature of 2°C (3.6°F).

EQUIPMENT AND INSTRUMENTATION

The specialized equipment used in avian critical care and emergency medicine is sufficiently important to warrant discussion. The following is a discussion of principles, not an endorsement of a specific product. Often several brands or manufactures of a product meet the recommendations.

Incubator, Baby Warmer, or Intensive Care Unit Cage

Thermal support is of utmost importance to the critically ill patient. The goal is to create an environmental temperature that is equal to or just below the normal body temperature of the patient, thereby eliminating heat loss. The heat should be supplied by conduction, convection, and radiation to minimize heat lost by these routes. The cage or chamber should have a heated floor and at least one heated wall. The heated surfaces supply heat by radiation and conduction, as well as through currents of warm air that heat the patient by convection as they rise from the floor and wall. A heated wall supplies a warm surface against which the bird may lean or huddle. The heated wall also creates a temperature gradient, warmer next to the wall and cooler away from it.

It is also important to humidify the air in the chamber to reduce heat lost by evaporation. An inexpensive chamber may be created by placing a circulating warm water blanket or heating pad under a glass or Plexiglas aquarium and up one side (Fig. 48–3). A small vessel of water or a moist cloth placed where it will not wet the patient supplies humidity. A commercial incubator is available with a jacket of water that extends under the floor of the patient chamber and up one side, which is heated with a submersible heater (Fig. 48–4). Humidity is supplied by a hole from the water compartment into the top of the animal chamber (Aqua-Brooder, D&M Bird Farm, San Diego, CA).

Incubators to avoid are those that have cold floors such as the outmoded human infant warmers and forced air units that supply heat only by con-

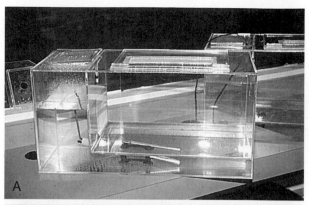

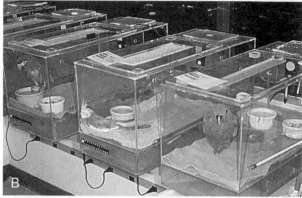

Figure 48–4

(A, B) An inexpensive commercial incubator (Aqua-Brooder, D&M Bird Farm, San Diego) is available with a jacket of water that extends under the floor of the patient chamber and up one side, which is heated with a submersible heater. Humidity is supplied by a hole from the water compartment into the top of the animal chamber. The low cost, ease of sterilizing, and small size of this incubator make it the favorite of the author.

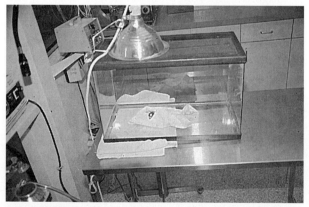

Figure 48–3

An incubator may be made by placing a heating pad under a glass or plexiglass aquarium illuminated by a 30- to 60-watt light above. Heat should be supplied by conduction, convection, and radiation to minimize heat lost by these routes.

vective currents. Controls should be easy to use and understand. The unit should have safety features that prevent or warn of overheating and failure, and the temperature should be easily monitored. Feedback units that are controlled by the body temperature of the animal in the unit, such as those used for laboratory animals (Harvard Apparatus, South Natick, MA), are impractical with most bird species when the animal is conscious. However, the units can be used for birds recovering from anesthesia or birds that are moribund. A portion of the unit should be transparent to facilitate observation of the patient. All parts of the unit must be easily cleaned and sterilized.

Many diseases, such as psittacine beak and feather disease, are transmitted by feather dust and respiratory secretions. If the unit is heated by forced or circulated air, it may require gas sterilization to ensure that it does not act as a fomite in disease spread.

The unit also should be oxygen-compatible. Electrical components that are not explosion-proof or designed to be used with oxygen are dangerous not only to the patient but also to personnel. A 40% O_2 saturation level is recommended for most patients with emergency or critical illnesses when in a chamber or incubator.

Parenteral Fluid Incubator and Fluid Warming Devices

An incubator to warm parenteral fluids ensures that they are available at body temperature at the time that they are needed (Fig. 48–5). A small microbiologic incubator has been used for this purpose in the author's practice for several years. The incubator should be large enough to hold various sizes of fluid bags or bottles. It must be easily cleaned and sterilized. Once opened, the fluid containers should be discarded if there is any chance that the sterile seal has been violated or if the fluids have been contaminated. Bacterial contaminants proliferate at a much higher rate at body temperature than at room temperature. Devices are available to keep

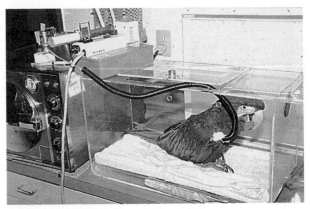

Figure 48–6

Green-winged macaw *(Ara chloroptera)* receiving fluids administered by a Razel syringe pump through an intraosseous catheter. The black "split loom" tubing prevents the bird from damaging the IV tubing.

fluids warm while they are being administered. Insulated "jackets" with chemical heating pads (Safe and Warm Intra-Therm and Reusable Instant Heat, Safe and Warm Incorporated, Boulder City, NV) or the heating pads alone may be used to wrap the syringe on a syringe pump.

Syringe and Infusion Pumps

The ability to administer intravenous or intraosseous fluids to a small patient over an extended period of time depends on equipment that allows a very low rate of administration along with a high degree of safety and accuracy. Intravenous infusion pumps work well for infusion rates higher than 60 to 100 ml/hour. Syringe pumps allow infusion rates much lower than those from infusion pumps (Fig. 48–6). It is possible to use a syringe pump to administer maintenance fluids to a budgerigar at 0.006 to 0.10 ml/hour through an intraosseous catheter.

Anesthesia Equipment

Anesthesia is discussed in Chapter 46; however, a brief mention of anesthetic equipment is important here. In some emergency and critical care situations it is preferable to use anesthesia rather than restraint to complete a procedure. Isoflurane is currently the anesthetic agent of choice because of its rapid

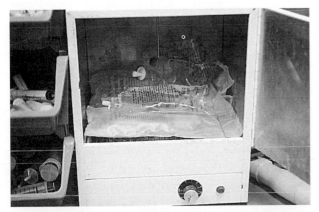

Figure 48–5

An incubator to warm parenteral fluids ensures that they are available at body temperature at the time when they are needed. A small microbiologic incubator has been used for this purpose in the author's practice for several years. The incubator should be large enough to hold several fluid bags or containers. It must be easily cleaned and sterilized.

Table 48-2

EQUIPMENT FOR AVIAN CRITICAL CARE

Isoflurane anesthesia machine (see text)	Blood filters, Hemonate (Fig. 48–10)
Ambu bag; those for neonates work better than those made for adult humans	Ball-tipped metal feeding needles (10–18 gauge) (Fig. 48–11)
Nebulizer (ultrasonic or disposable) (Fig. 48–7)	Red-rubber feeding tubes (3.5–14 Fr)
Cole and cuffed endotracheal tubes and small tubes made from feeding tubes, urinary catheters to size 3.5 Fr, modified to fit an endotracheal adaptor to be used as endotracheal tubes for tiny patients (Fig. 48–8)	Ball-tipped metal feeding needles (10–18 gauge)
Face masks for anesthetic induction	Parrot mouth speculums (Lafeber Co., Odell, Ill), or gauze for loops
Presterilized tubes for use as air sac (abdominal) airways	Bandage materials cut into small sizes, 0.25- to 1-inch widths (Fig. 48–12)
Cole endotracheal tubes, feeding tubes, etc.	Materials for collection of laboratory samples
Radiosurgical unit	Culturettes
Electrocardiography equipment	Mini-tip culturettes
Oscilloscope monitor	Microhematocrit tubes
Indirect blood pressure monitoring equipment, Doppler flow meter (see text)	Slides and cover slips
Rigid endoscopy equipment	Microtainers (Fig. 48–13)
Flexible endoscopy equipment	Incubators for various sized birds (see text)
Electronic thermometer (70–110°F)	Circulating warm-water blanket
Variety of syringes and small needles (including insulin syringes)	Heat lamps
Variety of spinal needles (18–25 gauge) (Fig. 48–9)	Fluid warming chamber
Small butterfly catheters (22–25 gauge) (Fig. 48–10)	Stethoscope with small (pediatric or infant) sized diaphragm and bell
Microdrip IV administration sets, 30-inch extension sets, extension set with Ts, and male adapter plugs (short)	Gram scale (see text)
Anticoagulant dextrose (ACD) buffer solution	Towels and washcloths for restraint
	Diagonal wire-cutting tool with fine sharp tip, two pairs of small Vice Grip pliers, and 18-inch bolt cutters to remove leg bands (Fig. 48–14)

induction and recovery times, lack of sensitization of the myocardium, and low toxicity. A newer agent, desflurane, may exceed the benefits of isoflurane; however, it may be some time before it is used in veterinary clinics and hospitals. Older agents, halothane and methoxyflurane, may be safe in experienced hands but pose a greater risk than isoflurane, especially when used with a patient in decompensated condition, and are not recommended. Anesthetic machines should therefore be equipped with an isoflurane vaporizer.

Flow rates may be critical, especially in birds with air sac breathing tubes. A flowmeter capable of delivering from 0 to 3 L/minute is recommended. Choose a nonrebreathing circuit to minimize deadspace, and use a reservoir bag (rebreathing bag) capable of handling peak respiratory flow rates but small enough so that respirations can be monitored and the bag safely used for respiratory assistance and positive pressure ventilation. A Normal elbow or Ayre's T system with an attached rubber party balloon as the rebreathing bag works well for this purpose. Conventional anesthetic machines can be modified easily to meet these requirements, often by simply adding a second flowmeter and nonrebreathing circuit. A simple system consisting of flowmeter, vaporizer, and nonrebreathing system is

recommended for practices with many avian and small exotic patients.

Other equipment and supplies advantageous to avian critical care in a small animal hospital are listed in Table 48–2 (Figs. 48–7 to 48–14).

Gram Scale

An accurate scale (one with an accuracy to ± 1 g) is important to calculate dosages based on an accurate

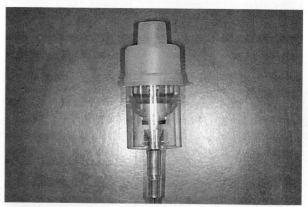

Figure 48-7

Disposable nebulizers like this Hudson unit are convenient and inexpensive.

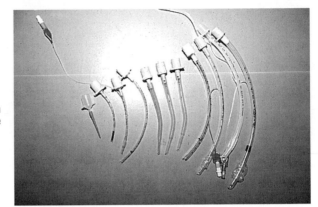

Figure 48–8

An assortment of endotracheal tubes used in avian patients. Those shown are cuffed, noncuffed, and Cole endotracheal tubes. The smallest are fashioned from rubber feeding tubes.

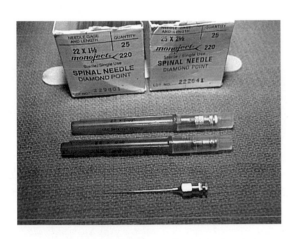

Figure 48–9

Spinal needles with steel hubs work well as intraosseous catheters and should be stocked in a variety of sizes.

Figure 48–10

Syringe, blood filter, and butterfly catheter used for administration of blood transfusion.

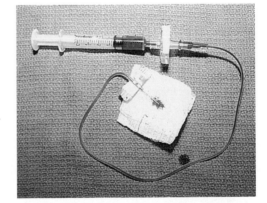

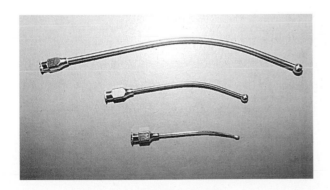

Figure 48–11

Ball-tipped steel feeding tubes in sizes from 10 to 18 gauge work well for tube feeding or administering oral medications to various avian species.

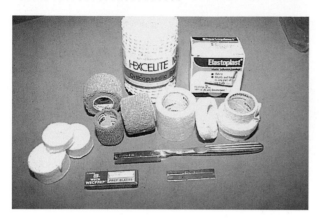

Figure 48–12

Bandage materials cut into ¼- to 1-inch widths. The author uses a single-edge blade in a dermatome handle to cut bandages.

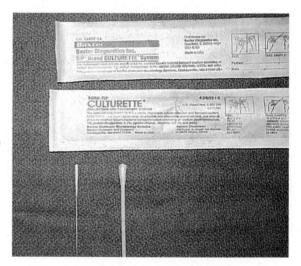

Figure 48–13

Sterile swabs with transport medium for the collection of materials for culture and cytologic testing should be available.

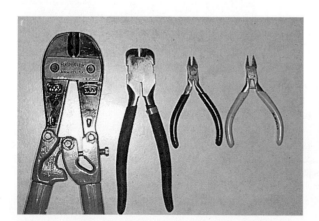

Figure 48–14

Equipment to remove leg bands: 18-inch bolt cutter, modified lineman's pliers, and diagonal wire cutting tools with fine sharp tips.

body weight and to monitor the progress of fluid therapy. A single gram may account for a significant weight change in very small birds. A scale that weighs in 0.1-g units is preferred when monitoring birds that weigh under 100 g. The scale should be easily zeroed or tared. A weighing basket or other container large enough to contain an unruly Moluccan cockatoo or macaw should fit on the scale, as should a perch.

Temperature Monitoring Devices

It is impractical, and in some cases even dangerous, to measure the body temperature of the average conscious avian patient. A critically ill patient is an occasional exception to that rule. Remote sensing constant readout thermometers (Fig. 48–15) are preferred by the author; however, conventional digital "rectal" thermometers work well. The thermometer should be small enough to pass easily into the cloaca to a depth that it will record an accurate temperature.

A good rule of thumb as to whether a bird's body temperature needs to be monitored is that when a bird attempts to remove the temperature probe or struggles during the procedure, monitoring the temperature is no longer needed.

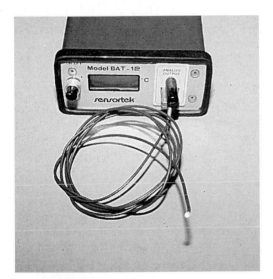

F i g u r e   4 8 – 1 5

Sensortec, Model Bat–12 (IITC, Inc., Wood Hills, CA), remote sensing, constant readout thermometer used in the author's practice. This unit is accurate to 0.1°C.

Electrocardiograph, Ultrasonic Imaging, and Ultrasonic Flow Doppler

Diagnostic imaging tools are unfamiliar to veterinarians but can provide significant information to the practitioner with a critically ill avian patient. Electrocardiography can be used as a diagnostic tool and as a monitor for critically ill patients. Surgical staples are placed at contact points in birds that require constant monitoring or repeated electrocardiographs. This allows leads to be clipped to the staples. The use of ultrasound imaging in avian medicine is becoming more widespread. Ultrasound technique can enhance diagnosis and hasten appropriate treatment. Dyspneic birds, especially those in which heart disease often occurs (e.g., toucans, mynahs,[9] lories, etc.), should be evaluated by electrocardiography and ultrasound. In cases of cardiac decompensation, diagnosis is critical. Radiology alone may not provide sufficient information. Ultrasound imaging with Doppler capabilities allows noninvasive evaluation of blood flow and tissue size, shape, and consistency.

Doppler flow detectors (Fig. 48–16) (Ultrasonic Doppler Flow Detector Model 811-B, Parks Medical Electronics, Aloha, OR) are used for measuring arterial blood pressure in small animals (dogs and cats).[10] Similar methods have been used to monitor rodents in laboratory environments (Model 129 Blood Pressure Amplifier, IITC, Inc., Woodland Hills, CA).[11] These automated units show great promise for noninvasive monitoring of avian patients during both critical care and anesthesia.

Dopplers may also be used, as with dogs and cats, to evaluate the effectiveness of cardiopulmonary resuscitation (CPR) in birds. They are similarly helpful in monitoring blood flow as a reflection of blood pressure and circulatory volume.

INFORMED CONSENT

A veterinarian should secure the owner's signature on a document of informed consent prior to providing any services. The key points of informed consent include information on medical and surgical alternatives, an explanation of the procedure, an explanation of the anticipated outcome, discussion of serious complications (including death), the type and extent of additional service that will be needed, and an estimate of fees and how payment must be

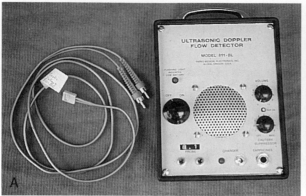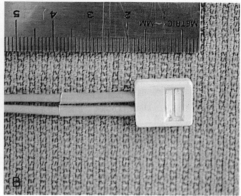

Figure 48-16

(A) Ultrasonic Doppler Flow Detector Model 811-B (Parks Medical Electronics, Inc., Aloha, OR). *(B)* Close-up of 8 MHz "infant flat" probe used to monitor blood flow in avian patients.

made. It is not always possible to include all of these points for informed consent during emergencies; however, they should be included once the patient is stable. The informed consent form used by the author's practice for emergency situations is shown in Table 48–3. The form should include the owner's name, address, and phone number, the signed authorization or "informed consent" to treat, and the patient's age and sex (if known).

TRIAGE

Assessment of a critically ill avian patient must progress rapidly; however, care must be exercised that

Table 48-3

(SAMPLE) EMERGENCY CARE RELEASE AND ESTIMATE

Please read carefully before you sign.

Your animal is in **critical condition.**

This special estimate and authorization is for **immediate** treatment to **attempt lifesaving** procedures. These procedures involve intensive and aggressive treatment and therefore can be costly. If there is any reason you do **not** want or cannot afford treatment, please do not sign this form of consent and inform the hospital staff immediately.

Estimate:

The estimate for these services is between **$250.00** and **$400.00.** If your animal can be stabilized, the veterinarian will prepare an estimate for further evaluation and treatment.

_____ Owner's/Agent's initials

Authorization:

I, the undersigned, owner, or authorized agent of the owner, of the below named patient, hereby authorize the veterinarian(s) and whomever they may designate as assistant(s) to administer such treatment as is necessary and such additional procedures as are considered therapeutically or diagnostically necessary on the basis of findings during the course of this **emergency and attempted life saving** evaluation and treatment. I hereby certify that I have read and fully understand the above authorization to perform emergency treatment, the reason that this treatment is considered necessary, that no guarantee or assurances have been made as to the results that may be obtained. I realize that with or without these procedures death may result. Further, I assume financial responsibility for all charges incurred by the patient and authorize direct payment by cash, check or bank card to the Avian & Exotic Animal Hospital.

Patient (Animal): _____

Owner/Agent: _____

Owner/Agent Signature: _____ **Date:**_____

Witness: _____ **Date:**_____

the examination be thorough. A minimum database of patient profile, physical examination, and laboratory samples should be collected prior to or coinciding with therapy. Include a brief history of the bird's origin, cage or aviary habitat, exposure to other birds (including boarding and grooming), a description of symptoms and their duration, and treatments given and results. Questions should be asked specific to organ systems: mental awareness; coordination; strength; problems walking, perching, or flying; and appetite. The presence of the following should also be noted: polyuria or polydipsia, change in color of droppings, regurgitation, bleeding, loss of coordination, or seizure activity.

The bird should be observed from some distance before restraint. Form a plan of action based on this initial observation, and gather necessary equipment and supplies. It is sometimes necessary to administer oxygen or allow the patient to gain strength before restraint is attempted.

Physical examination should include assessment of overall condition: mental attitude, state of hydration, color of mucous membranes, a brief palpation of body and limbs, auscultation of heart and airways, and examination of integument for signs of trauma or hemorrhage (Fig. 48–17). Special atten-

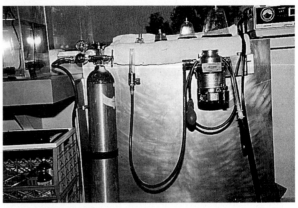

Figure 48–18

"Anesthesia stations," like the one pictured, are available in several locations in the author's practice where anesthesia may offer benefits over physical restraint. Isoflurane is currently the agent of choice because of its rapid induction and recovery times, lack of sensitization of myocardium, and low toxicity.

tion should be paid to the eyes and adnexal tissues. Head trauma commonly results in damage to the eye. Retinal detachment, luxation of the lens, and rupture of the pectin may result. Adnexal tissues should be examined for bruising or hemorrhage and presence of normal retrobulbar fat tissues. The turgor of the tissues of the eyelids along with the volume of tears produced in the eye may aid in the assessment of hydration. A neurologic examination, including assessment of cranial nerve function, should be done on birds with head trauma. Neurologic examination is reviewed in Chapter 27, The Nervous System.

The laboratory database varies with the condition of the bird and the presenting problem. However, a minimal database should include a blood smear, hematocrit or packed cell volume (PCV), and total solids. A diagnostic and therapeutic strategy must be devised. If possible, all procedures should be accomplished at one time to minimize the duration, and hence the stress, of restraint. With some critically ill patients it may be necessary to do the procedures in stages, allowing periods of rest along with supplemental oxygen between stressful restraint or painful treatment. Extremely dyspneic birds with respiratory obstructions may require placement of an abdominal air sac tube. Isoflurane anesthesia is preferred to protracted restraint in some critically ill birds (Fig. 48–18). Therapeutic priorities are the same for avian patients as for other

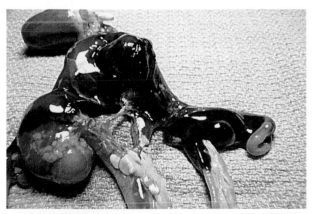

Figure 48–17

Hemorrhage resulting from significant trauma, such as from rupture of the liver as seen here, is immediately life-threatening. The first goal is to recognize the hemorrhage. Generalized clinical signs of blood loss include pallor of skin, nails, and mucous membranes; delayed capillary refill time; increased cardiac and respiratory rates; thin appearance to blood visible in peripheral veins (median ulnar and jugular veins); and generalized weakness, fear, and dyspnea, especially with restraint. More specific signs of hemorrhage depend on the location of the hemorrhage but may include bruising, distention or discoloration of the abdomen, and coolness of isolated limbs.

small animals: restore respiration; correct circulatory dysfunction; stop hemorrhage; treat neurologic injuries; stabilize fractures or luxations; and, finally, seek a definitive diagnosis.

The information obtained in these first few seconds to minutes should direct the initial treatment. Information from the patient's signalment and knowledge of disease trends may be lifesaving. A convulsing red-lored Amazon parrot (prone to epilepsy) should be approached differently than a convulsing African grey parrot (prone to hypocalcemia). Lead poisoning in Amazon parrots gives a presentation different from that in cockatoos or cockatiels. Drugs of very low pH (such as the doxycycline marketed in the US) given intravenously may be fatal to a hypotensive, anemic, and acidotic patient but may be tolerated by a bird with a lesser degree of decompensation.

PATIENT MONITORING

Advances in veterinary critical care and emergency medicine have made monitoring arterial pressure, central venous pressure, pulmonary capillary wedge pressure, oxygen saturation, and blood gases possible for the canine and feline patient. The instruments for these techniques, although very sophisticated, are not designed to use small sample sizes or measure the physiologic parameters of avian patients. Many avian patients, particularly psittacines, do not tolerate the use of invasive monitors. The conclusions of those using these instruments in dogs and cats is: "Despite this improved instrumentation and technology, the most important method of monitoring remains the physical examination. Noninvasive assessments and serial monitoring of temperature, pulse, respiration, urinary output, and cardiac rhythm gives clinicians valuable information about the status and progression of critical patients and their disease."[12] The same conclusion can be made for birds.

Body temperature is not commonly measured in birds; however, birds that are unconscious, either because of anesthesia, other therapy, or disease, may be unable to regulate their body temperature and should be both supported and monitored. A cloacal temperature of 38.3°C (101°F) should be maintained in these patients through a combination of radiant and conduction heat sources.

A subjective assessment of peripheral venous pressure can be made by observing the degree of distention of the basilic vein as it courses across the proximal ulna, capillary refill time, color of beak and mucous membrane, blood flow from a cut nail, and limb temperature. The basilic vein should be observed as part of a routine physical examination so that the clinician is familiar with its appearance. Light pressure may be placed on the rhamphotheca or toenails (if bone-colored) to blanch the underlying capillary bed, and the capillary refill time should be noted. The conjunctiva is also a good location to observe mucous membrane color. Centralization of circulation may also cause distal limbs to feel cool or clammy, and may induce slow bleeding from a cut toenail. (See Shock and Fluid Therapy, later.)

The heart rate can often be counted in the large avian species and is helpful in assessing response to therapy. Tachycardia may result from hypotension, hypoxia, anemia, and various other conditions. There may be an initial tachycardia caused by fear or excitement when the bird is first approached with a stethoscope. The heart rate often returns to "normal" and it may be counted after a short period of time. Electrocardiogram monitoring may demonstrate arrhythmias brought on by hypoxia, high circulating levels of catecholamine, and various metabolic, toxic, and other diseases. The electrocardiogram can also demonstrate heart rates too rapid to count.

Urinary output is a useful indicator of tissue perfusion and shock. The number of droppings in a cage should be recorded when the cage is cleaned. The number, size, and consistency of the droppings and urates can be monitored to provide a subjective assessment of urine production. The presence of feces in the droppings indicates that the bird is eating and digesting food and passing stool normally.

Serial accurate body weight measurements are critical for assessing continued fluid loss and response to fluid therapy. Birds receiving fluid therapy should be weighed at least twice daily. Passerines, small psittacines, and those too weak to perch may be weighed in a container or weighing pan (Fig. 48–19). Most pet psittacines will sit quietly on a perch fastened to a scale. Birds of prey often lie motionless when placed on their backs on a scale.

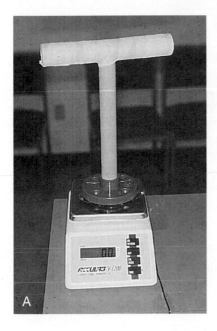

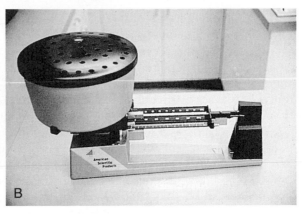

Figure 48-19

(A) Electronic or *(B)* mechanical scales may be easily modified to accept a perch or container to weigh avian patients.

This behavior is facilitated by covering the bird's eyes with a hood or small piece of cloth.

Hematocrit, or PCV, and total solids measurements are helpful indicators of blood loss and hydration. Serial measurements can be done on a small volume of blood and are beneficial in assessing response to therapy (Fig. 48–20). These measurements should be monitored on all but the smallest or most critically ill avian patients before initial treatment, and again 6 to 12 hours later. The PCV and total solids should be checked regularly in birds suffering from blood loss or severe dehydration until the condition is stable.

SHOCK AND FLUID THERAPY

Many of the physiologic changes observed in a critically ill patient are associated with shifts of fluids within the bird. Regurgitation, polyuria, diarrhea, and decreased water consumption lead to dehydration. Trauma or disease may result in internal hemorrhage. Stress from disease and trauma leads to centralization of blood away from limbs, gastrointestinal tract, and kidneys and redistribution of fluids to the heart and brain.[13] With significant trauma or hemorrhage, endocrine and metabolic changes result in the release of norepinephrine and epinephrine, causing large shifts in fluid to the central circulation.[14] Reduction of blood flow to the kidney causes endocrine changes that result in reduced urine formation and the retention of sodium and water.[3] The net result is the expansion of the vascular compartment at the expense of body tissues and kidney function.

Anesthetics affect fluid balance and blood flow. Tranquilizers and sedatives may affect neural controls of blood pressure and circulation, resulting in the resorption of interstitial fluids and hemodilution. Halogenated-ether inhalant anesthetics, halothane and isoflurane, cause some degree of respiratory depression and may profoundly affect the ventilatory response to hypoxia.[15] Isoflurane, the most commonly used avian anesthetic, causes a decrease in both respiratory rate and tidal volume that is proportional to the depth of anesthesia. Halothane and methoxyflurane have a depressant effect on cardiac tissue, leading to decreased cardiac output. Isoflurane has fewer myocardial depressant effects.[16]

The importance of maintaining fluid and electrolyte balance and blood volume is apparent, and correction of fluid shifts must be a priority. Most hospitalized patients undergoing brief or routine procedures can be given a replacement fluid volume during the treatment period, based on estimated losses from evaporation, hemorrhage, and presumed vasodilation.

The replacement fluid volume equates well to maintenance requirements, provided there is no significant blood loss and the bird is not regurgitating or polyuric. Calculated fluid replacement volumes for severely ill or traumatized patients must include fluids lost from the vascular compartment resulting from physiologic response to illness and fluids sequestered from the circulation as a result of trauma. Absolute losses (blood lost to hemorrhage) and fluid shifts into areas of injury, infection, or tissues with compromised blood flow must also be considered. The fluid deficit can be calculated based on body weight and perceived degree of dehydration with the following formula:

$$\text{Fluid deficit (ml)} = \text{degree of dehydration (\%)} \times \text{body weight (g)}$$

The degree of dehydration is estimated by evaluating subjective clinical signs. In general, dehydration should be assumed to be significant in any critically ill patient.[17] The patient must be reevaluated and fluid needs recalculated based on the effects of treatment and the response to supportive treatment.

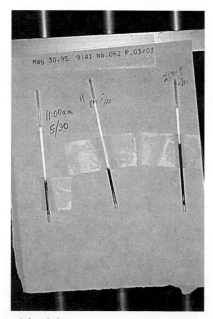

Figure 48–20

Hematocrit (PCV) and total solids measurements are helpful indicators of blood loss or hydration. Serial measurements can be done on a small volume of blood and are beneficial in assessing response to therapy. Posting tubes on the patient's cage enables all staff members working with the case to monitor progress.

Route of Fluid Administration

Oral fluids are inappropriate in critically ill birds. Oral fluids are not well absorbed, and debilitated birds are at serious risk of regurgitation and aspiration. Subcutaneous fluids are of little value in patients with decompensation from peripheral vasoconstriction. Intraosseous or intravenous administration is preferred in critically ill avian patients. Intraosseous catheters provide a rapid, stable, and accessible route for fluid therapy. The tibiotarsus or ulna may be used for catheter placement.[18] The use of an indwelling catheter in either the jugular vein[19] or the cutaneous ulnar vein also has been advocated.[20] A major disadvantage to the intravenous technique is the instability of the catheter, which requires restraint or extensive bandaging. Birds tolerate fluids well when given as a large bolus; however, infusion at a constant rate is preferable. (See Chapter 17 for the techniques of catheter placement.)

Choice of Fluids

Crystalloids are the fluid of choice for avian patients in a critical decompensated and dehydrated condition. Crystalloids are highly effective at replacing fluids within the interstitial compartments, expanding circulating fluid volume, and enhancing diuresis, which facilitates elimination of toxic byproducts. Crystalloid fluids rapidly leave the circulation and equilibrate in the interstitial fluid compartment. Only 25% of isotonic fluids, such as lactated Ringer's solution (LRS) or 0.9% saline solution, remains in the vascular compartment 30 minutes after administration.[21]

Many critically ill patients are acidotic for the reasons reviewed earlier. Lactated Ringer's solution is the fluid of choice for these patients, because lactate is metabolized to bicarbonate by the liver. In severe acidotic states, LRS should be supplemented with bicarbonate. (See Treatment of Acid-base Imbalances, later.) Hyperkalemia may result from severe tissue trauma or an extreme catabolic state. The amount of potassium in LRS is not great enough to endanger these patients; however, the addition of calcium gluconate at 5 mg/kg as a cardio-protectant and glucose, which facilitates the movement of potassium across cell membranes, is advisable.[17] Hypokalemia may result from persistent regurgitation or aggressive fluid therapy, requiring potassium supplementation. Potassium chloride can be added to LRS at a dose of 0.1 to 0.3 mEq/kg to a maximum of 11 mEq/day.[22] Infusion of large volumes of crystalloid fluids reduces colloid osmotic pressure and predisposes to pulmonary and peripheral edema and impaired peripheral tissue oxygen exchange.

Birds that are hypovolemic from blood loss may benefit from treatment with hypertonic (7.5%) saline or colloidal fluids. Hypertonic saline has been advocated as a replacement fluid therapy for mammals with acute hemorrhagic shock, endotoxic shock, and hypotension.[23] When given to mammals at 4 to 5 ml/kg, a rapid improvement in cardiovascular function and peripheral perfusion results. The vascular compartment is expanded as a result of fluid shifting from the interstitial and intracellular fluid compartments. Cardiac contractility and output increases from the expanded vascular volume and the direct inotropic effect on the heart. These benefits are transient, lasting up to 2 hours in dogs and only 15 to 20 minutes in cats.[26] The effects may be even shorter in birds. The addition of colloids (6% dextran 70) to the solution prolongs and enhances its beneficial effects.[23] Hypertonic saline is useful for hydropericardium, pulmonary edema, and increased intracranial pressure. It is contraindicated in dehydration, hypernatremia, and head trauma when intracranial hemorrhage may be present.[18] Synthetic colloids (hetastarch and dextrans) are polysaccharides of high molecular weight and particle size similar to albumin. Their effects are similar to those of hypertonic saline but with a longer half-life (24 hours in mammals). A dose of 10 to 20 ml/kg has been shown to be safe and effective in raptors.[22] Serum protein and albumin reserves may be severely compromised in massive hemorrhage and gastrointestinal or renal disease. Heterologous or homologous plasma has been poorly studied in avian medicine but may have advantages over synthetic colloidal fluids.

Blood Transfusion

Birds tolerate blood loss better than mammals. They may survive, at least for a short time, near total exsanguination. Transfusion should be considered, however, when blood loss is significant at surgery. In the author's opinion, birds rarely survive surgery if the hematocrit drops below 8 to 10%. Recently published research shows that some heterologous transfusions may be very short-lived;[25] therefore, species as closely related as possible are preferred. Anticoagulant citrate dextrose (ACD) solution (Formulation A, Baxter Healthcare Corp., Deerfield, IL) is recommended as an anticoagulant at a rate of 0.15 ml per milliliter of blood. A quantity equal to 1% of the bird's body weight may be collected safely from a donor, especially when that volume is replaced with fluids. Blood filters (Hemo-Nate filter no. HN-179; Gesco International, San Antonio, TX) should be used when administering transfusions, and the author prefers an intraosseous route. Fluids should be heated to body temperature so that they do not contribute to hypothermia.

Treatment of Acid-base Imbalances

When possible, bicarbonate deficit should be measured clinically to accurately determine metabolic acidosis.[17] Bicarbonate dose can then be calculated with the following equation:

Bicarbonate deficit = normal CO_2 value (as determined by the laboratory or use 20 mEq/l[26]) − measured value. Bicarbonate dose = deficit × 0.3

Alternatively, a dose of 1 mEq/kg every 15 to 30 minutes to a maximum of 4 mEq/kg may be given. Give the first dose intravenously followed by the remainder subcutaneously.[22]

RELIEF OF PAIN

Pain is poorly understood in avian species. The prevention and alleviation of pain are important for a number of reasons, including humane considerations and the prevention of undesirable metabolic and behavioral side effects. Answers to the following questions may be used to determine whether a patient is in pain: (1) Would the inciting surgical lesion be painful in humans? (2) Is the lesion damaging or crippling and to what degree? (3) Does the bird show *aversive* response to the lesion? Symptoms and signs that may indicate pain include change in temperament (aggressive or passive); appearance of being uncomfortable (unable to rest);

decrease in normal activity, especially grooming (often exhibited as fluffing, reluctance to perch); anorexia; lameness or dropped wing; guarding the back or splinting of the abdomen; and biting or chewing at the surgical site, sutures, or bandage. Rolling or thrashing may be a sign of severe pain but must be differentiated from seizures or rough recovery from anesthesia, especially if ketamine has been used.

Injuries that the author considers painful include burns, crushing trauma (especially those injuries involving long bones and large muscle masses), beak trauma, and abrasions or bruising of distal extremities, especially the scaled skin of the feet. Lacerations of the feathered skin and some simple fractures are not obviously painful. Pain may sometimes be alleviated by placing the bird in a warm environment with soft bedding, or protective or supportive bandaging. Analgesics have been poorly studied in birds, especially psittacines. The author has had good results with flunixin (Banamine, Schering, Kenilworth, NJ) at 1 to 5 mg/kg intramuscularly (IM) and butorphanol tartrate (Torbugesic, Fort Dodge Laboratories, Fort Dodge, IA) at 0.5 to 2.0 mg/kg IM. Buprenorphine hydrochloride (Buprenex, Rickitt & Colman, Hull, UK; distributed by Rickitt & Colman Pharmaceuticals, Richmond, VA) at a dose of 0.01 to 0.05 mg/kg IM also appears to be effective.

COMMON AVIAN EMERGENCIES

The Critically Ill Avian Patient

The most common avian emergency is the critically ill bird. Birds are often found on the bottom of the cage with little history of signs of illness. The signalment, visual examination, and initial diagnostic tests will often establish the direction of treatment and specific diagnostic tests. The following common problems are grouped by system.

Hypocalcemia Syndrome

African grey parrots, both Timneh and Congo subspecies, are sometimes affected by a hypocalcemic syndrome (although there appears to be a decreased frequency in our practice, perhaps because of increased awareness of nutritional needs). Young birds 2 to 5 years of age are most commonly affected. Signs may range from incoordination to status epilepticus. Hypocalcemia should be on the differential diagnosis of any grey parrot with neurologic signs. Birds presented in status epilepticus should be treated presumptively with calcium gluconate at 10 to 100 mg/kg IV slowly to effect, as well as with diazepam (Valium, Roche).

Respiratory Emergencies

Dyspnea is a common clinical sign in birds presented for emergency or critical care. After administering oxygen or establishing an airway and providing adequate ventilation, the bird's respiratory tract must be evaluated. The character of respirations may be helpful in making a diagnosis and determining appropriate treatment. Primary pulmonary disease (pneumonia, pulmonary congestion, or hemorrhage), upper airway obstruction, and abdominal disease that interferes with the filling of air sacs may all present as respiratory distress.

Pulmonary disease may result from a variety of causes including cardiac disease; mycotic, bacterial, viral, or parasitic pneumonia or pneumonitis; and airborne toxins. (See Chapter 25, Respiratory Disorders.) Symptomatic treatment should include oxygen, antibiotics, and possibly diuretics. The use of bronchodilators and corticosteroids is controversial. Nebulization of medication and humidification benefit some patients.

Upper airway obstructions are common avian emergencies. Inhaled foreign bodies (e.g., millet seeds inhaled by cockatiels), fungal and bacterial granulomas at the syrinx, and glottal papillomas may result in almost total obstruction. Birds may present with a history of acute onset of dyspnea, often with no previous sign of disease. An initial evaluation may show open-mouth breathing and inspiratory or expiratory stridor, or both. Musical squeak-like respiratory sounds originating at the glottis or syrinx, combined with cyanosis, are suggestive of upper airway obstruction. Cyanosis and signs of respiratory distress may become evident with stress or restraint. The decision when to intercede and cannulate the air sac should be based on whether the patient can tolerate diagnostic and therapeutic care without becoming extremely dyspneic. If the bird becomes dyspneic with or without restraint, cannulation should be considered.

Bleeding and Blood Loss

The sight of blood strikes fear in all bird owners and is a common emergency presentation (Fig. 48–21). Hemorrhage may result from numerous causes including trauma, infectious disease, metabolic and nutritional causes, and neoplasia. Trauma is the most common cause of hemorrhage. The hemorrhage from minor trauma can be easily treated. Broken and bleeding blood feathers, fractured or avulsed toenails and beaks, and traumatized wingtips make up the majority of these cases.

Bleeding blood feathers must be pulled. Even if the bleeding has stopped, it may resume if the tip of the growing feather brushes a perch or is groomed by the bird. If the feather appears to be gone but continues to bleed, look or gently palpate for a remnant of the feather shaft in the follicle.

After the feather is pulled, do not put hemostatic agents in the follicle! The bleeding will usually stop if the follicle is pinched closed for 60 to 90 seconds.

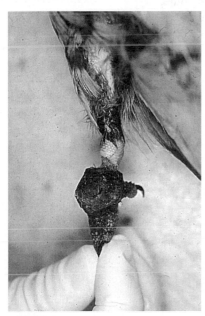

F i g u r e   4 8 – 2 1

Necrosis of the foot of a red lory *(Eos bornea bornea)* caused by a tight leg band. Although the lesion is chronic, the owner presented the bird for examination only after blood was seen.

If the hemorrhage continues, glue the follicle closed with a drop of tissue cement or place a 5–0 to 6–0 absorbable suture in the opening of the feather follicle. Bleeding toenails may be cauterized with a mild styptic such as ferric sub-sulfate, or the quick may be covered with a thin layer of cyanoacrylic tissue cement.

Broken beaks are occasionally difficult to stop from bleeding. This is particularly true with slab-type fractures of the tip of the rhinotheca (common with cockatoos and African grey parrots). These fractures may be difficult to diagnose because of blood spreading from the tip of the beak to the tongue, giving the appearance that the origin of the hemorrhage is elsewhere in the oral cavity. The bleeding often stops if the broken surface is filed or ground smooth. This also appears to make the broken tip less irritating to the bird. The tip of the beak may be cauterized with chemicals or (cautiously) with heat.

Hemorrhage resulting from significant trauma, such as lacerations of major vessels, hematoma, or fracture of a parenchymal organ, is immediately life-threatening. The first goal is to recognize the hemorrhage. This is not difficult when trauma results in external hemorrhage. The greater challenge is to recognize internal blood loss. The hemorrhage must be slowed or stopped and restorative therapy begun to prevent exsanguination and support vital organ function. As discussed earlier, birds tolerate hemorrhage better than mammals. The rate that blood is lost from the circulation is the determining factor in mortality. The loss of 20 to 25% of the blood volume over several minutes may be fatal, whereas the same volume lost over several hours is not. Clinical signs of blood loss include pallor of skin, nails, and mucous membranes; delayed capillary refill time; increased cardiac and respiratory rates, a thin appearance to blood visible in peripheral veins (median ulnar and jugular); generalized weakness; and dyspnea, especially with restraint. More specific signs of hemorrhage depend on the location of the hemorrhage but may include bruising, distention or discoloration (or both) of the abdomen, and coolness of isolated limbs.

A timely diagnosis may make the difference between life and death and should be aggressively pursued. If hemorrhage is not apparent in an animal with a history of recent trauma, internal hemorrhage should be assumed to be ongoing until proved otherwise.[2] Therefore, birds should be hospitalized for several hours after trauma for observation. External hemorrhage is usually apparent. The volume of blood loss may be estimated with the aid of the history and observation of blood on the cage or carrier floor papers or in the materials used to wrap the patient before presentation.

Diagnosis and assessment of internal hemorrhage is difficult. Birds with a history of trauma and signs of hypovolemia or hypotension should be assumed to have sustained internal hemorrhage. Hemorrhage into the coelom and osseofascial compartments is the most common in the author's experience. Discoloration or bruising of the abdominal wall, especially along the ventral midline or caudal ventral abdomen, may indicate hemorrhage. Radiographs and endoscopic examination may aid in locating the site. Removing the feathers from a traumatized limb or trunk may help to locate an area of hemorrhage. Bruised areas should be evaluated for increased size. Definitive location of internal hemorrhage may require exploratory surgery.

Treatment must begin early and progress rapidly. Apply direct pressure if it does not interfere with respiration. Clamp or suture vessels that are readily accessible. The application of counterpressure to pelvic limbs may increase systemic vascular resistance and venous return to the heart. The resulting influx of blood acts as an "autotransfusion" of blood pooled in the limbs. The degree of stress created by wrapping the limbs must be weighed against the benefits of increasing blood pressure. Counterpressure pneumatic "garments" (Vector, Inc., Milwaukee, WI) are not available for avian patients, and counterpressure cannot be applied to the abdomen of birds because of their need to expand abdominal air sacs for respiration. An intraosseous or intravenous catheter should be placed for the rapid administration of fluids. Whole blood, plasma, colloid plasma expanders, hypertonic (7.5%) saline or crystalloid solutions are recommended. (See Choice of Fluids, earlier.) Fluids should be continued until the distention of peripheral vessels (a subjective reflection of systemic blood pressure) is normal or slightly greater than normal. A single heterologous blood transfusion has been shown to be safe and anecdotally is reported to be efficacious.[26, 27] Recent studies of radioactive chromium (^{51}Cr)-labeled red blood cells administered as either homologous or heterologous transfusions have suggested the half-

life of the transfused cells to be substantially shorter than previously thought.[25] These studies imply that heterologous transfusions may be of no benefit and homologous transfusions of only limited benefit.

Anemia

A bird with signs of anemia must first be evaluated to determine the degree and site of blood loss. Gastrointestinal bleeding, genitourinary bleeding, and hemolysis may be difficult to diagnose. Hematochezia, typically from lesions in the lower gastrointestinal tract, and melena can be associated with gastritis, enteritis, gastrointestinal ulcers and foreign bodies, primary and secondary coagulopathies, and hepatopathies. Cloacal bleeding can be associated with severe cloacitis, cloacal or uterine prolapse, papillomas or other cloacal masses, and egg-laying. Heavy metal poisoning (see later) and chlamydiosis may result in hemolysis or depression anemia.

Bite Wounds

Scratches and bite wounds very often lead to a fatal septicemia if not treated aggressively. The bird should be evaluated for its overall condition and treated appropriately for blood loss or hypotension. The extent of the wounds should be evaluated. If the patient's condition allows, wounds should be thoroughly flushed and fractures stabilized. Aggressive antibiotic therapy should begin early in treatment. Piperacillin (Pipracil, Lederle) or cefotaxime (Claforan, Hoechst-Roussel Pharmaceuticals, Somerville, NJ) combined with amikacin (Amiglide-V, Fort Dodge, IA) or tobramycin (Nebcin, Eli Lilly) is a good choice and should be continued for a minimum of 5 days. If septicemia is suspected, begin treatment for septic shock (intravenous fluids, rapid-acting steroids, and intravenous bacteriocidal antibiotics).

Fractures

Fractures should be splinted to prevent further complication as soon as the bird's condition is stable. Simple bandaging techniques may be used to provide adequate stability until definitive treatment is possible. Fractures of the distal wing, including the radius and ulna, carpus, and manus, may be immobilized with a figure-eight bandage. Humeral fractures, shoulder luxations, and fractures of the shoulder girdle should be splinted to the bird's body with a figure-eight bandage, followed by wrapping the limb to the body to support the limb without restricting respiration or interfering with the movement of the legs. The opposing wing should be left out of the wrap. Fractures of the leg below the stifle may be immobilized with an Altman tape bandage or a modified Robert Jones bandage with or without an acrylic half cast. (See Chapter 47.) Fractures of the femur require a spica splint, if they are to be splinted externally, until surgical repair can be accomplished. (See Chapter 17, Hospital Techniques.)

Burns

Most burns result from contact with hot liquids, water (scalds), or cooking oil; electrical burns from chewing on electrical wires; or from hot formula fed to unweaned birds. Burns resulting from entrapment in burning buildings or inside containers (chick incubators with burning bedding) are rare and are much more difficult to treat because of the complication of smoke inhalation.

Burns may be classified by their severity as superficial, partial thickness, or full-thickness. Superficial burns, wherein only epidermis is affected, result in transient erythema and desquamation of epidermis, and the site is hyperesthetic. Clinical signs include hyperemia, desquamation, and pain. Partial-thickness burns extend to the mid-dermis. Loss of epidermis is complete, capillaries and venules in the dermis are dilated and congested, and the lesions exude plasma. Clinical signs include exudation, pain (especially in the feet, legs, and facial skin), and decreased sensitivity. Change in ease of feather pulling (as noted with hair in mammals) may not be affected because of the depth of the feather follicle.

Full-thickness burns result in coagulation of the epidermis and dermis so that they are no longer vital. Severe edema of the subcutis develops from the increased permeability of deep vessels. Necrosis of the damaged tissue occurs, resulting in a dry, leathery eschar. Feathers may be easily pulled if the burn is deep, and scaled skin may peel easily. Clinical signs include necrotic tissue without sensa-

tion, subcutaneous edema, little or no pain, and feathers that are easily pulled. Other signs of burns may include respiratory signs from smoke inhalation and carbon monoxide poisoning, hypovolemia and hypotension ("shock"), dehydration from loss of fluids, anorexia, or inability to eat in the case of crop burns.

Smoke exposure should be expected in situations when smoke accompanies the burn, especially in an enclosed space or involving materials with a likelihood of producing toxic fumes. A thorough physical examination may reveal the involvement of other organs. If greater than 50% of the body surface is involved with partial- or full-thickness burns, the prognosis is grave and the client may consider euthanasia. Advise the client that the condition of the bird may become much worse before it improves. Look for signs of hypovolemia or hypotension. Evaluate for signs of infection and pain. Diagnostic tests should include radiographs in birds exposed to smoke to evaluate pulmonary injury. Hematologic tests and measurement of serum electrolytes are indicated in severe or extensive burns.

Birds with severe or extensive burns need emergency treatment. Dyspneic birds often have laryngeal edema and accumulation of upper airway secretions and may benefit from an air sac tube and oxygen. An intraosseous catheter should be placed and the bird treated for shock. Administer an initial bolus of fluids equal to 2 to 3% of the bird's body weight (20–30 ml/kg) using LRS or some other balanced crystalloid electrolyte solution. Consider giving short-acting glucocorticosteroids such as hydrocortisone sodium (Na) succinate (Solu-cortef, Upjohn, Kalamazoo, MI) at 10 mg/kg IV or prednisolone Na succinate (Solu-delta-cortef, Upjohn) at 11 to 25 mg/kg IV. Begin systemic bacteriocidal antibiotics in birds with severe burns to prevent sepsis. Monitor PCV and total solids for hypoproteinemia and anemia. Plasma or colloidal fluids may be required when total solids and hence osmolality drop below 1.0 g/dl. Renal function should be monitored by the number of droppings and urine volume, uric acid concentration, and serum electrolytes. Continue fluids and diuretics (furosemide [Lasix, Hoechst-Roussel]) at 1–2 mg/kg (use lower dose in Loriidae, see Formulary). White blood cell counts commonly increase to very high levels in 24 to 48 hours and persist for 5 to 10 days (in the author's experience).

Analgesics are indicated in birds that appear to have pain (see earlier). If the burn is recent, treat the site with cold running water or cold compresses to minimize coagulation and decrease the burn depth by dissipating heat. Continue cold compresses for a period of 20 to 30 minutes after the time of the burn. Body temperature must be monitored during this procedure, especially in very small patients. Superficial burns should be gently cleansed using saline with 5% povidone iodine (Betadine) or chlorhexadine (Nolvasan, Fort Dodge) solution. Partial- and full-thickness burns should be gently cleansed and debrided daily and treated topically with a water-soluble antibiotic dressing such as silver sulfadiazine (Silvadine cream 1%, Marion Merrell Dow, Kansas City, MO). This procedure is very painful and should be done under general anesthesia. The lesions may be covered with a sterile dressing or left uncovered based on the likelihood of contamination and injury by the patient. Early surgical intervention may shorten the course of therapy of some small partial- and full-thickness burns.

Complications most likely to occur include circulatory collapse, oliguria, renal failure, and sepsis. Circulatory and renal complications are most likely to occur within the first 24 to 48 hours. This emphasizes the need to monitor hydration (PCV and total solids) and renal function (uric acid concentration, plasma electrolytes, and urinalysis). Infection is a common cause of death in birds surviving the initial injury. The most common microbial agents that infect the burns of mammals are opportunists and include *Pseudomonas, Streptococcus, Proteus,* and *Candida* species. Prevention of burn sepsis involves early wound cleansing and closure when indicated; topical antibiotics, isolation of the patient in a clean environment, and maintaining sterility of the burn site. Monitor the patient's white blood cell count and note any discharge or odor from the lesion. Wet dressings should be changed often with sterile technique. Parenteral antibiotics should be given if evidence of infection develops. Other potential complications include pneumonia, scarring, and difficulty in healing, especially around joints and areas of motion.

Crop (thermal) burns in young birds and chemical burns in adult birds are similar to other burns. Superficial burns may result in the chick refusing food and lead to secondary bacterial and fungal (yeast) infections. Partial- thickness and full-thickness burns may be identified early by edema of the tissue overlying the crop. Many partial-thickness burns result in the formation of an eschar that will later open to a fistula. Full-thickness burns may result in the death of the chick. Partial- and full-thickness crop burns should be treated as any other burn. (See also Chapter 6, Pediatrics.)

Poisonings

Poisonings are uncommon in avian emergency medicine, but do occur and involve a wide assortment of toxins. Heavy metal toxicosis is most common. In principle, the treatment of poisonings in birds is similar to that in other animals: treat the patient, not the toxin.[27, 28] The bird's condition should first be stabilized, an airway established, and respiration assisted if necessary. Cardiovascular needs should be addressed, and fluids and general supportive treatment given as needed. Further exposure and further absorption should be prevented or delayed. Soiled birds should be bathed, crops should be lavaged, and adbsorbents or cathartics administered. (Specific information on these products may be found in Chapter 35.) Specific antagonists or antidotes are available for a few toxins and should be used in those instances when a safe dosage is known. Treatments that may facilitate the removal of the toxin, such as diuresis, should be instigated.

Lead Poisoning

Lead poisoning adversely affects every body system to which the metal is distributed. Abnormalities and clinical signs may vary with species, dose, and duration of exposure. Signs may be vague and nonspecific, causing lead poisoning to be added to many lists of differential diagnoses. Neurologic, hematopoietic, gastrointestinal, renal, and immunologic systems are most often involved. Nervous system signs include dull or poorly responsive mentation, wing droop, incoordination, muscle twitches, and seizures. Central nervous signs are the result of perivascular edema, increase in cerebrospinal fluid, necrosis of nerves, and changes in neuronal metabolism. Peripheral neuropathy and associated muscular weakness may result from lead-induced demyelination in chronic cases.[29] (See also Chapter 35, Toxic Diseases.)

Lead damage to red blood cells results in anemia, polychromasia, and anisocytosis secondary to disruption of the formation of heme. Premature destruction of red blood cells results in biliverdinuria (yellow-green to green-black coloration of urine and urate). In Amazon parrots, and occasionally other species, hemoglobinuria, which presents as a classic "chocolate milk" to blood-colored droppings, may occur (Fig. 48–22).[30] With or without neurologic signs, lead toxicity should be suspected in these birds. Many birds with lead toxicity are polyuric from renal tubular damage caused by both the lead and hemoglobin. Gastrointestinal signs include anorexia, regurgitation, gastrointestinal stasis or paralytic ileus including proventricular dilatation. Gastrointestinal signs result from the local effects of the lead on the gastrointestinal tract and the neurologic effects.

Radiographic examination may or may not show metal in the ventriculus or elsewhere in the gastrointestinal tract. Hematologic effects of lead include mild to severe anemia, changes in red cell morphology, including margination of hemoglobin, polychromasia, and anisocytosis. Plasma biochemical test results may show elevations in concentrations of lactic dehydrogenase (LDH), aspartate aminotransferase (AST), creatine phosphokinase (CPK), and uric acid. (Blood lead levels higher than 20 μg/dl [0.20 ppm] are suggestive of lead toxicity; levels higher than 50 μg/dl are diagnostic.) Aminolevulinic acid dehydrase (ALAD) is inhibited by lead. (ALAD levels have been used to diagnose lead toxicity in waterfowl and occasionally in caged birds.) (See also Chapter 35.)

Initial therapy consists of supportive therapy along with chelation. Supportive therapy includes subcutaneous, IV, or intraosseous fluids, thermal support, and anticonvulsant medication, if needed. Chelation of lead forms nontoxic complexes that are excreted in the bile or by the kidneys. (See also Chapter 35). Calcium Disodium Versenate (CaEDTA) is the treatment of choice for initial therapy. A dose of 30 to 50 mg/kg IM or SC every 12 hours is recommended.[28, 29] D-penicillamine may be added to the therapy and has the advantage of oral administration. A dose of 55 mg/kg orally every 12 hours has been recommended.[28, 31]

Other chemical agents, diethylenetriamine pentaacetic acid (DTPA) and 2,3-dimercaptosuccinic acid (DMSA), have been investigated as treatments for lead intoxication, but there is little clinical experience in their use. Both DMSA and DTPA require a special Food and Drug Administration (FDA) permit. Therapies to remove metal fragments from the gastrointestinal tract have been suggested but have not proved successful. Cathartics, such as sodium sulfate (Gluuber's salts) or magnesium sulfate (Epsom salts) have been recommended to precipitate lead in the gastrointestinal tract. Large lead objects such as fishing sinkers or other large fragments may be removed with a rigid or (in large species) flexible endoscope once the patient's condition is stabilized. Surgical removal is indicated only as a last resort.

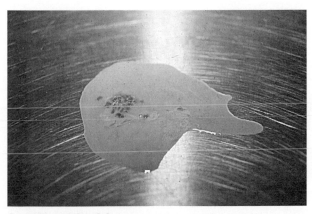

Figure 48–22

The classic "chocolate milk"- to blood-colored dropping characteristic of Amazon species poisoned with lead.

Zinc

Zinc toxicosis is similar to that of lead, and combined lead and zinc toxicosis does occur. Zinc toxicity differs from lead toxicosis in pathology and clinical signs in that the kidneys, liver, and pancreas are target organs for zinc. Often, poisoned psittacines show generalized weakness and no other signs. Tentative diagnosis is based on history and the presence of metal in the gastrointestinal tract on radiographs. Definitive diagnosis is made based on blood or tissue levels greater than 200 μg/dl and

75 μg/dl, respectively, although clinical signs may not be noticed until levels are as high as 1000 μg/dl. Samples should be submitted in plastic containers because the rubber stoppers may leach zinc from the sample, giving a false-low result. Treatment for zinc toxicosis is the same as for lead. In the author's practice, toxicosis resulting from zinc carries a poorer prognosis than that from lead intoxication.

Iron and copper toxicoses are rare in avian medicine.

Pesticides—Organophosphates and Carbamates

Pesticides implicated most often in avian emergency and critical care include insecticides and rodenticides. The most common insecticides are organophosphates including diazinon, dichlorvos, chloropyrifos and malathion, and carbamates (carbaryl). Intoxication generally results from ingestion through contamination of food or water, although secondary poisoning of wild insectivorous species may occur. Pathology and clinical signs result from binding of the insecticide to, and inhibition of, acetylcholinesterase and the resulting accumulation of acetylcholine at ganglia and neuromuscular junctions.

Organophosphate bonds are irreversible, but carbamate bonds are slowly reversible. Signs of toxicosis include anorexia, weakness, crop stasis, ataxia, muscular twitching, prolapsed nictitans, increased respiratory secretions, dyspnea, bradycardia, and death. Tentative diagnosis is based on history of exposure, clinical signs, and response to therapy. Bradycardia not responsive to atropine (0.02 mg/kg IV) is suggestive of toxicosis, but not established in avian medicine. Definitive diagnosis is based on cholinesterase assay from blood, plasma, or serum, paired with an analogous subject.

Specific therapy includes atropine at 0.20 mg/kg IM every 3 to 4 hours as needed to correct signs for organophosphate toxicosis. Pralidoxime chloride (2-Pam) (Protopam, Wyeth-Ayerst, Philadelphia, PA) is effective early in organophosphate toxicosis and should be given in birds that are presented soon after ingestion, at a dose of 10 to 20 mg/kg repeated in 10 to 20 hours, provided there is a positive response. 2-Pam is contraindicated in carbamate toxicosis and has been reported to be toxic in raptors.[32]

Anticoagulant Rodenticides

First-generation (warfarin) and second generation (brodifacoum and bromadoline) rodenticide toxicoses or suspected intoxications caused by both primary and secondary exposure (carnivorous birds) are sometimes seen, despite evidence that birds are less sensitive to their effects than some other animals. These agents are vitamin K antagonists that deplete and block the synthesis of prothrombin, and accessory factors VII, IX, and X. As noted earlier, birds rely principally on prothrombin for stimulation of clotting, and intrinsic clotting factors are not as important in avian patients. Clinical signs of toxicosis include depression, anorexia, feather follicle and subcutaneous hemorrhage, petechial hemorrhages of oral and cloacal mucosa, and bleeding from the nares. Many birds have no history of exposure and no specific symptoms. Once hemorrhage is noted, the prognosis is grave.

Treatment involves supplementation of vitamin K and, in critical cases, fresh whole blood transfusions. Vitamin K_1 is administered at 0.2 to 2.2 mg/kg sc or IM every 4 to 8 hours until stable, then the same dose is given sc, po, or IM daily[32] or fed in the diet at a rate of 800 g/kg of food. Intramuscular administration may result in hematoma formation in dogs with coagulopathy, but this may or may not occur in birds. Supplementation of menadione (K_3) is not effective in counteracting anticoagulants. Because of increased potency and slower metabolism (at least in mammals) of the second generation rodenticides it may be necessary to administer vitamin K for several weeks to control bleeding.

References

1. Murray MJ: Management of the avian trauma case. Semin Avian Exotic Pet Med 3(4):200–209, 1994.
2. Crowe DT: Triage and trauma management. In Murtaugh RJ, Kaplan PM (eds): Veterinary Emergency and Critical Care Medicine. St. Louis, Mosby YearBook, 1992, pp 77–121.
3. Sturkie PD, Griminger P: Body fluids: Blood. In Sturkie PD (ed): Avian Physiology. New York, Springer-Verlag, 1986, pp 102–129.
4. Kovach AGB, Szasz E, Mayer NPL: Mortality of various avian and mammalian species following blood loss. Acta Physiol Acad Sci Hung 35:109, 1969.
5. Zambraski EJ, Schuler R: Failure of prostaglandin inhibition to attenuate the tolerance to hemorrhage in the domestic fowl. Poult Sci 59:2567, 1980.

6. Fedde MR: Respiration. In Sturkie PD (ed): Avian Physiology. New York, Springer-Verlag, 1986, pp 191–220.

7. King AS, McLelland J: Integument. In Birds: Their Structure and Function. London, Baillière Tindall, 1984, pp 23–42.

8. Wittrow GC: Regulation of Body Temperature. In Sturkie PD (ed): Avian Physiology. New York, Springer-Verlag, 1986, pp 221–252.

9. Rosenthal K, Stamoulis M: Diagnosis of congestive heart failure in an Indian Hill Myna (Gracula religiosa). J Assoc Avian Vet 7(1):27–30, 1993.

10. Grandy JL, Dunlop CI, Hodgson DS, et al: Evaluation of the Doppler ultrasonic method of measuring systolic arterial blood pressure in cats. Am J Vet Res 53(7):1166–1169, 1992.

11. Bunag RD: Experimental and Genetic Models of Hypertension. Measurement of Blood-pressure in Rats. New York, Elsevier Science Publishers BV, 1984.

12. Kaplan PM: Monitoring. In Murtaugh RJ, Kaplan PM (eds): Veterinary Emergency and Critical Care Medicine. St. Louis, Mosby YearBook, 1992, pp 21–37.

13. Sturkie PD: Heart and circulation: Anatomy, hemodynamics, blood pressure, blood flow. In Sturkie PD (ed): Avian Physiology. New York, Springer-Verlag, 1986, pp 130–166.

14. Harvey S, Scanes CG, Brown KI: Adrenals. In Sturkie PD (ed): Avian Physiology. New York, Springer-Verlag, 1986, pp 479–493.

15. Pascoe PJ: Inhalants for avian anesthesia. Proc 18th Annual Veterinary Surgical Forum, Chicago, 1990, pp 112–114.

16. Thurmon JC, Benson GJ: Pharmacologic considerations in selection of anesthesics for animals. J Am Vet Med Assoc 191(10):1245–1259, 1987.

17. Hernandez M, Aguilar R: Steroid and fluid therapy. Semin Avian Exotic Pet Med 3(4):190–199.

18. Jenkins JR: Advanced avian techniques. In Manual of Avian Laboratory Procedures. Assoc Avian Vet, New Orleans, 1992, pp 87–92.

19. Bond MW, Wolf S: Intravenous catheter therapy. Proc Assoc Avian Vet, Nashville, 1993, pp 8–14.

20. Bond MW: In my experience: Intravenous catheter placement. J Assoc Avian Vet 6(1):40, 1992.

21. DiBartola SP: Introduction to fluid therapy. In Dibartola SP (ed): Fluid Therapy in Small Animal Practice. Philadelphia, WB Saunders, 1992, pp 321–340.

22. Redig PT: Fluid therapy and acid base balance in the critically ill avian patient. Proc Assoc Avian Vet, Toronto, 1994, pp 59–73.

23. Murr WW: Small volume resuscitation using hypertonic saline. Cornell Vet 80:7–12, 1990.

24. Muir WW, Sally J: Small-volume resuscitation with hypertonic saline solution in hypovolemic cats. Am J Vet Res 50(11):1883–1888, 1989.

25. Sandmeir P, Stauber EH, Wardrop KJ, Washizuka A: Survival of pigeon red blood cells after transfusion into selected raptors. J Avian Vet Med Assoc 204(3):427–429, 1994.

26. Altman RB: Heterologous blood transfusions in avian species. Proc Assoc Avian Vet, San Diego, 1983, pp 28–32.

27. Altman R: Transfusions. Proc 13th Ann Vet Surg Forum Seminar 10, Avian Surgery, 1985, pp 22–23.

28. LaBonde J: Avian toxicology. Vet Clin North Am 21(6):1329–1342, 1991.

29. McDonald SE: Lead poisoning in psittacine birds. In Kirk RW (ed): Current Veterinary Therapy IX. Philadelphia, WB Saunders, 1986, pp 713–718.

30. Woerpel RW, Rosskopf WJ: Heavy-metal intoxication in caged birds, I–II. Comp Cont Ed Pract Vet 4:9,10, 1982.

31. Mautino M: Avian lead intoxication. Proc Assoc Avian Vet, Phoenix, 1990, pp 245–247.

32. LaBonde J: Avian toxicology. Proc Am Board of Vet Practitioners, Chicago, 1994, pp 71–94.

Specific Species

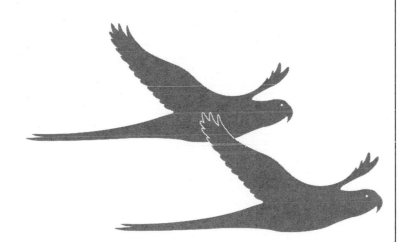

Gerry M. Dorrestein

49

Passerines

Passerines (songbirds) are increasingly presented for veterinary care as aviculturists recognize that successful medical and surgical treatment can be performed, even in these tiny patients.

The order Passeriformes contains over 4900 species, with body weights ranging from 4.8 to 1350 g. Compared with the other orders of the class Aves, passerines have an extremely high basal metabolic rate (K = 129, see Chapter 39A, Metabolism, Pharmacology, and Therapy).

Disease in these birds is very much influenced by nutrition, housing, and stress. For an optimal approach to veterinary problems, including diagnosis and treatment, it is necessary to become familiar with aviculture, housing, and husbandry of these species. Supportive care and measures to minimize stress are often needed to maintain the host's defense mechanisms.

Many veterinarians are relatively unfamiliar with the Passeriformes. The aviculture, diagnostic procedures, and common diseases and their treatment are discussed.

AVICULTURE

Species

The most common representatives of the passerines in captivity are canaries, finches, and mynahs. Canaries *(Serinus canaria)* are bred and kept for their song (e.g., the American singer), their color, or their build and shape (e.g., the border fancy and the Norwich canary). Their weight range is 15 to 25 g. The sexes are not sexually dimorphic, and their lifespan is 6 to 16 years. Canary fancy has a wide range of activities, ranging from preservation of some older and rarer breeds to the sphere of new color mutations that are constantly occurring. Showing is considered an important aspect of this fancy. Many people, however, take pleasure merely in their breeding or even in the possession of a single pet songster.[1]

There are several hundred species of finches, and they have a worldwide distribution. The more domesticated species have been bred in captivity for many decades. There is a fair amount of size disparity between the finches commonly kept as pets, from the small gold-breasted waxbill (7 g), to the large Java rice sparrow (20 g). Most common finches belonging to the families Fringillidae and Estrildidae, such as the zebra finch *(Poephila guttata),* Lady Gouldian *(Chloebia gouldiae)*, and parrot finch *(Erythrura psittacea)*, are kept for breeding but also as ornamental birds. Bengalese (or society) finches *(Lonchura striata domestica)* and zebra finches are used as foster parents for breeding Australian finches. This practice is problematic because these species can be carriers of diseases that can kill the foster-fledglings (i.e., cochlosomosis and *Campylobacter* infection).

Mynahs *(Gracula* species) are popular because of their ability to mimic the human voice. Therefore, they are usually kept as single pets. The veterinary approach to mynah birds is comparable to that for the psittacines, and they are not further discussed in this chapter.

Housing

Passerines are kept in captivity as individual pet birds and as flocks in aviaries. Two types of aviaries can be distinguished—mixed ornamental aviaries and breeding aviaries. The former is usually an outdoor aviary with different species housed together, mostly for ornamental purposes. In the latter, large numbers of the same species are kept, mostly indoors, for breeding. Breeders frequently show birds in competitions and often exchange birds (and possibly pathogens).

In mixed aviaries, the population is less dense than in breeding aviaries and usually consists of pairs of different species. Species-specific diseases are restricted to only a few of the occupants of the aviary. The birds are in the aviary year-round with a shed for shelter and a flight area outside. Planted aviaries are popular because the vegetation provides observers a more natural view of a bird's behavior. Disease control in planted aviaries can be difficult because of associated problems in control of microorganisms and in medicating individual birds.[2] Plantings, however, are often necessary for successful breeding.

In breeding aviaries, the housing depends on the season and climate. Canaries are usually bred indoors. Normally, canaries start breeding when the following conditions are met: maturity and good health, an accepted partner, a minimum length of day, presence of nest and nesting material, ample water and food, a minimum temperature, and photoperiod stimulation.[3] In the breeding season, the birds are mostly kept in pairs in small box-type cages (50 × 40 × 40 cm). Normally, pairs are bred two to three times before resting. The fledglings are housed in communal flights. In the winter season (resting season), the males and females are housed as separate groups in flight cages (Fig. 49–1). Singing canaries are housed individually in small sing cages (21 × 20 × 15 cm) for at least 5 months for training and to enter singing competitions.

Diet and Husbandry

Dietary and husbandry requirements are diverse. Most finch species are primarily seed-eating or granivorous and have been domesticated for centuries, whereas other passerine species are nectivorous, frugivorous, insectivorous, omnivorous, or carnivorous. Some species adapt readily to commercially available diets, whereas others may require live food.

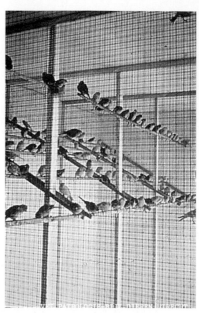

Figure 49–1

Canaries *(S. canaria)* after the breeding period separated in large flight pens.

The majority of commercially available passerine diets are seed mixes and therefore are multideficient. Because many disease problems, especially in tropical finches, are related to malnutrition, the diet history should be checked in every passerine that is admitted to a veterinarian. Knowledge of what and how much is actually consumed by the bird is important information for the owners to have. Often clients describe an impressive variety of food types that they offer their birds daily. When asked how much and what types of food their birds actually consume, they do not know. Actual consumption must be known if veterinarians are to make useful recommendations.

Common nutrient deficiencies of seeds include lysine, calcium, available phosphorus, sodium, manganese, zinc, iron, iodine, selenium, riboflavin, pantothenic acid, available niacin, choline, and vitamins B_{12}, A, D_3, E, and K. Nutritional inadequacies of a seed diet for growth apply also to reproduction and, to a lesser extent, to maintenance of adults.

The composition of the basic diet varies according to the species of bird. The following guidelines will serve as a general starting point for further diet modifications, depending on the species and individual birds involved. A good quality diet consists of an excellent seed selection and the addition of supplements to complete the deficient seed mixture. "Egg food" or "soft food" is commercially available as a supplement and is well accepted by canaries. Other finches usually do not accept these supplements readily. Adult "seed-eating" passerines should eat one part "soft food" and three parts of a good seed mixture. A calcium supplement should always be available, and fruit and vegetables are often a welcome addition.

All passerine species have a crop; the ceca are rudimentary. Granivorous birds are believed to need grit for digestion. Finches can consume up to 30% of their body weight in food daily. When recommended dietary levels of vitamins and minerals for poultry are followed, overdosage may occur, resulting in infertility, renal calcification, gout, and generally poor condition.[2] The daily water intake is 15 to 50% of the body weight, depending on species, diet, and environmental temperature. Desert birds (e.g., zebra finch) can survive on the water contents of dry seeds (maximum 16% water) and refuse drinking water when drugs are added.

DIAGNOSTIC PROCEDURES

Diagnostic and treatment options may be limited by owners' financial constraints and difficulties in collecting samples from small birds. Veterinary care in these species is frequently directed toward appropriate preventive husbandry measures and approaching medical problems from a flock perspective. The main clinical diagnostic procedures used in these small birds are history, examination of the cage, physical examination, and a limited number of clinical procedures. If possible, these procedures should be followed by a diagnostic necropsy, especially with flock problems.

Clinical Diagnostics

The history should include information on the species, age, symptoms, diet, and housing. A careful history will provide much information needed to arrive at a diagnosis.

Examination of the cage or aviary can provide much useful information. Note the droppings, the feed dishes, and the cage floor. Most breeders trans-

port their birds in small boxes or cages for examination. Birds should be put in a bird cage soon after arrival, even before the history is taken. The birds can acclimate then to the new surroundings, and fresh stool for examination is likely to be produced. Transport in their own cage is recommended whenever possible. "Light out/perches out" catching techniques are almost mandatory, and strong lighting in combination with a magnification device will greatly facilitate examination. When handling the birds, keep the windows closed!

The physical examination is limited, but nevertheless is very important. Most gram scales can provide an accurate weight if the finch is contained in a paper box or bag, but the container must be weighed or tared. The usual physical examination is performed as for any other bird.

Listen for respiratory sounds. Do not interfere with the movements of the sternum; this will inhibit normal respiration and could kill the patient. Note the state of molt, the pectoral muscle mass (chronic or acute disease), the abdomen (blow the feathers apart and look for an enlarged liver and dilatation of the gastrointestinal tract), and the skin (examine for pox lesions and parasites).

Routine Diagnostic Procedures

Fecal Examination

Helmintic infections are very rare in small passerines. Coccidia are excreted mainly between 2 PM and darkness. Yeasts and protozoal cysts (e.g., *Giardia* species) are found with direct wet preparations or after flotation techniques. The diagnosis of cochlosomosis in society finches or Australian finches can only be made by microscopic examination of direct wet mounts of fresh, warm stool without dilution. Passerines normally do not have resident gut flora; therefore, bacteria and other microorganisms should not be found in stained fecal smears. Routine microbiologic aerobic culture results should be negative. Microaerophylic strains (e.g., *Campylobacter jejuni*) can easily be recognized in stained fecal smears (DiffQuick or Gram's stain; see Chapter 15, Cytology).

Crop Swabs

Crop swabs are essential for the diagnosis of trichomoniasis and crop candidiasis.

Blood Samples

For additional information on individual birds, blood can be collected in heparinized capillary tubes after puncturing the medial metatarsal vein (Fig. 49–2). Some pressure with the thumb or a small piece of cotton wool stops the bleeding. The cotton wool must be removed the next day to prevent necrosis of the distal part of the leg. One drop of blood is used for a blood smear, which can be examined for blood parasites and, if present, for the type of anemia. The packed cell volume (PCV) normally ranges from 40 to 55%; any reading less than 35% indicates anemia. Total protein determinations provide a very significant diagnostic measure. A value below 3.5 g/dl may indicate a guarded prognosis. A buffy coat over 1 mm indicates leukocytosis. Lipemia is often seen, especially in fasting birds, but the significance of this finding is not clear. For the serologic diagnosis of paramyxovirus infections or toxoplasmosis, 0.5 to 1.0 ml blood can be collected from the right jugular vein. This is usually a terminal procedure prior to necropsy.

Diagnostic Necropsy

A necropsy should always be performed on birds that die from unknown causes so that flaws in management can be rectified and a possible epidemic can be forestalled. The necropsy is also the ultimate method to confirm a diagnosis. Tissues for histologic or electron microscopic examination can be fixed with as few postmortem alterations as possible.

Before starting the necropsy procedure, the packing in which the bird arrived should be inspected for the presence of mites or lice. These parasites leave the bird after death of the host. The bird itself is inspected for its nutritional condition. Atrophy of the pectoral muscle or the absence of body fat indicates a chronic problem.

For the necropsy procedure see Chapter 12, Diagnostic Necropsy and Pathology.

The following procedures can provide much additional information: direct wet preparations of the gut contents and of the coating of the serosa; scrapings from the mucosa of the crop, proventriculus, duodenum, and rectum; and contact or impression smears from a freshly cut surface of liver, spleen, lungs, and any altered tissues. The smears are stained routinely with Romanowsky stains (e.g., Giemsa) or quick stains (e.g., DiffQuick) and searched microscopically with oil immersion (see Chapter 15, Cytology). Special diagnostic techniques that may be used include bacteriologic, mycologic, virologic, serologic, and histopathologic examinations and immunodiagnostic techniques.

TREATMENTS

Passerines have a high body metabolic rate and drugs are eliminated very rapidly.[4] (See also Chapters 39A, 39B, Metabolism, Pharmacology, and Therapy and Formulary.) Effective blood levels after administration of drugs are of very short duration.

For parenteral administration (intramuscular or subcutaneous) in finches, a 27-gauge needle is required, and even these can cause significant hemorrhage if not used with caution. Intramuscular injections must be made more carefully than in other species. A small amount of alcohol (70%) with 10% glycerin is used for visualizing the site before attempting an injection. To minimize risk, the injection site should be located in the caudal third of the chest muscle. The needle is placed at an acute angle, and aspiration should be performed before injecting any drug to ensure that a blood vessel has not been cannulated. After the needle has been removed, a dry cotton-tipped applicator or a finger can be used to put pressure on the injection site if bleeding does occur.

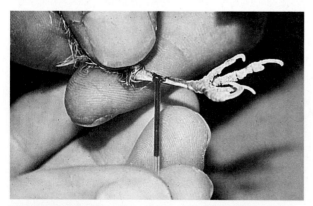

Figure 49–2

Canary *(S. canaria)*; blood sampling from the medial tarsal vein.

Table 49-1

DOSAGES FOR CHEMOTHERAPEUTICS AND ANTIBIOTICS IN CANARIES (Daily Water Intake, 250 ml/kg)

Drug	Concentration in Drinking Water (mg/l)	Concentration in Soft Food (mg/kg)
Amoxicillin	200–400	300–500
Ampicillin	1000–2000	2000–3000
Chloramphenicol	100–200	200–300
Chlortetracycline[1]	1000–1500	1500
Dimetridazole	100	
Doxycycline[1]	250	1000
Enrofloxacin[2]	200	200
Erythromycin	125	200
Furazolidone	100–200	200
Ivermectin[3]	800–1000	
Lincomycin	100–200	200
Ketoconazole	200	200
Metronidazole	100	100
Neomycin	80–100	100
Nystatin[4]	100,000 IU	200,000 IU
Polymyxin	50,000 IU	50,000 IU
Ronidazole	400	400
Spectinomycin	200–400	400
Spiramycin	200–400	400
Sulfachlorpyridazine	150–300	
Sulfadimidine	150	
Trimethoprim/sulfa[5]	50–100	100
Tylosin	250–400	400

[1]In case of ornithosis, 30 days.
[2]In case of ornithosis, 21 days.
[3]Concentration in µg/l alternative by topical application, one drop of 0.1% solution.
[4]For the treatment of *Candida albicans* for 3–6 weeks.
[5]This dosage is for the trimethoprim part alone.

Very active finches needing frequent treatments may be more easily caught in a small hospital cage (i.e., plastic-bottomed hamster cage). If such a cage is loaned to the owner, it may increase treatment compliance because it often lowers stress for the patient, and hence for owners. The number of birds returning for reexamination is increased as well.

Medication of the drinking water is a common route of drug administration in birds. Usually the water intake is reduced substantially. Water intake is normally irregularly spread over the day.[5] This results in very irregular or even inadequate blood levels of medication and therapeutic failure with the development of drug resistance. Water-administered medication is most successful in the treatment of mild gastrointestinal infections in which the drug may have a local effect in the gut.[6]

The drug should be administered at the same time in both drinking water and the soft or egg food to achieve better therapeutic results, with birds

performing self-medication several times a day (Table 49–1).

Because the elimination is so rapid, usually there are no measurable blood levels during the night. Water and food intake can be increased during the night by changing to a 24-hour light regimen, which will result in more evenly distributed blood levels over a period of 24 hours.[7] This change of day-night rhythm, however, will disturb breeding and can induce molting.

Antibiotics must be administered for at least 7 days, and bactericidal rather than bacteriostatic antibiotics are preferred.

Many drugs (i.e., dimetridazol [emtryl] and sulfa derivatives) cause toxic signs in passerines at doses used in poultry or pigeons.[4, 6, 8, 9] Canaries and finches normally drink 250 to 300 ml of water per kilogram of body weight and can ingest toxic amounts of drug.

Treatment of skin or leg lesions with ophthalmic ointments often results in toxicosis (Fig. 49–3). A few drops ingested during preening may cause the death of the bird. The owner should be instructed to apply the ointment very sparingly or put a collar on the bird.

COMMON DISEASES AND THEIR TREATMENT

A quick algorithm for determining a possible diagnosis based on the information collected and the

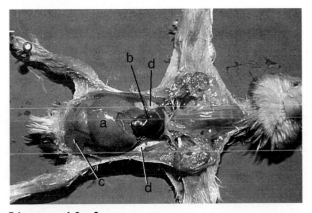

Figure 49-3

Canary *(S. canaria)*; severe liver degeneration after swallowing two drops of Panalog ointment. (a) pale liver; (b) heart; (c) duodenum with pancreas; (d) lungs.

most common diseases in passerines is presented in Table 49–2. Additional diagnostic tests and the differential diagnoses are listed in Table 49–3.

Problems in Mixed Aviaries

Nutritional problems, especially those resulting from an unbalanced diet, are often seen in mixed aviaries and with individual pet finches. The majority of the finches are granivorous and in captivity are fed either millet or canary seed or both,

with extras such as hemp, niger, and linseed. The seeding heads of panicum millet, called sprays, are greatly favored by nearly all finches; they consume large amounts. If these basic seeds are supplied ad libitum, most birds will not touch the other essential foods, such as green food (vegetables, herbs, etc.), grit, live food (insects, maggots, etc.) and soft food (mash fortified with vitamins and minerals). We believe in "controlled feeding," or "forcing" the birds by providing a daily measured amount of seed mix, supplemented with an adequate soft food. Even granivorous birds need a certain amount of

T a b l e   4 9 – 2

DIAGNOSTIC DETERMINATION TABLE

1. Species:
   Canary **2**
   Australian finch **12**
   Mixed aviary **7**
2. Age:
   Nestling **3**
   Juvenile, under 1 year of age **4**
   Any age **5**
3. Interior of the nests are yellow-stained by diarrhea of the nestlings, the feathers are sticky, the youngsters are stunted, and there is high mortality between 1 and 3 days of age .... *E. coli* **diarrhea**
   Very pale membranes are visible by opening their beaks and weak in stretching their necks. Females can be found dead sitting on the eggs .... **Blood-sucking mites**
4. The youngsters show huddling and ruffling of the feathers, debilitation, diarrhea, and sometimes neurologic signs (20%) and death. Mortality can be as high as 80%. .... **Atoxoplasmosis**
5. Respiratory distress **6**
   Respiratory symptoms not the main symptom **7**
6. Dyspnea, debilitation with scabs and pox lesions, especially on eyelids, and commissure of the beak and in feather follicles. Diphtheric lesions can be found in the mouth and the larynx. Birds of all ages can be affected, and the mortality is between 20 and 100%; the infection spreads quickly. .... **Avian pox**
   Severe respiratory signs, general illness, and central nervous symptoms and iridocyclitis, which often results in blind birds after 3 months due to a panophthalmia. .... **Toxoplasmosis**
   Minor to severe respiratory symptoms with anemia and sometimes a high mortality. The main complaint from the owner is usually a general depression in the bird. .... **Blood-sucking mites**
   Loss of voice, decline of physical condition, respiratory distress, wheezing, squeaking, coughing, sneezing, nasal discharge, head shaking, and gasping. The mortality is low. .... **Sternostomosis**
   Apathy, respiratory symptoms, regurgitation, blowing bubbles, and emaciation, but seldom diarrhea. .... **Trichomoniasis**
7. Diarrhea **8**
   Diarrhea not specific **9**
8. A general decline in the physical condition, huddling and ruffling of the feathers, debilitation, diarrhea, and emaciation. The mortality is low. .... **Coccidiosis**
   Several birds demonstrate a general malaise, with or without diarrhea, and some birds show conjunctivitis and rhinitis. Some birds may die. .... **Colibacillosis**

9. Obvious wasting **10**
   Sudden death of several birds **11**
10. Most infections are seen in winter. The clinical signs are apathy, decline in food and water intake, debilitation, emaciation, diarrhea, respiratory symptoms, ruffling of the feathers, and high mortality. .... **Pseudotuberculosis**
    Especially in outdoor aviaries, clinically indistinguishable from pseudotuberculosis, more often chronic .... **Salmonellosis**
    Apathy, diarrhea, debilitation, nasal exudate, and conjunctivitis. The mortality is usually less than 10% .... **Chlamydiosis**
11. Not specific. CNS symptoms, often obvious salivation and dyspnea or diarrhea in apathetic birds. .... **Toxicosis**
    Often after a weekend when someone other than the owner fed the birds. Sometimes black-stained droppings or diarrhea. Weakness is often interpreted as a CNS symptom. .... **Starvation**
12. Age:
    Nestlings and fledglings under the age of 3 months **13**
    All ages affected **16**
13. Bengalese or society finches as foster parents **14**
    Natural breed or foster parents **15**
14. From the age of 10 days until 6 weeks, there are debilitation, shriveling, and yellow-staining of the fledglings; difficulties with moulting; and parts of or whole seeds in the droppings. The foster parents show only watery droppings. .... **Cochlosomosis**
15. High losses of nestlings; adult Estrildidae can show apathy and yellow diarrhea or yellow solid droppings due to large amounts of undigested amylum. .... *Campylobacter*
    In nestlings there is crop bloating, and a thickened crop wall is relatively common. In weanlings and adult birds diarrhea and moulting problems are more prominent. .... **Candidiasis**
16. Respiratory distress **17**
    Respiratory signs not the main symptom **18**
17. Respiratory distress, wheezing, squeaking, coughing, sneezing, nasal discharge, loss of voice, head shaking, and gasping. The mortality is low. .... **Sternostomosis**
    Apathy, respiratory symptoms, regurgitation, blowing bubbles, and emaciation; sometimes diarrhea. .... **Trichomoniasis**
18. CNS symptoms **19**
    CNS-symptoms not the main symptom **7**
19. Torticollis is the main symptom. As long as birds with this symptom can still eat, mortality is low. .... **Paramyxovirus**
    Sudden death of several birds **11**

T a b l e 4 9 – 3

SPECIAL HINTS FOR FURTHER DIAGNOSTICS

Disease	Diagnostic Technique
Atoxoplasmosis	Necropsy; demonstration of the parasites in imprints of several organs
Avian pox	Necropsy and virus isolation
Mites	Demonstration of mites in the nest or bird-room crevices
Campylobacter	Demonstration of the microorganisms on fecal smears stained with DiffQuick; culture on special media
Candidiasis	Direct wet preparation and/or a stained smear fungal culture
Chlamydiosis	Necropsy and demonstration of the agent by staining, IFT, or ELISA
Coccidiosis	Fecal parasite examination of droppings collected between 2 and 6 PM
Cochlosomosis	Flagellates in a wet mount of fresh and body-warm feces
Colibacillosis	Assess other disease factors in combination with bacterial isolation
Helminthic parasites	Not important in small passerines; *Syngamus* occasionally
Toxicosis	Detailed case history A direct confirmation often impossible, if the toxin is not known
Paramyxovirus	Serologic and virologic screening Pancreatitis on histopathology
Pseudotuberculosis	Necrotic foci in liver and spleen; bacterial culture
Salmonellosis	Necrotic foci in liver and spleen; bacterial culture
Starvation	Hemorrhagic diathesis (bleeding into the gut)
E. coli diarrhea	Demonstration and isolation of bacteria in the feces
Sternostomosis	Diagnostic necropsy and demonstration of the parasite
Trichomoniasis	Demonstration of flagellates in crop swab Necropsy
Toxoplasmosis	Serology and demonstration of the parasite in brain smears, organ smears, or histologic sections

"softbill food," because an unbalanced diet may predispose them to problems with Enterobacteriaceae (e.g., *Escherichia coli, Klebsiella* species, *Enterobacter* species) and yeast infections (especially *Candida albicans*). The breeding results are also not optimal in birds with an unbalanced diet.

Most passerines relish an apple, orange, or green food whenever it is offered to them. This is the perfect vehicle for a vitamin or mineral supplement if "soft foods" are not accepted.

Specific deficiencies occur with vitamin D_3, calcium, and phosphorus, resulting in rickets and osteomalacia. By feeding rancid cod liver oil or mixing oil through the seed, encephalomalacia and fertility problems are seen because of vitamin E deficiency. Vitamin B deficiency can cause CNS disturbances, reduced hatching, stunting, and molting problems.

Other nutritional problems can include iron accumulation (hemochromatosis) in softbills (i.e., non–seed-eating Passeriformes) resulting in liver cirrhosis, and oversupplementation of vitamin A and D, which is associated with renal disease, infertility, and deaths.[2, 10]

Many problems in aviaries, however, are management and hygiene-related problems resulting from location of food and water containers. Overcrowding leads to aggression, and provision of insufficient nesting sites results in poor breeding outcomes. The control of ecto- and endoparasites must be constantly addressed.

Picking is a common problem in aviaries. This can range from a few feathers lost on the back of the head to cannibalism. Zebra finches are prone to this behavior. Picking can also be the result of inappropriate sexual behavior of one or more dominant male birds. Aggression is highest when aviaries are overcrowded or nesting sites or territory are involved. Sick birds may attract aggressive behavior; therefore, the attacked bird should be separated from others. Examine all picked birds and provide extra heat. Treat skin trauma or underlying disease. Corrective measures include providing adequate cage space, nests, nesting material, insect food or high protein food, and calcium. Provide multiple food and water containers and ample perches.

Fractures are relatively common in aviary birds. Affected birds have droppings on their backs and worn or frayed feathers (from floor sitting). Most fractures can be successfully treated with external fixation. A tape cast must be carefully applied with the leg in a flexed position, and the tape must be well trimmed to make it as small and light as possible. Elizabethan collars are not recommended in passerines.

Thread necrosis of the digits is more common in finches than in other pet birds, especially in nesting birds. Raw, unbleached, uncharted cotton in its natural form is the safest commercially available nesting material. Inflammations or abnormalities involving the foot of a nesting bird should be examined with a hand lens or other magnification. Always use magnification when locating and unwinding threads. Bandaging and antibiotics are recommended. Gangrenous necrosis may be irreversible if the injury is old. Hemorrhage is a serious complication, and an elastic band tourniquet is sometimes necessary for thread removal.

CANARIES

Other Noninfectious Disease Problems

Feather cysts ("lumps") are commonly found in Norwich canaries and Gloucester and dimorphic new color canaries (Fig. 49–4). A dysplastic feather syndrome is recognized that has been termed "straw feather disease." (See Chapter 32, Avian Dermatology.) Complete feather loss may also be related to irregular day (light) length.

In older canaries, cataracts and a syndrome of ataxia, head tilt, and body tremor of unknown etiology are sometimes seen.

Infectious Diseases in Canaries

Many infectious diseases are species-specific, although salmonellosis and pseudotuberculosis are exceptions. Coccidiosis is often diagnosed in canaries and finches. These coccidia were originally said to belong to the *Isospora lacazei* group.[11] Now it is

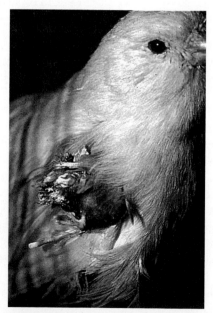

F i g u r e 4 9 – 4

Canary *(S. canaria)*; feather cyst ("lump").

believed that most species have their own coccidian species. For the canary these are *I. canaria* (intestinal coccidiosis) and *I. serini* (atoxoplasmosis).[12, 13]

Viral Diseases

Avian Pox

Avian pox is a viral infection seen almost exclusively in canaries and other *Serinus* species and occurs predominantly in the autumn and winter. Susceptible birds may show the cutaneous, diphtheric, or septicemic form of the disease. The septicemic or respiratory form causes a high mortality because of a severe tracheitis and occasionally pneumonic lesions around the bronchi.

Birds of all ages can be affected, and the mortality is between 20 and 100%. Infection spreads quickly. The most noticeable clinical signs are respiratory stridor, debilitation, and death. The infection is transmitted by insects and direct contact and indirectly through the food and the drinking water. A presumptive diagnosis is made on the appearance of signs and lesions. A positive diagnosis is made after virus isolation or histologic demonstration of the eosinophilic intracytoplasmic inclusion bodies in the epithelial cells.

Preventive vaccination is possible by the wing-web method (Fig. 49–5), preferable in early summer. Vaccination must be repeated once every year. In an epidemic all birds are caged individually, or, if this is impossible, in small groups. All clinically healthy birds should be vaccinated. Supportive treatment consists of the administration of antibiotics and multivitamin preparations. Two weeks after mortality has stopped, the birds can be housed again in the flight cages.

Recently a poxvirus has been demonstrated in masked bullfinches *(Pyrrhula erythaca)*, causing tumor-like lesions in the head region and inside the beak.[14]

Leukosis

An enlarged and pale liver and spleen are seen regularly at necropsy in some flocks. Histologic changes are identical to those of leukosis in poultry. The birds show primarily signs of respiratory distress, and morbidity is low (5–10%). A viral cause has not yet been proved.

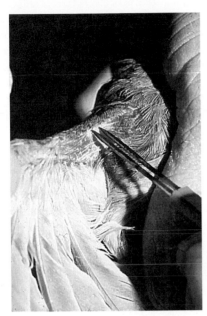

Figure 49–5

Canary *(S. canaria)*; vaccination against avian pox by the "wingweb" method.

Other Viral Infections

Newcastle disease (paramyxovirus 1) is occasionally seen in canaries, with watery diarrhea and respiratory signs. Torticollis (paramyxovirus 3) is a common disease in "tropical" finches. Infections with influenza virus have been reported. Recently a coronavirus has been demonstrated in the trachea of canaries with mild respiratory problems (unpublished data, GM Dorrestein).

Bacterial Infections

The following are brief descriptions of bacterial diseases that affect canaries. For more detailed information, see Chapter 18, Bacteriology.

Ornithosis *(Chlamydia psittaci)*

The annual incidence of ornithosis in canaries is between 0 and 1.4%. The symptoms are nonspecific and can include lethargy, diarrhea, debilitation, nasal exudate, and conjunctivitis. The mortality is usually less than 10%. The diagnosis is made at necropsy by demonstrating *Chlamydia* in impression smears from the air sacs and organs with special staining techniques or an enzyme-linked immunosorbent assay (ELISA) of swabs.

Treatment with chlortetracycline (30 days), doxycycline (30 days), or enrofloxacin (21 days) through drinking water and soft food is clinically effective.

Mycoplasma

Mycoplasma species have been isolated from canaries. Many canaries with conjunctivitis and upper respiratory disease respond to tylosin; however, there has been no conclusive evidence that *Mycoplasma* is associated with this syndrome. Tetracyclines and enrofloxacin may be effective against many *Mycoplasma* species as well as *Chlamydia* species.[2]

Yersiniosis (Pseudotuberculosis)

Disease caused by *Yersinia pseudotuberculosis* is regularly seen in winter months in canaries of all ages. The clinical signs are nonspecific: ruffling of the feathers, debilitation, and high mortality. At necropsy a dark, swollen, congested liver and spleen with small, yellow, focal bacterial granulomas are found. An acute catarrhal pneumonia and a typhlitis may be present. Many rod-shaped bacteria are seen in impression smears from all the organs. The diagnosis is confirmed after culturing the microorganisms. Treatment of choice is amoxicillin given in the drinking water and the soft food. The antibiotic may need to be changed once sensitivity test results are obtained. Cleaning and disinfection are essential to prevent a relapse after therapy has been completed.

Salmonellosis (Paratyphoid)

Infection with *Salmonella typhimurium* is identical to pseudotuberculosis both clinically and at necropsy (Fig. 49–6), although a chronic course is seen more often in salmonellosis. Existence of carriers is unknown in canaries. The diagnosis is confirmed after culture and identification of the microorganism.

Effective antibiotics include trimethoprim (with or without sulfa), amoxicillin, and enrofloxacin. Antibiotic therapy must be combined with good hygiene. Three to 6 weeks after therapy, a bacterial

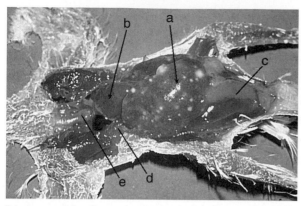

Figure 49–6

Canary *(S. canaria)*; bacterial granulomas in the liver *(Salmonella typhimurium)*. (a) liver with bacterial granulomas; (b) heart; (c) duodenum with pancreas; (d) lungs; (e) syrinx.

culture of a pooled fecal sample in enrichment medium should be done to evaluate the success of the therapy. When necessary, therapy as well as the hygienic measures are repeated until serial bacterial cultures are negative.

E. coli and Other Enterobacteriaceae

These bacteria are often isolated from the feces or the intestinal contents of diseased birds, with and without diarrhea. In general there is malaise, with some birds showing conjunctivitis and rhinitis; a few birds may die. These are secondary pathogens, however, and should be considered as a symptom of poor health or hygienic conditions. Possible causes are unbalanced diet, housing problems, or management-related problems. Other primary diseases may be present (e.g., atoxoplasmosis or coccidiosis). Treatment with antibiotics may cause temporary clinical improvement; the primary disease must be identified for successful therapy to be undertaken.

Enterobacteriaceae are regularly cultured from nestlings with diarrhea ("sweating disease"). The antibiotics of choice are neomycin or spectinomycin because they are effective and not absorbed from the gut. The drug is administered in the soft food. In fledglings, extra water, like green food, will prevent dehydration.

"Hemorrhagic enteritis" is diagnosed often at necropsy. This is not enteritis in the true sense, but is better described as a hemorrhagic diathesis (bleeding into the gut, Fig. 49–7). It is seen in small birds that are anorexic for over 24 hours, perhaps because of illness (e.g., an infection or toxicosis) or, more often, when they are offered the wrong food or no food at all (e.g., if the owner was away and someone else fed the birds). A typical sign is an empty stomach.

A similar interpretation should be given to swollen, white kidneys, which are the result of uric acid precipitation and stasis in the collection tubules that occur when birds do not drink (Fig. 49–8). This condition is often falsely called "renal gout," but it should not be interpreted as nephritis or gout. It should be differentiated from visceral gout that re-

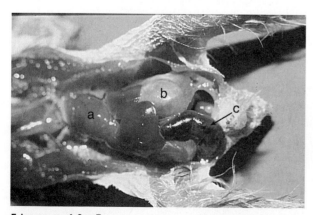

Figure 49–7

Chinese nightingale *(Leiothrix lutea)*; hemorrhagic diathesis caused by starvation. (a) heart; (b) gizzard; (c) hemorrhagic intestinal loop.

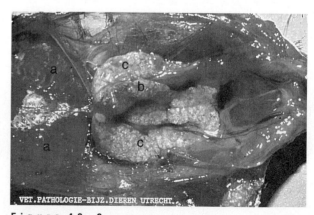

Figure 49–8

Canary *(S. canaria)*; uric acid precipitation in the kidneys caused by dehydration. (a) lungs; (b) inactive ovary; (c) kidney.

sults from impaired renal function or a high protein diet.

Cocci Infections

Infections with *Streptococcus* and *Staphylococcus* species are seen often. The clinical signs are abscesses, dermatitis, "bumble feet" and conjunctivitis, as well as, less often, sinusitis, arthritis, pneumonia, and death. Cocci are seen in the impression smears. Local and systemic treatment with ampicillin or amoxicillin is the therapy of choice.

Enterococcus faecalis has been associated with chronic tracheitis, pneumonia, and air sac infections in canaries. Clinically affected birds have harsh respiratory sounds, voice changes, and dyspnea.[15]

Pseudomonas Infections

Inexpertly prepared sprouted or germinated seeds and dirty drinking vessels or baths can be the source of *Pseudomonas* species infection, causing a foul-smelling diarrhea. A dirty flower spraying bottle, used for spraying the birds, can cause a severe necropurulent pneumonia and airsacculitis. Treatment includes identifying the source of the infection and administration of an antibiotic. Enrofloxacin is the drug of choice.

Avian Tuberculosis

The classic tuberculosis with tubercles in the organs is seldom seen in small passerines. Individual infections with acid-fast bacilli are seen relatively often. On histologic examination, macrophages loaded with acid-fast bacilli can be found in many organs. No alterations are apparent at necropsy, except perhaps a dark, slightly swollen liver.

Other Bacterial Infections

Gram-negative oviduct infections can cause high mortality in hens if untreated. This may occur in epidemic proportions in canary breeding establishments, usually affecting hens on their second clutch of eggs in the breeding season.[2] *Erysipelothrix rhusiopathiae, Listeria monocytogenes,* and *Pasteurella multocida* are occasionally isolated from diseased birds.

In canaries, infection with "megabacteria" of the

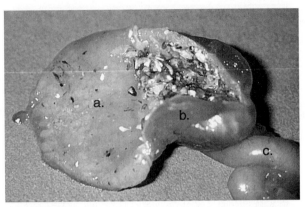

Figure 49–9

Canary *(S. canaria)*; thickened proventricular wall caused by megabacteria. (a) proventriculus; (b) gizzard; (c) duodenum.

proventriculus is very common. Affected birds show proventriculitis, and the pH in the lumen, originally 0.7 to 2.4, is increased to 7.0 to 7.4.[16] The birds are often debilitated; the morbidity is high, but the mortality is low. These microorganisms are seen in a smear from the thick, whitish mucus covering the mucosa (Fig. 49–9) and sometimes in fecal smears. Megabacteria are predominantly found on the mucosal surface and glandular ducts of the proventriculus.

Mycotic Infections

Mycotic infections are not a significant problem in canaries. Occasionally, cases of candidiasis are seen.

Protozoal Infections

The most important protozoal infections in canaries are atoxoplasmosis, coccidiosis, toxoplasmosis, and trichomoniasis.

Atoxoplasmosis

Atoxoplasmosis (formerly Lankesterella) is caused by *I. serini,* a coccidium with an asexual life cycle in the organs and a sexual cycle in the intestinal mucosa[12] (Fig. 49–10). Atoxoplasmosis is a disease of young canaries at the age of 2 to 9 months. The

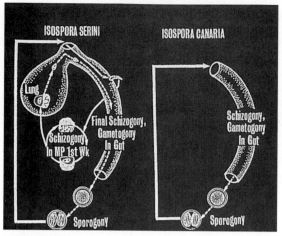

Figure 49-10

Life cycle of *I. serini* (atoxoplasmosis) and *I. canaria* (intestinal coccidiosis).

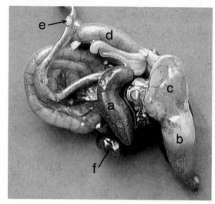

Figure 49-12

Canary *(S. canaria)*; splenomegaly caused by atoxoplasmosis. (a) spleen; (b) proventriculus; (c) gizzard; (d) duodenum; (e) rudimentary cecum; (f) liver.

clinical symptoms are huddling and ruffling of the feathers, debilitation, diarrhea, and occasionally neurologic signs (20%), and death. Mortality can be as high as 80%. An enlarged liver can be seen as a blue spot at the right side of the abdomen caudal to the sternum, referred to by fanciers as "thick liver disease" (Fig. 49–11). At necropsy an enlarged, sometimes spotted liver, in the acute phase with necrosis; a huge, dark red–colored spleen (Fig. 49–12); and often an edematous duodenum with vascularization are seen. In the imprints of the liver, spleen, and lungs the parasites are found in the cytoplasm of the monocytes. The nucleus of the host cell is crescent-shaped. Coccidia are seldom found in the feces or intestinal contents, because after the acute phase only a few coccidia (100–200/24 hours) are excreted.

Atoxoplasmosis is considered to be resistant to therapy.[2] In Europe, the treatment of choice is sulfachlorpyridazine (Esb3, Ciba-Geigy, or Vetisulid, Solvay), 150 mg/l in drinking water for 5 days a week. This treatment has to be repeated every week from the moment the diagnosis is confirmed until after molting. This approach is proven to be safe and effective,[17] but affects only the production of oocysts and does not influence the intracellular stages. It interrupts the infection cycle. Other coccidiostatics may be effective in interrupting the cycle as well.

Other improvements include feeding one part egg food and one part seed mixture until after molting, prevention of crowding, and better hygiene, especially after cleaning and changing the floor coating. These measures alone can prevent clinical outbreaks in infected canaries. Infection is also common in other European finches kept in captivity (e.g., goldfinch, siskin, greenfinch, and bullfinch).

Coccidiosis

Coccidiosis *(I. canaria)* can cause disease in any canaries older than 2 months. Clinical symptoms are diarrhea and emaciation. At necropsy the duodenum is edematous (Fig. 49–13), often with exten-

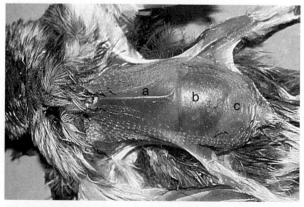

Figure 49-11

Canary *(S. canaria)*; "thick liver disease" caused by atoxoplasmosis. In the liver necrotic foci are visible. (a) sternum; (b) liver; (c) duodenal loop.

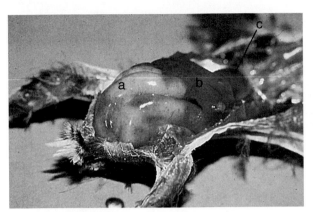

Figure 49–13

Black siskin (*Serinus* species); edematous duodenum caused by coccidiosis. (a) duodenum; (b) liver; (c) heart.

sive hemorrhages in the gut wall. In scrapings of the duodenal mucosa, trophozoites of the parasite can be found. In wet preparations from the droppings, large amounts of oocysts can be seen. Therapy consists of strict hygiene and treatment with coccidiostatic drugs. Amprolium solution has been recommended for the treatment of coccidiosis at a dosage of 50 to 100 mg/l for 5 days or longer.[9] Another therapy is sulfachlorpyridazine 300 mg/l in drinking water, 5 days a week for 2 to 3 weeks.

Toxoplasmosis

In the acute phase of toxoplasmosis, birds may show severe respiratory signs. Often this phase is not diagnosed, and the owner may not notice symptoms until several birds become blind many weeks after the infection. The route of infection is not known, but it is likely that oocysts excreted in feces of cats get into the aviary. At necropsy the canaries show, in the acute phase, hepatomegaly and splenomegaly, and sometimes a severe catarrhal pneumonia and a myositis of the pectoral muscle. The trophozoites are easily found in impression smears. The blind canaries have iridocyclitis or panophthalmia (Fig. 49–14), and trophozoites are found only in smears from the brains after a long search. In histologic slides from the brains, pseudocysts are relatively easy to find. Serologic test results, immunofluorescence on brain tissue slides, or inoculation of mice confirms the diagnosis. No effective treatment is known.

Trichomoniasis

Infections with this flagellate are seen sporadically in canaries. Birds of all ages can be affected. The clinical symptoms include respiratory changes, regurgitation, blowing bubbles, and emaciation. The diagnosis can be made in a live bird with a crop swab. At necropsy, trichomoniasis presents as a thickened, opaque crop wall.

Another flagellate is seen in the crop of canaries, causing the same clinical symptoms in adults and mortality in nestlings. The diagnosis can be made with a wet mount specimen, but the flagellates are difficult to recognize. The parasite does not move on the wet mount preparation, but "waves" with its flagella.[18]

Other Protozoal Infections

Plasmodium and other blood parasites have incidentally been reported in canaries.

Helminthic Parasitism

These parasites are of no significance in canaries or other finches. In outdoor aviaries, an infection with gapeworms *(Syngamus trachea)* occasionally is found. The symptoms include gasping for breath, and these small birds often die from occlusion of the trachea by the worms and the produced mucus. The diagnosis is confirmed by finding the eggs in the droppings and the worms in the trachea at necropsy (Fig. 49–15; see also Color Figure).

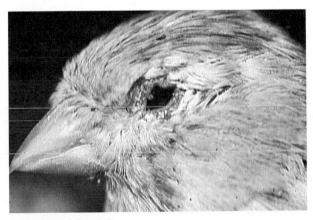

Figure 49–14

Canary *(S. canaria)*; one-sided panophthalmia caused by chronic toxoplasmosis.

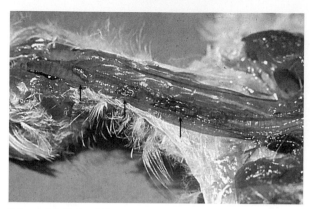

Figure 49–15

Canary *(S. canaria)*; trachea filled with *Syngamus* worms *(arrows).*

Arthropods

Ectoparasites and *Epidermoptes* species

Ectoparasites, including blood-sucking mites *(Dermanyssus gallinae* and *Ornithonyssus sylviarum)*, skin mites (e.g., *Backericheyla* species, *Neocheyletiella media* and *Epidermopetes* species) and feather mites (e.g., *Syringophylus* species and *Dermoglyphus* species) in the calamus (quill) of the feathers are found. Meal-mites *(Tyroglyphus farinae)* can cause unrest and irritation.

The red mite *(D. gallinae)* can cause high mortality among fledglings as well as adult birds. The invariable symptom is anemia. A bird with respiratory symptoms and a PCV less than 30% (Fig. 49–16) is suspected to have a severe infestation with blood-sucking mites. The main complaint from the owner is a general depression. The red mite spends the day in the nest (Fig. 49–17) or bird room crevices (Fig. 49–18) and ventures out at night to attack the birds. Treatment should be prompt and consists of dusting or spraying the victims with an insecticide, vacating the cage or room during the day, and thorough cleaning.

The white or Northern mite *(O. sylviarum)* increasingly is found to cause problems in aviaries. This blood-sucking mite spends its entire life cycle on the host. Dusting with insecticides can be hazardous, especially to nestlings. A relatively safe treatment is applying one drop of 0.1% ivermectin in propylene glycol on the bare skin; however, the mites are killed only after sucking blood.

Other ectoparasites cause no real disease prob-

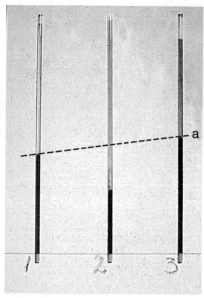

Figure 49–16

Canary *(S. canaria)*; blood capillary tube (middle) with PCV = 27% caused by blood-sucking mites. Left (PCV = 43%) and right (PCV = 53%) normal blood samples. (a) normal range.

lems except some irritation or feather damage. They are, however, considered a sign of inadequate hygiene and management.

Air Sac Mites *(Sternostoma tracheacolum)*

Air sac mites occasionally are found in canaries, but are seen most commonly in Australian finches.

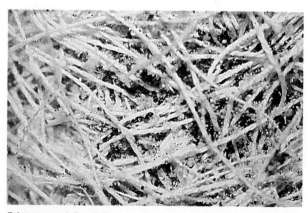

Figure 49–17

Canary *(S. canaria)*; nesting material infested with red blood mites *(Dermanyssus gallinae).*

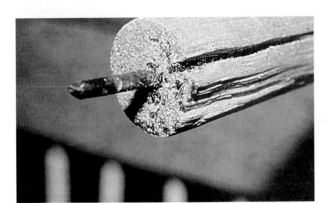

Figure 49–18

Perch with many red blood mites *(Dermanyssus gallinae).*

AUSTRALIAN AND TROPICAL FINCHES

Nutritional deficiencies are the primary cause of many problems in Australian and other tropical finches. Therefore, when treating disease problems in these birds, improvement of the diet is a primary objective. A diet consisting of three parts of a seed mix supplemented with one part soft food is recommended. Acceptance of the soft food is often a problem.

Viral Infections

Avian Pox

Avian pox infection is uncommon in these birds. A minor epizootic of poxvirus with no mortalities was reported in society finches.[10] Unilateral conjunctival inflammation and swelling were the principal signs.

Papovavirus

Papovavirus and polyoma-like virus infections occur in finch aviaries across Australia and the United States and are probably more common than the number of cases actually diagnosed would indicate. These infections are reported in many finch species, (such as Gouldian finches,[19, 20] painted finches,[21] and green finches.[22] The disease causes both young nestling mortality and a more chronic disease in which poor development and beak abnormalities

predominate. Secondary infections complicate the disease. Necropsy may reveal hepatomegaly. The predominant histologic lesion is hepatocellular necrosis with intranuclear inclusions. Myocarditis may be seen. The diagnosis is made by a specific fluorescent antibody test on liver and spleen impression smears. In an electron microscopic examination of the intranuclear inclusions, discrete, round to icosahedral (20 sides), electron-dense particles 45 to 50 nm in diameter can be found.

Paramyxovirus Infection

Paramyxovirus infection is common in many finches (e.g., African silver-bills, zebra finches, and Gouldian finches). Paramyxovirus, serotype 3, causes torticollis (Fig. 49–19), depression, and variable degrees of weight loss. The birds can be carriers for months before the clinical symptoms appear. Presumptive diagnosis is based on the clinical signs and can be confirmed by serologic testing and virus isolation. The necropsy findings are nonspecific. Severe pancreatitis is found on histologic examination (Fig. 49–20; see also Color Figure).

Antibiotic therapy produces no significant difference in survival rate or outcome. The disease must be differentiated from a vitamin E deficiency caused by feeding rancid cod liver oil or mixing oil through the seed.

Other Viral Infections

Several other viruses have been isolated from finches (e.g., herpesvirus and cytomegalovirus).[2]

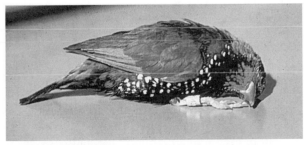

Figure 49–19

Emblema picta; torticollis caused by paramyxovirus type 3.

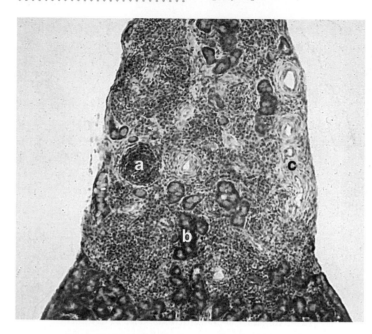

Figure 49-20

Sidney waxbill *(Aegintha temporalis)*; pancreatitis caused by paramyxovirus type 3. (a) lymph follicles; (b) exocrine pancreatic tissue; (c) area of fibrosis.

Bacterial Infections

E. coli septicemia is suspected as the major cause of epizootic mortality in new shipments of finches.[10] *Citrobacter* infection has also been reported as a cause of mortality in finches.[23] Gross necropsy findings can be unrewarding in either disease. The Enterobacteriaceae are more frequently secondary problems in finches than in canaries. The clinical symptoms and the gross necropsy results are non-specific. Bacterial cultures and sensitivity testing are necessary for diagnosis and selection of appropriate antibiotic therapy.

Salmonellosis and pseudotuberculosis are uncommon in Australian finches.

Tuberculosis (atypical *Mycobacterium avium*), as described under Canaries, is seen regularly in the Estrildidae.

Campylobacter *Infections*

Campylobacter fetus subspecies *jejuni* is commonly found in tropical finches, especially in Estrildidae.[24] Society finches often are asymptomatic carriers. Clinical signs include apathy, delayed molting, yellow droppings, and a high mortality rate, especially among fledglings. The yellow-colored droppings are caused by large amounts of undigested amylum

(ground seed) (Fig. 49–21). Sometimes undigested whole seeds or parts of seeds are found in the droppings. At necropsy the intestine is filled with a yellow liquid (amylum), or whole seeds are seen in the gut resembling the beads of a rosary (Fig. 49–22). Other postmortem findings include cachexia and a congested gastrointestinal tract. The diagnosis is confirmed by demonstrating the curved rods in stained smears from the droppings or gut contents, and culturing the bacteria on special microaerophilic media.

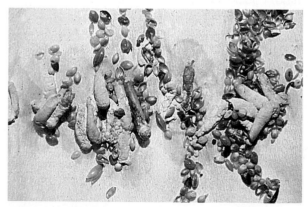

Figure 49-21

Pictorella finch *(Lonchura pectoralis)*; dry yellow feces caused by *Campylobacter* infection.

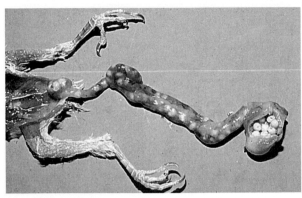

Figure 49-22

Lady Gouldian finch *(Chloebia gouldiae)*; whole seeds in the gut resembling the beads of a rosary caused by *Campylobacter* infection.

Mycotic Infections

Candidiasis

Candidiasis is a serious problem in finches and can be related to nutritional problems, poor hygiene, and the overuse of antibiotics. In nestlings and fledglings, crop candidiasis can occur with gas formation caused by fermentation. A thickened, opaque crop wall with a white coating on the mucosa is a common pathologic finding. Diarrhea and molting problems are more prominent in adult birds. The diagnosis is confirmed by identifying the budding yeasts in smears from crop swabs (Fig. 49–23) or feces. The birds are treated with nystatin

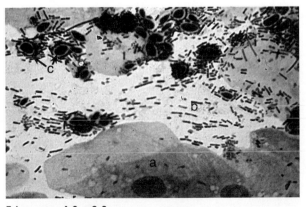

Figure 49-23

Parson finch *(Poephila cincta)*; *Candida* infection in the crop (Hemacolor ×1000). (a) squamous epithelial cell; (b) rod-shaped bacteria; (c) yeast cells. Notice the "halo" surrounding the yeast cells.

for 3 to 6 weeks at a dose of 100,000 IU/l of drinking water and 200,000 IU/kg of soft food. Predisposing factors should be corrected.

Protozoal Infections

Atoxoplasma-like infections and cryptosporidiosis are found occasionally in finches but are restricted to individual birds and do not occur as flock problems. Coccidiosis and trichomoniasis are common in these species; symptoms and treatment are similar to those discussed for canaries.

Cochlosomosis

Cochlosoma species is a flagellate that lives in the intestinal tract of society finches and can cause death among Australian finches that are fostered by these birds.[25] The problem is most severe in young birds from 10 days until 6 weeks of age. Typical symptoms are debilitation, shrivelling, and yellow staining of the fledglings; and difficulties with molting. The diagnosis is based on demonstrating the flagellates in fresh and body-warm feces from the finches. Treatment consists of ronidazole at 400 mg/kg of egg food and 400 mg/l of drinking water for 5 days. After a pause of 2 days, the regimen is repeated. This drug is relatively safe, and toxicity has not been seen. If dimetridazole is used, the concentration should not exceed 100 mg active drug per liter for 5 days. A sign of intoxication is torticollis, which disappears after the medication is stopped. Metronidazole has been reported to cause toxicity in finches.[26]

Helminthic Parasitism

Tapeworm infestations in insectivorous finches (particularly parrot finches and diamond firetails) are common. Occasionally, cestodiasis is seen as a recurring problem in the zebra finch.[2] At necropsy, the small intestines are sometimes literally packed with the tiny tapeworms. The typical hexacanth embryos are usually seen on fecal flotation.

Acuaria skrjabini infections of the gizzard with mucosal necrosis were reported in adult finches in Australia.[27] The mortality rate was 4 to 5%. Oral treatment with 80 mg levamisole or 50 mg fenben-dazole/l of drinking water for 3 days was effective.

Feeding live food (maggots, mealworms, or termites) or providing a compost heap in the aviary to attract live insect food are common management practices in Australia. These practices increase the likelihood of infection because insects are the intermediate hosts for gizzard worms and tapeworms.

Arthropods

Ectoparasites

The red mite is less common in aviaries with Australian finches than in those with canaries. Severe anemia and death caused by blood-sucking mites are possible.

Knemidokoptic mange and respiratory mites are both of importance in finches.

Knemidokoptes *pilae*

Knemidokoptes is occasionally seen on the base of the beak of finches. It is easily identified in scrapings from the altered beak. Local treatment with mineral oil or 0.1% ivermectin applied locally is effective. This infestation should not be confused with the "tassel foot" in European goldfinches (*Carduelis carduelis*), which is caused by a papillomavirus. Imported goldfinches occasionally are affected with tassel foot, in which smooth, hard projections arise from the plantar surface of the foot (Fig. 49–24).

Air Sac Mites

Air sac mites (*Sternostoma tracheacolum*) are found mainly in Gouldian finches and less frequently in canaries. This problem is also seen in wild Gouldian finches in Australia and may have been introduced through domestic canaries. The mites' life cycle is unknown, but it is thought that nestlings become infected from parents through regurgitation of food contaminated with mites. Adults may be infected via contamination of water and food by coughing or sneezing.

Clinical signs include physical debilitation, respi-

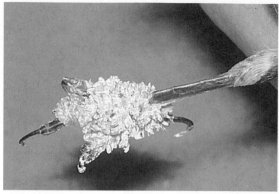

F i g u r e   4 9 – 2 4

European goldfinch *(Carduelis carduelis)* with a "tassel foot" caused by a papillomavirus.

ratory distress, wheezing, squeaking, coughing, sneezing, nasal discharge, loss of voice, head shaking, and gasping. Mortality is low. The diagnosis can sometimes be made by transillumination of the trachea in live birds, with the mites visible as tiny black points in the trachea. The throat of the bird must be wetted (e.g., with alcohol) and the feathers parted. Postmortem examination is more reliable and the condition is diagnosed by finding mites in the air sacs (Fig. 49–25; see also Color Figure), lungs, and trachea. Airsacculitis, tracheitis, and focal pneumonia can be found.

Several therapeutic regimens have been described for air sac mite infestations. Pest strips are a good preventative, provided the bird cannot get

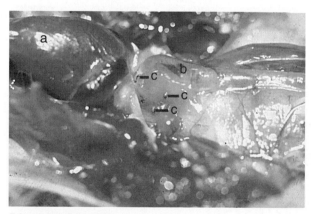

F i g u r e   4 9 – 2 5

Lady Gouldian finch *(Chloebia gouldiae)*; air sac mites *(Sternostoma tracheacolum)*. (a) heart; (b) syrinx; (c) mites.

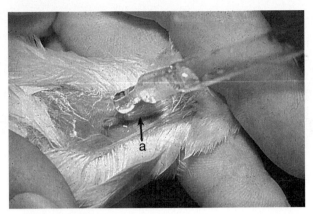

Figure 49-26

Canary *(S. canaria)*; spot-on of ivermectin. (a) right vena jugularis.

to the strips, and only if the bird is not held within a small enclosure. Ivermectin can be used for individual treatment by a spot-on method of one drop of 0.1% invermectin in propylene glycol, applied on the bare skin dorsolateral of the thorax inlet or on the chest (Fig. 49-26). A small amount of alcohol is necessary to view the site of application.

References

1. Dodwell GT: The Complete Book of Canaries. New York, Howell Book House, 1986.
2. MacWhirter P: Passeriformes. In Ritchie B, Harrison GT, Harrison LR (eds): Avian Medicine: Principles and Application. Lake Worth, FL, Wingers Publishing, 1994, pp 1172–1199.
3. Coutteel P: The importance of manipulating the daily photoperiod in canary breeding. Proc 3rd Conf Eur Assoc Avian Vet, Jerusalem, 1995, pp 166–170.
4. Dorrestein GM: Infectious diseases and their therapy in Passeriformes. In Antimicrobial Therapy in Caged and Exotic Pets. Int Sympos, Trenton, NJ, Veterinary Learning Systems, 1995, pp 11–27.
5. Dorrestein GM, Gogh H van, Wit P de: Blood levels of certain drugs administered via drinking water to homing pigeons *(Columba livia)*. Utrecht, The Netherlands, Unpublished thesis, 1986, pp 179–202.
6. Flammer K: Antimicrobial Therapy. In Ritchie B, Harrison G, Harrison L (eds): Avian Medicine: Principles and Application. Lake Worth, FL, Wingers Publishing, 1994, pp 434–456.
7. Bauck L, Hoefer HL: Avian antimicrobial therapy. Semin Avian Exotic Pet Med 2:17–22, 1993.
8. Debuf YM: Prescribing for exotic birds. In The Veterinary Formulary. London, The Pharmaceutical Press, 1994, pp 50–56.
9. Ritchie BW, Harrison GJ: Formulary. In Ritchie BW, Harrison GJ, Harrison LR (eds): Avian Medicine: Principles and Application. Lake Worth, FL, Wingers Publishing, 1994, pp 457–478.
10. Bauck L: Diseases of the finch as seen in a commercial import station. Proc Assoc Avian Vet, Seattle, 1989, pp 196–202.
11. Pellerdy LP: Coccidia and coccidiosis. Berlin, Verlag Paul Parey, 1974, pp 371–374.
12. Box ED: Life cycles of two *Isospora* species in the canary *(Serinus canaria* Linaeus). J Protozool 24:57–67, 1977.
13. Box ED: Isospora as an extraintestinal parasite of passerine birds. J Protozool 18:244–246, 1981.
14. Dorrestein M, Hage MH van der, Grinwis G: A tumour-like pox-lesion in masked bull finches *(Pyrrhula erythaca)*. Proc. 2nd Eur Assoc Avian Vet, Utrecht, 1993, pp 232–240.
15. Devriese LA, Uyttebroek E, Ducatelle R, et al: Tracheitis due to *Enterococcus faecalis* infection in canaries. J Assoc Avian Vet 4:113–116, 1990.
16. Herck H van, Duijser T, Zwart P, et al: A bacterial proventriculus in canary birds. Avian Pathol 13:561–572, 1984.
17. Dorrestein GM: Atoxoplasmosis in Passeriformes. Proceedings 1st Conference on Avian Diseases. München, 1979, pp 130–134.
18. van der Hage MH, Dorrestein GM: Flagellates in the crop of canary bird. Proc 1st Eur Assoc avian Vet, vienna, 1991, pp 303–307.
19. Forshaw D, Wylie SL, Pass D: Infection with a virus resembling papovavirus in Gouldian finches *(Erythrura gouldiae)*. Aust Vet J 65:26–28, 1988.
20. Marshall R: Papova-like virus in a finch aviary. Proc Assoc Avian Vet, Seattle, 1989, pp 203–207.
21. Woods L: Case report. Papova-like virus in a painted finch. Proc Assoc Avian Vet, Seattle, 1989, pp 218–219.
22. Sironi G, Rampin T: Papova-like splenohepatic infection in greenfinches *(Carduelis chloris)*. Clin Vet 110:79–82, 1987.
23. Gerlach H: Bacteria. In Ritchie BW, Harrison GJ, Harrison LR (eds): Avian Medicine: Principles and Application. Lake Worth, FL, Wingers Publishing, 1994, pp 948–983.
24. Dorrestein GM, Hage MH van der, Cornelissen JL: Campylobacter infections in cage birds—clinical, pathological and bacteriological aspects. Assoc Avian Vet Newsletter 5:89, 1984.
25. Poelma FG, Zwart P, Dorrestein GM, Lordens CM: Cochlosomose, een probleem bij de opfok van prachtvinken in volires. Tijdsch Diergeneesk 103:589–593, 1978.
26. Harrison GJ: Toxicology. In Harrison GJ, Harrison LR (eds): Clinical Avian Medicine and Surgery. Philadelphia, WB Saunders, 1986, pp 491–499.
27. McOrist S, Barton NJ, Black DG: *Acuaria skrjabini*-infection of the gizzard of finches. Avian Dis 26:957–960, 1982.

Jan Hooimeijer
Gerry M. Dorrestein

50

Pigeons and Doves

Estimates are made that pigeons comprise nearly 50% of all birds in captivity. Clearly there is a great disparity between the number of pigeons owned versus those presented in veterinary practice. There is a history of resistance to the use of veterinary services by pigeon breeders. Because of the huge percentage of the whole represented by pigeons, it is probably worth our effort to show pigeon fanciers what veterinarians can do for them. They need us as management and husbandry consultants, diagnosticians when management breaks down, and providers of hospitalization for individual pets and valuable breeding animals.[1-3]

As with other species, the more that is known about how birds are kept, bred, transported, shown, and flown, the better the ability to diagnose problems. Immersion in pigeon fancy allows one to gain knowledge of the culture, without which, in the opinion of some "pigeon veterinarians," one is somewhat handicapped (Table 50–1). On the other hand, part of the distance between veterinary medicine and the pigeon world has been created by veterinarians who are more pigeon fanciers than veterinarians.

In flock management, prevention of disease is far more rewarding than treatment. Regrettably, it often conflicts with common racing and homing, training, and showing practices. Training involves taking the kit of birds along with other club members' birds a distance away and releasing them to return home. Consequently, veterinary services will always be needed. Flock management requires attention to details of loft construction, husbandry, medical management, and vaccination protocol.

In many ways, medical management of pigeons differs from psittacine medicine. Husbandry practices, handling, and nutrition vary greatly, but veterinary care and client education are still essential elements of a winning loft. Making high quality veterinary care available to the pigeon fancier will foster clients and aid in improving the fancier-veterinarian relationship.

This chapter deals predominantly with the veterinary aspects of homing pigeons. There are many similarities in disease problems between ornamental pigeons and doves and homing pigeons. There are also many differences, especially in housing, feeding, and management. Differences in diseases also occur: for example, *Yersinia pseudotuberculosis* infection is very seldom seen in homing pigeons but is a very common problem in doves.

Table 50–1

GLOSSARY OF PIGEON TERMINOLOGY

Squab unfledged baby pigeon
Squeaker weaning or weaned fledgling with an immature squeaking voice
Young bird age between weaning and maturity, first-year fledged bird
Cock male bird
Hen female bird
Loft or coop the facility or cages where the birds are housed
Flights flight pens attached to the loft for captivity, outdoor exercise
Droppings the most common term used for fecal material
Billing or kissing exchange of crop contents between adults during courtship
Crop milk fluid/cells produced by ingluvial desquamation which is fed to the squab
Kit a group of 20 or fewer performing flying pigeons
Muffs feathers on the legs and feet
Slippered light feathering on the legs and feet
Frill a tuft of feathers that swirls on the breast; also a breed of pigeon
Crest a reversed swirl of feathers on the back of the head

From Rupiper DJ, Ehrenberg M: Introduction in pigeon practice. Main Conf Proc Assoc Avian Vet, 1994; pp 203–211.

BASIC INFORMATION

Pigeons are among the most ancient domesticated animals in the world. They were originally used as utility birds (meat, fertilizer, and feather products), and were later used for sport and as carriers of information and, more recently, as laboratory animals.[4]

The order Columbiformes consists of three families, pigeons (Columbidae), sandgrouses (Pteroclididae [two genera, 16 species]), and the extinct dodos (Raphidae). The family pigeons (Columbidae) is divided into green pigeons (Treroninae [nine genera, 26 species]), true pigeons (Columbinae [21 genera, 46 species of which one is extinct]), crowded pigeons (Gourinae [one genus, three species]), and tooth-billed pigeons (Didunculinae [one genus, one species]). The pigeons commonly kept by private owners are classified in the genera true pigeons (*Columba* [13 species, including the rock pigeon (*C. livia*)]), turtle doves (*Streptopelia* [eight species]), and ground doves (*Geopelia* [two species] and *Gallicolumba* [three species]).

The most popular pigeons kept as a hobby originate from the rock pigeon (*C. livia*) and include at least 800 varieties of homing or racing pigeons, fancy or ornamental pigeons, and tumbler pigeons (high flyers, sustained flyers, flying tipplers, purzulers, and rollers). The domesticated pigeons that have returned to the wild are also descended from the rock dove and are called city or street pigeons or, incorrectly, feral pigeons. The number of these city pigeons worldwide is estimated at approximately 500 million.[5]

Specific Anatomy and Physiology

The weight of pigeons ranges from 50 g (diamond dove, *Geopelia cuneata*) to 1300 g (crowded pigeon, Gourinae). The average weight of the homing pigeon is 400 g. Pigeons may live 20 to 30 years.[4-6]

In some pigeons there is a correlation between high powder production for maintenance of the condition of the feathers and reduction in size of the uropygial gland. The feather powder is composed entirely of keratin and is produced by pulviplumes (modified semiplumae). The powder is derived from cells that surround the differentiating cells of the barbules of a growing pulviplume. Powder is shed only while the feathers are emerging from their sheaths. Pulviplumes are characterized by a slow exsheathing process, decreased thickness of the rachis, and increased reduction of the barbules, resulting in larger quantities of powder.[4] Frequent exposure to feather powder has been associated with allergic alveolitis (pigeon breeder's lung) in susceptible humans.

Pigeons have a large bilobed crop. From 2 weeks before the squabs hatch until they are 10 to 16 days old, the mucosa of the crop of both genders proliferates, producing large amounts of exfoliated crop epithelial cells known as "crop milk" (Fig 50–1, A,B). This product contains many lipids and proteins (see Chapter 26).

In pigeons, the gallbladder is absent and the ceca are highly rudimentary.

From the cranium to the crop, both genders possess a vascular plexus in the cutis that is dorsally divided into left and right portions that are separated by a 1-mm-wide gap in the median plane. It is called the *plexus venosus intracutaneus collaris* and is used for sexual and territorial display and regulation of circulation and body temperature. Injections in or damage of this plexus, especially during display and hot weather, can cause a fatal hemorrhage. By administering injections only in the distal third part of the neck, dorsally, this problem can be prevented.[7]

The superficial breast muscle is vascularized only by three branches of the external thoracic artery. To prevent puncturing these vessels, an intramuscular injection should be given craniodorsally entering at two-thirds of the distance from the cranial point of the pectoral muscle, parallel to the keel. In racing pigeons, intramuscular injections in the pectoral muscle should not be given, because of risk of permanent damage. The existence of a renal portal system makes the effect of intramuscular injections in the leg muscles uncertain (see Chapter 39A, Pharmacology). Normally, in racing pigeons, the subcutaneous route, dorsally at the base of the neck, is preferred for injections.

The normal cloacal body temperature ranges from 39.8°C to 43.3°C and is dependent on the state of excitement, vigor of flight, and ambient temperature. The heart rate of homing pigeons ranges from 180 to 250 beats per minute.

Normal chemistry and hematologic values for

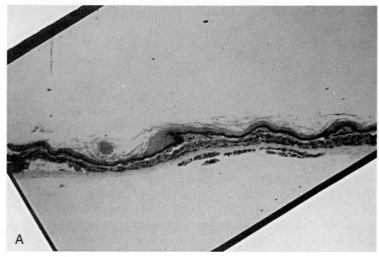

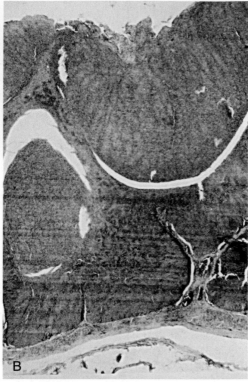

Figure 50–1

(A) Normal crop epithelium (hematoxylin and eosin stain). *(B)* Proliferated crop epithelium ("crop milk") (hematoxylin and eosin stain).

homing pigeons are listed in Table 50–2, and a practical formulary in Table 50–3.

For principles and physiology of navigation see Chapter 27.

HOUSING AND NUTRITION

Housing

Pigeons are rather aggressive, particularly during reproduction, and have no behavioral inhibitions against killing members of their own species, including their offspring. This behavioral trait should be considered when designing flight enclosures and constructing lofts. Birds should always have a place that they can use to escape from an aggressive male.

The construction of the lofts is adapted to the particular requirement of the individual pigeon varieties and the number of birds to be housed. Breeds maintained for their flying ability need the opportunity to fly freely to maintain a proper level of condition and health. Pigeons must be protected from

raptors, cats, dogs, foxes, opossums, raccoons, skunks, martens, weasels, and rats.

To be successful in pigeon racing, optimal environmental conditions are required. A loft should be warm, dry, and draft-free. This axiom is known by most fanciers but often is neglected. The climate in the loft should be kept as constant as possible without large fluctuations. Pigeons are very sensitive to drafts, but nevertheless they must have sufficient fresh air to keep them healthy. The loft should be dry with a relative air humidity of 60 to 70%. The temperature in the racing season is optimal at 20°C to 25°C, and the front of the housing should face southeast in moderate climate zones to get full benefit of the morning sun.

Extreme high temperatures and low humidities cause desiccation of mucous membranes, dust formation irritating the upper respiratory tract, polydipsia, anorexia, and loss of condition. Humidifying the air may help improve unsatisfactory conditions. In the winter, temperatures below zero in combination with dry weather are normally not associated with respiratory problems. When the racing season is approaching, the temperature during the night

Table 50-2

PLASMA CHEMISTRY REFERENCE VALUES FOR RACING PIGEONS

Parameter	$P_{2.5}$–$P_{97.5}$*
Sodium (mEq/L)	141–149
Potassium (mEg/L)	3.9–4.7
Calcium (mg/dl)	7.6–10.4
Magnesium (mg/dl)	2.7–4.4
Inorganic phosphorus (mg/dl)	1.8–4.1
Chloride (mEg/L)	101–113
Plasma iron (g/dl)	61–184
Iron binding capacity (μg/dl)	5.4–8.0
Osmolality (mOsm/kg)	297–317
Glucose (mg/dl)	232–369
Creatinine (mg/dl)	0.26–.04
Urea (mg/dl)	2.4–4.2
Uric acid (mg/dl)	2.52–12.86
Urea: Uric acid ratio	1.8 1.8 (mean sd)
CPK (U/L)	110–480
AP (U/L)	160–780
AST (U/L)	45–123
ALT (U/L)	19–48
GLDH (U/L)	0–1
LDH (U/L)	30–205
Bile acids (mol/L)	22–60
GGT (U/L)	0–2.9
Total protein (g/dl)	2.1–3.3
Albumin: Globulin ratio	1.5–3.6
Prealbumin (g/dl)	0.1–0.4
Albumin (g/dl)	1.3–2.2
Alpha globulin (g/dl)	0.2–0.3
Beta globulin (g/dl)	0.3–0.6
Gamma globulin (g/dl)	0.1–0.3

Adapted from Lumeij JT: PhD Thesis, Utrecht University, 1987.
*The inner limits are given for the percentiles $P_{2.5}$ and $P_{97.5}$ with a probability of 90%.

should be kept above 12°C with a humidity below 70%. In the Northern Hemisphere, this means good insulation, extra heating, and in some cases concentration of the birds in the loft. During the summer or in hot climate zones, optimal ventilation is essential. In those areas, the racing season is adapted to the "colder" periods of the year (autumn and spring).

Pigeon lofts or dovecotes should be partitioned so that several sections are provided (Fig. 50–2). There should be an entrance room that can be used for storage of equipment, tools, and feed. A new-bird isolation pen or flight, and one or more pens or sections for breeding pairs and different age groups, should be provided. After weaning, the squabs should be housed separately from the adult pigeons to prevent transmission of diseases. Ideally there should be an isolation loft to house sick birds and new birds. In some circumstances, the isolation loft may be used to house birds returning from shows and flights. The different sections should not be overcrowded during the racing season, and there should be sections for small groups of newly weaned birds. The ideal space requirement is 16 to 20 young pigeons in an area measuring $2 \times 2 \times 2$ m (two birds per m³). No more than one breeding pair, two hens, or one widower (single male) should be housed per cubic meter.

Excrement and discarded food should be removed on a daily basis. Dust production may be a problem with a completely dry and clean floor system. A vacuum cleaner can be used for cleaning. Sometimes the birds are placed on gratings so that the feces and food can drop through the openings.[4] However, grates have several disadvantages: They look animal-unfriendly, there is more dust production, and rodents are attracted by the dropped food. Mice can cause restlessness and may startle the pigeons during the night. This may be more damaging to the condition of racing pigeons than the risk of mice-vectored diseases. Sometimes chickens are kept under the loft to consume the dropped food to help prevent rodent infestations. One should realize that chickens can be carriers of diseases and therefore should be incorporated in the veterinary management. Other systems use dry litter, wherein the excrements are scraped loose but not removed. There is a real danger in this system of disease transmission and spread. A bedding material is sometimes used for young pigeons after weaning.

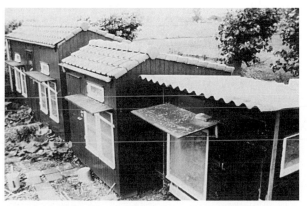

Figure 50-2

Typical small Dutch racing pigeon lofts with separate housing for different purposes.

T a b l e   5 0 – 3

FORMULARY OF DRUGS USED IN PIGEONS AND DOVES

Most drugs used in pigeons must be administered to the entire flock. Consequently, many of the drugs are administered in the food or water supply. Pigeons should be dosed based only on body weight (mg/kg). The calculated amount of drug for the total number of pigeons in a section should be administered in a portion of food or drinking water that is consumed in a short time. Many drugs will adhere to grains if mixed with buttermilk or syrup (see also Chapter 39A, Metabolism, Pharmacology, and Therapy). Intramuscular injections should not be given to racing pigeons during the racing season; instead, subcutaneous injections given dorsally at the neck base are preferred in most situations.

Drug	Dosage (mg/kg)	Frequency	Duration (d = days)	Route
Amikacin	15–20	BID	Maximum 5 d	IM, IV
Amoxicillin	100	BID	7 d	PO, IM, SC
Ampicillin	150–200	BID	7 d	PO, IM, SC
Amprolium	2.5	SID	5 d	PO
Atropine	0.5	q 4–8 hrs	As needed	IM, IV
Butorphanol	0.05–0.4	Once		IM
Calcium EDTA	30	BID	3–5 d	IM
Calcium gluconate	50–100	BID	1–2 d	IV
Carnidazole	20	Once		PO
Cefadroxil	100	BID–TID	7–10 d	PO, IM, IV
Cephalexin	100	BID	7–10 d	PO, IM, SC
Cephalothin	150	BID	7–10 d	IM, SC
Chloramphenicol palmitate	50	TID–QID	7 d	PO
Chlortetracycline[1]	50	SID–BID	7–45 d	PO
Ciprofloxacin	5–20	BID	4–7 d	PO
Clavamox	120	BID	7 d	PO
Dexamethasone sodium phosphate	1–4	SID–TID	1–2 d	IM, SC, IV
Diazepam	0.5–1.0		As needed	IM, IV
Dimetridazole	20–40	SID	5 d	PO
Doxycycline	50	BID	7–45[2] d	PO, IM, SC
Enrofloxacin	5–10	SID–BID	5–7 d	PO, IM, SC
Fenbendazole[3]	15–30	SID	3 d	PO
Furosemide	3	BID	As needed	PO, IM, IV
Injacom	0.33[4] ml/kg	Weekly	2–3 doses	IM, SC
Ipronidazol	5–10	SID	3–7 d	PO
Ivermectin,	0.2	Once	Repeat in 10 d	IM, SC
dilution 1:10	0.1 ml	Once		PO
Ketamine	25			IM, IV
Ketamine + diazepam	7.5 + 1.0			IM, IV
Ketoconazole	20–40	BID	15–60 d	PO
Levamisole	30	SID	1–3 d	PO

However, the use of moldy straw as bedding can cause problems with acute aspergillosis. Normally aspergillosis is very seldom found in racing pigeons.

Food and water containers should kept free of droppings and vermin. These and all other utensils should be cleaned regularly.

Nutrition

Homing pigeons eat 30 to 40 g of food (60–80 g/kg body weight) and drink 30 to 50 ml of water (60–100 ml/kg body weight) per day.

The natural feed of the Columbidae consists mainly of cereals, peas, beans, lentils, and oil-containing seeds.[5] Many free-ranging doves and pigeons feed on other cultivated plants, the seeds of weeds, green parts of many plants, berries, and other fruits and on animals (insects, snails, earthworms). Effective formulated diets are readily available for domesticated pigeons, and details of nutritional requirements are available in the literature.[4] These commercially available mixed seeds are often enriched by adding brewer's yeast, vegetables, and vitamin and mineral preparations.

Feeding methods vary considerably.[3] Typically, strenuously exercised performance pigeons are fed rations high in protein and fat. During long flights, pigeons mobilize fat depots stored in the pectoral

T a b l e 5 0 – 3

FORMULARY OF DRUGS USED IN PIGEONS AND DOVES *Continued*

Drug	Dosage (mg/kg)	Frequency	Duration (d = days)	Route
Lincomycin	70–100	SID	7–14 d	PO
Mebendazole[5]	10–20	SID	3–5 d	PO
	40	BID	5 d	PO
Metronidazole	10–20	SID	2 d	IM
Neo-calglucon	7 ml/kg	BID	As needed	PO
Nitrofurazone			Not recommended	
Nystatin	dose[6]	SID–BID	7 d	PO
Oxfendazole	10–40	Once		PO
Piperacillin	100–200	BID	7 d	IM, SC
Plaquenil[7]	10	SID	1 day	PO
Plaquenil + primaquine	10 + 1	SID	Weekly	PO
Praziquantel	5–10	Once		PO
Pyrantel pamoate[8]	100	Once	Yearly	PO
Ronidazole	6–10	SID	10 d	PO
Sulfachlorpyridazine	30	SID	5–(2)–5[9]	PO
Sulfamethazine	25	SID	3–(2)–3[9]	PO
Sulfamethoxine	25	BID	5 d	PO
Sulfaquinoxaline	10	SID	6–(2)–6[9]	PO
Tetracycline	100	SID	5–10 d	PO
Ticarcillin	200	BID–TID	7 d	IM, IV
Toltrazuril	7	SID	3 d	PO
Trimethoprim-S[10]	60	BID	7 d	PO
Tylosin	250	SID		PO
	25	QID	10–(5)–10[9]	IM, SC

Modified from Rupiper DJ, Ehrenberg M: Introduction in pigeon practice. Main Conf Proc Assoc Avian Vet, 1994, pp 203–211.

[1]Chlortetracycline. Grit should be removed during treatment. Poorly accepted in drinking water. A treatment period of 45 days is recommended for treatment of ornithosis (chlamydiosis).

[2]Doxycycline can be administered for 45 days to treat ornithosis. A common regimen in Europe is doxycycline (Vibramycin-IV) injections SC/IM, 75–100 mg/kg, at intervals of 7, 7, 7, 6, 5, and 5 days.

[3]Fenbendazole. During molt of young pigeons it will reduce growth and induce feather damage. Avoid in racing pigeons.

[4]Injacom 100, an aqueous multivitamin solution containing 100,000 IU vitamin A, 10,000 IU vitamin D3, and 20 IU vitamin E/ml.

[5]Mebendazole is toxic for pigeons at dosages of 30 to 40 mg/kg body weight.

[6]Nystatin 100,000–300,000 IU/kg.

[7]Plaquenil (hydrochloroquine), antimalarial drug. 200 mg tablet. Should be combined with primaquine. A safe regimen is chloroquine 10 mg/kg combined with primaquine 1 mg/kg po once a week during the malaria season to prevent clinical problems in infected pigeons.

[8]Pyrantel pamoate. The normal recommended dose is 4.5 mg/kg, once, repeated after 14 days.

[9]Regimen: days on medication–(days off medication)–days on medication.

[10]Trimethoprim/sulfa is the first choice of the authors for the treatment of *Salmonella* infections in pigeons. The duration of treatment is 3 weeks.

muscles. Thus, protein levels in pigeon rations may not be as important as once thought. The protein content of feeds varies from 12 to 20%, but usually is 13 to 16%. The average nonracing pigeon does well on a diet of 14% protein. The birds can be trained to accept pellets. Once-a-day feeding regimens are satisfactory, but twice-daily or free-choice feeding is also acceptable with show birds. In addition, birds pick small stones for grinding their seeds, and grit (oyster shells) should be supplied ad libitum as a calcium source.

The feed quality is of utmost importance. Grains, seeds, or formulated diets should be stored in a dry, clean, pest-free location. Fungi, particular mycotoxins, feed mites, and toxic seeds from weeds should be avoided.[5]

BASIC PRINCIPLES OF THE PIGEON SPORT

The principles of pigeon racing can look complicated and seem to have almost mysterious aspects to those unfamiliar with the sport.[4, 8, 9] There are basically three motivating and racing systems of "pigeon play"—the first two, "nestplay" and "widowhood", are played with adults and young birds (early fledged birds), and the third is "young-pigeon play" with only young pigeons. All systems are closely connected to the breeding system. The following description is based on the system in the Northern Hemisphere, where the racing season is from April to September. For other areas, these systems are adapted to local conditions and circumstances.

Breeding Systems

Classic Breeding

To prepare for racing with adult pigeons, the birds are paired for breeding in the beginning of February. The future "widowers" (older racing pigeons) are allowed to raise one nest of squabs, and with the second clutch the hens are removed on the tenth day of incubation. The cocks leave the nests spontaneously. The cocks are taken for their first short training flights in the beginning of April when there are two squabs in the nest.

The cocks are then, after the interruption of the breeding, taken on training flights of increasingly long distances. Every time the "widowers" return to the loft, their hen is in the nest box. They are allowed to spend a short time together, and then the hen is taken away. This is how birds are prepared for the "widower flights" that are held every week (Fig. 50–3). These flights are either short distance ("vitesse" races, 50–300 km), a longer interval ("minifond", 300–500 km) or "fond" races (500–1200 km). In the US, races are rated as short (up to 300 miles) and long (over 300 miles).

Winter Breeding

A more popular system than classic breeding is to start breeding in November or December. This will yield "early young pigeons" and few territorial problems with the cocks at the time of racing. At 14 days after hatching (early January) the squabs and hens are separated from the cocks. Shortly before the racing season starts (early March) the pigeons are paired again. After 10 days of sitting on the eggs, the hens are removed again, and the cocks are trained as widowers.

There are many variations on these basic breeding systems, depending on the moment of pairing—removing eggs instead of hens (for the long races), or allowing eggs to hatch and squabs to wean (nestplay with cocks and hens).

Playing or Racing Systems

Nestplay

This is the classic method of racing pigeons, which is replaced by "widowhood" by many fanciers. Nestplay uses the natural desire of pigeons to return to their nests. During the week the pairs stay together. Depending on the status of the nest, the hens or cocks are raced. Hens fly optimally when the eggs are about to hatch or when the squabs are 8 days past hatching. Cocks, however, perform best when a squab is over 14 days old. This is called "nestposition." One problem is that the pigeons start to molt with the second clutch. They molt one pair of primary remiges (PRs, wing feathers) each month, starting with PR 1. Therefore, nestplayers start breeding in March and race during the spring and early summer. In August, when PR 5 or PR 6 molts, the secondary remiges, rectrices (tail feathers), and covers start molting as well, and the pigeons can no longer participate in racing.

Widowhood

In widowhood the birds are separated by gender for the whole week during the racing season. Single widowerhood is played mostly with cocks only, but is also possible with hens. Widowhood hens do not perform as well as cocks on the long races (fond races). Double widowhood includes racing cocks and hens separately. This type of "play" requires much time, attention, and extra space. The different groups of pigeons (hens, cocks, young birds, and squeakers) have to loft-fly in rotation. The cocks

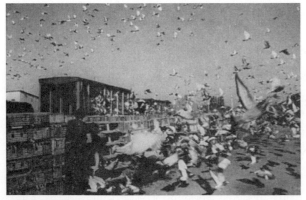

F i g u r e 5 0 – 3

Releasing racing pigeons to return to their lofts.

and hens are allowed to be together for a short time before and after the race.

Essential to single widowhood is the activity of the hens. They should show interest in the cocks. In some cases the hens start "calling" each other, lay eggs, and lose complete interest in their cocks. The widower will lose motivation for returning home quickly. These hens can be better used in the nestplay system.

The advantages of total widowhood are that the hens stay in optimal condition because of the daily training flights, the hens do not start producing eggs so readily, both cocks and hens can be selected for flying performances, and the total number of pigeons to be looked after with the same number of racers is lower. The biggest disadvantage is that the hen or cock can return after a race before the mate is home. Cocks have problems when they are not greeted by their hens. Therefore, some fanciers keep extra hens to "welcome" the cocks whose own hens are not yet home.

Both systems require much discipline and strict scheduling from the fancier. When not enough time can be spent with the pigeons, the results are disappointing. Lost pigeons (birds that do not return home) should never be "replaced" during the season. This induces territorial fights, and much energy is lost that should be available for racing.

Young-Pigeon Play

The play with young pigeons is different. Traditionally meant only to "teach" young pigeons how to fly, it has become an important discipline in the total racing sport. The simplest system is to fly the young birds to the "perch," the perch being the security of home, food, and the fancier.

These races are becoming an important part of the pigeon sport. Some pigeons (breeders that are often not used for racing themselves) are now allowed to raise three nests of two squabs. The first young pigeons will be trained together with the "early young pigeons" that the "widowers" were allowed to raise. They are trained in the second half of May with many short flights, and are trained to enter the loft when a signal is given, such as by a whistle or a bell. They are fed when they return to their loft. Sometimes both genders are housed in separate sections and are allowed to meet each other only the afternoon before the race ("open door play"). This is a kind of widower play. In other cases, young cocks selected for "half widower play" are paired with old hens, or old cocks are paired with young hens. They fly, however, only in young-pigeon races.

Because normally the molt of these young pigeons coincides with the most important races, the molt is often artificially delayed. This is done by darkening the loft from 7 PM until 7 AM.

The most important part of the young-pigeon flying is to train the birds frequently. This means taking the birds by car two to four times a week and letting them return home from some distance (50–60 km).

Darkening of Young Pigeons

Pigeons perform best when all feathers are intact. This means that they have "full feathers" and molting is minimal. In the adult pigeons that are supposed to participate in the important late and long races (fond races), molt is prevented by pairing them late in the season. Young pigeons normally molt at the end of summer. Two systems are used to prevent molt in these young pigeons.

1. The application of corticosteroids through eye drops, nasal drops, or in the drinking water. This may cause many secondary complications and may be detrimental to the health of the birds. Moreover, it is considered "doping" and is therefore illegal in many countries.

2. The day length is kept constant by darkening the lofts of the young pigeons for 10 to 12 hours a day. It is essential to adhere to the same schedule every day. An automatic system prevents mistakes. These pigeons molt their covert feathers, but not their remiges and rectrices. The "darkening" is best started after weaning and continued not later than the second half of May or, at a maximum, the first half of June. When the darkening is continued until after the last race in September, as done by some fanciers, several pigeons do not molt at all and enter the following season with "old" flight and tail feathers.

In general, darkened young pigeons cannot be used after racing for winter breeding, nor for shows in the autumn of the same year. Some fanciers also feel that darkened pigeons do not perform optimally the following year and are more sensitive to respiratory problems and diarrhea.

VETERINARY MANAGEMENT OF RACING PIGEONS

High demands are placed on performance of birds in pigeon racing. An intrinsic factor of pigeon racing is that the birds have frequent contact with pigeons of other fanciers and therefore are exposed to infectious agents in the transport baskets or crates (Fig. 50–4*A, B*). Free-ranging pigeons visit a loft regularly and can introduce diseases. For optimal condition, pigeons are trained every day by making them fly free, but contacts with feral birds expose the pigeons to contagious diseases. The latter factor includes also pigeons kept in outdoor flight pens.

All these factors require continuous alertness of the fancier to prevent the spread of infectious problems. The basis of preventive medicine is a "common sense" concept of knowing how to deal with pigeons, hygiene, and cleanliness. By the time the pigeons show clinical problems, infection has already occurred. Treatment will be too late to prevent damage and can only limit the damage for the racing season.

The aims of veterinary management are (1) prevention of (disease) problems; (2) improving performance; (3) timely and adequate adaptation to problems; (4) directed and efficient use of medications; (5) reduction of unwarranted drug use; (6) improving the position in racing with smaller numbers of pigeons. (This means that the fancier takes care of fewer birds but has more prize-winners.)

Veterinary management includes providing guidelines and requirements, regular contacts between veterinarian and fancier, regular disease surveillance, and preventive measures.

The guidelines include directives about loft construction, loft environment, number of pigeons per loft or section, composition of the group per flight or section, and selection or culling criteria. The fancier should be instructed to visually examine each bird every day to determine its overall state of health. Pigeons that appear abnormal should be isolated, observed, and evaluated by the veterinarian (Fig. 50–5). Birds that cannot be treated must be culled immediately and submitted for complete veterinary diagnostic tests and postmortem examination.[4]

Specific Preventive Medicine and Vaccinations

A fixed schedule for specific preventive medicine and vaccination for racing pigeons is not possible. A preventive medicine schedule should be tailored to the regional situation and depends on the schedule for breeding and racing. There are, however, some general guidelines:

1. Recently purchased birds must be placed in quarantine. *Trichomonas* infection, ecto- and endoparasites, and *Salmonella* infection should be con-

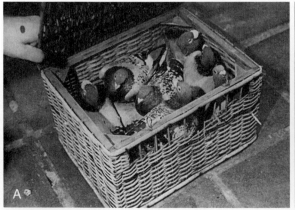
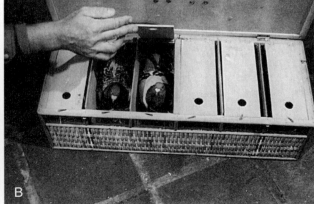

Figure 50–4

(A) Pigeons in a training basket (wrong). *(B)* Pigeons in a training basket (correct).

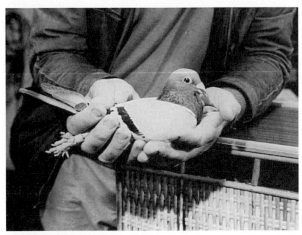

Figure 50–5

Holding a racing pigeon correctly. For examination pigeons should always be held with two hands, the thumbs on the wings, the legs between the index and middle finger, and the head pointing to the examiner's body.

trolled before adding the new birds to the flock. Separate vaccination is not necessary when the fancier performs routine vaccination of his flock.

2. A regular disease surveillance should take place, which includes a collective fecal examination (for endoparasites) and fecal bacterial culture (for *Salmonella typhimurium*), every time a new "pigeon season" starts. This means surveillance occurs before the breeding season, before the racing season, before the young-pigeon races, before molting, and again before the breeding season.

3. During the racing season, disease surveillance measures include regular diagnostic tests (every 6–7 weeks) to screen for endoparasites, ornithosis complex, *Salmonella,* and other problems based on symptoms.

4. *Trichomonas* infections are very common, and the risk for reinfection is present every week in the racing season. Common treatment regimens are 3 days every 3 weeks or every week on Saturday night and all of Sunday.

5. A complete examination of the birds is indicated at least twice a year: after the racing season (before breeding starts) and before the racing season. This includes crop swab, cloacal swab, ectoparasite examination, status of molt and feather quality, general condition and form of a selection of birds from the different sections. At the same time, the loft is evaluated for the climatologic situa-

tion. In some situations, necropsy is indicated for one or more of the culled pigeons after the last race.

6. All dead pigeons should undergo necropsy with complete histopathologic examination of tissue.

7. Important preventive measures include vaccinations for paramyxovirus, avian pox, and *Salmonella* (paratyphoid).

In regions where adenovirus infection is a problem, a vaccination schedule with egg drop syndrome vaccine is encouraged.[9] There is, however, no indication that this vaccine has any positive effect against pigeon adenovirus.

The authors use the following vaccination schedule:

1. Young pigeons (starting 3 weeks after hatching) can be first vaccinated for paramyxovirus before they start leaving the loft. When there is no direct danger of paramyxovirus infection, this first vaccination can be combined with *Salmonella* and pox vaccinations at 5 to 6 weeks after hatching. Before the *Salmonella* vaccination the pigeons should be fasted for ½ day and should be kept in the loft for 3 days. The pox vaccination is important, and will protect young pigeons for at least 2 years. The pigeons should not be allowed to bathe for 12 to 14 days after the pox vaccination. There is a practice of providing extra vitamins in the food for several days after vaccination.

2. All pigeons (adult and young pigeons) are vaccinated every year with paramyxovirus and *Salmonella* vaccines after molting, but not later than 3 weeks before pairing. In the case of winter breeding, the pigeons can be vaccinated with paramyxovirus while sitting on eggs. The disadvantage of vaccination when the pigeons are sitting on eggs is that no or only low paramyxovirus antibodies are present in the eggs and chicks.

Other Aspects of Veterinary Management

It should never be the aim of veterinary management to provide a pharmacy for the pigeon fancier. Differences among fanciers and lofts can be large. Gastrointestinal parasitism is a good example. Under optimal conditions, helminthic parasites are seldom seen and therefore treatment is not needed. Low coccidial counts are not treated. Pigeons improve with medication only when the treatment is directed at an actual problem. Unfortunately, often fanciers are encouraged to use many different products to improve their results. The advertisers anticipate fear and uncertainty of the pigeon fanciers. Good veterinary management includes treatment based only on clinical and laboratory results and actual situations.

The basic essentials for good racing results are: (1) quality of the pigeons, (2) quality of the fancier, (3) quality of the housing, and (4) quality of the veterinary support. Infectious disease is not the main factor affecting performance in pigeon racing. A restricted number of pigeons owned by the same fanciers perform best in pigeon racing and become the champions. The risk of contracting an infectious disease, however, is equal for pigeons of all fanciers. The quality of the pigeons, the fancier, and housing determine if and how these diseases influence the performance.

For good veterinary management the veterinarian should visit the loft regularly. On location, the different aspects that may influence racing success can be inspected. A general impression on the first approach is extremely important.[2]

The aspects to consider include cleanliness (loft, equipment), feeding systems, watering devices, outside exposure, position and direction of the loft, materials and construction of the loft, perches, litter, size, ratio of glass/mesh/wall of the front and roof, ventilation system, insulation, growth (trees, shrub), nest boxes, nesting material, and the number of pigeons in each flight.

The issues to be discussed during on-site evaluation include the type of racing system, breeding system, reproduction results, number of pigeons per section, selection criteria, results from the past, differences between the past and present, changes in housing or feeding, vaccination and medication history, and a tailored veterinary management program.

Specific Disease Problems

Many disease problems in pigeons are covered in Section 3 (Infectious Diseases) and Section 4 (Noninfectious Diseases) of this book. For therapy, see the Formulary (Section 5). Surgery is covered in Section 6. The basic principles of clinical examina-

tion and the procedures to reach a diagnosis and to select a treatment do not differ from methods accepted for other birds. Because in many situations there is a flock-related problem, necropsy is a very important tool to arrive at a quick and proper diagnosis.

This part of the chapter will help the veterinarian reach a diagnosis and presents pigeon-specific veterinary issues. The most common disease problems that are presented have a complex etiology and have been divided into separate headings.

Common Infectious Diseases

Infectious diseases of clinical importance are listed in Table 50–4. For a detailed description and treatment see the relevant chapters in this book or specific literature.

Principles of management of infectious diseases are as follows:

1. There are only a few bacterial infections of clinical importance in homing pigeons.

2. Many other bacteria may be identified, but they are mostly restricted to isolated disease problems.

3. Many viruses are isolated from pigeons, but only a few are important as disease agents.

4. However, many other viruses have been reported to occur randomly (Newcastle disease [PMV-1], infectious bronchitis, and infections with arbovirus, avian influenza A virus, reovirus, rotavirus, reticuloendotheliosis virus, and rubella virus). Not all are pathogenic, but nonprimary pathogenic viruses can make the bird more susceptible to other diseases.[10]

Problems Related to Homing Performances

When pigeons give disappointing race results without a specific pattern, it is essential that the veterinarian try to determine the underlying cause. In principle, the whole management system and the health status of the pigeons need evaluation. Based on those findings, corrective measures need to be taken. The following items should be considered: any disease or combination of diseases, flock management and play system, loft construction and climate, nutrition system, and ectoparasites.

T a b l e 5 0 – 4

THE MOST COMMON INFECTIOUS PROBLEMS IN RACING PIGEONS

Endoparasites
Nematoda *Ascaridia columbae*
          Capillaria obsignata
          Tetrameres spp[1]
          Acuaria spp[2]
Cestoda *Aporina delafondi*
          Hymenolepis spp
          Raillietina spp
Trematoda *Echinoparyphium paraulum*
          E. recurvatum
Protozoa *Elmeria labbeana*
          E. columbarum
          Trichomonas columbae
          Hexamita (Spiranucleus) columbae

Ectoparasites
  Columbicola columbae (slender pigeon louse)
  Campanulotes bidentatus (Goniocotis) compar (small pigeon louse)
  Falculifer rostratus (feather damaging mite)
  Megninia columbae (quill mite)
  Knemidokoptes laevis (depluming and scaly mite, seldom seen in
    pigeons)
  Dermanyssus gallinae (blood sucking mite)

Blood Parasites
  Haemoproteus spp
  Leucocytozoon spp
  Plasmodium spp

Bacteria
  Chlamydia psittaci
  Salmonella typhimurium
  Escherichia coli
  Streptococcus bovis

Viruses
  Pigeon paramyxovirus
  Pigeon pox
  Herpesvirus
  Adenovirus
  Circovirus

[1]In the proventriculus.
[2]Under the koilin layer of the gizzard; diagnosed in Europe, but are more common in U.S. and tropical areas.

Digestive System Problems

The main clinical sign indicative of a problem of the upper digestive tract is vomiting. Abnormal droppings (diarrhea) indicate an intestinal problem.

Vomiting and Regurgitation

Vomiting or regurgitation as a symptom in an individual pigeon is associated with a problem of the crop or upper gastrointestinal tract; however, as a flock problem it is a symptom of pigeon herpesvi-

rus, adenovirus, or *Escherichia coli* infection, hexamitiasis, or intoxications.

Normally, after eating, the crop is easily palpated through the skin. Six hours later the crop should be empty. Common causes of vomiting are listed in Table 50–5. The main infectious diseases that are associated with vomiting and regurgitation can be differentiated as listed in Table 50–6. The diagnosis is based on clinical signs, necropsy, histopathologic examination results (inclusion bodies), and isolation or demonstration of the agent. The diagnosis of hexamitiasis can be confirmed only by microscopic examination of a fresh, body-warm wet mount of the feces or small-intestinal contents, without adding water. Under the microscope the very small, quickly moving parasites can be seen.

Abnormal Droppings

The droppings are important for evaluating the health of pigeons. The fancier sees the feces every day and will notice any abnormalities.

T a b l e 5 0 – 5

COMMON CAUSES OF VOMITING AND REGURGITATION

Cause	Characteristics and Therapy
Crop stasis (sour crop)	The pigeon does not eat and the crop stays full. The fancier reports a foul-smelling odor from the beak. When more pigeons show the same problem, intoxication is suspected. Therapy consists of manual emptying and rinsing of the crop with an antibiotic or antimycotic solution.
Water-filled crop	In young pigeons a water-filled crop can be found. It is a common finding with paramyxovirus, adenovirus, acute enteritis, high salt concentrations in mineral blocks. Often this is also seen after ingestion of plant leaves or moss.
Trichomoniasis	A thick, firm crop indicates trichomoniasis. In the differential diagnosis, a tumor should be considered. The diagnosis is confirmed by taking a crop swab sample for a wet mount examination.
Overfilled crop	Incidentally seen in young pigeons that eat pebbles or, in autumn, acorns or beechnuts.
Crop fistula	Fistulas are seen after trauma or inadequate suturing of crop wounds.
Drugs	Vomiting is common after administration of levamisole tablets or suspension. Therefore, the manufacturer indicates that this drug should be given in an empty crop. A high oral dose of doxycycline can induce regurgitation.

Table 50–6

THE MAIN INFECTIOUS DISEASES ASSOCIATED WITH VOMITING AND REGURGITATION

Cause	Characteristics and Management	Cause	Characteristics and Management
Adenovirus	Anorexia, a watery overload of the crop with vomiting and diarrhea, is seen in young birds. The urine is discolored yellow to green, caused by liver damage. Mortality peaks 3–4 days after the beginning of the symptoms, usually stopping on the 5th day, but occasionally continuing for 2–4 weeks.	*E. coli* infection	Young pigeons show anorexia, sit fluffed, and are emaciated. There is a full crop, vomiting, polydipsia, and brown pulpy feces that eventually turn into green slimy to green watery stool. Probably a secondary pathogen to a viral infection. A differential diagnosis for diarrhea is hexamitiasis.
Pigeon herpesvirus	Vomiting is occasionally seen but predominantly in combination with trichomoniasis, which causes pseudomembranous membranes in the mouth, pharynx, esophagus, or larynx. Herpesvirus infection alone in young pigeons causes minor problems of the upper respiratory tract. Scattered losses occur mainly in young birds, often in relation to the first training flights.	Hexamitiasis	Clinical signs are seen only with a severe infection in young pigeons (up to 12 weeks). The birds have thin to very watery droppings, and show polydipsia, vomiting, and emaciation because of dehydration. Unexpected losses occur during the training of the young pigeons.

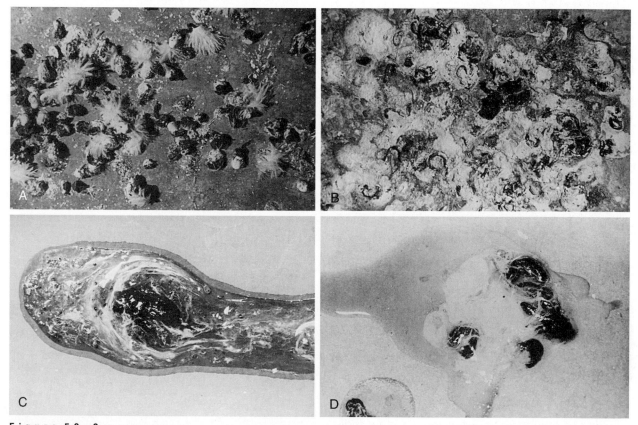

Figure 50–6

(A) Normal pigeon droppings in a loft covered with down feathers. *(B)* Abnormal droppings with diarrhea. *(C)* Watery droppings (diarrhea) typical of *Hexamita columbae* infection. *(D)* Droppings of a pigeon with acute salmonellosis with liver involvement (polyuria and yellow coloring of the urine fraction).

Normal feces in pigeons are dry droppings covered with a dry to slimy white layer of urates. In the loft, down feathers cover the droppings, indicating that the pigeons are healthy (Fig. 50–6*A*).

Abnormal feces are easily recognized by the fancier. Absence of down feathers covering the feces is a well-recognized sign of beginning problems. The combination of the two is very common (Fig. 50–6*B*).

Polyuria

A fecal examination begins with differentiating between diarrhea (Fig. 50–6*C*) and polyuria (Fig. 50–6*D*). Polyuria is recognized by normal feces surrounded by a large volume of water. The fancier, however, does not distinguish between the two; his complaint is abnormal droppings.

Differential diagnosis for polyuria is listed in Table 50–7.

The first clinical symptoms of paramyxovirus, after an incubation period of 10 to 12 days, are polydipsia and watery droppings (polyuria) in 20 to 70% of the unvaccinated birds. Feather changes are common in young and adult birds. Neurologic signs can follow, such as difficulty in flying, walking, or eating; ataxia; tremor of the head and neck; paresis or paralysis of one or both wings; and torticollis and circling, which are seen in 5 to 20% of affected pigeons (Fig. 50–7). A typical sign is pecking at food but missing it. Affected squabs have a high rate of mortality. Central nervous system signs are less prominent in paramyxovirus outbreaks now than in outbreaks in previous years. Acute mortality is associated with severely damaged kidneys in old pigeons. Respiratory signs are not observed.

Polyuria is often seen in squabs when they begin eating seeds. During this period the parents have a high water intake and feed this to the squabs. A

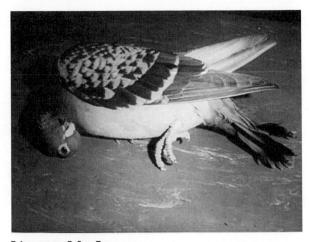

Figure 50–7

Pigeon with torticollis due to paramyxovirus.

high salt and mineral intake can also cause polyuria. Nervousness can lead to polyuria and is seen mostly in cocks. Polyuria is common in birds after transport to the veterinary hospital for examination.

In several gastrointestinal disease, polyuria is an accompanying symptom of diarrhea (e.g., hexamitiasis, *Streptococcus bovis* infection). Polyuria as a symptom of liver disease is seen with adenovirus infection. This symptom can also occur with *Salmonella* and *Chlamydia* infections with liver involvement, or with intoxications that affect the liver and kidneys.

Diarrhea

Intestinal Parasites

Digestive disturbances are recognized only with heavy infestations of *Eimeria, Ascaridia, Capillaria,* or *Hexamita* species, trematodes, or cestoda. In routine fecal examinations, these parasites can often be found without abnormal feces. Severe clinical problems with coccidiosis and worms are seen mostly in pigeons that are kept in flights. These pigeons are severely debilitated and may die.

Coccidial infections alone very seldom lead to clinical problems in pigeons. Low counts of coccidia (less than 3,000 oocysts per gram feces) in pigeons do not warrant treatment.[7] Pigeons with previously excellent performances perform less

Table 50–7

DIFFERENTIAL DIAGNOSIS FOR POLYURIA

Paramyxovirus
Change of food in squabs
A high salt or mineral intake
Nervousness
Gastrointestinal disease
Liver disease

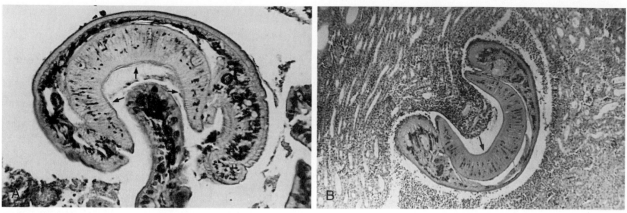

Figure 50–8

(A) A trematode (*Echinopariphium* species) "eating" an intestinal villus in a pigeon. *(B)* A trematode (*Echinopariphium* species) "eating" kidney parenchyma in a pigeon.

well when they shed coccidia. However, when these pigeons are given rest and proper care, without treating the coccidiosis, the rate of shedding drops.[8] Under normal conditions, coccidia induce immunity, preventing clinical coccidiosis. Shedding of coccidia should be considered a nonspecific sign of a health problem, and in many cases concurrent infectious diseases are present.[11]

Infections with helminthic parasites, however, should always be treated. There is no relationship between the number of eggs in the feces and the severity of infection in the pigeons. Parasitic infections are always a warning of poor hygiene.

Trematodes and cestodes need an intermediate host. Trematode infections are only a problem in areas with wetlands. The main disease problems are hemorrhagic droppings caused by damage of the intestinal villi (Fig. 50–8*A*) and renal disease caused by direct mechanical damage of the parenchyma (Fig. 50–8*B*).

Cestoda are mostly incidental findings, and flock treatment is seldom indicated.

Bacterial Infections

Bacterial infections, such as those caused by *S. typhimurium*, *E. coli*, *S. bovis*, *Clostridium* species, and *Chlamydia psittaci* occur frequently.

In young birds, clinical signs of salmonellosis are anorexia, greenish to yellow diarrhea, droopiness, and death within 2 to 3 days. Infected squabs are often retarded in growth, underweight, and exhibit a general depression and listlessness accompanied by a partial or complete inappetence. In a flock, signs include swollen joints (Fig. 50–9), wing paralysis, CNS signs, loss of weight or failure to thrive, diarrhea, and death. In groups of adult birds in a carrier state, individual birds may occasionally show a slimy, thin diarrhea.

The isolation of *S. typhimurium* var. Copenhagen is always to be followed by treatment of all pigeons and strict hygienic measurements. Only a small number of the pigeons in a loft develop clinical symptoms after a *Salmonella* infection. The majority are carriers. A major problem is the L-form, which cannot be cultured (see Chapter 18, Bacteriology). Serology testing does not identify carriers.

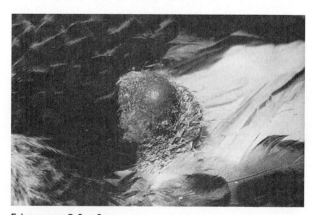

Figure 50–9

Swollen joint caused by a *Salmonella* infection.

E. coli diarrhea occurs in young pigeons after their first training flights and is called "young-pigeon diarrhea." It is primarily a problem in young pigeons (2 to 6 months old). However, adenovirus, *Hexamita,* herpesvirus, and other agents may be much more likely as primary causes.

S. bovis infection is characterized by sudden death in pigeons of all ages; inability to fly; lameness; emaciation; polyuria; and green, slimy droppings.

Clostridium species are sometimes found as a cause of enteritis in an individual bird.

Although chlamydiosis (ornithosis) is usually considered part of the respiratory disease complex of pigeons, certain strains (psittacine and turkey strains) are an important cause of diarrhea and weight loss in young birds.[11] Bacterial infections can also complicate the upper respiratory problems caused by pigeon strains.

Viral Infections

Viral infections include adenovirus and herpesvirus (influenza A virus). These infections are often complicated with secondary bacterial infections (*E. coli*), and parasitic infections can become apparent (hexamitiasis).

In complicated viral infections, antimicrobial or antiparasitic therapy does not solve the problem. The diagnosis often must be confirmed at necropsy after demonstration or isolation of the agent. Herpesvirus infections are mostly seen in association with *Trichomonas* infections, crowding, pigeons of different ages housed together, and poor climate conditions.

Intoxications

Intoxication most commonly results from eating in fields and gutters and eating moss.

Climate

Climatologic influences, such as wide variations in temperature and relative humidity, are thought to induce digestive disorders.

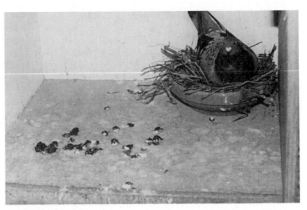

F i g u r e 5 0 – 1 0

Trampled and spread-out droppings in nest box in the morning as a result of restlessness and irritation caused by a severe infestation of ectoparasites.

Miscellaneous Changes

Abnormal color of the feces is seen regularly. A red or black color occurs after the intake of ground red brick or charcoal that is given to racing pigeons by some European fanciers. This practice should be discouraged.

Trampled and spread-out droppings in a loft or nest box in the morning are the result of restlessness and irritation caused by a severe infestation of ectoparasites (Figs. 50–10, 50–11). Abnormal droppings during the night only indicate poor housing. Abnormal droppings during the day are an indication of crowding or stress.

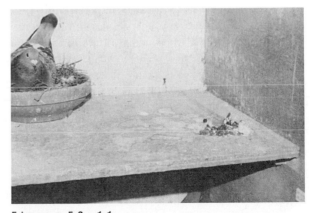

F i g u r e 5 0 – 1 1

Normal droppings in the morning in a nest box.

Respiratory Problems

Respiratory problems are the most important cause of disappointing performances and are difficult to approach diagnostically and therapeutically in pigeon medicine.

Management quality of the fancier and quality of loft construction, including climate and ventilation control, greatly influence the clinical presentation and spread of respiratory problems.

In pigeons that are presented for examination after poor performances in a race, slight respiratory symptoms or lesions are difficult to recognize. Even minor respiratory disease problems can influence homing performance. Most often a problem occurs throughout a flock, and many birds show symptoms. However, individual problems also are seen.

Birds do not have a diaphragm, and any space-occupying mass or disease process, in the thorax as well as the abdomen, can reduce the capacity of the air sacs and lungs and therefore reduce oxygen exchange. Therefore, not only changes in the respiratory system but also abdominal disease can cause signs of respiratory disease.

Anemia and pathology of the circulatory system also can provoke "respiratory symptoms."

Clinical Respiratory Signs

Abnormal Respiratory Sounds

Abnormal respiratory sounds must be localized to the upper (nose) or lower (trachea, bronchi) respiratory tract. Pressure on the sternum normally provokes sounds. Sneezing after pressure on the ceres, coughing produced by pinching the trachea, and grinding sounds after eating are considered normal.

Sneezing is always abnormal in pigeons that are in a transport basket or crate.

When respiratory symptoms are vague, the beak is held "in the ear" of the examiner. Breathing should not be heard. When breathing can be heard or other respiratory sounds are noticed, the pigeon is not fit for racing. These pigeons show "ears," or roughened head feathers. The pharynx is almost completely closed and swollen. Breathing of "good" pigeons that return home after a race cannot be heard "in the ear."

Slightly Open Beak

A slightly open beak is acceptable in roused pigeons, after training in hot conditions, in overweight pigeons, or in poorly trained birds. In birds at rest it should always be considered abnormal, unless the environmental temperature is very hot. However, pigeons that are fearful or nervous may sit with an open beak.

Scratching the Head

Scratching is sometimes seen in pigeons with severe coryza. Pigeons with fluid-filled sinuses or nares will shake their heads.

Wet Ceres

Small collections of purulent debris can be seen in the nasal openings of pigeons with rhinitis. With careful massage, fluid can always be milked out of the nose, but only a dirty-brown fluid indicates a pathology. Often the cere is discolored brown from exudate. This should not be confused with the normal dark cere in a young pigeon, a dirty cere caused by pair-feeding, or a feces-dirtied cere in a nervous pigeon with polyuria and polydipsia. Some nose drops are irritating and can induce abundant mucus production.

Progressive Erosion of Palatal Flap Papillae

Erosion is associated with *Trichomonas* infection. It is postulated that the "white points" or "sialolites" in the palatal flaps are associated with trichomoniasis or herpesvirus lesions. Both theories have never fully been proved. These "white points" represent chronic changes associated with small mucous glands that are blocked. Treatment for *Trichomonas* infection, unless the parasite is demonstrated, is not indicated. Erosion has no direct relationship with respiratory problems.

Yellow Flakes

Purulent material or diphtheric membranes in the beak or beak commissures are associated with *Trichomonas* infection. These lesions must be differentiated from lesions of pigeon pox (Fig. 50–12), which bleed during removal, and herpesvirus infection,

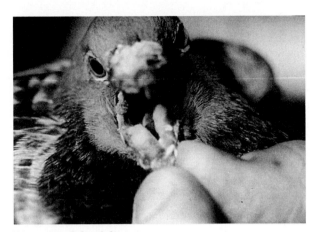

Figure 50-12

Proliferative beak lesions caused by pigeon pox.

which is rare, and involves the trachea. Yellow flakes and membranes next to the tongue and in the choanae often can be found after homing by the pigeon from a long-distance flight. Conjunctivitis-rhinitis-laryngitis (CRL) or coryza can cause yellow membranes on the palatum.

Severe Respiratory Distress

Respiratory distress in a pigeon is easily recognized by a stretched neck and forced abdominal and tail movements. Rarely, the mucous membranes appear cyanotic. The color of the mucous membranes and the amount and character of mucus are difficult to associate with specific respiratory problems.

Conjunctivitis

Bilateral conjunctivitis (including the "one-eye cold" [Fig. 50–13], that on closer inspection usually involves the other eye as well), and inflammation of the third eyelid should not always be associated with problems of the respiratory system. Unilateral eye lesions are the result of trauma often followed by an infectious conjunctivitis. The lacrimal gland and harderian gland should not be confused as a conjunctivitis lesion.

Pneumonia and Airsacculitis

Pneumonia and airsacculitis are always combined with general symptoms such as weight loss, dullness, depression, and ruffled feathers.

Different Presentations of Respiratory Problems

Respiratory Noises in the Squabs of Single Nests. No lesions are found in lungs or air sacs at necropsy. The signs usually resolve without treatment.

Respiratory Symptoms Spreading to Several Nests. There is retarded growth of the squabs, and feather damage is seen after the symptoms have disappeared. At necropsy, hepatomegaly, splenomegaly, and airsacculitis are found. The same disease complex is seen in early weaned squabs, and in crowded, humid, or drafty lofts. This problem is associated with the "ornithosis-complex."

Diphtheric Esophagitis, Laryngitis, and Pharyngitis. This is a rarely diagnosed disease complex seen predominantly in recently weaned squabs. Clinical symptoms are rhinitis, conjunctivitis, general depression, and mortality. In a flock, only a few birds may show the diphtheric lesions. These problems are associated with pigeon herpesvirus infection, possibly complicated by trichomoniasis.

Respiratory Problems in Young Pigeons After the First Few Races. Symptoms are not typical. Often the first complaint is reduced performance because of loss of condition. The pigeons return home late or not at all. The first subtle sign is the color of cere, which changes from white to grayish. A clinical symptom is often one wet eye (one-eye cold)—a minor conjunctivitis. The pigeon scratches the ear, eye, and nose. This is often mentioned by pigeon fanciers.

The symptoms can progress to a serous to puru-

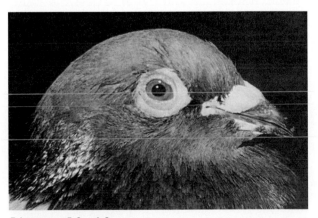

Figure 50-13

A pigeon with a one-eye cold.

lent conjunctivitis. The cere turns dark and moist, and the birds sneeze. Birds commonly shake their heads and the oral mucosa appears reddish-blue.

In other cases the ears are swollen and the cover feathers are erect; the fancier calls this "swollen head." Because of swollen mucosa, noises are heard during inspiration and expiration (rattle and rumble). The pigeons show severe dyspnea, are reluctant to fly, and keep their beaks opened. The breast muscle can turn blue (cyanosis).

Several pigeons are affected at one time or in succession, and adult pigeons can be affected as well. Losses are mostly related to "not homing."

This problem is often referred to as "chronic problems of the upper respiratory tract," coryza, CRL, or "ornithosis-complex." Often, *C. psittaci* is involved, especially in birds under 12 months of age,[11] but usually there is a combination of other agents such as *Mycoplasma* species, *E. coli, Haemophilus* species, or herpesvirus.

Differential diagnosis includes herpesvirus infection, pigeon pox, *Trichomonas* infection, and salmonellosis.

A common practice is to treat homing pigeons with large-scale drug and vitamin combinations on the day they return home. This practice should not be encouraged. Supportive treatment with high-energy foods, soya-milk, and vitamins on the day of arrival will reduce after-flight stress.

Severe Respiratory Distress. Severe dyspnea is seen with chlamydiosis, aspergillosis, abdominal tumor, egg binding, polyserositis caused by egg peritonitis, or a perforating corpus alienum through the gastrointestinal tract. Diseases of the circulatory system, heart failure, and visceral gout can cause severe respiratory symptoms.

Chlamydiosis is primarily a disease of the respiratory system, but often presents with clinical signs of enteritis and liver disease. There is evidence that in these cases virulent psittacine or turkey strains are involved. The so-called pigeon strains not only are less virulent for pigeons but also seem to play a minor role as a zoonotic agent. Problems are mostly seen in young birds. This disease has to be differentiated from pigeon herpesvirus infection and acute salmonellosis.

Mycotic infections are not important in pigeon medicine. Poor hygiene and moldy food, resulting in a high concentration of circulating spores in the air, can induce subacute mycotic pneumonia. In the winter, pea straw bedding sometimes is used and can be a source of *Aspergillus* spores.

Severe dyspnea can be seen in birds with an abdominal tumor, often complicated by ascites or egg binding. The clinical signs are dominated by general symptoms.

Most other problems are diagnosed at necropsy.

Treatment

Treatment of respiratory symptoms is guided by the diagnosis. *Trichomonas* infections are very common. During transport in trailers, the pigeons are watered by a common drinking system. Therefore, each week there is a real risk of a new infection. Parasitic infestations are commonly treated following a fixed schedule during the racing season. Regional resistance is seen against commonly used drugs.

Outside the racing season, drug treatment is indicated only when serious, treatable problems are diagnosed. A mild conjunctivitis or rhinitis is best left untreated; improvement of management, housing, loft climate, hygiene, and rest will "cure" these problems and leave the immunity of the pigeon "boostered."

During the racing season, treatment is selected based on the preliminary diagnosis and the severity of the problem. Individual sick animals should be isolated, and rest is very useful in therapy.

Preventive drug use after homing should be discouraged. A much better approach is to encourage health certification of pigeons before they are allowed to enter races or shows.

Important management measures to decrease the incidence and severity of respiratory problems are:

- Improvement of climatic and loft conditions. The ventilation system in lofts is often poor, resulting in temperature and humidity problems. During cold and humid weather there is too much ventilation; during warm and dry periods ventilation is often inadequate. The veterinarian can play an important role in managing ventilation. Principles of ventilation of poultry and swine facilities are valid in pigeon lofts also.
- The number of pigeons in a loft should be correct.
- Age differences between pigeons in each section should be minimal.

- Young pigeons with clinical signs of respiratory disease should be culled at the beginning of the young pigeon season. Normally more pigeons are bred and hatched than are kept, and 20 to 30% of young pigeons are culled. By removing those with signs of disease, the quality in the young pigeon loft is improved, and disease is less common.

- Only pigeons in top condition should be allowed to be "basketed" (participate in races). Each week only the best pigeons should be selected to race. By racing with only healthy pigeons in excellent condition, the chances of winning increase. The pigeons left at the loft will improve in condition to be fit for the next races. Pigeons in poor condition are more susceptible to infections from the transport trailers, and therefore are at high risk for introducing infections in the loft. The quality of a racing pigeon is in large part dependent on its resistance to diseases.

Reproduction and Reproductive Problems

Reproduction

In the wild, pigeons breed in caves; half-dark nests; or in open, poorly tended nests consisting of twigs or similar material. They normally lay two eggs.

In captivity, reproductive timing is almost completely related to the showing and racing season and the playing system. A nesting facility is provided in a nest box with a nonglazed terra cotta nest dish (Fig. 50–14).

All pigeons are considered monogamous, and the sexes cannot always be distinguished with certainty. However, pigeons often take a "French leave," and squabs of a hen can be conceived by the neighboring cock. Both partners share sitting on the eggs; the male prefers the daytime. The eggs hatch after 13 days for turtle doves and diamond doves and after 17 to 19 days for homing pigeons. The nestlings fledge after 3 to 4 weeks and are able to fly well after 35 days. The molt starts normally during the second nest and is complete after 3 to 4 months.[12] The chicks are sexually mature between 4 and 6 months of age, and reproduction continues until 10 years of age.

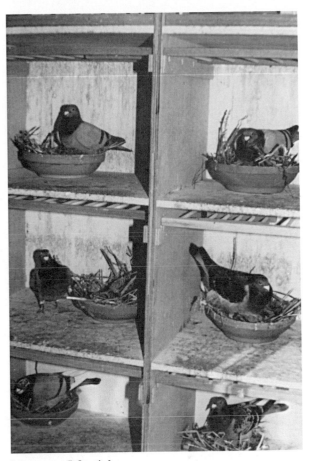

F i g u r e 5 0 – 1 4

Pigeon breeding boxes.

Infertility

Infertility is primarily a problem in old pigeons that are expected to produce fertile eggs. Old pigeons and late young pigeons, especially darkened pigeons, should not be paired for winter breeding. Fertility problems are more common in pigeons that are kept in flights. These pigeons are in poor condition because they cannot fly freely every day. During breeding, pigeons should be in a condition comparable to that required to be ready for a fond race.

"Poor" winters with little sunshine, relatively high temperatures, and high humidity are associated with more reproductive problems than freezing, dry periods with bright sunshine. A combination of reproductive problems and incomplete molt or malformed feathers often occurs. In these cases, subclinical paramyxovirus infection can be an under-laying cause of infertility.

Lack of egg production and sterility can be caused by many factors. Fertility problems have to be evaluated in males and females. Females normally only lay eggs when they can actually see the cocks. Management and food are important factors. Specific disease problems include paratyphoid, paramyxovirus, and herpesvirus infection, tumors, egg binding, oviductal abnormalities, fat accumulation, old age, hormonal imbalances, and pairing of two males. Heavy mite or lice infestation can negatively influence fertility because of restlessness. Laying or fertility problems are common in 8- to 10-year-old birds.

When the primary cause can be found and treated, often the problem can be solved. Hormone treatment (follicle stimulation hormone [FSH] or human chorionic gonadotropin [HCG]) are sometimes reported to be effective.

Normal egg production but no fertilization can result from problems in either bird in a pair. Changing of partners may help. An excessive growth of feathers is seen around the cloaca. The feces may be caked in this area, and cleaning or pulling the feathers may help. Cutting the feathers results in very hard, sharp stubbles. Disturbances of the incubation can cause infertility; therefore nest boxes should be closed.

During breeding, antihelmintic treatments should be avoided. Drugs can negatively influence fertility (such as benzimidazoles, 5-nitroimidazoles, nitrofuranes, and pyrimethamine). *Trichomonas* infection should be treated when the pigeons are sitting on the eggs.

Damaged eggs may result from territorial aggression, which can be prevented by providing more nest boxes and closing the nest box fronts. Toenail or broken leg feathers (muffs) may puncture the eggs if there is low calcium content in the shell. Soft-shelled eggs are caused by low calcium levels in the feed. When ground red brick or charcoal is provided by the fancier and the droppings turn red or black in combination with damaged eggs, this is an indication that there is a deficiency of calcium in the food. The pigeons compensate for this deficiency by overeating other products (pica).

Deformed eggs are primarily caused by hereditary predisposition. The pairs need to be separated.

Prolapse of the cloaca is most often seen in young pigeons after egg binding. After replacement

of the prolapse, the cloaca is sutured to the linea alba through the abdominal wall.

Sometimes a temporarily paralysis of the legs is seen after a pigeon lays a second egg; the condition is caused by low calcium levels in the diet (Fig. 50–15).

Disease Problems in Squabs and Young Pigeons

High mortality of squabs at 1 to 3 days after hatching is often difficult to account for. Hygienic problems and bacterial and yeast contaminations should be considered. Necropsy and microbiologic culture results may provide an answer.[3, 8] Sometimes the squeakers are chilled. Potential causes to be examined are loft construction, quality of nest material, and predators in the loft.

Mortality starting at day 4 after hatching can be associated with salmonellosis. This problem is only seen in heavily infected lofts. Treatment and cleaning are difficult, and without totally interrupting breeding relapses are commonly seen.

Squeaker mortality can be caused by cannibalism. Pairs should be separated and the young fostered or hand-fed. A problem with crowding may exist.

Infestations with ticks (*Argas* species) and blood-sucking mites (*Dermanyssus* species) can cause mortality. These ectoparasites hide under the nest dish and can cause anemia by blood sucking. The use of tobacco stems as nesting material may prevent problems with mite infestations.

Polyuria and polydipsia are commonly seen

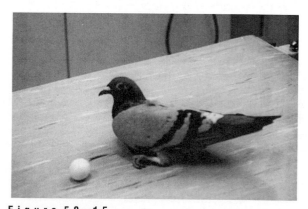

F i g u r e 5 0 – 1 5

A pigeon with egg paralysis.

when the squabs are switched from soft food to seeds (see earlier). Even after extreme illness, full recovery is seen after weaning. Polyuria and polydipsia can be related to paramyxovirus infection, hexamitiasis, or adenovirus infection. In hexamitiasis, the squabs languish starting 10 days after hatching, and the urates stay white. Adenovirus infection is sometimes difficult to differentiate from hexamitiasis. Typical of an adenovirus infection are yellow-green urates, a water-filled crop, and vomiting.

On very rare occasions, *Chlamydia* infections (ornithosis) can cause problems in nestlings or especially in early-weaned squabs. Diarrhea is a common symptom, and the chicks languish and should be euthanatized.

Abnormal respiratory sounds may be heard at the end of the nesting period until shortly after weaning. The cause is unknown and the squabs continue to grow normally.

Streptococcal septicemia is sporadically seen in individual squabs. Sometimes a hen sitting on eggs is found dead, with infection caused by *Streptococcus*.

Navel trichomoniasis can cause serious infections in nestlings. The infection can spread to the abdominal organs and air sacs. Involvement of the pharynx, crop, and liver is seen only after weaning.

Severe pigeon navel pox infections are sometimes seen in the summer and can cause multiple lesions in squabs that cover the head, navel, and legs. Older pigeons show only single lesions.

Severe rickets is seen only in neglected animals that were not provided with minerals. Curved keels of the sternum are seen also in well-managed lofts and do not seem to influence racing performances.

Coccidial oocysts are rarely seen in squabs. The clinical meaning of oocysts for this age group is under debate.

Problems of Skin and Feathers

General abnormalities of feathers and skin are discussed in Chapter 32, Avian Dermatology. Disease problems are presented here that are specific for pigeons.

Pigeon Pox

Pigeon pox causes characteristic lesions in the skin. Exudative lesions appear on the upper surface of

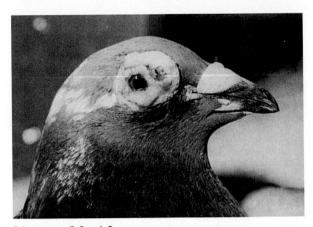

F i g u r e 5 0 – 1 6

Pigeon pox lesions on the eyelid.

the skin of the eyelids (Fig. 50–16) and the base of the beak, feet, and legs, but other parts of the body (e.g., the ears) also can show these lesions. They start as small, whitish, blister-like foci that rapidly increase in size within a week and become yellowish. These form warty growths, which join and form large, rough, brownish scabs that usually last 3 to 4 weeks. This form is known as the *skin form*. In squabs the navel and cloaca can be affected, and in severe infections fledglings can be covered with pox lesions, as is seen in canaries. If the dried scab is removed, the undersurface may be oozing, moist, and bleeding. If the scab falls off, a smooth scar may be present.

The *diphtheric form* can be found on mucous membranes of the mouth, throat, crop, eye, or trachea. Diphtheric raised, yellowish-gray, soft, curdy masses of adherent dead tissue appear on the mucous membranes and can block the trachea. The corners of the mouth are often affected first. In the eye, a cheesy, yellow, swollen mass may replace the eyeball.

The disease often appears as a combined skin and mucous membrane infection. Secondary signs include anorexia and weight loss; sticky, viscid, cheesy material in the eyes; and stained hackle (neck) feathers.

Atypical Pox

Atypical pox or *blood tumors* occur usually as solitary lesions (Fig. 50–17). Histologically, these le-

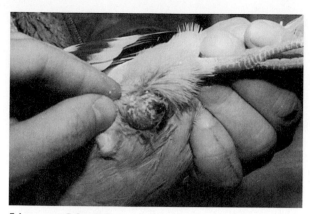

Figure 50-17

Atypical pox or blood tumor.

sions are associated with poxvirus and are characterized by a melanin accumulation. The lesion cannot be transmitted experimentally, and the poxvirus cannot be isolated.

Pruritus and Automutilation

Pruritus and automutilation are rare problems in pigeons. The automutilation is mostly located on the breast or bilaterally around the uropygial gland. It has been associated with the mite *Ornithocheyletia hallae,* but this is not proved. The prognosis is poor.

Xanthomatous Skin

Xanthomatous skin is also called orange-peel skin. It is seen in association with lipomas. Often, resection is possible.

Bare Breast

Some pigeons damage the breast feathers over a surface of 4 cm, producing a bare breast. Only broken feathers are left. There are several theories concerning the cause:

1. Mite infestation. This can be confirmed by microscopic examination, but normally there are no broken feathers.

2. Trauma. This is seen only in pigeons that have an abnormal, very excited drinking behavior. When more pigeons in one loft show the same problem, there is often a family relationship (e.g., an old cock and his two young sons).

3. Unknown. The feather quality may be related to nutrition.

Broken feathers need to be pulled; after 14 days new feathers will appear.

Bad Feathers

Bad feathers and "old" down are the appearance of malformed, broken, bent, dirty, stained, or unusually colored feathers and should be considered abnormal. As a result of a strenuous flight or straying for some days, growing remiges and rectrices are disturbed. This results in "stress marks"—segmental discoloration, black lines, or transparent areas across the vane.

Sometimes the growth is permanently stopped. This causes an irregular wing shape, which therefore influences performance. This growth stoppage is always caused by disease, intoxication, or feeding problems. Sometimes it is seen after vaccination. At the same time, the down molt stops. Normally in a loft, the feces are covered by down feathers.

In spring and summer, so-called old down can be noticed. It is recognized as dark small feathers

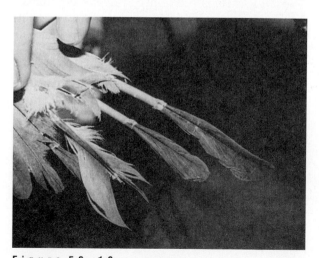

Figure 50-18

Chronic illness or subclinical paramyxovirus infections in the autumn during the molt leads to formation of pin feathers.

(in other birds called definitive down feathers) at the base of the coverts. These should be absent in pigeons. Their presence means that the pigeon had problems in the winter period. Experience has taught that these pigeons will not be top flyers in that season and should not be used for this purpose.

Starvation Feathers

Starvation, pin, and blood feather conditions give much information about the health status and flying condition of the bird. Illness (e.g., salmonellosis, paramyxovirus) during growth of the feathers leads to "working" or "starvation" feathers. Chronic illness or subclinical paramyxovirus infection in the autumn during the molt leads to pin feathers (Fig. 50–18). A rupture of the blood vessels inside the pin feather creates a blood feather. These feather injuries are sometimes seen when oil-adjuvant vaccines are used for paramyxovirus protection in pigeons.

Stress Feathers

Stress feathers are sometimes seen in the secondary feathers of pigeons that are top performers. During the homing season, the first three secondaries are molted. When the "old" feather loosens during the flight, it can damage the follicle.

Mechanical Damage

Mechanical damage of feathers is not uncommon, but usually is not a serious problem. Pathologic conditions and ectoparasites must be excluded. Small holes in the vanes of the remiges and rectrices are associated with louse flies that suck blood from developing feather follicles.

Malformation

Malformation may be seen after a paramyxovirus infection in the autumn and after drug treatment during molting (fenbendazol, sulfa preparations). Intoxications and iatrogenic hypercorticosteroidism are other causes of malformation. Sometimes congenital malformations are seen.

References

1. Hooimeijer J: Principles of veterinary support in racing pigeons. Proc Assoc Avian Vet, 1993, pp 151–155.
2. Rupiper DJ, Ehrenberg M: Introduction in pigeon practice. Main Conf Proc Assoc Avian Vet, 1994, pp 203–211.
3. Rupiper DJ, Ehrenberg M: Diagnostic proceedures for pigeon loft management. Main Conf Proc Assoc Avian Vet, 1994, pp 225–230.
4. Vogel C, Gerlach H, Löffler M: Columbiformes. In Avian Medicine: Principles and Application. Ritchie BW, Harrison GJ, Harrison LR (eds): Lake Worth, FL, Wingers Publishing, 1994, pp 1200–1217.
5. Vogel C, Vogel M, Detering W, Löffler M: Tauben. Berlin, Deutscher Landwirtschafts Verlag, 1992.
6. Abs M: Physiology and Behaviour of the Pigeon. London, Academic Press, 1983.
7. Brückner D: Topography of the blood vessels of head and neck in pigeons and their meaning for injections of paramyxovirus-1-vaccine. Proc Eur Sympos Birds Diseases. Beerse, Belgium, 1987, pp 46–57.
8. Devriese L: Diseases of ornamental birds and pigeons. State University of Ghent, Dept of Poultry Pathology, Bacteriology and Infectious Diseases, ed 3. 1986.
9. Stam JWE, Sluis J van der: Handbook for Pigeon Racing. Maarsen, The Netherlands, Janson, 1994.
10. Dorrestein GM: Viral infections in racing pigeons. Proc Assoc Avian Vet, 1992, pp 244–257.
11. Pennycott TW: Pigeon diseases—Results from a Scottish diagnostic laboratory. Main Conf Proc Assoc Avian Vet, 1994, pp 231–239.
12. Kummerfeld N: Pigeon. In: Gabrisch K, Zwart P (eds): Diseases of Small Pet Animals, ed 3. Hannover, Germany, Schlütersche Verlaganstalt und Druckerei GmbH, 1995, pp 569–624.

Amy B. Worell

51

Toucans and Mynahs

Toucans and mynahs are often grouped together as "softbilled birds" but are from two very different families. Toucans are members of the order Piciformes, family Ramphastidae, and are found in Central and South America. Mynahs are members of the order Passiformes, family Sturnidae, and originate in India, Southeast Asia, and Indonesia.

TOUCANS

The family Ramphastidae is composed of six genera and approximately 35 species. Toucans are grouped into three general categories; the large toucans, the smaller toucanettes, and the small and slender aracaris. Ramphastids are distinguished by a large, elongated bill, which varies in coloration from black to multicolored. The bill is thought to aid in species recognition and to facilitate food procurement.

The vast majority of captive ramphastids are kept as aviary birds in breeding situations (see Color Fig. 51–1). Most of these birds are wild-caught individuals, although the captive populations of some species are now composed of mostly captive-reared birds. Ramphastids, primarily hand-reared young birds, are seldom seen in the pet trade. Hand-reared toucans can make wonderful pets, whereas wild-caught toucans are difficult to tame and are more suitable for aviaries. The most common species in the pet trade are the toco toucan (*Ramphastos toco*) and the sulfur-breasted or keel-billed toucan (*Ramphastos sulfuratus*). Toucans are very active and entertaining and enjoy interaction with their owners. Food items as well as toys are commonly carried in the bill and become objects for play.

Dietary Recommendations

In the wilds of Central and South America, ramphastids are known to eat various foods, including fruits; small vertebrates such as lizards, rodents, and small birds; and various insects.

Dietary recommendations for captive ramphastids revolve around concern for diet-induced iron storage problems or hemochromatosis. Certain species of toucans appear to be susceptible to this devastating condition, and current recommendations thus center around diets that are essentially low in iron. Whether dietary iron is significant in the development or exacerbation of hemochromatosis is unknown. In human medicine, wherein idiopathic hemochromatosis is a well-studied entity, it has been demonstrated that dietary iron levels do not contribute to or augment the disease state.[1, 2]

Diets now recommended for captive toucans include a small-size kibbled dog food or commercial softbill pellets, in addition to a variety of diced fruits. Until further research demonstrates otherwise, the dog food or softbill pellets should contain a low iron level. Dietary iron recommendations for poultry are between 40 and 60 parts per million (ppm), and these levels can be used as guidelines for levels that may be appropriate in ramphastids. However, manufacture of diets containing below 100 ppm of iron can be difficult. The author recommends that the iron level in the kibbled or pelleted component of the diet be less than 150 ppm (ideally less than 100 ppm), and that the use of certain dry kibbled dog foods is preferable. (The only dog food recommended by the author is Waynes Bites, Pet Products Plus, 1-800-592-6687, iron level 90 ppm). Kibble or pellets should be offered dry on an ad lib basis. Fresh fruits, such as papaya, grapes, berries, and melons, or ½ to 1 cup of diced fruit should be offered per bird per day.

Medical Problems in Ramphastids

Ramphastids are very hardy birds and appear to be unaffected by many common avian diseases. Medications can be easily administered by several methods. Parenteral administration through intramuscular injections in the breast muscle is rapid and relatively nonstressful. Oral medications can be administered directly, by metal or rubber gavage tube, or by placement of a desiccated form (tablet or granules) in the center of a grape. Administration of medication in the drinking water is not recommended in ramphastids because they generally do not consume large quantities of water. They obtain most of their daily fluid requirement from fruit. In addition, some toucans choose to bathe in their water containers when size permits.

Infectious Diseases

Documented cases of viral, chlamydial, and fungal infections in ramphastids are essentially nonexistent. It is not uncommon to identify the yeast *Candida albicans* in cultures or cytology specimens of the gastrointestinal tract. This organism may be found in clinically healthy birds and in clinically ill individuals. It may also be found in underweight, slow growing, or unthrifty chicks.

The incidence of internal parasitism in captive ramphastids is quite low. *Giardia* species, ascarids, coccidia, *Capillaria,* and gizzard worms are occasionally noted in fecal examinations or identified on postmortem examination. Recently imported toucans may be heavily parasitized, both internally with coccidia and externally with lice. Parasiticides used in other avian species are also useful in ramphastids. As in other species, *Capillaria* and *Giardia* may be difficult to eliminate from affected birds.

Pathogenic bacteria are more common than other disease agents, but the overall incidence is still quite low. The majority of the bacterial infections in ramphastids involve either the upper respiratory or gastrointestinal systems. Most potentially pathogenic bacteria are gram-negative organisms. *Escherichia coli* is frequently isolated in large numbers from both the upper and lower gastrointestinal tracts of toucans. The importance of these isolates should be considered in light of the total clinical picture. In clinically healthy toucans, *E. coli* should be considered a normal inhabitant and as a potential pathogen in ill birds.

Other conditions occasionally identified in ramphastids include digital necrosis (constricted toe syndrome)[3] in hand-fed toucans, avian tuberculosis, and yersiniosis.[4, 5]

Traumatic Injuries and Deaths

Traumatic injuries, some of which are fatal, are not uncommon when dealing with captive ramphastids. The most common injuries are beak injuries, fractures, trauma to the tarsometatarsal joint, and eye injuries. Aggression between birds often results in trauma.

Beak injuries occur most frequently in young birds that are learning to fly or in juveniles that have been recently introduced into a new flight. The majority of these injuries involve the distal tip of the upper bill and do not require surgical intervention. Occasionally birds are presented with entire sections of the lateral bill missing. Repair of these lesions with various dental materials has resulted only in short-term success, because the repaired area eventually separates from the bill. Similarly, many prosthetic devices, including those involving wires or pins, demonstrate varying degrees of success. These birds are quite adaptable, however, and many individuals manage quite well even with significant defects of the distal bill.

Fractures are infrequently encountered. Birds affected with metabolic bone disease often have multiple fractures. Trauma to the tarsometatarsal joint is frequently encountered and is often related to injuries received during transit. Many of these birds have sustained damage to the joint in the past, and there is a dramatically reduced range of motion in the affected joint. Varying degrees of ankylosis, bony proliferation or severe osteomyelitis, and soft tissue swelling are usually present. In early cases, wrapping the joints and applying topical dimethyl sulfoxide (DMSO) may reduce the chance of permanent damage or tendinitis. If extensive soft tissue swelling is present, the birds should be sedated and the joint opened, cultured, and cleaned. Long-term antibiotic therapy based on culture and sensitivity test results may be indicated. Treatment of advanced cases is generally unrewarding.

Eye injuries ranging from mild superficial corneal abrasions to panophthalmitis and atrophy of the globe are often encountered in recently imported birds. Treatment, when possible, is related to the severity and nature of the injury. Shipping ramphastids in individual carriers helps to prevent injury from fighting.

Intraspecies aggression occurs most frequently during the breeding season when a male attacks or kills its mate (see Color Fig. 51–2). Aggression resulting in severe injury or fatality may occur when two males of any species are housed together in one enclosure. Toucans may drown in rainstorms when rain accumulates in large puddles in aviaries. Affected birds are found dead in the unabsorbed puddle. Unacclimated toucans may be very susceptible to hypothermia, especially if allowed to get wet and cold. Toucans have no down and frequently sunbathe to increase body temperature. Acclimated toucans, however, may be able to withstand cold.

Diabetes Mellitus

Diabetes mellitus is most frequently diagnosed in toco toucans and keel-billed toucans. Affected birds demonstrate classic signs, including weight loss, polydipsia, polyuria, lethargy, anorexia, and hyperglycemia. Although the hyperglycemia may be specifically related to defective glucagon metabolism rather than to lack of insulin production, affected individuals may respond to daily or intermittent insulin injections.

Hemochromatosis

Hemochromatosis or iron storage disease results when excessive amounts of iron accumulate in various body tissues. Cellular damage may or may not result from iron deposition and replacement of normal tissue with iron pigment. When cellular damage does occur, organ dysfunction and illness or death may result.

The etiology of iron storage disease in avian spe-cies is unknown and perhaps it varies significantly with different species. The clinical manifestation varies somewhat in those species affected by the disease.[2, 6, 7, 8] The condition may be a genetically transmitted metabolic disorder, as is the case with idiopathic hemochromatosis in man.[1, 9, 10] Idiopathic hemochromatosis in man is not thought to be related to the amount of iron in the diet because large amounts of available iron in the diet of unaffected individuals do not produce the disease.[1] Potentially, then, dietary iron may be insignificant and noncontributory to the development, progression, and manifestation of the disease in susceptible species of ramphastids.

The signs of iron storage disease are usually subclinical. Affected birds are often found dead without apparent clinical abnormalities. Ongoing clinical trials comparing hematology, serology, and liver biopsy results indicate that liver biopsy is the most reliable means of in vivo diagnosis of hemochromatosis. Liver samples can be examined both histologically and for measurable iron content to reach a diagnosis.[11] Iron storage disease has been reported in 13 species of ramphastids. The three species most commonly affected by hemochromatosis are also the three most common species in captivity—the toco, keel-billed, and the red-billed toucan (*Ramphastos tucanus;* Table 51–1).

Postmortem examination of affected birds frequently demonstrates iron deposition only in the liver. Grossly evident changes may include hepatomegaly and an orange discoloration of the hepatic parenchyma. Microscopic changes often include iron deposition in hepatocytes and Kupffer cells,

T a b l e 5 1 – 1

SPECIES OF RAMPHASTIDS AFFECTED WITH HEMOCHROMATOSIS

Channel-billed toucan	*Ramphastos vitellinus*
Toco toucan	*Ramphastos toco*
Keel-billed toucan	*Ramphastos sulfuratus*
Red-billed toucan	*Ramphastos tucanus*
Ariel toucan	*Ramphastos vitellinus ariel*
Choco toucan	*Ramphastos brevis*
Plate-billed Mt. toucan	*Andigena laminirostris*
Pale mandible toucanet	*Pteroglossus erythropygius*
Chestnut-eared aracaris	*Pteroglossus castanotis*
Black-necked aracaris	*Pteroglossus aracari*
Spot-billed toucanet	*Selenidera maculirostris*
Saffron toucanet	*Baillonius baillioni*
Emerald toucanet	*Aulacorhynchus prasinus*

and varying degrees of iron replacing normal hepatic tissue.

Periodic phlebotomies are recommended for treatment of affected birds. Excessive iron should be mobilized from the liver for production of red blood cells to replace those lost by phlebotomy. Blood removal at the rate of 1% of the bird's body weight, on a weekly basis, has been used for periods of longer than 1 year. Progress should be monitored by serial hepatic biopsies.[12]

Interactions between some nutrients may be important in the etiology of iron storage disease. Deficiencies of specific amino acids or vitamins or imbalances in dietary mineral composition may influence iron metabolism and storage.[13] Inclusion of food items containing ascorbic acid in the diet of susceptible species may enhance the bioavailability of iron; hence, the widespread recommendation that citrus fruits not be included in the diet of toucans.[13, 14]

Tannins or tannic acids theoretically have a protective effect and may reduce the incidence of iron storage disease. Tannins are naturally occurring compounds in certain trees that accumulate in some tropical river waters where free-living ramphastids drink. Tannins theoretically act as natural mineral chelating agents, hence affording a natural counter to iron overload in susceptible species. The addition of tea to the drinking water of ramphastids is thought to replicate the protective effects of tropical river water. Interestingly, no reports of tropical river tannin levels or hepatic iron samples from clinically healthy ramphastids are available in the literature.

A prevalent theory associates the development of iron storage disease to stress in captive birds. This theory holds that stresses such as breeding, captivity, and environmental influences lead to the increased and abnormal storage of iron in susceptible species. This theory seems implausible because most wild-caught ramphastids show fewer signs of stress in captive environments than many species of psittacines, such as wild-caught African gray parrots or cockatoos.

Another theory presumes a relationship between the development of hemochromatosis and intestinal parasitism. Research in poultry has shown that the absorption of numerous minerals, including copper, cobalt, and iron, is affected by intestinal parasitism. Several studies have demonstrated an increased concentration of iron in the liver of growing chicks infected with *Eimeria acervulina*.[15, 16] This occurred only when excess iron (1000 to 1500 ppm) was supplemented in the diet.[15] Although hepatic and tissue levels of iron increased in chicks with coccidiosis and fed diets heavily supplemented with iron, the intestinal iron content itself decreased, which was thought to be the result of destruction of intestinal absorptive cells by the parasitizing coccidia.[15, 16] Some newly imported ramphastids have in the past had positive test results for intestinal coccidiosis, but it is hard to draw valid conclusions as to its significance in iron formation or iron storage.

A retrospective study of iron storage disease involving tanagers at the National Aquarium in Baltimore involved 19 birds, some wild-caught and some captive-bred. All 19 birds had histologic evidence of hemochromatosis. Ten of these individuals had concomitant diseases that contributed to their death, three of which included coccidiosis. In these three individuals, the microscopic changes referable to iron deposition were rated mild to moderate. Several other individuals that did not have intestinal coccidiosis had severe microscopic changes. Interestingly, all birds were on a diet that could be considered excessive in iron. The diet included a large number of items, including mynah pellets, which were analyzed to contain 1230 ppm of iron.[2]

Sex Determination

The majority of ramphastids are phenotypically monomorphic; only a few species are dimorphic. Dimorphic birds include the lowland toucanets of the genus *Selenidera,* and two of the aracaris, *Pteryglossus viridis* (green aracaris) and *Pteryglossus inscriptus* (lettered aracaris). In *Pteryglossus* species, gender is apparent as soon as developing head feather coloration is discernible. Males have prominent black head feathering, and females have brown heads. In *Selenidera culik* (Guyana toucanet) the female has a black cap, chestnut nape, and gray underparts, whereas the male is black in all of these parts.

Two other species demonstrate very slight dimorphism. Males of *Pteryglossus aracari* (black-necked aracaris) and *P. plurinctus* (many-banded aracaris) typically have chestnut-colored ear covert feathers, whereas the females lack this coloration and have black feathers instead.

Males generally have a longer, narrower beak than females of the same species. This difference may be quite apparent when several individuals can be compared, but beak morphology cannot be relied upon for accurate sex determination. Measurement of the upper bill (tomium maxillare) from its origination with the facial skin to the tip may also be helpful in determining sex. In mature toco toucans, birds with tomium maxillare length less than 15½ cm are usually females, but if the length exceeds 16 cm the bird is usually a male.

Definitive sex determination in ramphastids is possible through surgical sexing and chromosome sexing. Sexing by DNA probe was not available at the time of this writing.

Gonadal morphology of ramphastids is similar to that of psittacines. Certain individuals may have darkly pigmented gonads, as are often seen in cockatoos. Specially designed elongated anesthetic masks are necessary to accommodate those species with lengthy beaks. As an alternative, a large Ziploc plastic bag may be used to elongate a standard anesthetic mask and seal against the escape of anesthetic gases. Pre-anesthetic fasting for at least 4 hours is suggested because a distended proventriculus and intestinal loops make the procedure more difficult. The author uses a surgical approach to the birds in a slightly different location than is used in psittacines—the surgical site for sexing psittacines is located cranial to the distal end of the proximal third of the left femur when the left leg is extended caudally. The best surgical approach is more dorsal, near the distal end of the proximal third of the left femur, in ramphastids. This location avoids food-filled intestinal loops.

Ramphastid Pediatrics and Hand-Feeding

The majority of ramphastids are now parent-raised. Some are removed from the nest when young and are commonly removed after mutilation or parent consumption of nest mates. This behavior occurs most often in smaller species and often becomes habitual. With such pairs, fostering or hand-rearing is necessary.

Incubation of ramphastid eggs is not commonplace among aviculturists, and the eggs that are incubated have a low rate of hatchability. Ramphastid chicks can be treated similarly to psittacine chicks in regard to brooders, temperature recommendation, substrates, container needs, and basic visual parameters for health. Ramphastid chicks do not have a crop. They open their eyes at approximately 3 weeks of age. They temporarily have a spurred heel pad on the caudal surface of the proximal tarsometatarsal bone. This heel pad disappears at about 3 weeks of age, coinciding with the eyes opening. The pad is thought to serve as a stabilizing apparatus when the bird is young and sightless (see Color Fig. 51–3).[17]

Ramphastid chicks must be observed very closely for dehydration, which is common in hand-fed chicks. Normal, healthy, well-hydrated chicks are pink with smooth soft skin (see Color Fig. 51–4). Dehydrated babies may be dark pink to purple in color; have dry, cracked, and flaky skin; and look parched. Oral rehydration fluids, subcutaneous fluid administration, and increased brooder humidity may be necessary.

Nutritional requirements for optimal growth and health in young ramphastids are not known. Various diets have been used, including those prepared from pulverized softbill pellets, soaked dog or cat foods, pinkie mice, and homemade combinations of pureed food mixtures. Pureed food mixtures may be composed of applesauce, papaya, baby food, and ground dog food. This type of liquid mixture can easily be fed with a pipette, syringe, or stainless steel feeding tube that is gently inserted into the esophagus. Pureed mixtures such as commercially available parrot hand-feeding preparations seem to work best for very small chicks, although tiny pieces of whole food can also be offered. Pureed or liquid diets can be continued until weaning, or the diet can be changed to include small pieces of whole food items.

Whole food items such as pinkie mice, soaked or softened dog or puppy kibble, and various types of diced fruit can also be fed. A feeding response is easily elicited in healthy youngsters with gentle pressure of the feeding apparatus on the tip or the commissures of the bill. A feeding tube, a pipette, or a small piece of moist food can then be placed in the back of the chick's mouth. Food passes directly into the upper esophagus and proventriculus. The abdomen of a full chick feels turgid, and the chick will refuse food or may regurgitate. Feeding small amounts frequently is preferable to feeding large quantities quickly, as with psittacine chicks.

Neonates should be fed every 2 to 4 hours, even if only a few morsels are accepted at each feeding.

As toucan babies grow and learn to perch, small pieces of freshly diced fruits and dry or soaked kibble or pellets can be placed in the cage. Most chicks wean easily.

Chicks that have poor daily weight gain or poor feeding response should be examined for potential bacterial or yeast overgrowth. Gram's stains or cultures of the upper esophagus and cloaca should be performed. *E. coli* and *C. albicans* are most commonly associated with failure to thrive. Although the significance of these organisms is unknown, their presence in such a chick warrants treatment with appropriate antibiotics and antifungal drugs.

Severe metabolic bone disease is often observed in ramphastid chicks. Babies may refuse to eat kibble, in preference to the apparently tastier fruit. Close attention must be given to relative amounts of fruit versus kibble in the diet of chicks.

MYNAH BIRDS

Mynahs are members of the family Sturnidae and originate in Southeast Asia and India. The mynahs are divided into at least eight genera, with one genus having at least 10 species. The most common mynahs in the US are the *Gracula* species (hill mynahs), *Leucospar rothschildi* (Bali or Rothschild's mynah) and *Acridotheres* species (common mynahs).

Adult hill mynahs can be recognized by their beautiful iridescent black plumage accented by yellow feet, legs, and fleshy wattles ventral to the eyes. Equally striking is the snow white plumage of the Bali mynah, which is accented by black tips on the wings and tail and a bright blue mask around the eyes.[18]

Captive mynahs are uncommon in the US, the most common being the lesser and greater hill mynahs and the Java hill mynahs. Most are wild-caught and many were imported while still being hand-fed. Many of these birds did not survive for long, and most entered the pet trade rather than aviculture. Mynahs are often considered difficult avicultural subjects, although many breed quite well in captivity. Hand-fed mynahs make good pets, with exceptional ability to talk or mimic words and sounds. Mynahs are often considered the best of the talking birds.

Dietary Recommendations

Wild mynahs consume various foods including fruits, insects, and small vertebrates such as lizards. Diets low in iron are recommended for captive mynahs because of the potential for iron storage disease, even though it is unknown whether dietary iron is significant in the development or exacerbation of the disease. Small kibbled dog food (so that it is easily swallowed whole) or commercial softbill diets should be fed in addition to a variety of diced fruits. Until further research demonstrates otherwise, the dog food or softbill diet should contain less than 150 ppm (ideally less than 100 ppm) of iron. If dietary iron recommendations for poultry are considered, a diet containing approximately 60 ppm (mg/kg) of iron is desirable. Some "mynah bird pellets" in the past have contained as much as 2000 ppm or iron. Water should be available at all times, and a powdered vitamin-mineral mixture can be sprinkled on the fruit each day.

Medical Problems

Many of the medical problems described in mynahs are related specifically to conditions of imported wild-caught birds documented in quarantine or holding facilities. General practitioners may not have exposure to these problems.

Three different ocular problems have been described in imported *Gracula* species—corneal scratches, keratitis, and chronic keratoconjunctivitis. No specific etiology was identified. Corneal scratches were related to injuries during shipping or with multiple birds in a cage and were traumatic in origin. Most healed rapidly without permanent effects. Keratitis, conjunctivitis, eyelid depigmentation, and lid distortions were identified in young Indian hill mynahs infected with avian pox virus.[19, 20]

A number of paramyxoviruses have been reported in mynahs, including PMV-1 (Newcastle disease), PMV-2, and PMV-3.[21, 22] Avian influenza type A has been isolated from imported mynahs. Postmortem lesions included hemorrhagic tracheitis, pneumonia, and air sacculitis (see Color Fig. 51–5).

Avian poxvirus infection has been identified in mynahs. Typical pox lesions, including eye lesions, and scabs on the head, beak, and eyelids were observed.[20–22]

Avian cholera, caused by *Pasteurella multocida,* resulted in a fatal septicemia in mynahs. Postmortem lesions, including hemorrhages on viscera and pulmonary edema, were similar to clinical signs observed in poultry. *Campylobacter* species has also been isolated from cloacal swabs from newly imported mynahs.[18] Parasites reported in imported mynahs include *Toxoplasma gondii, Tetrameres,* and coccidia.[21, 22]

Medical Problems of Captive Mynahs

The two most common medical problems affecting captive mynahs are upper respiratory infections and hepatic disorders, particularly hemochromatosis. Avian pox has been diagnosed in Bali mynahs kept in outdoor flights. The source of the virus was thought to be feral starlings. Typical pox lesions were observed.[23, 24]

Fatal septicemias have been associated with the following bacteria: *Salmonella* species, *Yersinia pseudotuberculosis, Klebsiella pneumoniae, E. coli,* and *Mycobacterium.*[18, 19] Fatal toxoplasmosis has been reported in young mynahs. Clinical signs included weight loss, respiratory disease, and death.[21, 25–27] A number of hepatic disorders occur in mynahs with some regularity, including hepatocellular carcinoma, lymphosarcoma, adenocarcinoma, and hemochromatosis.[21–23, 28–304]

Hemochromatosis

Hemochromatosis is a well documented entity in both starlings[2, 6, 28] and mynahs.[2, 21–24, 28, 29] Affected birds may simply be found dead in their cages or may be presented with clinical signs such as cachexia, abdominal swelling due to ascites and/or hepatomegaly, and dyspnea. Histopathology routinely demonstrates deposition of iron pigment in hepatocytes and usually in hepatic Kupffer cells. In addition, iron is frequently deposited in the spleen, myocardium, kidney, and pancreas.

The exact etiology of iron storage disease is unknown. Treatment includes abdominocentesis, di-

uretics, and phlebotomies. Whether formulated diets with low iron content are beneficial is currently unknown. A recent study involving mynahs concluded that the iron intake from a controlled and analyzed diet was not excessive and that the excessive iron loading was potentially the result of enhanced intestinal absorption, as is the case with humans with idiopathic hemochromatosis. The prognosis in affected birds is extremely guarded.

Miscellaneous Conditions

Congestive heart failure accompanied by clinical signs similar to those observed in mammals has been documented in mynahs. Idiopathic seizure disorders have also been described. Respiratory infections, involving both the upper and lower respiratory tract, have been described in mynahs. The etiology is varied and often multifactoral, involving stress, bacterial agents, fungal agents, and species susceptibility. Pulmonary aspergillosis was very common in some lots of imported mynahs.

References

1. Niederau C, Stremmel W, Strohmeyer G: Hemachromatosis. Ergrbniddr Jder Inneren Medizin und Kinderheilkunde 117–148, 1987.
2. Kincaid A, Stoskopf M: Passerine dietary iron overload syndrome. Zoo Biol 6:79–88, 1987.
3. Worell AB: Suspected ergotism in hand-fed Toucans. Proc Thirty-Sixth Western Poult Dis Conf, 1987, pp 113–135.
4. Dhillon A, Shafer D: *Yersinia pseudotuberculosis* infection in two toco toucans and a touraco. Proc First Int Conf Zoo Avian Med 1987, pp 37–38.
5. Jawetz E, Melnick J, Adelburg E: Review of Medical Microbiology, ed 19. Los Aetos, CA, Lange Medical Publications, 1991.
6. Lowenstein L, Petrak ML: Iron pigments in the livers of birds. In Montali RJ and Myaki G (eds): Comparative Pathology of Zoo Animals. Washington DC: Smithsonian, 1979.
7. Worell AB: Management and medicine of toucans. Proc Assoc Avian Vet, 1988, pp 253–262.
8. Hill JE, Bruke DL, Rowland GN: Hepatopathy and lymphosarcoma in a mynah bird with excessive iron storage. Avian Dis 30(3):634–636, 1986.
9. Weintraub LR, Edwards CQ, Krikker M (eds): Annals of The New York Academy of Science, Hemochromatosis: Proceedings of the First International Conference. New York, New York Academy of Sciences, 1988.
10. Bothwell TH, Charleton RW, Cook JD, Finch LA: Iron overload—general considerations. In: Iron Metabolism, 1979.
11. Worell AB: Further investigations in ramphastids concerning hemochromatosis. Proceedings Annual Conference AAV, Nashville, TN, 1993, 98–107.

12. Worell AB: Phlebotomy for treatment of hemochromatosis in two sulfur-breasted toucans. Proceedings Annual Conference AAV, Chicago, IL, 1991, 9–14.
13. Dierenfeld ES, Sheppard CD, Pini M: Investigations of hepatic iron levels in captive avifauna. Unpublished work, 1994.
14. Worell AB: Personal communication with aviculturists.
15. Bafundo KW, Baker DH, Fitzgerald PR: The zinc-iron interrelationship in the chick as influenced by *Eimeria acervulina* infection. J Nutrition 114:1306–1313, 1984.
16. Southern LL, Baker DH: Iron status of the chick as affected by *Eimeria acervulina* infection and by variable iron ingestion. J Nutrition 112:2353–2363, 1982.
17. Personal communication with Jerry Jennings, 1994.
18. Schroeder D: Bali (Rothschild's) mynah. AFA Watchbird XVIII:4–7, 1991.
19. Karpinski LG, Clubb SL: Clinical aspects of ophthalmology in caged birds. Proceedings Annual Conference AAV, San Diego, CA, 1983, 216–227.
20. Karpinski LG, Clubb SL: An outbreak of pox in imported mynahs. Proceedings Annual Conference AAV, Houston, TX, 1986, 35–37.
21. Panigraphy B, Senne DA: Diseases of mynahs. J Am Vet Med Assoc 199:35–38, 1991.
22. Dorrestein GM: Veterinary problems in mynah birds. Proceedings Annual Conference AAV, Miami, FL, 1988, 263–274.
23. Rosskopf WJ, Woerpel RW: Pet avian conditions and syndromes. 1989 update, Proceedings Annual Conference AAV, Seattle, WA, 1989, 394–424.
24. Gerlach H: The so-called iron storage disease in mynahs. Proceedings International Conference Zoo & Avian Medicine, Oahu, HI, 1987, 19–85.
25. Partington CJ, Gardiner CH, Fritz D, et al: A toxoplasmosis in bali mynahs (*Leucospar rothschildi*). J Zoo Wildlife Med 20:328–335, 1989.
26. McMillan MC, Petrak ML: Retrospective study of aspergillosis in pet birds. J Assoc Avian Vet 3:211–215, 1989.
27. Hasholt J, Petrak ML: Diseases of the urinary system. In Petrak ML (ed): Diseases of Cage and Aviary Birds, 2nd ed. Philadelphia, Lea & Febiger, 1982, 449–457.
28. Dierenfeld ES, Sheppard CD, Pini M: Unpublished material.
29. Morris PJ, Avergis SE, Baumgartner RE: Hemochromatosis in a greater Indian Hill mynah (*Gracula religiosa*): Case report and review of the literature. J Assoc Avian Vet 3:87–89, 1988.
30. Gosselin SL, Kramer LW: Pathophysiology of excessive iron storage disease in mynah birds. J Am Vet Med Assoc 183:1238–1240, 1983.
31. Ward RJ, Iancu TC, Henderson GM, et al: Hepatic iron overload in birds: Analytical and morphological studies. Avian Pathol 17:451–464, 1988.

Patrick T. Redig

52

Raptors

APPROACH TO MEDICAL CONDITIONS OF RAPTORS (FALCONRY BIRDS)

Trained and wild raptors are afflicted by a relatively small number of diseases, most of which are well-recognized entities in the falconry literature. The principal problems are oral trichomoniasis, aspergillosis, bumblefoot, herpes virus hepatitis, cutaneous pox, malaria, coccidiosis, intestinal parasites, and low condition with secondary sour crop. There are also typical injuries occurring as a consequence of handling, training, and utilization as hunting hawks in the sport of falconry (e.g., jess injuries to legs, broken legs [especially the tibiotarsus], bites from prey [especially squirrel bites], torn crops from fighting with pheasants, broken coracoid bones from forceful collisions with prey, and miscellaneous injuries to wing bones and joints [especially in young birds]) (Figs. 52–1 to 52–3). Some obscure upsets of the gastrointestinal tract cause loss of appetite, vomiting, and diarrhea; these require further research to determine their cause. For now, such problems are treated symptomatically. Some species of raptors are more prone to certain diseases than others. For instance, most are susceptible to frounce (trichomoniasis), although peregrine falcons *(Falco peregrinus)* are more resistant than others. Most prairie falcons *(Falco mexicanus)* taken from the wild have air sac worms *(Serratospiculum* species). Passage red-tailed hawks *(Buteo jamaicensis)* and goshawks *(Accipiter gentilis)* are prone to have or soon develop aspergillosis, and most will be harboring *Capillaria* species when trapped. Chamber-raised birds of any species may have coccidiosis as youngsters. Gyrfalcons *(Falco rusticolus)* have the least resistance to the most

devastating diseases and conditions, including bumblefoot, aspergillosis, malaria, and herpes virus infections.

Diseases of raptors fall into the following major

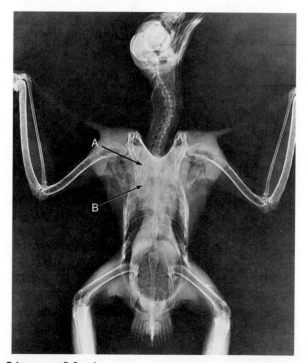

F i g u r e 5 2 – 1

A trained prairie falcon *(Falco mexicanus)* has the neck of a pheasant lodged in its esophagus. The outlines (A, B) of the cervical vertebrae can be seen tracking from the crop through the thoracic inlet and into the proventriculus. This problem may occur when the falcon picks the neck up in the midsection and swallows it like a horseshoe. Signs include persistent movements of the head and neck as the bird attempts to mechanically drive the mass into the proventriculus. These birds typically become anorectic and often develop a stasis-related inflammation of the upper gastrointestinal tract (sour crop).

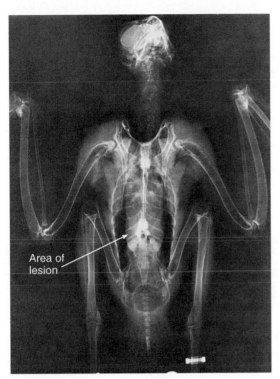

F i g u r e   5 2 – 2

A juvenile peregrine falcon in which osteomyelitis has developed in the region of the vertebral column where the lumbar vertebrae join the synsacrum. In due course, the process of bone necrosis and inflammation led to spinal cord injury. The falcon presented with an acute flaccid paralysis of both pelvic limbs.

categories: Infectious (including parasitic), management-related, toxic, and idiopathic.[1, 2]

1. The major infectious diseases that affect raptors are aspergillosis, trichomoniasis, herpes virus inclusion body hepatitis, cutaneous pox, malaria, and coccidiosis.

2. The major management-related diseases that affect raptors are low condition, coccidiosis, candidiasis, and bumblefoot.

3. The major toxicities encountered in raptors are lead poisoning, exposure to cholinesterase-inhibiting compounds, and exposure to anticoagulants or other rodenticides.

4. The major idiopathic, idiosyncratic problems seen are obscure gastrointestinal upsets, unattributable to any of the above-mentioned etiologies, resulting in anorexia, weight loss, vomiting, and depression. True diarrhea usually does not accompany this problem.

Group and species differences exist among raptors used for falconry in terms of disease susceptibility. Some of these differences are related to geographic origin of the species and some presumed naiveté to certain pathogens (malaria, herpes virus, and aspergillosis). Other differences are related to temperament and fractiousness and the management problems they pose. The latter also involves the skill, temperament, and fundamental character of the falconer. Temperament of the bird is in turn influenced by chronologic age, age at which it was taken from parent birds, and sex. These differences have been long recognized in the literature of falconry and a whole terminology system has evolved.[3] Important terms are listed in Table 52–1.

The following generalizations can be made about states of health and disease in captive raptors:

1. Tiercels (males) tend to be more difficult to manage than falcons (females).

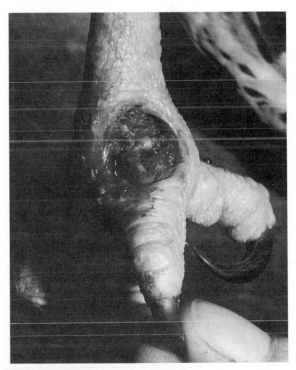

F i g u r e   5 2 – 3

The dorsal aspect of the halux of a prairie falcon that features an ulcerated epithelial wound accompanied by transsection of the extensor tendon. The lesion occurred as a result of ice and snow building up underneath the leather anklet (Aylmeri jess) typically worn by trained raptors (not shown here). The ice ball, which is formed by thawing and freezing of snow, can lead to pressure necrosis of the underlying tissues.

Table 52-1

TERMS USED IN CLASSIFICATION OF RAPTORS KEPT IN CAPTIVITY WITH BEHAVIORIAL IMPLICATIONS

Eyas (pl. eyasses). A young raptor removed from parent birds and taken up for conditioning and training before it is capable of flight. Typically refers to birds taken before 15 days of age, at which time they will imprint upon human handlers. They become very tame and they are easily trained, but they can become very demanding, often developing habitual screaming and aggressiveness toward people, particularly when hungry.

Branchers. A subcategory of eyas, these are young raptors taken from the nest when they are nearly feathered, very ambulatory, but not yet capable of flight. They will become tame, but will not imprint.

Chamber-raised birds. A phenomenon of captive propagation, these are young that are left in the breeding chambers with adult parents until well after they can fly. They tend to be very wild and much more difficult to train.

Passage birds. These are fledged, free-flying young of the year raptors that are trapped on their first migration (hence, passage). They become tame, but do not imprint. They have some survival savvy (hence, if lost, have a reasonable chance of surviving), good manners, and some knowledge of flying and hunting. On the other hand, a fair proportion of these birds are caught because they are at low weight from lack of hunting success, many are heavily parasitized, and some have aspergillosis.

Haggards. These are free-flying wild birds that have matured to their adult plumage in the wild. Present-day regulations prohibit their being taken for falconry purposes. They possess great flying and hunting skills and are relatively disease-free, having survived most of the problems that are fatal to younger birds. However, rehabilitators often see old haggards in debilitated condition because of age-related organ failure (e.g., hypothyroidism).

Falcon. A term used to refer to the female of a species, particularly among long-wings. "Hen" is also used.

Tiercel. A term referring to the male, who is about ⅓ smaller than the female in most instances.

Teenager. Refers to imprinted young, whether domestically raised or taken from the wild, during the period of life when wild-reared birds would be learning to fly and gain independence (between 6 and 16 weeks of age). It is a time period of psychologic maturation and adaptation to the environment, which may be frustrated in the captive environment.

---

2. Teenagers, especially tiercels, can be very unpredictable in their behavior and have the greatest susceptibility to management-related and infectious diseases, partially as a result of the generalized state of stress they seem to endure as they go through stages of psychologic maturation in the late summer of their first year.

3. Passage birds tend to have a window of susceptibility to diseases during the first 6 weeks of captivity. Many are taken from the wild with, and perhaps as a result of, ongoing disease. They are most likely to have either heavy intestinal parasite burdens (especially *Capillaria* species) or aspergillosis.

TREATMENT AND OTHER DETAILS OF PRINCIPAL PROBLEMS

Aspergillosis

This fungal disease of the respiratory system is the most commonly occurring disease among raptors held in captivity. Although it may occur in individuals of virtually any species, hawk or owl, there are clearly species predilections (Table 52–2). Keymer[4] reported it as a common cause of death among owls in the London Zoo, but the near-complete lack of occurrence of aspergillosis in the more than 3000 owls handled at The Raptor Center (TRC) leads me to believe this situation represented a unique exposure problem.

Diagnosis

Diagnosis is based upon clinical suspicion (signs, species, sex, time of year), antibody detection (enzyme-linked immunosorbent assay [ELISA*]), tracheal culture, blood work, and endoscopy. Radiology is generally of limited value as a diagnostic tool during stages of development where treatment is a reasonable possibility. Clinical suspicion coupled with positive tracheal culture (taken from deep within the trachea with a nasopharyngeal swab [sterile nasopharyngeal calcium alginate–tipped applicators, Hardwood Products, Guilford, ME]) and an elevated white cell count (15,000 to 20,000 ml/mm^3+) is taken as circumstantial evidence of occurrence and the basis upon which to commence treatment.

Treatment

Options for aspergillosis treatment are limited. Drugs used in treatment of aspergillosis have in-

---

Aspergillus ELISA testing, NCACS, in care of The Raptor Center, 1920 Fitch Avenue, St. Paul MN 55108.

T a b l e 5 2 – 2

RAPTORS AND OTHER AVIANS WITH APPARENT RISK FOR DEVELOPING ASPERGILLOSIS

Gyrfalcons *(Falco rusticolus)*
Goshawks *(Accipiter gentilis)*
Rough-legged hawks *(Buteo lagopus)*
Golden eagles *(Aquila chrysaetos)*
Immature red-tailed hawks *(Buteo jamaicensis)*
Snowy owls *(Nyctea scandiaca)*
Eider ducks
Loons
Trumpter swans (especially with lead poisoning)
African grey parrots

cluded 5-fluorocytosine (5FC) (Ancobon, Hoffman-LaRoche, Nutley, NJ), itraconazole (Sporanox, Janssen, Piscataway, NJ), fluconazole (Diflucan, Pfizer, New York), clotrimazole (clotrimazole, 10% in PEG, Island Pharmaceutical, Woodruff, WI), and amphotericin B (Fungizone, Squibb, Princeton, NJ). Only the latter is fungicidal. Amphotericin, along with 5FC, itraconazole, and clotrimazole, have documented efficacy in treating known cases of aspergillosis; diflucan appears to be ineffective.

In individuals with elevated ELISA titers or vague signs of illness that are attributable to aspergillosis based on clinical suspicion, tracheal culture and elevated white cell count, 5FC (75 mg/kg/day in two or three divided doses) has been effective in a large number of cases over the last 15 years. With the recent availability of itraconazole (10 mg/kg once or twice daily), it is now supplanting 5FC in this use. Recently, the combination of clotrimazole nebulized in polyethylene glycol with orally administered itraconazole has been found effective in recovering some birds with very severe cases of pulmonary and air sac aspergillosis.[5, 6] This treatment and other modalities have been comprehensively reviewed by Aguilar and Redig.[7]

Clearly aspergillosis is to be *prevented* or treated while subclinical. Prophylactic treatment with 5FC or itraconazole is recommended for newly captured, newly admitted birds of species that have an established track record of susceptibility. The usual program is to give 5FC at 75 mg/kg twice daily (bid) or itraconazole at 10 mg/kg bid for 2 weeks. This approach should also extend to individuals of highly susceptible species that are undergoing change of management (e.g., transfer to new owner or new enclosure), regardless of age or other cir-

cumstance. Domestically reared gyrfalcons and gyrhybrids should be provided with this prophylactic regimen from a period beginning at 45 days of age through 75 days of age. If extreme heat conditions prevail during the months of August and September in a locale, young gyrfalcons should be provided with extended prophylactic treatment during this time.

Vaccination

Vaccination for aspergillosis is clearly needed to replace these extensive prophylactic treatment programs. Presently none is available. Vaccination would probably be useful in treating clinically ill birds as a means of boosting the immune system.

Malaria

Once diagnosis is established by finding *Plasmodium* species organisms on a blood film in correlation with clinical signs, management may be attempted according to the following approach, which has been excerpted from Redig.[8]

Treatment

The goals of treatment in avian malaria are: (1) to eliminate erythrocytic forms; (2) to eliminate or reduce tissue forms; (3) to provide protection from massive rupture of infected red blood cells resulting from stress during treatment; and (4) if necessary, to provide the bird with a supply of functional red blood cells through transfusion, which not only improves oxygen carrying capacity, but also can help reduce the number of infected erythrocytes. Other supportive care such as provision of fluids and easily digested food are a matter of routine.

Two agents are effective for treatment: chloroquine and primaquine (Aralen, Sanofi Winthrop, New York).[9] The former is effective against erythrocytic forms and the latter against the tissue forms. The two drugs are combined for administration. The target dose for chloroquine is 15 mg/kg/dose and the target for primaquine is 0.75 to 1.0 mg/kg/dose. Preparation of the proper dose is complicated by the nature of the compound as supplied. A 500-

mg tablet contains 325 mg of active base; dosages are based upon the patient receiving a prescribed amount of the active base.

One tablet of each drug is ground with a mortar and pestle, then weighed out in the appropriate amount of the two-drug mixture on a precision balance and loaded into a #2 gelatin capsule. Alternatively, whole tablets of each compound can be crushed and mixed with 10 ml of water, which will yield a final concentration of approximately 30 mg/ml chloroquine and 1.5 mg/ml primaquine. A 0.5-ml aliquot of this mixture will then yield 15 mg of chloroquine and 0.75 mg of primaquine. The drugs do not dissolve in water; hence, the suspension must be well agitated just prior to administration. This method of administration is preferred in critically ill patients, because absorption of the drugs, which is rapid and enhanced by food, will be greatly expedited.

Despite reasonable success in treating clinical cases, it is clear that the parasite is not cleared from the system in all cases treated. Indeed, it appears that most recovered birds may have lifelong infections. Evidence for this condition derives from reports of periodic recrudescence in treated birds, as well as experimental expression of latent parasitemias by glucocorticoid injection into recovered birds.[10]

Prevention

Prevention of malaria is based upon two approaches: (1) vector exclusion, and (2) prophylactic treatment. The latter is not entirely effective without the former. Where susceptible species are housed at a time of the year and a place where vectors (*Culex* mosquitoes) and reservoirs (waterfowl, blackbirds, robins, crows, and sparrows) are present, raptors must be protected from insects during the time of day when vectors are active.[10] Maintenance in or movement to a tightly screened enclosure is desirable for adult birds and essential for nestlings and juveniles. Prophylactic treatment consists of a once-weekly, single treatment either with primaquine or chloroquine/primaquine combination commencing 1 month before and continuing 1 month after the insect season. The dose of the combination drug is 25 mg/kg, and appropriate amounts can be taken from Table 52–3. Periodic

Table 52–3

DOSES OF CHLOROQUINE, PRIMAQUINE, AND THE COMBINATION OF THE TWO FOR TREATING AVIAN MALARIA

Bird Weight (mg)	Chloroquine* (mg)	Primaquine† (mg)	Combination (mg)
100	2.50	0.13	2.63
150	3.75	0.20	3.95
200	5.00	0.26	5.26
250	6.25	0.33	6.58
300	7.50	0.39	7.89
350	8.75	0.46	9.21
400	10.00	0.52	10.52
450	11.25	0.59	11.84
500	12.50	0.65	13.15
550	13.75	0.72	14.47
600	15.00	0.78	15.78
650	16.25	0.85	17.10
700	17.50	0.91	18.41
750	18.75	0.98	19.73
800	20.00	1.04	21.04
850	21.25	1.11	22.36
900	22.50	1.17	23.67
950	23.75	1.24	24.99
1000	25.00	1.30	26.30
1050	26.25	1.37	27.62
1100	27.50	1.43	28.93
1150	28.75	1.50	30.25
1200	30.00	1.56	31.56
1250	31.25	1.63	32.88
1300	32.50	1.69	34.19
1350	33.75	1.76	35.51
1400	35.00	1.82	36.82
1450	36.25	1.89	38.14
1500	37.50	1.95	39.45
1550	38.75	2.02	40.77
1600	40.00	2.08	42.08
1650	41.25	2.15	43.40
1700	42.50	2.21	44.71
1750	43.75	2.28	46.03
1800	45.00	2.34	47.34
1850	46.25	2.41	48.66
1900	47.50	2.47	49.97
1950	48.75.	2.54	51.29
2000	50.00	2.60	52.60
2050	51.25	2.67	53.92

*500 mg chloroquine tablet containing 300 mg active base.
†26 mg primaquine tablet containing 15 mg active base.

blood samples (e.g., 4- to 6-week intervals) should be taken for monitoring purposes.

Trichomoniasis

This protozoan infection of the oral pharynx was among the first diseases of raptors for which the etiology was clearly established and effective treatments developed. The disease presents as caseous lesions of varying size and location in the oral pharynx. Lesions are usually found around and under the tongue or on the palate, occasionally extending into the crop and respiratory system. The progression of the disease is slow. Among captive birds, detection occurs at a stage when lesions are small and relatively innocuous. Because the disease causes no systemic effects, debilitation and death occur as a result of a progressive inability of the affected bird to manipulate and swallow food. Therefore, among wild birds, the typical presentation is that of an extremely debilitated individual with well-developed lesions in the mouth. Cases have been seen where the palate is completely destroyed by a large caseous lesion extending from border to border and invading the ventral cranium. In addition, lesions have been found encircling the inside of the mandible, in one case lysing the mandibular bone itself. Clearly, such cases have an extremely poor prognosis.

The disease is transmitted from a pigeon that is eaten by a raptor. Incubation is about 10 days, after which small, raised, white plaques may be seen in the mouth of the patient. The organism is fragile and generally dies soon after the body of the dead pigeon cools. The appearance of the lesions is generally sufficient for diagnosis, but diagnosis may be confirmed by scraping portions of the lesion at the mucosal interface, placing the material in a warm drop of saline on a slide, and examining the specimen under 40x magnification. With reduced light, motile protozoa can be seen moving in and about the debris. Better definition can be obtained by staining the preparation with trichrome stain.

Treatment

Treatment is accomplished by the administration of metronidazole (Flagyl) at 40 mg/kg bid for 3 to 5 days. An alternative treatment is carnidazole (Spartrix, Janssen, distributed by Wildlife Laboratories, Fort Collins, CO), a drug used in pigeons. It is given at 30 mg/kg bid for 3 to 5 days. In most cases, the lesions disappear within 24 to 48 hours of the initiation of treatment.

There is variation among raptors regarding their susceptibility to this disease and variation in the

virulence of different strains. Peregrine falcons, although not totally immune, do develop the disease much less frequently than expected, given the numbers of pigeons consumed by them. Additional information may be obtained from referenced material.[11]

NUTRITIONAL DEPLETION (LOW CONDITION)

Severe debilitation resulting from insufficient food intake is the most common emergency encountered among raptors kept for falconry.[12] It occurs most frequently among males during the peak of their first season in the field. Trained raptors are managed by controlling their weight to a greater or lesser extent, and idiosyncratic responses to weight control as well as variations in the degree of weight control exerted by individual falconers are initiating factors in the problem (Table 52–4). Although trained birds seldom encounter the prolonged fasts that injured wild birds do, nevertheless, trained birds are kept in a state of a lean body mass for extended periods, during which catabolism of body proteins occurs. The problem is exacerbated in Northern climates by the increased energy requirements of winter's cold. Afflicted birds are presented in states of extreme weight loss, severe anemia, dehydration, and depression. They may have less

T a b l e 5 2 – 4

METABOLIC BODY MASSES (MBM) FOR SELECTED RAPTORS

Species	Weight (g)	MBM (kg)
Saw-whet	60	0.120
Kestrel	100	0.180
Sharpy	150 (f)	0.240
Merlin	200	0.300
SEO/LEO	350	0.460
Peregrine	500 (m)	0.590
Peregrine	750 (f)	0.810
Red-tailed hawk	1000	1.00
Osprey	1500	1.360
GHO/Snowy	1900	1.620
Bald eagle	3000 (m)	2.280
Bald eagle	5000 (f)	2.830

From Bates G: Hyperalimentation in Birds. Unpublished data.
GHO = Great horned owl, SEO = short-eared owl, LEO = long-eared owl, Snowy = snowy owl, Saw-whet = Saw-whet owl, Sharpy = sharp-shinned hawk, f = female, m = male.

T a b l e   5 2 – 5

HYPERALIMENTATION SCHEDULE SAMPLE

Juvenile Red-tailed Hawk
Assume weight of 1000 g

Energy requirement $= 200 \times$ MBM/day (see Table 52–4)
$\qquad\qquad\qquad = 200 \times 1.0 = 200$ kcal/day
Water requirement $= 80$ ml $\times$ MBM $= 80$ ml/day

> 30% Nutrical (Evsco, IGI Inc, Buena, NJ) in electrolyte contains 650 kcal/l
> With Gerber baby food—**2 volumes** contains 1000 kcal (strained beef, veal, chicken, or turkey–2nd food)
> Combined solution has 1650 kcal/l = 1.65 kcal/ml
> (Water content is about 880 ml/l = 0.8 ml/ml)

How much to give:

$$\frac{\text{kcal requirement}}{\text{Energy content}} = \frac{200 \text{ kcal/day}}{1.65 \text{ kcal/ml}} = 121 \text{ ml/day}$$

> This would also give 97 ml of water/day, which is more than the calculated amount of 80 ml/day.

Treatment protocol: Give 40 ml of 2:1 Nutrical (30%) and baby food three times/day. If food is vomited, reduce volume, but increase frequency of feeding.

---

than 24 hours to live at the time of presentation, and yet they may have put in a reasonably normal performance in the field as recently as the day before.

The following is a list of *behavioral* signs of a bird in low condition, listed in order of frequency of occurrence.

1. Change in behavior
   a. Refusing quarry
   b. Half-hearted chases
   c. Pole or tree sitting
2. Weakness to wing beat—characterized as a "butterfly" wingbeat
3. "Almond-eyed" appearance rather than a bright, perfectly round eye in a healthy bird
4. "Blank gaze" or hazy cornea; dry membranes in mouth
5. Minor tremor or shaking, fixed gazes, flicking of nictitans
6. Sudden increase in prominence of the keel in the preceding 24 hours and concomitant weight loss
7. Sleeping during the day, especially after a drop in ambient temperature
8. Convulsion and seizures due to hypoglycemia (rare)

Similarly, the *clinical* signs of a raptor in low conditions are:

1. Profound dehydration
2. Low packed cell volume (PCV), typically between 15 and 20%
3. Low total plasma solids, typically off the scale of the refractometer
4. Nonregenerative anemia
5. Complete blood count (CBC) results are normal, except as noted in 1 and 2

The elements of treatment for a raptor in low condition[12] are:

Agent	Dosage Schedule
1. Intravenous fluids	Lactated Ringer's solution given as a bolus at 30 ml/kg
2. Iron dextran	10 mg/kg, intramuscularly (IM), one dose
3. B-vitamin complex	Equivalent to 10 mg thiamine content, IM
4. Steroids	Dexamethasone, 2 mg/kg
5. Warm environment	Warm slowly to avoid "reheating shock," use heating pad on low setting
6. Feed easily digestible items for first 1–3 days, depending on progress	See the hyperalimentation schedule, Table 52–4. Feed only small amounts of food at any one feeding, even if the bird appears to have a voracious appetite
7. Full recovery will require about 3 weeks	Recovery is complete when PCV has returned to near normal conditions

Some occurrences of low condition are accompanied by crop stasis or "sour crop." The problem is often further complicated by the tendency of bird owners to "feed up" a hawk that they suddenly realize has gotten too low in weight. Although the bird may ingest food, it is not passed from the crop. Secretions accumulate and bacteria proliferate in the static organ, leading to the development of a foul-smelling, swollen, fluctuant crop. (This condition occurs in some birds that are not in poor nutritional state, apparently from unknown causes that cause crop stasis, e.g., undefined bacterial or viral agents.) Treatment consists of removing crop contents, either by massaging them out the mouth or through ingluviotomy. Metoclopramide dosed at 0.1 ml/kg (Smith and Nephew, Franklin Park, IL) is very effective in stimulating motility and should be administered as part of the treatment protocol outlined earlier. It may have to be repeated at 4- to 6-hour intervals during the first day of treatment. Once there is evidence of motility and black fecal material is produced, treatment may be discontinued.

PRINCIPAL MEDICAL PROBLEMS OF RAPTORS AND APPROPRIATE DIAGNOSTIC PROCEDURES*

Principal Signs	Possible Problems	Possible Causes	Primary Diagnostics	Secondary Diagnostics
All cases			History, physical examination	CBC Radiograph
Raised scabby lesions on unfeathered skin	Pox	Pox virus	Light microscopic examination of skin scraping	Electron microscopic examination

Respiratory Signs
Voice change, croaking sound when flying
Nasal discharge
Increased respiratory effort
	Upper airway blockage
	
	Sinusitis
	1. Pulmonary disease (early stages)
	2. Air sac disease (early stages)
	3. Airway obstruction
	4. Carbon monoxide
		Aspergillus granuloma in trachea or syrinx
		Various bacteria/fungi[14]
		1,2. Aspergillosis[7]
		1,2. Pneumonia
		3. Granulomatous airway blockage
		3. Airway stricture
		1,2. Rarely, *Chlamydia* or tuberculosis infection
			Tracheal endoscopy
			
			Nasal flush and culture
			1,2,3. PCV/TP
			  1,2. Radiographs ventrodorsal/ lateral
			    3. Tracheal culture or wash grown on Sab-Dex
			    1. ELISA[15] for aspergillus
				Radiographs (ventrodorsal and lateral)
				
				Chlamydia culture or latex agglutination test

Respiratory difficulty with anorexia, lethargy, exercise intolerance, passing lime green stools	As above, except later stages	1. Pulmonary aspergillosis[7] 2. Lead poisoning[16]	1. ELISA test 2. Lead level (atomic absorption)	Porphyrin levels Radiographs
As above, but passing jade green stools, acute onset (species = gyrfalcons, prairie falcons, and hybrids thereof)	Intravascular hemolysis	*Plasmodium* infection[8] (malaria)	Blood film examination, serum chemistry, direct stool examination	
Gastrointestinal Signs Flicking of food	Prehension impairment	1. Trichomoniasis 2. Sinew or tendon wrapped around tongue	1,2. Oral examination 1. Scraping of lesions	1. Bacterial cultures 2. Blood work

Unproductive head and neck movements for aboral food movement	Obstruction of esophagus	1. Trichomoniasis[9]
		2. Trapped food item (e.g., chicken neck, see Fig. 52–1)
		3. Inflammatory stricture of esophagus (e.g, grass awn penetration)
			1. Lesion scrape
			    2. Palpation
			  1,2. Radiograph
			1,2,3. Endoscopic examination
				1. Cultures
				2,3. Explorative surgery

Anorexia	1. Obstruction 2. Inflammation resulting from systemic disease	1. Candidiasis 2. Coccidia[17] 3. Aspergillosis	1. Pharyngeal cultures 2. Fecal examination	3. *Aspergillus* ELISA

Vomiting	1. Obstruction, inflammation, irritation occurring anywhere in GI tract
	2. Secondary to systemic problem
		1. Primary causes
		  a. Bacterial infection of ventriculus or proventriculus
		  b. Antibiotic or other drug intolerance
		  c. Candidiasis
		  d. Lead poisoning
		  e. Intussusception arising from parasitic infection[18]
		2. Secondary causes
		  a. Aspergillosis
		  b. Coccidiosis
		  c. Motion sickness (especially peregrine falcons)
			1abc. Pharyngeal and cloacal cultures—bacteria and yeast
			1d. Blood lead
			1e. Contrast radiography, exploratory surgery, fecal examination
				1d. Blood lead
				2. *Aspergillus* ELISA
				3. Endoscopic examination of GI tract

Crop stasis (sour crop)	1. Loss of motility in upper GI tract 2. Bacterial infection	1. Secondary to low condition[2] 2. Bacterial infection (nonspecific) contaminated food	1. Physical examination 2. Crop culture	
Stool Variations Emerald green stools	Unutilized bile in stool	Normal situation seen a few hours before a bird is fed when GI tract is otherwise empty		
Well formed with black fecal center surrounded by watery white urates	Normal stool			

Table continued on following page

PRINCIPAL MEDICAL PROBLEMS OF RAPTORS AND APPROPRIATE DIAGNOSTIC PROCEDURES *(Continued)*

Principal Signs	Possible Problems	Possible Causes	Primary Diagnostics	Secondary Diagnostics
Lime green stools	Alterations in motility and absorptive processes	1. Aspergillosis 2. Lead poisoning 3. Coccidia 4. Anaerobic GI infection 5. Nonspecific GI tract infection	1. ELISA *(Aspergillus)* 2. Blood lead 3. Fecal examination 4,5. Cloacal culture	1. Blood work 2. Radiographs
Jade green stools	Increased biliverdin production from hemolysis	1. *Plasmodium*—erythrocytic stages	1. Examine blood film	
Brown, sticky stools	High fat content in stool	1. Feeding day-old chicks with high yolk content 2. Pancreatic insufficiency	1. Normal stool on high fat diet 2. Fat and starch stains on stool	2. Treat food with pancreatic enzymes
Mucus in stool	Severe intestinal insult	1. Coccidia infection 2. Other problem of unknown etiology	1. Fecal examination	1,2. CBC, cultures
Stools with granular consistency, often yellowish-tinged	Cloacal uroliths	1. Dehydration 2. Renal and/or urinary tract infection 3. Secondary to prolonged recumbency 4. Loss of lower urinary and GI tract motility as with back injuries 5. Kidney failure, usually resulting from drug toxicity (e.g., aminoglycosides[20])	1. Physical examination PCV/ TP determination 2. Cloacal cultures	3,4. Neurologic examination[19] 5. Serum chemistry
Clotted blood in stools	Intestinal bleeding	1. Duodenal ulcers resulting from lead poisoning[21]	1. Blood lead 2. General examination	
Diarrhea	Inflammation	1. *Coccidia* 2. *Salmonella*	1. Fecal examination 2. Fecal culture	1,2. CBC

Musculoskeletal/Neurologic Problems Excluding Obvious Traumatic Injury

Principal Signs	Possible Problems	Possible Causes	Primary Diagnostics	Secondary Diagnostics
Acute unilateral lameness	Fracture	1. Midshaft fracture of tibiotarsus 2. Other leg bone fracture	1. Radiograph	
Slow-onset lameness	Arthritis	1. Femoral head necrosis from extended air sac infection—*Aspergillus* sp. typical	1. Radiograph	1. Trephine and tap marrow cavity for a culture

Musculoskeletal with Possible Neurologic Component

Principal Signs	Possible Problems	Possible Causes	Primary Diagnostics	Secondary Diagnostics
Reluctance or inability to fly	1. Fracture or avulsion 2. Arthritis 3. Soft tissue problem 4. Cardiac pathology	1a. Shoulder or elbow separation 1b. Coracoid fracture 2. Humeral head necrosis 3. Dorsal root avulsion or neuritis[22] 4. Conduction problems of unknown etiology, occasionally associated with lead[23]	1,2. Radiograph 3. EMG† 4. ECG	4. Palpation of muscle
Loss of proprioceptive and locomotor function in legs	1. Neurologic problem	1. Osteomyelitis of lower vertebral column (see Fig. 52–2)	1. Radiograph	1. Neurologic examination
Convulsions or seizures	Neural toxicity	Organophosphate or carbamate toxicity	Cholinesterase activity	
Star-gazing, torticollis	1. Neurologic dysfunction	1. Thiamine deficiency 2. Aberrant sarcocystoid infection[24]	1. Response to treatment 2. None	
Undercurling of rear toe	Soft tissue injury from equipment	1. Inflammation of extensor tendon 2. Tearing of flexor tendon	1,2. Examination	
Ulceration of dorsal halux	Severe damage to extensor talon	Accumulation of ice under jess anklet	Visual observation	

Information is exclusive of traumatic injuries.
*Based on more than 7000 raptors seen in the last 20 years by the author.
†Radiographically, denervation injuries often present as detectable areas of muscle atrophy.

SYMPTOMATIC TREATMENT OF UNDIAGNOSED INTESTINAL UPSETS

Vomiting and occasionally diarrhea not attributable to identifiable pathogens other than the ubiquitous *Escherichia coli* (a normal inhabitant of the gastrointestinal tract of carnivorous birds) may occur, especially in young birds. There is some evidence to suggest that various anaerobic bacteria may be involved. Despite limited knowledge about the cause, treatment is successfully accomplished by the administration of kaolin preparations (Pepto-Bismol, Procter & Gamble, Cincinnati, OH), along with metronidazole (orally) and piperacillin (Piperacil, Lederle, Carolina, Puerto Rico) (100 mg/kg qid, parenterally). Nutrition and hydration are maintained through application of the hyperalimentation protocol (Table 52–5). The course of treatment typically runs for 4 to 6 days.

BUMBLEFOOT

Aside from traumatic injuries resulting in fractures and soft tissue injuries, and the specific problems mentioned in this section, the remaining major problem of raptors that veterinarians may be called upon to treat is bumblefoot. Much has been written about causes and treatment, but it all condenses to a simple concept. That is, following trauma to the bottom of the foot from wear associated with poor perching surfaces, bruising from bating onto hard surfaces, or puncture with a sharp talon, the tissues become infected with a bacterial agent, usually *E. coli* or *Staphylococcus aureus*, and an inflammatory condition develops.[13] Treatment consists of establishing and maintaining drainage; protective bandaging; treatment with appropriate systemic antibiotics; and local treatment with a cocktail of dimethyl sulfoxide (DMSO), dexamethasone, and a suitable antibiotic, typically piperacillin.[5] With time, good management, and persistence, most cases can be successfully treated. Typical duration of treatment is 8 to 10 weeks.

CONCLUSION

Despite the carnivorous nature of raptors, they have medical conditions not dramatically different from those seen in other avian species. Analysis of presenting signs and problems leads to many of the same disease syndromes and treatment approaches seen elsewhere in avian medicine. However, the conditions, management, and metabolic state in which raptors kept for falconry purposes are found generate some unique circumstances (Table 52–6). The practitioner who aspires to treat such birds has to acquire a good knowledge base in both avian medicine and the sport and art of falconry.

This chapter is an attempt to provide some insight into the basic aspects of falconry and how they are related to problems and disease syndromes encountered in these birds. In that light, I would recommend reading first the referenced material about falconry, then commencing with a review of the specific medical literature about raptors.

References

1. Cooper JE: Infectious and parasitic diseases of raptors. In Fowler ME (ed): Zoo and Wildlife Medicine: Current Therapy. Philadelphia, WB Saunders, 1993.
2. Redig PT: Medical Management of Birds of Prey. St. Paul, MN. The Raptor Center at the University of Minnesota, 1993.
3. Beebe FL, Webster HA: North American Falconry and Hunting Hawks. P. O. Box 1484 Denver, CO, 1994.
4. Keymer IF: Diseases of birds of prey. Vet Rec (90)21:579, 1972.
5. Redig PT: Bumblefoot. In Fowler ME (ed): Current Therapy in Zoo and Wild Animal Medicine, ed 3. Philadelphia, WB Saunders, 1993.
6. Pokras MA, Karas AM, Kirkwood JK, Sedgwick CJ: An introduction to allometric scaling and its uses in raptor medicine. In Redig PT, Cooper JE, Remple JD, Hunter DB (eds): Raptor Biomedicine. Minneapolis, University of Minnesota Press, 1993.
7. Aguilar RF, Redig PT: Diagnosis and treatment of avian aspergillosis. In Banagura JD, Kirk RE (eds): Current Veterinary Therapy XII. Philadelphia, WB Saunders, 1995, pp 1294–1299.
8. Redig PT: Avian malaria: A review of 3 cases and the pertinent literature. Proc Assoc Avian Vet, Nashville, 1993, pp 173–180.
9. Remple JD: Avian malaria with comments on other haemosporidia in large falcons. In Cooper JE, Greenwood AG (eds): Recent Advances in the Study of Raptor Diseases. Keiglley, West Yorkshire, England, Chiron Publications, 1981.
10. Cranfield MR, Shaw M, Beall F, et al: A review and update of avian malaria in the African Penguin *(Speniscus demersus)*. Proc Am Assoc Zoo Vet, 1990, pp 243–248.
11. Pokras MA, Wheeldon EB, Sedgwick CJ: Trichomoniasis in owls: Report on a number of clinical cases and a survey of the literature. In Redig PT, Cooper JE, Remple JD, Hunter DB (eds): Raptor Biomedicine. Minneapolis, University of Minnesota Press, 1993.
12. Redig PT: Management of medical emergencies in raptors.

In Kirk RE: Current Veterinary Therapy XI. Philadelphia, WB Saunders, 1992.

13. Remple JD, Al-Ashbal AA: Raptor bumblefoot: Another look at histopathology and pathogenesis. In Redig PT, Cooper JE, Remple JD, Hunter DB (eds): Raptor Biomedicine. Minneapolis, University of Minnesota Press, 1993.

14. Bauck L: Mycoses. In Ritchie BW, Harrison GJ, Harrison LR (eds): Avian Medicine: Principles and Application. Lake Worth, FL, Wingers Publishing, 1994.

15. Redig PT, Post GS, Concannon TM: Development of an ELISA test for the diagnosis of aspergillosis in avian species. Proc Assoc Avian Vet, Miami, 1986, pp 165–178.

16. Redig PT: The diagnosis and treatment of lead poisoning in bald eagles and trumpeter swans. Proc First Int Conf Zool Avian Med, Oahu, 1987, pp 401–403.

17. Cawthorn RJ: Cyst-forming coccidia of raptors: Significant pathogens or not? In Redig PT, Cooper JE, Remple JD, Hunter DB (eds): Raptor Biomedicine. Minneapolis, University of Minnesota Press, 1993.

18. Cooney JC, Redig PT: Intussusception in a kestrel arising from intestinal fluke infestation. Manuscript in preparation.

19. Bennet RA: Neurology. In Ritchie BW, Harrison GJ, Harrison LR (eds): Avian Medicine: Principles and Application. Lake Worth, FL, Wingers Publishing, 1994.

20. Flammer K: Antimicrobial therapy. In Ritchie BW, Harrison GJ, Harrison LR (eds): Avian Medicine: Principles and Application. Lake Worth, FL, Wingers Publishing, 1994.

21. Degernes LA, Frank RK, Freeman ML, Redig PT: Lead poisoning in trumpeter swans. Proc Assoc Avian Vet, Seattle, 1989, pp 144–157.

22. Smith SA: Diagnosis of brachial plexus avulsion in three free-living owls. In Redig PT, Cooper JE, Remple JD, Hunter DB (eds): Raptor Biomedicine. Minneapolis, University of Minnesota Press, 1993.

23. Burtnik NL, Degernes LA: Electrocardiography on fifty-nine anesthetized convalescing raptors. In Redig PT, Cooper JE, Remple JD, Hunter DB (eds): Raptor Biomedicine. Minneapolis, University of Minnesota Press, 1993.

24. Aguilar RF, Shaw DP, Dubey JP, Redig PT: Sarcocystis-associated encephalitis in an immature northern goshawk. J Zoo Wildl Med 22(4):466–469, 1991.

Robert Stonebreaker

Ratites

The ratite classification includes the African ostrich (*Struthio camelus*), the South American rhea (*Rhea americana* and *Pterocnemia pennata*), the Australian emu (*Dromaius novae-hollandiae*), the Australian cassowary (*Casuaris* spp.), the New Guinea archipelago, the Central and South American tinamou (*Eudromia* spp.), and the New Zealand kiwi (*Apteryx* spp.). Ratites are flightless birds that have evolved from flighted ancestors. Their name is derived from the Latin word *ratis,* meaning raft, to which their flat sternum bears a resemblance.

Breeding of ratites has rapidly developed into a worldwide industry. It is being promoted as an alternative form of agriculture, with meat, leather, oil, and feathers as the main products. With the increase in the number of these birds, there is a growing demand for veterinary services related to their health care and husbandry. Client education in flock health management and disease prevention is the key role for veterinary practitioners who treat ratites.

STRESS

Stress is an extremely important consideration in ratite management. Any change to a ratite is a stressor. Chicks do no tolerate change well. Anything that upsets them can influence their overall metabolism and cause severe sequelae. Stress can cause inappropriate ingestion, diarrhea, aberrant neurotic behavior, and immune suppression.

Reduce stress by gradually introducing birds to a new area or situation and avoid complete social isolation. Calming ratites by confinement in dark-ness for ease of handling and examination is recommended. It is common practice to place a hood over the head of an ostrich to be handled. This makes the bird more amenable to handling; however, hoods do not work well with other ratite species.

NUTRITIONAL DISEASES

Nutritional diseases may be related to over- or underfeeding, or a deficiency or imbalance of individual vitamins, essential amino acids, or minerals. The specific dietary requirements of ratites are unknown, but guidelines have been extrapolated from that which is known for chickens and turkeys. Several commercial ratite feeds are available that apparently satisfy the nutritional needs of these birds. Marginal dietary deficiencies are likely to occur especially for growing chicks and for breeding stock, which are under considerable nutritional stress when in full production (Fig. 53–1).

Several dietary deficiencies have been identified in ratites. Vitamin A deficiency has been described in rhea chicks. Clinical signs are ocular discharge, oral abscesses on the palate, and stunted growth.[1]

Vitamin D_3 deficiency is most likely to occur when a high-fat diet is fed. Diets containing over 10% fat should be considered excessive. Vitamins A, D, and E are fat-soluble and can be bound by dietary fat to prevent absorption from the intestinal tract. Clinical signs of deficiency are rickets, which include enlarged joints and epiphyses, lameness, and pathologic fractures. Angular leg deformities may also be seen.

Vitamin E and selenium deficiencies have been

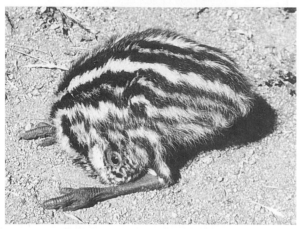

Figure 53–1

A condition in which the head tucks under the body between the legs may be observed in young emu chicks. When attempting to move, they may jump forward and tumble over or walk backward. Most cases recover spontaneously, although treatment with various vitamins and minerals has been used.

suspected of causing muscle degeneration. Dietary deficiency or excessive destruction of vitamin E results in muscle necrosis; increased destruction of erythrocytes; and degenerative lesions in the brain, blood vessels, skeletal muscle, heart, and gizzard muscle. Vitamin E deficiency is manifested as encephalomalacia in poultry chicks, exudative diatheses, muscular degeneration, decreased hatchability of eggs, early embryonic death, and testicular degeneration.

Important B vitamins in ratites are thiamine (B_1), riboflavin (B_2), biotin, and pantothenic acid. Thiamine deficiencies are thought to cause "stargazing." Riboflavin deficiencies may be a cause of curled toe deviation. Pantothenic acid and biotin deficiencies affect epithelial tissues causing curling of the feathers and hyperkeratosis of the skin around the beak, eyes, feet, and neck (Fig. 53–2).[2] Vitamin B_6 supplementation was used as therapy for a goose-stepping gait syndrome in young rheas.[1]

Calcium and phosphorus, together with vitamin D_3, are necessary for the mineralization of bones. It is essential that they be provided in the correct ratio in the diet. The calcium-to-phosphorus ratio should be approximately 2:1. Rickets is caused by a lack or imbalance of calcium and phosphorus, or a vitamin D_3 deficiency. Oversupplementation with calcium (i.e., with oyster shells) is common, resulting in phosphorus deficiency (see Vitamin D_3 Defi-

ciency). Clinical signs include limb deformities, especially rickets and bowed legs.

TOXIC DISEASES

Many toxicity problems can occur in ratites. Most toxins also affect other birds and mammals. Specific treatment is the same as in other species. General treatment of ingested toxins includes giving activated charcoal and intravenous fluids, sedation if the bird is convulsing, and general supportive care

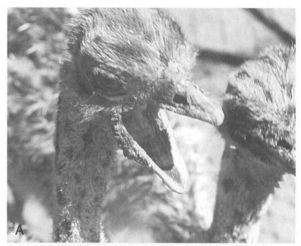

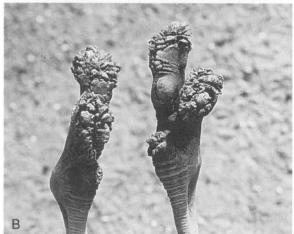

Figure 53–2

Hyperkeratosis of the skin in and around the face and feet is highly suggestive of pantothenic acid and biotin deficiencies in young ostriches. *(A)* Marked proliferation and hyperkeratosis of the eyelids and skin of the mucocutaneous junction at the commissures of the beak. *(B)* Severe hyperkeratosis and cracking of the plantar surfaces of the feet.

while the body metabolizes the toxin. Chelation therapy is indicated in a heavy metal toxicity.

Mycotoxins may be a problem on farms where feed is stored in bulk containers. Toxins such as aflatoxin, ochratoxin, T-2 toxin, and zearalenone may be produced.[2] These products cause kidney and liver damage, diarrhea, and immunosuppression. Each toxin tends to have its own clinical manifestation. Confirmation of mycotoxin toxicity can be quite difficult in ratites.

Nitrofurazone toxicity caused by incorrect administration of furazolidone in the drinking water is a major cause of intoxication. Furans are generally used as water-soluble treatments for coccidiosis and enteritis. Intoxication causes hyperexcitability, loss of neuromuscular control, and death.

Heavy metal toxicities usually originate from the propensity of ratites to peck and swallow foreign objects. They have a particular interest in bright, shiny objects, which is a general description of most metals. Lead toxicosis frequently causes neurologic signs. Toxicity may be manifested by incoordination, depression, and fasciculations. Although zinc, copper, and iron have been reported as toxic agents in ratites, they do not produce substantial neurologic signs.

Monensin toxicity caused by accidental overdosing of a feed additive may cause paralysis, poor hatchability in breeding birds, or death. Monensin is commonly used as a feed additive in ruminant and poultry diets.

Selenium toxicity is caused by overzealous administration of selenium to prevent or treat white muscle disease. Birds may die acutely from pulmonary edema.

Benzene hexachloride is highly toxic and may kill birds even when correctly mixed for ectoparasites. Death may occur up to 96 hours after spraying. Chlorinated hydrocarbon solutions should not be used on ratites.

Cantharidin toxicity is caused from the consumption of beetles containing high levels of cantharidin. Clinical signs include collapse, vomiting, and acute death. Mortality levels of 25% were reported in a group of emus that consumed three-striped beetles that were attracted to a barn light.[3]

PARASITE PROBLEMS

Numerous parasitic infections have been identified in ratite species. Several of these parasites can cause serious disease. The prevalence of parasites is relatively low and currently does not play a major role in ratite production in North America.

Intestinal protozoa associated with diarrhea in ratites include *Balantidium, Cryptosporidium, Giardia, Histomonas, Toxoplasma*, and *Trichomonas* species. The pathogenesis is unclear but warrants treatment when identified. Metronidazole (Flagyl, Searle) is an effective treatment for some of these protozoa at 1.25 g/l of drinking water for 7 to 10 days. Coccidiosis is occasionally diagnosed and is manifested by diarrhea and malaise in juvenile birds. Oocysts can be easily observed by fecal flotation techniques. An unnamed *Eimeria* species has been found in ostriches, emus, and rheas in North America. Trimethoprim sulfadiazine (Bactrim, Roche) given orally at a dose of 10 mg/kg twice a day (bid) for 5 to 7 days has been an effective treatment. *Leucocytozoa* and *Plasmodia* species have been identified as blood parasites in ostriches.

Libyostrongylus douglassi, also referred to as wire worm, is the most significant parasite of ostriches. This small nematode causes a verminous gastritis in young ostriches referred to as "vrotmaag" or rotten stomach. It is associated with high chick mortality. The adult parasites are found in the glandular crypts of the proventriculus where they suck blood and cause a severe inflammatory reaction and anemia. The clinical symptoms are those of gastric stasis, similar to those of impaction and megabacteriosis. Anemia can be detected as paleness of the buccal mucosa. Diagnosis is made by examination of fecal flotation specimens. This parasite produces large numbers of drought-resistant eggs. The recommended treatment is with fenbendazole (Panacur, Hoechst-Roussel) at a dosage of 15 mg/kg.[4] Ivermectin (Ivomec, Merck-Agvet) at 0.2 mg/kg is also considered effective. Levamisole hydrochloride (Levisole, Pittman Moore) given at 30 mg/kg has been used for a number of years against this parasite. However, treatment has resulted in the development of resistant strains.[5]

The tracheal worms *Syngamus trachea* and *Cyanthostoma bronchialis* have been associated with hemorrhagic tracheitis in emus.[6]

Filarid nematodes *Chandlerella quiscali* have been found to cause verminous encephalitis in emu chicks.[7] Grackles are the normal host for *C. quiscali*, which is transmitted by *Culicoides* gnats. In the emu, the larval stages of this parasite migrate destructively through the spinal cord and subdural regions. Clinical signs include ataxia, torticollis, abnormal gait, recumbency, and death. There is no known treatment for this parasite once it has entered the spinal cord. Ivermectin (Ivomec, Merck-Agvet), given at a dosage of 0.2 mg/kg administered every 4 weeks, may be effective in preventing larval migration to the central nervous system. The raccoon roundworm *Baylisascaris procyonis* has also been shown to cause neurologic signs in emus.[8] (See Neurologic Disorders.)

The ostrich tapeworm *Houttynia struthionis* inhabits the small intestine, causing unthriftiness and high mortality in young birds. The infestation is diagnosed by the presence of proglottids in the feces. The intermediate host of this parasite is still unknown. Both praziquantel (Droncit, Haver-Diamond) at 7.5 mg/kg and fenbendazole (Panacur, Hoechst-Roussel) at 15 mg/kg are effective in eliminating the infestation.

Arthropod parasites seldom cause serious disease in ratites. The ostrich louse, *Struthiolipeurus struthionis*, feeds on body scales and feather matter, causing considerable damage. The economic loss resulting from feather damage should make this parasite a cause for concern. Signs include excessive grooming and ruffled and frayed feathers. Infestations are easily diagnosed by observing the mites adherent to the barbs along the feather shafts. Control is achieved with appropriate application of pyrethrins or 5% carbaryl at 2-week intervals. Quill mites live in the ventral longitudinal shaft groove and bore into the feather shaft, where they feed on the gelatinous contents of the growing feather, deleteriously affecting its normal growth. They can cause a mange-like condition with severe pruritus. Control is achieved with ivermectin and synthetic pyrethroids.

Tick infestation is an ectoparasitic problem of great concern. The preferred site of attachment of ticks is under the chin. Infestation of chicks with *Hyalomma truncatum* can cause paralysis. Tick bite marks can produce blemishes on skins and cause their downgrading. Ticks are also potential carriers of human and livestock diseases. The United States Department of Agriculture imposed an immediate ban on the importation of ratites in 1989 because of the discovery of ticks on newly imported ostriches that carried *Cowdria ruminantium*, the rickettsial organism that caused heart-water disease in ruminants.[9, 10] Removal of ticks can be easily accomplished by thorough dusting of the animal with 5% carbaryl (Sevin, Southern Agriculture Insecticides).

Certain free-flying biting insects have been known to cause problems in ratites, particularly *Simulium* species (black flies) but also *Culicoides* species (gnats) and mosquitoes. They can cause a great deal of annoyance, causing birds to run and injure themselves, become unthrifty, and fail to eat or drink adequately. When they attack in large numbers they can cause a significant amount of blood loss in small chicks and actually may result in anemia and secondary death. Biting insects are also potential vectors of viral, bacterial, and parasitic infections. Ants (especially fire ants) have killed small chicks; even only one bite can kill chicks. This may be a result of an anaphylactic-type reaction or toxin. Clinical signs may be incoordination, weakness, frothing of the mouth, submandibular edema, or peracute death. Use of dexamethasone (Azium, Schering) at 2 mg/kg intramuscularly (IM) or intravenously (IV) has been a very effective treatment. Problems have also resulted from bee stings and the consumption of toxic beetles (see Toxic Diseases).

CONJUNCTIVITIS

Conjunctivitis may be precipitated by primary irritants such as dust, alfalfa, or flies. Several bacterial species are often secondary invaders that further complicate the conjunctivitis. Staphylococcal infections of the eyes are frequently seen. *Pseudomonas* species and other gram-negative bacteria cause inflammation of the eyes and respiratory tract in ratites. Serous to purulent frothy discharge of the eyes may be seen. These problems often appear bilaterally. Cytology and culture examinations are necessary for an accurate diagnosis. Treatment includes isolation of sick birds and use of topical ophthalmic antibiotics. Prevention includes good ventilation and reduced airborne debris.

Lacerations, abrasions, ulcerations, or foreign bodies may cause ocular discharge and blepharospasms. In these cases, the discharge is serous and often only unilateral. The diagnosis is made by a thorough ocular examination and fluorescein staining. Treatment is determined according to the findings.

Eye flukes, *Philophthalmus gralli*, were found in large numbers in the conjunctival sacs of young ostriches in Florida that suffered from severe conjunctivitis. Physical removal of the trematodes under anesthesia and additional carbamate treatment resulted in their elimination.[11] Flukes may also be removed from the eyes by rinsing the eyes with salt water.

NEUROLOGIC DISORDERS

Nervous system diseases can be caused by bacteria, viruses, fungi, or parasites. Encephalitis may occur as an extension of a rhinitis and sinusitis or septicemia. Various bacteria have been cultured from these cases. Noninfectious causes of nervous system diseases include storage disease, overheating, hypoglycemia, trauma, or toxins.

Viscerotrophic velogenic Newcastle disease (VVND) virus affects the central nervous system in certain species. An outbreak in ostriches resulted in up to 80% mortality. VVND virus has been eradicated from the US. Vaccination for Newcastle disease using a modified live vaccine is common in other countries where the disease is endemic.

Eastern equine encephalitis (EEE) and Western equine encephalitis (WEE) viruses have been identified as viral pathogens of emus. EEE virus has been isolated from several disease outbreaks in emus in the southwestern and Gulf Coast regions of the US. Severe enteric and neurologic signs are most commonly seen. High WEE virus titers have been found in emus that have died after an acute illness. Some affected birds may recover with supportive care. Vaccination of emus against both of these viruses is recommended in endemic regions. An inactivated equine vaccine has shown good efficacy in preventing the disease in emus. Two or three vaccinations are administered to emus 3 months of age and older at 30-day intervals. Subsequent booster injections are recommended at 6-month intervals. Written client consent and insurance carrier clearance are necessary before vaccination that is an unapproved (off-label) use of the vaccine.[12]

Verminous encephalitis has been reported in emus and an ostrich as a result of migration of the larvae of *Baylisascaris* species and *Chandlerella quiscali*.[20] (See Parasite Problems.) Ratities serve as aberrant hosts of these nematodes. Clinical signs of ataxia and incoordination, characterized by a wobbly gait, splayed legs, and frequent falling over are common. Some birds may lose balance and walk backwards. No effective treatment is currently available for birds already showing neurologic signs. The use of ivermectin administered at 4-week intervals to reduce non-neural tissue migration by this parasite is recommended.

Lysosomal storage disease is a neuronal storage disease occurring in young growing emus 5 to 11 months of age. Clinical signs are ataxia, anorexia, wasting, recumbency, tremors, and terminal convulsions. Histologically, nerve cell bodies in the brain and spinal cord are enlarged with foamy cytoplasm and Purkinje cells are decreased in the nuclei. This condition is generally hereditary and progressive.

Young chicks left in pens in the sun without shade may be found ataxic, seizuring, or prostrate. Other chicks in the flock may be panting and have their wings extended. Circumstantial evidence indicates the cause to be heat stroke. Too much heat is a constant concern in the summer months. Birds easily overheat, with fatal results. Treatment consists of cold water baths and treatment for shock. Chicks may also show signs similar to heat stroke because of water intoxication (drinking too much water).

Hypoglycemia can be seen in anorectic chicks. Some chicks will not eat. Birds may lose their appetite from other disease processes, impactions, stress, or trauma. Obvious clinical signs are weight loss, weakness, and empty intestines upon abdominal palpation. Treatment includes dextrose IV, orally, intraosseously (io), or subcutaneously (SC) and tube feeding with a high carbohydrate gruel at 20 ml/kg body weight two to four times daily. The chick may need to be trained to eat. Newly hatched chicks may need to be kept with slightly older chicks who are already feeding.

Trauma is generally self-induced but can be inflicted by predators. Injuries to the brain or spinal cord can lead to ataxia or seizures. Cases are cared for in a similar manner to that for most other animals with neurologic involvement. The bird should be kept quiet and prevented from thrashing about. The use of anti-inflammatory medications may be indicated.

There are many sources of toxins that can cause CNS symptoms including toxic plants, insecticides, endotoxins produced by bacteria, insect bites, and the overconsumption of water with electrolytes resulting in sodium toxicity.

AORTIC RUPTURE

Aortic rupture occurs in both growing and adult birds. The wall generally ruptures at the aortic arch. The cause is unknown but is related to a degeneration of the arterial wall, which is then weakened. The condition appears to be more common in overweight birds. In pigs and turkeys, copper deficiency is one predisposing cause to a similar condition; however, in affected emus and ostriches, liver copper levels have been normal. The bird is usually found dead and the mucous membranes are extremely pale. Upon postmortem examination, free blood is present throughout the abdomen. Tears in the artery can usually be identified. Prevention is to provide adequate exercise and limit overfeeding.

FRACTURES

Fractures and dislocations of the legs and wings are common in ratites. Fractures usually occur in the long bones. Long bone fractures involving the legs are nearly always associated with extensive soft tissue damage. Fractures of the legs usually respond poorly to splinting, casting, or surgical fixation because of the tremendous force exerted on the legs (similar to that in horses). Bone plating may be attempted, but the stress on the bone and its poor texture for holding fixation materials make recovery difficult.[13] Therefore, ostriches with leg fractures usually have to be euthanized. In smaller birds, fixation is easier but their very rapid growth requires splints and casts to be changed frequently. Birds may be suspended in a sling until the leg is healed; however, only the emu tolerates slings well. Tibiotarsal fractures are best repaired with a Kirschner apparatus. Tarsometatarsal fractures are usually compounded, and the bird hobbles around with the stump exposed and contacting the ground. There is no treatment for this other than euthanasia. Fractures of the lower extremities can be managed with acrylic or fiberglass casts.

Fractured wings may be easily stabilized by splinting or taping the wing to the body in a natural position for 4 to 6 weeks. Wing fractures are usually of little importance in emus because of the relatively small size of the wing. Fractures and dislocations of the wing can be resolved by surgical removal of the wing, or, in the case of fractures, by surgical plating, pinning, or Kirschner fixation of the broken bone.

Fractures of either the upper or lower beak can be quite serious, making eating and drinking difficult.[14] Good results have been accomplished with a combination of Kirschner wires and dental acrylic fixation.

EGG BINDING

Ratite hens may become egg-bound, which is thought to be caused by genetic factors, poor nutrition, cold weather, or lack of exercise.[15] Other possible factors related to egg binding include first-time layers, eggs too large, oviduct infections, and presence of soft-shelled eggs. The history may consist of nesting activity and previous egg-laying. Clinical signs may include cessation or failure to lay eggs, lethargy, anorexia, straining, passing pieces of broken eggshell, or vaginal prolapse. Some hens may exhibit no clinical signs. The diagnosis may be made by palpating the retained egg in the caudal abdomen; otherwise, radiology or ultrasound examinations may be required. Egg binding may be treated medically or surgically. The medical management involves placing the hen in a warm environment with the administration of multivitamins, calcium, and oxytocin. Intravenous fluids with glucose may be needed if the hen is weak. A gentle warm enema or lubrication of the bird's cloaca with K-Y jelly or mineral oil may also be effective. If none of these work, surgical intervention is necessary. Ovocentesis therapy is not recommended with egg-bound ratites. The procedure is much more difficult in these species, and the risk of tearing the oviduct and producing peritonitis is a major concern.

PROLAPSED OVIDUCT/CLOACA

Oviduct prolapses usually occur as a result of underlying metritis or egg retention. Excessive contraction of the abdominal muscles, exacerbated by poor physical condition and malnutrition, may cause these prolapses. Various portions of the oviduct and uterus protrude through the cloaca, often together with a partial prolapse of the vagina and cloaca. Oviduct prolapses have been associated with deformed and soft-shelled eggs. Timely, aggressive therapy is necessary to prevent devitalization of uterine tissues and secondary infections. All exposed tissue should be thoroughly cleaned with a sterile saline solution and kept moist. Topical antibiotics containing dimethyl sulfoxide (DMSO) can be used to reduce swelling so that prolapsed tissues can be replaced. Repeated replacement of tissues may be required, because prolapses often recur. Stay-sutures placed in the cloaca or percutaneous retention sutures generally prevent further prolapsing while uterine tissues regress in size, abdominal tissues regain structural integrity, and the hen has a chance to regain normal muscle tone and strength.[16] The prognosis for birds with oviduct prolapse is good as long as the condition is treated immediately.

PROLAPSE OF THE PHALLUS

Adult male ostriches may develop partial or complete prolapses of the phallus. The exact etiology is unknown, but prolapse occurs frequently as a result of trauma, infection, or extreme weather fluctuations.[15] Infections may occur after mucosal irritation from excessive mating, vent sexing, or by fecal contamination. The phallus may become enlarged and ulcerated. Frostbite or necrotizing dermatitis may occur as a result of prolapse. In severe cases of phallic prolapse, the rooster may be depressed, anorexic, and uninterested in copulation. Permanent infertility may occur as a sequela. Exposed tissue should be thoroughly washed and cleaned with a sterile saline and betadine solution. Traumatized tissue is debrided carefully and an antibiotic cream is applied. Topical DMSO may help reduce swelling and inflammation, making replacement of the phallus easier and more permanent. Daily therapy and cloacal purse-string suture may be necessary to prevent recurring prolapses. Systemic antibiotics should be administered to prevent ascending urogenital infections. Nonsteroidal anti-inflammatory agents are also indicated. If large areas of necrosis are present, surgery is necessary to debride the wound.

SALPINGITIS AND METRITIS

Oviduct infections are common in ratites. Salpingitis may occur from air sacculitis, pneumonia, liver disease, migrating foreign body, or retrograde infections of the lower reproductive tract. Salpingitis has been associated with impactions of the oviduct and egg-related peritonitis. Excessive abdominal fat has been associated with many cases of salpingitis in domestic fowl.[17] Metritis is a localized problem within the uterine portion of the oviduct. It can be a sequela to dystocia, egg binding, or chronic oviduct impaction. Bacterial metritis is often the result of systemic infections.[18] Metritis may affect shell formation or uterine contractility or may cause embryonic death or neonatal infections (weak chicks). Metritis can also cause egg binding, uterine rupture, peritonitis, and septicemia. Common isolates on culture are *Escherichia coli*, *Acinetobacter*, *Corynebacterium*, *Klebsiella*, *Pseudomonas*, and *Salmonella* species and other gram-negative bacteria. *Mycoplasma* species, paramyxovirus, and papillomavirus have been isolated from the reproductive tracts of ratites, but their clinical significance has not been determined.

Depression, anorexia, weight loss, and abdominal enlargement may occur with salpingitis. A foul-smelling discharge from the cloaca may also occur. An affected ratite hen may have a history of erratic production, malformed or odoriferous eggs, or a sudden drop in production. Abnormally shelled eggs such as eggs with rough-textured surfaces, ridges, a lack of mucin coat, or soft shells may be an indication of metritis. Cessation of breeding may be the only clinical sign occurring with metritis. Affected hens often have elevated white blood cell counts with pronounced heterophilia in acute cases to lymphocytosis in chronic cases. Serum chemistry test results are generally unremarkable. Radiographs often reveal indistinct abdominal detail. Ultrasonography is most useful in determining the degree of exudate in the oviduct. Abdominocentesis is indicated to assess the nature of the abdominal fluid.

Metritis and salpingitis are treated aggressively with parenteral antibiotics, supportive care, and therapy for shock. Antibiotic therapy should be based on culture and sensitivity test results for the organism. The oviduct may be flushed with sterile saline (with or without antibiotics) in cases of exudate in the oviduct. This may be accomplished by placing a catheter in the uterus and performing a retrograde lavage. In nonresponsive cases, a laparotomy may be necessary to remove necrotic tissue, inflammatory exudate, or egg material.

EGG YOLK PERITONITIS

Egg yolk peritonitis occurs most frequently in hens that are overweight (too fat). It may have multiple etiologies and may be part of several syndromes, including ectopic ovulation, ruptured oviducts, and salpingitis. It is unclear which component of the egg is most important in inducing peritonitis, but it is most likely to be the yolk that has become secondarily contaminated with bacteria.

Clinical signs include sudden death, abdominal swelling, depression, anorexia, ruffled feathers, and cessation of egg production. The hemogram may show a severe inflammatory response. Radiology, ultrasonography, abdominocentesis, and laparotomy are helpful diagnostic aids. Septic peritonitis leading to severe debilitation, sepsis, and death can occur if the yolk is contaminated with bacteria. Peritonitis may lead to secondary infection of other abdominal organs; and in advanced cases, extensive adhesions may form in the abdomen. Treatment consists of antibiotics, anti-inflammatory agents, and supportive care. Long-term antibiotic therapy is necessary, and dietary correction is advised. In most cases, surgery is required to remove egg material and perform abdominal irrigation. An early diagnosis is essential.

NEONATAL AND PEDIATRIC PROBLEMS

Edematous Chicks

Chicks that do not lose enough moisture during incubation often are edematous upon hatching. This condition can occur in eggs that are too large and do not allow adequate water loss and in eggs with poor eggshell quality, such as low pore density or excessively thick shells. It may also be associated with high incubation humidity.[3]

The chicks have generalized edema especially noticeable in the feet and legs, abdomen, and head. These chicks are weak and may need assistance in hatching. They may not be able to stand or walk for several days after hatching. Spraddle legs is common in edematous chicks. Because of edema, the chick is often unable to adduct the legs. Application of a hobble with rubberbands between the legs helps the chicks stand.

Most chicks lose the edema within several days after hatch. Diuretics have been used to treat this condition, but they are unnecessary. The best guide for prevention is to adjust the incubation relative humidity to achieve a 12 to 15% egg weight loss.

Yolk Sac Retention and Infection

One of the most common problems encountered in chicks younger than 3 weeks of age is retention of the yolk sac, with or without infection. The yolk sac should be totally utilized by 2 weeks of age, but in certain instances yolk digestion and absorption slows or ceases. A retained yolk sac is one that has not been properly absorbed by the chick and is larger than it should be for the chick's age. A retained yolk sac may or may not be infected; however, *E. coli, Campylobacter jejuni, Klebsiella pneumoniae, Pseudomonas aeruginosa, Clostridium, Proteus,* and *Salmonella* species, and various other bacteria have been isolated from infected yolk sacs.

Causes of yolk sac retention are numerous and poorly understood. It is generally associated with stress, improper incubation parameters, insufficient exercise, environmental temperature extremes, too much handling, systemic diseases, or excessive vitamins. Infections of the yolk sac are caused by improper storage and handling of eggs, washing of eggs, infections or malnutrition of the hen, contamination during assisted hatches, and systemic infectious disease processes (septicemia and viremia such as from coronavirus and adenoviruses).

Clinical signs of chicks with yolk sac retention or infection include continued weight loss beyond the normal weight loss seen the first 4 to 5 days after hatch, weakness, depression, lethargy, dyspnea, inappetence, failure to grow, isolation from the other chicks, erratic pecking behavior, and abdominal distension. There may be no clinical signs in some chicks before death.

Diagnostic tests include abdominal palpation, radiography, and ultrasonography. A doughy abdominal mass can usually be palpated. Radiographs and ultrasound recordings reveal an enlarged mass displacing the abdominal viscera cranially.

Treatment for yolk sac retention or infection is surgical removal of the yolk sac. Replacement fluid therapy along with high energy nutrition and appropriate antibiotic therapy are recommended. Retained or infected yolk sacs may represent 15 to 40% of a chick's total body weight. Broad-spectrum antibiotic therapy is indicated, pending culture and sensitivity results with trimethoprim-sulfa at 10 to 20 mg/kg bid or Amikacin, 5 mg/kg bid. The prognosis is poor with a high mortality rate because of the deteriorated and often moribund condition of the chicks at presentation.

Prevention is accomplished by identifying the cause and eliminating the source of infection. To help prevent infections, an antibiotic ointment is applied to the umbilicus immediately upon hatching. If infectious agents cannot be cultured from the yolk sac, improper incubation is suspected.

Umbilicus Problems

Failure of the umbilicus to close properly results in protrusion of the yolk sac from the abdomen. Causes of this condition include too-high incubation temperature, poor gas exchange, egg infections, and too-early assisted hatch. The yolk sac may protrude from the umbilicus. Treatment in mild cases is to carefully replace the externalized yolk into the abdomen, then cover the umbilicus with an antibiotic ointment and gauze and wrap the abdomen. In cases with a large quantity of the yolk sac protruding or the umbilicus already sealed, surgical removal of the yolk sac is recommended. In all cases, systemic antibiotic therapy should be initiated as soon as possible. The prognosis is guarded. Prevention is the critical key for this condition. Careful evaluation of the incubation and hatching parameters best determines the cause.

Diarrhea

Diarrhea is the most frequently observed clinical symptom in ostrich chicks between 2 weeks and 4 months of age. Emus have consistently loose droppings, which may be difficult to discern from diarrhea. Diarrhea often presents as a flock problem because symptomatic chicks are not isolated. Chicks are notoriously coprophagic, and therefore transmission is rapid.

Diarrhea can be caused by bacteria, viruses, parasites, diet, or environmental stressors. A wide range of enteric bacterial organisms has been tied to outbreaks of diarrhea. *Clostridium perfringens* is commonly isolated and has caused large outbreaks of necrotic enteritis. *Clostridia* are toxin-producing bacteria and therefore cause lesions with multiple characteristics. This makes the diagnosis of clostridial infections difficult. In addition, *Clostridia* are anaerobic bacteria and consequently are difficult to culture. Salmonellosis is probably the enteric infection of greatest concern in ratites. *Salmonella* has been associated with high mortality in chicks because of diarrhea and dehydration. *Salmonella* species can be harbored by carrier birds for long periods of time. Carriers shed the bacteria sporadically but particularly when stressed. Outbreaks of salmonellosis in artificially incubated chicks have been traced back to infected hens, particularly in rheas. A necrotizing typhlitis associated with spirochetes has been reported in young rhea flocks. These birds also have been infected with a *Trichomonas*-like species. *E. coli* can be a pathogen but it is also overrepresented as the cause of disease in ratite chicks. Viruses associated with diarrhea are adenovirus and coronavirus.

Stress is important in initiating diarrhea. Chicks that are maintained in a hot or humid environment, especially if they are kept indoors with inadequate ventilation and lack of exercise, develop with diarrhea. Improper use of antibiotics or sudden dietary changes also cause diarrhea.

Providing warmth and rehydration of affected chicks is critical. Appropriate antibiotic selection should be dictated by culture and sensitivity test results of the pathogenic bacteria. Transfaunation by the use of feces from a healthy bird has been practiced but is not recommended. The use of commercially prepared digestive bacteria such as Bene-Bac (Pittman Moore) or Fast Track is a safe method of transfaunation in ratites and may help re-establish the normal digestive flora or reduce the overgrowth of pathogens.

Impactions

Impactions are probably one of the most common problems seen in ratites, especially the ostrich. Impactions may occur at any age, but are most common during the first 6 months. Proventricular impactions are most common but impaction of the ventriculus can also occur. Impactions may be acute or chronic, partial or complete, and primary or secondary. Impactions are considered management-related problems. Chicks do not adapt well to being moved and handled. The stress associated with a change in environment, substrate, or diet places the chicks at high risk for impactions. Consumption of large quantities of inappropriate substances can cause mechanical obstruction. Impactions can also result from other diseases that create paralytic ileus in the gastrointestinal tract.

The clinical presentation varies depending upon whether the impaction is partial or complete. Ratites with partial impactions may show poor appetite, chronic weight loss, and firm or pelletized feces. Chicks affected by partial impactions become lethargic and stunted. Affected birds may not rise or may be reluctant to move because of weakness or pain. Cloacal prolapse may occur from straining. Ratites with complete impactions show rapid weight loss and dehydration. They may pass only urates or scant amounts of dry pelletized feces and death may ensue very quickly.

Impactions of the proventriculus can frequently be palpated on the left side of the abdomen. Impactions with rocks or sand can be easily detected, whereas impactions caused by grass, hay, or leaves may be difficult to palpate (Fig. 53–3). Radiography, ultrasound, and gastroscopy are effective for diagnosis.

Early or mild cases of impactions may be managed with psyllium fiber laxatives and supportive therapy. When an impaction does occur, surgical repair is typically the only successful treatment. Proventriculotomy may be the only means to relieve impactions, but the debilitated condition of many of these birds precludes surgical intervention. Medical therapy for 1 to 2 days usually provides for a better anesthesia and surgical risk. The procedure for proventiculotomy is well described.[19, 20] It is important that an impaction problem be diagnosed and surgically corrected early to ensure a good prognosis. Chronic and severe distension of the proventriculus may cause a permanent loss of muscle tone that is irreparable. A common secondary manifestation to impaction is an intussusception. Postoperatively, broad-spectrum antibiotics should

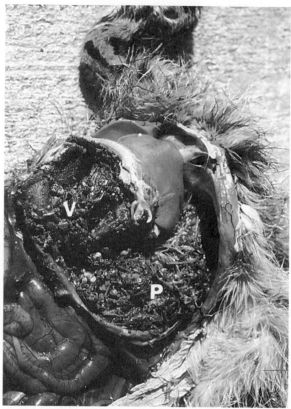

Figure 53–3

Impaction of the proventriculus (P) and ventriculus (V) with grass and alfalfa stems in an ostrich chick. The proventriculus is a large, thin-walled, distensible structure that is easily accessible surgically because it extends caudal to the ventriculus.

be administered for 5 to 7 days. Nonsteroidal anti-inflammatory drugs appear to improve the patient's well-being. For debilitated birds, nutritional and fluid therapy can be administered through esophagostomy tubes.

Cloacal Prolapse

Cloacal prolapses are common in chicks. It is important to determine the exact nature of the everted tissue as well as the underlying cause before taking the appropriate course of action. Cloacal prolapses are generally the result of other problems, such as proventricular or intestinal impactions, large bowel torsions, excessive straining associated with diarrhea, distended abdomens associated with excessive water drinking during hot weather, enteritis from infection, inappropriate diet, sand irritation, and rough cloacal sexing.

Mild cases may be treated by simply replacing the cloaca through the vent. Most cases require retention sutures for 3 to 5 days in conjunction with necessary nutritional management changes. More severe cases necessitate an exploratory laparotomy to identify and correct impactions, foreign bodies, or intestinal torsions. Amputation of the prolapse, as in mammals, is generally contraindicated because of the potential for obstruction of the urinary and reproductive systems. If the prolapsed tissue has become extensively necrotic, surgical debridement may be required.

Gastric Foreign Bodies

Ingestion of foreign bodies is a common malady in ratites. Anyone working around ratites must be aware that any object dropped into the bird's pen may be consumed. Ratites are especially attracted to bright, shiny objects. Common objects are bottle caps, glasses, gloves, keys, locks, nails, rocks, sand, sticks, tools, and almost anything the bird can get its beak on (Fig. 53–4).

Metal objects dissolve fairly rapidly within the proventriculus because of its low pH. Nails and other sharp objects frequently remain within the proventriculus without perforating the wall. If these objects work into the ventriculus, they can be impelled into the muscular wall by the organ's grinding and constricting action. If there is perforation or leakage into the peritoneal cavity, it can cause acute peritonitis and rapid death. Impactions can occur as a result of a foreign body. This occurs when food or grass material is wrapped around the foreign body. A foreign body can cause a bleeding ulcer by the constant grinding upon the stomach wall.

The clinical signs can include lethargy, inappetence, weight loss, reluctance to rise or move, isolation from the flock, or possibly impaction. Birds known to have swallowed objects have been watched closely without incidence.

The diagnosis is made through the history, clinical signs, palpation, complete blood count, radiographs, ultrasound, or abdominal paracentesis. In most cases, swallowed objects need to be removed. Surgical treatment through a proventriculotomy is indicated. Certain objects can evidently be dissolved or ground down to a small enough size to be passed out without surgical removal. Serial radiographs can be instrumental in recording the number of objects to be removed or passed.

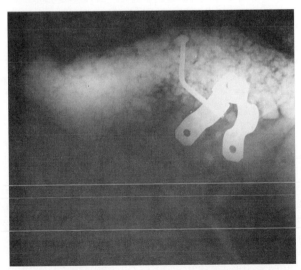

F i g u r e 5 3 – 4
Abdominal radiograph of a 3-month-old ostrich chick reveals multiple metallic foreign bodies in the proventriculus. The large amount of stones and grit material also present in the proventriculus is a normal finding in ratites.

Rhinitis and Sinusitis

Upper respiratory tract infections are observed most commonly when chicks are confined in poorly ventilated areas. These infections are usually caused by bacteria, but may also be caused by fungi (*Aspergillus* species), *Mycoplasma*, or viruses. These organisms are highly transmissible and flock spread is rapid. Gram-negative bacteria such as *E. coli, Pasteurella multocida, Pseudomonas, Klebsiella, Bordetella,* and *Haemophilus* species are common isolates. *Chlamydia psittaci* has been isolated from ostrich chicks. Newcastle disease has also been reported to cause rhinitis.

Clinical signs include ocular or nasal discharge, dyspnea, open-mouthed breathing, sneezing, head-shaking, stretching of the neck, excessive yawning, and periophthalmic or sinus swellings. Affected birds should be isolated immediately.

The diagnosis is made through the history, physical examination, evaluation of environmental conditions, and various laboratory tests. The database for respiratory problems includes results of cytology, culture and sensitivity, complete blood count, radiographs, and, when indicated, rhinoscopy tests. Special diagnostic testing for *Chlamydia* should be considered. A sinus aspirate is important in determining the cause of sinusitis.

Treatment is based on etiology. In refractory cases, it may be necessary to surgically drain and flush the sinuses. Prevention includes good ventilation, minimizing airborne debris, and appropriate use of antibiotics.

Pneumonia and Air Sacculitis

Pneumonia and air sacculitis are associated with poor ventilation, stress, and exposure to cold, wet environments. They are most commonly caused by bacteria or *Aspergillus* species.

Clinical signs include labored respiration, coughing, exercise intolerance, change in vocalization, proventricular impaction, and weight loss. A complete blood count generally reveals a persistent leukocytosis with a heterophilia. Laparoscopy or tracheoscopy may be helpful in the diagnosis. Serologic tests for *Aspergillus* may be useful. Treatment is based on cytology or culture and sensitivity test results from a transtracheal lavage. Aspergillosis has been associated with acute death and high mortality in ratite chicks. Antifungal drugs are of variable effectiveness. The most effective has been itraconazole (Sporanox, Janssen) at 10 mg/kg every 12 hours orally for several months.

Prevention is the key to these infections, including providing good ventilation, eliminating organic debris and contamination, minimizing stress, and avoiding cold, wet climates and prolonged or inappropriate antibiotic use that predisposes the bird to secondary bacterial or fungal infections.

Spraddle Leg

Newly hatched ratite chicks are prone to the development of deviations of the legs. Spraddle leg is thought to be caused by an abnormality of the coxofemoral joint. This prevents the legs from being adducted. Birds with this condition have one or

both legs directed laterally, resulting in the inability to stand. This condition is generally found in edematous chicks. Suggested etiologies include nutritional deficiencies, trauma, poor footing, improper incubation conditions, and genetic defects. Hobbling the legs together with elastic tape until they are able to stand on their own is usually an effective treatment. As an alternative, the chick is placed in a restrictive container that forces the legs together. The problem can be prevented by ensuring proper incubation conditions.

Rolled Toes

Rolled toes is a common condition in young chicks, especially edematous chicks. It is usually seen before the second week of age. The main (medial) toe is rotated off the center line, causing the toenail to point laterally or medially. The chick may walk on the side of the toe and not on the foot pad.

The cause is unlikely to be related to riboflavin deficiency, which produces curly toe paralysis in poultry. In ratites, rolled toes may be caused by improper substrates during brooding, improper incubation conditions, genetics, and dietary deficiencies of the hen. In most cases, incubation conditions appear to have the most influence. In chicks housed on concrete floors, the nails touching the floors may encourage rolled toes. Trimming the nails may reduce the incidence of this condition.

Toe deformities may be easily corrected with a variety of splints on young chicks if done early. The author prefers dental acrylic casts. Surgical correction may be required on older chicks with severe deviations.

Slipped Tendons

Slipped tendons occur in all ratite species, and are more common in chicks than adults. This condition results when the gastrocnemius tendon slips out of its groove on the distal tibiotarsus. The retinacula sheath that holds the tendon in place generally tears on the medial aspect, causing lateral tendon slippage. This is clinically very much like perosis in poultry. It has therefore been suggested that manganese deficiency may be a predisposing factor. The tendon generally slips to the lateral side of the hock, causing the leg to angle sharply medially at the hock while the foot and toe point laterally.

This condition is usually associated with trauma or angular limb deformities. The leg undergoes rapid pathologic changes once it begins to deviate. Bandaging or splinting the leg is usually unsuccessful. This support can often prevent total joint luxation. Surgical correction is generally required. Trochlear grooving or transplantation of the tendon medially has been attempted. Open reduction and stabilization of the luxated tendon are successful in some cases. Tendon contracture is often a limiting factor. When a bird is presented with slipped tendons and opened wounds over the hocks, the prognosis is guarded because generally the cruciate and the lateral collateral ligaments have ruptured. If multiple cases occur in a flock, management practices and feed quality should be evaluated.

Leg Deformities

Ratite chicks are prone to the development of deformities of the legs. The percentage of chicks affected may range from 5 to 30%. The etiology seems to be multifactorial, but there is a certain nutritional orientation. Deficiencies of vitamin E and selenium and manganese have been suggested, and total food intake has also been implicated. High protein levels in starter feeds have also been reported to cause leg deformities. Understanding the growth rates of these long-legged birds may be the first step toward solving leg deformities. Results of feeding studies with rheas suggest that if the growth rate is reduced, leg problems are less likely to result.[21]

Incubation in excessive humidity may lead to edematous chicks with leg bones that develop out of alignment. Trauma of a growth plate or epiphyseal injury can readily cause one side of the bone to grow too fast or too slow, creating rotational deformities. The incidence of leg deformities is increased with a lack of sufficient exercise. Observations also suggest a genetic predisposition.

Bowed legs is a condition wherein the toes or feet still point forward but the legs bow inward (varus) or outward (valgus). It is generally seen as an outward bowing and appears to be caused by chicks that are too heavy for the soft growing bones that support their weight. The growth areas of the bones often appear thickened. It is observed in chicks that receive excessive vitamin and protein supplements. Weight restriction can be helpful, but there is little therapy if the condition is severe. If oversupplementation is the problem and is withdrawn soon enough, the bowing may cease and the legs tend to realign with growth and aging.

Rotated legs are a condition wherein one or both legs rotate laterally at the distal tibiotarsus, causing the toes to point laterally. Onset may be sudden with rotation exceeding 90° of normal (Fig. 53–5). The rotation is usually obvious, and affected chicks are lame and linger in the back of the flock. They generally lose condition and eventually become recumbent. Leg rotations are progressive, and affected chicks ultimately have to be destroyed. Several procedures have been tried to treat tibiotarsal rotations. These include derotational osteotomies; periosteal stripping; and various splinting, casting, hobbling, and slinging techniques. A high recurrence of rotation follows surgery. The splints, casts, hobbles, and slings are generally too stressful and confining for chicks.

Rotational and angular leg deformities are the result of improper management. Most important is providing sufficient exercise from an early age. Avoid overfeeding and rapid weight gains. The protein content of chick diets should not exceed 18 to

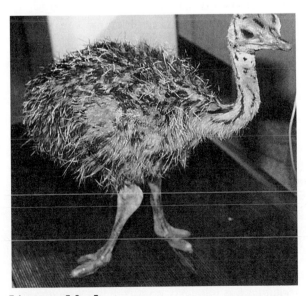

Figure 53–5

Rotational limb deformities are a common problem in all ratite chicks. A leg may rotate laterally, exceeding 90° of normal. The prognosis is poor, and these birds should be condemned.

20%. Restrict vitamin supplementation. Adjust dietary levels of calcium, phosphorus, and vitamin D_3 as necessary. Correct possible incubation problems to reduce the occurrence of weak or edematous hatchlings. The provision of a nonslippery surface is an additional factor in the prevention of these deformities.

Degenerative Myopathy

Degenerative myopathy appears to be primarily a disease of young ratites. A deficiency of vitamin E and possibly selenium is the most probable cause; however, histologically lesions could not be distinguished from capture myopathy, or from furazolidone, ionophore, or *Cassia* species toxicity.[22] The possibility of intoxication must be considered in all cases of degenerative myopathy, but the clinical history should rule it out. Some authors believe that capture myopathy may be an acute manifestation of a subclinical deficiency of vitamin E or selenium.[23] Clinical signs often involve depression, reluctance to rise or move, paresis, and rapid progression to death. Myopathy may variably affect skeletal, cardiac, or gizzard muscle. Gross lesions are often lacking or too subtle to detect unless the degenerating muscle is calcified. There may be paleness and possibly white streaks in the muscles. Histologic examination is necessary to confirm the diagnosis. Clinical pathology findings include elevations of aspartate transaminase (AST) greater than 1200 u/l, and creatinine phosphokinase (CPK) greater than 40,000 u/l.

Serum or plasma levels of vitamin E in ratites could be a useful diagnostic tool for the monitoring of the nutritional status, but normal values have not yet been established in all species. Additional research on serum and organ levels of vitamin E and selenium in ratites and its correlation with degenerative myopathy, diet, and health is necessary.[24] Once these levels are determined, the diagnosis of impending degenerative myopathy may be achieved, and prompt effective treatment administered.

Vitamin E is relatively nontoxic, but selenium can be toxic at relatively low levels. Therefore, dietary supplementation with vitamin E appears to be a safer and more cautious method of treatment and

prevention. Treatment with 300 IU of vitamin E orally followed by immediate correction of the diet is recommended for affected birds.[25] Another treatment regimen is with injectable vitamin E (Rocavit E, Roche) at a dose of 5 mg/kg IM every other day until the condition is clinically resolved. Then an oral formulation of vitamin E in the drinking water (Rocavit E-40%, Roche) or in the feed (vitamin E-20, Leo Cook Co.) at the rate of 100 IU/kg of feed is used for maintenance therapy.[24]

The following recommendation for prevention of myopathy is vitamin E and selenium injections (Bo-Se, Burns Biotec) given at 2 days of age, then weekly for a total of three injections at a dosage of 3.0 mg of vitamin E and selenium 0.06 mg/kg of body weight.[18] To prevent deficiency diseases for domestic poultry, a dietary vitamin E level of 10 to 25 IU/kg of food is recommended. Recent information on exotic avian species suggests that they may need up to 100 to 250 IU vitamin E/kg of dry matter feed to prevent deficiency disease.[23]

References

1. Flieg GM: Nutritional problems in young ratites. Int Zoo Yearbook 13:158–163, 1973.
2. Perelman B: Proc 3rd Ann Conf Ostrich Med Surg, College Station, TX, Texas A&M University, 1991.
3. Wade JR: Ratite pediatric medicine and surgery. Proc Assoc Avian Vet, 1992, pp 340–353.
4. Fockena A, Malan FS, Cooper GG, et al: Anthelmintic efficacy of fenbendazole against *Libyostrongylus douglassi* and Houttuynia struthiones in ostriches. J S Afr Vet Assoc 56(1):47, 1985.
5. Malan FS, Grass B, Roper NA, et al: Resistance of *Libyostrongylus douglassi* in ostriches to levamisole. J S Afr Vet Assoc 59(4):202, 1988.
6. Watter CE, Joyce KL, Heath SE, Kazacos KR: Cyathostoma infections as the cause of respiratory distress in emus. Proc Assoc Avian Vet, 1994, pp 151–155.
7. Blue-McLendon AR, Graham DL, Ambrus SI, et al: Cerebrospinal nematodiasis in Emus. Proc Assoc Avian Vet, 1992, pp 326–327.
8. Smith DA, Wiecien JM, Smith-Maxie L: Encephalitis in emus resulting from migration of Baylisascaris sp. Proc Assoc Avian Vet, 1993, pp 301–303.
9. Grow B: Exotic ticks on imported ostriches. Foreign Anim Dis Report 7:5, 1989.
10. Mertins JW, Schlater JL: Exotic ectoparasites of ostriches recently imported into the United States. J Wildl Dis 27:180–182, 1991.
11. Greve JH, Harrison GJ: Conjunctivitis caused by eye flukes in captive-reared ostriches. J Am Vet Med Assoc 177(9):909–910, 1980.
12. Tully TN, Shane SM: Eastern equine encephalomyelitis in emus. Proc Assoc Avian Vet, 1992, pp 316–317.
13. Bruning DF, Dolensek EP: Ratites. In Fowler ME (ed): Zoo

and Wildlife Medicine, ed 2. Philadelphia, WB Saunders, 1986, pp 277–291.

14. Jensen JM, Johnson JH, Werner, ST: Husbandry and medical management of ostriches, emus and rheas. College Station, TX, Wildlife and Exotic Animal TeleConsultants, 1992.

15. Hicks KD: Ratite reproduction. Proc Assoc Avian Vet, 1992, pp 318–325.

16. Martin HD: Avian reproductive emergency surgical management. Vet Med Rep 2:250–253, 1990.

17. Peckham M: Reproductive disorder. In Biester HE, Peckham MC (eds): Diseases of Poultry, ed 5. Ames, Iowa State University Press, 1965, pp 1201–1205.

18. Rosskopf WJ, Woerpel RW: Pet avian obstetrics. Proc 1st Int Conf Zool Avian Med, 1987, pp 213–231.

19. Honnas C, Jensen J, Cornick JL, et al: Proventriculotomy to relieve foreign body impaction in ostriches J Am Vet Med Assoc 199(4):461–465, 1991.

20. Stewart JS: A simple proventriculotomy technique for the ostrich. J Assoc Avian Vet 5(3):139–141, 1991.

21. Bruning D: Breeding and rearing rheas in captivity. Int Zoo Yearbook 13:163–167, 1973.

22. Julian RJ: Poisons and toxins. In Calnek BW, Helmbolt CF, Reid WM, et al (eds): Diseases of Poultry, ed 9. Ames, Iowa State University Press, 1991, pp 863–884.

23. Dierenfeld ES: Vit E Deficiency in Zoo Reptiles, Birds and Ungulates. J Zoo Wild Med 10:3–11, 1989.

24. Rae M: Degenerative myopathy in ratites. Proc Assoc Avian Vet, 1992, pp 328–335.

25. Wallach JD, Boever WJ: Disease of Exotic Animals. Philadelphia, WB Saunders, 1983, pp 947–950.

Helga Gerlach

54

Galliformes

The order Galliformes includes common poultry species such as chickens, turkeys, and quail, as well as popular game birds and exotic Galliformes that may be found in specialized avicultural collections and zoos (Table 54–1). Poultry diseases and medicine are covered extensively in poultry texts. The avian practitioner, however, may be presented with problems in backyard poultry and exotic Galliformes.

GENERAL CHARACTERISTICS

Gallinaceous birds have nidifugous chicks that hatch with a downy plumage. Most species molt once a year, but retain their ability to fly.[1] Galliformes fly at low levels, flap their wings at high frequency, and tire easily. Surgically rendering birds flightless (pinioning) may be necessary in restricted enclosures.[2, 3]

Bacterial Diseases

Bacterial diseases are similar to those in other avian groups, including salmonellosis, yersiniosis, pasteurellosis and erysipelas (Figs. 54–1 to 54–5). Antibiotic dosages are similar to those used in domestic poultry. *Mycobacterium avium* causes the granulomatous form of tuberculosis. Coligranulomatosis must be ruled out for gallinaceous birds. For duck septicemia and borreliosis in Galliformes, refer to Chapter 55.

Viral Diseases

Viral diseases are much more species-specific than bacterial diseases. Except for avipoxvirus (histo-

pathologic demonstration of the pathognomonic Bollinger bodies), diagnosis is made either by virus isolation or demonstration of antibodies.[4, 5] Supportive therapy is the main treatment. It should include application of para-immune inducers (Baypamun 1 ml/kg body weight [BW], three times in 2 days) or vitamin C (50 mg/kg BW). Antibiotics are given only if bacteria are secondary invaders, and only according to sensitivity testing, because of the high immunosuppressive effect of these drugs. Gallinaceous birds are generally highly susceptible to Newcastle disease, and vaccination is recommended. Inactivated adjuvanted vaccines are recommended, which are injected subcutaneously to avoid local irritations or necrosis in the breast muscles.[4, 5]

Chlamydia and *Mycoplasma*

Chlamydia psittaci is present in many avian species causing no clinical disease, but it may be a triggering factor under stressful conditions. In the US, turkey strains may be highly infectious for humans.

Mycoplasma and other mollicutes play an important role in chickens and turkeys. For show chickens the problems may be less severe because of small flock sizes. *Mycoplasma* are also significant pathogens in exotic Galliformes (Fig. 54–6).[4, 5]

Many gallinaceous birds may be part of the infectious chain of *Rickettsia* infection, but there are no known clinical diseases, except for *Aegyptianella pullorum*. Morphologically, confusion with *Plasmodium* is possible. Therapy is effected by application of tetracyclines.[4, 5]

T a b l e 5 4 – 1

NAMES OF BIRDS MENTIONED IN THE TEXT

Common Name	Scientific Name	Common Name	Scientific Name
Australian brush turkey	*Alectura lathami*	Lady Amherst's pheasant	*Chrysolophus amherstiae*
Black grouse	*Lyrurus tetrix*	Mikado pheasant	*Calophasis mikado*
Blood pheasant	*Ithaginis cruentus*	Mongolian pheasant	*Phasianus colchicus mongolicus*
Blue grouse	*Dendragapus obscurus*	Painted quail	*Coturnix chinensis*
Bobwhite quail	*Colinus virginianus*	Plumed guineafowl	*Guttera plumifera*
Bronze-tailed peacock pheasant	*Polyplectron chalcurum*	Prairie chicken	*Tympanuchus cupido*
California quail	*Callipepla californica*	Red grouse	*Lagopus lagopus scoticus*
Capercaillie	*Tetrao urogallus*	Red junglefowl	*Gallus gallus*
Cheer pheasant	*Catreus wallichii*	Red-legged partridge	*Alectoris rufa*
Chukar partridge	*Alectoris chukar*	Ring-necked pheasant	*Phasianus colchicus*
Common quail	*Coturnix coturnix*	Rock partridge	*Alectoris graeca*
Common partridge	*Perdix perdix*	Rock ptarmigan	*Lagopus mutus*
Common turkey	*Meleagris gallopavo*	Roulroul	*Rollulus roulroul*
Congo peafowl	*Afropavo congensis*	Ruffed grouse	*Bonasa umbellus*
Crested argus	*Rheinardia ocellata*	Sage grouse	*Centrocercus urophasianus*
Crested guineafowl	*Guttera pucherani*	Salvadori's pheasant	*Lophura inornata*
Gambel's quail	*Callipepla gambelii*	Sand partridge	*Ammoperdix heyi*
Golden pheasant	*Chrysolophus pictus*	Siamese fireback	*Lophura diardi*
Great argus	*Argusanius argus*	Silver pheasant	*Lophura nycthemera*
Green pheasant	*Phasianus colchicus tenebrosus*	Spruce grouse	*Falcipennis canadensis*
Helmeted curassow	*Pauxi pauxi* or *Pauxi unicornis*	Stone partridge	*Ptilopachus petrosus*
Helmeted guineafowl	*Numida meleagris*	Swinhoe's pheasant	*Lophura swinhoii*
Japanese quail	*Coturnix japonica*	Willow ptarmigan	*Lagopus lagopus*
Koklass	*Pucrasia macrolopha*		

Data from Wolters HE: Die Vogelarten der Erde. Hamburg, Paul Parey, 1975–1982.[45]

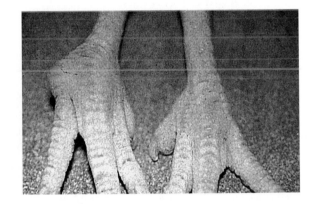

F i g u r e 5 4 – 1

Actinobacillus arthritis is found primarily in domestic chickens.

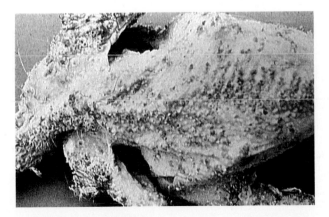

F i g u r e 5 4 – 2

Staphylococcus dermatitis in a backyard chicken.

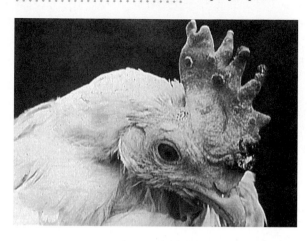

F i g u r e 5 4 – 3

Staphylococcus dermatitis in a backyard chicken.

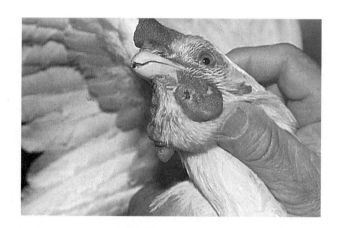

F i g u r e 5 4 – 4

Chronic pasteurellosis (wattle disease) in a backyard chicken.

F i g u r e 5 4 – 5

Tuberculosis in a backyard chicken.

F i g u r e 5 4 – 6

Mycoplasmosis in a chukar (rock partridge).

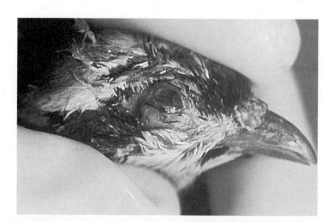

Fungal Diseases

Fungi (yeasts, *Aspergillus, Mucor,* or *Penicillium*) can cause mycosis. Mycosis is always a secondary disease. For successful treatment and prophylaxis, the triggering factor needs to be recognized and eliminated, which may be difficult. *Aspergillus fumigatus,* the most frequent invader, produces mycotoxins (gliotoxin) within the host that cause severe nephro- and hepatopathies and immune suppression in the birds, further reducing their chances of successful treatment.

Parasites

Flagellates (*Histomonas* species, *Trichomonas* species, rarely *Chilomastix* species) are seen in many species. For diagnosis, swabs from live birds must be examined within 1/2 to 1 hour of collection. For therapy, various imidazole derivatives can be used. Hygienic methods are used for control, including the cleaning of the gutters for *Trichomonas* and the treatment for *Heterakis* (fenbendazole) to break the life cycle of *Histomonas.*

Blood protozoa (*Plasmodium, Leukozytozoon,* and *Haemoproteus* species) can be recognized on stained blood smears and should be expected in birds in outdoor aviaries at the flight season of the insect vectors. Anemia as a clinical sign is difficult to ascertain, but affected birds may show somnolence, apathy, and emaciation. Differential diagnoses include *Aegyptianella* infection, borreliosis, and anemia of another etiology.

Coccidiosis can occur in many gallinaceous birds. *Eimeria* species predominate, and they are very host-specific.[5] Diagnosis is by fecal flotation tests. Species diagnosis is difficult because the range of colonization in the intestine is taxonomically important. Coccidiostats are toxic in some species. Sulfonamide with bi- or trimethoprim, and amprolium with or without ethopabate are the most frequently used drugs in gallinaceous birds other than chickens or turkeys. For control it is advisable to allow low numbers of coccidia in the environment to procure some immunity, while reducing the number of environmental oocysts by means of good hygiene. Few disinfectants are efficacious. Flame or steam is recommended to reduce environmental contamination.

Worm infestations are common in gallinaceous birds kept in captivity (Fig. 54–7). Most common are infestations of cestodes and nematodes. Trematodes are rare in gallinaceous birds.

Demonstrating cestodes in live birds is not easy. For unknown reasons, fecal flotation or sedimentation may fail to reveal eggs. Taxonomy and biology including intermediate hosts are not yet described for all cestodes in gallinaceous birds. Praziquantel is the drug of choice for therapy. Toxicity is unknown, but care should be taken when treating rare and endangered birds. Intermediate hosts should be restricted or eliminated for control.

Nematodes of the genera *Ascaridia, Heterakis, Thomix, Capillaria, Trichostrongylus, Eucoleus, Syngamus,* and *Dyspharynx* can be diagnosed from eggs in fecal samples by using flotation or sedimentation tests.[4, 5] Egg morphology is not sufficient for the species diagnosis in many cases. Detection of parasitism may be difficult in the prepatent period. This is particularly important with *Syngamus* infections in the spring, when birds have eaten the transport hosts (earthworms) and die from hemorrhage of the lung caused by larval migrations. In small birds one specimen that is still within the prepatent period may be enough to cause severe dyspnea or asphyxiation. Fenbendazole is recommended for treatment. Acanthocephalosis is rare in gallinaceous birds (See Chapter 55.)

Many ectoparasites (including the scaly-leg mite) seen in gallinaceous birds are aptly described.[4, 5] Drugs recommended for treatment in chickens or turkeys may be too toxic for many exotic gallina-

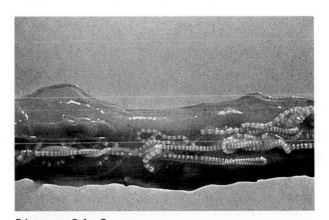

F i g u r e　5 4 – 7

Raillietina in a backyard chicken.

ceous birds. Carbamate and organophosphorus can be used, if the antidote (atropine) is ready for use.

CHARACTERISTICS AND MAJOR DISEASES OF GALLIFORM TAXA

Megapodes (Megapodiidae)

The megapodes (seven genera, 12 species) live on the floor of primeval forests of Australia, New Guinea, and the eastern islands of Indonesia. The birds have very large feet, which they use to scratch for feed and for building large incubation mounds for their eggs. Megapodes do not brood their own eggs, but have them incubated by solar heat, fermentation heat, or geothermal heat. The eggs are large (up to 17% of the body mass of the hen) and thin-shelled, and they contain a large fatty yolk. The mound is constructed by the cocks or both genders when the environmental conditions are right (temperature, humidity, etc.). The eggs do not have a fixed air chamber or chalacae and are not turned during incubation.

Hens lay eggs every 2 or 3 days with the pole pointed downward into preformed holes that are immediately covered. The parents monitor the temperature in the mound with their tongue or beak, maintaining temperatures around 34°C. Cooling is achieved by scratching holes in the mound, which, at the same time, allows for gaseous exchange. The incubation period varies between 45 and 90 days and is correlated with the temperature inside the mound. The chicks leave the mound some hours after hatching. They are able to fly immediately and fend for themselves together with some hatch mates. By 1 year of age, the birds are sexually mature. For the differentiation of genders, endoscopy may be necessary.

The monogamous Australian brush turkey is the most common species kept in captivity. It can be fed commercial poultry diets. Some megapodes have completely featherless heads and/or necks or featherless patches in these regions, the skin of which may be colored. Some species also have colored integumental appendages. The four toes are on the same plane.[1] Little is known about specific diseases in megapodes.[1]

Fowl (Phasianidae)

Fowl are composed of 15 subfamilies, 70 genera, and 203 species.

Guineafowl (Numininae)

Domesticated guineafowl (four genera, six species) were derived from the helmeted guineafowl, which originated in Northern Africa. Reproduction in guineafowl is similar to that in chickens, except hatching is accomplished at lower humidity. Incubation periods vary between 23 and 27 days. Guineafowl are monomorphic, but the cock's call has three syllables and the hen's only two. Guineafowl of all ages can be fed commercial turkey pellets for the appropriate ages. Coccidiostats must be used with caution because of potential toxicity. Only amprolium, DOT (Zoalen, [dinitrotolmid], Dow Chemical, Salisbury), and Lerbec (combination of methichlorpindol and methylbenzoquate = 100 parts + 8.3 parts [100–110 ppm of the mixture], Dow Chemical) may be used for treatment.

Some species have a helmet of spongy bone covered with corium and keratinized epidermis situated near the junction of the upper bill with the cranium. The wattles are white to light blue and, as the helmet, are larger in cocks than in hens. Guineafowl can be noisy, particularly during the breeding season. Crested and plumed guineafowl have an elongated trachea that loops before entering the thoracic inlet.[2]

Many diseases in guineafowl resemble chicken or turkey diseases. Avipox has been described in guineafowl, but few details are available. Adenovirus group 1 produces necrotic pancreatitis and air sacculitis.[6] Adenovirus group 2 causes acute pulmonary edema, splenomegaly, and pathologic lesions similar to the marble spleen disease of pheasants or splenomegaly in chickens. The virus is probably identical to or at least closely related to turkey group 2 strains.[7] Adenovirus group 3 has been demonstrated in flocks with soft shell problems. The disease could be reproduced with the agent of the adenoviral salpingitis in chickens.[8]

A rotavirus is known as the etiologic agent of a transmissible enteritis of short duration (5–8 days), which is self-limiting.[9] Guineafowl from the age of 3 days onward can suffer from enteritis and hepatopancreatitis when infected with a coronavirus distinct from the chicken infectious bronchitis virus. In addition, emaciation and dehydration can be seen.[10, 11]

Guineafowl are highly susceptible to Newcastle disease and develop a systemic constellation (peracute to acute) with fever, lassitude, dull plumage, edema of the eyelids and face, severe dyspnea caused by pulmonary edema and fibrous or catarrhal tracheitis, and watery diarrhea. Mortality can approach 50 to 90% in 4 to 8 days. Vaccination with inactivated vaccines is recommended.

Orthomyxovirus strains from the helmeted guineafowl are not pathogenic for chickens or ducks, but cause mainly a 30 to 40% decrease in egg production and hatchability. Egg-layers with no clinical signs or only listlessnes and cyanosis can be observed.[12]

Osteopetrosis can be caused in the chicks of guineafowl by a chicken-derived avian type C retrovirus. Besides typical bone lesions, the birds develop epithelial tumors of the pancreas and the duodenal mucosa.[13]

Mycoplasmosis in guineafowls can be caused by *Mycoplasma gallisepticum* and *M. synoviae*. The latter disease shows no sinusitis but rather joint lesions as in chickens or turkeys. In addition, guineafowl develop severe amyloidosis.[14]

Peafowl (Pavoninae)

Peafowl (two genera, three species) originate from India and Southeast Asia; only the Congo peafowl comes from tropical Africa. The hens lay small clutches of three to five eggs that are incubated 26 to 30 days, depending on the species. The monogamous Congo peafowl nests in trees and needs a nest box that is about 1.50 meters high, stuffed with hay or foliage and covered from easy sight. Some slanted boughs should provide easy access to the nest. Hens reach maturity in the second and cocks in the third year of life. Peafowl can be highly aggressive, even attacking humans, and very noisy during the breeding season. Commercial turkey pellets can be fed according to the appropriate ages. Peafowl need perches about 3 to 4 meters above the ground to accommodate their tail feathers. Cocks have spurs that are osseous protuberances originating from the tarsometatarsus and covered

with a keratinized epidermis; they may serve as weapons. Annual rings are formed toward the base of the spurs that can be used for determining the minimum age of the bird.[15] If hens have spurs, they are smaller and without an osseous base.[16]

The ornamental feathers of the cocks, which are used for courtship, develop from tail coverts. Peafowl do not have after-feathers (hypopennae). Peafowl live approximately 20 years.

The diseases of peafowl are similar to those of chickens and turkeys. Following infection with *Mycobacterium avium*, granulomas develop also in the trachea causing respiratory signs similar to those of foreign bodies. Peafowl can contract avipoxvirus and develop a disease as seen in chickens. Vaccination with chicken vaccine does not protect peafowl against peafowl strains of avipoxvirus. For clinical signs of Newcastle disease refer to Guineafowl.

M. gallisepticum causes depression in peafowl. Birds shake their heads to remove sticky nasal exudates. The infraorbital sinuses are swollen, and the birds display gurgling respiratory sounds. Latency is possible.[17]

Peafowl are prone to infection with *Histomonas meleagridis* and develop typhlohepatitis (blackhead disease). Invasions with *Heterakis* species trigger the infection and occurrence of the disease.

Turkeys (Meleagridinae)

Turkeys (one genus, two species) are common in North and Central America. The domesticated turkey originated from the common turkey (*Meleagris gallopavo*). Female turkeys select their mate. Hens produce clutches of eight to 15 eggs that are incubated 28 days. Because of the great difference in body weight and the tendency for males to injure hens, artificial insemination is the rule with domesticated breeds. Free-ranging turkeys have a brain volume about 35% larger than that of domesticated birds, and they behave quite differently. Free-ranging turkeys fly well, at 15 mph (24 km/hour), even through the forest. Poults are able to fly at 2 weeks of age. Commercial feeds are available for all age and utility groups.

Skin appendages on the head and neck do not have an elastic intermediate layer like in chickens but have a superficial muscular and vascular layer. The dewlaps are smooth, can change color, and are of alternating size, as is the single snood on the forehead. Numerous red caruncles can be found on the bluish, poorly feathered skin of the head. In the distal part of the ventral neck region, a "beard" is found typically in males. It consists of a tuft of stiff keratinous filaments pointing downward.[16] The common turkey has only seven air sacs (the paired caudal thoracic air sacs are not developed).

The diseases of domesticated turkeys are very aptly covered in two textbooks (Fig. 54–8).[4, 5] A new disease in turkeys has been described in which 1 to 3% mortality, disturbance of the general condition, listlessness, rough plumage, reduced water and feed intake, and dyspnea with severe coughing are observed.[18] At necropsy, fibrinopurulent pneumonia and lung edema as well as fibrinous pericarditis, air sacculitis, and peritonitis are observed. The causative agent is *Ornithobacterium rhinotrachealis* and is a nonfermenter, growing only on blood agar in tiny colonies resembling *Moraxella*.[18] Further genetic and taxonomic studies are under way.

Peacock Pheasants (Argusianinae)

Peacock pheasants (three genera, eight species) are found in Southeast Asia including many islands, and in India up to the Himalayas. Hens lay only two eggs that are incubated between 23 and 25 days.

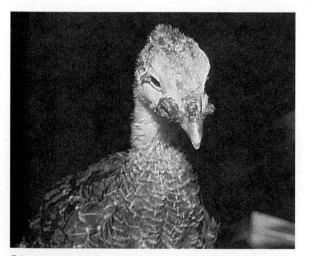

Figure 54–8

Pox virus infection in a turkey.

The bronze-tailed peacock pheasant and the crested argus nest in trees like peafowl. They require high perches to prevent damage to their tails. Generally, both genders of the peacock pheasants establish a territory that is defended. Males should be introduced to females only in the beginning of the breeding season to avoid aggression and injuries.

Peacock pheasants require a high-protein diet. Commercial high-protein turkey or pheasant mixtures, mealworms, chopped hard-boiled chicken eggs, chopped meat with fruit, and a small amount of grain may compose the feed. Green plants probably will not be eaten. The chicks of some peacock pheasants do not pick downward during the first days of life. Hens feed their chicks from their beaks. Chicks of the great argus start to pick at live feed (mealworms) sooner than at other food particles. Gender differentiation is difficult in mature birds of the genus *Polyplectron*, where the plumage of the hen is much duller than that of the cock, and the cock has spurs.

Peacock pheasants have no preen glands. Ornamental feathers develop from rectrices. When frightened or shocked (faced by predators, caught by humans) peacock pheasants can release their feathers. A half-naked bird escapes.

Special care must be taken when handling these species. Little is known about the diseases of these birds. Blackhead can be a problem (see Turkeys).

True Pheasants (Phasianinae)

Pheasants (eight genera, 21 species) originate from Central and East Asia up to the Himalayas and from the tropical islands of the Southeast. Depending on the species, the clutch sizes are five to 15 eggs, and incubation times vary between 22 and 26 days. The common pheasant in captivity can lay up to 60 eggs annually, but this species is an unreliable brooder in captivity. The Mikado pheasant and Salvadori's pheasant nest in trees (see Peafowl). For many gallinaceous birds, in particular for the Phasianinae, the removal of the first clutch provokes a second and sometimes even a third. Artificial or foster incubation is necessary. Chinese silk fowl and bantams make good foster parents. For tropical species, moistening of the eggs during the last week of incubation may be necessary. For artificial incubation it appears advantageous to increase carbon dioxide levels to around 1% to ensure the pipping of the chicks ready to hatch. The normal air supply should be restored after pipping.[2]

Most pheasants are polygamous, but the free-ranging golden pheasant is monogamous and can be kept in small groups in captivity. Eared pheasants (genus *Crossoptilon*) and cheer pheasants use the upper beak to search for roots and insects in the soil. If kept on concrete or other hard surfaces, the beaks have to be trimmed regularly by the caretaker.

Commercial feed mixtures for pheasants, even for their chicks, are available. Chicks can also be fed small seeds and commercial feed for insectivores. When chicken or turkey feeds are used, beware of halofuginone (Stenorol, Roussel), which is toxic for the common pheasant.

Some species have ornamental appendages on the head and the neck including featherless, colored patches of skin frequently used only for mating display. Cocks have spurs that can be used for the determination of the minimum age. Ornamental feathers can originate from the rectrices. Golden pheasants show polychromatism of the plumage.[1, 2]

Phasianinae are reasonable flyers and attain a speed of 20 mph (33 kmh). The common pheasant flies straight up when startled; therefore, the top netting of the aviary should be flexible or padded to avoid injuries.

Many diseases are known and are covered in other textbooks.[4, 5]

Haemophilus other than *H. paragallinarum* may cause sinusitis and a diphtheroid inflammation of the oral mucosa in the golden pheasant, and necrosis of lung tissue in the Siamese fireback.

The common pheasant is susceptible to tularemia. Clinical signs and pathology resemble pasteurellosis or yersiniosis.[4, 5] The causative agent, *Francisella tularense*, needs special cultural methods.

Aviadenovirus has been isolated from Phasianinae, but no typical signs of disease have been described. It is mainly a latent infection, except for pheasant adenovirus 1, which in the common pheasant causes marble spleen disease. The virus is closely related or identical to the agent of the hemorrhagic enteritis in turkeys. The incubation period is about 6 days. Clinical signs are sudden death or a short disease with anorexia and dyspnea caused by severe pulmonary edema. At postmortem examination, splenomegaly is present with a mottled surface and multiple grayish confluent foci. For prophylaxis, splenic homogenisates from turkeys with hemorrhagic enteritis have been taken in the drinking water (one spleen for 10,000 birds), but because turkeys are rather frequently infected with retrovirus, these practices are discouraged. The use of turkey vaccines has not been reported in pheasants. For diagnosis refer to other textbooks.[4, 5]

Orthoreovirus has been reported from pheasants, causing immunosuppression with no recognizable clinical disease. Rotavirus has been associated with catarrhal enteritis. A coronavirus deviating from the chicken strains has been isolated from birds with reduced egg production, poor egg quality, and slight to moderate respiratory signs. A low mortality is associated with egg peritonitis, urolithiasis, visceral gout, or swollen kidneys. In 8- to 10-week-old birds, mortality can be up to 40% with renal lesions the most conspicuous.[19] Phasianinae are susceptible to infectious laryngotracheitis.[4, 5]

Eastern or Western equine encephalomyelitis can cause clinical signs such as depression, incoordination, paresis, paralysis, torticollis, tremor, polydipsia, and somnolence. Chicks become resistant after they are 28 days old.[20] In pheasants the virus is not only spread by insect bites but also by feather picking and other forms of cannibalism. The virus also occurs in the feather quills. Debeaking may limit the horizontal distribution of the virus.[20] Formalin-inactivated vaccine for horses (five pheasants are given one horse dose) is reported efficacious, whereas formalized bivalent chicken embryo vaccine protects only 65% of the vaccinated birds when challenged.[20]

The common pheasant is also susceptible to louping ill, the causative agent being a member of the Flavoviridae. Central nervous system signs are rarely observable.[21]

Pheasants are extremely susceptible to Newcastle disease (see Guineafowl), but wild-living birds rarely contract the disease. They are unable to stand and refuse feed. Dyspnea can be distinct (acute tracheitis) or totally absent. Hemorrhagic diarrhea may occur.

Influenza A/pheasant/Washington/1985 (H9N9) has been isolated from 2- to 8-week-old common pheasants with a mortality rate of 25 to 35%. The adult breeder birds did not show any clinical signs, although they were infected and excreted the virus.

The sick birds revealed severe air sacculitis, catarrhal tracheitis, purulent rhinitis, fibrinopurulent polyserositis, and splenomegaly.[22] The strain was nonvirulent for chickens and domesticated ducks.

Avian type C retrovirus subgroup F has been isolated from the common pheasant and the green pheasant and subgroup G from the Lady Amherst's pheasant, golden pheasant, and silver pheasant. Retrovirus (not classified) has been recognized in the Mongolian and Swinhoe's pheasant. (For clinical signs, pathology, diagnosis, and control refer to the section on chickens.) A reticuloendothelosis of the Twiehaus type is described and could be experimentally reproduced.[23] The virus of avian encephalomyelitis (picornavirus) has been demonstrated in pheasants with no clinical signs.

Phasianinae are susceptible to *Rickettsia* (no clinical disease) and *Mycoplasma gallisepticum* but also have their own strains.[17] Chicks at the age of 2 to 8 weeks succumb to the disease, particularly when raised in large flocks. Adults rarely show clinical signs. Morbidity is high, and mortality, depending on secondary factors, varies between 30 and 90%. Blinking and scratching at the eyelids are the first signs. Deteriorating general condition, photophobia, swollen eyelids followed by exudation and blepharoconjunctivitis (probably keratitis) are observed. Death by cachexia can be the result of blindness. A voluminous expansion of the infraorbital sinus with little exudate may be seen. The birds show dyspnea, particularly when agitated.[17]

Severe cecal lesions with up to 10 times enlargement of the organs followed by death are caused in many Phasianinae by *Heterakis isolonche* (Fig. 54–9). The coprologic diagnosis is complicated by the close resemblance of the eggs with *Ascaridia* eggs (*H. isolonche* is smaller in width and length). It takes some experience to see the difference. Because *H. isolonche*, especially the pathogenic larvae, are resistant to piperazine, treatment with fenbendazole (10–40 mg/kg) is recommended whenever eggs are found that resemble *Heterakis* or *Ascaridia*.

Monals (Lophophorinae)

Monals (one genus, three species) live in the Himalayas and northwest China. The clutch of four to five eggs is incubated for 27 days. The upper beak

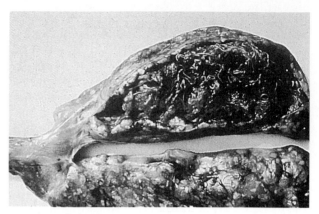

Heterakis isolonche in the cecum of a common pheasant.

of the monal is used in searching for roots and insects in the soil. The beak must be trimmed regularly if the bird cannot use it naturally. Monal chicks pick at the toes of their siblings when fed mealworms. Specific diseases are unknown.

Koklasses (Purcrasiinae)

The Koklasses (one genus, one species) live in China and the Himalayan region. Hens of the monogamous birds lay five to seven eggs that hatch after 20 to 21 days of incubation. The genders are dimorphic. Koklasses are strict vegetarians and should not be fed commercially available pellets and similar feeds. Koklasses naturally feed on ferns, grasses, leaves, mosses, buds, and berries. In captivity they should be given soft green plants, fruits, berries, and no grains. During summer, feed grasses and lucerne as well as fruits and berries, and in winter a variety of vegetables can be used as substitutes.

The birds are difficult to keep healthy, and it is even more difficult to raise the chicks. No formula for chick feed is available. Specific diseases are unknown. Most mortality seems to be the result of nutritional deficiencies.

Blood Pheasants (Ithagininae)

Blood pheasants (one genus, one species) live at an altitude of 3500 to 5000 meters. During winter they can be found living at 2500 meters. The polygamous birds lay a clutch of five to 12 eggs that is incubated 27 days. Free-ranging blood pheasants feed on mosses, lichens, ferns, grasstips, and conifer needlebuds. They feed constantly in planted aviaries.

The birds are difficult to keep healthy. There are no successful formulas for raising the chicks. They can probably be fed like the koklasses. Most diseases are caused by malnutrition.

Junglefowl (Gallinae)

Junglefowl (one genus, four species) originated in the tropical regions of India and Southeast Asia. The red junglefowl is the ancestral stock from which the domesticated chicken was derived. Free-living species lay clutches of five to eight eggs, which hatch following 19 to 21 days of incubation, depending on the species. Commercial feed mixtures are available for all age and utility groups.

The heavy "Asian breeds" such as Brahmas, Cochins, Faverolles, and the large fighting cock breeds have a high protein requirement and should be given chopped meat in addition to the "normal" diets.

Wild junglefowl and domesticated breeds are characterized by an unpaired fleshy comb that has an intermediate layer consisting of a fibrillar network filled with mucus-like substances. This material gives elasticity to the comb, which is covered by a heavy vascularized corium and epidermis. The morphology of the comb has changed considerably in domesticated breeds. Paired wattles of the same structure as the comb are present, and under the influence of sexual hormones are larger in cocks than in hens. Paired cheeks or earlobes can be found ventral to the auditory canal; they are colored red or whitish (if subepithelial sinusoids are absent).[16] Cocks have spurs, and some domesticated breeds may have feathers around the toes and tarsometatarsus. Breeds such as the Houdans, Faverolles, Dorkins, and Chinese silk fowl have five digits, the fifth near the first mediocaudally.[8] Normally, domesticated cocks have typical dimorphic plumage, but in some breeds the cocks carry the feather morphology typical of female plumage.

For diseases, refer to other textbooks.[4, 5]

Tragopans (Tragopaninae)

Tragopans (one genus, five species) originate in the Himalayas and the mountainous countryside of Assam, Burma, and Southeast China. Tragopan hens lay four to 10 eggs that hatch after 28 to 31 days of incubation. Tragopans are tree-breeders and need sheltered baskets or boxes high above the ground. Tragopans are primarily vegetarians and eat bamboo sprouts, grasses, mosses, acorns, berries, and a few insects. In captivity, grasses, lucerne, apples, cucumbers, and various berries can be given as well as some small seeds, but not common grains.[2] It is rather difficult to raise the chicks. There are no chick formulas. It appears best to release the clucking hen with the chicks into a portable pen, with young grasses (and some ants and other small insects) and each day give them a new patch to fend for themselves. A heated shelter is necessary, and the chicks should be kept dry.

Little is known about diseases in these birds. One of the principal problems is obesity caused by malnutrition and small aviaries. Large enclosures planted with grasses, bushes, and shrubs are recommended.

Spurfowl (Galloperdicinae)

Spurfowl (one genus, three species) live in India, Nepal, and Ceylon. The clutch of two to five eggs hatch after 23 days of incubation. No further information is available.

Stone Partridges (Ptilopachinae)

Stone partridges (one genus, one species) range from Senegal and Ethiopia south to Kenya. No other pertinent information is available.

Snowcocks, Partridges, and Quail (Perdicinae)

All (27 genera, 98 species) are Old World species, and with the exception of the snowcocks that dwell in mountains, most live in semi-arid countrysides or bush lands. Only the common and the Japanese quail are truly migratory. Many species have camouflaging plumage. The birds crouch, immobilized on the ground, if a predator approaches, flying up at the last moment. Many species are pure ground-dwellers and do not require perches. They can be kept in aviaries together with species that prefer to live mainly on perches. Using audible signals, Japanese quail chicks can synchronize their hatch. Japanese quail in captivity are considered to be domesticated and reach sexual maturity at the age of 6 weeks.

Most of these birds are omnivorous. Commercially available feed for Japanese quail, pheasants, chickens, and turkeys can be supplemented with green plants, silage, or shortly cut grasses. **Attention!** Beware of halofuginone because it is toxic for the common partridge. The roulroul has a high protein requirement and is therefore fed commercial soft feed for insectivorous birds together with live insects and chopped meat or hard-boiled eggs. This diet may result in odoriferous feces.[2] Snowcocks eat mainly grasses and leguminous plants. Grains or pellets should be limited or excluded from the diet. Snowcock chicks start feeding on plants immediately after hatching. Turkey pellets with antiflagellates may be life-threatening because of the presence of symbiotic flagellates in the ceca.

Snowcocks need large rocks for perching and sharpening their beaks. Because of the high content of crude fibers in their diet, they have highly developed ceca and a heavily muscled ventriculus. A crop is not visible and is just a bulge in the diameter of the esophagus.

The sand partridge has salt glands located in osseous indentations above the eyes, which empty into the nasal cavity.[24] These glands enable them to use salty waters in arid environments.

Diseases caused by avipoxvirus are seen in Japanese quail (cross-immunity with fowlpox makes it possible to vaccinate) as well as in the common partridge (no details known, strain not well examined). Japanese quail are susceptible to Marek's disease virus, but outbreaks of the disease following natural infections are not well documented. An adenovirus has been isolated from chicks of the Japanese quail with central nervous system signs. Nucleic acid analysis showed that the strain is closely related to fowl adenovirus (FAV-4).[25] Rotavirus has been shown to be the cause of scour, stunting, and mortality (up to 30%) in several partridges, especially when they are infected as chicks.[26] A

corona-like virus has been isolated from Japanese quail with respiratory signs.[27] Serologically the strains are not related to other avian or mammalian strains.

Outbreaks of Eastern and Western equine encephalomyelitis are seen in chukar partridges and Japanese quail with mortality up to 80 to 90%, depending on the age. Clinical signs are the same as in pheasants.

Israeli turkey meningoencephalitis from a virus belonging to the Flaviviridae can be infectious for Japanese quail, which may show progressive paresis or paralysis, beginning with incoordinated movements. Mortality can approach 10 to 30%.

Perdicinae are highly susceptible to the Newcastle disease virus and develop an acute disease with high mortality (see Guineafowl). Orthomyxovirus can be the cause of disease in chukars and many quail.[28, 29] As described in Japanese quail, influenza A/quail (Italy/1117/65) results in mortality of between 15 and 80%, depending on age and environmental conditions. Clinically, somnolence, sneezing, nasal discharge, swelling of the infraorbital sinus, lacrimation, and dyspnea are seen. Central nervous system signs are present in 1 to 2% of the birds.

Antibodies to avian type C retrovirus, subgroups A and B, are found in many Perdicinae. Japanese quail serve as experimental animals for research. Subgroup H consists of an endogenous virus isolated from a common partridge. A nonclassified endogenous virus was isolated from a painted quail. Lymphoid leukosis is the most common form, but other expressions may occur. (Leukosis of all forms seems to be increasing in captive birds.) Clinically a massively distended liver or ascites is sometimes palpable. Neoplastic blood cells or their precursors are seldom present in blood smears because avian leukosis is rarely leukemic. The virus causes a variety of non-neoplastic conditions, including immunosuppression and reduced thyroid function (stunting in chicks). A retained bursa of Fabricius is indicative. For details, refer to other textbooks.[4, 5]

Japanese quail also suffer from reticuloendotheliosis (Twiehaus-type strains). In contrast to other avian groups, the disease appears shortly after sexual maturity, causing thickenings and nodular foci along the digestive tract (crop, proventriculus, ventriculus, intestine, and ceca). Lesions may be observed in other organs, but with less frequency.

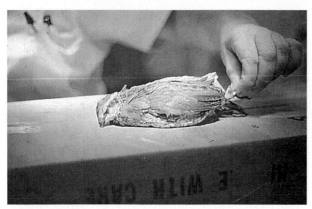

Figure 54–10

Vitamin E deficiency in a bobwhite quail. The bird is paralyzed and unresponsive to stimulation.

Mortality may approach 100%.[30] The picornavirus of avian encephalomyelitis has been demonstrated by antibodies in the rock partridge and red-legged partridge without clinical signs.

Quail (*Coturnix* species) can be infected with *Aegyptianella pullorum*, which may cause anemia, icterus, hepatomegaly, and splenomegaly in young birds. Infections with other *Rickettsia* are possible, but do not cause clinical disease. *Mycoplasma gallisepticum* can be found in Japanese quail, which has a subclinical course. Infected chickens may be the source. Egg transmission is possible. Partridges are supposed to harbor the same strains as pheasants, but there is no seasonal peak. In contrast to pheasants, partridges have a fibrinous-cheesy exudate in the swollen infraorbital sinus. Rock partridge show clinical disease only in chicks. Emaciation and swollen sinuses are the main symptoms. Isolates assumed to be *M. gallisepticum* are experimentally apathogenic for chickens and turkeys. In the red-legged partridge, the disease resembles that of other partridges. Strains are assumed to be identical to strains from pheasants. Free-living adults become sick in August and December.[17]

New World Quail (Odontophorinae)

Quail (nine genera, 31 species) are distributed over many parts of the New World. Most are ground-dwellers and do not need perches. Bobwhite quail are domesticated and have clutch sizes between seven and 28 eggs; other members of the subfamily have four to 17 eggs. Incubation periods vary between 22 and 30 days, depending on the genus.[2] New World quail are generally monogamous, and both genders build nests and brood the chicks. Bobwhite quail can be kept in groups of one cock and two hens. In the nonbreeding season, New World quail live together in family groups, but older cocks become aggressive toward youngsters at the beginning of the new breeding season. Sexual maturity is reached at 1 year of age (or even earlier), and in aviaries pairs must be separated to avoid injuries.[2, 31] New World quail are unreliable breeders in captivity. Fostering eggs (bantams) or artificial incubation is necessary. New World quail are primarily seed-eaters (Figs. 54–10, 54–11). Forest-adapted species are more insectivorous and have a higher and more specified requirement for proteins. The lower beak is serrated or slightly toothed.

Diseases of New World quail are not much different from those of other avian groups, except for ulcerative enteritis in bobwhite quail and other Odontophoridae caused by *Clostridium colinum*. Sick birds show an acute to prolonged course with bloody diarrhea and polydipsia, depending on age. Birds that die suddenly or emaciated birds that finally die display ulcers in the mucosa of the upper jejunum on postmortem examination. Clindamycin (100 mg/kg BW), or spiramycin (up to 200 mg/kg) can be tried. For control, 200 ppm bacitracin zinc is given as a feed additive.

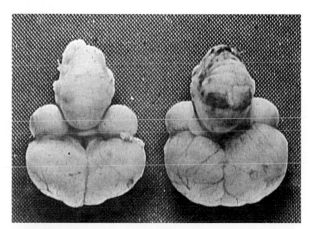

Figure 54–11

Hemorrhages of the brain, particularly of the cerebellum, associated with vitamin E deficiency in bobwhite quail.

Avipoxvirus is seen in captive and free-ranging bobwhite quail (and probably also in California and Gambel's quail) as a severe disease (wet form) at the height of the mosquito season (Fig. 54–12). Mortality is mainly the result of the inability to see, because the eyelids become pasted together. The virus is not related to fowlpox, and vaccination with fowl vaccine is of no avail.[32, 33] A herpes virus related to the crane herpes virus was isolated from bobwhite quail, together with *Clostridium*. The bobwhite quail herpes virus caused an inclusion body hepatitis, but because of the simultaneous infection with *Clostridium*, no description of the untriggered infection is available. Bobwhite quail is the only species susceptible to the so-called quail bronchitis (QB) caused by an aviadenovirus.[34] The virus is serologically an FAV-1 serotype, but nucleic acid analysis has revealed genetic differences.[25] QB is highly infectious, and is spread mainly by contact, causing mortality up to 90% in bobwhites up to 6 weeks. Vertical transmission is suspected, but no evidence has been furnished to date. Clinical signs are sudden death, respiratory rales, coughing, ballooning of the skin over the infraorbital sinus, sneezing but no nasal discharge, lacrimation, and conjunctivitis. Histologic diagnosis by demonstration of intranuclear inclusion bodies in the tracheal and bronchial epithelium is possible 2 to 5 days after infection. Proliferation of lymph follicles and lymphocytic infiltrations are evident.

In contrast to other aviadenoviruses, the QB virus is difficult to propagate. Many adaptation passages are necessary because of slow replication in chicken embryos and chicken embryo cell cultures. Vaccination with chicken embryo lethal orphan-type vaccines is of no avail.

Quail are known to be infected with the virus of Eastern and Western equine encephalomyelitis but, as a rule, do not develop clinical disease. An endogenous avian group C retrovirus subtype I has been isolated from Gambel's quail.[4, 5]

Cryptosporidiosis is a severe disease in bobwhite quail chicks. Frequently the disease begins between 9 and 14 days of life; chicks show diarrhea and die shortly afterward. Mortality may approach 80 to 90%. Chicks surviving the 21st day have a chance of normal development; however, mortality continues up to 7 weeks. At necropsy, a catarrhal enteritis (mainly caused by secondary invaders), particularly of the upper jejunum, is observed, but the cryptosporidia can only be demonstrated about 1/2 hour postmortem, in the middle of the jejunum. There is no therapy. For disinfection, chlorine-releasing compounds can be tried.[35, 36]

Bobwhite quail kept on farms frequently suffer from crop capillariosis. The worms are located in the multilayered squamous epithelium of the ingluveal mucosa. Their eggs are laid into the epithelium and are released into the crop lumen with the desquamation of the epithelium. The crop wall is thickened, and the birds suffer from chronic emaciation. The *Capillaria* species has no valid name.[35]

Grouse (Tetraoninae)

Grouse (nine genera, 16 species) inhabit mountainous countrysides or subarctic regions in the Northern Hemisphere. Some species are well adapted to cold. Feet and toes are covered with feathers, and in ptarmigans the plantar surface of the foot is also covered. Long nails and keratinous pin-like protrusions on both sides of the digits make it easier to move on snow. Particularly dense plumage and a subcutaneous layer of fat serve as further protection. Hair-like feathers cover the nostrils. Ptarmigans shiver to increase body temperature at ambient temperatures below −12°C.[2, 37, 38]

Ptarmigans, ruffed grouse, hazelhens, spruce grouse, and blue grouse are monogamous. Cocks must be housed so that they cannot see or hear other cocks. Hazelhen males attack hens when a rival can be heard but not seen.

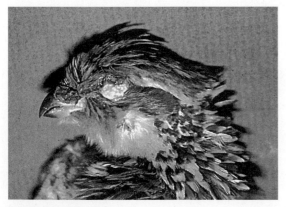

F i g u r e 5 4 – 1 2

Naturally occurring avipox in a bobwhite quail.

Other grouse are polygamous. Females select from displaying males. When genders are of different body weight, hens can be protected from cocks by housing them in aviaries divided into different pens. Small holes between the pens allow the female to go to the cock for mating, but to retreat if the cock is molesting her. Hens breed best when allowed to choose from two or more cocks. One cock can be the choice of several hens. Crossbreeding between several genera and species can be seen in natural habitats.[2, 37, 38]

Sage grouse and other North American species have a diverticulum in the middle of the esophagus that they use for territorial display (and perhaps for amplifying the voice). This diverticulum is inflated with air to expose a featherless, brightly colored skin. Clutch sizes are five to 12 eggs, depending on the genus. Eggs hatch following 20 to 27 days of incubation.[2] Grouse have strong beaks for cutting tough greenage.[37, 38] Many grouse species consume only one or two plant species during winter. Spruce grouse and capercaillies feed almost exclusively on conifer needles, black grouse on birch buds, and ptarmigans on buds from birch, alder, and willow trees. Sage grouse live mainly on the leaves and buds of the North American big sagebrush. Accordingly, the ceca and ventriculus are well developed. In capercaillies, it has been shown that birds in captivity (with more or less artificial diets) have intestinal flora more like that of chickens than that of free-raging specimens.[39] The tannins and essential oil content of the natural diet are assumed to allow an autochthonous intestinal flora free of Enterobacteriaceae, which is typical for all Tetraoninae.[40]

Captive grouse should receive as much natural feed as possible. A high percentage of crude fiber is important. Commercial poultry pellets should be limited. Turkey feeds can contain antiflagellates, which may be inhibitory to the cecal flora and life-threatening in species that depend on this function. Many grouse are unable to synthesize vitamin C because of sufficient content in the natural feed.

Grouse have no spurs. Many grouse species have red-colored supraocular comb-like structures that are swollen during mating display.[37, 38] Ornamental feathers develop from the chin feathers. Willow ptarmigan that live in a subarctic habitat molt three times a year, with the winter plumage being almost pure white. Capercaillies even molt the rhampho-theca of the beak piece by piece after the breeding season. Ptarmigans also replace their nails.[38] Grouse, like pheasants, are prone to shock or stress molt. The capercaillie has a looped elongated trachea.

Colibacillosis is the most common bacterial disease in grouse and is probably the result of malnutrition. Ulcerative enteritis is another problem in grouse. Capercaillies in their natural habitat have no demonstrable clostridia in their fecal flora.[40] *Clostridium perfringens* is the main agent in Europe. Vaccination with a human toxoid vaccine has been successful. For clinical signs and treatment, see the section on bobwhite quail. Grouse, particularly blue grouse, are susceptible to aspergillosis.[37]

Fowlpox has been described in blue grouse, sage grouse, black grouse, ruffed grouse, and prairie chickens. Vaccination with fowlpox vaccine is possible. A disease caused by a virus supposed to be an aviadenovirus with a course comparable to the marble spleen disease in pheasants has been observed in blue grouse. The virus so far has not been isolated. Clinical signs are apathy, rough plumage, foamy, watery feces, and sudden onset with acute mortality. Only a few birds show rales or other respiratory symptoms. Interstitial pneumonia, fibrinous pleuritis, and splenomegaly are the main lesions.[41]

Louping ill has been described in willow grouse, red grouse, rock ptarmigan, capercaillie, and black grouse. Whereas the latter two species, which live in woodlands and forests, react mildly to the infection with louping ill virus, the other three species with moorland and tundra as their habitat usually respond with central nervous system signs.[21]

Grouse are very susceptible to Newcastle disease, to which their reaction is similar to that of guineafowl. Only willow grouse react with conjunctivitis and impairment of general condition. Blindness is observed in black grouse and capercaillie when they are raised in the proximity of fowl chicks vaccinated against avian encephalomyelitis (Picornaviridae).

Grouse suffer from blackhead disease (refer to Turkeys) and coccidiosis.[2] For therapy, amprolium and ethopalat (Merck Sharp & Dohme) 6 ml/l drinking water or one of the various sulfonamides (2 g/l drinking water) are given. If birds refuse medicated water, give 0.4 ml sulfadimidine sodium (20%)/kg BW intramuscularly for 5 days.[37]

Guans and Curassows (Cracidae)

All cracid species (10 genera, 43 species) originate in the tropical forests of Central and South America. They are all endangered. Guans are active tree climbers and nest in trees. They are monogamous. Most lay only two eggs, which are incubated only by the hen for 28 to 30 days. In captivity guans are unreliable breeders. Artificial incubation appears to be successful, but no details are published. Chicks are ready to fly 3 to 4 days after hatching and are able to climb trees immediately.

Cracids are mainly vegetarians. They can be fed pellets with 21% crude protein and fruits, but no grains. During the breeding season the diet is supplemented with soybean paste, chopped meat and hard-boiled eggs, or mealworms.[42, 43]

Guans do not have spurs. Caruncles and helmets are developed in many species. The toes of the cracids are on the same plane. Many guans, particularly the helmeted curassow, have a looped trachea that extends almost to the cloaca before entering the thorax. The function of this tracheal development is not known, but it may be used for producing deep and loud voices. Two-thirds of the beak may be covered by the cere.[2] Guans do not have crops but have only a slight bulge in the esophagus.

Little is known about the diseases of cracids. They are susceptible to paramyxovirus-1-pigeon and develop a central nervous system disease resembling Newcastle disease.[44]

References

1. Spearman RIC, Hardy JA: Integument. In King AS, McLelland J (eds): Form and function in birds, vol. 3. London, Academic Press, 1985, pp 1–56.
2. Raethel HS: Hühnervögel der Welt. Melsungen, Neumann-Neudamm, 1988.
3. Franchetti DR, Klide AM: Restraint and anesthesia. In Fowler ME (ed): Zoo and Wild Animal Medicine. Philadelphia, WB Saunders, 1978, pp 303–304.
4. Calnek BW (ed): Diseases of Poultry, ed 9. London, Wolfe Publishing, 1991.
5. Heider G, Monreal G, and Mészáros J (eds): Krankheiten des Wirtschaftsgeflügels—Ein Handbuch für Wissenschaft und Praxis. Band I and II. Jena, Stuttgart, Gustav Fischer Verlag, 1992.
6. Pascucci S, Rinaldi A, Prati A, et al: CELO virus in Guineafowl: Characterization of two isolates. Proc 5th Int Congress WVPA, vol. II, 1973, pp 1524–1531.
7. Cowen BS: A case of acute pulmonary edema, splenomegaly, and ascites in Guineafowl. Avian Dis 32:151–156, 1988.
8. Guittet M, Picault JP, Bennejean G: Experimental soft shelled

9. Pascucci S, Misciratelli EM, Giovannetti L: Transmissible enteritis of Guineafowl: Electron microscopic studies and isolation of a Rotavirus strain. Proc 7th Int Congress WVPA, 1981, p 57.
10. Andral B, et al: Maladie foudroyante de la pintade: Recherche étiologique. LaPoint Veterinaire 19:515–520, 1987.
11. Fleury HJA, et al: Unidentified viral particles could be associated with enteritis of various commercial bird species. Ann Inst Pasteur/Virol 139:449–453, 1988.
12. Tányi J, Klaczinski K: Influenzavirus-A-Infection. In Heider G, Monreal G (eds): Krankheiten des Wirtschaftsgeflügels, ein Handbuch für Wissenschaft und Praxis. Jena, Stuttgart, Gustav Fischer Verlag, 1992, pp 669–682.
13. Kirev TT: Neoplastic response of Guinea Fowl to osteopetrosis virus strain MAV-2(0). Avian Pathol 17:101–112, 1988.
14. Maestrini N, Pascinci S: Amiloidosi nella gallina faraona. Atti della societa Italiana della Scienza Veterinarie 24:485–486, 1970.
15. Keller H: Hornringe am Sporn der Hühnervögel zur Altersbestimmung. Lebensmitteltierarzt 5:11, 1954.
16. Vollmerhaus B, Sinowatz F: Haut und Hautgebilde. In Nickel R, Schummer A, Seiferle E (eds): Lehrbuch der Anatomie der Haustiere. Band V. Anatomie der Vögel. Berlin, Verlag Paul Parey, 1992, pp 16–49.
17. Gerlach H: Infektionen durch Mollicutes bei Vögeln. In Gylstorff I (ed): Infektionen durch Mycoplasmatales. Infektionsifkrankheiten und ihre Erreger. Band 21 Jena, VEB Verlag Gustav Fischer, 1985, pp 448–491.
18. Hafez HM, Kruse K, Emele J, Sting M: Eine Atemwegsinfektion bei Mastputen durch pasteurella-ähnliche Erreger: Klinik, Therapie und Diagnostik. Potsdam, Proc DVG/WVPA Int Fachtagung Geflügelkrankheiten, 1993.
19. Spackman D, Cameron FRD: Isolation of infectious bronchitis virus from pheasants. Vet Rec 113:354–355, 1983.
20. Ritchie BW: A review of Eastern equine encephalomyelitis in pheasants. Assoc Avian Vet Today 1:152–154, 1987.
21. Reid HW, Buxton D, Pow F: Experimental Louping-ill virus infection of Black Grouse (*Tetrao tetrix*). Arch Virol 78:1983.
22. Dhillon AS, Wallner-Pendelton AE: Mortality in young pheasants and avian Influenza infection. Proc 35th West Poult Dis Conf, 1986, p 38.
23. Drén, Cs N, Sághy E, Glávits R, et al: Lymphoreticular tumours in pen-raised pheasants associated with reticuloendotheliosis-like virus infection. Avian Pathol 12:55–71, 1983.
24. Vollmerhaus B, Sinowatz F: Atmungsapparat. In Nickel R, Schummer A, Seiferle E: Lehrbuch der Anatomie der Haustiere. Band V. Berlin, Verlag Paul Parey, 1992, pp 159–175.
25. Logemann K, Bauer A, Bauer H-J: Vergleichende Untersuchungen zur Charakterisierung aviärer Adenoviren von Wachteln und Hühnern. München, DVG VII. Tagung Vogelkrht, 1990, pp 294–297.
26. Gough RE, Collins, MS, Alexander DJ, Cox WJ: Viruses and virus-like particles detected in samples from diseased game birds in Great Britain during 1988. Avian Pathol 19:331–342, 1990.
27. Pascucci S, Cordioli P, Giovannetti L, Gelmetti D: Characterization of a Coronavirus-like agent isolated from Coturnix Quail. Proc 8th Int Cong WVPA, Jerusalem, 1985, p 52.
28. Rinaldi A, Nardelli C, Pereira HG, Mandelli GC: Atti della Societa Italiana della Scienza Veterinariae 22:777–782, 1968.
29. Castro AE, Peter D, Webster RG, et al: Isolation and identification of a strain of avian Influenza Virus A/Quail/California/4794/90 (H4N6) antigenically similar to A/Duck/Czechoslo-

vacia/56 (H4N6) from a quail flock in California. Proc West Poult Dis Conf 1991, pp 42–44.

30. Carlson HC, Seawright GL, Pettit JR: Reticuloendotheliosis in Japanese Quail. Avian Pathol 3:169–175, 1974.

31. Johnsgard PA: The quails, partridges, and francolins of the world. Oxford, Oxford University Press, 1988.

32. Reed WM: Characterization of pox viruses isolated from recent outbreaks of avian pox. Proc West Poult Dis Conf [Suppl] 1991, pp 11–12.

33. Reed WM: Pathogenicity and immunologic relationship of quail and mynah pox viruses to fowl and pigeon pox viruses. Proc 37th West Poult Dis Conf 1988, pp 5–8.

34. Olson NO: A respiratory disease (bronchitis) of quail caused by a virus. Proc 54th Ann Meet US Lifst San Assoc 1950, pp 171–174.

35. Gerlach H: Gesundheitsprobleme bei farmmäBaig gehaltenen Virginischen Baumwachteln (Colinus virginianus). Tierarzt Prax 67:212–213, 1986.

36. Tham C, Gosyo M, Uwemura T: Cryptosporidiosis in quails. Avian Pathol 11:619–626, 1982.

37. Aschenbrenner H: RauhfuBahühner. Hannover, Verlag Schaper, 1985.

38. Johnsgard PA: The Grouse of the World. Croom Helm, University of Nebraska Press, 1983.

39. Schales C: Untersuchungen über die antibakterielle Wirkung ätherischer Öle und hydrophiler Inhaltsstoffe aus Koniferennadeln auf Bakterien aus dem Kot von in Gefangenschaft gehaltenen Auerhühnern (Tetrao urogallus L., 1758) in vitro. Diss Med Vet München, 1992.

40. Schales C: Untersuchungen über die aerobe Flora und Clostridium perfringens. im Kot von freilebenden und in Gefangenschaft gehaltenen Auerhühnern Tetrao urogallus L., 1758). Diss Med Vet München, 1992.

41. Gylstorff I: Adenoviridae. In Gylstorff I, Grimm F: Vogelkrankheiten. Stuttgart, Eugen Ulmer, 1987, pp 275–278.

42. Rüttgers A (ed): Enzyklopädie für den Vogelliebhaber.I.-if Band. Verlag "Littera Scripta Manet." Holland, Grossel, 1966–1970.

43. Lopez JE: The cracidae. Avic Mag 85:210–215, 1979.

44. Schneeganss D, Korbel R: Zum aktuellen Vorkommen aviärer Paramyxovirosen. Tierarztl Prax 16:156–160, 1988.

45. Wolters HE: Die Vogelarten der Erde. Hamburg, Berlin, Paul Parey, 1975–1982.

Helga Gerlach

55

Anatiformes

Anatiformes are cosmopolitan in distribution, except for the Antarctic. They colonize a wide variety of aquatic habitats. Taxonomy is controversial and often confused by hybridization (Table 55–1).[1–4]

GENERAL CHARACTERISTICS

The body shape is elongated and roundish, an adaptation to aquatic life. Walking on land is awkward. Male Anatiformes have a copulatory organ analogous to the mammalian penis that can be retrieved from the inner cloaca manually from the first day of life onward for sex determination. There are special designations for gender and offspring:

Female	Male	Chick or Juvenile
Goose	Gander	Gosling
Duck	Drake	Duckling
Swan	Cob	Cygnet

The bill is broad or conical with serrated lamellae inside that vary anatomically as an adaptation to feeding habits. The "nail," a shield-like formation at the tip of the upper bill, is used for grazing or catching mollusks. It has hundreds of sensory nerve endings, and its removal to inhibit feather-picking is cruel.

Anatiformes have strong, fully scaled legs. The hind toe may be reduced or elevated and the three forward toes are joined by webs. Wings are very strong because the bodies are relatively heavy. Pinioning is recommended for captive birds, and chicks should be pinioned during the first days of life.[5]

Anatiformes have a thick, well developed plumage with dense down that is carefully preened and oiled from the feather-tufted preen glands for waterproofing. Down feathers from domesticated geese, ducks, and eiders are used for making pillows and quilts. Most wild-ranging species molt their flight feathers simultaneously and become temporarily flightless until the new feathers have been hardened enough to sustain the body weight (3–4 weeks). All species have salt glands, although they are well developed only in birds living in brackish or sea water. The glands remove excess salt from the blood and excrete it as concentrated fluid dripping off the tip of the bill. Males have an osseous or cartilaginous bulla syringis of asymmetric and varying shape that functions as a tube for intensifying the voice.[6]

Chicks are nidifugous and leave the nest shortly after hatching. For proper husbandry, both adults and chicks need reliable sources of water and shelter with dry litter that enables the birds to sit with their abdomen on a dry surface. The litter must be changed or overstrewn regularly to remove defecation.

A peculiarity of Anatiformes is that prior to death central nervous system (CNS) abnormalities are frequently seen, which, upon histopathologic examination are found to be related to edema in the brain. It is therefore difficult to recognize specific CNS signs associated with a specific disease. Another peculiarity is the frequent development of amyloidosis in association with chronic infectious diseases.

Furan derivatives are rather toxic to Anatiformes. The mechanism is unknown, although reabsorption from the intestinal tract may approach 70 to 90%, compared with 7% in various mammals. The younger the birds, the more toxic the drug may

Table 55–1

NAMES OF BIRDS MENTIONED IN THE TEXT

Common Name	Scientific Name
American wigeon	Anas americana
Andean goose	Chloephaga melanoptera
Bewick's swan	Cygnus bewickii
Black swan	Chenopis atrata
Black-necked swan	Cygnus melancoryphus
Bar-headed goose	Eulabeia indica
Bufflehead	Bucephala albeola
Canada goose	Branta canadensis
Canvasback	Aythya valisineria
Cape Barren goose	Cereopsis novaehollandiae
Cinnamon teal	Anas cyanoptera
Comb duck (knob-billed duck)	Sarkidiornis melanotos
Common eider	Somateria mollissima
Common goldeneye	Bucephala clangula
Common pintail	Dafila acuta
Common shel duck	Tadorna tadorna
Common teal	Nettion crecca
Coscoroba swan	Coscoroba coscoroba
Crested fireback	Lophura ignita
Domesticated duck	Anas platyrhynchos var. dom.
Domesticated goose	Anser anser var. dom.
Egyptian goose	Alopochen aegyptiacus
European pochard	Aythya ferina
Freckled duck	Stictonetta naevosa
Goosander	Mergus merganser
Greater nene	Aythya marila
Greylag goose	Anser anser
Hawaiian goose	Branta sandvicensis
Magpie goose	Anseranas semipalmata
Mallard	Anas platyrhynchos
Mandarin duck	Dendronessa galericulata
Muscovy duck	Cairina moschata
Musk duck	Biziura lobata
Mute swan	Cygnus olor
Northern shoveler	Anas clypeata
Red head	Aythya americana
Ring-necked duck	Aythya collaris
Snow goose	Chen caerulescens
Spur-winged goose	Plectropterus gambensis
Swan goose	Anser cygnoides
Tufted duck	Aythya fuligula
White-fronted goose	Anser albifrons
Whooper swan	Cygnus cygnus
Wood duck	Aix sponsa

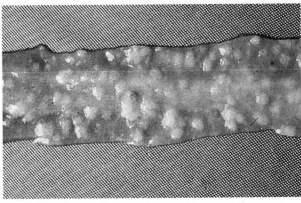

Figure 55–1

Chronic salmonellosis in the intestines of a goose.

BACTERIAL DISEASES

Bacterial diseases are similar to those of other avian groups (Fig. 55–1). *Clostridium botulinum* affects Anatiformes frequently. Botulism is a nutritional neurogenic intoxication caused by exotoxins (mainly type C but also A and E) of *C. botulinum*. Sources of the toxin are cadaverous proteinaceous feed including plants, fly maggots, and other invertebrates that are resistant to the toxin. Drought or flooding can enhance anaerobic conditions necessary for the propagation of *C. botulinum*. Toxic feed shows no change in smell or taste. Clinical signs include flaccid paralysis of the skeletal musculature including the tongue and the muscles of deglutition (Fig. 55–2). In addition, bulbar paralysis,

become. The application of therapeutic agents in feed or water is not recommended, because of the habit of ducks to dabble their food in water prior to swallowing. Intramuscular or subcutaneous administration of drugs is recommended, or a moistened medicated mash may be offered in the absence of water. Using medicated pellets is also possible.

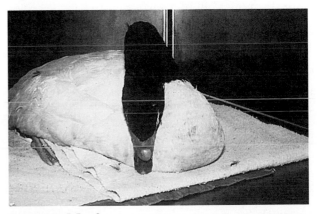

Figure 55–2

Flaccid paralysis of neck muscles associated with botulism in a black-necked swan.

loss of feathers, and diarrhea are seen. Severely ill birds die, but depending on the type and dose of the toxins, spontaneous recoveries occur. Diagnosis requires demonstration of the toxin. Toxin breaks down at room temperature; therefore, samples of feed, water, liver, and kidneys should be submitted frozen. *Aeromonas hydrophila* must be ruled out (refer to Geese). Treatment can be attempted in early cases by parenteral application of antitoxin and oral administration of a laxative such as sodium sulfate. Guanidine (30 mg/kg body weight [BW]) is supposed to counteract the effect of the toxins at the neuromuscular junction. For control carcasses are removed and waters kept aerated and at an even level.

Anatiformes can harbor *Vibrio* species, but mainly the NAG strains, which can cause only a mild intestinal disease in humans.[7] Borreliosis, caused by *Borrelia anserina* and transmitted by ticks, affects Anatiformes and several Phasianiformes. Affected birds are febrile and show anorexia, cyanosis, yellowish diarrhea, somnolence, ataxia, and paralysis. Morbidity is high, and mortality varies between 1 and 100%, depending on the host species. The course is prolonged, and affected birds show anemia and dyspnea. Serum albumin, alkaline phosphatase, total lipids, and cholesterol decrease, and aspertate aminotransferase increases.

Diagnosis can be carried out by Giemsa-stained blood smears or darkfield microscopy. Antibodies are present at between 4 and 30 days post infection. For treatment, tylosin and spectinomycin are recommended. Ticks are controlled by insecticides and the removal of bushes around aviaries and premises. In some tropical areas, strain-specific vaccines are available, which provide protection for about 1 year.

Anatiformes are highly susceptible to *Pasteurella multocida*, and the agent can survive in natural bodies of water for more than 1 year.[8] The conditions required for an enzootic outbreak are not yet known. Clinical signs are like those in other birds.[9, 10] Vaccination is recommended, according to the literature, although the results are not satisfactory, possibly because of the serovariability of the strains. Therapy with hyperimmune serum and antibiotics may be efficacious.[9, 10] Generally, diagnosis is made by culture results, and hygienic methods are used for control.

Duck septicemia (new duck disease) is caused by a member of the Cytophaga group named *Riemerella anatipestifer (Moraxella anatipestifer,* or *Pasteurella anatipestifer).*[11, 12] The host spectrum includes most Anatiformes, although domesticated ducks are most susceptible, and pheasants can be affected. The microorganism forms at least 19 serovars, serovars 1 to 3 being predominant in Europe, serovars 1, 2, and 5 in the US, and serovar 3 in Australia. The portal of entrance is the respiratory tract. Strain virulence and predisposing factors are variable. The egg-transferred disease causes high mortality. Peracute death is seen in ducklings at about 2 weeks of age (up to 75%). In acute cases, exudates from the nares and the conjunctiva, some coughing, and diarrhea are observed. Two days later, neurologic signs (tremor, ataxia) may develop. At necropsy, a fibropurulent polyserositis is characteristic and may serve as an indicator for the diagnosis. Isolation and identification require a specialized laboratory. Serologic flock control is possible via enzyme-linked immunosorbent assay (ELISA). Antibiotic therapy should start as soon as possible; in case of known egg transmission, therapy should begin within the first week of life before the onset of clinical signs. Experiments with vaccines have shown that the protection is serovar-specific. In contrast to Phasianiformes, where salpingitis is frequently caused by Enterobacteriaceae, in Anatiformes *P. multocida* and *P. anatipestifer* play an important role in enzootic outbreaks of the disease.[12]

VIRAL DISEASES

Avipox is occasionally seen in Anatiformes. Lesions can be recognized mainly on the webs between the toes. As a rule, only skin lesions occur and the birds survive spontaneously after some weeks. Vaccination with fowlpoxvirus does not fully protect all birds.

Duck plague (DP), also called duck virus enteritis, is caused by a herpes virus, occurs worldwide (possible exception, Australia), and infects wild as well as domesticated birds. The virus belongs to the alpha-Herpesviridae, is serologically uniform, and has no close relations to other members of the group. The disease is characterized by vascular damage resulting in tissue hemorrhage, free blood in body cavities, and typical lesions (band formation) in the digestive mucosa and lymphatic tissue.[9, 10]

Susceptibility is variable, but mallards, common teal, and common pintail ducks are the main reservoirs. The host spectrum includes the mute swan, black swan, black-necked swan, white-fronted goose, Canada goose, Egyptian goose, common shelduck, Muscovy duck, wood duck, Mandarin duck, American wigeon, canvasback, redhead, ring-necked duck, tufted duck, greater scaup, common eider, bufflehead, common goldeneye, and gosander.[13] Intermittent viral shedding in clinically healthy birds has been observed for 5 years. Outbreaks in duck farms have been traced to wild-ranging birds.[7] Once infected, domesticated stock can maintain the infection in the absence of wild birds.

The virus can be egg-transmitted but egg production ceases immediately in sick birds. Transovarially infected offspring usually die during the first 2 weeks of life. Clinically healthy survivors are partially immunotolerant and excrete large quantities of virus for up to 6 months. It is still unknown why in some farms DP may kill only single birds, whereas in others cases mortality may be up to 100%. The virus is infectious in water for 2 months at 4°C or 1 month at 22°C. Close connections can be observed between DP and climatic factors such as heat and cold, for example; tropical species are far more susceptible to disease in northern areas.

Clinical signs are peracute death without any signs; polydipsia, photophobia, nasal discharge, serous to hemorrhagic lacrimation, anorexia, cyanosis, and greenish, watery, occasionally hemorrhagic diarrhea, inability to fly, swimming in circles, and paralysis of the phallus. Convulsions or tremors of the neck and head muscles are observed rarely. Wild birds can be seen on the water with their neck and head in extreme extension. Mature birds generally show a more protracted course.[14] Differential diagnoses include the rare clinical forms of avian influenza, in ducklings duck hepatitis, and in goslings goose hepatitis. Diagnosis is by culture in embryonated chicken or duck embryos, chick embryo fibroblasts, or duck embryo fibroblasts. For viral identification and serologic screening virus neutralization is recommended. For control of the disease, wild Anatiformes must be excluded from the premises. Live attenuated vaccine strains are available.

Anatiformes are susceptible to Newcastle disease virus, but disease rarely develops. The birds are latently infected even with velogenic strains that propagate and are shed in geese for only 3 days. Spontaneous disease is without respiratory signs (except in geese). Disturbed mobility and local paresis may be seen. In geese, spontaneous drowning is typical. Ducks may develop CNS signs. Most species develop humoral antibodies, but some wild-living duck species are assumed to be refractory. For virus isolation, at least two to three passages are necessary. Vaccination is not necessary and not recommended.

Anatiformes are relatively resistant to avian influenza and are considered to be the natural reservoir.[15] About 25 to 30% of all free-ranging ducks and geese in the Northern Hemisphere carry avian influenza A virus (AIV) with a high variability of hemagglutinins and neuraminidases. Infected birds shed the virus from the fifth day post-infection for several weeks. Local replication of AIV takes place in the mucosa of the caudal intestinal tract. Many birds develop no humoral antibodies, which allows the conclusion that the antigen has had no contact with the cells of the immune system.[16]

Clinical signs occur following stressors (other infections, transport, etc.) and in growing birds. Poor condition, anorexia, dyspnea, swelling of the infraorbital sinuses, lacrimation, diarrhea, and, rarely, CNS signs are seen. Mortality can reach 40% during 3 weeks. For diagnosis, isolation of the virus is necessary.[9, 10] Vaccines are available but not recommended for Anatiformes.

Avian type C retrovirus group causes lymphoid leukosis in Anatiformes. Clinical signs and pathology are not essentially different from those of other avian species.[9, 10]

Chlamydia and *Rickettsia*

Chlamydia psittaci (ornithosis) usually results in latent infections in Anatiformes. Transmission is oral (rarely leading to disease), airborne (high dosage of a virulent strain is likely to develop disease), or vertical (only in ducks). In domesticated ducks and geese, conjunctivitis may be the only clinical sign, although ducklings can show a mortality rate between 10 and 80%.[17] Treatment includes tetracyclines (100 mg/kg BW), or enrofloxacin. In Europe, humans can become infected and diseased by duck strains, particularly in processing plants.

Rickettsia do not play a role, although anatiformes are known to be susceptible (Q-fever and *Aegyptianella pullorum*).[18, 19] Treatment is with tetracyclines.

For details of fungal infections, refer to Chapter 54, Galliformes. Subarctic species, such as eiders, are most susceptible to these infections.

Parasites

Flagellates (mainly *Chilomastix gallinarum*) cause listlessness, anorexia, ruffled plumage, diarrhea with whitish-yellow to bloody discharge, and emaciation particularly in growing birds. (For diagnosis, see Chapter 54, Galliformes.) For therapy, 50 mg metronidazole/kg BW (or another imidazole derivative) is recommended. Stable cysts produced by the agent ensure recurrences of the disease. Contamination of the premises or aviary is self-limiting if they are left unused for at least 3 weeks. The efficacy of disinfectants on the cysts is unknown. For other flagellates, refer to other textbooks.[9, 10]

Blood protozoa (*Plasmodium, Leucocytozoon, Trypanosoma,* and *Haemoproteus* species) are recognizable on blood smears stained according to Pappenheim, Giemsa, and other techniques. Infection can be expected in outdoor premises during the vector season. Anemia is seen with mass infections. (See Chapter 39.) Differentials include *Aegyptianella* (see Chapter 54, Galliformes) and borreliosis.

Coccidiosis is far less important than in gallinaceous birds, with the possible exception of renal coccidiosis in geese. *Eimeria boschadis* lives in renal epithelium of ducks, but is considered of low pathogenicity. *Tyzzeria* and *Wenyonella* occur.[10] Beware of prophylactic coccidiostats in chicken and turkey feed. Incompatibilities are known: halofuginone (Stenorol, Roussell) for geese and ducks, narasin (Monteban, Eli Lilly) for ducks, and nitrofuran (several producers) for ducks. Aprinocid (Aprocox, Merck Sharpe & Dohme) causes severe malformation of the bill in growing ducklings.[20] Ionophoric compounds should not be combined with sulfonamides, pleuromutilin, or erythromycin. Nothing is

known about coccidiosis and control or therapy in swans. The use of anticoccidial drugs in Anatiformes should not be encouraged unless careful studies on the compatibility in the species in question have been carried out.

Worm infestations are not as common as in captive gallinaceous birds. Because of the aquatic habitat, parasites with intermediate hosts in the biologic cycle occur more frequently.

For details on trematodes (*Bilharziella, Notocotylus, Catatropis;* Echinostomatidae; *Metorchis, Opisthorchis, Prosthogonimus*), refer to other textbooks.[9, 10] As a rule only heavy infestations lead to clinical disease. Eggs can be demonstrated in the feces (in most instances), but identification requires expertise.

Therapy for some of the parasites is unknown. Drugs active against trematodes in mammals are more likely to be efficacious against avian cestodes and vice versa. Niclosamide is toxic for geese. Rafoxanide (50 mg/kg BW) or praziquantel (10–40 mg/kg BW) may be tried. Control of intermediate hosts is vital. It may be necessary to keep birds seasonally off a natural body of water infested with infected intermediate hosts.

Anatiformes are infested with cestodes mainly of the Hymelolepidae.[9, 10] Clinical outbreaks are seen mainly in youngsters and with heavy parasitic loads. (For diagnosis and therapy, refer to Chapter 54, Galliformes, control as for trematodes.)

Nematodes of the genera *Capillaria, Thomix, Trichostrongylus,* and *Heterakis* can be found in Anatiformes, but only heavy infestations produce clinical disease.[9, 10] Nematodes of the genera *Amidostomum, Echinuria, Tetrameres,* and *Streptocara* live in the proventriculus, and can cause severe lesions even if their numbers are small to medium. *Amidostomum* and *Streptocara* destroy the koilin layer of the gizzard beginning at the junction between the gizzard and proventriculus. The inability to grind feed properly (mainly plant material) inhibits proper digestion and absorption from the intestinal tract causing stunting and emaciation.

Echinuria is found in the heavily mucus-covered mucosa of the proventriculus. The helminths are surrounded by connective tissue–forming nodules with the worms inside. Intermediate hosts are water fleas. Eggs do not survive the winter, and breeder birds are the source of infection for their offspring. Ducklings and goslings should be raised apart from mature birds.

Tetrameres invade the mucosa of the proventriculus. Males live on the surface of the mucosa. Females are transformed into bloody-red cyst-like forms that can be recognized best from the peritoneal surface of the proventriculus. The species mentioned with stomach disorders belong to the suborder Spirurina, and members of this suborder are difficult to treat because no effective drug is available. Fenbendazole can be tried. Control of the intermediate hosts depends on local circumstances.

Cyathostoma is a parasite of the main bronchi (analogous to *Syngamus* in gallinaceous birds). Clinical signs depend on the size of the birds and the number of worms (larvae). Treatment with ivermectin was unsuccessful in the Hawaiian goose.[21]

Acanthocephalosis by the genera *Polymorphus* and *Fillicollis* can cause disturbance of the nutritional reabsorption in the intestine by means of inflammatory processes originating from the attachment of the probosci to the mucosa. Diagnosis is by fecal sedimentation. Adult worms found on postmortem examination should be morphologically differentiated from cestodes. Therapy is still a problem; no controlled experiments have been reported with modern drugs.

Ectoparasites are far less common than in gallinaceous birds.

CHARACTERISTICS AND MAJOR DISEASES OF ANSERIFORMES FAMILIES

Ducks and Geese (Anatidae)

Ducks and geese constitute 69 genera and 151 species.

Magpie Geese (Anseranatidae)

Magpie geese (one genus, one species) live in Australia and southern New Guinea. They live on flood plains of tropical rivers, feeding on grass, seeds, bulbs, and roots, the latter two being dug up by use of the hooked bill. Magpie geese migrate according to feed and water availability. Polygamous colony nesting with one male mated to two females has been observed. The nest is a floating mound of vegetation. Clutch sizes of five to 11 eggs hatch after 23 to 25 days of incubation. Sexual maturity is reached in females after 2 years, in males after 3 to 4 years. Little is known on diseases.

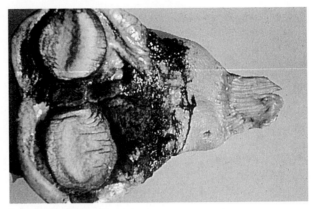

Figure 55–3

Typical hemorrhages undermining the koilin layer of the ventriculus associated with blood feeding of the parasite *Amidostomum anseris*.

Whistling Ducks (Dendrocygninae)

Most species (two genera, nine species) inhabit tropical and subtropical parts of the New World, East Asia, Australia, and Africa. Whistling ducks are nocturnal and perch in trees. They are generally monogamous and nest singly or in small groups in tree hollows, tree nests, or on the ground, depending on water levels. Clutch sizes are four to 16 (mean nine) eggs that hatch after between 24 and 36 days of incubation. In captivity the ducklings need dry litter beds to sleep on and protection from drafts. The feed consists mainly of greens supplemented in most species by invertebrates such as snails, worms, crustaceans, and larvae. Feeding is mainly by dabbling, rarely diving. Specific diseases affecting them are unknown.

Freckled Ducks (Stictonettinae)

Freckled ducks (one genus, one species) originate in southeast and southwest Australia. The bowl-shaped nest consists of woven twigs among reed beds or on water with a clutch of five to 10 eggs that are incubated for 26 to 31 days. They are mainly vegetarians and feed on algae, seeds, green parts of aquatic plants, and some invertebrates, mainly insects. Diseases affecting them are unknown.

Geese and Swans (Anserinae)

The Anserinae comprise 11 genera and 23 species. Geese inhabit the Northern Hemisphere, whereas swans are found in North and South America, Australia, and New Zealand. The greylag goose was domesticated in Europe and parts of Asia around the same time the swan goose formed the base for domesticated geese in East Asia. The latter is characterized by a large bill knob in both genders, a swan-like neck, and a more erect posture.

Many geese occupy subarctic regions, where they breed and during the winter migrate in large flocks south to aquatic habitats. Geese construct shallow nests lined with down feathers. Nests are located in depressions on the ground or above. The monogamous birds lay three to eight eggs that hatch after 21 to 30 days depending on the species.[2] Most pairs breed singly or in loose colonies. Geese are essentially vegetarians and feed on grass and aquatic plants. During winter migration they also eat roots, rhizomes, and grains from cultivated lands.

Swans have exceptionally long necks used for "upending" (bringing the body into a vertical position with the head underwater searching for feed). Most swans are monogamous and protect a territory year-round. The whooper swan migrates regularly in winter to more southern regions. Swans breed singly or in small groups. Their nests are constructed from plant material and situated on reedbeds and like habitats. Clutch sizes are four to nine eggs, which are incubated between 33 and 40 days. Swans are very aggressive during the breeding season. They are mainly vegetarians and feed on grass and aquatic plants (leaves, roots, stems) supplemented with invertebrates, larvae from insects, and fish spawn. Cygnets need higher protein feed than adults.

Geese and swans may show a knob-like protuberance on the upper bill temporarily or permanently in both sexes. The horny or fleshy tissue of the protuberance is covered by the cere and is smaller or absent in females.

The bar-headed goose lives at an altitude of 4000 to 5000 m and migrates in winter in lower regions. The Hawaiian goose has receded webs as an adaptation to the life on volcanic slopes at an altitude of 1500 to 2500 m. This species is not migratory, but is endangered in its natural habitat. Coscoroba

swans are unreliable breeders in captivity, abandoning their eggs if disturbed. Eggs may be fostered under chickens or turkeys. The goslings are difficult to raise. They need short fresh grasses and duckweeds (Lemaceae). Black-necked swans cannot be kept together with common shelducks because of aggression possibly resulting from similar coloration.

Some diseases of domesticated geese are included in other textbooks,[9, 10] particularly the problems with fattening geese, producing fat livers for liver pâté, and hybrid lines.

A nontuberculous form of mycobacteriosis is caused by *Mycobacterium avium* in geese. In most cases only the lungs display necrotic areas, which can be overlooked as a mycobacteriosis. Geese generally are more susceptible to pneumonia than other avian species. Erysipelas occurs in geese mainly during winter in aquatic habitats where the causative agent is surviving or even enriching. Clinical signs include sudden death, which may be preceded by somnolence, weakness, green droppings, or nasal discharge. In the rare chronic course, leather-like dermal patches (the agent is found only in these areas), serofibrinous arthritis, or valvular endocarditis may be found. Diagnosis is by examination of culture specimens. Serologic means are unreliable, because cell-mediated reactions are the main immunologic response. Pasteurellosis (fowl cholera) must be ruled out.[9, 10] The agent is sensitive to penicillin, and intramuscular injections are recommended (beware of procaine preparations, which may be toxic). Hyperimmune serum can be given simultaneously with the antibiotics. Adjuvanted vaccines are available, but they may merely sensitize the host, and provoke disease rather than protect after contact with field strains. Birds should be kept away from infected soil or water, and rodents must be controlled.

Wild-ranging swans and geese seem to be predisposed to infections with *Pseudomonas* species and *Aeromonas hydrophila*, particularly during the summer (rule out botulism). Both are considered secondary invaders, but because of their toxins, the host may die. Clinically, septicemia with toxic strains causes severe general signs combined with diarrhea, dyspnea, dehydration, and respiratory symptoms. Edematous or necrotizing lesions of the skin can be observed following trauma. Treatment can be tried with enrofloxacin or polymyxin B.

Captive geese and swans should be kept off natural bodies of water with temperatures exceeding 20°C.

In domesticated geese, *Actinobacillus* causes an egg-transmissible disease in goslings (stunting, arthritis, septicemia during the first week of life, and increased embryonic mortality), which has to be treated shortly after hatching with tetracyclines or other drugs according to sensitivity testing. The organism is difficult to culture; it requires blood agar plates and serum or blood in the media for biochemical tests.[22] *Haemophilus* species other than *H. paragallinarum* can cause rhinitis, hemorrhages, and jejunitis. Special culture methods are necessary for isolation.[9, 10] Sulfonamides are the drugs of choice. Additional vitamin A is recommended.

Three different serotypes of aviadenovirus have been recognized in goslings. The strains are related to FAV.[23] No clinical or pathologic lesions could be reproduced experimentally, but an inclusion body hepatitis with high mortality is described in goslings.[24] Adenovirus-like particles are seen in hepatocytes.

The causative agent of the goose parvovirus infection (also known as Derzsy's disease, or goose hepatitis) occurs in all major goose farming countries in Europe and Asia. The natural host is probably the domesticated goose, but the Canada goose, snow goose, and the Muscovy duck are also susceptible to the disease, whereas the cygnet of the mute swan can be infected experimentally. The virus is considered serologically uniform and is highly infectious. It is transmitted orally, nasally, or transovarially with freshly infected, nonimmune breeder geese. Latent infections in adult geese are epornitically important. It is a disease of goslings, the intensity, course, and mortality of which are governed by maternal immunity. There is a pronounced age resistance beyond the age of 4 to 6 weeks that is independent of maternal antibodies (half-life of the maternal antibodies is only 2.5–3 days).[25]

Goose parvovirus infection starts with anorexia and polydipsia followed by cessation of water intake and increased need for warmth. Conjunctivitis, diarrhea, and fibrinous material on the tongue may be seen at this point. Somnolence and giddiness occur prior to death (up to 100%). In older surviving birds, the down feathers fall off at various body regions, revealing reddened skin and swollen uropygial glands (Fig. 55–4). The more chronic course shows stunting, difficulties with standing and walk-

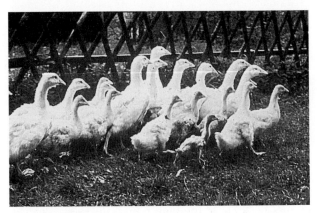

Figure 55–4

The small, naked geese are survivors of goose hepatitis and are the same age as the other geese in the flock.

ing, and occasionally convulsions. Ascites causes a penguin-like posture. If new feathers grow, they are rather brittle.[26–28]

Clinical and pathologic signs vary with age and immune status as well as by secondary invaders. Infections with orthoreovirus and "nephroenteritis" must be ruled out. Age, clinical signs, and pathology test results are indicative for diagnosis. For culture, geese or Muscovy duck embryos, or the respective fibroblasts are necessary. The virus replicates from the second passage onward also in chicken embryo rough cells, causing a cytopathic effect in the form of cellular syncytia. Cell cultures must be infected early because the virus needs propagating host cells for its own replication. Virus can be identified by virus neutralization, enzyme-linked immunosorbent assay (ELISA), or immunofluorescence (IF). Humoral antibodies appear 5 to 10 days post-infection and persist for approximately 1 year. Day-old goslings can be protected with subcutaneous injection of 1 ml reconvalescent serum.

To control the infection, vaccination of breeder geese at least 6 weeks before the beginning of egg production is recommended. An attenuated strain is available (apathogenic mutant) and must be given intramuscularly only. Breeder geese without humoral antibodies should be vaccinated twice. Booster vaccination may be necessary for the second half of the breeding season, depending on the number of eggs laid.

Infectious myocarditis in domesticated geese (and Muscovy ducks) is caused by an orthoreovirus.

Ducklings show no clinical signs, but the virus replicates in the intestinal tract. Goslings become sick at between 5 and 21 days of age (later age resistance). Sudden death, or somnolence, anorexia, increased water consumption, mild nasal discharge, conjunctivitis, dyspnea, and rarely watery grayish-whitish feces are observed. The body temperature decreases to 38°C. The skin at the bill and the feet peels off, weakness of the legs is caused by myositis, and occasionally paresis or tremor of the neck muscles occurs. Survivors are stunted.[29] Reo-chicken vaccines should only be tried in controlled experiments because of the high risk of disease.

The Canada goose is a carrier of California encephalitis virus, a member of the Bunyaviridae.[30]

Reticuloendotheliosis of the Twiehaus-type strain has been described in domesticated geese.[31] The disease starts around 17 weeks of age, and mortality approaches 40% by the end of the 22nd week. Clinical signs include listlessness, emaciation, ruffled plumage, and frequently lameness, but no CNS signs. On necropsy, the spleen and liver are usually diffusely enlarged, and histologic amyloidosis is seen occasionally.

Nephroenteritis of the domesticated goose is a disease of unknown etiology, although a virus is highly suspected.[26, 32, 33] Clinically, goslings seem to develop normally. The watery feces (often overlooked) at the onset of the disease are followed by certain weakness and malodorous, fibrinous, or bloody feces 8 to 10 hours before death (up to 100%). In natural outbreaks, peak mortality occurs between 18 and 21 days of age; however, in contrast to goose hepatitis and goose myocarditis, mortality in contact birds can be observed beyond 6 weeks of age. On necropsy, mucoid fibrinoid-necrotizing enteritis, hemorrhagic nephritis, and visceral gout are found. Diagnosis is confirmed by histopathology examination, and the disease can be reproduced with filtered tissues from kidneys and intestine.[33]

Mycoplasma and other mollicutes are important pathogens in geese. *M. gallisepticum* can be isolated from domesticated geese and Canada geese, *M. gallinarum* from domesticated geese and Bewick's swans, and *M. iners* and *M. synoviae* from domesticated geese, but they are not considered to be pathogenic.[34] A unidentified mycoplasma strain (nonpathogenic) has been isolated from a white-fronted goose.

Infections in domesticated geese with mixed cultures of mostly *M. cloacale*, but also *M. anseris* one unnamed taxon, and *Acholeplasma laidlawii*, cause cloacitis and inflammation of the phallus. Lesions of the phallus are characterized by a serofibrinous inflammation of the mucous membrane of the lymph sinus, the glandular part of the phallus, and sometimes the peritoneum and the cloaca. Necrosis of the phallus may be effected by secondary invaders. Mortality is less than 1%, but the incidence in a flock may be 40 to 100% of all ganders. Infertility and increased embryonic death result from this phallic disease. *Mycoplasma* species can be isolated from the phallic lymph, testes, spleen, air sacs, liver, and peritoneum.[35, 36]

A. axanthum is pathogenic in domesticated geese, causing embryonic death (up to 60%) around the 13th day of incubation. *A. axanthum* can be isolated from breeder flocks that have a high incidence of fibrinous salpingitis, peritonitis, and air sacculitis. Goslings hatched from infected flocks suffer from air sacculitis.[35] The pathogenicity of *A. axanthum* can be triggered by simultaneous infection with parvovirus, although there may be no clinical outbreaks of goose hepatitis.[37] Culture requires a specialized laboratory and use of a transport medium containing penicillin. No commercial antigens are available for serology testing. Tylosin or pleuromutilin, preferably in moistened soft feed, is recommended for therapy.

Eimeria truncata is the causative agent of renal coccidiosis in geese. Goslings are most susceptible. Clinical signs are depression, weakness, polyuria, polydipsia, dehydration, and anorexia. The birds may show vertigo and CNS signs prior to death. The tubuli are marked with pin-head sized, grayish-white foci containing the various forms of the endogenous biocycle. Oocysts can be found in the urine and in the ureters at necropsy. Survivors develop immunity to reinfection. For therapy only sulfonamides potentiated by pyrimidine derivatives are recommended, although generally sulfonamides because of their side effects are not given during kidney diseases. Some mortality is expected from therapy, depending on the severity of the disease.

Cape Barren Geese (Cereopsinae)

Cape Barren geese (one genus, one species) originate in southern Australia, where they enter water only during molt and while raising goslings. Breeder pairs live singly and defend a territory. The clutch of three to six eggs is incubated for 34 to 37 days. The birds are specialized grazers and feed on grasses, sedges, and other plants with high water content. Specific diseases are unknown.

Shelducks and Allies (Tadorninae)

Some members of this subfamily (seven genera, 14 species) are called "geese," others "ducks." They are distributed worldwide. The goose-like species are mainly vegetarians and have specialized habitats (the Andean goose lives at an altitude of >3300 m), whereas the duck-like members are omnivorous and live in brackish or salty water habitats.

Goose-like pairs are rather aggressive and defend a territory. Nests lined with down are built on the ground or in tree hollows. Clutch sizes are three to 12 eggs that are incubated for approximately 30 days.

The duck-like members form single pairs that build down-lined nests in old mammalian burrows, tree hollows, or on cliffs. Clutches contain six to 10 eggs, which hatch after 28 to 31 days of incubation. One specific disease is known, the visceral lymphomatosis of the common shelduck caused by an avian reticuloendotheliosis virus.[38] Clinical signs and pathology examination results resemble those of lymphoid leukosis in other avian species. Diagnosis is by histopathologic examination.

Spur-winged Geese (Plectropterinae)

Spur-winged geese (one genus, one species) occupy Central and South Africa but avoid arid and semi-arid regions. They carry a strong spur in the region of the elbow joint. Single pairs construct down-lined nests on the ground or in tree hollows. Geese lay six to 14 eggs that are incubated for 30 to 33 days. They are vegetarian and nocturnal. Specific diseases are unknown.

Ducks (Anatinae)

The subfamily (46 genera, 102 species) can be divided into five tribes and 46 genera. Adornments in the form of colored bare facial skin between bill and eye are shown during mating displays. Frontal knobs (fleshy protuberances covered by epidermis) and caruncles as well as colored bills are seen mainly in drakes and are used in the mating display. A distensible gular skin (very small in females) becomes turgid in drakes during display. The tribe aythyini are specialized divers. They are omnivorous and feed on water plants and aquatic invertebrates.[2, 3]

Many merganser species have "sawbills" with distinctly serrated lamellae to retain fish and other slippery feed components safely. They are also good divers but swim with their head underwater for catching prey. The ruddy ducks and stiff-tails have very pointed tails that are carried pointed forward close to the back while displaying.

Domesticated ducks are derived from mallards (*Anas platyrhynchos*-type) and Muscovy ducks (*Cairina*-type). The crosses, mullards, are infertile. Because Muscovy ducks are tropical birds, they are not adapted to cold and frostbite must be differentiated from exogenous staphylococcosis.[10]

Ducks infected with *Mycobacterium avium* may show lung lesions, as with geese, but a nontubercular form can also develop with or without ascites that can be overlooked on postmortem examination (among others, in the cinnamon teal). (For erysipelas, refer to Geese.) Salmonellosis can cause CNS signs in ducks, which result in swimming with an inverted keel ("keel disease"). Ducks are especially susceptible to *Salmonella* (Arizona strains) and frequently develop ocular lesions. Chronic *Yersinia pseudotuberculosis* causes tarsitis deformans in ducks, with yellow exudate in the joint cavity. Organic granulomas can also be found. Mycobacteriosis must be ruled out. Special cold enrichment is recommended for culture.[39]

Y. pseudotuberculosis is a competent pathogen for humans. (For *Pseudomonas* and *Aeromonas*, refer to Geese.) Muscovy ducks can suffer from *Haemophilus* infections other than that from *H. paragallinarum*, showing rhinitis and sinusitis. (For diagnosis and treatment, refer to Geese.)

An aviadenovirus group I (new serotype) is described as the cause of an epornitic infection in Muscovy ducks. Affected animals are lame and emaciated. Acute mortality starts at the age of about 35 days.[40] Tracheitis occasionally associated with bronchitis and pneumonia has been seen in about

10% of 2- to 3-week-old Muscovy ducklings that had adenovirus-like particles within the epithelial cells of the trachea.[41] Aviadenovirus group III seems to have an asymptomatic reservoir in various ducks in Europe and Asia. Domesticated geese and Muscovy ducks may also be infected.

Two different parvovirus strains cause disease in Muscovy ducklings, the agent of the goose hepatitis and a newly recognized taxon that is hardly pathogenic for geese. Clinically, Muscovy ducklings become ill at 6 weeks of age. They huddle together for warmth, are unable to walk, and drag their legs behind them. Enteritis can be seen, but in contrast to goose hepatitis, there is no feather loss. The main pathologic finding is hepatopathy. An inactivated vaccine was tried in the field in France.

Pekin ducks have been considered as a reservoir for the agent Hepadnavirus of the human B hepatitis. Meanwhile, it could be shown that ducks harbor only strongly host-specific avihepadnavirus, posing no danger to humans. The avihepadnavirus strains are distributed worldwide in commercial duck and goose farms. Generally, the infection causes no lesions. Transmission is vertical and leads to chronic viremia without production of humoral antibodies. Avian strains are less oncogenic than mammalian strains and need co-carcinogens such as mycotoxins. Avihepadnavirus is also known as a triggering factor for duck septicemia. In chronic infected birds the virus is directly demonstrable from the blood (titer 10^{11} particles per 1 ml serum).[42]

Orthoreovirus different from the myocarditis virus of geese is the causative agent of two rather similar diseases in Muscovy ducks. Growth inhibition and impaired development of the plumage is seen in 3-week-old ducklings. Mortality can approach 90%.[43] On necropsy, pericarditis and air sacculitis are the main lesions. The other disease causes liver necrosis in Muscovy ducklings between 10 days and 6 weeks old. Experimentally infected domesticated geese and Pekin ducks do not succumb to disease.

The ducklings of mallards and domesticated ducks are susceptible to disease following natural infections with the virus of Eastern or Western equine encephalomyelitis only during the first 18 days of life.

The rhabdovirus causing rabies has been isolated from ducks.[44] Clinical signs begin with a short excitable period during which jumping, crying, trying to flee, aggressiveness toward humans, and epileptiform convulsions can be observed. About 24 hours later ataxia, weakness of the limbs, falling on the flanks, and later flaccid paresis (including the head and neck) can be seen. Two weeks afterward, somnolence, apathy, compulsive movements, and death or spontaneous healing can occur.[45] Negri bodies are not found regularly. Diagnosis requires specialized laboratories (and vaccination of the personnel).

Avian reticuloendotheliosis virus (REV) can cause several diseases in ducks that are diagnosed by histopathologic examination. For isolation and identification of these strains, specialized laboratories are necessary. The Twiehaus-type strains affecting chickens are transmissible to ducks, which show nonspecific signs such as apathy and ruffled plumage. Mortality can approach 25%. Tumors can be found in the heart, skeletal muscles, and many other internal organs.[38]

Duck infectious anemia is transmitted by *Plasmodium lophurae*, one of the avian malaria agents (its main host is the crested fireback). The disease is rare and non-neoplastic.[46] The anemia can be severe and is frequently fatal, even if the *Plasmodium* infection has been treated successfully. The virus can be neutralized by antiserum.

Duck spleen necrosis virus is transmitted by direct contact. After a 7- to 10-day incubation period, affected ducks show apathy and anorexia followed rapidly by death. On necropsy, hemorrhages and splenic necrosis are the main lesions.

An unclassified REV-like virus is considered the causative agent of a neoplastic disease in 6-month-old Muscovy ducks.[47] About 10% of the flock died within 1 week. After 1 year a new outbreak coinciding with the new laying period was observed. In blood smears from sick birds, large numbers of undifferentiated blast cells, assumed to be of the lymphatic series, were prominent. On necropsy, tumors of the thymus were seen at a rate of 40%, but other organs are involved as well.[47]

Duck virus hepatitis can be divided into three types. Type I, a member of the Picornaviridae, is distributed worldwide causing high mortality (up to 100%) in domesticated ducklings during the first week of life. Chicks die showing no clinical signs. A distinct age resistance (3–6 weeks) is seen, but young birds can be protected by maternal antibodies. In Europe, where chlamydial infections in ducks are endemic, the typical course of the disease may be altered because *C. psittaci* can overcome immunity to duck hepatitis in ducklings older than 4 weeks. The liver is no longer the main locus of lesions. Duck fatty kidney syndrome and focal pancreatic necrosis are part of the disease.[48] Mallard ducklings are susceptible to infection but show no signs of illness. The virus has been isolated from a variety of ducks in zoo collections, but has not proved to be the cause of death. The virus does not seem to be uniform; two variant strains are described. Vaccines for breeder flocks are available. Freshly hatched ducklings can be treated with reconvalescent serum. A live avirulent vaccine can also be used in ducklings in the face of an outbreak.[49]

Type II has so far occurred only in East Anglia, UK. In contrast to types I and III, it is an astrovirus (antigenically different from chicken and turkey strains), and may cause 10 to 50% mortality in ducklings, depending on the age. All reported outbreaks concern birds kept in open fields, and free-ranging birds are suspected to be the vectors.[49] Type III is caused by a picornavirus and has only been isolated in the US. The disease is less severe than type I, and losses range around 30%. Ducklings of the *Anas*-type have been the only susceptible species to date.[49]

M. gallisepticum and *M. synoviae* are considered nonpathogenic in ducks. *M. cloacale* can be isolated from the domesticated duck, tufted duck, European pochard, and Muscovy duck, but the typical lesions as in geese are not known in these ducks. *M. anatis* (nonpathogenic for geese) is supposed to cause rhinitis, sinusitis, and air sacculitis in domesticated ducks, the greater scaup, common and other teals, and common shoveler. However, experimental investigation shows that this is only the case if the infection is triggered by influenza A virus.[50, 51] In ducks, at least seven other *Mycoplasma* strains are known and may cause mild respiratory signs. *M. anatis* associated with influenza virus may cause morbidity of between 50 to 80%, but mortality is below 5%. Affected ducklings usually recover spontaneously, without therapy. But most of the strains described cause increased embryonic mortality.

References

1. Wolters HE: Die Vogelarten der Erde. Hamburg, Berlin, Paul Parey, 1975–1982.
2. Carboneras C: Anseriformes. In Handbook of the Birds of the World, vol I. Barcelona, Lynx Edicions, 1992, pp 536–628.
3. Rüttgers, A: Enzyklopädie für den Vogelliebhaber. I. Band. Verlag Littera Scripta Manet. Holland, Gorsel, 1966–1970.
4. Wobeser GA: Diseases of Wild Waterfowl. New York, Plenum Press, 1981.
5. Franchetti DR, Klide AM: Restraint and anesthesia. In Fowler ME (ed): Zoo and Wild Animal Medicine. Philadelphia, WB Saunders, 1978.
6. Vollmerhaus B, Sinowatz E: Atmungsapparat. In Nickel R, Schummer A, Seiferle E: Lehrbuch der Anatomie der Haustiere. Band V, 2. Auflage, Berlin, Paine Parey, 1992, pp 165–166.
7. Bisgaard M, Kristensen KK: Isolation, characterization and public health assets of Vibrio cholera NAG isolated from a Danish duck farm. Avian Pathol 4:271–276, 1975.
8. Bredy JP, Botzler RG: The effects of six environmental variables on Pasteurella multocida populations in water. J Wild Dis 25:232–239, 1989.
9. Calnek BW (ed): Diseases of Poultry, ed 9. London, Wolfe Publishing, 1991.
10. Heider G, Monreal G, Mészáros J: Krankheiten des Wirtschaftsgeflügels. Ein Handbuch für Wissenschaft und Praxis. Band I + II. Jena, Stuttgart, Gustav Fischer Verlag, 1992.
11. Piechulla K, Pohl S, Hannheim W, et al: Phenotypic and genetic relationships of so-called Moraxella (Pasteurella) anatipestifer to the Flavobacterium/Cytophaga group. Vet Microbiol 11:281–270, 1986.
12. Bisgaard M: Salpingitis in web-footed birds. Prevalence, etiology and possible pathogenesis. Proc DVG/WVPA Internationale Fachtagung Geflügelkrankheiten, Potsdam, 1993.
13. Weingarten M: Entenpest: Klinik, Diagnose, Bekämpfung, VI. München, DVG, Tagung Vogelkrht, 1988, pp 197–203.
14. Leibovitz L: Duck virus enteritis (duck plague). In Calnek BW (ed): Diseases of Poultry, ed 9. London, Wolfe Publishing, 1991, pp 609–618.
15. Ottis K, Badmann PA: Isolation and characterization of ortho- and paramyxovirus from feral birds in Europe. Zentralbl Vet Med [B] 30:22–35, 1983.
16. Kosters J: Personal communication, 1993.
17. Strauss J: Microbiology and epidemiologic aspects of duck ornithosis in Czechoslovakia. Am J Ophthalmol 63:1246–1259, 1967.
18. Gothe R, Kreier JRP: Genus II. Aegyptianella (Carpano, 1929). In Bergey's Manual of Systematic Bacteriology, vol 2. Baltimore, Williams & Wilkins, 1986, pp 722–723.
19. Gylstorff I: Rickettsiales. In Gylstorff I, Grimm F: Vogelkrankheiten. Stuttgart, Verlag Eugen Ulmer, 1987, p 317.
20. Siebentritt M: Die Wirkung von Aprinocid 9-[(2-chlor-6-fluorphenyl)-methyl]-9H-purin-6-amin auf die Entwicklung junger Enten (Anas platyrhynchos var. domestica). München, Diss Med Vet, 1982.
21. Gassmann-Duvall R: An acute Cyathostoma bronchialis outbreak in the Hawaiin Goose and other parasitic findings. Proc 1st Int Conf Zoo Avian Med, Oahu, 1987, pp 61–68.
22. Gerlach H: Infection with the so-called Haemophilus septicaemiae anseris in geese. Proc VIIth Int Congress WVPA, Oslo, 1981, p 80.
23. Zsak L, Kisary J: Characterization of adenoviruses isolated from geese. Avian Pathol 13:253–264, 1984.
24. Riddell C: Virus hepatitis in domestic geese in Saskatchewan. Avian Dis 28:774–782, 1984.
25. Schettler CH: Virus hepatitis of geese. 3. Properties of the causal agent. Avian Pathol 2:179–193, 1973.
26. Schettler CH: Die Virushepatitis der Gänse. München, Vet Hab Schrift, 1973.

27. Gylstorff I: Derzsy's Krankheit—Hepatitis der Gänse. In Gylstorff I, Grimm F: Vogelkrankheiten. Stuttgart, Verlag Eugen Ulmer, 1987, pp 279–280.

28. Gough RE: Goose parvovirus infection. In Calnek BW (ed): Diseases of Poultry. London, Wolfe Publishing, 1991, pp 684–690.

29. Gylstorff I: Reoviridae. In Gylstorff I, Grimm F: Vogelkrankheiten. Stuttgart, Verlag Eugen Ulmer, 1987, pp 257–259.

30. Gerlach H: Vögel als Reservoire und Verbreiter von Krankheitserregern. Ber. Münch. Tierarztl. Wochenschr 92:169–173, 1979.

31. Drén Cs N, Németh I, Sári I, et al: Isolation of a reticuloendotheliosis-like virus from naturally occurring lymphoreticular tumours of domestic goose. Avian Pathol 17:259–277, 1988.

32. Bernath S, Szalai F: Investigations for clearing the etiology of the disease appeared among goslings in 1969. I. Animal infection experiments. Az Allatgyogyaszath oltoanya-gellenörzö intezet Evkönyve, 1968–1972, Budapest, 1972, p 38.

33. Trötschel, A.: Pathomorphologie der akuten Form der Nephro-Enteritis der Junggänse. München, Diss Med Vet, 1973.

34. Buntz B, Bradbury JM, Vuillaume A, Rousselot-Paillet D: Isolation of Mycoplasma gallisepticum from geese. Avian Pathol 15:615–617, 1986.

35. Stipkovits L, El-Ebeedy AA, Kisary J, Varga L: Mycoplasma infection in geese. I. Incidence of Mycoplasmas and Acholeplasmas in geese. Avian Pathol 4:35–43, 1975.

36. Varga ZS, Stipkovits L, Dobos-Kovacs M, Czifra G: Biochemical and serological study of two Mycoplasma strains isolated from geese. Arch Exper Vet Med 43:733–736, 1989.

37. Kisary J, El-Ebeedy AA, Stipkovits L: Mycoplasma infection in geese. II. Studies on pathogenicity of mycoplasmas in goslings and goose and chicken embryos. Avian Pathol 5:15–20, 1976.

38. Gylstorff I: Retroviridae. In Gylstorff I, Grimm F: Vogelkrankheiten. Stuttgart, Verlag Eugen Ulmer, 1987, pp 259–260.

39. Gerlach H: Diagnose der Pseudotuberkulose bei lebenden Vögeln. München, DGV-Tagung Vogelkrht, 1979, pp. 76–101.

40. Bouquet JF, Moreau Y, McFerran JB, and Connor TJ: Isolation and characterization of an Adenovirus isolated from Muscovy ducks. Avian Pathol 11:301–307, 1982.

41. Bergmann V, Heidril R, Kindes E, et al: Pathomorphologisch und elektronenmi kroskopische Feststellung eimner Adenovirus-Tracheitis bei Moschusenten (Cairina moschata). Mh Vet Med, 40:313–315, 1985.

42. Will H, Kaleta EF: Hepatitis-B-Virus-Infektion der Enten. In Heider G, Monreal M, Mészáros J (eds): Krankheiten des Wirtschaftsgeflügels. Stuttgart, Gustav Fischer Verlag Jena, 1992, pp 361–367.

43. Gaudry D, Tektoff J: Essential characteristics of three viral strains isolated from Muscovy Ducks. 5th Intkong WVPA, 1973, pp 1400–1405.

44. Kronberger HH, Schüppel KF: Ergebnisse der postmortalen Untersuchungen von 4000 Vögeln. 14th Int Symp Erkrankungen d Zootiere, Wroclaw, 1972, pp 85–87.

45. Gylstorff I: Rhabdoviridae. In Gylstorff I, Grimm F: Vogelkrankheiten. Stuttgart, Verlag Eugen Ulmer, 1987, pp 256–257.

46. Ludford CG, Purchase GH, Cox HW: Duck infectious anemia virus associated with Plasmodium lophurae. Exp Parasitol 31:29–38, 1972.

47. Malkinson M: An outbreak of an acute neoplastic syndrome accompanied by undifferentiated leukemia in a flock of Muscovy Ducks. Proc 31st West Poult Dis Conf, 1982, p 110.

48. Farmer H, Chalmers WSK, Woolcock PR: Aspects of the pathogenesis of duck viral hepatitis. Proc 8th Int Cong WVPA, Jerusalem, 1985, p 38.

49. Woolcock PR, Fabricant J: Duck virus hepatitis. In Calnek BW (ed): Diseases of Poultry. London, Wolfe Publishing, 1991, pp 597–608.

50. Bencina D, Dorrer D, Tadina T: Mycoplasma species from six avian species. Avian Pathol 16:653–664, 1987.

51. Poveda JB, Carranzs J, Miranda A, et al: An epizootiological study on avian mycoplasma in Southern Spain. Avian Pathol 19:627–633, 1990.

Glenn H. Olsen
James W. Carpenter

56

Cranes

Long-legged, long-necked cranes (order Gruiformes, family Gruidae) live throughout the world with the exception of Central and South America, Oceania, and Antarctica, and are one of the oldest bird species. Of the 15 species in the Gruidae family, nine species or subspecies are endangered (Appendix I, Convention on International Trade in Endangered Species of Wild Fauna and Flora, 50 CFR 23.23, Feb. 20, 1990). Two species of cranes native to North America, the whooping crane *(Grus americana)* and the sandhill crane *(Grus canadensis)*, may be encountered in wildlife rehabilitation work. Whooping crane numbers were reduced to 15 birds in 1942, but through concerted efforts of conservationists, they have increased to about 250 today, 150 in the wild, the remainder in captive breeding programs. There are six subspecies of sandhill cranes: Canadian, greater, lesser, Florida, Mississippi, and Cuban, with the last two considered endangered.

The whooping crane stands over 1¼ m high and has a wing span of 2½ m. The sandhill crane is generally smaller, standing 1 m high with a wing span of 2 m. Cranes, heavier than herons (order Ciconiiformes), fly in a **V** formation, with their necks and legs extended, similarly to geese. Once they have attained altitude, cranes make extensive use of thermals and gliding flight. The color of a crane's plumage ranges from black through various shades of gray to startling white. They have a stately walk, moving with three toes facing forward, while their tertial wing feathers tuft out over their rump. Many crane species expand or contract vivid red, warty skin on the head or face to indicate various behavioral moods. Their convoluted trachea makes a loop within the sternum, allowing them to make loud, piercing or bugling calls. This looping trachea occurs only in cranes and swans (Anatidae subfamily Cygninae). Coupled with their exceptional height, cranes have a powerful beak, which they frequently use as a weapon of self-defense. In addition, some cranes jump up and lash out with their feet, causing injuries with the sharp nails on their innermost toes. During restraint, a crane may struggle and injure itself, or a handler, with the sharp nails.

Numerous successful captive crane breeding programs exist, and there has been increasing interest in crane management and husbandry. Cranes can live 50 years or more in captivity. The propagation of cranes succeeds through appropriate health monitoring and disease and parasite control procedures. This involves routine observations and clinical examinations of the birds with the initiation of prophylactic or therapeutic medication when indicated. The veterinarian needs to know the clinical pathology of cranes, chemical restraint procedures, surgical procedures, and common diseases. Of utmost importance to a high-quality crane breeding and management program is the design and implementation of a preventative health program.

HOUSING

Cranes generally adapt well to captivity, and even wild-caught cranes have adjusted to pen situations. Chicks are extremely aggressive and are generally held separately until they are juveniles, when they can be socialized as a group. However, as cranes mature (2–5 years, depending upon the species), they form pairs and aggressively defend their territory against former penmates. Therefore, adults are best housed only as mated pairs. At the authors' center (Patuxent Environmental Science Center, Laurel, MD), adult cranes breed in large chain-link enclosures (9 × 18 m). A fence that is 2.1 m high can prevent the escape of flight-restrained birds. Fully flighted birds can be kept in pens that are 2.4 m high and are covered with nylon netting. Pens need to have a shelter for the feed container, a shade shelter, and a source of fresh water. Cranes learn to drink from a bucket, water cup, or water trough, but may prefer a wet area such as a small pond as a water source, a place to bathe, an area to probe for food, and a place for protection from predators. Unfortunately, shallow ponds in captive environments lead to fecal contamination, and parasite control is difficult.

In northern climates, provide indoor facilities for cranes during the coldest part of the winter, although cranes tolerate snow and cold weather quite well if open water and shelter from the wind are provided. Smaller crane species and those from tropical climates require the greatest protection in cold climates because frostbitten feet can be a problem in these areas.

DIET

Cranes eat various foods ranging from grains and peanuts to fish, amphibians, rodents, mollusks, and insects. Feeding a natural diet to cranes in captivity has proved impractical, leading to the development of commercially formulated diets.[1, 2]

Feed crane chicks a starter diet of 24% protein, 5% fat, and not more than 6% fiber, from hatching until they are 40 to 50 days old, or until their primary feathers are fully emerged. Reduce the sulfur-containing amino acids (methionine and cysteine) in the starter diet to levels of 0.7%. Without this reduction in sulfur-containing amino acids, crane chicks in captivity, especially those raised by hand, grow too rapidly and develop deformities in their limbs. As the chicks mature, a maintenance diet of 14% protein and 3.5% fat supplies the cranes' energy needs, especially during the cooler months of the year. Two months before breeding, cranes start egg production, and they are given a breeder diet containing a higher protein level (22%), plus additional calcium (3% as compared with 1.4% in the

starter diet and 0.8% in a maintenance diet). Vitamin supplements are added to all three diets, but levels are higher in the starter and breeder diets than in the maintenance diet (Table 56–1).

BLOOD COLLECTION

Collect blood samples from either the right jugular or the medial metatarsal vein. Hold the bird securely to prevent struggling and collect the sample rapidly. Cranes have died when the jugular vein was accidentally lacerated during venipuncture procedures. Blood is not commonly obtained from the ulnar or brachial veins because of difficulties encountered in restraining all but sedated or the most feeble cranes in a position appropriate to obtain a sample. Normal hematologic values are summarized in Table 56–2. Methodology and characteristics of crane hemograms have been previously discussed.[3, 4]

T a b l e 5 6 – 1

CRANE DIETS*

	Diet		
Calculated Analysis	**Starter (Crumble or Pellet)**	**Maintainer (Pellet)**	**Breeder (Pellet)**
Protein %	23.8	15.0	22.0
Metabolizable energy (kcal/kg)	2689.0	2873.0	2677.0
Methionine and cysteine (%)	0.7	0.6	0.8
Lysine %	1.3	0.7	1.2
Calcium %	1.4	0.8	3.0
Phosphorus	0.9	0.5	0.8
Niacin (mg/kg)	66.0	22.0	66.0
Riboflavin (mg/kg)	11.0	3.3	4.4
Menadione (mg/kg)	2.2	2.2	3.3
Biotin (mg/kg)	0.22	0.11	0.11
Folic acid (mg/kg)	4.4	1.1	2.2
Insitol (mg/kg)	138.0	137.5	137.5
Ethoxyquin (mg/kg)	125	125	125
Vitamin B_{12} (mg/kg)	0.0066	0.003	0.009
Ascorbic acid (mg/kg)	110	110	110
Para-aminobenzoic acid (mg/kg)	22	22	22
Choline (mg/kg)	440	250	250
Vitamin A (IU/kg)	16,500	6630	6630
Vitamin D_3 (IU/kg)	1650	1320	1650
Alpha-tocopheroyl IU/kg	11	22	33
Manganous oxide (mg/kg)	375	166	166
Iron carbonate (mg/kg)	99.0	83.3	83.3

Data from Zeigler Bros., Inc., PO Box 95, Gardners, PA 17324.
*Diets formulated and fed to cranes at various stages in their life cycle. Pellets are 5 mm diameter, 7 mm long (³⁄₁₆-inch commercial pellet).

Table 56-2

HEMATOLOGIC AND SERUM BIOCHEMICAL REFERENCE RANGES FOR CAPTIVE SANDHILL AND WHOOPING CRANES

Measurement	Sandhill Crane		Whooping Crane	
	Mean	Range	Mean	Range
Hematology				
Packed cell volume (%)	43	37–49	42	38–48
Hemoglobin (g/dl)	13.5	10.5–18.7	14.4	13.0–16.7
Red blood cells ($\times 10^6/\mu l$)	2.5	1.9–3.3	2.2	1.8–2.6
White blood cells ($\times 10^3/\mu l$)	13.0	6.2–22.6	18.2	12.2–25.1
Chemistry				
Albumin (g/dl)	1.5	1.0–4.5	1.5	1.2–1.7
Albumin/globulin	0.63	0.38–1.32	0.65	0.57–0.76
Alkaline phosphatase (U/L)	164	34–423	46	28–72
Alanine aminotransferase (ALT) (U/L)	50	19–162	53	42–71
Aspartate aminotransferase (AST) (U/L)	181	16–260	261	133–612
Calcium (mg/dl)	9.7	8.8–10.9	9.1	8.3–9.7
Chloride (mEq/L)	108	101–115	107	102–113
Cholesterol (mg/dl)	128	87–187	148	96–200
Creatinine (mg/dl)	0.7	0.4–1.2	0.6	0.4–0.8
Globulin (g/dl)	2.3	1.8–3.4	2.3	1.8–2.8
Glucose (mg/dl)	247	87–323	232	210–267
Lactic dehydrogenase (U/L)	278	108–488	440	178–975
Phosphorus (mg/dl)	3.6	1.7–5.4	2.8	2.0–4.1
Potassium (mEq/l)	3.4	2.2–4.8	3.4	2.6–4.2
Protein, total (g/dl)	3.9	2.9–7.9	3.8	3.1–4.4
Sodium (mEq/L)	148	142–160	147	140–152
Uric acid (mg/dl)	9.7	4.1–24.6	8.1	6.5–10.2

From Carpenter JW: Cranes (Order Gruiformes). In Fowler ME (ed): Zoo and Wild Animal Medicine. Philadelphia, WB Saunders, 1986, pp 315–326.

DISEASES AND MANAGEMENT OF CRANE CHICKS

Reproduction

Wild cranes normally lay two eggs in a ground or floating nest built with dead vegetation (Fig. 56–1). The precocial young hatch in about 30 days. Often the young are extremely aggressive toward their siblings, which can result in the death of one or both chicks. As the chicks fledge, this aggressive tendency disappears, and cohorts of immature cranes form during the winter and spring.[5]

In captivity, cranes can be induced to mate, nest, and rear young. Large cranes (whooping cranes and greater sandhill cranes at the author's center, for example) are frequently incapable of mating if not fully flighted. If a crane's wing is crippled from an injury or because of previous flight-restraining

surgery (such as tenectomy), it still may be possible to use the crane in a breeding program by artificial insemination. The crane pair can incubate their own eggs, or the eggs can be given to a surrogate crane pair or moved to a mechanical incubator. Although mechanical incubators are successful, parental incubation is better. Artificial incubation is most successful at a temperature of 37.35°C (99.15°F) and a relative humidity of 57%.

Hatching takes 12 to 24 hours from pipping to breaking free. The newly hatched chick requires several hours to dry and gain strength. Generally, a chick remains relatively immobile and close to the nest for the first day or two. Crane chicks do not feed well for the first 2 to 3 days, relying instead on their yolk sac. The typical chick may lose 10% of its hatch weight during its first 3 days. In the wild or with chicks being reared by parent cranes, the adult birds (especially the female) coax the chick and offer it pieces of food. Cranes reared by hand do better if they are frequently (sometimes hourly) offered food until they begin eating on their own.

To avoid imprinting hand-reared crane chicks on people, two methods are commonly used. In the first, the chick is exposed to a taxidermy brooder model made from a dead crane and a puppet head also made from the head and neck of a crane (Fig. 56–2). The person working with the puppet head

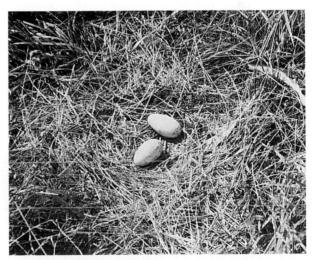

Figure 56–1

Typical sandhill crane nest. Cranes are provided with clean straw to build the nest. In the wild, plant material for nests is readily obtained in marshes or wet meadows where cranes typically nest.

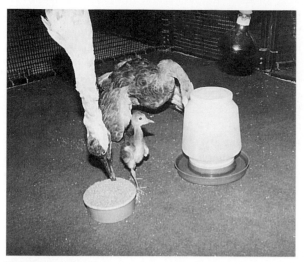

Figure 56-2

Hand-rearing a young sandhill crane with a brood model (with heat lamp placed above it) and a feeding puppet on a string worked from outside the enclosure.

hides behind an opaque screen to minimize human contact. In the second rearing technique, the person providing for the chick dresses in a costume (gray for sandhill cranes, white for whooping cranes) and works with the chick directly in the pen (Fig. 56–3). With both techniques, crane chicks are exposed to conspecific adults in an adjacent pen to ensure proper imprinting. Crane chicks raised by screened handlers have proved suitable as captive breeders or for exhibit. Crane chicks reared by costumed personnel have been successfully released into the wild.

Exteriorized Yolk Sac

At hatching, the medical problem seen most frequently (3% of hatching chicks at the authors' center) is an exteriorized yolk sac. The degree of exteriorization varies; however, treatment remains essentially the same. Clean the yolk sac with povidone iodine (1%) solution and then gently manipulate it into the abdominal cavity using cotton-tipped applicators moistened with saline. Once the yolk sac is completely within the abdomen, close the umbilicus with 4–0 polyglycolic acid suture in a simple interrupted or pursestring pattern. Occasionally the yolk sac cannot be manipulated back into

the abdomen or the umbilicus has started to seal, creating a necrotic yolk sac remnant. In either case, tie a ligature around the yolk sac close to the umbilicus and allow the necrotic piece to fall off or remove it. Maintain chicks with yolk sac problems on antibiotics (gentamicin 5 mg/kg twice a day [q12h]), and keep the area clean with applications of a povidone iodine solution (1%) two or three times daily for up to 5 days. Chicks with umbilical problems must be reared alone because other chicks may peck at an exposed yolk sac remnant or surgical site. Chicks with yolk sac problems must be carefully monitored for lethargy or weakness, which may indicate omphalitis. Occasionally, omphalitis develops even in chicks without exposed yolk sacs, and it is often associated with gram-negative organisms, particularly *Escherichia coli*. As a preventive measure, hatch crane chicks in a clean environment, treat the umbilicus with topical povidone iodine (1%), and give the chick gentamicin (5 mg/kg intramuscularly [IM] q12h for the first 3 days. In cases of nonresponding omphalitis or retained

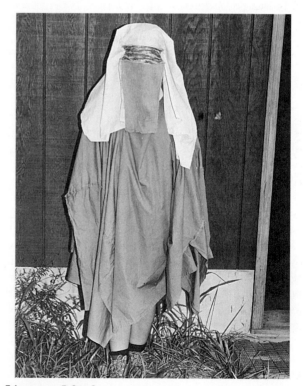

Figure 56-3

Costume worn by a technician while working with hand-reared crane chicks to avoid imprinting.

yolk sac, removing the yolk sac by surgical means is an option, but survival is low.[6]

Respiratory Diseases

Respiratory diseases are common in young crane chicks. Typical signs include a click heard on auscultation, open-mouthed breathing (gaping), raspy breathing, lethargy or dullness, and cyanotic or pale mucous membranes. For the first 2 weeks after hatching, bacterial pathogens cause most respiratory disease, but after day 14, disseminated visceral coccidiosis and fungal diseases (especially aspergillosis) also become common causes. Treatment consists of antibiotics, coccidiostats, or antifungal medications as appropriate, plus nebulization therapy and good supportive care. Young crane chicks between days 3 and 6 commonly develop diarrhea, usually associated with heavy growth of *E. coli*. Treat these chicks against the ensuing dehydration and give antibiotic therapy, based on sensitivity test results when possible, and kaolin-pectin by mouth. It is critically important to keep chicks that are younger than 15 days old warm, because chilling is often associated with subsequent diarrhea.

Heat Stress

During the hotter days of summer, especially in southern latitudes, crane chicks more than 30 days old and adults are susceptible to heat stress and heat prostration. Whooping crane chicks appear to be more susceptible than other crane species. Signs of heat stress include gaping or open-mouth breathing, panting, staggering, rapid breathing, and wings held away from the body and drooping. If the chick's body temperature remains elevated, brain damage and death may follow. Cool the bird with cool water or place it in a swimming pool. Fluids help to counteract the stress and shock associated with heat prostration. Schedule all necessary handling during the cooler early morning hours.

Orthopedic Conditions

Several orthopedic problems may develop in crane chicks. Severe deformities can develop in chicks fed diets too high in sulfur-containing amino acid (see Diet, earlier). When hand-rearing chicks, excessive weight gain during the first 4 weeks can lead to leg deformities.[2] Detection involves observing the chick's gait and monitoring weight gain daily. Alleviate the problem by increasing the amount of exercise the chick receives and reducing food consumption. Two methods of increasing exercise are to place the food and water in opposite ends of a long pen, or to swim the chick in a small pool twice daily for 10 to 30 minutes. In cases when weight gain continues to be excessive (>10% per day), withhold food. Make food available overnight, but only for four 15-minute periods during the day. Chicks must always have unlimited access to drinking water.

Hock rotation, another serious problem, is first seen when the middle toes are no longer parallel to one another when the chick is walking forward. Rotational problems result from injury, improper handling, excessive weight gain, malpositioning at hatching, improper bedding, or lack of exercise. If rotation is observed, swimming exercise coupled with food withholding to control excessive weight gain give the best chance of arresting the problem. Injury, improper handling, malpositioning at hatch, or genetic predisposition may contribute to hock and leg injuries. Slippery substrates often lead to injury. Frequently, swimming exercise is the best therapy for the growing chick.

Correct deviated or crooked toes, frequently encountered in young chicks, as soon as they are discovered. Make a splint from a thin wooden dowel, such as a cotton-tipped applicator stick, and tape it to the outside of the curvature of the toe. The splint should remain in place for only 24 to 48 hours. If required, reapply the splint until the problem is corrected. Tape with low-tack adhesive, such as reinforced packing tape (strap tape), works well for this type of splint and is easily removed without damaging the skin.

Beak, Wing, and Feather Conditions

Crane chicks suffer from problems observed in other species. Correct beak deformities by judicious trimming or applying a splint to the beak for all or part of a day. However, the beak may always remain deformed. Sometimes a drooping or twisted wing, called "angel wing," occurs in older chicks when muscular development fails to keep pace with the development of primary and secondary feathers and subsequent increased weight of the wing. Bandaging the affected wing into a normal position for 3 to 5 days generally corrects the problem. Young chicks may break new flight feathers. Removing the broken quill stops bleeding.

THERAPEUTIC TECHNIQUES

Basic Supportive Care

Many medical treatment principles developed for use in domestic animals or other avian species apply to cranes. Although specific medications (including drug selection, dosage, and route of administration) and treatment regimens depend on diagnosis of the disease and evaluation of the patient's condition by a veterinarian, the following procedures can generally be followed.

When disease or injury occurs in a captive crane, the individual may need to be isolated from other birds for protection, because cranes kept in groups often attack a weak or injured flock member. However, for established crane pairs, the continued presence of the mate is beneficial and often less stressful than separation. Treat an injured, sick, or debilitated crane to reduce stress, prevent further injury, and reduce infection. Hospitalization permits intensive care and reduces the opportunities for disease transmission and intraspecific aggression. Most sick birds require supplemental heat (air temperature at 29–30°C), which can be provided by a heater, heat lamp, or incubator (if the patient is a chick). Frequent observation is required to monitor the patient's condition and evaluate its response to treatment.

In cases involving dehydration, emaciation, shock, stress, and electrolyte imbalance, supportive care includes fluid therapy (i.e., 2.5% dextrose and Ringer's solution, lactated Ringer's solution, 5% dextrose, normal saline, or maintenance and replacement electrolyte solutions).[7] Fluid type, volume, frequency, and route of administration (oral, intravenous, or subcutaneous) vary with the patient's condition. A crane needs 44 ml/kg of fluid daily; this need increases in cases of dehydration and diarrhea. In situations when the bird is drinking,

administer some medications and vitamin supplements such as vitamin D_3 through the drinking water to reduce handling stress. Other medication, such as pills or small amounts of powder, can be administered inside a small fish or dead mouse.

Cranes may require antibiotic therapy (Table 56–3) for bacterial diseases or for cases when the opportunity for secondary bacterial infection exists. When possible, base antibiotic therapy on crane pharmacokinetics (i.e., rate of appearance, plasma concentration, and biologic half-life). Without specific pharmacokinetic information for cranes, extrapolate the dosage and frequency of administration of medications from those parameters for other bird species or by metabolic scaling. Administer antibiotics orally (through the drinking water, feed, gavage, or as a bolus) or parenterally (subcutaneous, intravenous, or intramuscular). Administering antibiotics in the feed or water, however, is less desirable to other routes because of variability in dose levels consumed.

Nebulization can be supportive and therapeutic in the treatment of some respiratory infections. Depending on the cause of the disease, cranes respond best when either gentamicin (1 ml) or tylosin (2 ml) is used in combination with 1 ml acetylcysteine in 15 ml normal saline.[7] With a 1 to 2 liter low flow of oxygen, administer the medications for 20 minutes three times daily. For aspergillosis, 3 ml of 10 mg/ml clotrimazole in glycerol glycolate nebulized for 20 minutes three times daily is helpful. Although the value of nebulization therapy is difficult to assess, it appears to be useful in some instances.

High-quality nutrition is a critical component of supportive care. Feed an anorexic or starving bird by gavage (tube feeding). Because many sick cranes suffer from some degree of nutritional deficiency and usually eat less than normal when hospitalized, forced feeding is essential for recovery. Cranes respond well to forced feeding when given a mixture consisting of crane pellets softened in water (750 ml total volume pellets and water), liquid hypoallergenic soybean food (Isomil concentrate, Ross Laboratories, Columbus, OH, 25 ml), a concentrated energy source (Nutri-cal, Evsco Pharmaceutical Corp., Buena, NJ, 5 ml), infant instant rice cereal (30 ml), multiple vitamins (including D_3 and B complex), vegetable oil (30 ml), and mineral supplements.[7] Administer the mixture slowly (to reduce the possibility of regurgitation) with a 60-

T a b l e 5 6 – 3

DRUGS COMMONLY ADMINISTERED TO CRANES*

Drug	Indications	Route of Administration	Dose mg/kg	Frequency of Administration
Antibiotics				
Amikacin	Broad-spectrum aminoglycoside, especially effective against gram-negative rods; often used in conjunction with piperacillin to increase spectrum; maintain good hydration	IM or SQ	10	q12h
Ampicillin	Broad-spectrum antibacterial drug; gram-negative and gram-positive bacteria, including several pathogenic enteric organisms	IM	20	q12h
Carbenicillin	Especially effective against gram-positive bacteria; good only for 3 days after mixing; synergistic with aminoglycosides	IM or IV	100	q12h
Cefotaxime sodium	Broad-spectrum; sometimes used in conjunction with aminoglycosides	IM	50–100	q8h
Cephalexin	Broad-spectrum; effective against most gram-positive organisms and some gram-negative organisms, including various enteric organisms	PO	35–50	q6h
Cephalothin	Same as cephalexin	IM or SQ	100	q6h
Enrofloxacin	Broad-spectrum antibiotic; also for *Chlamydia*, *Mycoplasma*	IM or PO	8–15	q12h
Piperacillin	Broad spectrum, bacteriocidal	IM	100	q12h
Antifungals				
Amphotericin B	For treatment of aspergillosis	IV	1.5	q8h
		Nebulization	10 ml in 15 ml H_2O	q8h for 20 minutes
Flucytosine	For treatment of aspergillosis	PO	100	q8–12h
Itraconazole	For treatment of aspergillosis and *Candida*	PO	5–10	q12h
Nystatin	For treatment of *Candida*	PO	3	q12h
Clotrimazole	For treatment of aspergillosis	Nebulization	30 (3.0 ml)	q8h for 20 minutes
Antiparasitic				
Fenbendazole	For nematodes	PO	100	Repeat in 14 days
	For *Syngamus*	PO	100	For 5 days then repeat in 14 days
Ivermectin	For nematodes, mites	SQ	0.4	Repeat in 14 days
Levamisole	For nematodes, especially *Capillaria*	IM	20–40	Repeat in 14 days
Amprolium	Control of coccidia	In feed or add to only source of drinking water	2.2 ppm	Free choice
Monensin	Control of coccidia	In feed	90 g/ton	Free choice
Sulfachlorpyridazine	Control of coccidia	Add to only source of drinking water	1 tsp/gal	For 7–14 days
Thiabendazole	For nematodes	PO	100	Repeat in 14 days
Miscellaneous				
Calcium gluconate	Egg binding	IM or SQ	50–100	Once 15 minutes before oxytocin
Oxytocin	Egg binding	IM	0.2–0.5 ml (20 units/ml)	Once
Calcium glycerophosphate/ lactate	Egg binding	IM or SQ	1–5 ml	Once 15 minutes before oxytocin
Furosemide	Excessive fluid especially in respiratory system	IM	0.15	q12h
Dexamethasone	For treatment of shock	IV or IM	2–8	q8–12h, reducing dosage
Prednisolone sodium succinate	For treatment of shock	IV	30	Once
Vitamin A/D	Supplement	IM	0.3–1.0 ml/kg	Once every 7 days
Vitamin E/selenium	Capture myopathy	IM	0.06 selenium	q3days

*Data from references 7, 12, 19, 38, 39, 40, 41, 42.
IM = intramuscular; SQ = subcutaneous; IV = intravenous; PO = oral

ml catheter-tipped syringe (for adult cranes) and a flexible feeding tube at a rate of 12 ml/kg body weight three times daily (more frequently if indicated). For chicks, the pellet mixture must be strained with a fine-mesh sieve, and small syringes (3–6 ml) and gavage tubes are used. The bulk and caloric content of the mixture can be increased during the recovery period.

Restraint

Physical Restraint

Careful handlers can avoid injuring themselves and the crane's long legs, wings, and neck during capture and restraint. The easiest way to capture a bird is to herd it into a corner or another confined space. With the crane's head in the corner, grasp the secondary and tertial flight feathers with one hand to maintain the wings in a closed position. Then place the other arm over the bird's body and wings while directing the bird's head and neck behind the handler's back. From this point the bird can be restrained in two different positions. Immediately grasp the hocks of both legs (one or two fingers are placed between hocks) with the hand of the arm over the bird. The hand holding the wings can be released after picking up the bird and, with aggressive birds, used to hold the bird's head behind the handler's back. In the second position, with the hand of the arm over the bird and supporting the keel, the hand holding the wings can be released and used to grasp the hocks. The bird can then be picked up and the legs can be extended parallel to the ground. If a bird is facing the handler during capture, grab it by the neck and quickly manipulate it into the restraint position just described. In addition to reducing stress to the bird, this technique reduces risk to the handler. Safety glasses or goggles offer eye protection to the handler and are highly recommended.

Chemical Restraint

Chemical restraint is frequently required for extensive handling and for certain diagnostic and surgical procedures. A mixture of ketamine and xylazine or diazepam, 10 to 15 mg/kg ketamine hydrochloride and 1 mg/kg xylazine hydrochloride or 0.2 to 0.5 mg/kg diazepam, serves as a preanesthetic agent and for sedation before surgery or manipulation of short duration. Diazepam alone (0.5–1 mg/kg) also provides short-term sedation. Local infiltration of areas with lidocaine is also useful in small laceration repairs, tenotomies, and other procedures, thereby avoiding general anesthesia.

For longer procedures, the authors recommend that the preanesthetic be followed by intubation and administration of isoflurane (AErrane, Anaquest, Madison, WI), a compound with a wide margin of safety and low toxicity. Isoflurane administration permits more precise and immediate control over the plane of anesthesia. Isoflurane can be used for induction of anesthesia (4–5%) by a face mask made from a 60-ml plastic syringe case. The closed end is cut open to accept the tube from the nonrebreathing apparatus on the anesthetic machine. The open end is partially closed with padded tape (Microfoam Surgical Tape, Medical Products Division/ 3M, St. Paul, MN) to form a tight fit around the crane's face. After intubation, maintain the crane at a surgical anesthetic plane with 2 to 3% isoflurane and an oxygen (O_2) flow rate of 1–2 l/minute. If inhalant anesthesia is not available, use a mixture of ketamine at 22 mg/kg and xylazine at 1 mg/kg for surgical procedures.

Monitor vital signs and maintain the corneal and palpebral reflexes during anesthesia. To reduce the chance for injury to a crane during recovery, place the bird in a warm, dark, quiet recovery pen, or, preferably, hold the crane until it can stand on its own, usually about 10 minutes after ending anesthesia.

COMMON DISEASES

Little is known about the incidence and pathogenic effects of infectious and parasitic diseases in free-roaming cranes. Wild cranes are difficult to study (they generally seek dense cover when ill or become vulnerable to predation), and studies of captive birds form the basis for much of the existing literature on crane diseases. Most infectious bacterial diseases in cranes occur sporadically and primarily in birds that have been predisposed to infection by environmental or population stresses.[7] Although various viral agents have been identified in cranes, their occurrence, distribution, and frequency are less well understood. Parasites are probably present in most wild and captive cranes in small numbers. Because parasites are opportunistic, the parasite burden increases in captivity and in areas where wild cranes congregate. Parasitism generally increases the susceptibility of an individual to other mortality factors and reduces the bird's chances of survival during times of stress.

Because infectious and parasitic diseases can be detrimental to the health and productivity of cranes, early detection and diagnosis of disease are important. Start treatment early to alleviate the impact of the disorder and reduce recovery time. Observe captive cranes daily for indications of health problems as evidenced by reduced physical activity, decreased food consumption, or other clinical signs of disease.[7] Establish routine monitoring procedures as part of the facility's regular care. Procedures should include frequent fecal parasite monitoring, annual physical examinations, and blood chemistry testing.

Bacterial Diseases

At least 20 species or subspecies of bacteria have been isolated as apparent pathogens from cranes; they include *Salmonella* species, *Pasteurella multocida, Mycobacterium avium* and *M. tuberculosis, Clostridium* species, *Erysipelothrix,* and numerous members of the Enterobacteriaceae. The significance of most of these organisms in cranes is not known, although some are known pathogens of other species of birds.

Viruses

Several viral diseases, including avian pox and Newcastle disease, have been identified in cranes, but their occurrence, distribution, and significance are not well documented. Two viral diseases, inclusion body disease of cranes virus (IBDCV) and eastern equine encephalitis (EEE), are especially pathogenic. IBDCV, a herpesvirus, has caused the death of 18 captive cranes of four species. Nondescript clinical signs, including anorexia, lethargy, weakness, and breathing difficulties, are observed for several days before death. Pathologists isolated

the herpesvirus from the liver and spleen of some of the cranes and observed inclusion bodies in these organs. It is not known if IBDCV is endemic in wild crane populations or occurs only in captive flocks, because it has only been isolated from captive cranes. Similar viruses can produce latent infections during which the virus apparently disappears from affected individuals for long periods of time. This latency aids in spreading the virus, especially when translocating captive cranes to other facilities or for release to the wild.

EEE virus infects a wide variety of indigenous bird species. Mortality is generally restricted to introduced birds, such as pheasants, pigeons, house sparrows, and chukar partridges. This virus is found primarily in the eastern and north central US and adjacent areas of Canada, in parts of Central and South America, and in the Caribbean.[8] The enzootic cycle involves transmission of virus between wild birds by mosquitoes, with occasional outbreaks in equines and, rarely, in humans. The principal vector for the virus, the mosquito *Culiseta melanura,* breeds in wooded swamps and primarily feeds on birds. An outbreak of EEE virus infection in 1984 resulted in the deaths of 7 of 39 captive whooping cranes (primarily adult females) at the Patuxent Environmental Science Center.[7, 9] Four birds were found dead without any clinical signs, and three showed signs of lethargy, ataxia, and neck and leg paresis before death. The EEE virus was isolated from tissues from embryonated egg inoculations and tissue culture. Fourteen (44%) of the 32 surviving whooping cranes had antibodies to the EEE virus present in their serum. Clinical signs of EEE virus infections in birds may vary from inapparent disease to acute death. In general, EEE viral infections in birds are primarily found in the liver rather than the central nervous system (CNS). In cases when the virus successfully invades the CNS, affected birds become depressed, lethargic, uncoordinated, and paralyzed, and they assume abnormal postures, especially of the head and neck.

The epizootic of EEE virus in captive whooping cranes represents a potential risk to the recovery of this species. Vaccination with formalin inactivated human EEE viral vaccine elicits antibody response ($\geq$1:10) in whooping cranes.[10] Whether whooping cranes are protected against natural infection has not been determined. However, the level of EEE viral neutralizing antibody induced by the vaccine indicates a protective state and may minimize the risk of captive cranes to EEE viral infection. The vaccine is readily available, inexpensive, and has not caused any apparent adverse side effects in cranes when administered intramuscularly. Antibody response can be elicited in the cranes by a primary inoculation followed by a 30-day booster injection and can be sustained by only one or two annual booster injections. In 1989, EEE was detected at Patuxent through virus isolation from mosquitoes and seroconversion in sentinel bobwhites.[11] This has provided an indirect means of assessing the efficacy of the vaccination program, which appears successful, because none of the vaccinated whooping cranes died from EEE.

Mycotic Diseases

Few mycotic infections other than aspergillosis have been reported in members of the family Gruidae. However, aspergillosis has been diagnosed in both young and adult captive cranes. *Aspergillus* species has caused the deaths of numerous crane chicks, some as young as 9 days. Treatment with various antifungal products to achieve 0.1 to 1.0 μg/ml blood levels is desired. Currently at Patuxent, itraconazole is given at a dosage of 10 mg/kg q12h. The itraconazole comes as beads in small capsules (100 mg). Each bead represents approximately 0.153 mg of the drug. The appropriate number of beads are mixed with 1 to 3 ml of orange juice and given by tube orally. In addition, we often nebulize with amphotericin B at a dose of 5 to 10 mg in 15 ml of saline, or 3 ml of a 10 mg/ml solution of clotrimazole in glycerol glycolate, in individual treatments for a total of 60 minutes per day. Treatment with a variety of antifungal agents has been unrewarding once clinical disease becomes severe.

Parasitic Diseases

Crane parasites, like parasites in other birds, are usually opportunistic. Therefore, sanitation and sound husbandry practices such as pen rotation reduce the impact of parasitism, whereas stress, unsanitary conditions, and overcrowding compound it. Clinical signs of parasitism are usually inapparent and when they occur are frequently nonspecific (i.e., mild anorexia, poor weight gain, lethargy, diarrhea, and dyspnea). Parasites generally increase the susceptibility of an animal to disease, predation, malnutrition, and other mortality factors and reduce the bird's chances of survival during times of stress.[12]

At least seven species of protozoa infect cranes, including those of the genera *Haemoproteus* and *Leucocytozoon*. The coccidia *Eimeria gruis* and *E. reichenowi* are common parasites of sandhill and whooping cranes. Although coccidiosis is generally recognized as a disease of the intestinal tract, *Eimeria* infections in sandhill and whooping cranes are especially pathogenic because infection can become systemic with widespread dissemination of developmental stages extraintestinally.[13–15]

Disseminated visceral coccidiosis caused by *Eimeria* species was first recognized as a disease entity in captive cranes at the Patuxent Environmental Science Center in 1978 to 1979.[13–15] In disseminated visceral coccidiosis, granulomatous nodules may form in many tissues and organs or may result in bronchopneumonia, hepatitis, myocarditis, splenitis, and enteritis (Figs. 56–4, 56–5).

The basic host response to disseminated visceral coccidiosis in young sandhill and whooping cranes is granulomatous inflammation.[16] Changes in the respiratory system are primarily the result of infiltration of lymphoid cells laden with developing asexual stages of *Eimeria*.[17] The consequent rupture and death of infected cells initiates a necrotizing or granulomatous pneumonia, tracheitis, and airsacculitis. In experimentally infected sandhill crane chicks, morbidity and death occurred at the peak of merogony (9 to 11 days post-infection). The widespread merogony is directly responsible for the development of clinical disease and mortality in young cranes of both species in the wild. By 14 days after infection, gamonts and oocysts are present in respiratory epithelium, indicating that crane coccidia can complete their life cycle in both the respiratory and digestive tracts.[17]

In adult sandhill cranes, focal aggregates of lymphoid cells and granulomatous nodules in many tissues, including the lungs, air sacs, trachea and nares, are the main lesions (Figs. 56–6, 56–7, 56–8).[17] Because cranes, as they mature, appear to tolerate the coccidia, a chronic infection may develop, but death is rare. The inherent ability of the crane coccidia to complete their life cycle in

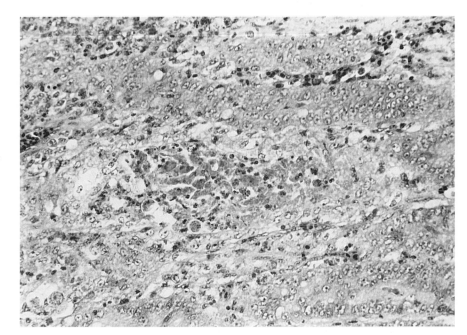

Figure 56–4

Section of duodenal mucosa from a sandhill crane with disseminated visceral coccidiosis. Note the necrosis and desquamation of enterocytes associated with gametocytes and oocysts. (Hematoxylin-eosin stain.)

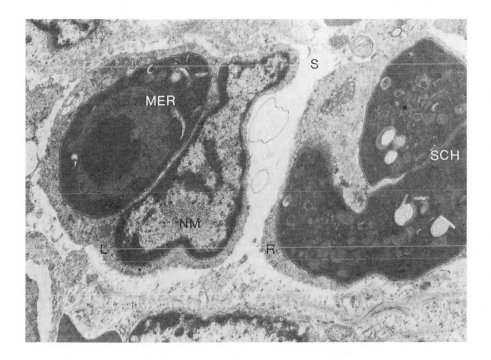

Figure 56–5

Electron micrograph of spleen specimen from a whooping crane chick, showing 2 macrophages (L, R) within a sinus (S) harboring parasites. The left macrophage contains a merozoite (MER) indenting the macrophage nucleus (NM), and the right macrophage contains a developing schizont (SCH), apparently in the process of division. (Uranyl acetate and lead citrate stain; × 14,970) (From Carpenter JW, Spraker TR, Novilla MN: Disseminated visceral coccidiosis in whooping cranes. J Am Vet Med Assoc 177:848, 1980.)

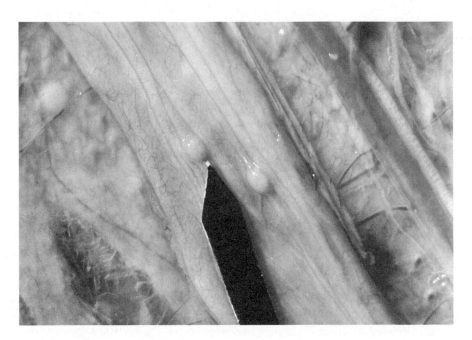

Figure 56–6

Multiple nodules (one at end of pointer) in the mucosa of the esophagus of a captive sandhill crane with disseminated visceral coccidiosis. (From Carpenter JW, Novilla MN, Fayer R, Iverson GC: Disseminated visceral coccidiosis in sandhill cranes. J Am Vet Med Assoc 185:1344, 1984.)

Figure 56–7

Multiple nodules in the proventriculus mucosa of a sandhill crane with disseminated visceral coccidiosis. (From Carpenter JW, Novilla MN, Fayer R, Iverson MS: Disseminated visceral coccidiosis in sandhill cranes. J Am Vet Med Assoc 185:1344, 1984.)

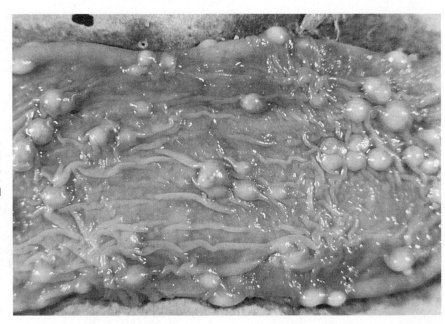

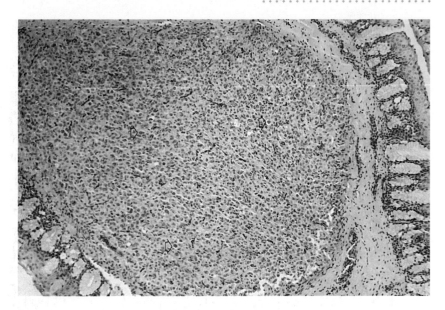

Figure 56–8

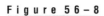

Section of an esophageal granuloma from a wild sandhill crane with disseminated visceral coccidiosis. (Hematoxylin-eosin stain, × 68) (From Carpenter JW, Novilla MN, Fayer R, Iverson GC: Disseminated visceral coccidiosis in sandhill cranes. J Am Vet Med Assoc 185:1344, 1984.)

extraintestinal sites, and the establishment of a chronic infection tolerated by migratory hosts, reflect adaptation that may be necessary for the coccidia to survive in nature.[17]

Although *Eimeria* species occur in free-ranging cranes, they represent a special problem for crane chicks raised in captivity. Concentrations of these parasites in the soil may increase substantially where cranes are held in close confinement. Infections of extraintestinal coccidia represent a significant health problem for captive cranes. In captivity, some control of coccidia can be augmented by pen rotation, parasite surveillance, and separation of cranes by age class. Use of proper medications also is an integral part of a coccidia control program. Monensin, a polyether, carboxylic ionophorous antibiotic, is an effective coccidiostat in cranes and acts primarily against intraluminal stages of coccidia.* Monensin (90 g/ton [99 ppm][18]) can be given to cranes in feed throughout the year, or for 2 months before and 2 months after the chick-rearing season.

Endoparasites, including at least 25 species of acanthocephalans, cestodes, trematodes, and nematodes, infect cranes.[7, 19] Although some of these parasites cause illness in other birds and may cause illness in cranes under certain conditions, the overall impact in wild and captive cranes is probably not significant. Two groups of nematodes, *Capillaria* species and gapeworms (*Syngamus* species and *Cyathostoma* species), are pathogenic, occasionally resulting in debility or death. Gapeworms may obstruct the trachea, resulting in pneumonia and asphyxiation. Ivermectin and fenbendazole are effective for treatment (see Table 56–3 for dosage recommendations).

Five species of mites (order Acarina) and four species of biting lice (order Mallophaga) have been reported in cranes. These ectoparasites are probably of little pathologic significance, although they can contribute to a crane's debilitated condition or may serve as vectors of disease. A 5% carbaryl powder is an effective treatment.

In summary, parasitic diseases can be detrimental to the health and productivity of captive cranes. Control of parasites includes providing cranes with a nutritionally balanced diet, good hygiene, therapeutic and prophylactic administration of parasiticides (see Table 56–3), and limited stress. Parasite control also requires pen rotation, quarantining new birds, and separation by age class (juveniles, paired adults, unpaired adults, etc.).[12]

Traumatic Conditions

Intraspecific aggression is the leading cause of traumatic injury in captive cranes. Aggression in cranes is often associated with the formation of dominance

---

*Carpenter JW, Novilla MN, Hatfield JS, unpublished data, 1989.

hierarchies and the mate selection process, including defense of territory, food, or water.[7, 20] Any act that disrupts an established social order can also result in aggression, including moving a new crane into an established pen or a crane accidentally jumping or flying into an occupied pen. Usually the new crane in the social hierarchy will be the victim of the aggression. One recommendation is to form a new social group in a new pen any time two groups of cranes need to be combined or even to introduce a single individual. Sometimes introducing the single individual crane into an adjacent pen for a few weeks before allowing it to join a group is also effective. At the Patuxent Environmental Science Center during one 15-year period, 7.3% of whooping crane deaths resulted from aggression.[20]

Aggression usually results in soft tissue trauma to the head and neck, plus skull fractures. Often the crane is in a deep state of shock after the attack. Administer corticosteroids (dexamethasone 2–8 mg/kg or prednisolone sodium succinate 30 mg/kg), intravenous fluids, and antibiotics immediately. Treat the wounds, and take radiographs to determine the extent of skull damage when the crane is in stable condition. Cranes given supportive care during the first 24 hours, and surviving beyond the initial 24 to 48 hours, usually recover. Often permanent scarring of the head or neck results.

In another form of aggression, parents attack their chick. Usually there is an underlying cause such as a sick or lethargic chick, parental disturbance (redirected aggression), or an abnormal appearance (wounded or deformed chick). In these cases, parents often kill the chick.

Occasionally ruptured air sacs result in subcutaneous emphysema in both chicks and adults. Often minor cases resolve without medical intervention, but severe cases can result in extensive subcutaneous emphysema over the entire body including up along the neck and over the top of the head. Air can be withdrawn with a syringe, needle, and three-way valve. If the affected area is limited, a pressure bandage may prove helpful. In the most severe cases, however, surgical insertion of Penrose drains or setons through the skin into the air-filled subcutaneous spaces is required to resolve the problem. Place the crane on antibiotics and clean the drains with diluted povidone iodine solution (1%) twice daily. After 1 to 2 weeks the drains can be removed.

Lacerations are common injuries. Causes vary from aggression, to collision with sharp objects, to self-inflicted wounds. A struggling crane can lacerate itself with a sharp toenail while being captured. Treatment varies with the extent of injury and ranges from minor cleaning to surgical repair of the wound.

Frequently, captive cranes injure their beaks. Minor fractures of the tip of the beak are not repaired. Instead, the two ends of the beak are trimmed evenly. This technique works well for fractures of the distal 2 to 3 cm of the beak. Fractures close to the head require some type of medical or surgical repair. Lang's dental acrylic and K-wires can be used to create a splint around the fractured beak. The splint is left in place for 3 to 4 weeks and removed after healing has occurred.

Nontraumatic Conditions

Several neoplasms, although relatively rare, have been reported in cranes. These neoplasms include renal adenocarcinoma,[21, 22] renal carcinoma,[22] lymphocytic leukemia,[22] granulocytic leukemia,[23] and metastatic cholangiocarcinoma.[24] A hematopoietic stem cell neoplasia was seen in one Florida sandhill crane. A high incidence of adenocarcinoma exists in wild Mississippi sandhill cranes, but not in captive cranes of the same endangered subspecies, leading to speculation that there is an environmental link to the neoplasm.

Crane mortalities resulting from toxic substances such as famphur and lead have been reported. Cranes in Georgia have died from exposure to famphur,[25] an organophosphorus compound. Famphur is known to be extremely toxic to wildlife, especially avian populations, by inhibiting cholinesterase in the nervous system and disrupting synaptic transmission of nerve impulses, leading to failure of the brain respiratory center and death by asphyxiation. Both wild and captive sandhill cranes have died from lead poisoning. Sources of the lead range from fishing weights and bullets[26] to lead-based paint.[27]

An estimated 9500 sandhill cranes died in Texas and New Mexico between 1982 and 1987 because of mycotoxins produced by *Fusarium* species growing on unharvested peanuts.[28] Poisoned cranes were unable to hold their heads straight or erect while flying or standing. The lesions most commonly seen at necropsy were multiple muscle hemorrhages and submandibular edema. Increasing fall tillage of peanut fields has reduced crane mortality in recent years. Other sources of mycotoxin toxicity are possible. Cranes may be more sensitive to these toxins than other birds. Approximately 4% of the sandhill and whooping cranes at Patuxent Environmental Science Center died in 1987 from deoxynivalenol poisoning associated with pelleted feed. The toxin was present in extremely low levels of 0.4 ppm, in combination with the mycotoxin T-2 at 1 to 2 ppm.[29]

Cranes, because of their inquisitive, probing nature, pick up small metal objects and may ingest them. These objects then lodge in the ventriculus producing "hardware" disease. Clinical signs reported for sarus cranes *(Grus antigone)* that ingested foreign metallic objects included difficulty in standing, sitting on hocks, and diarrhea.[30] One whooping crane died at Patuxent from an ingested nail that punctured the ventriculus, and at least two others have had surgery to successfully remove objects from the abdomen.

To remove foreign objects, perform surgery under general anesthesia, after fasting the patient for 24 hours. Place the patient in right lateral or dorsal recumbency and incise the skin and muscle parallel to the last rib. Exteriorize the ventriculus and make an incision through the musculus intermedin at the posterior end of the ventriculus. After removing the foreign objects, close the ventriculus with a three-layer closure, mucosa and submucosa with simple interrupted sutures of 4–0 absorbable suture material, ventriculus muscle wall with horizontal and vertical mattress sutures of 3–0 or 4–0 nylon, and adventitia with an interlocking continuous suture pattern with 4–0 absorbable suture. Close the abdominal air sac with 4–0 absorbable suture and the muscle wall and skin with 3–0 or 4–0 nonabsorbable suture. Reduce food intake for 5 days after surgery and continue antibiotic and fluid therapy. Feces should return to normal within 10 days after surgery.[30] To avoid "hardware" disease, sweep all new pens, or pens undergoing renovation, with a metal detector before introducing cranes.

Capture myopathy, also known as exertional myopathy or exertional rhabdomyolysis, occasionally occurs in domestic and wild mammals following trapping and transportation and, in some cases, has been associated with chemical immobilization. Although not commonly reported in wild or captive birds, capture myopathy has been observed in East African crowned cranes *(Balearica rugelorum gibbericaps)*,[31] a greater sandhill crane,[32] and an endangered Mississippi sandhill crane *(G. canadensis pulla)*.[33] Clinical signs include peracute death from cardiac failure, or pain, stiff movement, swollen hard muscles that are warm to the touch, and trauma to the limbs from struggling. High serum biochemical concentrations of creatinine kinase, lactic dehydrogenase, and aspartate aminotransferase are useful in diagnosing the condition.[31] Subsequent elevations in uric acid and creatinine can result from increased uric acid production, myoglobinuria, or impaired mobility with subsequent dehydration. Because of the susceptibility of long-legged birds to capture myopathy, special care must be taken when trapping, handling, chemically immobilizing, and transporting cranes.[31]

Prevention of capture myopathy by minimal, but proper, handling and shipping of cranes is extremely important. Treatment, which is not always successful, consists of supportive care with intravenous fluids, corticosteroids, vitamin E and selenium, antibiotics, and good nursing care. If blood pH levels are below normal, intravenous sodium bicarbonate should be administered. If blood pH levels are unavailable but acidosis is still suspected, give sodium bicarbonate 4 to 6 mEq/kg body weight.

Other conditions seen in cranes, such as egg retention (egg binding), prolapsed cloaca, pododermatitis, aspiration pneumonia, ophthalmic disorders, frostbite, and hypo- and hyperthermia, all occur with some frequency. Treatment of these maladies in cranes is similar to that for other species of birds.

SPECIAL PROCEDURES

Flight Restraint

When keeping cranes in open or uncovered pens, flight must be restrained in some manner. Four forms of flight restraint have proven useful at Patuxent Environmental Science Center: (1) wing (feather) clipping, (2) vane trimming, (3) brailing, and (4) tenotomy.[34] Each technique is used for a specific purpose.

Wing clipping keeps immature birds flightless for

a year. The cranes regain their ability to fly after new feathers replace the clipped feathers. In this technique, similar to that used in other birds, cut the rachis of all primaries and three or more secondaries on one wing about 2 cm out from the skin. Leave the outermost two or three primaries intact to prevent a bird from injuring another bird with the sharp hard rachis tip when wings are extended.

Use brailing primarily to restrain birds for short periods, such as fledglings that will later be placed in flight (netted) pens or released, or for intact adult cranes when it is necessary to keep them in open pens for short periods. Begin brailing the fledgling when the blood-filled zone of the rachis extends less than 4 cm from the skin of the wing. Construct the brail from 1-mm thick flexible clear plastic material cut into strips of 2 × 40 cm (Fig. 56–9). Punch holes in the plastic strip at 2.5-cm intervals. Run the brail between the bases of the third and fourth primaries and then around the radial/ulnar section of the wing. Form the strap into a loose loop with the wing folded. With a commercially available rivet gun, secure a rivet with one washer on the outside, through two of the pre-punched holes on the top surface of the wing (where the two ends of the plastic loop meet). Next, run the rivet through the open space between the carpal and radial/ulnar sections of the folded wing and secure through another hole in the plastic strip on the underside of the wing, again using a washer on the outside surface of the plastic. The resulting two loops should be about equal size and loose enough to allow two fingers to pass under each loop. After brailing, cranes may strain at the braile and groom or preen the area extensively for several hours. After this initial interest, the birds return to normal. On birds intended for future flight, change brailes regularly at 2- to 3-week intervals, alternating the wing used.

Perform a tenotomy on the outer surface of the carpal joint using local anesthesia (1 ml of 2% lidocaine hydrochloride). Remove the feathers from the surgical site and prepare the area with a povidone iodine solution (1%). Radiosurgery is used to make a skin incision and to incise the tendo longa of the musculus tensor propatagidalis and the tendonous attachment of the musculus extensor metacarpi radialis as they pass over the carpal joint.[34] In addition, open the underlying synovial capsule. Apply a topical antibiotic to the resulting wound and tape the wing in a folded position for 5 to 6 weeks, during which ankylosis of the joint takes place.[35] About 5% of tenotomized birds retain enough flight capability to clear a 2.4-m fence. Clip the primary feathers on one wing to restrict flight capabilities of these cranes.

Any flight restraint may have an adverse effect on the ability of cranes to breed naturally, and this is particularly true in large crane species.

Orthopedic Procedures

Fractures of the long bones are a serious problem in cranes. In the period between 1984 and 1992, long bone fractures and complications were the cause of 8% (n=5) of deaths in the Mississippi sandhill crane (*G. canadensis pulla*) at the Patuxent Environmental Science Center.[36] In an 11-year period, fractures contributed to the death of 10% (n=11) of cranes at the International Crane Foundation in Baraboo, WI.[37] Tibiotarsal fractures are the most common type of long bone fracture and have the highest failure rate, with 90% of cranes dying or being euthanatized because of complications![36]

Various surgical techniques are used to repair fractures in cranes (Table 56–4). Techniques for fracture repair are similar to those used in other avian species and are covered in other chapters.

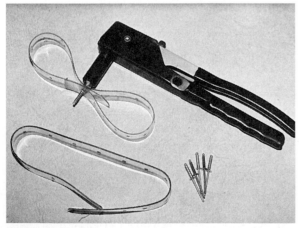

F i g u r e 5 6 – 9

Brail of clear flexible plastic 1 mm thick applied to the wing of a sandhill crane for flight restraint. Rivet used to form two loops, one around the radial/ulnar section of the wing and the other around the metacarpus.

Table 56-4

ORTHOPEDIC TECHNIQUES USED FOR FRACTURE REPAIR IN CRANES 1987–1994 AT THE PATUXENT ENVIRONMENTAL SCIENCE CENTER, LAUREL, MD

Repair Method	Number Seen	Percent Healed	Mean Healing Time—Days (Range)
Bandage, figure-8	4	75	65 (39–79)
IM pin	5	80	62 (39–93)
IM pin and cerclage wire	9	55	48 (20–84)
Cerclage wire alone	1	0	———
External splint	3	67	42
Amputation	4	75	18 (14–27)
Femoral head ostectomy	1	100	18

Revised from Olsen GH: Orthopedics in cranes: Pediatrics and adults. Semin Avian Exotic Pet Med 3:73–80, 1994.
IM = intramedullary

Bandaging and splinting are useful techniques for fracture stabilization in cranes. Use a figure-eight bandage of nonadhesive elastic bandage material (Vetrap, 3M Health Products, St. Paul, MN) to immobilize the wing. For fractures of the radius or ulna and metacarpal fractures, a figure-eight wrap alone is often sufficient for stabilization and healing. Humeral fractures and combined radial/ulnar fractures require internal fixation. Often, a figure-eight bandage is used for additional stabilization and support.

Splints are used successfully for fractures of the digits, tibiotarsus, and tarsometatarsus. Mason-meta splints and Schroeder-Thomas splints are most commonly used. Fractures of the femur, tibiotarsus, and occasionally the tarsometatarsus require additional support using intramedullary pins.

At least two sandhill cranes have been fitted successfully with leg prostheses made from lengths of polyvinyl chloride (PVC) pipe. Both cases involved extensive fractures of the tarsometatarsus, resulting in loss of the leg below the fracture site. With thin-walled PVC pipe (2.54 cm outside diameter, 2.38 inside diameter) cut a piece the appropriate length for the leg up to just below the hock. Wrap the stump of the leg in gauze padding extending 2 to 3 cm above where the PVC pipe will rest below the hock. Fit the PVC pipe onto the leg, and tape the pipe to the hock, continuing the tape 3 to 4 cm above the hock to provide additional support and to prevent the prosthesis from slipping. Change the prosthesis at 4- to 8-week intervals.

Cranes are very dependent on two properly functioning legs because they spend a large portion of their time on the ground. If an injury affects one or both legs it may become necessary to provide supplemental support for the crane during recovery. Construct a framework of PVC pipe (Fig. 56–10) and attach a sling of a strong fabric material. A crane in a sling should be restrained to prevent further injury and will continue to be a management problem. Initially the crane may refuse to eat or drink under such confined conditions. Some cranes continue to struggle with the constraining support system and may require light sedation at first. Careful observation and management of a crane in a sling is important to ensure recovery, and may require 24-hour care. Birds have been successfully held in such a device for as long as 5 to 6 weeks to allow a fracture to heal.

Repair of Fractured Beaks

Serious fractures of the beak often can be repaired with self-curing dental acrylics. The crane is given general anesthesia and the fracture site is cleaned and treated appropriately if an open wound is present. Align the fracture and cover the beak with an initial layer of self-curing dental acrylic (Lang's Jet Acrylics, Lang Dental Manufacturing Company, Chicago, IL). The acrylic usually needs additional reinforcement in this application. Therefore, after the

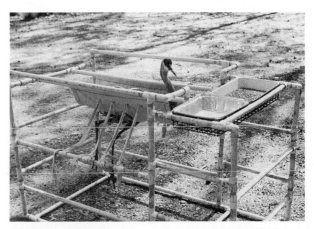

Figure 56-10

A sling constructed of PVC pipe and fabric used to support cranes with severe leg or spinal cord injuries. Food and water are placed in front of the crane, and the bird is initially monitored 24 hours daily.

first layer of acrylic has hardened, place Kirschner wires along the beak over the acrylic to act as reinforcing rods. Then apply a second layer of acrylic over the wires and first layer. As the acrylic cures, it generates heat, so surround the area with ice packs to help dissipate the heat. As a final step, smooth the outside surface of the acrylic splint and shape to eliminate sharp projections. To add stability, implant one or more Kirschner wires at right angles through the acrylic splint and beak. Satisfactory healing normally takes place in 4 to 6 weeks, at which time the wires and acrylic splint are removed. In young, growing birds, change the splint more frequently (every 3–5 days in some cases).

References

1. Serafin JA: Influence of dietary energy and sulfur amino acid levels upon growth and development of young sandhill cranes. Proc Am Assoc Zoo Vet 1980, p 30.
2. Serafin JA: The influence of diet composition upon growth and development of young sandhill cranes. Condor 84:427–434, 1982.
3. Gee GF, Carpenter JW, Hensler GL: Species differences in hematological values of captive cranes, geese, raptors, and quail. J Wildl Manag 45:463–483, 1981.
4. Hawkey C, Samour JH, Aston DG, et al: Normal and clinical hematology of captive cranes (Gruiformes). Avian Pathol 12:73–84, 1983.
5. Erickson RC: Captive breeding of whooping cranes at the Patuxent Wildlife Research Center. In Martin RD (ed): Breeding Endangered Species in Captivity. New York, Academic Press, 1975, pp 99–114.
6. Kenny D, Cambre RC: Indications and techniques for the surgical removal of the avian yolk sac. J Zoo Wildl Med 23(1):55–61, 1992.
7. Carpenter JW: Cranes (Order Gruiformes). In Fowler ME (ed): Zoo and Wild Animal Medicine. Philadelphia, WB Saunders, 1986, pp 315–326.
8. Monath TP: Arthropod-borne encephalitides in the Americas. Bull WHO 53:513–533, 1979.
9. Dein FJ, Carpenter JW, Clark GG, et al: Mortality of captive whooping cranes caused by eastern equine encephalitis virus. J Am Vet Med Assoc 189:1006–1010, 1986.
10. Clark GG, Dein FJ, Crabbs CL, et al: Antibody response of sandhill and whooping cranes to an eastern equine encephalitis virus vaccine. J Wildl Dis 23:539–544, 1987.
11. Pagac BB, Turell MJ, Olsen GH: Eastern equine encephalomyelitis virus and *Culiseta melanura* activity at the Patuxent Wildlife Research Center, 1985–90. J Am Mosquito Control Assoc 8(3):328–330, 1992.
12. Carpenter JW: An outline of the treatment and control of crane parasites. In Lewis JC (ed): Proceedings of the 1978 Crane Workshop. Fort Collins, Colorado State University Press, 1970, pp 101–108.
13. Carpenter JW, Spraker TR, Gardiner CH, Novilla MN: Disseminated granulomas caused by an unidentified protozoan in sandhill cranes. J Am Vet Med Assoc 175(11):948–951, 1979.
14. Carpenter JW, Spraker TR, Novilla MN: Disseminated visceral coccidiosis in whooping cranes. J Am Vet Med Assoc 177(9):845–848, 1980.
15. Carpenter JW, Novilla R, Fayer R, Iverson C: Disseminated visceral coccidiosis in sandhill cranes. J Am Vet Med Assoc 185(11):1342–1346, 1984.
16. Novilla MN, Carpenter JW, Spraker TR, Jeffers TK: Parenteral development of eimerian coccidia in sandhill and whooping cranes. J Protozool 28(2):248–255, 1981.
17. Novilla MN, Carpenter JW, Jeffers TK, White SL: Pulmonary lesions in disseminated visceral coccidiosis of sandhill and whooping cranes. J Wildl Dis 25(4):527–522, 1989.
18. Carpenter JW, Novilla MN, Hatfield JS: The safety and physiologic effects of the anticoccidial drugs monensin and clazuril in sandhill cranes (Grus canadensis). J Zoo Wildl Med 23(2):214–221, 1992.
19. Carpenter JW: Infectious and parasitic diseases of cranes. In Fowler ME, (ed): Zoo & Wild Animal Medicine. Current Therapy III. Philadelphia, WB Saunders, 1993, pp 229–237.
20. Carpenter JW, Derrickson SR: Whooping crane mortality at the Patuxent Wildlife Research Center, 1966–1981. In Lewis JC (ed): Proceedings of the 1981 Crane Workshop. New York, National Audubon Society, 1981.
21. Decker RA, Hruska JC: Renal adenocarcinoma in a sarus crane (Grus antigone). J Zoo Anim Med 9:15, 1978.
22. Montali RJ: An overview of tumors in zoo animals. J Am Vet Med Assoc 171:531, 1977.
23. Wei YC: Three cases of granulocytic leukemia in the red crested crane. Chin J Zool 21:32–33, 1986.
24. Allen JL, Martin HD, Crowley AM: Metastatic cholangiocarcinoma in a Florida sandhill crane. J Am Vet Med Assoc 187:1215, 1985.
25. White DH, Hayes LE, Bush PB: Case histories of wild birds killed intentionally with famphur in Georgia and West Virginia. J Wildl Dis 25:184–188, 1989.
26. Windingstad RM, Kerr SM, Locke LN: Lead poisoning of sandhill cranes (Grus canadensis). Prairie Naturalist 16:21–24, 1984.
27. Kennedy S, Crisler JP, Smith E, Bush M: Lead poisoning in sandhill cranes. J Am Vet Med Assoc 171:955–958, 1977.
28. Windingstad RM, Cole RJ, Nelson PE, et al: *Fusarium* mycotoxins from peanuts suspected as a cause of sandhill crane mortality. J Wildl Dis 25:38–46, 1989.
29. Olsen GH, Carpenter JW, Gee GF, et al: Mycotoxin-induced disease in captive whooping cranes (Grus americana) and sandhill cranes (Grus canadensis). J Zoo Wildl Med 26:569–576, 1995.
30. Bush M, Kennedy S: Ventriculostomy for removal of foreign bodies from sarus cranes. J Am Vet Med Assoc 173:1107–1110, 1978.
31. Brannian RE, Graham DL, Creswell J: Restraint associated myopathy in East African crowned cranes. In Fowler ME (ed): Proc Am Assoc Zoo Vet, Seattle, 1981, pp 21–23.
32. Windingstad RM, Hurley SS, Sileo L: Capture myopathy in a free-flying greater sandhill crane (Grus canadensis tabida) from Wisconsin. J Wildl Dis 19:289–290, 1983.
33. Carpenter JW, Thomas JJ, Reevers S: Capture myopathy in an endangered sandhill crane (Grus canadensis pulla). J Zoo Wildl Med 22(4):488–493, 1979.
34. Ellis DH, Dein FJ: Flight restraint techniques for cranes. In Proceedings International Crane Workshop, Oiqihar, Peoples Republic of China. International Crane Foundation, Baraboo, WI, 1991, pp 447–451.
35. Miller JC: The importance of immobilizing wings after tenectomy and tenotomy. Vet Med Small Anim Clin 73:35–38, 1973.

36. Olsen GH: Orthopedics in cranes: Pediatrics and adults. Semin Avian Exotic Pet Med 3:73–80, 1994.
37. Hartman L: Summary of mortality of 14 species of cranes at the International Crane Foundation, 1972–1982. In Archibald GW, Pasquier RF (eds): Proc 1983 Crane Workshop, International Crane Foundation, Baraboo, WI, 1983.
38. Locke D, Bush M, Carpenter JW: Pharmacokinetics and tissue concentrations of tylosin in selected avian species. Am J Vet Res 43(10):1807–1810, 1982.
39. Bush M, Locke D, Neal LA, Carpenter JW: Gentamicin tissue concentrations in various avian species following recom-

mended dosage therapy. Am J Vet Res 42(12):2114–2116, 1981.
40. Bush M, Neal LA, Custer RS: Preliminary pharmacokinetics studies of selected antibiotics in birds. Proc Am Assoc Zoo Vet, 1979, p 45.
41. Custer RS, Bush M, Carpenter JW: Pharmacokinetics of gentamicin in blood plasma of quail, pheasants, and cranes. Am J Vet Res 40(6):892–895, 1979.
42. Bush M, Locke D, Neal LA, Carpenter JW: Pharmacokinetics of cephalothin and cephalexin in selected avian species. Am J Vet Res 42(6):1014–1017, 1981.

The Human-Avian Bond

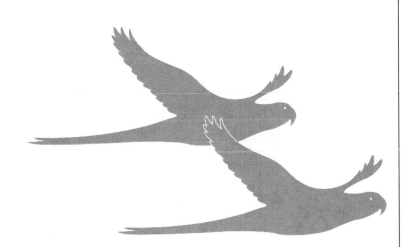

57

The Human-Avian Bond

HISTORY OF THE HUMAN-AVIAN BOND

Prehistory

There is ample evidence in archeologic material and at archeologic sites that *Homo sapiens* was interested in avian species. Numerous examples exist of pottery decorated with bird motifs. The decorations did not improve the function of the pot: it held water or stored food whether it was decorated or not. Perhaps decorating the object made it more visible so that clumsy cave-dwellers did not trip over it and break it, but one must suspect that the decoration served to satisfy early humans' aesthetic sense, connect them with the living environment in which they existed, and perhaps imbue some mystic or magic reference. Land-bound humans have always been fascinated with flying species and flight itself. In many cultures, birds were symbols of deities or were considered to be deities themselves.

Primitive Societies

There are vast numbers of examples of the relationship of primitive societies and birds. To many tribes of native North America, birds represented and still represent guardian spirits, totems, and the possessors of magic powers. Eagles, ravens, hawks, loons, and parrots are some examples of totem birds with perceived magic powers. Naked primitive people also adorned their bodies with feathers. Perhaps they were jealous of the birds' beautiful plumage and tried to emulate them by adorning their own bodies with feathers. Examples of the use of feathers for adornment and images of birds as totem figures, fertility objects, and connections with the spirit world are plentiful in South America, Africa, Melanesia, Polynesia, and Asia.

Contemporary Societies

Modern technologic society also uses feathers for adornment. Decoration on both men's and women's hats are common to this day. At one time the use of feathers in the fashion industry (e.g., on dresses, hats, and boas) was so popular that it led to the passage of avian protection laws in this country early in the 20th century.

In addition to the aesthetic and mystic connections with birds, we must also be reminded of the practical use of birds and their parts by humans, both primitive and contemporary. Birds were and are hunted and eaten. During the Middle Ages, the pigeon was a main source of protein in the late winter months. Most castles had connected dovecotes. Raptors have been humans' hunting partners for several millennia. Native Americans made whistles of the wing bones of birds. The Inuit crafted sewing needles from bird bones. Well before recorded history, humans took the jungle fowl and by careful selection created the domestic chicken, an efficient converter of surplus grain to protein and a major source of protein for contemporary society. Homing pigeons are also used in the delivery of messages and material such as raptor semen between raptor breeding programs.

TYPES OF CONTEMPORARY HUMAN-AVIAN INTERACTIONS

Contact with Nature

Urban society, often cut off from the living environment, longs for its roots and contact with nature.

Birds kept in cages and aviaries or viewed through binoculars afford urban humans a window on nature. People visit zoologic parks, wildlife centers, and sanctuaries or travel to the surrounding countryside to see and observe birds. "Bird watching" is an increasingly popular pastime, and for some a lifetime passion.

Intellectual Curiosity

Some individuals keep birds to observe their behavior—courting, breeding, nestling, and chick-rearing activities. The birds may be selected for their interesting biology, behavior, or appearance.

Aviculture

Many species of birds that have no value as food are kept and bred today. They may be kept and bred for commercial purposes such as the pet trade. Canaries, budgerigars, finches, quail, parrots, macaws, and cockatoos are some of the types of birds reared for this purpose. Many aviculturists have become sensitized to habitat destruction and species decimation and are breeding birds to maintain captive gene pools. This activity, once confined to zoologic facilities, is now spilling into the private sector and has been very successful in the captive propagation of many species. In some cases these captive populations are all that remain of a species that is extinct in the wild. It is hoped that aviculture will be the future source of all birds destined for the pet trade. Aviculture can also preserve a gene pool for some species for eventual release back into protected preserves of natural habitat.

Companionship

There is no question that the majority of families in the US and the Western world that keep birds do so for companionship. A singing canary to cheer a "shut-in" or a psittacine bonded to a person or family can be an ideal companion and an integral part of a family system. Some birds are more suitable than others as feathered companions.

Alternate Companionship

In some cases, birds may not have been the owner's preference for companionship, but space constraints and medical considerations, such as hypersensitivity to mammals on the part of family members, make the bird a suitable family addition.

Surrogate Roles

With the decline of the traditional nuclear family and the shift from rural or suburban location to urban life, companion animals, including birds, often assume surrogate roles. Practitioners should not be surprised at these nonconventional bonds. Examples of surrogate roles that birds assume are child substitutes, spouse substitutes, surrogate lovers, and parent substitutes.

Assume a nonjudgmental attitude and assist clients in maximizing the potentials of the relationship for both bird and human. Be sensitive to the potential for problems when the bond is broken. (See Chapter 58, Grief and Bereavement.)

THE PRACTITIONER'S ROLE

Selection for Species, Space, and Habitat Considerations

It appears that birds are here to stay and are rapidly increasing in numbers as one of the life forms with which contemporary society has chosen to share its space. "Doctor, we are considering acquiring a companion pet and would like a bird. What type would you recommend?" Practitioners are in a unique position to counsel and advise clients in this process. We must strive to offer preacquisition consultations resulting in satisfactory human-avian bonds, rather than playing fireman after the fact.

Native wild birds must not be kept. It is illegal to possess native species in the US without special permits. In addition, it is highly stressful for wild-caught birds to be held in captivity in confined spaces. Raptors are also unacceptable as "pets." In the hands of a licensed falconer, they are hunting partners but should not be in the hands of the general public.

Many species are available for companionship.

Passerines are acceptable as companions. They can be kept as single caged birds (canaries) or as multiple caged or aviary birds (finches). Although they do not usually bond strongly to their human stewards, they do habituate to the presence of people, often completing their life cycle in close proximity to the family. Some finches are quite territorial and, regardless of space, exhibit aggression toward other birds. Others do well in colonies. Practitioners can advise clients on appropriate mixes of species to minimize problems with selection.

Columbiformes can be acceptable companions. The smaller doves such as diamond doves are satisfactory aviary birds, but are very nervous and flighty. Larger doves like the ring-neck are peaceful, quiet birds that do well in roomy cages or enclosures. They breed well in captivity and have been placed in classrooms and institutional settings. The common rock dove (pigeon), originating in North Africa and now found worldwide, bonds well to people and is a gentle species.

Galliformes are kept for companionship. Miniature quail make good aviary birds. Chickens and turkeys are often found in "schoolyard farms" in schools and other institutions with outside facilities. They do not make good house or apartment companions. Eggs are a bonus to anyone keeping chickens. Unfortunately, roosters are not acceptable in urban areas. Although desensitized to diesel buses and the cacophony of other urban sounds, urbanites appear to be totally intolerant of crowing at sunrise.

Anseriformes (ducks, geese, swans) are most suitable for facilities with available bodies of water if they can be housed outside. To maintain normal plumage, these birds must have access to water for swimming on a daily basis. Because they have messy droppings, they do not make suitable apartment or house pets even if adequate water is available. They bond exceptionally well to people, and ducks also supply eggs.

Toucans and mynahs are not suitable birds for companions. Although mynahs are exceptionally good at mimicking their human stewards, their loose projectile droppings are incompatible with most people's perceptions of an acceptable pet. In addition, they have a propensity to develop hepatic problems. Toucans also have a high incidence of hepatic disease, and their specialized requirements for housing, care, and diet generally preclude their use as human companions.

Psittaciformes represent the group of avian species with the greatest potential for companionship. They are naturally gregarious and have a strong sense of attachment to a conspecific or alternately to a human. Domestic-bred, hand-reared birds make ideal companions. Nestlings that have been hand-fed by humans are "little people" with avian qualities, some of which must be modified and controlled.

Psittacines have a wide range of adult weights, from less than 30 g to more than 1500 g. Cage or enclosure dimensions must be adequate for the bird's size. Some psittacines are quiet and gentle; others are vocal, raucous, and raspy. Some have better language learning skills than others. Most have high levels of cognitive ability. The hookbills need to exercise their beaks, one of nature's most remarkable tools. They need to have the opportunity to chew with all the variations of splitting, cracking, prying, and splintering.

Of all the birds, canaries, budgies, hand-raised cockatiels, and some of the larger psittacines make the best avian companions.

Maintaining the Relationship

To maintain the human-avian bond, veterinary practitioners must set an example and teach responsible stewardship. Stewardship is the contemporary alternative to dominion. Responsible, dedicated caring rather than owning is the basis for stewardship. Knowledge is essential to provide proper care. The primary role of the veterinarian in the relationship with clients is that of teacher. What species of bird would be appropriate for the client? What basic information on avian species does the client need to have? What are the specialized requirements of the avian species in question? What zoonotic diseases should the client be aware of? This material can be discussed with clients during office visits and augmented with brochures and recommended reading lists. By facilitating the client's decision-making process, veterinarians further enhance the human-avian relationship. When should the bird be examined and how often? Should wings be clipped? Should the bird be sexed? Should the bird have a mate? These and many more issues presented by clients give the clinician an opportunity to provide information and educate clients to become better stewards of birds.

Maximizing the Potentials of the Bond

In addition to basic education and the teaching of stewardship, the human-avian bond will never reach its maximum potential if the bird is not healthy or has undesirable behavior problems. Unacceptable behavior may be the single greatest reason for the breaking of the bond. Rather than being reactive and remedial in our advice, let us strive to be proactive and prevent undesirable behaviors from developing in the first place. Excessive screaming, aggression, destructiveness, self-mutilation, insecurity, and fear responses are all undesirable behaviors. (See Chapter 7, Behavior.)

Identifying Special Bonds

As mentioned earlier, avian companions often assume surrogate roles. In most of these situations the clinician, if attentive, will recognize clear signs of these nonconventional relationships. "He's like my child" or "Be careful of my baby" are clear statements pointing to the avian patient as a child substitute. Clients who speak "motherese" to their birds also consider the bird as they would a child. "He courts me each morning when I come down to the kitchen." This statement by a widow who

acquired her macaw 18 years earlier, a week after her husband died, points to a bird as a spousal substitute. Last-link pets also are special bonds. "Tweety was my late wife's companion" is a revealing statement that the practitioner needs to note on the records for future use. The bird that was "rescued" is also of special interest. It may have been found on the street or "saved" from the pet shop. The loss of these last-link and rescued birds is a devastating experience for clients. This phenomenon and appropriate actions are discussed in Chapter 58, Grief and Bereavement.

References and Reading List

1. Anderson RS (ed): Pet Animals and Society. London, Bailliere Tindall, 1975.
2. Arkow P (ed): Dynamic Relationships in Practice: Animals in the Helping Professions. Alameda, CA, Latham Foundation, 1984.
3. Beck A, Katcher A: Between Pets and People: The Importance of Animal Companionship. New York, Putnam and Sons, 1983.
4. Bustad L: Animals, Aging, and the Aged. Minneapolis, University of Minnesota Press, 1980.
5. Cusack O, Smith E: Pets and the Elderly: The Therapeutic Bond. New York, Haworth Press, 1984.
6. Fogle B (ed): Interrelations between People and Pets. Springfield, IL, Charles C Thomas, 1981.
7. Forshaw JM: Parrots of the World. Neptune, NJ, TFH Publications, 1977.
8. Katcher A, Beck AM (eds): New Perspectives on Our Lives with Companion Animals. Philadelphia, University of Pennsylvania Press, 1983.
9. Lawrence EA: Wild Birds: Therapeutic Encounters and Human Meanings. Anthrozoos III-2:111–118, 1989.
10. Sussman MB (ed): Pets and the Family. New York, Haworth Press, 1985.

James M. Harris

58

Grief and Bereavement

Living things die. None is immortal. *Homo sapiens* is a long-lived species and with few exceptions should expect to outlive avian companions. The life expectancy of avian species ranges from a few years to many decades. In the wild, creatures rarely die from natural causes in old age because predators take the weak and aging. Captive birds are protected from predation and, if properly nourished and cared for, can be expected to live to their full life expectancy.

TYPES OF LOSS

Natural Causes

All living things age and eventually die. Organ function decreases below the point of sustaining the organism. The immune system fails, allowing lurking opportunists to take over, or neoplastic processes are triggered by a variety of causes. For most, death from natural causes is an acceptable event.

Diseases

There are many factors that affect and control populations and their numbers: space, food supply, population density, climatic conditions, and the like. With reasonable care captive birds in cages or indoor aviaries, whether kept singly or in groups, are generally protected from excess population densities, inadequate food supply, and adverse climatic conditions. Poor management and ignorance on the part of avian caretakers can result in the introduction of disease with both morbidity and mortality.

Chlamydiosis, salmonellosis, mycobacteriosis, psittacine beak and feather disease, and others are examples of infections that should be excluded from the aviary.

Trauma ("Things That Go Bump in the Night")

Aberrant stimuli can startle avian species. Earthquakes, sudden noises, and flashes of light can all result in a sudden fright and flight response. For a caged bird this means potential head, body, and feather trauma, often resulting in death. Cage doors are often slammed shut on birds, and birds not acclimated to a particular space may fly into windows, walls, mirrors, or objects such as ceiling fans. Predatory household pets can traumatize accessible birds.

Disasters

In recent times earthquakes, hurricanes, floods and fires have devastated areas of the US and other parts of the world. The destruction of structures often results in loss of life, both human and nonhuman.

Lost Birds

A bird that flies out an open window or door or takes flight from the owner's shoulder while outside creates additional issues of loss. The owner is often unable to establish closure. There is hope that the bird will one day come back or be found. If the client had a particularly strong attachment to the lost bird it can be difficult to obtain a new bird and establish a new relationship.

Euthanasia

The decision to end the life of a creature, even when there is suffering, poor quality of life, or a hopeless medical situation, is accompanied by some degree of guilt.

FACTORS INFLUENCING RESPONSE TO LOSS

Contemporary relationships, both intraspecies and interspecies, can be very complex. We are an urban society somewhat isolated from the living environment, in which we struggle for both physical and emotional survival. Companion species have become integral parts of family systems and in some cases make up an individual's whole family.

To paraphrase the British psychiatrist Keddie, people who insist on a special relationship with a pet can be expected to have a rather sharp reaction at the loss of that pet. Special relationships include surrogate roles: children, spouse, siblings, family, and friends. The companion bird of a deceased partner, last-link pets, and sudden unexpected death will influence the response to loss. Unresolved grief from prior losses or piggyback loss (multiple losses within a short period of time) affect and influence the response to the demise of a bird companion or on occasion an aviary bird.

Death of a bird as the first loss experience of a client is not so unusual today. In past decades children were exposed to the death of grandparents, parents, other relatives, friends, or childhood pets and had the opportunity to practice grieving. With increased longevity, many adults have avoided any prior losses. The number of creatures kept by a client also influences the response at a time of loss. The intensity of the response is inversely proportional to the number kept. I have had the personal experience of working with clients who had no childhood pets and no family deaths. These clients were quite traumatized by the death of the

companion bird and had no idea how to cope with their feelings.

The rescue syndrome is familiar to mental health professionals. Clients who inform us of their rescuing the patient are at great risk from a mental health standpoint at the time of loss.

STAGES OF GRIEF

Kübler-Ross pioneered the study and understanding of grief. She observed that the grieving process involves various stages. These stages progress and, except in pathologic situations, eventually resolve. When this occurs the client has established closure. The stages are denial, anger, depression, acceptance, and recovery. These stages do not have fixed time schedules and may vary in duration and intensity from person to person. Sometimes clients experience slipping back to a previous stage before moving on again. Grief becomes pathologic when a client gets stuck in a stage, cannot move forward, and becomes nonfunctional.

STRATEGIES FOR THE PRACTITIONER

We are family practitioners. We care for families. Our patients are part of family systems. We are often the only ones privy to the emotions, feelings, and priorities of our clients. As such, we can help and be successful facilitators at the time of loss. Granted, at times death can be an unpredicted occurrence. Often we are aware of the possibility of death and owe an early warning to our clients. Being proactive is more effective than being reactive or taking no action at all.

Tell clients presenting newly acquired birds of the realistic life expectancy of the species. A thorough client questionnaire helps identify clients at risk. Singles, childless couples, and the like should be noted. Clients who verbally state the presence of surrogate roles placed on their birds are likewise at risk. Clients who use baby talk or "motherese" with their avian companions give a clear signal to the clinician to prepare in advance for troubled waters when death approaches or occurs.

When patients are hospitalized it is imperative that both day and night contact phone numbers are obtained from the client. Any change in condition may signal deterioration and should be reported to the client. If death does occur, the client must be immediately notified by the practitioner in a sensitive and tactful manner.

When death occurs, give clients options for the care of the bird's remains. Consider and comply with all special requests, if reasonable. When death occurs in the absence of the client, offer the client the opportunity to view the remains. When children are involved this action is vital to help them establish closure. If necessary, hold remains until the client can decide on the final deposition of the bird. Sometimes it is best to hold a family conference and poll the family members on their wishes. Do not rush clients in their decision-making. Whereas one may need to have a speedy decision with the body of a Saint Bernard in the middle of the summer, the remains of avian patients can certainly be kept refrigerated for periods of time without taking up much space. Offer your time to discuss issues and choices.

When the client is single and/or advanced in age it is supportive to make a personal telephone contact on the evening of the day the bird dies. Checking in on a client and telling them that you were thinking of them, that you just wanted to know if they were all right, and that you were available if they want to talk is most appreciated by clients.

Encourage clients to memorialize their deceased pets. Enlarging and framing a favorite photograph of the bird or planting a tree or flowering perennial in its honor are two ways a client can create a positive reminder of the relationship they had.

If a postmortem examination is desired and the client wants to view the remains or to take them home for burial, a cosmetic post mortem must be done. All patient deaths should be followed up with a handwritten condolence card. The personal touch is most comforting to clients. This is especially so when a euthanasia decision had been made. Thanking clients for their unselfish kindness and reassuring them that they made a proper decision helps to assuage the guilt feelings that inevitably accompany euthanasia. Clients sometimes request that they be present for euthanasia service. Offer them that choice. Large birds can have euthanasia solution administered by direct intravenous injection. Small and very debilitated birds may need intracardiac or intracoelomic injections. This form of administration may appear brutal to clients. In this case, preanes-

thesia with inhalation anesthetics followed by an injection is cosmetically appropriate.

Euthanasia should not be accomplished by decapitation. A number of veterinary practitioners who have used decapitation have been successfully sued by clients who have asked for their bird's remains for burial at home. In one instance, the client decided to open the box to view the bird's remains before burial and found the head separated from the body.

Clients sometimes request cremation, and in most areas this service is available. It is appropriate to know the providers of this service and to check on their credibility.

When should a client obtain a new bird? Practitioners are often asked this question. There is no certain answer. Clients with multiple birds generally have a less traumatic response to loss. Birds that die that were perceived to have a special relationship with clients may trigger an overt response, even if multiple birds are in the household. It is always appropriate to identify the person who has the primary relationship with the patient. Be sure that the person is included in all decisions on euthanasia and care of the remains.

If a child is involved and the bird dies while the child is in school or away, discourage parents from buying a replacement. It is improper to do so because the child needs to be given time to grieve. Slipping a substitute in the cage during the child's absence is a disservice. It does not promote a reverence for life. Children are not fooled and invariably are aware of the fact that the "Tweety" in the cage when they return from school is not the same bird that was there earlier in the day. The anger generated by this action will remain for years afterward. Remember that the loss of a pet allows a child to practice grieving and prepares children to work through future losses that will occur.

Last-link pets are also a special circumstance that require special sensitivity on the part of the practitioner. A late spouse's bird is often the last connection with the departed family member, and the loss of that pet may exacerbate unresolved grief for the loved one. The contract does not end when the pet dies. Family members still need care.

ALTERNATIVE ACTIONS

At times the practitioner must refer clients for outside assistance. Clients may need counseling or support that the veterinarian cannot provide. Make a reading list of suitable material available for both children and adults. If available, a social worker can be consulted. Refer clients to a pet loss support group that functions in the community.

Identify private therapists and counselors in the community who specifically work with issues of loss, grief, and bereavement. Contact them and ask if they take referrals. When appropriate, offer to provide clients with a list of these therapists.

The breaking of bonds is as much a part of our professional work as the making of bonds. Heal sometimes, but always offer compassionate support.

References and Reading List

1. Doyle P: Grief Counseling and Sudden Death: A Manual and Guide. Springfield, IL, Charles C Thomas, 1980.

2. Keddie KMG: Pathological Mourning after the Death of a Domestic Pet. Br J Psychiatr 131:21–25, 1977.
3. Kosins MS: Maya's First Rose. Royal Oak, MI, Open Sky Books, 1992.
4. Kübler-Ross E: On Death and Dying. New York, Macmillan, 1969.
5. Kushner HS: When Bad Things Happen to Good People. New York, Avon Books, 1981.
6. Lemieux CM: Coping with the Loss of a Pet. Reading, PA, Wallace R. Clark, 1992.
7. Mellonie B, Ingpen R: Lifetimes. New York, Bantam Books, 1983.
8. Nieburg HA, Fischer A: Pet Loss: A Thoughtful Guide for Adults and Children. New York, Harper & Row, 1982 (out of print).
9. Quackenbush J, Graveline D: When Your Pet Dies: How to Cope with Your Feelings. New York, Simon & Schuster, 1985 (out of print).
10. Sibbitt SB: Oh, Where Has My Pet Gone? Wayzata, MN, Libby Press, 1991.
11. Stearns AK: Living Through Personal Crisis. New York, Ballantine, 1984.
12. Viorst J: The Tenth Good Thing About Barney. Hartford, CT, Aladdin Books, 1975.
13. White EB: Charlotte's Web. New York, Harper & Row, 1952.

Appendices

Appendix I

Hematology/Biochemical Reference Ranges

Appendix IA

HEMATOLOGIC AND PLASMA BIOCHEMICAL REFERENCE RANGES OF
COMMON PSITTACINE SPECIES

Table 1
HEMATOLOGIC REFERENCE RANGES OF COMMON PSITTACINE SPECIES*

Value	African Grey Parrot	Amazon Parrot	Budgerigar	Cockatiel	Cockatoo	Conure	Eclectus Parrot	Jardine's Parrot	Lovebird	Macaw	Pionus	Quaker Parrot	Senegal Parrot
Hematocrit (%)	38–48	37–50	38–48	36–49	38–48	36–49	35–47	35–48	38–50	35–48	35–47	35–46	36–48
	42–53†	43–49†	44–54†	43–58†	42–51†	43–56†	43–50†		43–55†	43–54†	43–54†		
Red blood cells (×10⁶/μl)	2.4–3.9	2.4–4.0	2.4–4.0	2.2–3.9	2.2–4.0	2.5–4.0	2.4–3.9	2.4–4.0	2.3–3.9	2.4–4.0	2.4–4.0	2.3–4.0	2.4–4.0
	2.80–3.36†	2.33–2.95†	3.90–4.70†	3.8–4.58†	2.50–2.95†	3.13–3.94†	2.7–3.1†		2.63–3.50†		2.7–3.5†		
Hemoglobin (g/dl)	11.0–16	11.0–17.5	12–16	12–16	11.5–16	12–16	11.5–16	11–16	13–18	11–16	11–16	11–15	11–16
	15.1–16.9†	14.4–16.7†	13.4–15.3†	12.1–14.6†	12.0–14.8†	12.1–14.8†	14.1–16.0†		11.9–15.1†		14.2–15.5†		
Mean corpuscular volume (fl)	90–180	85–200	90–200	90–200	85–200	90–190	95–220	90–190	90–190	90–185	85–210	90–200	90–200
	143–155†	163–170†	115–124†	128–142†	154–170†	135–147†	157–170†		155–166†		154–164†		
Mean corpuscular hemoglobin (g/dl)	28–52	28–55	25–60	28–55	28–60	28–55	27–55	26–56	27–59	27–53	26–54	26–55	27–55
	32.3–45.6†	49.8–58.2†	25.9–30.9†	24.9–36.0†	45.0–55.5†	30.0–40.1†	51.3–54.2†		40–48†		41.4–46.0†		
Mean corpuscular hemoglobin concentration (g/dl)	23–33	22–32	23–30	22–33	21–34	23–31	22–33	21–33	22–32	23–32	24–31	22–32	23–32
	23.16–31.78†	32.8–35.31†	19.80–26.75†	18.91–25.61†	24.12–32.91†	23.5–28.6†	31.2–34.0†		21.9–29.3†		25.8–28.7†		
White blood cells (×10³/μl)	5.0–11.0	6.0–11.0	3.0–8.5	5.0–10.0	5.0–11.0	4.0–11.0	4.0–10.0	4.0–10.0	3.0–8.5	6.0–12.0	4.0–11.5	4.0–10.0	4.0–11.0
	6.0–13.0†	5.0–12.5†	3.0–8.0†	5.0–9.0†	5.0–12.0†	4.0–9.0†			3.0–8.0†	7.0–12.0†			
Heterophils (%)	55–75	55–80	50–75	55–80	55–80	55–75	55–70	55–75	50–75	58–78	50–75	55–80	55–75
	45–72†	32–71†	41–67†	47–72†	45–72†	45–72†			41–71†	48–72†			
Lymphocytes (%)	25–45	20–45	25–45	20–45	20–45	25–45	30–45	25–45	25–50	20–45	25–45	20–45	25–45
	25–50†	20–65†	22–58†	27–58†	20–50†	22–49†			28–52†	18–52†			
Monocytes (%)	0–3	0–3	0–2	0–2	0–1	0–2	0–2	0–2	0–2	0–3	0–2	0–3	0–2
	0–1†		0–2†	0–1†	0–1†	0–1†			0–1†	0–1†			
Basophils (%)	0–1	0–1	0–1	0–2	0–1	0–1	0–2	0–1	0–1	0–1†	0–1	0–2	0–1
	0–1†		0–2†	0–1†	0–1†	0–2†			0–1†				
Eosinophils (%)	0–2	0–1	0–2	0–2	0–2	0–2	0–1	0–1	0–1	0–1	0–2	0–1	0–1
	0–1†	0–0.05†	0–0.05†	0–2†	0–2†	0–1†			0–1†	0–1†			

*Except where noted by (†) values from the Avian and Wildlife Laboratory, University of Miami School of Medicine, Miami, FL 33136. Hematologic determinations were done by Unopette method (Becton-Dickerson, Rutherford, NJ) from EDTA samples 24 hours after collection. Slides for the differential cell count were made at the time of collection.
†Values from the California Avian Laboratory, Citrus Heights, CA 95621.

Table 2
PLASMA BIOCHEMICAL REFERENCE RANGES OF COMMON PSITTACINE SPECIES*

Value	African Grey Parrot	Amazon Parrot	Budgerigar	Cockatiel	Cockatoo	Conure	Eclectus Parrot	Jardine's Parrot	Lory	Lovebird	Macaw	Pionus	Quaker Parrot	Senegal Parrot
Alanine aminotransferase [ALT]/(U/L)	5.0–12.0	5.0–11.0	—	5.0–11.0	5.0–11.0	5.0–13.0	5.0–11.0	—	—	—	5.0–12.0	—	—	—
Albumin (g/dl)	1.57–3.23†	1.90–3.52†	—	0.7–1.8† 0.3–0.9‡	1.8–3.1† 0.3–0.9‡	1.9–3.6† 0.3–0.9‡	2.3–2.6†	1.85–2.23†	1.26–1.96†	2.0–2.8† 0.3–0.9‡	1.24–3.11†	2.19–3.19†	1.26–2.52†	1.45–2.28†
Alkaline phosphatase (U/L)	20–160	15–150	10–80	20–250	15–255	80–250	150–350	—	—	10–90	20–230	—	—	—
Amylase (U/L)	210–530	205–510	—	—	—	100–450	150–645	—	—	—	150–550	—	—	—
Aspartate aminotransferase [AST] (U/L)	100–365 112–339‡	130–350 155–380‡	145–350 160–372‡	95–345 130–390‡	145–355 145–346‡	125–345 147–360‡	120–370	150–275	150–350	110–345 130–343‡	100–300 60–165‡	150–365	150–285	100–350
Bile acids (μmol/L)	13–90 12–85‡	18–60 35–144‡	15–70 35–110‡	20–85 45–105‡	25–87 37–98‡	15–55 35–90‡	10–35	25–65	20–65	13–65 34–88‡	6–35 30–80‡	14–60	25–65	20–85
Blood urea nitrogen [BUN] (mg/dl)	3.0–5.4	3.1–5.3	—	2.9–5.0	3.0–5.1	2.8–5.4	3.0–5.5	—	—	—	3.0–5.6	—	—	—
Calcium (mg/dl)	8.5–13.0 8.3–11.7†	8.5–14.0 8.5–13.0‡	6.5–11.0 8.5–11.0‡	8.0–13.0 8.3–10.9‡	8.0–13.0 8.4–11.0‡	7.0–15.0 8.4–11.0‡	7.0–13	7.0–13	6.5–13	8.0–14.0 8.6–11.5‡	8.5–13.0 8.3–11.0‡	7.0–13.5	7.0–12.0	6.5–13.0
Carbon dioxide [CO₂], total (mmol/L)	13–25	13–26	14–25	13–25	14–25	14–25	14–24	—	—	14–25	14–25	—	—	—
Cholesterol (mg/dl)	160–425	180–305 150–220‡	145–275 120–220‡	140–360 90–195‡	145–355 90–200‡	120–400 83–190‡	130–350	—	—	95–335 125–195‡	100–390	130–295	—	—
Creatine kinase [CK] (U/L)	165–412 120–410‡	55–345 120–410‡	90–300 120–360‡	30–245 167–420‡	95–305 150–400‡	35–355 150–397‡	220–345	—	—	52–245 160–320‡	100–300 90–360‡	—	—	100–330

Analyte	1	2	3	4	5	6	7	8	9	10	11	12	13	14
Creatinine (mg/dl)	0.1-0.4 / 0.1-0.5‡	0.1-0.4	0.1-0.4	0.1-0.4 / 0.1-0.5‡	0.1-0.4 / 0.1-0.8‡	0.1-0.4 / 0.1-0.8‡	0.1-0.4	—	—	0.1-0.4 / 0.1-0.8‡	0.1-0.5 / 0.1-0.7‡	0.1-0.4	—	0.1-0.4
Gamma glutamyl-transferase [GGT] (U/L)	1-10	1-12	1-10	1-30	1-45	1-15	1-20	—	—	2.5-18.0	1-30	—	—	1-15
Globulin (g/dl)	—	—	—	2.5-3.8‡	2.5-3.8‡	2.5-3.8‡	—	—	—	2.5-3.8‡	—	—	—	—
Glucose (mg/dl)	190-350 / 280-354‡	190-345 / 250-370‡	190-390 / 210-450‡	200-445 / 230-440‡	185-355 / 210-410‡	200-345 / 230-400‡	145-245	200-325	200-300	195-405 / 210-390‡	145-345 / 210-360‡	125-300	200-350	140-250
Glutamate dehydrogenase [GLDH] (U/L)	0-9.9	0-9.9	0-9.9	0-9.9	0-9.9	0-9.9	0-9.9	—	—	0-9.9	0-9.9	—	—	—
Lactate dehydrogenase (U/L)	145-465 / 154-380‡	155-425 / 160-360‡	145-435 / 162-380‡	120-455 / 125-374‡	220-550 / 200-400‡	120-390 / 210-390‡	200-425	—	—	105-355 / 230-345‡	70-350 / 70-210‡	—	—	—
Lipase (U/L)	35-350	35-225	30-280	30-280	25-275	30-290	35-275	—	—	—	30-250	—	—	—
Phosphorus (mg/dl)	3.2-5.4 / 3.5-6.9‡	3.1-5.5	3.0-5.2 / 3.7-7.1‡	3.2-4.8 / 4.0-7.7‡	2.5-5.5 / 4.2-7.8‡	2.0-10.0 / 4.0-7.9‡	2.9-6.5	—	—	2.8-4.9	2.0-12.0 / 4.0-7.8‡	2.9-6.6	—	—
Potassium (mmol/L)	2.9-4.6	3.0-4.5	2.2-3.9	2.4-4.6	2.5-4.5	3.4-5.0	3.5-4.3	—	—	2.1-4.8	2.0-5.0	3.5-4.6	—	—
Protein, plasma (g/dl)	3.0-4.6 / 3.2-4.5†§	3.0-5.0 / 3.2-4.5†§	2.5-4.5 / 3.0-4.4†§	2.5-4.5 / 2.9-4.2†§	3.0-5.0 / 3.1-4.4†§	3.0-4.2 / 3.2-4.4†§	2.8-3.8	2.8-4.0	2.0-3.5	2.8-4.4 / 3.2-4.4†§	2.1-4.5 / 2.7-4.7†§	2.2-4.0	2.8-3.6	3.5-4.4
Sodium (mmol/L)	157-165	125-155	139-165	130-153	130-155	135-149	130-145	—	—	132-168	140-165	145-155	—	—
Thyroxine [T4] (μg/dl)	0.3-2.1	0.1-1.1	0.5-2.1	0.7-2.4	0.7-4.1	0.5-2.0	0.5-3.5	—	—	0.2-4.3	0.5-2.3	—	—	—
Triglycerides (mg/dl)	45-145	49-190	105-265	45-200	45-205	50-300	70-410	—	—	45-200	60-135	—	—	—
Uric acid (mg/dl)	4.5-9.5 / 1.9-9.7†	2.3-10.0 / 2.3-9.8‡	4.5-14.0 / 4.0-12.2‡	3.5-10.5 / 3.5-10.4‡	3.5-10.5 / 3.6-10.7‡	2.5-11.0 / 2.7-10.2‡	2.5-11.0	2.5-12.0	2.8-11.5	3.5-11.0 / 3.2-10.2‡	2.5-11.0 / 1.5-11.0‡	3.5-10.0	3.5-11.5	2.3-10.0

*Except where noted by (‡), values are from the Avian and Wildlife Laboratory, University of Miami School of Medicine, Miami, FL 33136. All biochemical determinations at this laboratory were done by Kodak Ektachem and Dupont Analyst systems. Analysis was done 24 hours after sample collection into lithium heparin. Samples were centrifuged and separated at time of collection.
†Plasma protein electrophoresis measured by the Beckman Paragon system.
‡Values from the California Avian Laboratory, Citrus Heights, CA 95621.
§Measured by temperature compensated refractometer.

Table 3

PLASMA PROTEIN ELECTROPHORESIS REFERENCE RANGES OF COMMON PSITTACINE SPECIES*

Value	African Grey Parrot	Amazon Parrot	Cockatiel	Cockatoo	Conure	Eclectus Parrot	Jardine's Parrot	Lory	Lovebird	Macaw	Pionus	Quaker Parrot	Senegal Parrot
Prealbumin (g/dl)	0.03–1.35	0.35–1.05	0.8–1.6	0.24–1.18	0.18–0.98	0.4–1.04	0.18–0.32	0.48–0.76	0.6–1.2	0.05–0.7	0.19–0.93	0.48–1.13	0.19–0.64
Albumin (g/dl)	1.57–3.23	1.90–3.52	0.7–1.8	1.8–3.1	1.9–2.6	2.3–2.6	1.85–2.23	1.26–1.96	2.0–2.8	1.24–3.11	2.19–3.29	1.26–2.52	1.45–2.28
Alpha-1 (g/dl)	0.02–0.27	0.05–0.32	0.05–0.40	0.05–0.18	0.04–0.23	0.09–0.33	0.04–0.15	0.04–0.14	0.08–0.21	0.04–0.25	0.10–0.16	0.04–0.25	0.02–0.20
Alpha-2 (g/dl)	0.12–0.31	0.07–0.32	0.05–0.44	0.04–0.36	0.08–0.26	0.11–0.27	0.08–0.15	0.04–0.23	0.08–0.25	0.04–0.31	0.08–0.15	0.05–0.28	0.08–0.16
Beta (g/dl)	0.15–0.56	0.12–0.72	0.21–0.58	0.22–0.82	0.07–0.47	0.17–0.43	0.18–0.38	0.15–0.58	0.19–0.40	0.14–0.62	0.08–0.45	0.20–0.55	0.26–0.58
Gamma (g/dl)	0.11–0.71	0.17–0.76	0.11–0.43	0.21–0.65	0.12–0.61	0.18–0.55	0.12–0.26	0.13–0.29	0.18–0.45	0.1–0.62	0.18–0.40	0.13–0.48	0.14–0.23
A/G ratio	1.6–4.3	1.9–5.9	1.5–4.3	2.0–4.5	2.2–4.3	2.62–4.05	2.9–3.5	2.3–4.0	2.5–4.6	1.6–4.3	3.4–5.5	2.2–3.2	2.2–3.9

*Values from the Avian and Wildlife Laboratory, University of Miami School of Medicine, Miami, FL 33136. Protein electrophoresis was done with the Beckman Paragon system.

Appendix IB

HEMATOLOGIC AND SERUM BIOCHEMICAL REFERENCE RANGES OF SELECTED SPECIES: JUVENILES

Table 1

HEMATOLOGIC REFERENCE RANGES FOR JUVENILE COCKATOOS (*Cacatua* spp.)*

	30-day Mean Range (n = 58)	60-day Mean Range (n = 44)	90-day Mean Range (n = 29)	180-day Mean Range (n = 21)	All Mean Range (n = 152)
RBC ($\times$ 10^6/μl)	1.96 1.5–2.5	2.7 2–3.6	2.84 2–4	3.38 2–4	2.53 1.5–4
HB (g/dl)	8.12 6.5–10	12.76 10–16	14.04 12–17	14.22 12–16	11.43 6.5–17
HCT (%)	30.1 25–36	44.6 34–59	47.6 39–56	47.2 42–52	39.7 25–59
MCV (fl)	155 130–200	167 120–215	172 130–215	141 120–175	160 120–215
MCH (pg)	38.9 31–50	47.9 36–60	49.0 38–65	42.7 35–55	43.8 31–65
MCHC (g/dl)	24.6 24–33	28.8 24–33	28.5 27–33	30.1 28–33	27.2 24–33
WBC ($\times$ 10^3/μL)	13.7 5.5–25.0	13.4 6.0–25.0	10.0 6.0–15.0	13.5 8.0–25.0	12.9 5.5–25.0
BAND (%)	1.3 0–6	1.8 0–7	1.3 0–6	0.3 0–2	1.3 0–7
HET (%)	54.8 36–74	51.9 27–77	49.0 33–65	39.6 15–64	50.8 27–74
LYMPH (%)	36.4 20–53	39.1 16–62	43.6 27–61	55.9 29–83	41.2 17–65
MONO (%)	6.9 1–12	6.0 1–12	4.9 0–12	3.5 0–9	5.8 0–12
EOS (%)	0	0	0	0	0
BASO (%)	0.6 0–2	1.2 0–4	1.2 0–4	0.9 0–3	0.9 0–4
BAND (cells/μl)	150 0–1000	245 0–1200	130 0–1400	45 0–1000	160 0–1400
HET (cells/μl)	7800 2200–18000	6800 2000–17000	4400 2800–10000	5400 2200–13000	6500 2000–18000
LYMPH (cells/μl)	4900 1800–10000	4600 2000–8500	3900 2200–8000	6800 4500–10000	4900 1800–10000
MONO (cells/μl)	880 0–2000	680 0–1600	440 0–1200	500 0–1600	690 0–2000
EOS (cells/μl)	0	0	0	0	0
BASO (cells/μl)	67 0–500	140 0–500	115 0–500	115 0–500	100 0–500
HET:LYMPH (ratio)	1.6 0–3	1.6 1–4	1.2 0–2	0.8 0–2	1.4 0–3

*From Clubb SL, Schubot RM, Joyner K, et al: Hematologic and serum biochemical reference intervals in juvenile cockatoos. J Assoc Avian Vet 5(1):20–23, 1991.

RBC = red blood cells; HB = hemoglobin; HCT = hematocrit; MCV = mean corpuscular volume; MCH = mean corpuscular hemoglobin; MCHC = mean corpuscular hemoglobin concentration; WBC = white blood cells; HET = heterophils; LYMPH = lymphocytes; MONO = monocytes; EOS = eosinophils; BASO = basophils; HET:LYMPH = heterocytes to lymphocytes.

T a b l e 2

HEMATOLOGIC REFERENCE RANGES FOR JUVENILE UMBRELLA COCKATOOS (*Cacatua alba*)*

	30-day Mean (n = 22)	60-day Mean (n = 43)	90-day Mean (n = 16)	180-day Mean (n = 30)	All Mean (n = 111)
RBC ($\times 10^6/\mu$l)	1.98	2.69	2.75	3.23	2.54
HB (g/dl)	7.9	12.3	14	14.3	11.6
HCT (%)	29.5	41.6	46.9	47	39.3
MCV (fl)	151	158	175	147	158
MCH (pg)	35.3	46.7	51.9	44.7	43.6
MCHC (g/dl)	21.8	29.6	29.9	30.3	27
WBC ($\times 10^3/\mu$l)	20.3	17.9	10.2	14.7	16.6
BAND (%)	1	1.88	1.93	0	1.31
HET (%)	58.4	57.4	50	44.1	54.1
LYMPH (%)	34.4	33.7	41.2	50.5	38.1
MONO (%)	5.77	5.59	5.29	4	5.35
EOS (%)	0	0	0.07	0	0.02
BASO (%)	0.45	1.29	1.43	1.33	1.03
BAND (cells/μl)	185	353	192	0	202
HET (cells/μl)	12041	10523	4465	6440	8917
LYMPH (cells/μl)	6893	5836	3663	6072	5695
MONO (cells/μl)	1118	955	492	607	843
EOS (cells/μl)	0	0	0	0	0.00011
BASO (cells/μl)	83	224	137	147	143
HET:LYMPH (ratio)	1.83	2	1.33	1	1.64

*From Clubb SL, Schubot RM, Joyner K, et al: Hematologic and serum biochemical reference intervals in juvenile cockatoos. J Assoc Avian Vet 5(1):20–23, 1991.
RBC = red blood cells; HB = hemoglobin; HCT = hematocrit; MCV = mean corpuscular volume; MCH = mean corpuscular hemoglobin; MCHC = mean corpuscular hemoglobin concentration; WBC = white blood cells; HET = heterophils; LYMPH = lymphocytes; MONO = monocytes; EOS = eosinophils; BASO = basophils; HET:LYMPH = heterophils to lympchocytes.

Table 3

SERUM BIOCHEMICAL REFERENCE RANGES FOR JUVENILE COCKATOOS (*Cacatua* spp.)*

	30-day Mean Range (n = 58)	60-day Mean Range (n = 44)	90-day Mean Range (n = 29)	180-day Mean Range (n = 21)	All Mean Range (n = 152)
NA (mEq/L)	139	145	150	152	145
	135–145	141–150	145–155	145–155	135–155
K (mEq/L)	4.0	3.3	3.1	3.6	3.6
	2.5–5.5	2.5–5.5	2.5–4	3–5	2.5–5.5
CL (mEq/L)	105	109	115	115	110
	97–112	104–115	109–120	110–120	97–120
CA (mg/dl)	9.2	9.9	9.5	9.9	9.6
	8–10	9–11	7–11	8–11	8–11
PHOS mg/dl)	7.0	6.4	5.1	4.8	6.1
	6–8	5–8	3.5–7	3.5–6.5	3.5–8
UREA (mg/dl)	1.6	2.1	2.6	2.4	2.0
	0–5	0–6	0–6	0–6	0–6
CREAT (mg/dl)	0.31	0.37	0.42	0.46	0.4
	0.3–0.5	0.2–0.7	0.2–0.5	0.2–0.7	0.2–0.7
UA (mg/dl)	1.2	2.7	5.1	4.5	2.9
	0.2–3.2	0.4–6.5	2.0–8.5	2.0–8.5	0.2–8.5
CHOL (mg/dl)	165	320	350	202	251
	100–250	180–450	150–500	150–300	100–500
GLUCOSE (mg/dl)	247	259	249	262	253
	200–300	200–300	200–300	200–300	200–300
LDH (U/L)	393	338	367	386	371
	150–1000	130–1000	150–1000	150–1000	150–1000
AST (U/L)	98	139	195	195	143
	50–175	80–250	150–400	120–320	50–400
ALT (U/L)	2	3	3	2	2
	0–13	0–13	0–12	0–5	0–13
ALP (U/L)	593	714	478	407	579
	280–1000	400–1000	280–800	200–850	200–1000
GGT (U/L)	2.35	3.00	2.79	1.81	2.55
	0–6	0–6	1–5	0–4	0–6
CK (U/L)	595	615	368	267	510
	300–1000	170–1000	170–600	140–410	140–1000
TP (g/dl)	2.2	3.1	3.1	3.2	2.8
	1.5–3	1.5–4	2–4	2.6–4	1.5–4
ALB (g/dl)	0.8	1.2	1.2	1.4	1.1
	0.3–1.2	0.6–1.5	0.7–1.6	1.0–1.6	0.3–1.6
GLOB (g/dl)	1.3	1.9	1.9	1.8	1.7
	0.8–1.2	1.2–2.5	1.5–2.5	1.5–2.5	0.8–2.5
A:G (ratio)	0.6	0.6	0.6	0.8	0.6
	0.38–0.8	0.45–0.85	0.5–0.85	0.6–1	0.38–1
Protein electrophoresis					
PRE-ALB (g/dl)	0.4	0.5	0.5	0.5	0.5
	0.2–0.6	0.2–1	0.2–0.8	0.3–0.6	0.2–1.0
ALB (g/dl)	1.1	1.7	1.7	1.9	1.5
	0.5–1.8	1.1–2.3	0.2–2.3	1.6–2.3	0.5–2.3
ALPHA GLOB (g/dl)	0.2	0.2	0.3	0.4	0.2
	0.1–0.3	0.1–0.5	0.1–0.5	0.1–0.5	0.1–0.5
BETA GLOB (g/dl)	0.3	0.4	0.3	0.3	0.3
	0.1–0.7	0.1–0.8	0.2–0.5	0.2–0.4	0.1–0.8
GAMMA GLOB (g/dl)	0.2	0.3	0.3	0.5	0.3
	0.1–0.4	0.2–0.8	0.1–0.4	0.5–0.5	0.1–0.8

*From Clubb SL, Schubot RM, Joyner K, et al: Hematologic and serum biochemical reference intervals in juvenile cockatoos. J Assoc Avian Vet 5(1):20–23, 1991.

NA = sodium; K = potassium; CL = chloride; CA = calcium; PHOS = phosphorus; CREAT = creatinine; UA = uric acid; CHOL = cholesterol; LDH = lactate dehydrogenase; AST = aspartate aminotransferase; ALT = alanine aminotransferase; ALP = alkaline phosphatase; GGT = gamma glutamyltransferase; CK = creatine kinase; TP = total protein; PRE-ALB = prealbumin; ALB = albumin; GLOB = globulin; A:G = albumin to globulin.

Table 4

SERUM BIOCHEMICAL REFERENCE RANGES FOR JUVENILE UMBRELLA COCKATOOS (*Cacatua alba*)*

	30-day Mean (n = 22)	60-day Mean (n = 43)	90-day Mean (n = 16)	180-day Mean (n = 30)	All Mean (n = 111)
NA (mEq/L)	139	145	149	152	145
K (mEq/L)	4.23	3.13	3.13	3.42	3.54
CL (mEq/L)	107	108	115	116	111
CA (mEq/L)	9.64	10.16	9.43	9.93	9.77
PHOS (mg/dl)	6.5	5.88	4.7	4.49	5.55
UREA (mg/dl)	1	1.31	1.94	2.8	1.61
CREAT (mg/dl)	0.34	0.4	0.33	0.44	0.37
UA (mg/dl)	0.83	2.11	4.95	3.98	2.73
CHOL (mg/dl)	180	351	427	199	291
GLUCOSE (mg/dl)	244	248	236	250	244
LDH (U/L)	326	257	341	410	325
AST (U/L)	84	115	187	192	136
ALT (U/L)	1.8	2.27	2.69	1.6	2.11
ALP (U/L)	426	520	404	394	440
GGT (U/L)	1.95	3.56	2.81	2.4	2.66
CK (U/L)	629	653	395	271	517
TP (g/dl)	2.47	3.38	3.25	3.26	3.03
A:G (ratio)	0.6	0.62	0.62	0.76	0.64
Protein electrophoresis					
PRE-ALB (g/dl)	0.43	0.44	0.49	0.44	0.45
ALB (g/dl)	1.27	1.91	1.86	1.98	1.69
ALPHA GLOB (g/dl)	0.17	0.22	0.29	0.52	0.26
BETA GLOB (g/dl)	0.39	0.45	0.34	0.33	0.38
GAMMA GLOB (g/dl)	0.23	0.35	0.31	—	0.29

*From Clubb SL, Schubot RM, Joyner K, et al: Hematologic and serum biochemical reference intervals in juvenile cockatoos. J Assoc Avian Vet 5(1):20–23, 1991.

NA = sodium; K = potassium; CL = chloride; CA = calcium; PHOS = phosphorus; CREAT = creatinine; UA = uric acid; CHOL = cholesterol; LDH = lactate dehydrogenase; AST = aspartate aminotransferase; ALT = alanine aminotransferase; ALP = alkaline phosphatase; GGT = gamma glutamyltransferase; CK = creatine kinase; TP = total protein; PRE-ALB = prealbumin; ALB = albumin; GLOB = globulin; A:G = albumin to globulin.

T a b l e 5

HEMATOLOGIC REFERENCE RANGES FOR JUVENILE MACAWS (*Ara* spp.)*

	30-day Mean Range (n = 32)	60-day Mean Range (n = 37)	90-day Mean Range (n = 30)	180-day Mean Range (n = 14)	All Mean Range (n = 113)
RBC ($\times 10^6$/μl)	1.9 1.5–2.5	2.7 1.9–3.4	3.7 2.6–4.5	3.7 2.7–4.5	2.9 1.5–4.5
HB (g/dl)	7.7 7–9.5	11.2 9.6–13	15.4 14–17	16.0 15–17	12.3 7–17
HCT (%)	30.9 25–35	40.0 35–45	49.5 45–53	51.1 47–55	41.7 25–55
MCV (fl)	165.5 130–200	150 112–200	137 115–185	140 125–170	149 112–200
MCH (pg)	41.7 32–51	42.0 32–55	42.8 36–55	44.0 36–55	42.3 32–55
MCHC (g/dl)	25.1 22.5–27.5	28.1 25–30	31.1 28–33	31.4 29–35	28.7 22.5–35
WBC ($\times 10^3$/μl)	19.3 11.0–30.0	22.2 10.0–30.0	17.7 10.0–30.0	14.9 7.0–22.0	19.2 7.0–30.0
BANDS (%)	0.8 0–5	0.6 0–5	0.3 0–5	1.0 0–5	0.6 0–5
HET (%)	58.9 43–75	56.5 43–70	53.9 37–65	48.3 40–60	55.3 37–75
LYMPH (%)	33.8 20–45	38.1 21–52	41.6 26–55	46.6 35–60	39.0 20–60
MONO (%)	5.9 1–10	4.2 1–10	3.6 1–8	3.7 1–8	4.4 1–10
EOS (%)	0 0–0	0 0–0	0.1 0–1	0.1 0–1	0 0–1
BASO (%)	0.7 0–3	0.6 0–3	0.6 0–3	0.1 0–1	0.5 0–3
BANDS (cell/μl)	134 0–800	119 0–1000	59 0–1000	143 0–500	110 0–1000
HET (cells/μl)	10200 5000–20000	11600 5000–20000	9400 5000–16000	7400 3000–13000	10100 3000–20000
LYMPH (cells/μl)	5500 3000–11000	7800 3000–13000	7000 3000–12000	6700 3000–11000	6800 3000–13000
MONO (cells/μl)	910 300–18000	784 200–13000	627 200–14000	555 200–13000	750 200–14000
EOS (cells/μl)	0 0–0	0 0–0	9.3 0–275	17.1 0–240	4.6 0–275
BASO (cells/μl)	115 0–500	111 0–600	75 0–400	18.5 0–200	91 0–600
HET:LYMPH (ratio)	2.0 0.95–4.0	1.6 0.75–3.50	1.4 0.6–3.0	1.1 0.6–1.75	1.6 0.6–4.0

*From Clubb SL, Schubot RM, Joyner K, et al: Hematologic and serum biochemical reference intervals in juvenile macaws. J Assoc Avian Vet 5(3):158–161, 1991.
RBC = red blood cells; HB = hemoglobin; HCT = hematocrit; MCV = mean corpuscular volume; MCH = mean corpuscular hemoglobin; MCHC = mean corpuscular hemoglobin concentration; WBC = white blood cells; HET = heterophils; LYMPH = lymphocytes; MONO = monocytes; EOS = eosinophils; BASO = basophils; HET:LYMPH = heterophils to lymphocytes.

Table 6

HEMATOLOGIC REFERENCE RANGES FOR JUVENILE BLUE AND GOLD MACAWS (*Ara ararauna*)*

	30-day Mean (n = 16)	60-day Mean (n = 17)	90-day Mean (n = 10)	All Mean (n = 43)
RBC ($\times 10^6/\mu$l)	1.9	2.8	3.5	2.7
HB (g/dl)	7.9	11	15	11
HCT (%)	30	40	48	40
MCV (fl)	163	144	137	149
MCH (pg)	43	40	41	38
MCHC (g/dl)	26	28	31	25
WBC ($\times 10^3/\mu$l)	19.2	21.5	16.6	18.9
BAND (%)	0.36	0	0	0.12
HET (%)	57	52	48	52
LYMPH (%)	37	44	47	42
MONO (%)	5.3	3.6	3.8	4.3
EOS (%)	0	0	0	0
BASO (%)	0.9	0.8	1.1	0.9
BANDS (cells/μl)	0.36	0	0	0.12
HET (cells/μl)	11000	11000	8100	10000
LYMPH (cells/μl)	7000	9600	7700	8000
MONO (cells/μl)	949	686	639	756
EOS (cells/μl)	0	0	0	0
BASO (cells/μl)	194	145	156	154
HET:LYMPH (ratio)	1.75	1.26	1.19	1.38

*From Clubb SL, Schubot RM, Joyner K, et al: Hematologic and serum biochemical reference intervals in juvenile macaws. J Assoc Avian Vet 5(3):158–161, 1991.

RBC = red blood cells; HB = hemoglobin; HCT = hematocrit; MCV = mean corpuscular volume; MCH = mean corpuscular hemoglobin; MCHC = mean corpuscular hemoglobin concentration; WBC = white blood cells; HET = heterophils; LYMPH = lymphocytes; MONO = monocytes; EOS = eosinophils; BASO = basophils; HET:LYMPH = heterophils to lymphocytes.

Table 7

SERUM BIOCHEMICAL REFERENCE RANGES FOR JUVENILE MACAWS (*Ara* spp.)*

	30-day Mean Range (n = 32)	60-day Mean Range (n = 37)	90-day Mean Range (n = 30)	180-day Mean Range (n = 14)	All Mean Range (n = 113)
NA (mEq/L)	137 135–139	144.2 140–152	151.1 148–156	151 148–156	145 135–156
K (mEq/L)	3.3 2.7–4.2	2.6 1.9–3.7	2.7 2.0–4.7	2.8 2.2–3.9	2.9 2.0–4.2
CL (mEq/L)	101 96–110	105 100–108	112 108–118	110 105–113	106 96–118
CA (mg/dl)	9.5 8.5–10	10 9.2–10.8	10 9.1–10.8	10 9.5–10.5	9.9 8.5–10.8
PHOS (mg/dl)	7.3 6.4–8.4	6.9 6.2–7.5	5.6 4.7–6.9	5.2 4.6–6.4	6.5 4.6–6.9
UREA (mg/dl)	1.0 0–4	2.1 0–5	3.4 0–6	4.5 0–6	2.4 0–6
CREAT (mg/dl)	0.4 0.3–0.4	0.4 0.3–0.5	0.4 0.3–0.6	0.6 0.5–0.6	0.4 0.3–0.6
U.A. (mg/dl)	0.6 0.2–1.5	1.5 0.7–2.8	3.9 2.5–6.0	4.2 1.0–6.0	2.3 0.2–6.0
CHOL (mg/dl)	119 75–160	144 85–215	231 140–300	178 100–300	165 75–300
GLUCOSE (mg/dl)	264 225–330	285 240–325	290 245–325	292 280–320	281 225–330
LDH (U/L)	132 35–275	176 50–275	114 40–275	98 40–250	138 35–275
AST (U/L)	84 60–120	92 60–120	127 90–180	123 90–180	104 60–180
ALT (U/L)	3 0–9	4 1–9	4 1–9	3 0–5	3 0–9
ALP (U/L)	1072 675–1600	1205 750–1600	786 475–1200	431 290–750	970 290–1600
GGT (U/L)	2.0 0–4	1.9 0–4	1.2 0–4	2.0 0–4	1.8 0–4
CK (U/L)	596 250–1000	714 250–1200	442 215–1000	256 180–500	550 180–1100
TP (g/dl)	1.7 1.5–2.2	2.7 2.1–3.2	3.0 2.4–3.5	3.1 2.7–3.5	2.6 1.5–3.5
ALB (g/dl)	0.7 0.6–0.9	1.2 0.9–3.2	1.4 1.2–1.7	1.5 1.3–1.7	1.2 0.6–1.7
GLOB (g/dl)	0.8 0.8–1.3	1.4 1.1–1.9	1.5 1.3–1.9	1.8 1.3–1.9	1.3 0.8–1.9
A:G (ratio)	0.7 0.5–0.9	0.9 0.6–1	0.9 0.7–1	0.8 0.7–1	0.8 0.5–1
Protein electrophoresis					
PRE-ALB (g/dl)	0.2 0.1–0.3	0.3 0.2–0.4	0.5 0.3–0.6	0.4 0.3–0.6	0.3 0.1–0.6
ALB (g/dl)	1.0 0.5–1.5	1.6 1.2–1.9	1.8 1.2–2.4	1.8 1.4–2.2	1.5 0.5–2.2
ALPHA GLOB (g/dl)	0.2 0.1–0.3	0.3 0.1–0.4	0.3 0.2–0.4	0.3 0.1–0.4	0.3 0.1–0.4
BETA GLOB (g/dl)	0.3 0.1–0.4	0.3 0.2–0.6	0.4 0.2–0.5	0.4 0.2–0.6	0.3 0.1–0.6
GAMMA GLOB (g/dl)	0.2 0.1–0.3	0.3 0.2–0.4	0.3 0.2–0.4	0.3 0.2–0.4	0.3 0.1–0.4

*From Clubb SL, Schubot RM, Joyner K, et al: Hematologic and serum biochemical reference intervals in juvenile macaws. J Assoc Avian Vet 5(3):158–161, 1991.

NA = sodium; K = potassium; CL = chloride; CA = calcium; PHOS = phosphorus; CREAT = creatinine; UA = uric acid; CHOL = cholesterol; LDH = lactate dehydrogenase; AST = aspartate aminotransferase; ALT = alanine aminotransferase; ALP = alkaline phosphatase; GGT = gamma glutamyltransferase; CK = creatine kinase; TP = total protein; PRE-ALB = prealbumin; ALB = albumin; GLOB = globulin; A:G = albumin to globulin.

SERUM BIOCHEMICAL REFERENCE RANGES FOR JUVENILE BLUE AND GOLD MACAWS (*Ara ararauna*)*

	30-day Mean (n = 16)	60-Day Mean (n = 17)	90-Day Mean (n = 10)	All Mean (n = 43)
NA (mEq/L)	136	143	150	142
K (mEq/L)	3.20	2.41	2.20	2.71
CL (mg/dl)	98.8	104	111	104
CA (mg/dl)	9.7	10.2	10.2	10
PHOS (mg/dl)	7.2	6.7	5.6	6.6
UREA (mg/dl)	1.2	1.9	2.5	1.9
CREAT (mg/dl)	0.3	0.4	0.4	0.4
UA (mg/dl)	0.6	1.6	3.4	1.9
CHOL (mg/dl)	114	151	251	164
GLUCOSE (mg/dl)	266	301	299	288
LDH (U/L)	136	189	97	144
AST (U/L)	88	98	127	101
ALT (U/L)	3	5	4	4
ALP (U/L)	1225	1475	950	1200
GGT (U/L)	2.0	1.9	0.9	1.7
CK (U/L)	498	763	330	540
TP (g/dl)	1.7	2.7	2.9	2.5
ALB (g/dl)	0.7	1.3	1.4	1.2
GLOB (g/dl)	0.8	1.4	1.4	1.3
A:G (ratio)	0.8	0.8	0.9	0.8
Protein electrophoresis				
PRE-ALB (g/dl)	0.2	0.3	0.5	0.3
ALB (g/dl)	1.0	1.6	1.8	1.5
ALPHA GLOB (g/dl)	0.2	0.3	0.3	0.3
BETA GLOB (g/dl)	0.3	0.3	0.4	0.3
GAMMA GLOB (g/dl)	0.2	0.3	0.3	0.3

*From Clubb SL, Schubot RM, Joyner K, et al: Hematologic and serum biochemical reference intervals in juvenile macaws. J Assoc Avian Vet 5(3):158–161, 1991.

NA = sodium; K = potassium; CL = chloride; CA = calcium; PHOS = phosphorus; CREAT = creatinine; UA = uric acid; CHOL = cholesterol; LDH = lactate dehydrogenase; AST = aspartate aminotransferase; ALT = alanine aminotransferase; ALP = alkaline phosphatase; GGT = gamma glutamyltransferase; CK = creatine kinase; TP = total protein; PRE-ALB = prealbumin; ALB = albumin; GLOB = globulin; A:G = albumin to globulin.

T a b l e   9

HEMATOLOGY REFERENCE RANGES FOR JUVENILE ECLECTUS PARROTS (*Eclectus roratus*)*

	30-day Mean Range	60-day Mean Range	90-day Mean Range	180-day Mean Range	All Mean Range
RBC ($\times\ 10^6/\mu$l)	1.95 1.5–2.5	2.74 2–3.5	3.22 2.5–4	3.38 2.7–3.8	2.69 1.5–4.0
HB (g/dl)	8.83 6.5–10.5	12.82 10.5–14.5	15.42 13.5–18	14.91 13.5–16	12.46 6.5–18
HCT (%)	33.7 26–40	44.5 40–50	53.8 43–58	48.6 45–55	43.8 26–58
MCV (fl)	174 125–215	165 125–215	169 125–200	145 125–175	166 125–215
MCH (pg)	43.9 36–62	46.2 36–62	49.1 35–62	41.7 40–50	45.5 35–62
MCHC (g/dl)	26.1 23–32	28.1 25–32	28.7 25–32	28.6 29–32	27.7 23–32
WBC ($\times\ 10^3/\mu$L)	18.5 8.0–25.0	10.6 5.5–18.0	10.9 6.5–18.0	15.0 9.0–20.0	13.7 5.5–25.0
BANDS (%)	0.2 0–0	1.1 0–5	0.4 0–5	0.0 0–0	0.5 0–5
HET (%)	62.8 50–75	51.9 40–75	52.1 36–65	41.9 35–50	53.9 35–75
LYMPH (%)	30.4 20–42	41.0 20–55	40.8 28–57	53.8 45–65	39.5 20–65
MONO (%)	5.5 1–0	5.1 1–11	5.2 1–10	3.1 1–7	5.0 1–11
EOS (%)	0.0 0–1	0.0 0–1	0.1 0–1	0.2 1–1	0.1 0–1
BASO (%)	1.2 0–3	0.7 0–3	1.5 0–3	1.1 0–3	1.1 0–3
BAND (cells/μl)	34 0–1000	144 0–800	48 0–400	0.0 0–0	70 0–1000
HET (cells/μl)	11800 4400–17000	5600 2600–9000	5900 3000–12000	6800 2800–9000	7700 4400–17000
LYMPH (cells/μl)	5500 2500–8800	4200 2500–6400	4200 2600–5300	7600 5800–10000	5100 2500–10000
MONO (cells/μl)	930 200–2000	526 200–1200	532 0–1200	454 0–900	639 0–2000
EOS (cells/μl)	0 0–0	3 0–100	9 0–200	34 0–300	8 0–300
BASO (cells/μl)	209 0–500	82 0–500	175 0–500	161 0–400	152 0–500
HET:LYMPH	2.2 1–4	1.4 1–3	1.4 1–3	0.9 1–2	1.6 1–3

From Clubb SL, Schubot RM, Joyner K et al: Hematologic and serum biochemical reference intervals in juvenile *Eclectus* parrots *(Eclectus roratus)*, J Assoc Avian Vet 4(4):223–224, 1990.

*RBC = red blood cells; HB = hemoglobin; HCT = hematocrit; MCV = mean corpuscular volume; MCH = mean corpuscular hemoglobin; MCHC = mean corpuscular hemoglobin concentration; WBC = white blood cells; HET = heterophils; LYMPH = lymphocytes; MONO = monocytes; EOS = eosinophils; BASO = basophils; HET:LYMPH = heterocytes to lymphoctes.

T a b l e 1 0

SERUM BIOCHEMICAL REFERENCE RANGES FOR JUVENILE ECLECTUS PARROTS (*Eclectus roratus*)*

	30-day Mean Range	60-day Mean Range	90-day Mean Range	180-day Mean Range	All Mean Range
NA (mEq/L)	141 138–144	148 145–152	154 150–158	153 150–158	148 138–158
K (mEq/L)	2.9 2–4.6	2.8 2–4	2.7 2.2–4.6	3.1 2.2–4.6	2.8 2.0–4.6
CL (mEq/L)	105 100–108	112 108–116	115 110–120	116 112–120	111 100–120
CA (mg/dl)	9.5 9–10.2	9.4 8.8–10.2	9.1 8.5–9.8	9.3 8.8–9.8	9.3 8.5–10.2
PHOS (mg/dl)	7.9 6.5–9	7.2 6–9	5.7 5–8	5.5 4.5–7	6.8 4.5–9
UREA (mg/dl)	1.5 0–6	1.4 0–6	2.0 0–6	2.3 0–6	1.7 0–6
CREAT (mg/dl)	0.3 0.2–0.4	0.4 0.2–0.5	0.4 0.4–0.5	0.5 0.4–0.5	0.4 0.2–0.5
UA (mg/dl)	0.8 0.2–1.2	1.6 0.6–3.2	3.9 18–6.5	2.7 0.7–5.0	2.0 0.2–6.5
CHOL (mg/dl)	181 125–275	326 190–450	300 200–450	266 220–325	268 125–450
GLUCOSE (mg/dl)	249 220–285	263 240–285	265 240–300	258 225–300	258 220–300
LDH (U/L)	235 130–250	218 125–250	268 250–400	178 100–280	228 100–400
AST (U/L)	85 65–120	130 90–180	216 180–260	160 135–230	140 65–260
ALT (U/L)	4 0–10	4 0–10	7 0–13	2 0–5	4 0–10
ALP (U/L)	421 260–570	540 350–750	565 360–900	407 200–750	489 200–900
GGT (U/L)	5 0–7	4 1–7	2 0–5	4 1–5	4 0–7
CK (U/L)	555 350–1000	773 400–1600	643 400–1200	362 200–625	616 200–1600
TP (g/dl)	2.6 1.8–3.2	2.9 2–3.4	2.9 2–3.4	3.4 2.8–3.8	2.9 1.8–3.8
ALB (g/dl)	1.2 0.8–1.5	1.3 1–1.6	1.3 1–1.6	1.7 1.4–1.8	1.3 0.8–1.8
GLOB (g/dl)	1.3 0.8–1.7	1.6 1.2–2.0	1.6 1.2–2.0	1.7 1.3–2.3	1.5 0.8–2.2
A:G (ratio)	0.9 0.7–1.1	0.9 0.6–1.1	0.8 0.6–1.0	0.9 0.6–1.1	0.9 0.6–1.1
Protein electrophoresis					
ALB (g/dl)	1.8 1.5–2.3	2.2 1.7–2.6	2.1 1.5–3.0	2.5 2.1–3.0	2.2 1.5–3.0
GLOB (g/dl)	0.7 0.5–1.2	0.8 0.5–1.2	0.7 0.5–1.2	0.9 0.6–1.2	0.8 0.5–1.2

*From Clubb SL, Schubot RM, Joyner K, et al: Hematologic and serum biochemical reference intervals in juvenile *Eclectus* parrots *(Eclectus roratus).* J Assoc Avian Vet 4(4):223–224, 1990.

NA = sodium; K = potassium; CL = chloride; CA = calcium; PHOS = phosphorus; CREAT = creatinine; UA = uric acid; CHOL = cholesterol; LDH = lactate dehydrogenase; AST = aspartate aminotransferase; ALT = alanine aminotransferase; ALP = alkaline phosphatase; GGT = gamma glutamyltransferase; CK = creatine kinase; TP = total protein; PRE-ALB = prealbumin; ALB = albumin; GLOB = globulin; A:G = albumin to globulin.

Appendix IC

HEMATOLOGIC AND SERUM BIOCHEMICAL REFERENCE RANGES OF RATITES

Table 1

HEMATOLOGIC REFERENCE RANGES OF RATITES*

Value	Ostrich Adults		Emu Adults	
	Mean	*Range*	*Mean*	*Range*
Red blood cells ($\times 10^6/\mu$l)	1.8	—	1.85	—
Hematocrit (%)	45	41–57	47.4	39–57
Hemoglobin (g/dl)	16.92	—	16.04	—
Mean corpuscular volume (fl)	212	—	219	—
Mean corpuscular hemoglobin (pg)	82.19	—	86.51	—
Mean corpuscular hemoglobin concentration (g/L)	37.65	—	39.37	—
Red blood cell distribution width percentage† (%)	11.11	—	10.9	—
White blood cells ($\times 10^3/\mu$l)	18.65	10.0–24	14.87	8–21
Heterophils (%)	75.1	58–89	78.8	54–88
Lymphocytes (%)	24.1	12–41	19.8	10–44
Monocytes (%)	0.2	0–2	0.1	0–1
Basophils (%)	1.36	0–3	0.2	0–1
Eosinophils (%)	2.16	0–4	2.58	0–6

*Values from the California Avian Laboratory, Citrus Heights, CA 95621. Values were calculated from samples collected in field conditions and vary somewhat from previously published ranges.

†Red cell distribution width (RDW) percentage is a numerical expression of the coefficient of variability of the mean corpuscular volume, calculated by automated erythrocyte analysis (laser flow cytometry). An increase in RDW percentage denotes an increase in anisocytosis; a decrease in RDW percentage denotes a decrease in anisocytosis, as seen in nonregenerative anemia.

Table 2

SERUM BIOCHEMICAL REFERENCE RANGES OF RATITES*

Value	Ostrich Adults		Emu Adults	
	Mean	*Range*	*Mean*	*Range*
Albumin (g/dl)	1.72	1.1–2.3	1.7	1.2–2.4
Aspartate aminotransferase [AST] (U/L)	447.9	226–547	227.2	80–380
Bile acids (μmol/L)	21	2–30	18	2–34
Calcium (mg/dl)	10.7	8.0–13.6	11.1	8.8–12.5
Cholesterol (mg/dl)	103	39–172	122	68–170
Creatine kinase (U/L)	3702	800–6600	428.8	70–818
Creatinine (mg/dl)	0.26	0.1–0.7	0.22	0.1–0.4
Globulin	2.21	1.4–3.1	2.23	1.4–3.2
Glucose (mg/dl)	217	164–330	134.1	101–243
Lactate dehydrogenase (U/L)	970	408–1236	778.1	318–1243
Phosphorus (mg/dl)	5.33	2.9–7.7	5.7	3.8–7.2
Plasma protein (g/dl)	3.93	2.4–5.3	3.93	3.4–4.4
Total protein (g/dl)	4.47†	2.5–5.2†	4.26†	2.5–5.6†
Uric acid (mg/dl)	8.62	1–14.5	6.3	1–13.7

*Values from the California Avian Laboratory, Citrus Heights, CA 95621. Values were calculated from cases sampled in field conditions and vary somewhat from previously published ranges.

†Measured by temperature-compensated refractomer.

Appendix I D

HEMATOLOGIC, BIOCHEMICAL, AND MORPHOMETRIC REFERENCE RANGES OF SELECTED RAPTOR SPECIES

T a b l e 1

HEMATOLOGIC REFERENCE RANGES OF SELECTED HEALTHY ADULT CAPTIVE RAPTORS*

Value	Red-Tailed Hawk (n = 10)	Great-Horned Owl (n = 10)	Bald Eagle (n = 8)	Peregrine Falcon (n = 14)	Gyrfalcon (n = 12)
PCV (%)	44.6 (2.6)†	43.3 (2.9)	44 (4)	44 (4)	49 (2)
Total protein (g/dl)	4.3 (0.5)	5.1 (0.6)	4.0 (1)	2.65 (1.18)	2.94 (0.38)
White blood cells (× 10³/µl)	6.0–8.0	6.0–8.0	12.8 (4.8)	8.7 (2.2)	4.6 (1.7)
Heterophils (%)	35 (11.1)	47 (10.7)	75 (13)	65 (12)	51 (5)
Lymphocytes(%)	44 (8.9)	27 (7.0)	18 (10)	35 (13)	47 (5)
Monocytes (%)	6 (3.2)	9 (3.6)	3 (3)	0 (0)	1 (1)
Basophils (%)	2 (1.3)	Rare	Rare	0 (0)	Rare
Eosinophils (%)	13 (3.8)	1 (1.2)	4 (3)	0 (1)	1 (1)

*From Dr. P. Redig, The Raptor Center, University of Minnesota, St. Paul, MN 55108.
†Standard deviation in parentheses.

T a b l e 2

HEMATOLOGIC AND MORPHOMETRIC MEASUREMENTS OF WILD RED-TAILED HAWK NESTLINGS*

Stage of Development	Primary Feather Length (cm)	Central Tail Feather Length (cm)	PCV (%)	Total Protein (g/dl)	RBC (× 10⁶/µl)	Hemoglobin (g/dl)
Early (n = 5)	0–10	0–8	28 (1)†	3.4 (0.1)	1.74 (0.09)	8.79 (0.40)
Late (n = 5)	11–18	9–16	33 (1)†	4.0 (0.1)	2.35 (0.03)	10.98 (0.14)

*From Dr. P. Redig, The Raptor Center, University of Minnesota, St. Paul, MN 55108.
†Means ± standard deviations in parentheses.

T a b l e 3

SERUM BIOCHEMICAL REFERENCE VALUES OF SELECTED RAPTOR SPECIES*

Value	Bald Eagle (n = 8)	Peregrine Falcon (n = 14)	Gyrfalcon (n = 12)	Red-Tailed Hawk (n = 10)	Great-Horned Owl (n = 10)
Acetylcholinesterase (delta pH units/h)	0.16 (0.06)	—	—	—	—
Alanine aminotransferase [ALT] (U/L)	25 (13)	62 (56)	—	31 (5)	39 (14)
Albumin (g/dl)	1.09 (0.18)	0.96 (0.13)	0.73 (0.09)	1.34 (0.41)	1.27 (0.35)
Alkaline phosphatase (U/L)	57 (12)	99 (44)	257 (61)	53 (18)	31 (7)
Amylase (U/L)	1158 (376)	—	—	—	—
Aspartate aminotransferase [AST] (U/L)	218 (63)	78 (31)	97 (33)	303 (22)	287 (65)
Bilirubin, total (mg/dl)	0.31 (0.08)	4.57 (2.04)	—	0.16 (0.08)	0.07 (0.06)
Blood urea nitrogen [BUN] (mg/dl)	3.10 (2.47)	3.25 (1.39)	4.67 (0.82)	4.67 (0.47)	5 (2.94)
Calcium (mg/dl)	9.94 (0.45)	8.93 (0.46)	9.61 (0.24)	—	10.19
Chloride (mmol/L)	120 (3)	114.38 (43.36)	125 (2)	125 (3)	122
Creatine kinase (U/L)	383 (300)	783 (503)	402 (163)	1124 (251)	977 (407)
Creatinine (mg/dl)	0.70 (0.26)	0.51 (0.22)	—	—	—
Glucose (mg/dl)	302 (25)	366 (29)	318 (39)	356 (16)	356
Osmolality (mmol/kg)	319 (6)	—	—	—	—
Phosphorus (mg/dl)	3.03 (0.51)	3.35 (0.70)	3.57 (1.13)	3.14 (0.5)	4.34
Potassium (mmol/L)	3.0 (0)	2.04 (0.81)	1.99 (0.56)	2.42 (0.73)	2.8
Protein, total (g/dl) (biuret)	3.51 (0.75)	2.63 (0.48)	2.89 (0.31)	4.17 (0.69)	4.33
Sodium (mmol/L)	156 (4)	143 (54)	160 (3)	157 (1)	156
Uric acid (mg/dl)	5.07 (3.33)	4.50 (4.24)	13.93 (5.64)†	10.84 (5.1)†	13.7 (10.8)†

*From Dr. P. Redig, The Raptor Center, University of Minnesota, St. Paul, MN 55108. All samples were collected from healthy adult birds—either display/education or breeders or birds flown in falconry. All samples were collected after the birds had been anesthetized for a minimum of 10 minutes with isoflurane.
†Postprandial samples.

Appendix IE

HEMATOLOGIC AND SERUM BIOCHEMICAL REFERENCE RANGES OF SELECTED NON-PSITTACINE AVIAN SPECIES*

Table 1

HEMATOLOGIC AND SERUM BIOCHEMICAL REFERENCE RANGES OF SELECTED NON-PSITTACINE AVIAN SPECIES*

Measurement	Canary	Finch	Greater Indian Hill Mynah	Toucan	Domestic Duck
Hematology:					
PCV (%)	45–60 37–49†	45–62	44–55	45–60	30–43
Red blood cells ($10^6/\mu l$)	2.5–4.5 2.5–3.8†	2.5–4.6	2.4–4.0	2.5–4.5	2.3–3.5
White blood cells ($10^6/\mu l$)	4–9 4–9†	3–8	6–11	4–10	4.5–13.0
Heterophils (%)	20–50 50–80†	20–65	25–65	35–65	30–70
Lymphocytes (%)	40–75 20–45†	20–65	20–60	25–50	20–65
Monocytes (%)	0–1 0–1†	0–1	0–3	0–4	0–3
Eosinophils (%)	0–1 0–2†	0–1	0–3	0–1	0–4
Basophils (%)	0–5 0–1†	0–5	0–7	0–5	0–5
Chemistries:					
Alkaline phosphatase (U/L)	146–397 20–135†	—	—	—	—
Aspartate aminotransferase [AST] (U/L)	45–170 145–345†	150–350	130–350	130–330	5–100
Calcium (mg/dl)	5.1–13.4 5.5–13.5†	—	9–13	10–15	10–18
Creatinine (mg/dl)	0.1–1.0 0.1–0.4†	—	0.1–0.6	0.1–0.4	0.1–0.5
Glucose (mg/dl)	291–391 205–435†	200–450	190–350	220–350	150–300
Lactate dehydrogenase (U/L)	1300–1816 120–350†	—	600–1000	200–400	150–800
Phosphorus (mg/dl)	1.6–5.6 2.9–4.9†	—	—	—	—
Potassium (mmol/L)	2.7–4.8 2.2–4.5	—	0.3–5.1	—	3.0–4.5
Protein, total (g/dl)	2.0–4.4 2.8–4.5†	3–5	2.3–4.5	3–5	2.5–6.0
Sodium (mmol/L)	125–154 135–165†	—	136–152	—	130–155
Thyroxine [T_4] ($\mu g/dl$)	0.7–3.2†	—	—	—	0.8–3.3
Uric acid (mg/dl)	4.3–14.8 4.0–12.0†	4–12	4–10	4–14	2–12

*Except where noted, adapted from Carpenter JW, Mashima TY, Rupiper DJ: Exotic Animal Formulary. Manhattan, KS, Greystone Publications, 1996, p 156.
†Values from Avian and Wildlife Laboratory, University of Miami School of Medicine, Miami, FL 33136.

Appendix IF

PLASMA BIOCHEMICAL REFERENCE RANGES
FOR RACING PIGEONS

Table 1

PLASMA BIOCHEMICAL REFERENCE RANGES
FOR RACING PIGEONS

Parameter	$P_{2.5} - P_{97.5}$*
Sodium (mEq/L)	141–149
Potassium (mEq/L)	3.9–4.7
Calcium (mg/dl)	7.6–10.4
Magnesium (mg/dl)	2.7–4.4
Inorganic phosphorus (mg/dl)	1.8–4.1
Chloride (mEq/dl)	101–113
Plasma iron (g/dl)	61–184
Iron binding capacity (μg/dl)	5.4–8.0
Osmolality (mOsm/kg)	297–317
Glucose (mg/dl)	232–369
Creatinine (mg/dl)	0.26–.04
Urea (mg/dl)	2.4–4.2
Uric acid (mg/dl)	2.52–12.86
Urea: Uric acid ratio	1.8 1.8 (mean sd)
CPK (U/L)	110–480
AP (U/L)	160–780
AST (U/L)	45–123
ALT (U/L)	19–48
GLDH (U/L)	0–1
LDH (U/L)	30–205
Bile acids (mol/L)	22–60
GGT (U/L)	0–2.9
Total protein (g/dl)	2.1–3.3
Albumin: Globulin ratio	1.5–3.6
Prealbumin (g/dl)	0.1–0.4
Albumin (g/dl)	1.3–2.2
Alpha globulin (g/dl)	0.2–0.3
Beta globulin (g/dl)	0.3–0.6
Gamma globulin (g/dl)	0.1–0.3

From Lumeij JT: PhD thesis, Utrecht University, 1987.
*The inner limits are given for the percentiles $P_{2.5}$ and $P_{97.5}$ with a probability of 90%.

PROCEDURES FOR CONDUCTING AVIAN WHITE BLOOD CELL COUNTS*

UNOPETTE METHOD FOR INDIRECT DETERMINATION OF THE TOTAL WHITE BLOOD CELL COUNT (TWC) (PHLOXINE DILUENT)†

1. Count the number of stained cells in each of the four corner squares on both sides of the hemacytometer.

2. Average the counts from the two sides.

3. Multiply the average count $\times$ 80 = the number of granulocytes/μl of blood.

4. Conduct a differential count on a Diff-Quik stained smear.

5. Add the percentages of heterophils, eosinophils, and basophils for the total percentage of granulocytes.

6. % heterophils + % eosinophils + % basophils $\times$ total WBC/μl = number of granulocytes.

7. Therefore, total WBC/μl = number of granulocytes $\div$ by % granulocytes.

ESTIMATED WHITE BLOOD CELL COUNT METHOD‡ (AFTER L. McENTEE)

1. Count all WBCs in five to eight high dry microscopic fields (40$\times$).§

2. Divide the total WBCs counted by the number of fields counted for the average number of WBCs/field.

3. Multiply the average $\times$ 2000 for the total estimated WBCs/μl.

4. To correct for an abnormal PCV, the WBC count is adjusted in the direction of the change in PCV. The formula for this adjustment is:

Divide the observed PCV by the normal PCV and multiply by the total estimated WBC count. This gives you the corrected amount.

Example: Forty WBCs are counted in eight high dry fields and the PCV is 35%.

$^{40}\!/_8 = 5 \times 2000 =$ estimated WBC = 10,000

$^{35}\!/_{40} \times 10,000 = 8500$ (corrected WBC)

RECIPES FOR FREQUENTLY USED HEMATOLOGIC STAINS

Wright's Stain for Avian Blood

Dry Wright's stain—3 g
Giemsa stain—1 g

Add to 4 quarts of **acetone-free** methanol. Begin agitation immediately for several minutes. Continue with intermittent agitation for 10 days. Filter before use.

Wright-Giemsa Buffer

106.08 g KPO_4 anhydrous monobasic
51.20 g Na_2PO_4 anhydrous dibasic

Dilute to 16 liters in distilled water. Adjust pH to 6.8.

$\downarrow$ pH—add dibasic
$\uparrow$ pH—add monobasic

---

*From Dr. P. Redig, The Raptor Center, University of Minnesota, St. Paul, MN 55108.

†Unopette, test 5877, Becton-Dickinson, Rutherford, NJ 07070.

‡(This determination is predicated on the fact that birds with normal PCVs have approximately 2–4 million RBCs/μl and one leukocyte per 1000 RBCs. There are 1000 RBCs in five to eight high dry fields prepared from avian blood. Therefore, the estimate gives you the average number of leukocytes/μl. This is also based on the assumption that a monolayer blood film area of a properly prepared slide or coverslip is evaluated.)

§Typically done on a "stat"-stained slide using Diff-Quik (Harleco, Gibbstown, NJ) or Hema3 (Curtin-Mathisen, Houston, TX).

Conversions to Système International (SI) Units*

Table 1

HEMATOLOGY

Component	Conventional Unit	Conversion Factor	SI Unit Symbol	Significant Digits†
Hemoglobin	g/dl	10	g/L	XXX
Mean corpuscular hemoglobin concentration	g/dl	10	g/L	XXO
	pg	1	pg	XX
Mean corpuscular volume	μm^3	1	fL	XXX
Red blood cell count	$10^6/mm^3$ or $10^6/\mu L$	1	$10^{12}/L$	X.X
Reticulocyte count	$/mm^3$ or $/\mu L$	0.001	$10^9/L$	XX
Thrombocytes	$10^3/mm^3$ or $10^3/\mu L$	1	$10^9/L$	XXX
White blood cell count	$/mm^3$ or $/\mu L$	0.001	$10^9/L$	XX.X

*Modified from the American Medical Association Manual of Style, ed 8. Baltimore, Williams & Wilkins, 1989.

†Significant digits refers to the number of digits used to describe reported results. XX means that results expressed to the nearest whole number are meaningful; XXO means that results are meaningful when rounded to the nearest 10. Results reported to lower numbers or decimal points are beyond the sensitivity of the test.

T a b l e   2

CLINICAL CHEMISTRY

Component	Conventional Unit	Conversion Factor	SI Unit Symbol	Significant Digits*
Alanine aminotransferase (ALT)	U/L	1	U/L	XX
Albumin	g/dl	10	g/L	XX
Amylase	U/L	1	U/L	XXX
	Somogyi units/dl	1.850	U/L	XXO
Alkaline phosphatase	U/L	1	U/L	XXX
Aspartate aminotransferase (AST)	U/L	1	U/L	XX
Bile acids (total)	mg/L	2.547	μmol/L	X.X
Bilirubin	mg/dl	17.1	μmol/L	XX
Calcium	mg/dl	0.2495	mmol/L	X.XX
Calcium, ionized	mEq/L	0.5	mmol/L	X.XX
Carbon dioxide content (bicarbonate + CO_2)	mEq/L	1	mmol/L	XX
Chloride	mEq/L	1	mmol/L	XXX
Cholesterol	mg/dl	0.02586	mmol/L	X.XX
Cortisol	μg/dl	27.59	nmol/L	XXO
Creatine kinase (CK)	U/L	1	U/L	XXX
Creatinine	mg/dl	88.40	μmol/L	XXO
Electrophoresis, protein	%	0.01	1	X.XX
	g/dl	10	g/L	XX
Fibrinogen	mg/dl	0.01	g/L	X.X
γ-Glutamyltransferase (GGT)	U/L	1	U/L	XX
Glucose	mg/dL	0.05551	mmol/l	XX.X
Globulins	mg/dl	0.001	g/L	XX.XX
Insulin	μU/ml	7.175	pmol/L	XXX
	μg/L	172.2	pmol/L	XXX
Iron	μg/dl	0.0179	μmol/L	XX
Lactate dehydrogenase	U/L	1	U/L	XXX
Lipase	U/L	1	U/L	XXO
Magnesium	mg/dl	0.4114	mmol/L	X.XX
	mEq/L	0.5	mmol/L	X.XX
Phosphate	mg/dl	0.3229	mmol/L	X.XX
Potassium	mEq/L	1	mmol/L	X.X
	mg/dl	0.2558	mmol/L	X.X
Protein (total)	g/dl	10	g/L	XX
Sodium	mEq/L	1	mmol/L	XXX
Thyroxine	μg/dl	12.87	nmol/L	XXX
Triglycerides	mg/dl	0.01129	mmol/L	X.XX
Triiodothyronine	ng/dl	0.01536	nmol/L	X.X
Urate (as uric acid)	mg/dl	59.48	μmol/L	XXO
Urea nitrogen	mg/dl	0.3570	mmol/L	X.X

*Modified from the American Medical Association Manual of Style, ed 8. Baltimore, Williams & Wilkins, 1989.

†Significant digits refers to the number of digits used to describe reported results. XX means that results expressed to the nearest whole number are meaningful; XXO means that results are meaningful when rounded to the nearest 10. Results reported to lower numbers or decimal points are beyond the sensitivity of the test.

Appendix III

Adult Bird Weights

Psittaciformes

Cockatoos	Citron	283–514 g*
	Goffin's	221–386 g
	Greater Sulphur-Crested	608–1200 g
	Lesser Sulphur-Crested	251–412 g
	Major Mitchell's	300–452 g
	Moluccan	640–1025 g
	Palm (Goliath)	990–1057 g
	Rose-Breasted	281–390 g
	Umbrella	458–756 g
Macaws	Blue and Gold	892–1294 g
	Buffon's	1080–1534 g
	Green-Winged	1058–1529 g
	Hyacinth	1185–1529 g
	Military	774–1065 g
	Scarlet	1058–1464 g
	Yellow-Collared	223–308 g
Parrots	African Grey	300–380 g
	Blue-Fronted Amazon	275–510 g
	Blue-Headed Pionus	238–278 g
	Double Yellow-Headed Amazon	545 g
	Eclectus	383–524 g
	Hispaniolan Amazon	268 g
	Mealy Amazon	600–685 g
	Orange-Winged Amazon	440–470 g
	Senegal	125–150 g
	Yellow-Fronted Amazon	260–460 g
Smaller Species	Budgerigar	30–60 g
	Blue-Crowned Conure	84–96 g
	Jandaya Conure	118–128 g
	Pennant's Parakeet	180–200 g
	Red-Crowned Parakeet	60–75 g
	Love Birds (various species)	50–70 g

Anseriformes	Domestic Duck	2–3 kg
	Domestic Goose	4–5 kg
	Canada Goose	3.5–4.5 kg
Apodiformes	Hummingbirds	2.5–5 g
Columbiformes	Collared Dove	150–220 g
	Diamond Dove	40 g
	Domestic Pigeon	260–350 g
Falconiformes	Harris Hawk	574–1000 g
	Kestrel	145–282 g
	Peregrine Falcon	560–1500 g
	Red-Tailed Hawk	698–1350 g
	Sparrow Hawk	150–300 g
Galliformes	Domestic Fowl	1.75–4 kg
	Domestic Turkey	4–15 kg
	Japanese Quail	18–42 g
Gruiformes	Crowned Crane	3.5–4 kg
Passeriformes	Canary	12–29 g
	English Robin	20–30 g
	Glossy Starling	74–82 g
	Goldfinch and Green Finch	15–20 g
	Greater Indian Hill Mynah	180–240 g
	House Sparrow	25–30 g
	Java Sparrow	24–30 g
	Zeba Finch	10–16 g

(Data from Schubot RM, Clubb K, Clubb SL: Psittacine Aviculture, pp 14–19. Loxahatchee, FL, Avicultural Breeding and Research Center, 1992; Arnall L, Keymer IF: Bird Diseases, p 482. Neptune City, NJ, T.F.H. Publications Inc, 1975; Coles BH: Avian Medicine and Surgery, pp 209–213. London, Blackwell Scientific Publications, 1985.)
*Weights are the lowest female weight to the highest male weight.

Appendix IV

Scientific Names of Common Psittacine Species

Amazon
Blue-fronted	*Amazona aestiva*
Cuban	*A. leucocephala*
Green-cheeked	*A. viridigenalis*
Hispaniolan	*A. ventralis*
Lilac-crowned	*A. finschi*
Mealy	*A. farinosa*
Orange-winged	*A. amazonica*
Red-lored	*A. autumnalis autumnalis*
Tucuman	*A. tucumana*
White-fronted	*A. albifrons*
Yellow-crowned	*A. ochrocephala ochrocephala*
Yellow-headed	*A. ochrocephala oratrix*
Yellow-naped	*A ochrocephala auropalliata*
Yellow-shouldered	*A. barbadensis*

Budgerigar — *Melopsittacus undulatus*

Caique
Black-headed	*Pionites melanocephala*
White-bellied	*P. leucogaster*

Cockatiel — *Nymphicus hollandicus*

Cockatoo
Ducorp's	*Cacatua ducorps*
Galah	*Eolophus roseicapillus*
Gang-gang	*Callocephalon fimbriatum*
Goffin's	*Cacatua goffini*
Lesser sulphur-crested	*Cacatua sulphurea*
Major Mitchell's	*Cacatua leadbeateri*
Palm	*Probosciger aterrimus*
Red-tailed	*Calyptorhynchus magnificus*
Red-vented	*Cacatua haematuophygia*
Salmon-crested	*Cacatua moluccensis*
Sulphur-crested	*Cacatua galerita*
White	*Cacatua alba*

Conure
Austral	*Enicognathus ferrigineus*
Aztec	*Aratinga nana astec*
Black-capped	*Pyrrhura rupicola*
Blue-crowned	*Aratinga acuticaudata*
Dusky-headed	*Aratinga weddellii*
Finsch's	*Aratinga finschi*
Golden	*Aratinga guarouba*
Golden-capped	*Aratinga auricapilla*
Green	*Aratinga holochlora*
Green-cheeked	*Pyrrhura molinae*
Jandaya	*Aratinga jandaya*
Maroon-bellied	*Pyrrhura frontalis*
Mitred	*Aratinga mitrata*
Nanday	*Nandayus nenday*
Olive-throated	*Aratinga nana nana*
Painted	*Pyrrhura picta*
Patagonian	*Cyanoliseus patagonus*
Peach-fronted	*Aratinga aurea*
Red-masked	*Aratinga erythrogenys*
Slender-billed	*Enicognathus leptorhynchus*
Sun	*Aratinga solstitialis*
White-eyed	*Aratinga leucophthalmus*

Corella
Little	*Cacatua sanguinea*
Long-billed	*Cacatua tenuirostris*

Kea — *Nestor notabilis*

Lory

Chattering	*Lorius garrulus*
Black	*Chalcopsitta atra atra*
Black-capped	*Lorius lory*
Blue-streaked	*Eos reticulata*
Dusky	*Pseudeos fuscata*
Duivenbode's	*Chalcopsitta duivenbodei duivenbodei*
Papuan	*Charmosyna papou papou*
Rainbow	*Trichoglossus haematodus haematodus*
Red	*Eos bornea*
Tahitian	*Vini peruviana*

Lorikeet

Goldie's	*Trichoglossus goldiei*
Iris	*T. iris*
Musschenbroek's	*Neopsittacus musschenbroekii*
Red-flanked	*Charmosyna placentis*

Lovebird

Black-cheeked	*Agapornis nigrigenis*
Fischer's	*A. fischeri*
Grey-headed	*A. cana*
Masked	*A. personata*
Nyasa	*A. lilianae*
Peach-faced	*A. roseicollis*

Macaw

Blue and yellow	*Ara ararauna*
Buffon's	*A. ambigua*
Caninde	*A. caninde*
Chestnut-fronted	*A. severa*
Green-winged	*A. chloroptera*
Hyacinth	*Anodorhynchus hyacinthinus*
Illiger's	*Ara maracana*
Military	*A. militaris*
Red-bellied	*A. manilata*
Red-fronted	*A. rubrogenys*
Red-shouldered	*A. nobilis*
Scarlet	*A. macao*
Yellow-collared	*A. auricollis*

Parakeet

Alexandrine	*Psittacula eupatria*
Blossom-headed	*P. roseata*
Canary-winged	*Brotogeris versicolorus*
Cobalt-winged	*Brotogeris cyanoptera*
Derbyan	*Psittacula derbiana*
Grey-cheeked	*Brotogeris pyrrhopterus*
Monk	*Myiopsitta monachus*
Plum-headed	*Psittacula cyanocephala*
Rose-ringed	*P. krameri*
Slaty-headed	*P. himalayana*
Tui	*Brotogeris sanctithomae*

Parrotlet

Blue-winged	*Forpus xanthopterygius*
Green-rumped	*F. passerinus*
Mexican	*F. cyanopygius cyanopygius*
Pacific	*F. coelestis*

Parrot

African Grey	*Psittacus erithacus*
Amboina King	*Alisterus amboinensis amboinensis*
Australian King	*A. scapularis*
Blue-crowned	*Loriculus galgulus*
Blue-naped	*Tanygnathus lucionensis*
Bourke's	*Neophema bourkii*
Bronze-winged	*Pionus chalcopterus*
Brown-headed	*Poicephalus cryptoxanthus*
Cape	*P. robustus*
Desmerest's fig	*Psittaculirostris desmarestii desmarestii*
Double-eyed fig	*Opopsitta diophthalma*
Dusky	*Pionus fuscus*
Edward's fig	*Psittaculirostris edwardsii*
Grand Eclectus	*Eclectus roratus roratus*
Great-bill	*Tanygnathus megalorynchos*
Hawk-headed	*Deroptyus accitrinus*
Jardine's	*Poicephalus gulielmi*
Meyer's	*P. meyeri*
Pileated	*Pionopsitta pileata*
Plum-crowned	*Pionus tumultuosus*
Princess	*Polytelis alexandrae*
Red-bellied	*Poicephalus rufiventris*
Red-rumped	*Psephotus haematonotus*
Red-sided Eclectus	*Eclectus roratus polychlorus*
Regent	*Polytelis anthopeplus*
Rock	*Neophema petrophila*
Salvadori's fig	*Psittaculirostris salvadorii*
Scarlet-chested	*Neophema splendida*

		Rosella	
Scaly-headed	*Pionus maximiliani*		
Senegal	*Poicephalus senegalus*	Adelaide	*Platycercus adelaidae*
Tanimbar Eclectus	*Eclectus roratus riedeli*	Crimson	*P. elegans*
Thick-billed	*Rhynchopsitta pachyrhn-*	Eastern	*P. eximius eximius*
	cha pachythncha	Northern	*P. venustus*
Vasa	*Coracopsis vasa*	Pale-headed	*P. adscitus*
White-crowned	*Pionus senilis*	Western	*P. icterotis*

Index

Psittacine(s) *(Continued)*
feeding volumes for, 81–82, *82*
femur rotational deformity in, 82, *82*
flock behavior of, 97, 98
folding fractures in, 91
food-borne contamination of, 75–76
foreign body pneumonia in, 88
formula for, 79
fostering of, 73–74
fractures in, 91–92
gout in, 92
growth of, assessment of, 76, *76*
rates for, 75, *75*
gut transit time in, 87–88
hand-feeding of, 80t–81t
hand-rearing of, 75
hematologic reference ranges for, 1005t
hepatic hematoma in, 89, *89*
husbandry for, 73–100
problems in, 82–88
infections in, 74, 94
insect infestation in, 74–75
intestinal microflora of, bacteriology of, 78–79
intestinal stasis in, 88–89
kidney disease in, 92, *92*
laboratory tests in, 78–79
lateral maxillary deviation in, 84–85, *85*
leg deformities in, 82–84, *82–84*
braces for, 83, 83–84, *84*
packing for, 82–83, *83*
surgery for, 84
"lockjaw" syndrome in, 94
mandibular prognathism in, 85, 85–86, *86*
maxillary brachygnathism in, 85–86, *86*
maxillary fracture in, 90, *90*
monogamous behavior of, 98
natural environment of, 97
neck deformities in, 86, *87*
neonatal assessment in, 75–79
neonatal mortality in, 74
nursery management for, 75
nutrient levels for, 81–82
nutritional deficiencies in, 74
oral examination in, 77
organ examination in, 77
parasites in, 74
parenteral therapy for, 88–89
parent-reared chicks of, 73–75
pharyngeal puncture in, 91
plasma biochemical reference ranges for, 1004t, 1006t–1007t
plasma protein electrophoresis reference ranges for, 1008t
red mites in, 74
regurgitation in, 88
reproductive failure in, 103, 103t
restraint of, 132, *132*
retained yolk sac in, 86–87, *87*
scientific names of, 1029–1031
"scissors beak" in, 84–85, *85*
skin color in, 76, *76*
splay leg deformity in, 82, *82*
stifle luxation in, 84, *84*, 91

Psittacine(s) *(Continued)*
stunting in, 76, *76*, 77, 82
toe deformities in, 86
trauma in, *89–91,* 89–92
urate deposition in, 92, *93*
water-borne contamination of, 76
wild-caught vs. domestically bred, 97
Psittacine beak and feather disease, 284–288
acute signs of, 285–286
adult, 291
beak lesions in, 284–285, *285*
beak powder absence in, 284, *284*
biology of, 286–287
control of, 287–288
diagnosis of, 287
dysplastic feathers in, 284, *285,* 287
immune function alterations in, 285
in lovebirds, 291
necropsy of, 162, *163*
polymer chain reaction assay in, 287
presentation of, 284–286
Psittacine beak and feather disease virus, incubation periods for, 287
prevention of, 288
replication of, 286–287
testing for, 287–288
transmission of, 286
Psittacine mutilation syndrome, 558–559
Psittacine proventricular dilatation syndrome, 312
biology of, 313–314
central nervous system disease in, 312
diagnosis of, 314–315, *315*
dilatation in, 313, *313–315,* 314
leukocytosis in, 313
muscle wasting in, 312
presentation of, 312t, 312–313
radiography of, 313, *313, 314*
synopsis of, 312–313
treatment of, 315
Psittacosis. See *Chlamydiosis.*
Pteryglossus, sex determination in, 913
Ptilopachinae, 953
Ptosis, in microphthalmos, 568–569
Pubis, anatomy of, 522
Pulpitis, bacterial, feather mutilation in, 549
Pulse deficit, in heart disease, 493
Puncture, esophageal, 427
pharyngeal, 427
Pupil, 565, *565*
Purcrasiinae, 952
Purulent reaction, 215
Pygostyle, 518, *519*
Pyoderma, bacterial, 554
Pyrantel pamoate, 681t
Pyrethrins, 681t
Pyridoxine, deficiency of, reduced hatchability from, 64
requirements for, 34
Pyrimethamine, 681t

Quadrate bone, 517, *518*
Quail, 953–954

Quail *(Continued)*
diseases of, 954–955
New World, 955
diseases of, *955,* 955–956
Quarantine, for viral disease, 281–282
in aviculture, 105
in bird importation, 49
Quinacrine, 681t

Rabies, zoonotic, 357–358
Radial nerve, 458
Radiation, in thermoregulation, 843
Radiation therapy, 601–602
Radiography, 170–198
anesthesia for, 171, 824
cardiovascular, *176–180,* 177–178
in disease, 188–189
CC view in, 173
contrast, 181, 183, *184–185,* 186, 186t
exposures in, 170–171
film in, 170
gastrointestinal, *176–179,* 178–179, *183*
in disease, 189, *189–191,* 192, *193–197*
lateral view in, 172–173
normal anatomy in, 173–181, *173–183*
of appendicular skeleton, 175–176, *180–182*
of axial skeleton, 173–174, *173–180*
of metabolic bone disease, 186, *187*
positioning in, 172–173
respiratory, 176–177
in disease, 187–188, *188, 189*
restraint for, 171–172
skeletal, in disease, 186–187, *187*
techniques in, 170–173
urogenital, *177,* 179–181, *180*
in disease, 194, *197, 198*
VD view in, 172–173
Radiology, 170–198
Radiosurgery, 767–772
advantages of, 769
cautions for, 769–770
current in, 768
disadvantages of, 769
equipment care in, 771–772, 772t
frequency in, tissue effects of, 768, *768*
fulguration in, 769
fully rectified unfiltered current in, 768–769
ground plate in, 768
history of, 767–768
lateral heat in, 769
partially rectified unfiltered current in, 769
radiowave in, 768
technique for, *770,* 770–771
unit for, *767*
wave forms in, 768
Radius, anatomy of, 521
fracture of, external fixation of, *746*
treatment of, 750–752, *751*
radiography of, 175, *181*

ISBN 0-7216-5446-0

90069

9 780721 654461